AF566937

IMAGING OF CARDIAC DISORDERS

VOLUME 2: ACQUIRED DISORDERS

IMAGING OF CARDIAC DISORDERS

VOLUME 2: ACQUIRED DISORDERS

Benigno Soto, M.D.
Professor of Radiology
Director of Cardiopulmonary Radiology
University of Alabama at Birmingham School of Medicine
Birmingham, AL

E. George Kassner, M.D.
Director of Diagnostic Radiology
Kings County Hospital Center
Professor of Radiology
State University of New York
Health Science Center at Brooklyn
Brooklyn, NY

William A. Baxley, M.D.
Professor of Medicine
Division of Cardiovascular Disease
University of Alabama at Birmingham School of Medicine
Birmingham, AL

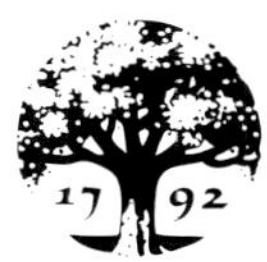

JB Lippincott • Philadelphia
Gower Medical Publishing • New York • London

LIBRARY OF CONGRESS CATALOGING-IN-PUBLICATION DATA
Soto, Benigno, 1929–
Imaging of cardiac disorders / Benigno Soto, E. George Kassner, William A. Baxley.
p. cm.
Includes bibliographical references and index.
Contents: v. 1. Congenital disorders — v. 2. Acquired disorders.
ISBN 1-56375-093-7 (v. 1). — ISBN 1-56375-094-5 (v. 2)
1. Heart—Imaging—Atlases. 2. Pediatric cardiology—Diagnosis—-Atlases. 3. Heart—Interventional radiology—Atlases.
I. Kassner, E. George. II. Baxley, W. A. (Williams A.) III. Title.
[DNLM: 1. Cardiovascular Diseases—diagnosis—atlases.
2. Diagnostic Imaging—atlases. 3. Heart Defects, Congenital—-diagnosis—atlases. WG 17 S7181]
RC683.5.I42S67 1991
616. 120754—dc20

91-22715

BRITISH LIBRARY CATALOGUING IN PUBLICATION DATA
Imaging of cardiac disorders.
Vol. 2 : Acquired disorders.
I. Benigno, Soto II. Kassner, E. George, 1937-
III. Baxley, William A.
616.120757

ISBN 1563750945

DISTRIBUTED IN USA AND CANADA BY:
JB Lippincott Company
East Washington Square
Philadelphia, PA 19105, USA

DISTRIBUTED IN THE REST OF THE WORLD (EXCEPT JAPAN) BY:
Gower Medical Publishing Ltd.
Middlesex House
34-42 Cleveland Street
London W1P 5FB, UK

DISTRIBUTED IN JAPAN BY:
Nankodo Co., Ltd.
42-6, Hongo 3-Chome
Bunkyo-Ku
Tokyo 113, Japan

ISBN 0-397-44678-0 (Set)
ISBN 1-56375-093-7 (Volume 1)
ISBN 1-56375-094-5 (Volume 2)

10 9 8 7 6 5 4 3 2 1

ILLUSTRATORS: Wendy Jackelow, Patricia Gast (line tracings)
ART DIRECTOR: Jill Feltham
INTERIOR DESIGN AND LAYOUT: Jeff Brown
COVER DESIGN AND LAYOUT: Selina Waxman

Printed in the United States by Arcata Graphics/Kingsport

Dedicated to the patients
who suffer from the
cardiac diseases described
in this book, and to their
families.

CONTRIBUTORS

William A. Baxley, M.D.
Professor of Medicine
Division of Cardiovascular Disease
University of Alabama at Birmingham School of Medicine

Vera A. Bittner, M.D.
Assistant Professor of Medicine
Division of Cardiovascular Disease
University of Alabama at Birmingham School of Medicine

Robert C. Bourge, M.D., F.A.C.C.
Associate Professor of Medicine and Radiology
Division of Cardiovascular Disease
University of Alabama at Birmingham School of Medicine

Edward C. Colvin, M.D.
Associate Professor of Pediatrics
Division of Pediatric Cardiology
University of Alabama at Birmingham School of Medicine

Gregory B. Cranney, M.D.
Assistant Professor of Medicine
Division of Cardiovascular Disease
Clinical Director, Cardiovascular NMR Laboratory
University of Alabama at Birmingham School of Medicine
Clinical Director, Cardiovascular NMR Laboratory
University of Alabama Hospitals
Birmingham, Alabama

Milena J. Henzlova, M.D., F.A.C.C.
Assistant Professor of Medicine
Division of Cardiovascular Disease
University of Alabama at Birmingham School of Medicine

E. George Kassner, M.D., F.A.C.P.
Professor of Radiology
State University of New York Health Science Center at Brooklyn
Director of Diagnostic Radiology, Kings County Hospital Center
Head of Section of Pediatric Radiology, University Hospital
Brooklyn, New York

William R. Morrow, M.D.
Assistant Professor of Pediatrics
Division of Pediatric Cardiology
University of Alabama at Birmingham School of Medicine

Navin C. Nanda, M.D.
Professor of Medicine
Division of Cardiovascular Disease
University of Alabama at Birmingham School of Medicine
Director, Heart Station and Echocardiography-Graphics Laboratories
University of Alabama Hospitals
Birmingham, Alabama

Benigno Soto, M.D.
Professor of Radiology
University of Alabama at Birmingham School of Medicine
Director of Cardiopulmonary Radiology, University of Alabama Hospitals
Birmingham, Alabama

Isidre Vilaicosta, M.D.
Associate
Division of Cardiovascular Disease
University of Alabama at Birmingham School of Medicine
Assistant Professor
Division of Cardiology
University Hospital "San Carlos"
Madrid, Spain

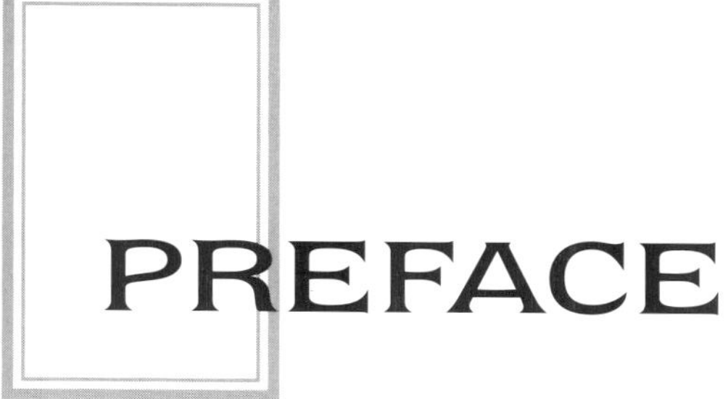

PREFACE

BEFORE THE TWENTIETH CENTURY, cardiovascular diagnosis was based on clinical observation and physical diagnosis. In the early years of this century, this limited armamentarium was augmented by plain radiography and fluoroscopy of the chest and by electrocardiography. Objective evaluation of cardiovascular physiology in vivo became possible in 1941 when Cournand demonstrated that intravascular exploration, using percutaneously introduced catheters, was both feasible and safe. Cardiac catheterization was soon followed by the advent of angiocardiography, which made it possible to identify morphologic abnormalities of the heart and great vessels in the living patient. The precise physiologic and anatomic data provided by cardiac catheterization and angiocardiography led to rapid advances in the field of cardiac surgery.

The past two decades have seen revolutionary advances in diagnostic imaging. The introduction of noninvasive (or minimally invasive) modalities such as echocardiography, nuclear cardiology, computed tomography, and magnetic resonance imaging has dramatically altered the diagnostic approach to the patient with cardiovascular disease. In some instances, sophisticated noninvasive techniques have decreased (or eliminated) the need for invasive diagnosis. In others, noninvasive techniques have provided new insights into the pathophysiology and natural history of cardiovascular disease. The ability of these modalities to detect cardiac disease in its earliest stages (e.g., silent ischemia, subclinical diastolic dysfunction) has important implications for the clinician. Rapid advances in interventional cardiology—coronary balloon angioplasty in particular—have stimulated major advances in imaging technology. Digital subtraction and other image enhancement techniques that provide high-resolution instant replay images are now available in all state-of-the-art interventional laboratories.

Imaging of Cardiac Disorders represents an effort to bridge the gap between introductory texts and more encyclopedic and highly specialized works on cardiology and specific imaging modalities. The emphasis is on plain radiography and angiocardiography, which continue to be the pillars of cardiac diagnosis; however, the newer modalities are extensively discussed and illustrated.

As the scope of the book widened, and production costs increased, the publisher suggested publishing it as a two-volume set. The authors agreed, since the two-volume format would make the book available to a wider audience (each volume can be purchased separately). Volume I discusses congenital heart disease in the child and adult. [A chapter on fetal cardiac diagnosis ("Imaging the Fetal Heart"), added because of the importance of sophisticated fetal cardiac diagnosis for pediatricians and pediatric cardiologists, appears as Chapter 15A.] Acquired heart disease in the child and adult, including ischemic heart disease resulting from congenital anomalies of the coronary arteries, is discussed in Volume II. A series of introductory chapters on imaging techniques and electrocardiography appears in both volumes. (Not included in the initial numbering scheme, a chapter on nuclear cardiology has been added as Chapter 4A.) Invasive catheter techniques employed in the treatment of congenital and acquired heart disease are discussed in Volume I and Volume II, respectively. Embolization techniques used in the treatment of congenital heart disease are discussed in Volume II.

The authors are indebted to their colleagues at the University of Alabama Medical Center and elsewhere who contributed chapters in their areas of expertise and provided images that appear throughout the book. We also wish to thank Abe Krieger and his team at Gower, who have captured our highly visual discipline in this beautifully produced book.

E. GEORGE KASSNER, M.D.

Contents

VOLUME 2: ACQUIRED DISORDERS

Chapter 27 ... 276
Diseases of the Thoracic Aorta

Chapter 28 ... 304
Trauma to the Heart and Great Vessels

Chapter 29 ... 318
Acquired Heart Disease in Children

Chapter 30 ... 338
Treatment of Ischemic Heart Disease with Catheter Techniques and Surgery

Chapter 31 ... 362
Balloon Valvuloplasty, Embolization Therapy, and Valve Replacement

CHAPTER 1

Noninvasive Radiologic Techniques and Electrocardiography

CHEST RADIOGRAPHY AND FLUOROSCOPY

The initial radiologic examination in any patient with suspected heart disease consists of frontal and lateral radiographs of the chest. This simple, inexpensive technique provides important information about the size and configuration of the heart, atrial and visceral situs, the great arteries, and the pulmonary vasculature. The high-kilovoltage (140–160 kVp) technique normally used in adults usually provides excellent visualization of the trachea, bronchi, mediastinal structures, and pulmonary vasculature (Fig. 1.1). The ultra-high kilovoltage/magnification technique may be helpful when atrial situs is uncertain or when compression or displacement of the trachea is suspected (Fig. 1.2). Although no longer employed routinely, the four-film "cardiac series" is useful for evaluating the size of the cardiac

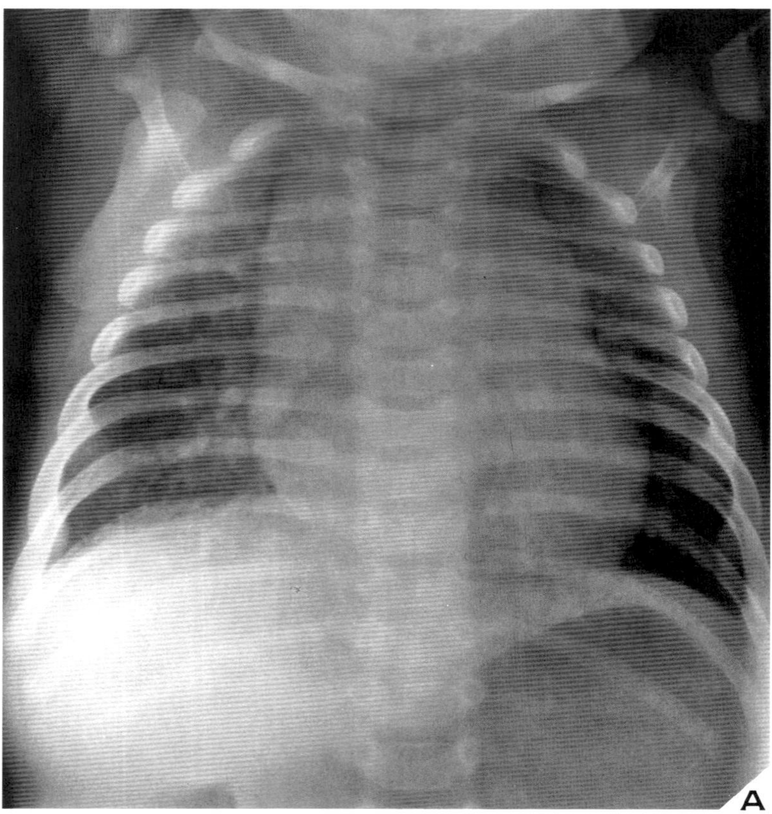

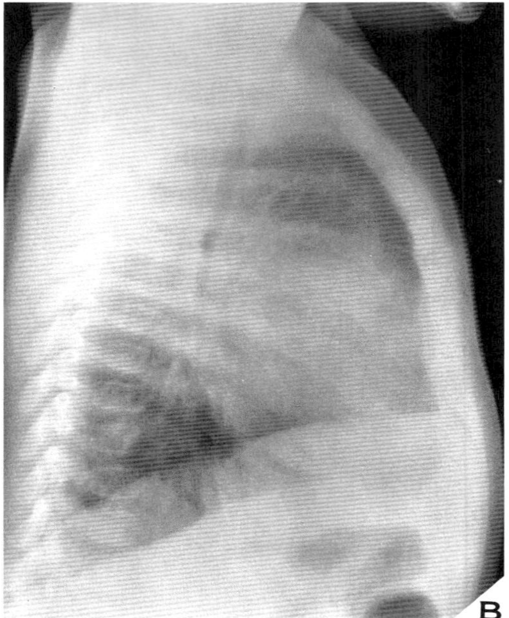

Fig. 1.1 High-kilovoltage chest films. (A) Frontal and (B) lateral chest films of an infant with transposition of the great arteries, obtained with 160 KVp using a very short exposure, clearly demonstrate the trachea, bronchi, mediastinal structures, and cardiovascular silhouette. The plethoric pulmonary vasculature is well demonstrated.

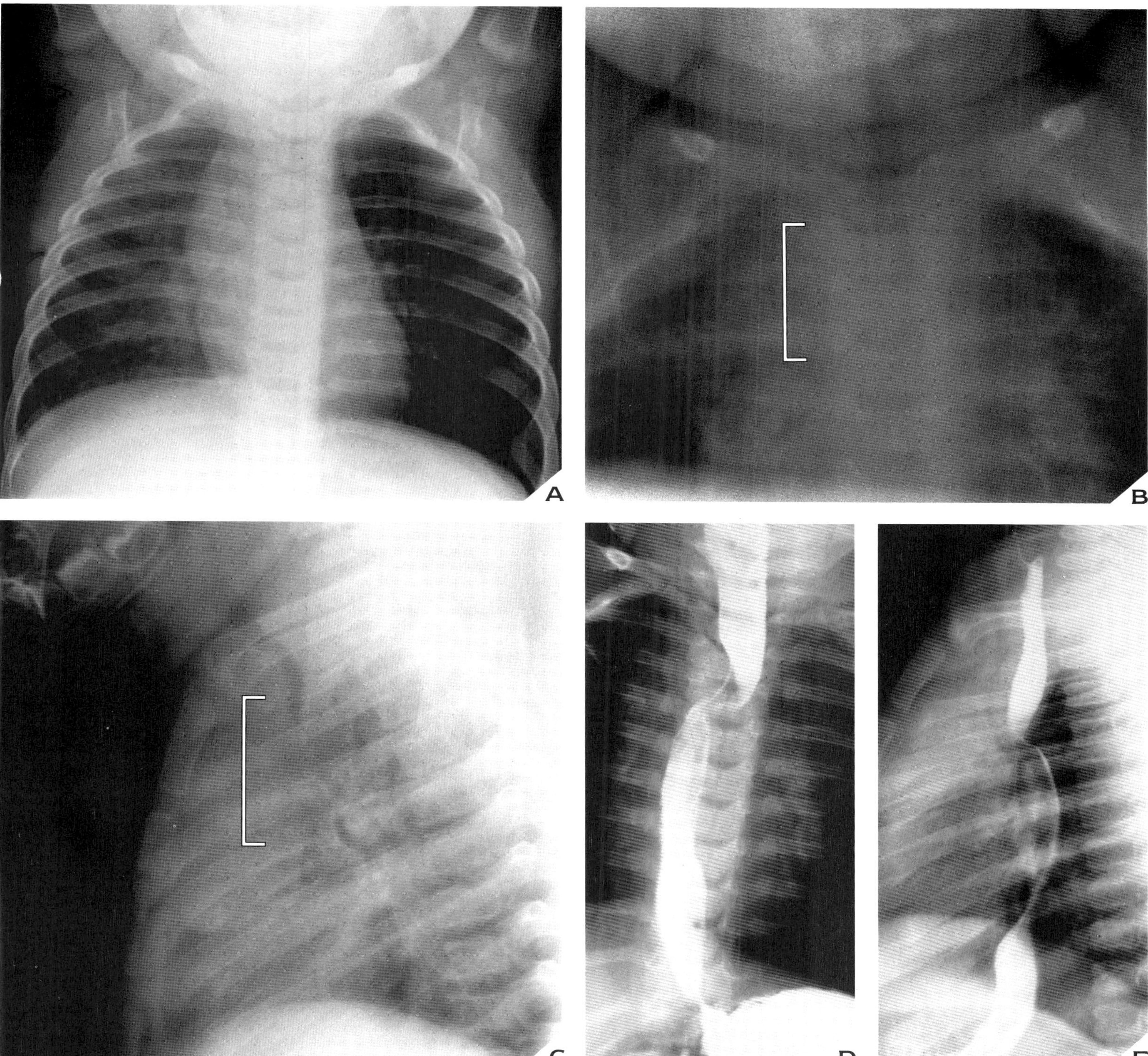

Fig. 1.2 Ultra-high kilovoltage/magnification technique and barium esophagram in investigation of vascular ring. Infant with stridor and feeding difficulty associated with a vascular ring (right aortic arch and left descending thoracic aorta). (A) Frontal chest film shows hyperlucency of the left lung. The tracheal air column cannot be identified. (B) Ultra-high kilovoltage magnification film shows absence of the tracheal air column ("empty segment sign") between the carina and the thoracic inlet (*brace*). (C) Conventional lateral chest film shows anterior displacement of the thoracic segment of the trachea, with complete effacement of its lumen. (D) Frontal and (E) lateral projections of esophagram show characteristic indentations of the right and posterior aspects of the esophagus produced by the vascular ring.

In the ultra-high kilovoltage/magnification technique illustrated in B, a Thoreus (tin–copper–aluminum) filter is placed in the X-ray beam to "harden" the radiation to an effective peak kilovoltage of about 300 kVp. At this energy, Compton scattering predominates and photoelectric interactions are relatively insignificant. The probability of photoelectric interactions between X-rays and the inner orbital electrons of the calcium atom is greatest on the low-kilovoltage films; consequently, the trachea and main bronchi are often obscured by overlying bony structures in infants' chest films. Because Compton scattering is related to electron density (which is approximately the same in bone and soft tissue), the ultra-high kilovoltage technique largely negates the "hiding" power of the thoracic and cervical vertebrae. Because electron density of soft tissue is much greater than that of air, there is excellent contrast between the tracheal air column and the surrounding soft tissues. The presence of an "empty" segment implies narrowing of the trachea by intrinsic or extrinsic pathology (in this instance, a tight vascular ring).

chambers (particularly the left atrium) and great arteries (Fig. 1.3). The barium esophagram is invaluable in patients with suspected vascular rings or aortopulmonary collaterals, which produce characteristic impressions on the barium-filled esophagus (see Fig. 1.2). With the advent of echocardiography, cardiac fluoroscopy is no longer performed routinely; however, it remains the most sensitive means of detecting calcifications of the cardiac valves and coronary arteries. Certain classical findings (eg, the "hilar dance" of pulmonary vavular insufficiency) can be detected only by fluoroscopy.

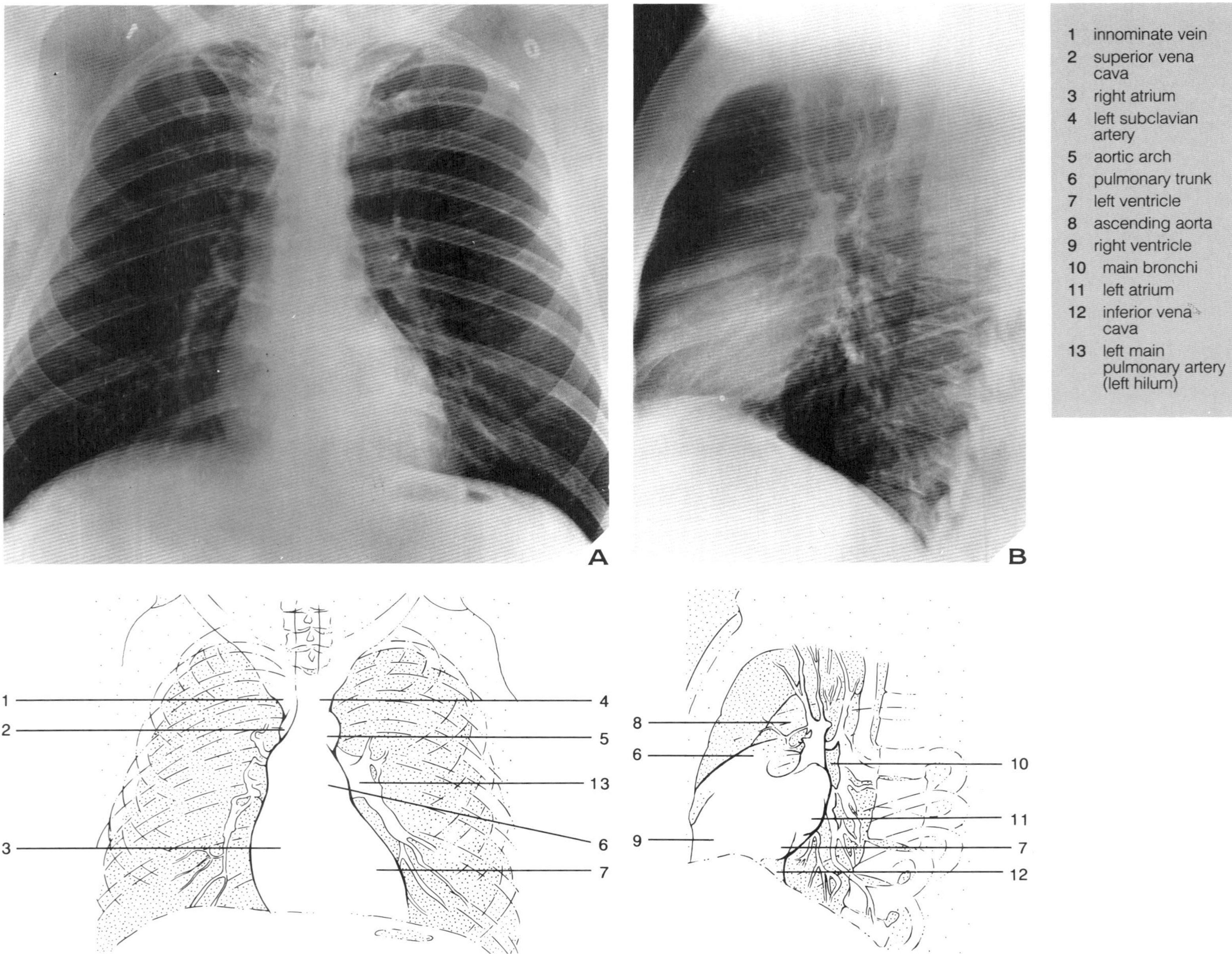

Fig. 1.3 Normal cardiac series. The standard cardiac series consists of four projections: posterior (PA), lateral, 60° left anterior oblique (LAO), and 45° right anterior oblique (RAO). (A) Posteroanterior (PA) projection. The right border of the cardiovascular silhouette is formed (from above downward) by the innominate vein, superior vena cava, and right atrium. The border-forming structures on the left are (from above downward) the left subclavian artery, left aortic arch, pulmonary trunk, and left ventricle. The left atrial appendage normally does not contribute to the left heart border; in patients with an enlarged left atrium the left atrial appendage appears as a discrete bulge between the pulmonary trunk and the left ventricle. The left pulmonary artery, which forms the central portion of the left hilum, lies posterior to the pulmonary trunk and is distinctly separate from it. (B) Lateral projection. The anterior border of the cardiovascular silhouette is formed (from above downward) by the ascending aorta, pulmonary trunk, and right ventricle. Normally, the ascending aorta and pulmonary trunk are not well visualized in the lateral projection. The lower one third of the right ventricle normally makes contact with the anterior chest wall. The posterior border of the cardiovascular silhouette extends from the inferior margin of the mainstem bronchi and extends to the diaphragm; the border-forming structures are (from above downward) the left atrium, left ventricle, and inferior vena cava. (C) 60° left anterior oblique (LAO) projection. In this projection the anterior border of the cardiovascular silhouette is formed (from above downward) by the right innominate vein, superior vena cava, right atrium, and right ventricle.

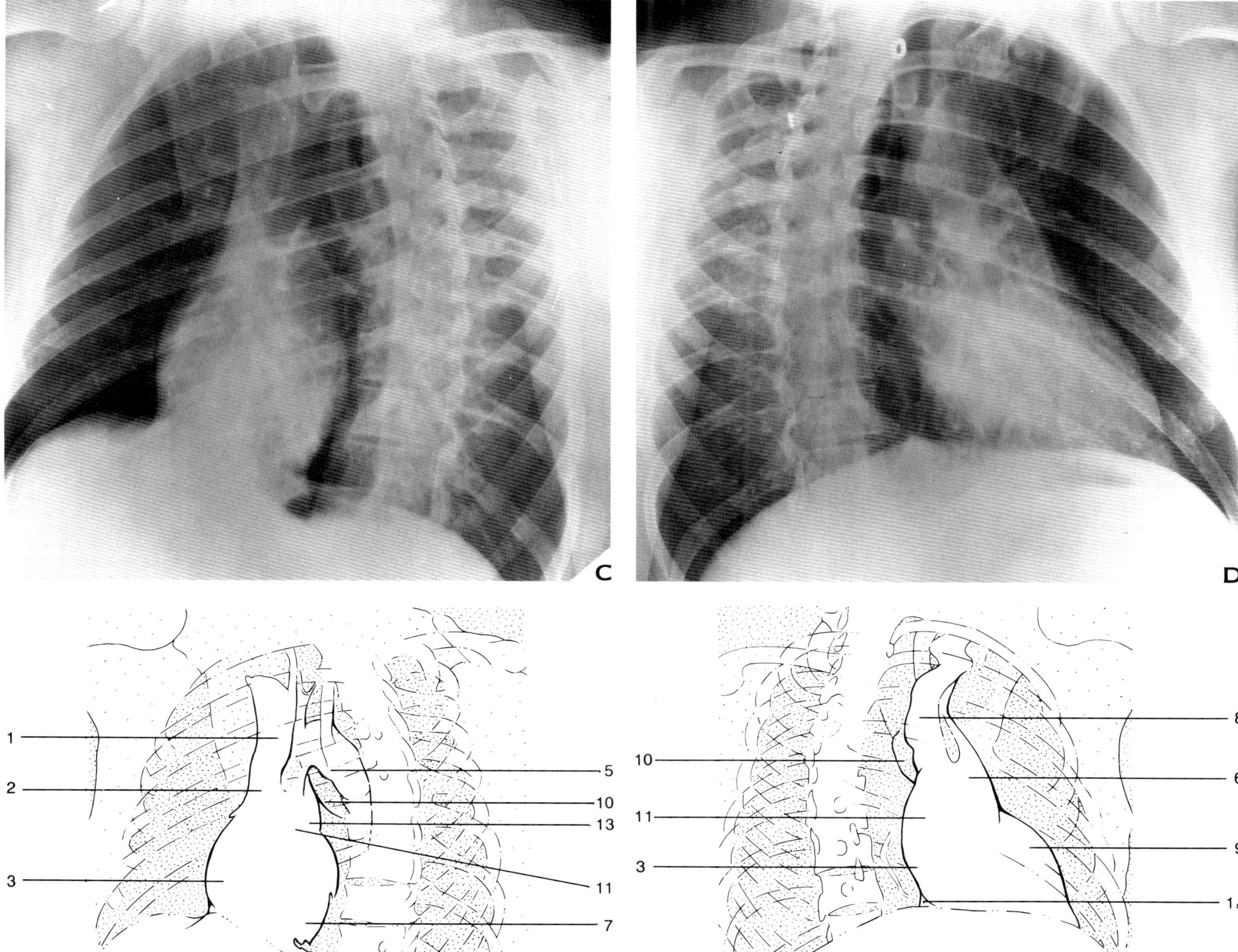

Depending on its size, the ascending aorta may or may not contribute to the contour anterior contour in this projection. An enlarged or tortuous ascending aorta appears as a discrete structure between the superior vena cava and the right atrium. The right ventricle is usually not visualized in this projection; however, in some individuals the inlet portion of the right ventricle is border forming. On the left, the border-forming structures are the left atrium, the upper margin of which lies just below the left main bronchus, and the left ventricle, which extends to the level of the diaphragm. The inferior aspect of the aortic arch and the upper aspect of the left pulmonary artery are separated by a clear space, the aortopulmonary window. (In this example, the left main bronchus is projected over the aortopulmonary window.) Enlargement or displacement of either (or both) of these structures may narrow or obliterate the aortopulmonary window. (D) 45° right anterior oblique (RAO) projection. The anterior border of the cardiovascular silhouette is formed (from above downward) by the ascending aorta, the pulmonary trunk, and the right ventricle. The posterior border is formed by the left atrium (just beneath the main bronchi) and the right atrium.

Administering barium paste to opacify the esophagus facilitates identification of an enlarged left atrium (in the RAO and lateral projections) or dilated descending aorta (in the PA and lateral projections).

COMPUTED TOMOGRAPHY

Unlike plain films and angiography, CT is capable of displaying anatomic structures without overlapping. The standard study consists of a set of contiguous transverse slices. To evaluate the heart and great vessels, rapid-sequence images are obtained after an intravenous bolus injection of contrast material (Fig. 1.4). By adjusting window and level settings, it is possible to create images with a wide range of contrast.

Whereas most thoracic structures, including the great vessels, are adequately visualized on conventional contrast-enhanced CT scans, motion artifacts often severely degrade images of the

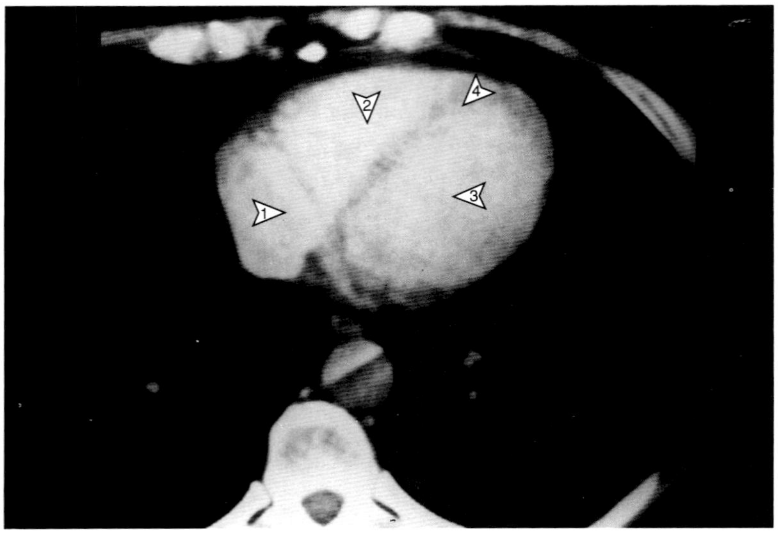

Fig. 1.4 Conventional CT of the heart. Nongated axial image at the level of the ventricles. The right ventricle is anterior and to the right of the left ventricle. The left atrium is not included in this section.

1 right atrium
2 right ventricle
3 left ventricle
4 ventricular septum

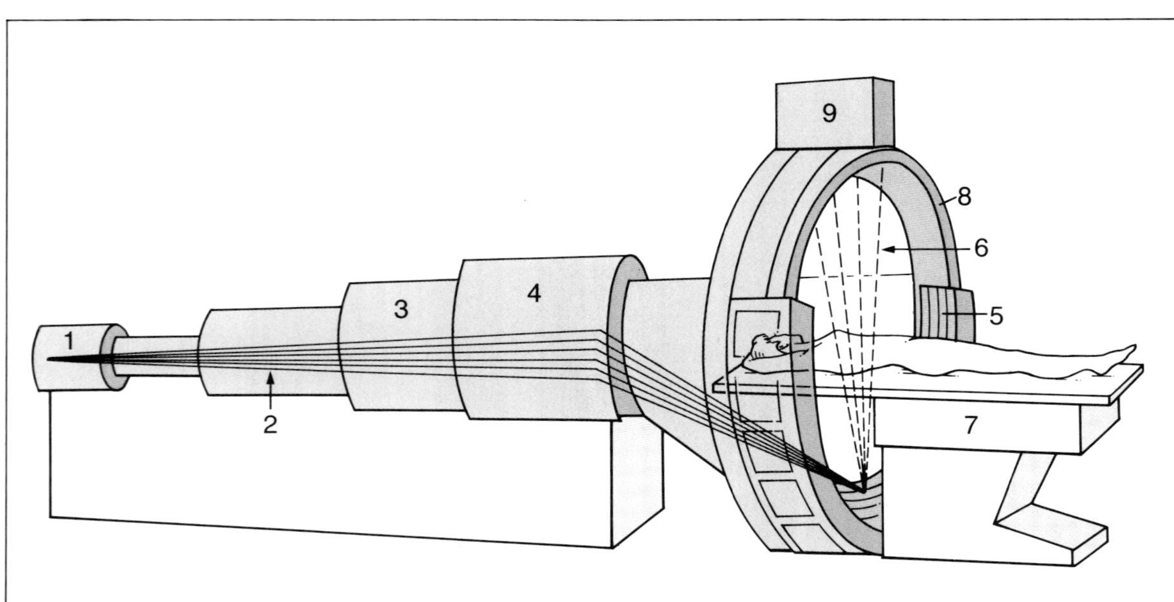

1 electron gun (cathode)
2 electron beam
3 focusing coil
4 deflector coil
5 tungsten target ring (anodes)
6 fan-shaped X-ray beam
7 patient couch
8 detectors
9 data acquisition system (computer)

Fig. 1.5 Cine CT scanner. Schematic cross-section of the Imatron C-100 cine CT scanner. In this device a focused beam of electrons originating in the cathode ("electron gun") is accelerated by electromagnetic fields and directed to four fixed tungsten targets (anodes), which are arrayed in a semicircle beneath the patient. The fan-shaped beam of radiation emitted by the tungsten targets passes upward through the patient and is collimated by the detector array, which comprises two rows of stationary detectors located above the patient. The detectors, which consist of scintillation crystals coupled to photodiode arrays, feed the data into an acquisition system which digitizes and stores information at the rate of eight million 16-bit words per second. The reconstructed images are similar to those of a conventional CT scan. Unlike a conventional CT scanner, which depends on the mechanical motion of a motorized gantry, the cine CT scanner has no moving parts. By minimizing the constraints imposed by heat loading in a conventional CT scanner, the cine CT scanner allows a rapid scanning speed (short exposure time), multiplanar images, and continuous multilevel scanning.

heart. Therefore, conventional CT is largely limited to the evaluation of pericardial disease and mediastinal masses contiguous with the heart and great vessels.

A "cine" CT scanner, which produces very short (millisecond) exposures, overcomes most of the problems associated with conventional CT. Unlike conventional CT scanners, which employ X-ray tubes, the cine CT scanner employs an electron gun and accelerator to generate a beam of electrons, which is steered magnetically to four tungsten cathode rings (targets) located beneath the patient. Each target generates a fan beam of photons which pass through the patient and activate a double ring of stationary detectors arranged in a semicircle overhead (Fig. 1.5). Because cine CT does not employ moving parts or X-ray tubes, it is not limited by mechanical inertia or tube heating capacity.

Three modes of cardiac cine CT are currently available. In the *cine mode*, electrocardiographically triggered images are created at a rate of 17 images per second on each target ring. Such images clearly depict changes in the ventricular chamber and wall thickness throughout the cardiac cycle (Fig. 1.6). In the *flow mode*, electrocardiographically gated images are acquired at each of two to eight levels; at each level the data are acquired at precisely the same point in the cardiac cycle. A computer-generated time-density curve, which correlates with cardiac output, is used to measure blood flow in a region of interest (cardiac chamber, vessel, or myocardium). In the *volume mode*, rapid scanning on two target rings is combined with automated movement of the patient couch at 17 cm/sec, generating 80 contiguous slices covering an area of 64 cm^2. The images are reformatted to display the entire ventricular cavity in systole and diastole. Using these images, it is possible to measure end diastolic volume, ejection fraction, and ventricular wall motion. The quantitative assessment of ventricular function provided by cine CT correlates well with data obtained from combined cardiac catheterization and angiocardiography, which remains the "gold standard."

Although cine CT provides valuable structural and functional data, it may be superseded by advances in echocardiography and magnetic resonance imaging (MRI) (see Chapters 2 and 4). At present, cine CT is available in only a few centers; whether it will assume a major role in cardiac diagnosis remains to be seen.

ELECTROCARDIOGRAPHY

The electrocardiogram (ECG) detects the electrical activity of the heart. It is an essential part of the work-up of patients with both congenital and acquired heart disease.

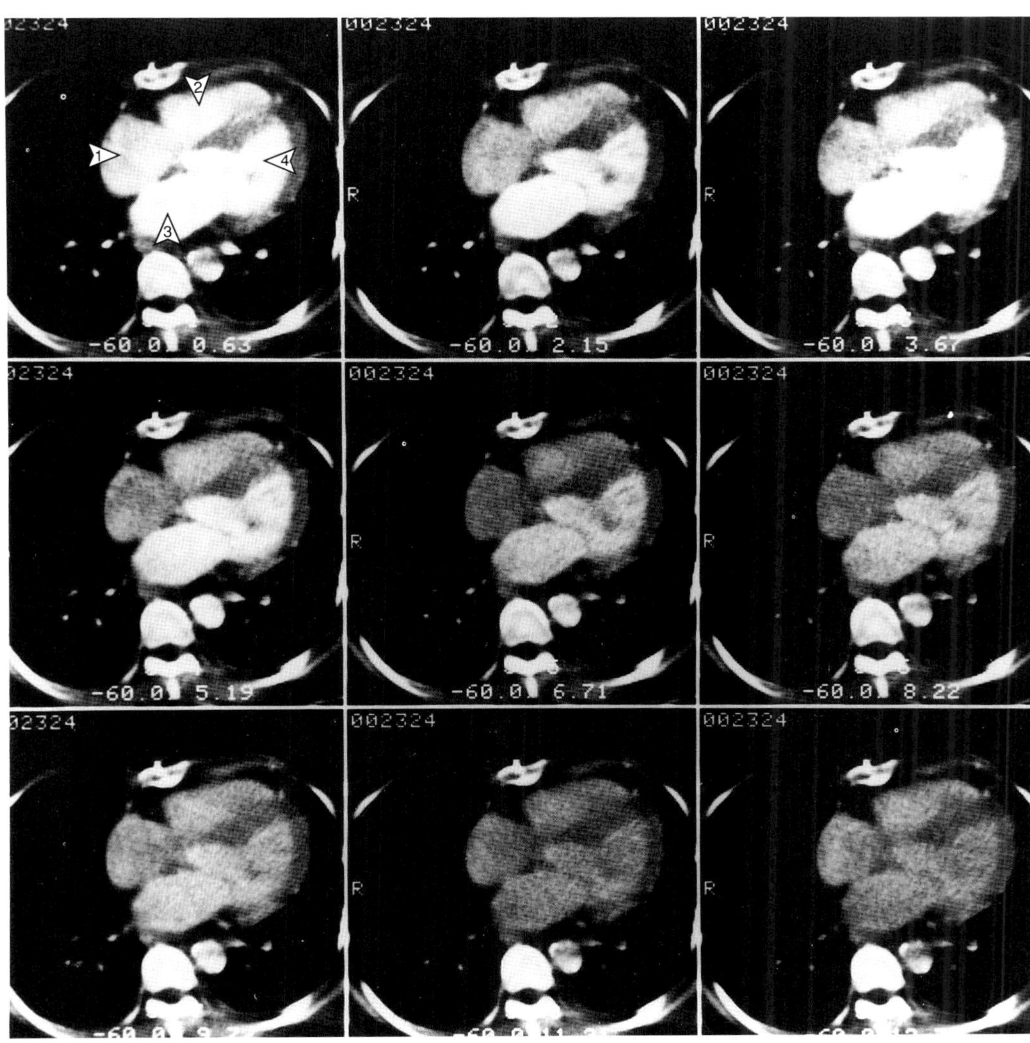

Fig. 1.6 Cardiac cine CT. Rapid-sequence images through midportion of the heart. The first frame is at the top left, the last is at the bottom right.

1 right atrium
2 right ventricle
3 left atrium
4 left ventricle

EXTERNAL ELECTROCARDIOGRAPHY

The normal external ECG consists of a series of waves which represent cardiac electrical activity (Figs. 1.7 and 1.8). The P-wave reflects electrical activity during atrial depolarization. The T-wave is produced by repolarization of the atria. The Q-wave (negative deflection), R-wave (positive deflection), and S-wave (negative deflection) result from ventricular depolarization. The time needed for atrial depolarization and subsequent atrial repolarization, as well as for conduction through the atrioventricular node, is indicated by the PR-interval (the inter-

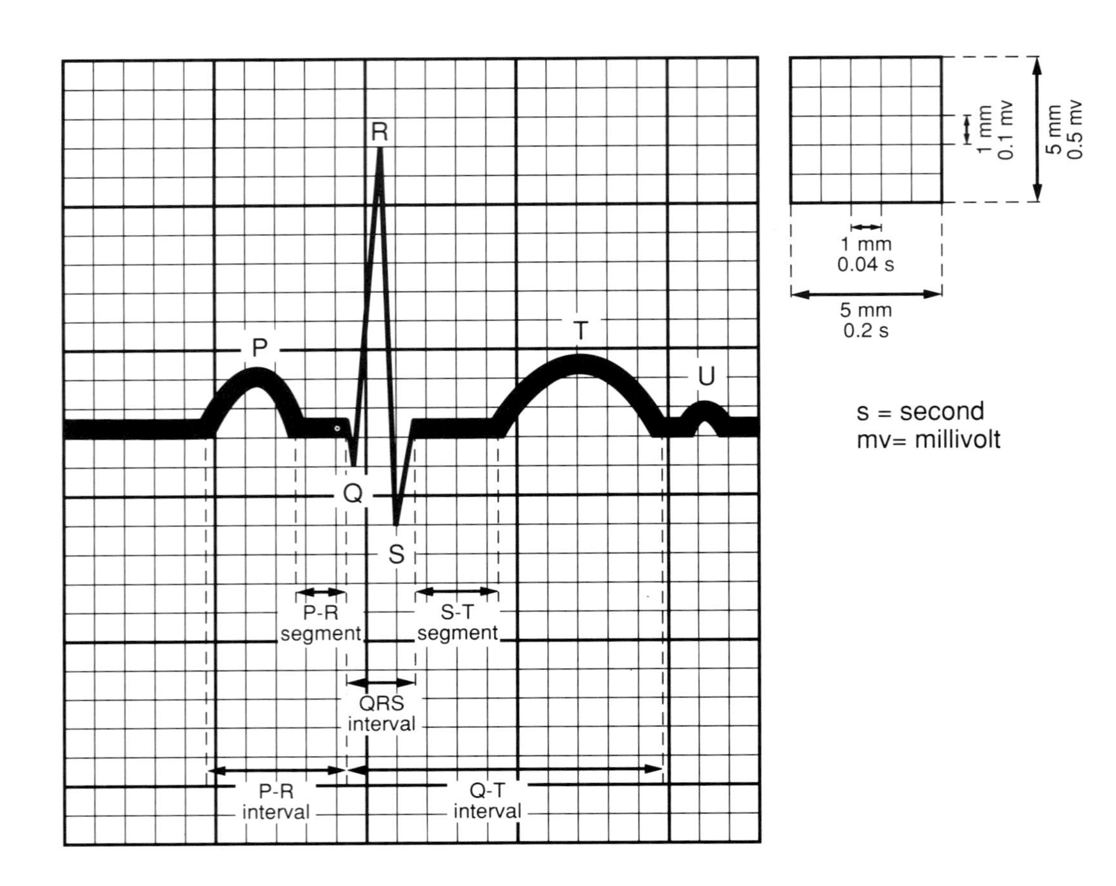

Fig. 1.7 Normal electrocardiogram (schematic).

NORMAL RANGES				
	P-R Interval (seconds)	QRS Interval (seconds)	Rate	Q-T Interval (seconds)
ADULTS	0.12-0.20	0.07-0.10	60	< 0.42
			70	< 0.40
			80	< 0.37
			90	< 0.35
			100	< 0.34
			120	< 0.31

val between the P-wave and the initial deflection of the QRS complex). Ventricular repolarization occurs during the ST-segment and T-wave. (The junction between the end of ventricular depolarization and the ST-segment is known as the J-point.) The fetal ECG normally exhibits considerable variation in voltage and duration of electrical activity. This normal variability persists throughout infancy, childhood, and adolescence.

INTERNAL ELECTROCARDIOGRAPHY

Electrophysiological abnormalities that are not apparent on the external ECG can be quantitated by mapping the endocardium electrophysiologically with an intracardiac electrode ("electrophysiologic study"). Such abnormalities include aberrant con-

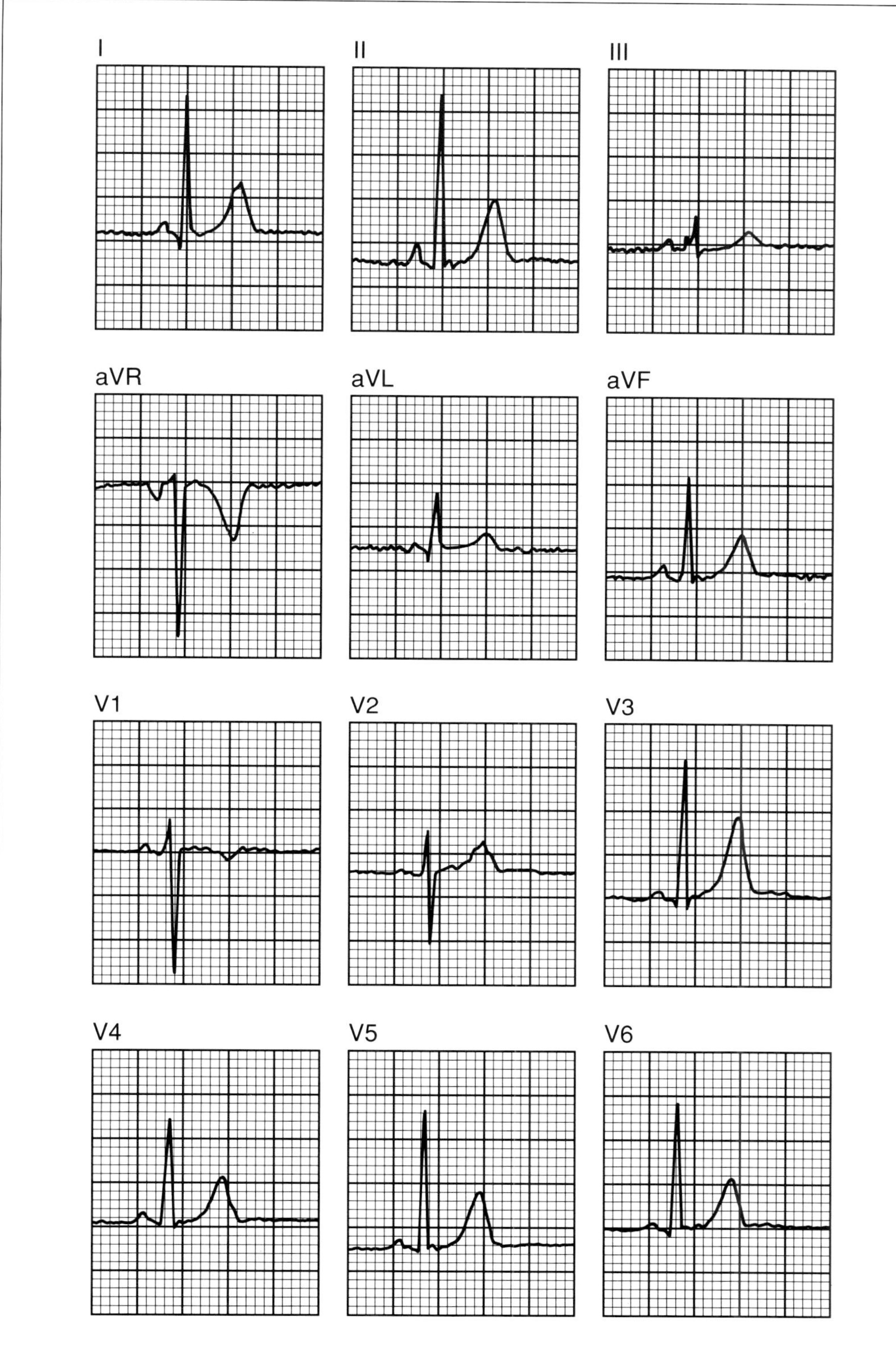

Fig. 1.8 Normal electrocardiogram. In this normal subject the ventricular rate is 75 beats/minute; the PR-interval is 112 milliseconds; the QRS duration is 68 milliseconds; and the P, R, and T axes are 57, 38, and 39, respectively.

duction pathways, ectopic foci, and gaps in the intraventricular conduction system (Fig. 1.9). Intracardiac electrodes can also be used therapeutically. For example, by applying a strong electrical pulse it is possible to excise ectopic foci, which can lead to dramatic improvement in patients with severe arrhythmias caused by an ectopic focus or an aberrant conduction pathway.

CONTINUOUS MONITORING

The Holter system, which enables the cardiologist to monitor electrical activity for prolonged periods, is commonly used in the diagnosis and management of intractable arrhythmias (Fig. 1.10). Continuous monitoring is also used to diagnose ar-

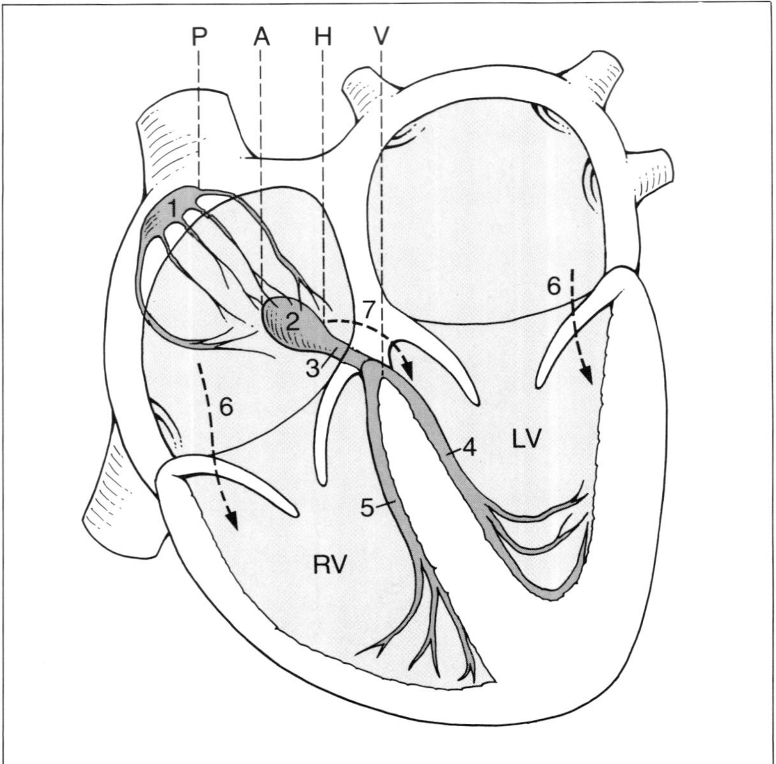

Fig. 1.9 Electrophysiological mapping of the endocardium. Tracings obtained at the superior vena cava–right atrial junction reflect the electrical activity of the sinus node. The electrical activity of the atrioventricular node, the bundle of His, and bundle branches is monitored by moving the electrode to the appropriate position. The P-A interval indicates the intraatrial conduction time (normal, 5–40 milliseconds). The A-H interval indicates the transit time between the atrioventricular node and the bundle of His (normal, 50–150 milliseconds). The His–ventricular (H-V) interval is a parameter of ventricular depolarization (normal, 30–55 milliseconds). By recording and stimulating different segments of the endocardium, it is possible to detect aberrant connections such as Kent's fascicle or the bundle of Mahaim.

1	sinus node	LA	left atrium
2	atrioventricular node	RA	right atrium
3	bundle of his	LV	left ventricle
4	left bundle branch	RV	right ventricle
5	right bundle branch	P-A	interval intra-atrial conduction
6	Kent's fascicle	A-H	atrioventricular node transit
7	bundle of Mahaim	H-V	ventricular depolarization

Strip #	Time	Date	Marker	Arrhythmia	Symptoms/Activities
1	09:46:40	07-SEP-90		Couplet	
2	10:19:50	07-SEP-90		Couplet	
3	11:30:00	07-SEP-90	*	Isolated PVC	Palpitations
4	11:30:16	07-SEP-90		Couplet	
5	12:00:00	07-SEP-90	*	Isolated PVC	Palpitations
6	12:49:34	07-SEP-90		Isolated PVC	
7	15:00:00	07-SEP-90	*	Bigeminy	Palpitations
8	15:49:56	07-SEP-90		VTACH, 7 bts, 168 BPM	
9	16:43:17	07-SEP-90		VTACH, 4 bts, 103 BPM	
10	17:00:00	07-SEP-90	*	Isolated PVC	Palpitations
11	18:14:10	07-SEP-90		VITACH, 4 bts. 106 BPM	
12	18:14:13	07-SEP-90		VTACH, 4 bts, 106 BPM	
13	18:54:48	07-SEP-90		HR 109	
14	19:30:00	07-SEP-90	*	Isolated PVC	Palpitations
15	21:00:00	07-SEP-90	*	Couplet	Palpitations
	21:00:00	07-SEP-90	*	Couplet	Palpitations
16	22:12:41	07-SEP-90		VTACH, 4 bts, 128 BPM	
17	23:13:59	07-SEP-90		VTACH, 4 bts, 126 BPM	
18	02:31:40	08-SEP-90		HR 51	
19	03:49:20	08-SEP-90		HR 51	
20	05:39:14	08-SEP-90		Isolated PVC	
21	06:00:00	08-SEP-90	*	Couplet	Palpitations
22	06:06:03	08-SEP-90		Isolated PVC	
23	06:06:07	08-SEP-90		Couplet	
24	07:48:43	08-SEP-90		VRHY, 3 bts, 53 BPM	

A

Fig. 1.10 Holter monitoring system. This system enables one to obtain a continuous record of the electrical activity of the heart over a prolonged period. The example shown is from a 60-year-old patient with dilated cardiomyopathy. (A) The time of abnormal electrical activity (arrhythmia) is indicated.

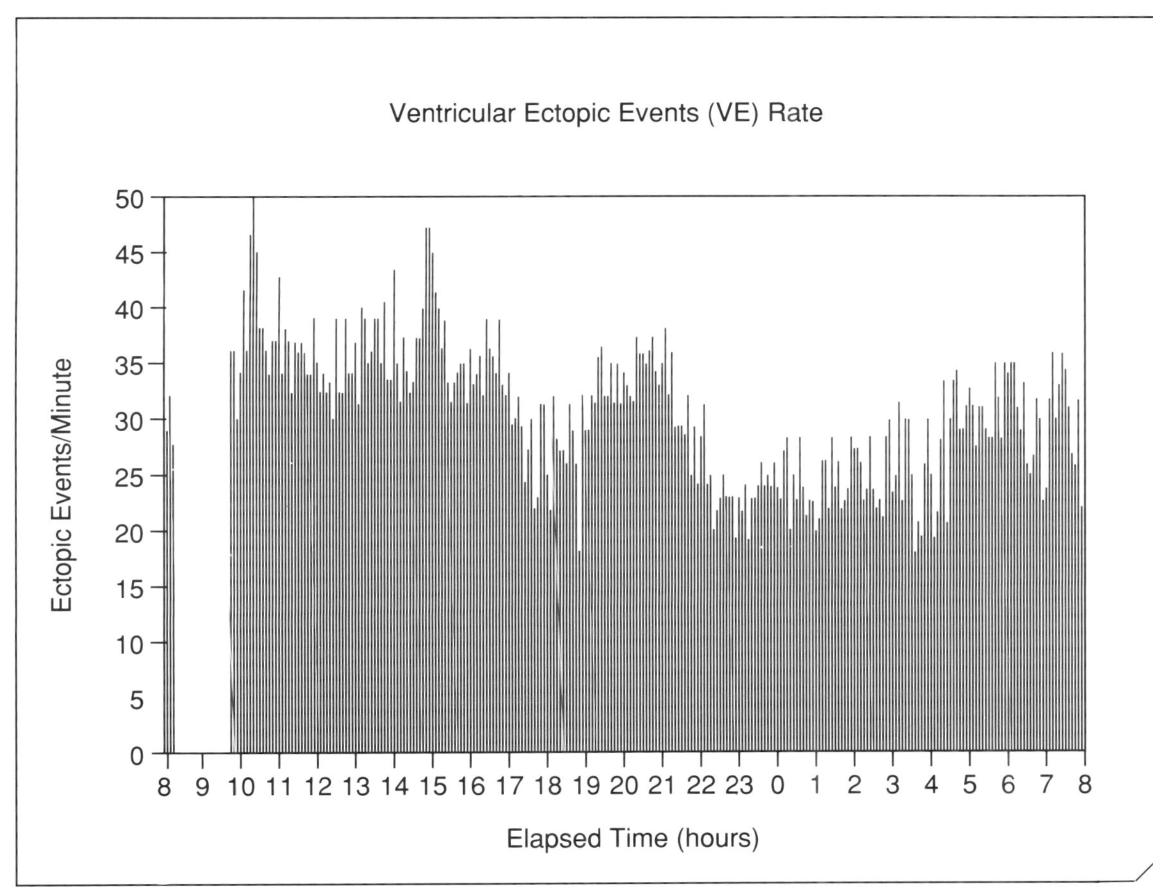

Fig. 1.10 (continued) (B) The frequency of ventricular ectopic events is displayed graphically. The vertical axis indicates the number of ectopic events per minute and the horizontal axis indicates elapsed time in hours. (C) The summary indicates that this patient has a severe arrhythmia characterized by couplets, premature ventricular contractions (PVCs), isolated PVCs, bigeminy, ventricular tachycardia, and bradycardia. Altogether, ventricular ectopic events account for 31 percent of the QRS complexes. These detailed data are very helpful in assessing the severity of the arrhythmias in a given patient.

104085 QRS complexes

32641	Ventricular	ectopics which represent	31% of total QRS complexes
194	Supraventricular	ectopics which represent	1% of total QRS complexes
	Paced QRS complexes	which represent	% of total QRS complexes

Ventricular Ectopy

16157 Isolated
1805 Bigeminal Cycles
7974 Couplets
174 Runs
536 Beats in Runs
7 Beats LONGEST at 168 BPM at 15:49:55 07-SEP-90
7 Beats FASTEST at 168 BPT at 15:49:55 07-SEP-90

Supraventricular Ectopy

165 Isolated
5 Couplets
4 Runs
19 Beats in Runs
7 Beats LONGEST at 80 BPM at 06:06:03 08-SEP-90
7 Beats FASTEST at 80 BPM at 06:06:03 08-SEP-90

Heart Rates

49 MIN at 07:48:43 08-SEP-90
76 AVG
109 MAX at 18:54:48 07-SEP-90

S-T Levels Channel

mm at
mm at

C

rhythmias that are intermittent or occur during physical activity or emotional stress, and to monitor the response to medical therapy.

ELECTROCARDIOGRAPHY IN CONGENITAL HEART DISEASE

The external ECG provides information about heart rate, rhythm, abnormalities of the conduction system, and chamber enlargement in patients with suspected or documented congenital heart disease; it can also be used to monitor ventricular function over time. Hypertrophy of one or both ventricles is a feature of many congenital defects (Fig. 1.11). Certain cardiac malformations [eg, atrioventricular septal defect (endocardial cushion defect), corrected transposition of the great arteries, univentricular atrioventricular connection] are associated with abnormal patterns of depolarization and repolarization. The atrioventricular node and penetrating bundle (of His), which are abnormally positioned in these malformations, are likely to be injured during corrective surgery. Certain malformations (eg, Ebstein's malformation, right ventricular dysplasia) are associated with accessory conduction pathways (Fig. 1.12).

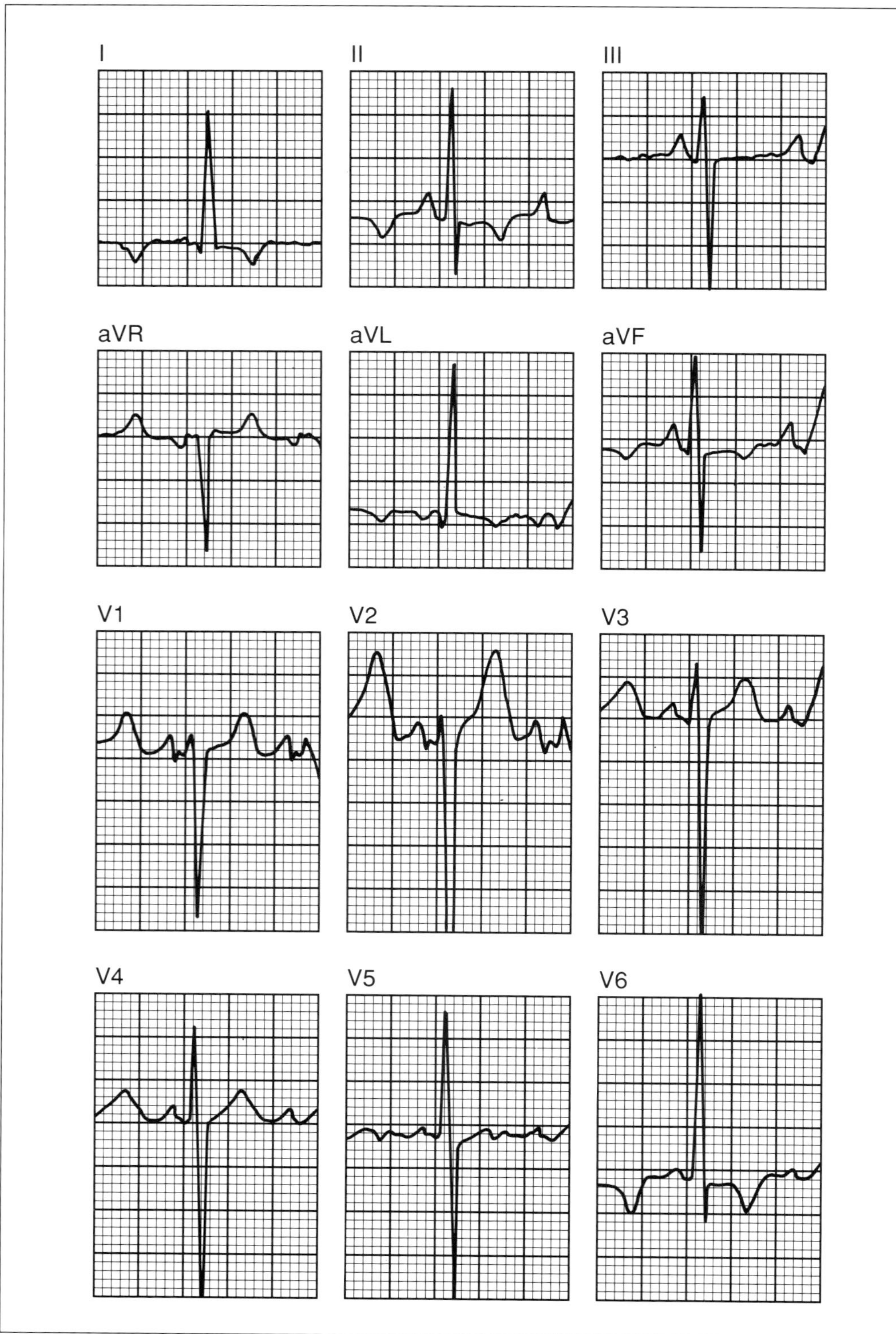

Fig. 1.11 Electrocardiographic findings in left ventricular hypertrophy. Note the small R-wave in V1 and V2, the tall R-wave in V5 and V6, and the absence of S-wave in V5 and V6.

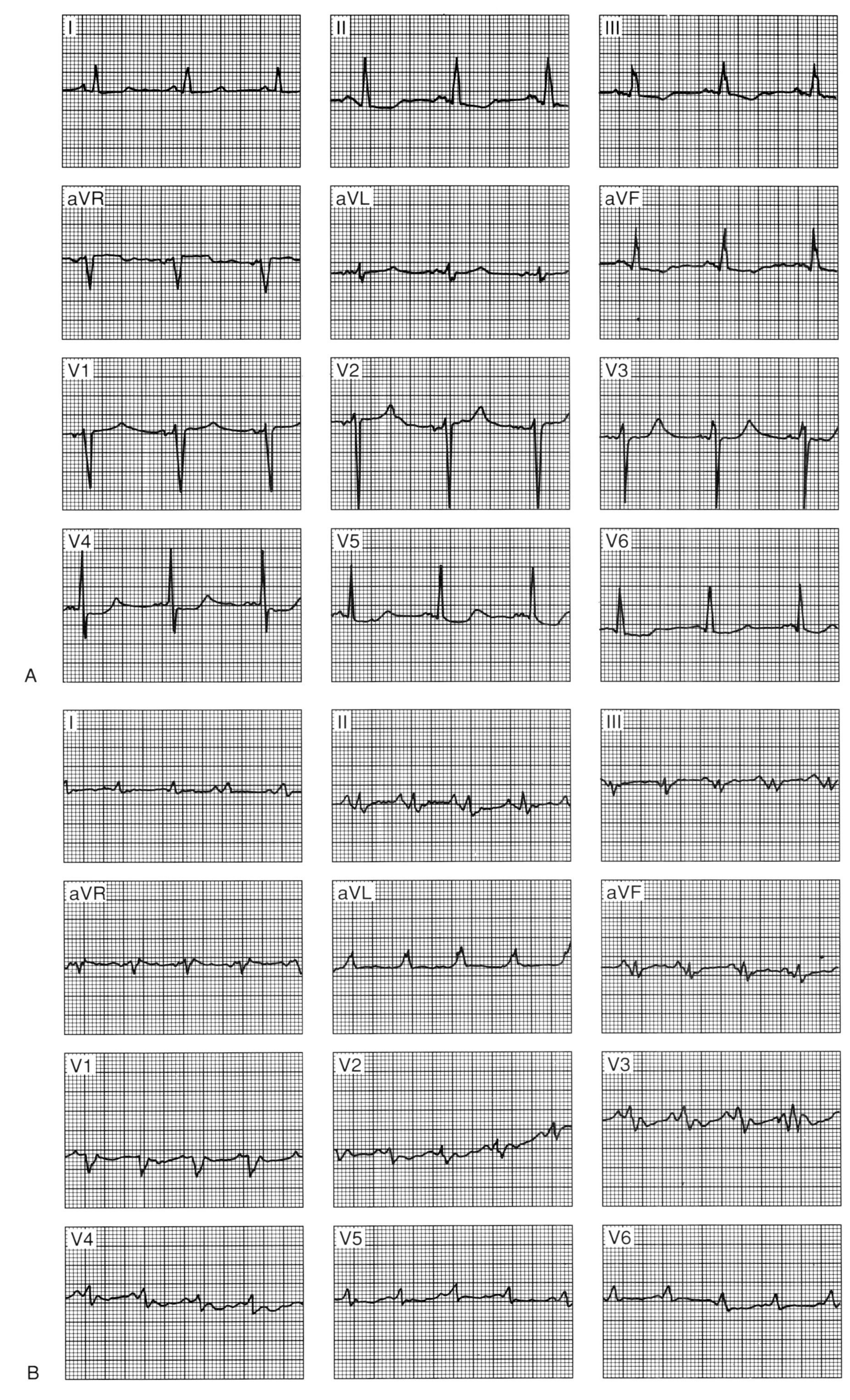

Fig. 1.12 Arrythmia due to congenital heart disease. This man with Ebstein's malformation of the tricuspid valve had experienced repeated episodes of supraventricular tachycardia. (A) ECG demonstrates typical features of the Wolff–Parkinson–White syndrome (type B): a short P-R interval and slurring of the initial inscription of the QRS complex, producing a delta wave that is directed superiorly, posteriorly, and to the left. (B) A subsequent tracing in the same patient demonstrates peaked P-waves (indicating right atrial overload) and low-voltage "splintered" QRS complexes (indicating right ventricular conduction delay). This pattern is typical of Ebstein's malformation (see Chapter 12).

Patients with these anomalies tend to develop ectopic foci of electrical activity, which can lead to an intractable arrhythmia. Such pathways can usually be detected with an electrophysiologic study.

ELECTROCARDIOGRAPHY IN ACQUIRED HEART DISEASE

The electrocardiographic findings in patients with acquired heart disease are quite variable and depend on the portion of the heart affected. Valvular disease is usually associated with pressure or volume overload, which may affect one or more chambers. Abnormal myocardial perfusion secondary to ischemic heart disease is manifested electrocardiographically by altered depolarization and repolarization.

Increased right atrial pressure and right atrial volume overload are manifested on the ECG by tall, peaked, and narrow P-waves ("P-pulmonale"), which are best seen in leads II, III, and aVf.

Left atrial enlargement secondary to mitral stenosis or mitral insufficiency is manifested electrocardiographically by wide, notched P-waves ("P-mitrale") in leads II and V6. The abnormal P-waves are typically 0.11 seconds or longer in lead II.

Right ventricular hypertrophy is manifested electrocardiographically by QR forces that are directed to the right. The R-waves are abnormally tall in leads V1 and V2, and there are deep S-waves in leads V4 and V5. Characteristically, the direction of the ST-segments and T-waves is opposite to that of the widest portion of the QRS complex.

Left ventricular hypertrophy causes distortion of the QRS loop in the direction of the left scapula. This is manifested on the ECG by small R-waves and deep S-waves in leads V1 and V2, and tall R-waves and small or absent S-waves in leads V5 and V6. The ST-segment and T-wave are positive in V1 and negative in V6 (see Fig. 1.10).

The transmission of electrical activity through the heart is altered in many types of acquired heart disease (Figs. 1.13 to 1.15). Conduction defects (eg, complete atrioventricular disso-

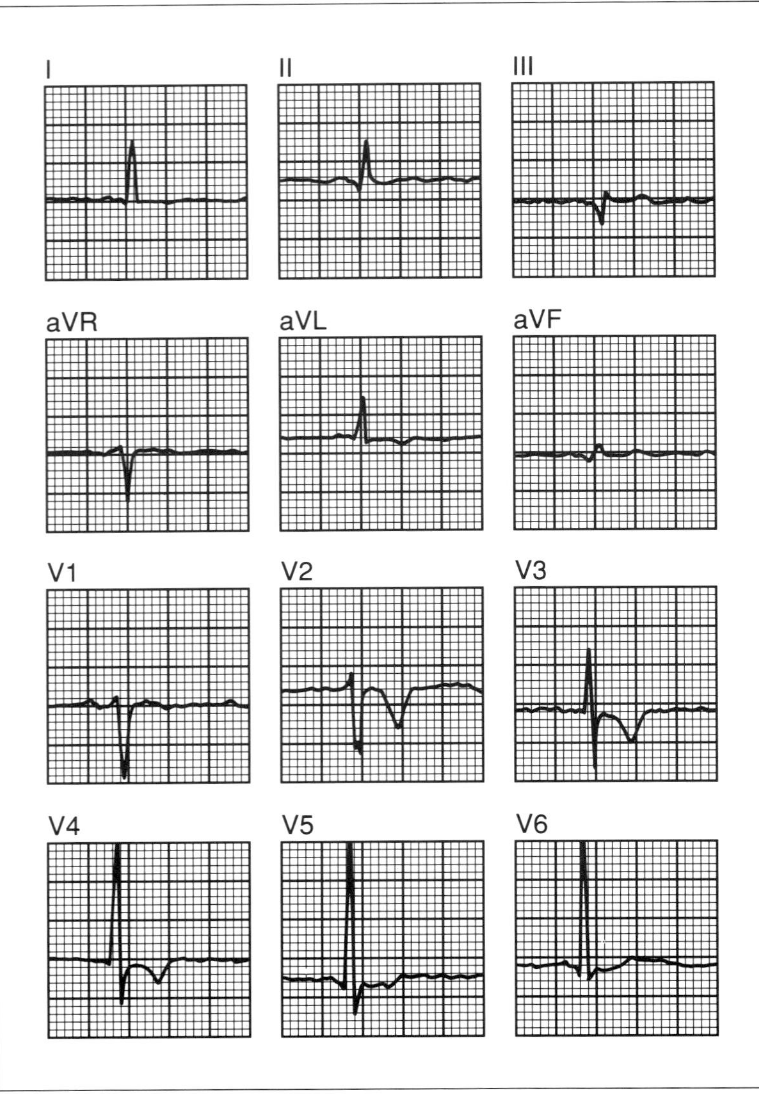

Fig. 1.13 Anterior myocardial infarction. ECG of a 72-year-old patient demonstrates inverted T-waves in leads I, aVl, V5, and V6; poor progression of the R-wave; and Q-waves in V1, V3, and V4. The QRS is prolonged (128 milliseconds). These ECG findings are typical of an anterior wall infarction of the left ventricle.

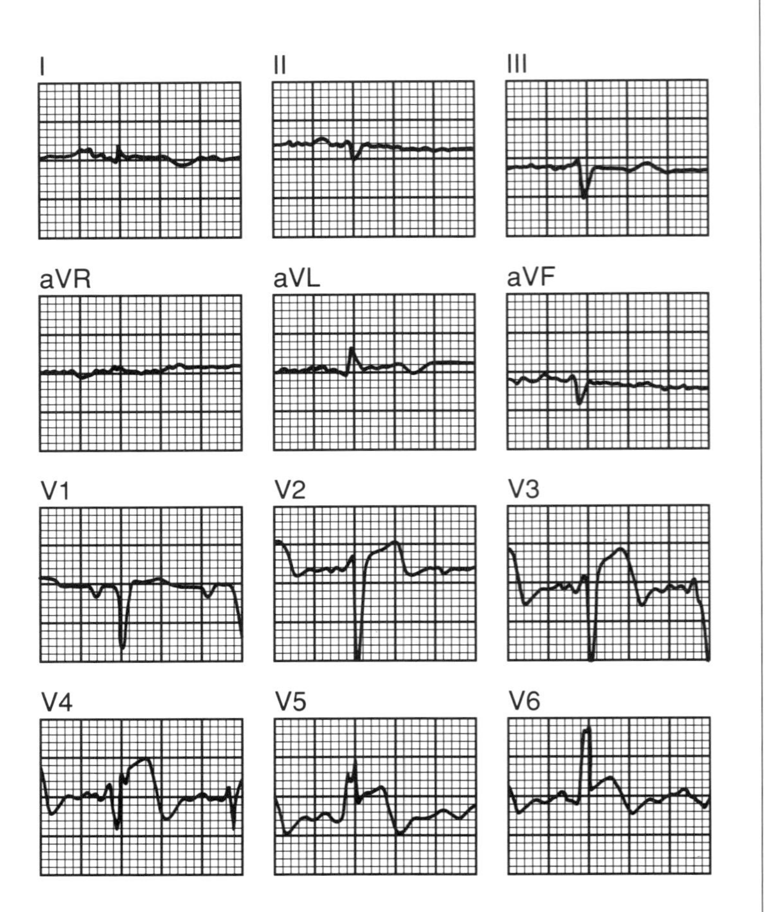

Fig. 1.14 Anteroseptal myocardial infarction. ECG of a 50-year-old man shows absence of the R-wave in V1 through V4 and T-wave inversion in I, aVl, V5, and V6. This pattern is typical for an anteroseptal infarction of the left ventricle.

ciation, bundle branch block) are quite common in patients with ischemic heart disease.

Altered transmission through branches of the conduction system (bundle branch block) is common in patients with acquired heart disease. It can affect the left ventricle, right ventricle, or both. When the duration of the QRS complex is moderately prolonged (0.1–0.12 seconds) the conduction disturbance is called an incomplete bundle branch block; when the QRS complex is longer than 0.12 seconds, it is called a complete bundle branch block (Fig. 1.16). In patients with a right bundle branch block, the first 0.04 seconds of the QRS complex are normal in configuration but the last part is abnormal. In patients with a left bundle branch block the entire QRS complex is "written" by an abnormal depolarization wave, resulting in a markedly abnormal tracing.

Some individuals have accessory conduction pathways between the right atrium and the ventricles. One anomaly, which is manifested electrocardiographically by a short PR-interval and an abnormally wide QRS complex, is known as the *Wolf–Parkinson–White complex* (see Fig. 1.12). Clinical manifestations include atrial tachycardia and other arrhythmias.

Acquired heart disease is associated with a wide variety of arrhythmias. One of the most common is atrial fibrillation, which is typically associated with mitral stenosis (Fig. 1.16).

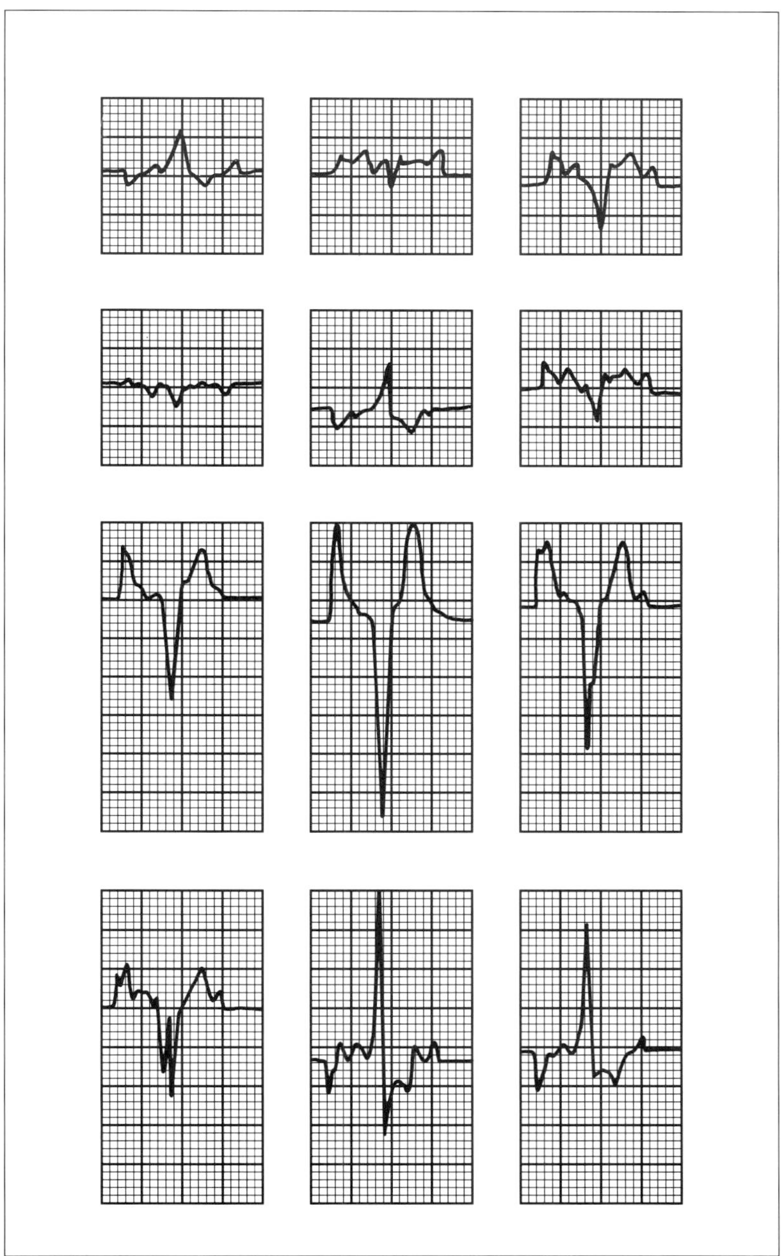

Fig. 1.15 Inferoseptal myocardial infarction. ECG of a 72-year-old patient shows a sinus tachycardia (154 beats/minute) and an abnormally short P-Q interval (104 milliseconds). Abnormal repolarization is seen in leads V5, V6, I, and aVl. This pattern meets the criteria for an inferoseptal infarction of the left ventricle.

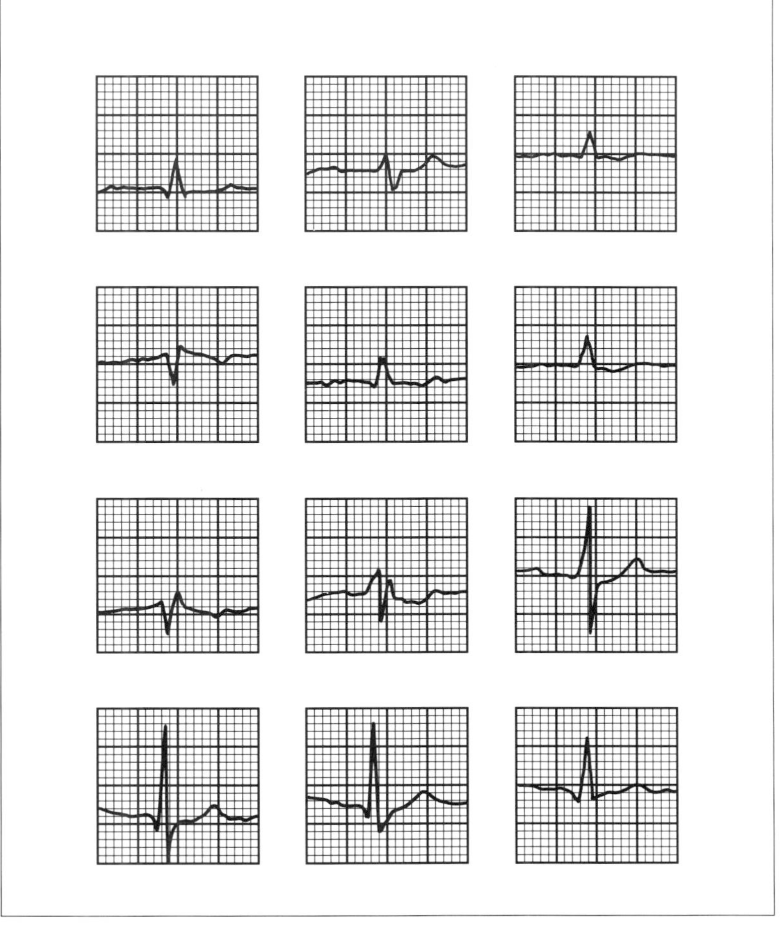

Fig. 1.16 Atrial fibrillation and right bundle branch block. ECG of a 72-year-old patient shows an irregular rhythm with a ventricular rate of 102 beats/minute. P-waves are absent. There is left axis deviation of 30°, as well as a right bundle branch block.

CHAPTER 2

Echocardiography

ISIDRE VILAICOSTA, M.D.
NAVIN C. NANDA, M.D.

The piezoelectric effect was first described by Curie. Rhythmic changes in the shape of a piezoelectric crystal are induced by an alternating electric current. Because of their frequency of occurrence, these changes generate high-frequency sound waves in material with which the crystals are in contact. The ultrasonic waves, when directed at a target object, are reflected owing to the difference of acoustic impedance between the transmission medium and the object. These units were initially used in medical practice to produce energy for application of local heat in the treatment of different pain syndromes and for fragmentation of renal calculi.

In 1954, Edler and Hertz were the first scientists to image, using A-mode ultrasound, a rheumatic mitral valve with an ultrasonic transducer placed over the precordium. This achievement led to the development of M-mode echocardiography in the mid 1960s. In the early 1970s, rapid technologic advancement expanded M-mode echocardiography into two-dimensional echocardiography. The ability to measure the depth of an ultrasound interface is utilized in echocardiography to depict anatomic structures as they produce signals at a given distance from the transducer. This technique has a high degree of resolution and overcomes many of the limitations of the M-mode technique by enabling tomographic sections of the heart to be displayed, depicting cardiac structures in an approximation of real time. Since 1976 this modality has been improved dramatically with ongoing new developments in technology.

Two-dimensional imaging can depict the spatial orientation of the cardiac structures and provides the opportunity to image slices of the heart from multiple transducer positions. The resultant picture is a circular arc sector format displaying a tomographic section of the heart. The use of the Doppler shift in reflected ultrasound beams to measure the velocity of blood flow within the heart began to have clinical application during the late 1970s. A new technique for real-time imaging of intracardiac blood flow, color Doppler imaging, was separately and independently developed in 1982 by two groups: Namekawa, Kasai and Koyano, and Bonner and Miller. Finally, in the 1980s, images representing real-time blood flow could be obtained from third-generation echocardiographic equipment.

INSTRUMENTATION AND TECHNIQUES

Both the instrumentation and the techniques for cardiac ultrasonography have evolved rapidly over the past 20 years. Echocardiography, which initially consisted only of the single-beam M-mode technique, now encompasses two-

CHAPTER LABELING KEY			
RA	right atrium	RV	right ventricle
LA	left atrium	LV	left ventricle

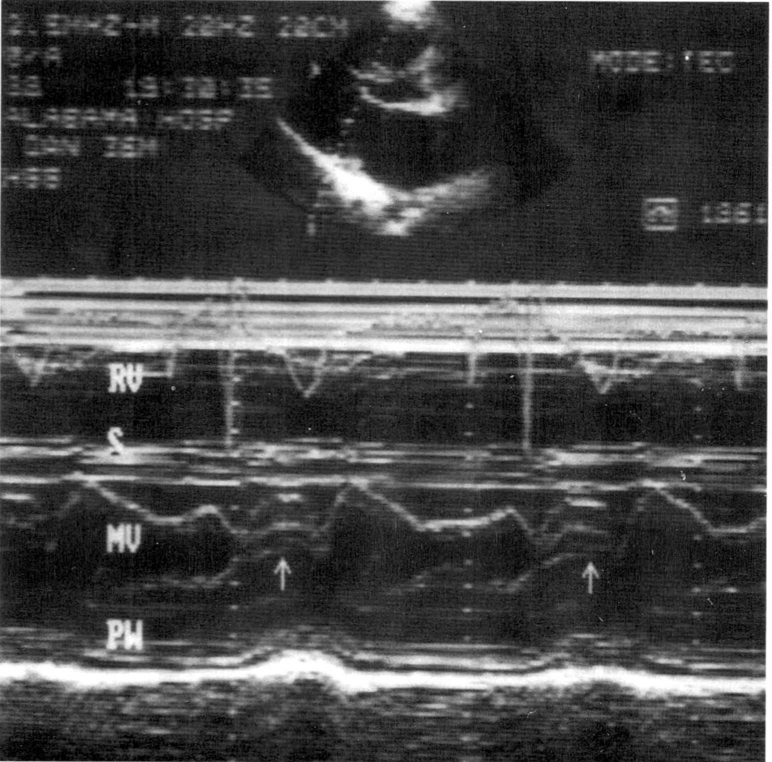

Fig. 2.1 Parasternal long-axis plane with M-mode cursor at the level of the left ventricular inlet. The inferior tracing represents the free wall of the left ventricle, the middle tracing represents the septum, and the segment immediately above it the right ventricular cavity. The lines between the septum and posterior wall of the left ventricle represent the anterior and posterior leaflets of the mitral valve. Note that the anterior leaflet of the mitral valve contacts the septum during systole, indicating anterior systolic motion in this patient with obstructive hypertrophic cardiomyopathy.

S	ventricular septum	PW	posterior wall of left ventricle

dimensional echocardiography, pulsed and continuous-wave Doppler, and color Doppler imaging.

The ultrasonic transducers contain the piezoelectric crystals that generate ultrasonic waves at 2.25 to 5 mHZ. The hand-held transducer is usually placed on the surface of the chest, and the ultrasonic beam is directed towards the part of the heart to be scanned. Trained physicians or technologists can aim these ultrasonic waves at specific cardiac structures. No preliminary preparation of the patient is required for an echocardiographic study, and the test can be easily performed at the bedside. The images can be recorded on videotape for analysis and playback. Stop-action frames are photographed as still images.

M-MODE TRACING

M-mode echocardiography provides an "ice pick" view of the heart, displaying instantaneously the depth of cardiac structures from the chest wall throughout the cardiac cycle. This display is not a one-dimensional recording of the heart because time is the second dimension on M-mode tracings (Fig. 2.1). The amount of information obtained can be increased by changing the direction of the ultrasonic beam. M-mode echocardiography is useful for analyzing the motion of cardiac structures in real time, and, to some extent, for dimension measurement, but is quite limited for investigating cardiac anatomy.

TWO-DIMENSIONAL ECHOCARDIOGRAPHY

Cross-sectional echocardiographic techniques reconstruct an image of the heart from multiple individual ultrasonic scan lines. Most two-dimensional echocardiographs move the ultrasonic beam so that approximately 30 scan lines are obtained per second. The ultrasonic beam can be moved mechanically by oscillating one or more crystals through space, or by sequentially firing a series of crystals.

Two-dimensional echocardiography classically images the heart from several different conventional locations or echocardiographic windows: parasternal, apical, subcostal, and suprasternal (Fig. 2.2). In the parasternal window, the transducer is placed along the left or right parasternal area with the patient supine and slightly tilted into the left or right lateral

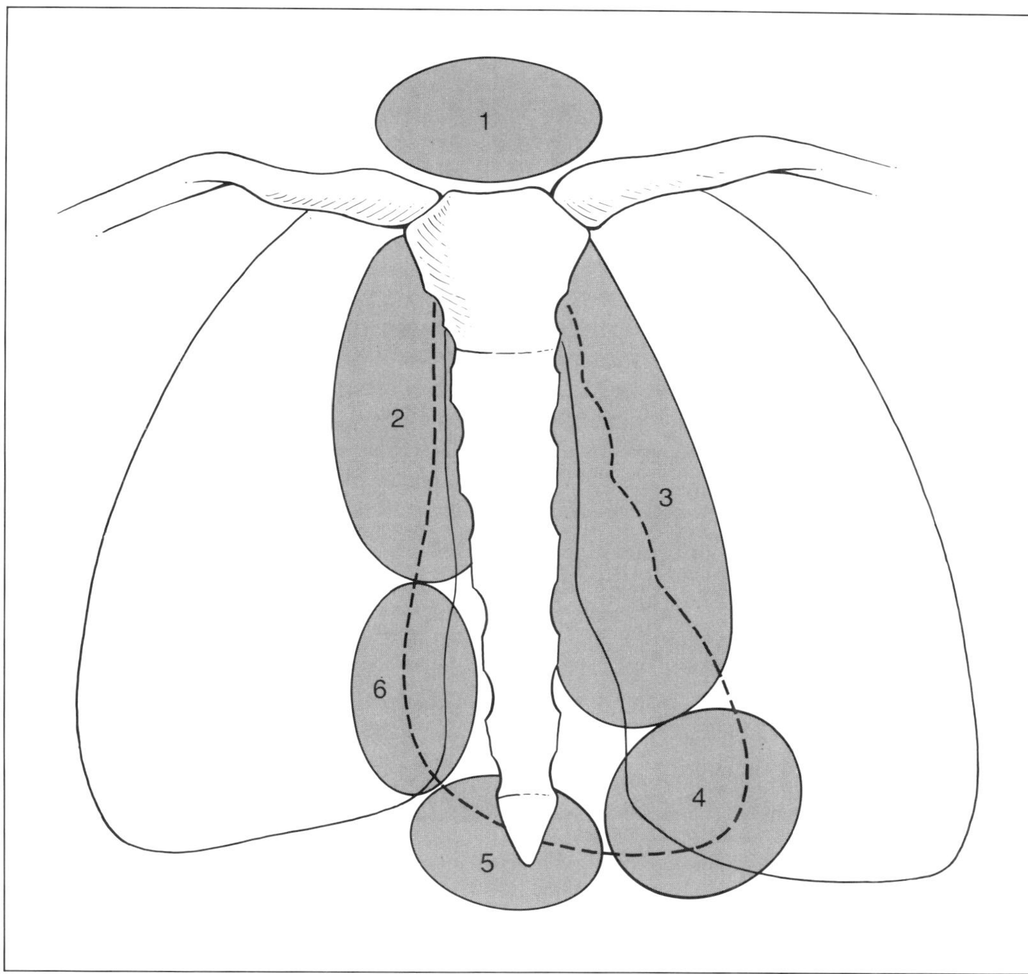

Fig. 2.2 Scanning windows for echocardiography. Schematic representation shows the placement of the transducer in the anterior chest wall for obtaining various echocardiographic projections.

1	suprasternal	4	apical
2	right parasternal	5	subcostal
3	parasternal	6	right apical

decubitus position. This creates tomographic sections that transect the heart parallel to its long axis (Figs. 2.3 and 2.4). The same parasternal window also yields tomographic sections perpendicular to the long axis of the heart (short-axis tomographic views), transecting the heart at several levels from the apex (Figs. 2.5 and 2.6) to the base (Figs. 2.7 and 2.8).

The apical planes are obtained by placing the transducer near (usually inferior to) the palpable cardiac apex while the patient is in the left lateral decubitus position. The apical

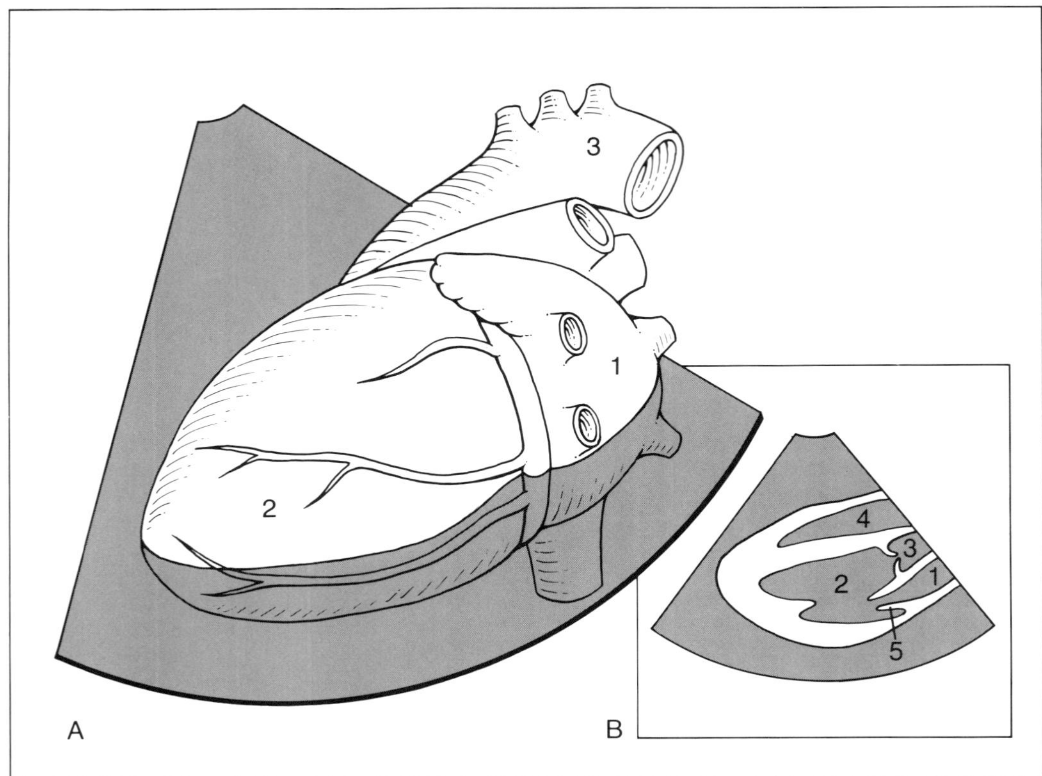

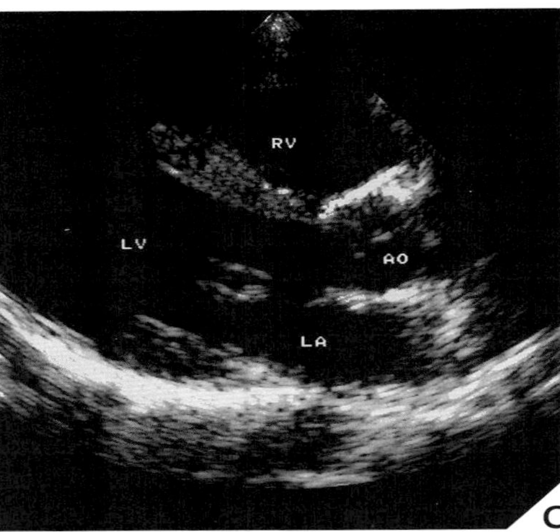

1 left atrium
2 left ventricle
3 aorta
4 right ventricle
5 mitral valve

Fig. 2.3 Normal heart in parasternal long axial plane. (A) Schematic representation shows the parasternal long-axis plane, which passes through the heart, including the two ventricular chambers, arteries, and part of the septum. (B) Schematic representation shows the heart through this view. (C) Parasternal long-axis echocardiogram, in which the echocardiographic section passes through the heart such that it exposes the posterior aspect of the right and left ventricles, left atrium, and aorta.

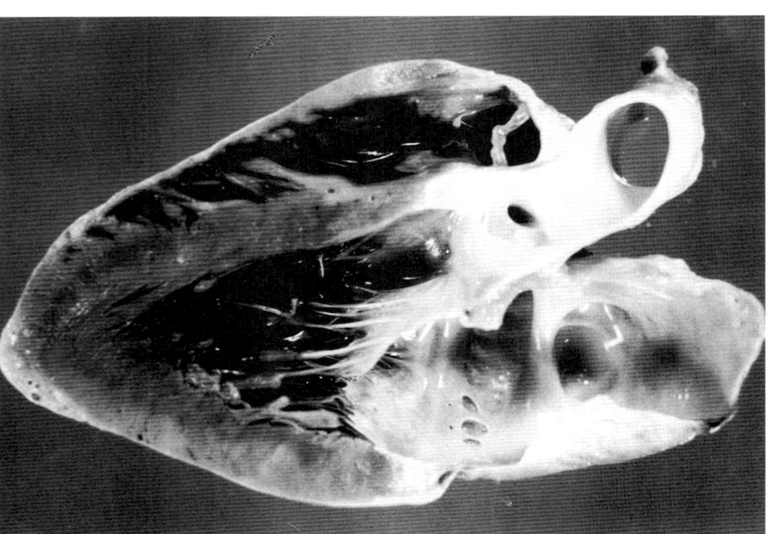

Fig. 2.4 Section of the heart using the same plane as in echocardiography long-axis view.

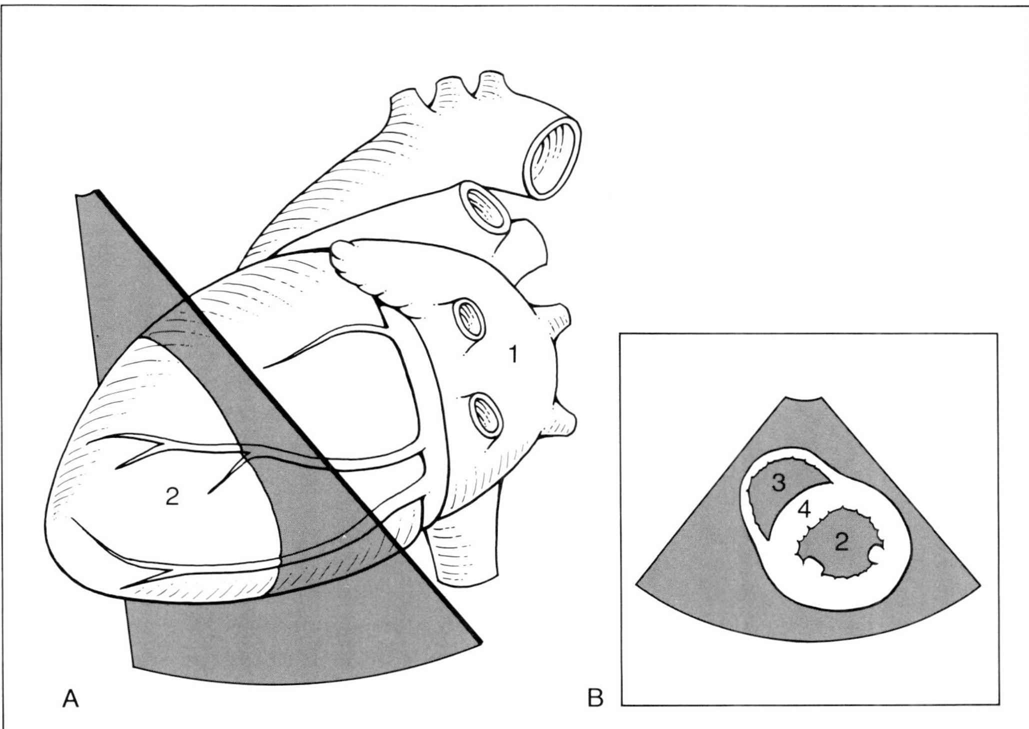

Fig. 2.5 Schematic representation of the plane used for short-axis view at the middle portion of the ventricular chambers; parasternal window. (A) Diagram of the approximate plane, as seen from outside of the heart, is shown. (B) Representation of the ventricular chamber morphology is shown, as seen from this view. (C) An echocardiogram through the base of the left ventricle is shown.

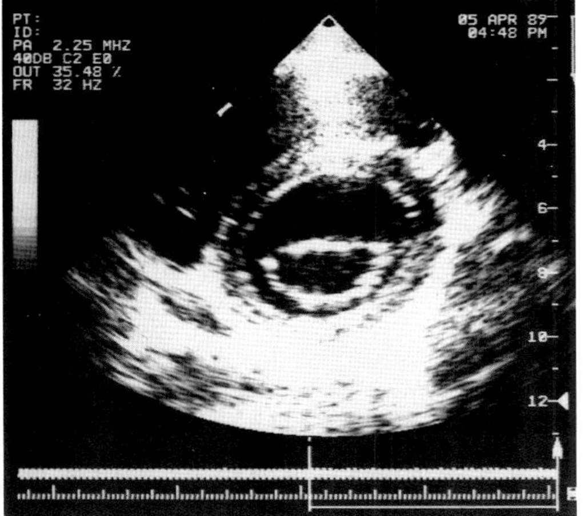

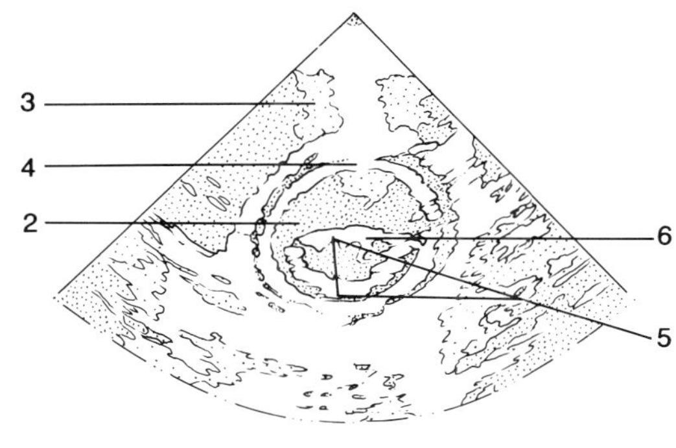

1 left atrium
2 left ventricle
3 right ventricle
4 ventricular septum
5 mitral valve
6 anterior mitral leaflet

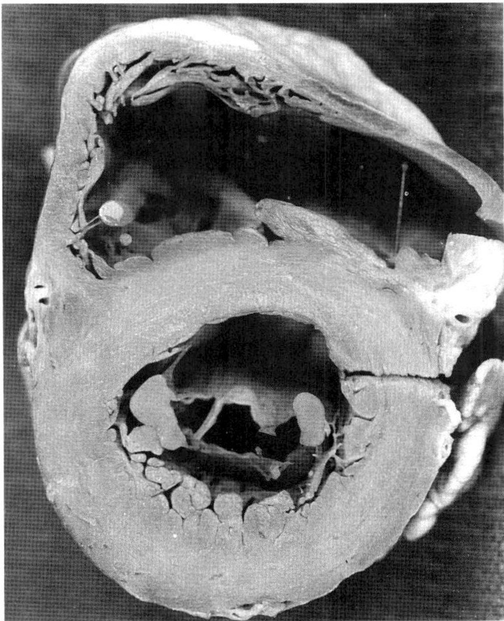

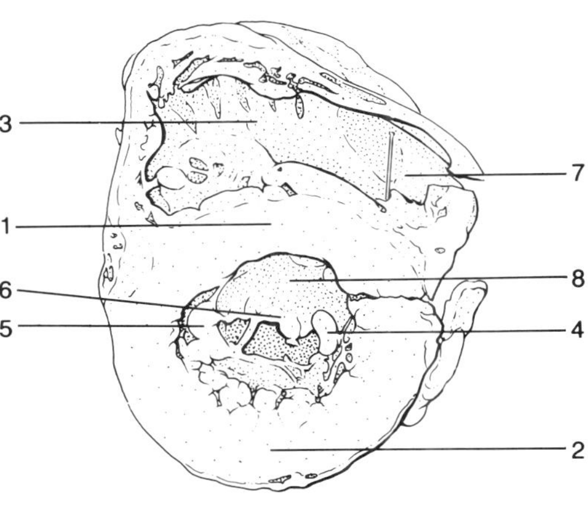

Fig. 2.6 Section of the ventricular chamber as seen through a short axis at the level of the atrioventricular valves. Left ventricle has a circular appearance; the right ventricle makes a semicircle around the left ventricle in its upper and right aspects.

1 ventricular septum
2 free wall of the left ventricle
3 right ventricle
4 anterior papillary muscle
5 posterior papillary muscle
6 anterior mitral leaflet
7 right ventricular outflow tract
8 left ventricular outflow tract

window enables one to obtain four-chamber tomographic sections (Figs. 2.9 and 2.10), apical long-axis views, two-chamber views of both sides of the heart, and a variety of short-axis views of the ventricles.

In the subcostal window, the transducer is placed just under the subxiphoid process, allowing visualization of the four chambers of the heart, the interatrial septum along its entire length, and a variety of short-axis planes, as well as depiction of the systemic venous drainage.

For the suprasternal window, the patient should be supine with a pillow under the shoulders so that the head and neck are slightly hyperextended. This position gives the operator

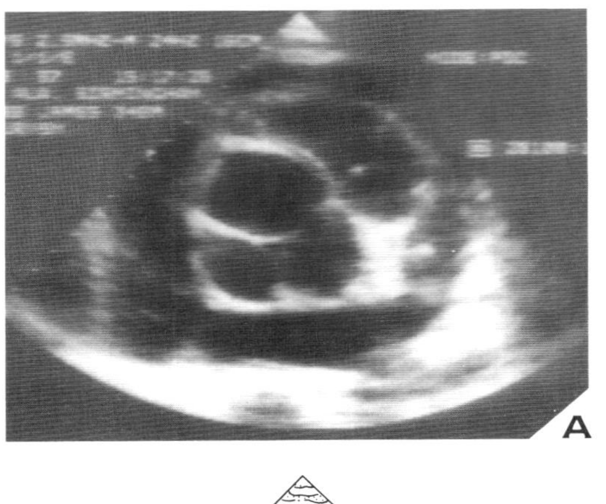

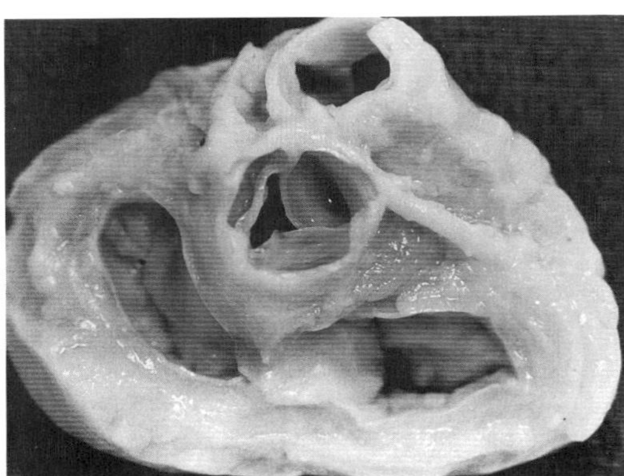

Fig. 2.8 Short-axis, section of the heart, 2-D echocardiographic plane, at the aortic level. The aortic valve lies between the right ventricular outflow tract and the left atrium.

Fig. 2.7 Short-axis 2-D echocardiographic plane of the heart at the level of the aortic valve obtained through transesophageal approach. (A) Diastolic frame and (B) systolic frame are shown. The aorta lies between the right ventricular outflow tract and the left atrium.

1 pulmonic valve
2 right ventricular outflow tract
3 aortic valve with:
3.1 right coronary cusp
3.2 noncoronary cusp
3.3 left coronary cusp
4 position of membranous septum

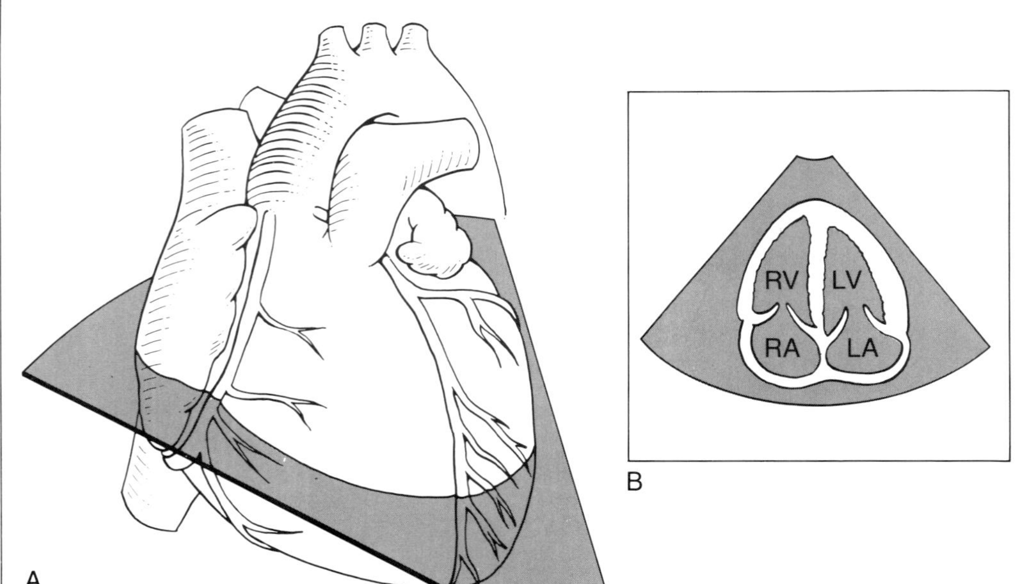

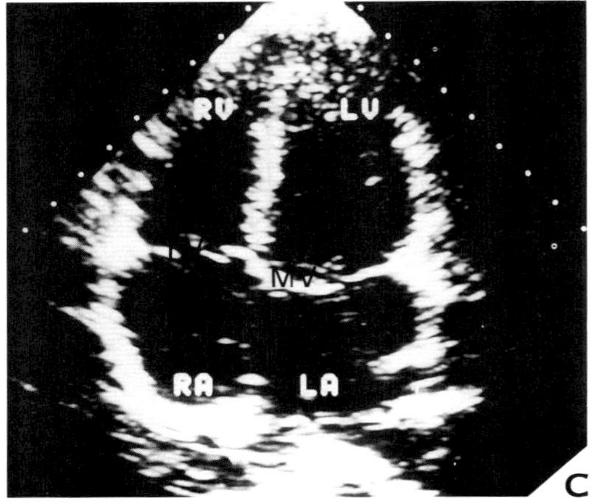

TV tricuspid valve MV mitral valve

Fig. 2.9 Schematic representation of 2-D echocardiography obtained in four-chamber view. (A) Apical approach is shown. (B) Schematic represents the cardiac chambers in this view. (C) Normal echocardiogram of a normal heart is shown. The echocardiographic section is through the atria and ventricles separated by septal structures. The four cardiac chambers are well demonstrated; the septal mitral leaflet is higher than the septal tricuspid leaflet, delineating a portion of the septum between them, the so-called "atrioventricular septum".

better access to the suprasternal and/or supraclavicular spaces and can provide tomographic sections of the ascending aorta, aortic arch, descending aorta, superior vena cava, pulmonary trunk, and main pulmonary arteries. A properly performed two-dimensional echocardiographic study permits a comprehensive and precise three-dimensional anatomic study of the heart (Fig. 2.11).

DOPPLER ECHOCARDIOGRAPHY

Doppler echocardiography uses ultrasound to evaluate the direction, velocity, and character of blood flow within the cardiovascular system. All Doppler instruments work on the *Doppler principle,* which states that the frequencies received from an energy source differ from those sent according to the

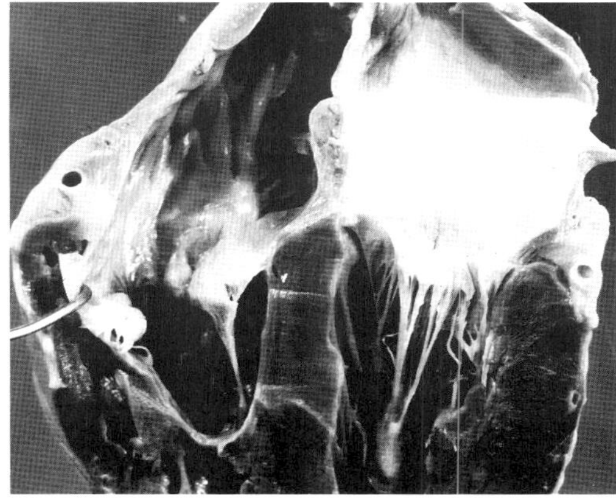

Fig. 2.10 Section of normal heart as seen on four-chamber view, similar to that observed in Fig. 2.9. Note the different level of implantation of the septal leaflets of the tricuspid and mitral valves.

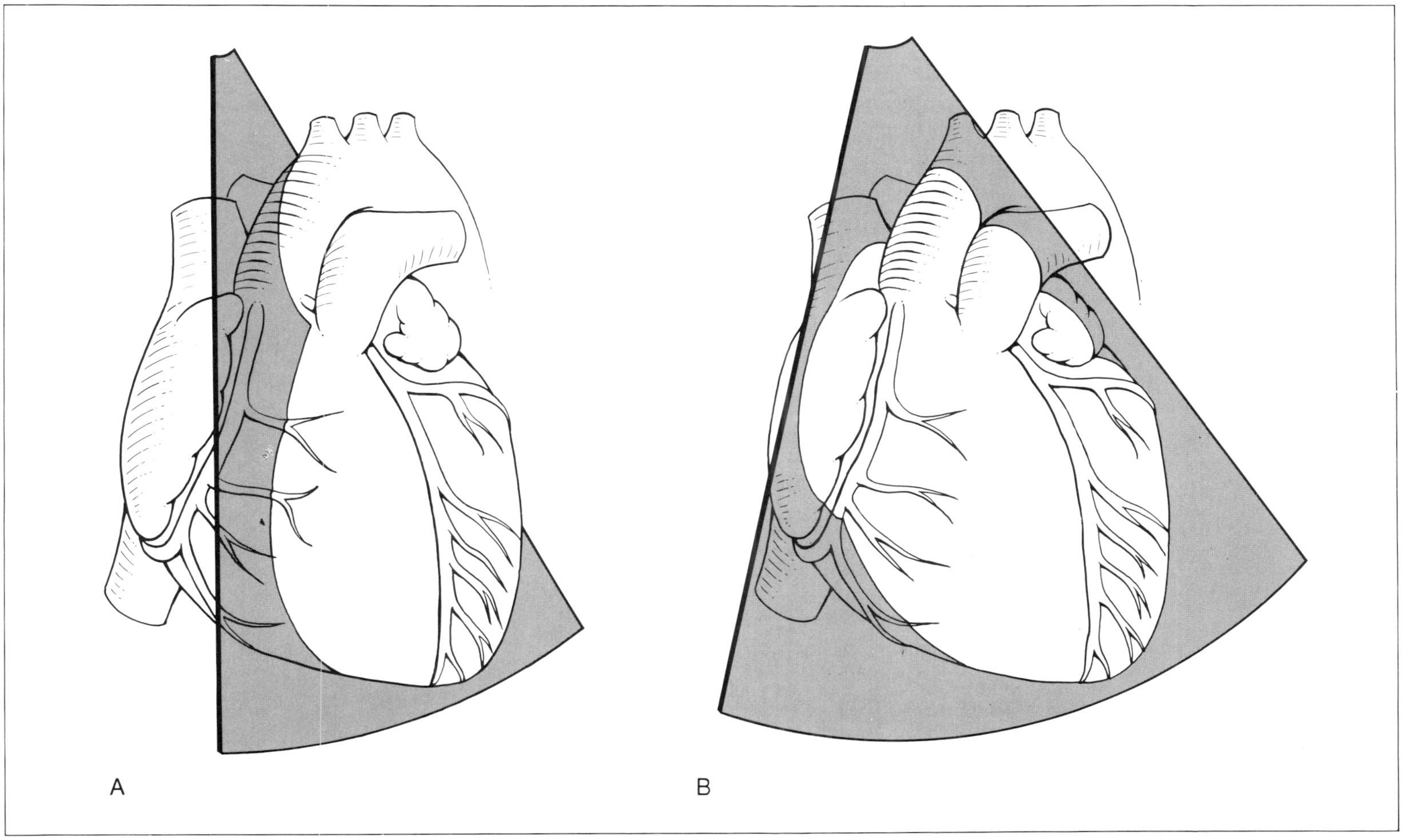

A

B

Fig. 2.11 Schematic representation of orientation of the sections when the transducer is in a suprasternal location. (A) Suprasternal long axial view. (B) Suprasternal short-axis view.

direction and velocity of motion relative to the receiver. If an ultrasonic beam is reflected by a stationary object, the transmitted frequency (F_0) and the received frequency (F_1) are equal. However, if the target reflecting the ultrasonic energy is moving towards the transducer, the received frequency is greater than the transmitted frequency. When the target is moving away from the transducer, the received frequency is less than the transmitted frequency. The difference between the reflected and transmitted frequency represents the *Doppler frequency shift.* By knowing the degree of shift, it is possible to calculate the velocity of the moving target, which is the red blood cells. The Doppler equation can be summarized by

$$V = \frac{C}{2F_o} \cdot \frac{f}{(\text{Cos } \phi)}$$

where Doppler blood flow velocity is f ($F_1 - F_0$), the velocity of sound in tissue (c), the frequency of transmitted sound is (F_0), and the cosine of the ultrasound beam is the angle of incidence. The velocity of the sound in soft tissue and blood is assumed to be 1540 cm/sec. From this equation, for clinical evaluation the ultrasonic beam must be almost parallel to the direction of blood flow to obtain an accurate determination of the blood flow. The cosine functions, however, allow variations between the Doppler beam and the velocity axis to result in minor changes in the calculated velocity.

There are two basic modes of Doppler interrogation: continuous-wave Doppler and pulsed Doppler. The former mode was the first mode of Doppler interrogation; it requires separate transmission and reception elements so that one piezoelectric element continuously transmits ultrasonic energy and the other continuously and passively receives the reflected sound. The continuous-wave Doppler technique is capable of resolving very high velocities. In this mode, the sound energy is processed for the Doppler frequency shift along the course of the beam; however, this technique is limited by its inability to interrogate and characterize flow in specific regions.

The pulsed Doppler mode employs only one crystal. Crystal deactivation between pulses for specific periods of time enables a temporal gate to be established so that reflections from blood flow at a specific distance from the transducer can be analyzed for Doppler shift. Changes in duration of the reactivation period prior to the next pulse allow selection of the size of the specific region to be interrogated (the *sample volume*). Because the *Nyquist limit* (the highest frequency shift that can be unambiguously resolved) is equal to one half the pulse repetition frequency, the long interval necessary between pulses with the pulsed Doppler mode interferes with velocity determination. However, pulsed Doppler's primary utility is to locate and characterize blood flow; continuous-wave Doppler, with its extremely high pulse repetition frequency but poor range gating capability, can be used for high-velocity determination.

A third mode of pulsed Doppler ultrasound, called *high pulse repetition frequency* Doppler, uses multiple range gates. By sacrificing unambiguous range gating, this system allows the resolution of higher velocities than is usually possible with conventional pulsed Doppler.

Conventional Doppler visual display is in the form of an analog trace or a Fast Fourier Transform (FFT) spectral trace, both of which are graphic, with time along the X-axis and frequency shift (or velocity) along the Y-axis. FFT spectral trace is the more common mode of display presently in use. This mode displays, insofar as possible, all frequency shifts present over time. The analog trace displays the modular (mean) frequency shift over time linearly (Fig. 2.12, Appendix). Because the Doppler frequency shifts fall within the range of human hearing, an audio signal is usually available as an adjunct to the visible graphic trace, and represents an important aspect of the Doppler examination.

COLOR DOPPLER IMAGING

A standard echocardiographic transducer is used and the returning signals are split after being received. One part of the signal is used to create a standard black and white two-dimensional echocardiographic tomogram and the other part is evaluated for Doppler phase shift information analogous to conventional Doppler frequency shift, which is subsequently encoded in color and superimposed on the black portions of the two-dimensional echocardiographic image. Because color Doppler imaging is analogous to conventional pulsed Doppler, it is susceptible to all the constraints of pulsed Doppler. However, the velocity display modes are somewhat different. Conventional pulsed Doppler provides a display of the full spectrum of velocities within a single sample region, whereas color Doppler provides an estimate of the mean velocity for multiple sample volume sites. In addition, pulsed Doppler provides information for one sample volume site along one beam path, and Doppler flow mapping provides information regarding multiple sample sites along multiple beam paths, allowing a semblance of real-time two-dimensional display of the signals (Fig. 2.13, Appendix).

The velocity data are depicted for each site in terms of two characteristics: direction and relative velocity of blood flow. These parameters are displayed in color: flow towards the transducer is depicted in red, and flow away from the transducer in blue (Fig. 2.14, Appendix). Color brightness is increased in proportion to flow velocity. This is done using standard television technology; green is added to the primary direction color in proportion to the degree of phase shift. The more green, the lighter the shade of the color. Most instruments also add green as a distinct color when there is evidence of disturbed blood flow. In contrast to Doppler spectral recordings, flow mapping provides measurements only of the mean velocity within a sample volume site, and also allows excellent two-dimensional orientation, as the flows are displayed directly within the chambers and vessels.

TRANSESOPHAGEAL ECHOCARDIOGRAPHY

Although advances in two-dimensional echocardiography, pulsed and continuous-wave Doppler, and color Doppler imaging have revolutionized noninvasive assessment of cardiac disorders, a major limitation of transthoracic echocardiography is its inability to obtain consistently high-quality imaging of the heart and aorta in all patients. Transesophageal echocardiography overcomes this limitation and opens up "a new window to the heart." This new and rapidly expanding technique allows ultrasonic imaging of the cardiac structures and great vessels via the esophagus. The transesophageal approach uses a 3.5 or 5.0 mHZ transducer fixed to the tip of a modified flexible gastroscope without fiberoptics. The probe is passed into the esophagus and manipulated in a manner similar to that in gastrointestinal endoscopy. A transverse view can be obtained at any given level with the conventional uniplanar transesophageal probe. Recently, a transesophageal biplanar probe has been developed; transverse and longitudinal transducers are mounted side by side, 1.5 mm apart on the same transesophageal shaft. This arrangement enables transverse and longitudinal views to be obtained. This new technique provides ultrasonic access to the heart and thoracic aorta from the esophagus without being restricted by lung tissue or bone, and the proximity of both structures allows the use of high-frequency, near-focused transducers, resulting in better image quality (Fig. 2.7). Transesophageal echocardiography can be performed in an outpatient setting for ambulatory patients, intraoperatively for patients undergoing cardiac or noncardiac surgery, or at the bedside for those in intensive care units.

ASSESSMENT OF VENTRICULAR PERFORMANCE

One of the most valuable clinical applications of two-dimensional and Doppler echocardiography is the evaluation of left ventricular performance by assessment of both systolic and diastolic function. M-mode echocardiography permits an accurate measurement of left ventricular dimension and wall thickness. Precise endocardial definition and correct orientation of imaging planes with regard to internal landmarks is required. The rapid sampling rate provides a continuous record of the motion of the ventricular septum and the left ventricular free wall, allowing determination of chamber dimension, wall thickness, and rate of change of these variables over the course of the cardiac cycle. The most commonly used echocardiographic indexes of left ventricular performance are dimensional fractional shortening, fractional area change, and ejection fraction.

$$\text{fractional shortening} = \frac{\text{end diastolic dimension} - \text{end systolic dimension}}{\text{end diastolic dimension}}$$

$$\text{fractional area change} = \frac{\text{end diastolic area} - \text{end systolic area}}{\text{end diastolic area}}$$

$$\text{ejection fraction} = \frac{\text{end diastolic volume} - \text{end systolic volume}}{\text{end diastolic volume}}$$

Under certain conditions, these indexes provide a reliable and reproducible estimate of ventricular performance. Determination of left ventricular muscle mass is the accepted standard for identifying the presence or absence of left ventricular hypertrophy. M-mode and two-dimensional echocardiography have been shown to be reliable noninvasive methods for determining left ventricular mass (LVM).

$$\text{Anatomic LVM} = 1.04\,[(\text{LVID} + \text{PWT} + \text{IVST})^3 - (\text{LVID})^3] - 13.6\ \text{gm}$$

Altered geometry of the cavity due to an aneurysm, localized thinning from myocardial infarction, and asymmetrical or segmental hypertrophy limit the accurate determination of left ventricular volume and mass. The American Society of Echocardiography recommends that left ventricular volume be computed from the dimensions and area measurements obtained from four-chamber and two-chamber views using the modified Simpson's rule or "method of discs," which treats the ventricle as a stack of discs or slices. This algorithm is recommended because it is independent of preconceived ventricular shape (Fig. 2.15). The noninvasive determination

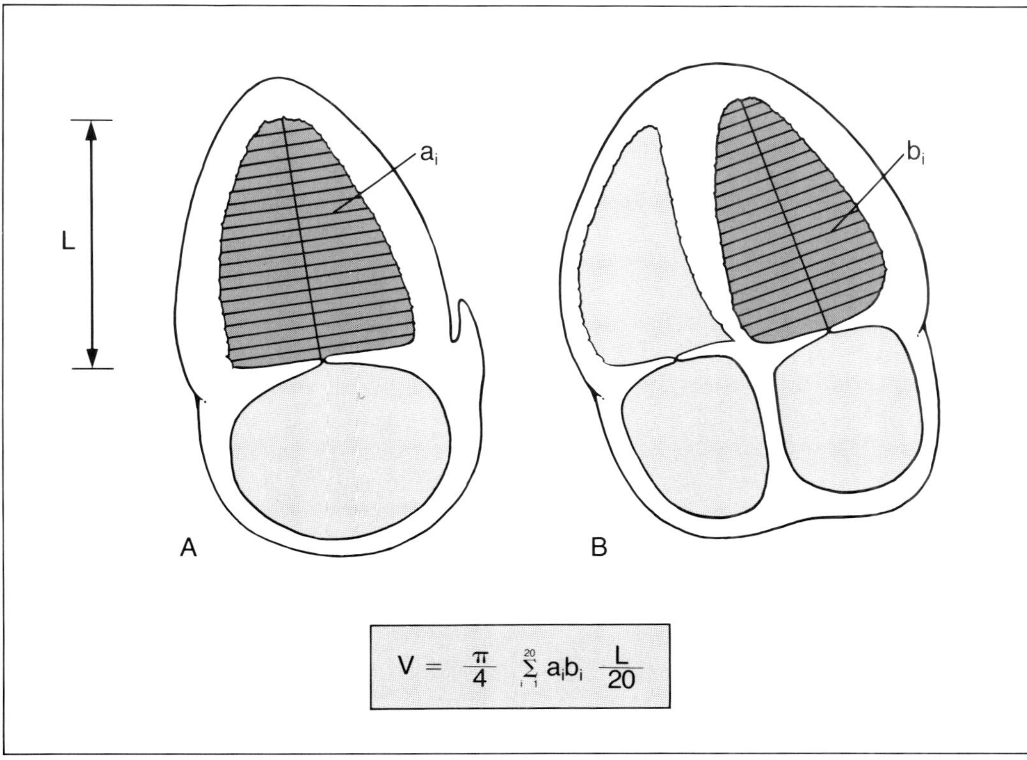

Fig. 2.15 Biplanar method of discs (modified Simpson's rule) from apical two- and four-chamber views. Calculation of volume (formula) results from summation of areas from diameters a_i and b_i of 20 cylinders of discs of equal height.

of left ventricular wall stress has been validated. The force per unit area, or "stress," acting along the circumference of the left ventricle at its minor axis is directly dependent on intracavitary pressure and radius of curvature, and is inversely dependent on wall thickness.

As a real-time tomographic technique, two-dimensional echocardiography is especially suitable for study of regional wall motion. The American Society of Echocardiography recommends a 16-segment model (Fig. 2.16) based on the following considerations: anatomic logic, easy identification of the segments using internal anatomic landmarks, relationship of the segments to known coronary arterial supply, and a uniform scoring system for grading the severity of segmental wall motion abnormalities.

Doppler echocardiography has been used in many clinical studies to assess left ventricular diastolic function by evaluating the ventricle's diastolic filling characteristics. Diastolic time intervals, peak flow velocities, and the proportion of flow during the various phases of diastole can be accurately measured from the Doppler recording with the pulsed-wave sample volume positioned properly in the left ventricular inflow tract. Abnormal patterns of diastolic filling include: delayed onset of flow, with resultant decreased total duration of diastolic filling; decreased velocity and total volumetric flow during the early rapid filling phase; prolonged time to early peak filling; decreased rates of left ventricular relaxation; increased velocity and total volumetric flow during late diastolic (atrial) filling (A wave); abnormal E/A flow ratios; and decreased or absent atrial filling despite sinus rhythm. Diastolic filling of the heart is a complex sequence of interrelated events. Therefore, attempts to interpret these Doppler findings should take into consideration the complex nature of the subject.

ECHO DOPPLER IN MANAGEMENT OF PATIENTS WITH VALVULAR HEART DISEASE

Echocardiographic visualization of each of the four cardiac valves can identify specific anatomic abnormalities characteristic of each type of valvular heart disease. Optimal echocardiographic evaluation of a patient with valvular heart disease requires determination of the following issues: detection of the particular valve lesion, its etiology and severity; valve morphology; complications of disease such as left atrial

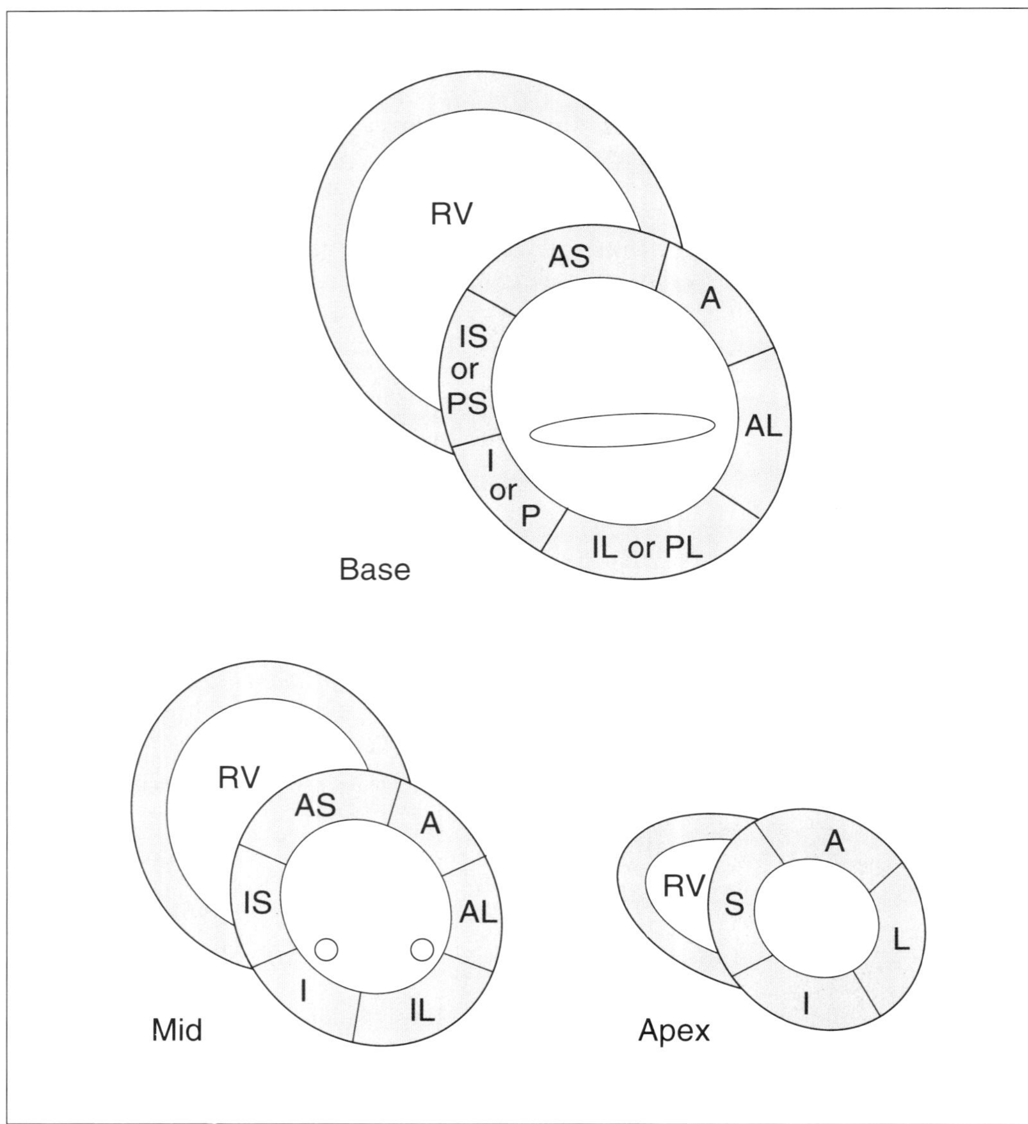

Fig. 2.16 Proposed 16-segment model for wall motion analysis.

A	anterior	IS	inferior septum
I	inferior	PL	posterior lateral
P	posterior	PS	posterior septum
AL	anterior lateral	S	septum
AS	anterior septum	L	lateral
IL	inferior lateral		

thrombus and endocarditis; presence of pulmonary hypertension; presence of other congenital or acquired heart lesions; and assessment of ventricular function.

One of the most important contributions to the usefulness of Doppler ultrasonography for the quantitative assessment of pressure gradients across stenotic valves has been the application of the modified Bernoulli equation. This equation is based on the Bernoulli principle for short segment stenosis and states

$$P = P/2 \times (V_2^2 - V_1^2)$$

where P is the pressure drop in mm Hg, P is the mass density of blood, V_2 is the velocity distal to an area of obstruction, and V_1 is the velocity proximal to it, both measured in meters per second. The equation has generally been further modified to yield the pressure drop: $P = 4 \times V_2^2$. If the proximal velocity rises to values of 2 meters per second or more, it must also be considered in the equation as $P = 4 \times (V_2^2 - V_1^2)$. When the Doppler velocity is defining a pressure difference from a jet, the pressure differences are assessed instantaneously. These are referred to as *peak instantaneous gradients*. The measurement of all the pressure drops during the ejection phase of the cardiac cycle divided by the ejection times yields the mean gradient. Mean pressure gradients calculated by Doppler ultrasonography appear to correlate better with those measured at cardiac catheterization than do peak pressure gradients. The examination of peak jet velocity must be performed from many transducer locations. Obtaining the highest velocity indicates that the jet and transducer are closely aligned.

A combination of two-dimensional and Doppler parameters is used to calculate the valvular area with the simplified continuity equation. The continuity equation states that because flow (Q) is a product of mean velocity and cross-sectional area, the product of the proximal mean velocity (V_1) and the proximal area (A_1) equals the product of the distal velocity (V_2) and the distal area (A_2), which is the valve area. Therefore, the valve area can be calculated from $A_2 = (V_1 \times A_1)/V_2$. In atrioventricular valve stenosis, the concept of *pressure half-time* has been applied to calculate the valvular area on the basis of hemodynamic studies in patients with mitral stenosis. Pressure half-time is the time taken for the initial maximum diastolic gradient to drop to one half; it is prolonged in atrioventricular valve stenosis, and the degree of prolongation is proportional to the severity of stenosis. Hatle et al. noted that mitral valve area was 1 cm^2 at a pressure half-time of 220 msec; therefore, mitral valve area can be calculated by the formula MVA = 220/pressure half-time in msec. Valvular regurgitation is mainly assessed either by pulsed Doppler echocardiography or color Doppler mapping; both are equally able to detect the regurgitant flow (Fig. 2.17, Appendix). The size of the regurgitant jet can be determined more easily and accurately with color Doppler mapping.

Doppler echocardiography has also been useful for noninvasive estimation of pulmonary artery pressure. Tricuspid regurgitation is fairly common in adults (Fig. 2.18, Appendix). The difference between right ventricular and right atrial pressure can be calculated from the transtricuspid velocity using the modified Bernoulli equation. Right ventricular systolic pressure is then approximated by adding the right atrial mean pressure to the pressure drop across the tricuspid valve. In the absence of pulmonary stenosis, this is a very reliable method for calculating the systolic pulmonary artery pressure.

In the past decade, echocardiography has been used increasingly in patients with bacterial endocarditis, as this technique can detect vegetations, delineate valvular lesions, and document progression of the disease. The presence of vegetations is of prognostic importance in patients with subacute bacterial endocarditis, as it is correlated with a higher rate of complications. Ultrasonographic detection of vegetations, in general, is limited by the size of the vegetation (lesions as small as 2 mm in diameter can be resolved) the relative echogenicity of the lesion, the presence of preexisting valvular disease, the timing of the examination in relation to the course of the illness, the sensitivity of the instrument used, and the skill of the operator. Transesophageal echocardiography can be performed in patients with suspected SBE but may yield equivocal results as compared with transthoracic echocardiography. In addition, prosthetic valve endocarditis, often difficult to evaluate by precordial echocardiography, may be more reliably assessed with transesophageal echocardiography.

ASSESSMENT OF PROSTHETIC HEART VALVE FUNCTION

All prosthetic valves are mildly stenotic as well as insufficient. Likewise, all are subject to such complications as thrombosis, infection, degeneration, dehiscence, fibrous ingrowth, and embolization, all of which may lead to hemodynamically significant insufficiency or obstruction (Fig. 2.19). Doppler

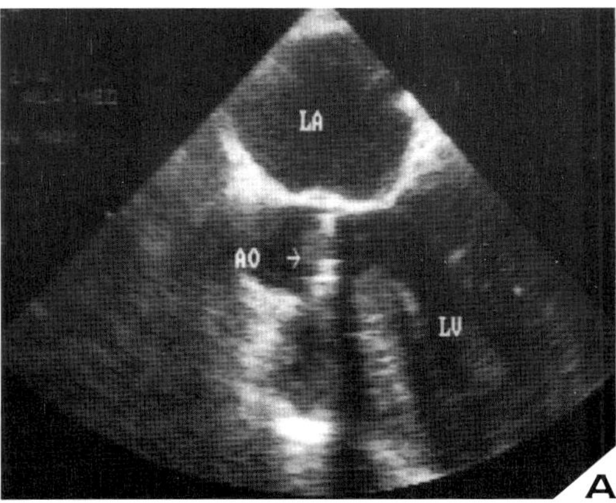

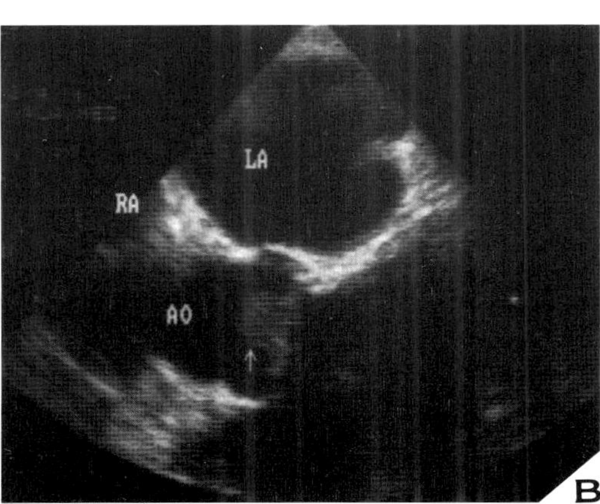

Fig. 2.19 Short axis of the heart at the level of the aorta in a patient with prosthetic Bjork–Shirley valve. The support of the valve is positioned in anterior–posterior direction. The disk is in open position in A and in closed position in B. (AO = aorta)

echocardiography is the procedure of choice for evaluation of the patient with suspected prosthetic heart valve dysfunction. An excellent correlation has been demonstrated between Doppler and catheterization techniques for both peak instantaneous and mean pressure gradients. In evaluation of patients with suspected prosthetic valve stenosis, if the interrogating Doppler beam is carefully aligned parallel to flow, the peak and mean transvalvular pressure gradients can be accurately measured by applying the modified Bernoulli equation. Physiologic insufficiency is detected in a higher percentage of patients with prosthetic heart valves. The regurgitant jet has a relatively small area, usually confined to within a centimeter of the valve plane, and a weak Doppler signal. Paravalvular leaks are much more readily identified using color Doppler mapping techniques. Several studies have demonstrated the high sensitivity and specificity of Doppler echocardiographic diagnosis of significant prosthetic valve insufficiency, particularly in the presence of an aortic prosthesis. Demonstration of mitral prosthetic insufficiency has been slightly more difficult, mainly owing to technical factors such as increased distance of the left atrium from the transducer and masking of the regurgitant signal by the prosthetic valve. Transesophageal echocardiography has been shown to be very helpful in this regard.

ECHOCARDIOGRAPHY AND DOPPLER TECHNIQUES IN EVALUATION OF PERICARDIAL DISEASES

Echocardiography has proved to be an important diagnostic tool for assessment of pericardial disease. As a semiquantitative technique, two-dimensional echocardiography has become the procedure of choice for detection and serial follow-up studies of pericardial effusion. A small amount of pericardial fluid (ie, 30 to 50 mL) can be accurately detected. The echocardiographic hallmark of pericardial effusion is the presence of an echo-free space posterior to the heart. M-mode echocardiography is usually adequate for the diagnosis of pericardial effusion in most patients; however, two-dimensional echocardiography provides valuable additional information. Precise quantitation of pericardial fluid is not extremely accurate, and most laboratories roughly estimate the size of an effusion as minimal, small, medium, or large. In large pericardial effusions the heart tends to move freely within the pericardial cavity; this type of motion has been called *swinging heart sign.* Using multiple tomographic sections, one can obtain a precise idea of the distribution of pericardial fluid and thereby determine the safest approach for pericardiocentesis.

Cardiac tamponade is an abnormal hemodynamic state resulting from impaired diastolic filling of the heart, usually due to a large collection of pericardial fluid under pressure. Cardiac tamponade should probably be defined in hemodynamic and clinical terms. A variety of M-mode, two-dimensional, and Doppler echocardiographic findings have been reported; among them, right atrial collapse and right ventricular collapse are very sensitive indicators. Pericardial constriction is accompanied by thickening, fibrosis, and calcification of the pericardium, with fusion of the epicardium and parietal pericardium and ensuing visceral constriction. A high index of suspicion is required to diagnose pericardial thickening. Among the echocardiographic features of constrictive pericarditis are rapid early and flat mid-diastolic motion of the posterior wall of the left ventricle, abnormal early diastolic ventricular septal motion, atrial systolic notch on the interventricular septum, a dense, rigid shell of pericardium, enlarged atria, ventricular septal bulging towards the left ventricle during inspiration (septal bounce), dilated inferior vena cava and hepatic veins, and marked inspiratory decrease in mitral "E" velocity. Characteristic echo Doppler features differentiate constrictive pericarditis from restrictive cardiomyopathy. The echocardiographer should have a high index of suspicion and should utilize the various M-mode, two-dimensional, and Doppler echocardiographic features to make the diagnosis of constrictive pericarditis. Total or partial absence of the pericardium is a rare congenital anomaly and is usually asymptomatic; M-mode and two-dimensional echocardiography may show features of right ventricular volume overload. Pericardial cysts, usually asymptomatic and typically located at the right costophrenic angle, can be accurately diagnosed by two-dimensional echocardiography.

ECHOCARDIOGRAPHY FOR ASSESSMENT OF INTRACAVITARY MASSES

Adequate identification of the nature of an intracavitary mass (eg, ventricular thrombus, primary cardiac tumor, metastatic tumor, hydatid cyst, vegetations) is mandatory before appropriate therapy can be undertaken. Two-dimensional echocardiography, the procedure of choice for detection of cardiac masses, yields precise anatomic information regarding the morphology of the mass, its attachment, mobility, location, and its relation to cardiac structures. The procedure can be repeated as often as necessary. With this technique, previously unrecognized intracavitary lesions can now be diagnosed, the natural history of vegetative endocarditis can be better defined, and the incidence of left ventricular thrombi accompanying myocardial infarctions can be ascertained. Transesophageal echocardiography yields images of cardiac structures that are superior in quality and structural resolution to two-dimensional echocardiography; the detailed anatomic visualization of the atrial chambers, interatrial septum, and atrial appendages makes this technique a superb tool for evaluation of atrial masses.

ECHOCARDIOGRAPHY FOR ASSESSMENT OF CONGENITAL HEART DISEASE

The instrumentation used in infants and children includes either phased-array or mechanical sector scanners and high-resolution, medium-focused 3.5 and 5.0 mHZ transducers. In addition to the standard parasternal long- and short-axis, apical, and suprasternal notch windows, infants and young children have an excellent subxiphoid window that enables intracardiac anatomy to be assessed. Ultrasonographic techniques now allow examination of human fetal cardiac development and function in utero. Diagnostic quality images of the fetal heart in utero can be obtained as early as 16 weeks of gestation, thus delineating congenital heart defects.

Analysis of the morphology and function of the fetal heart during the second and third trimesters of pregnancy enables cardiologists to counsel prospective parents and to formulate management plans for pregnancy, delivery, and the immediate postnatal period. It appears clear, for example, that nonimmune fetal hydrops often represents end-stage fetal cardiac decompensation. Pulsed Doppler examination of the fetus supplements the echocardiographic findings in identifying the responsible defects. Fetal cardiac echocardiography is of particular importance in analyzing disturbances of fetal cardiac rhythm.

To assess intracardiac anatomy and to obtain detailed morphologic information, a segmental approach to echocardiographic examination should be employed. The three cardiac segments are the atria, ventricles, and great arteries. *Atrial situs* describes the arrangement of the atrial chambers within the chest. The atria are identified by defining the morphology of the atrial appendages. A transverse cross-section of the abdomen displaying the liver, inferior vena cava, and aorta is useful to define the situs. To define ventricular position, ventricular morphology must be assessed. The morphologic characteristics of the right ventricle include a coarse trabecular pattern, a pyramidal shape with a moderator band and a crista supraventricularis, and a discrete outlet portion (ie, the arterial and atrioventricular valves are not in continuity). In contrast, the morphologic left ventricle has a prolate elliptical shape, a thin trabecular pattern, and no discrete outlet portion (ie, arterial valve is in fibrous continuity with the atrioventricular valve). There are two distinct papillary muscle masses, one in the anterior lateral position and one in the posterior medial position. Finally, it is important to note that the tricuspid valve rests in a slightly more apical position than the anatomic mitral valve. The great arteries are considered to be normally connected with the ventricles when the aorta exits the morphologic left ventricle and the pulmonary trunk exits the morphologic right ventricle. These arteries are normally related when the pulmonary artery lies anterior and to the left of the aorta.

Echocardiographic diagnoses that can often be made with certainty include: aortic valvular, subvalvular, and supravalvular stenosis; aortic coarctation; hypoplastic left heart syndrome; atrial, ventricular, and atrioventricular septal defects; cor triatriatum; tricuspid atresia; Ebstein's anomaly; valvular and subvalvular pulmonic stenosis; univentricular–atrioventricular connection; double-outlet right ventricle; transposition of the great arteries; patent ductus arteriosus; tetralogy of Fallot; truncus arteriosus; anomalous pulmonary venous connection; and pulmonary atresia. Color Doppler imaging is extremely useful for detection and assessment of cardiac shunts. Using Doppler echocardiography it is possible to measure gradients across stenotic valves, to calculate cardiac output, to identify blood flow patterns in the cardiac chambers and great arteries, and to estimate the size of a shunt. Many methods use Doppler echocardiography to quantitate pulmonary to systemic flow ratios (Q_p/Q_s). This requires sampling of a Doppler flow velocity profile in the pulmonary artery and the aorta, and calculation of mean flow velocity. In these methods, the area beneath the flow velocity curve is measured by planimetry. The cross-sectional area of the vessel is calculated according to the following formula: vessel area = πr^2, where r = radius of the vessel. Pulmonary flow can be calculated from the equation: flow = mean pulmonary artery velocity × pulmonary artery vessel area × right ventricular ejection time × heart rate. Systemic flow can be calculated by the equation: flow = mean aortic velocity × aortic root area × left ventricular ejection time × heart rate. The ratio between pulmonary and systemic flow (Q_p/Q_s) can then be calculated.

The interventricular systolic pressure drop across ventricular septal defects can also be evaluated using the modified Bernoulli equation (Fig. 2.14). Correct alignment of the transducer with the jet is quite critical. The transducer must be axial to the direction of the jet across the ventricular septal defect to obtain an accurate velocity signal (this can be best achieved by color Doppler mapping). In many circumstances, a fair estimate of the interventricular pressure difference can be assessed. A peak velocity across a ventricular septal defect of 3.5 meters per second or more suggests that the defect is restrictive in nature.

DISEASES OF THE AORTA

A portion of the ascending aorta is imaged in the parasternal and the apical long-axis views; however, right parasternal, supraclavicular, and suprasternal notch imaging is required to image the entire ascending aorta, transverse aortic arch, and part of the descending aorta. With routine parasternal imaging, the descending aorta is visualized posterior to the left atrium and left ventricle (it should not be mistaken for the echo-free space in the atrioventricular groove region produced by the coronary sinus). Dilatation and aneurysms of the ascending aorta can usually be diagnosed from the parasternal long-axis position.

Aneurysms of the sinuses of Valsalva are well depicted on parasternal and apical views. Color Doppler imaging is valuable for identifying any rupture site and blood flow into the recipient chamber. Although the diagnosis of dissecting aortic aneurysm can be made by M-mode echocardiography, it is more clearly defined with two-dimensional imaging. The echocardiographic hallmark of aortic dissection is the demonstration of an abnormal linear echo in the lumen of the aorta in more than one scan plane. Color Doppler imaging provides comprehensive evaluation of flow dynamics in aortic dissection. Transesophageal echocardiography yields accurate anatomic information in patients with aortic dissection, and is becoming the diagnostic technique of choice in this disease.

CHAPTER 3

Invasive Cardiac Diagnosis

THE CARDIAC CATHETERIZATION LABORATORY

IMAGING EQUIPMENT

Sophisticated imaging equipment is essential for proper performance of cardiac catheterization and angiography. Most invasive cardiologists prefer 35-mm techniques for angiocardiography and coronary arteriography. (Large-format roll- or cut-film is usually preferred for studies of the aortic arch and great vessels.) Both biplane and single-plane systems are available in a variety of designs, most of which employ movable floor mounts or cantilever tables (Fig. 3.1). Useful enhancements include a video recording system and a digital subtraction system that allows selective magnification and computerized image enhancement and image analysis. A power injector and film processing equipment complete the imaging component of the cardiac catheterization suite.

Modern angiocardiographic systems, which operate at low peak kilovoltage (kVp) and high milliamperage (mA), have high photon flux (photons/frame). The resulting cine images have high resolution with wide contrast latitude (long gray scale), which enhances slight differences in radiographic density.

Cardiac catheterization and angiocardiography often entail extensive, time-consuming catheter manipulations; therefore, they may expose the patient, as well as the operating personnel, to a significant radiation hazard. The danger is greatest for children, owing to their longer life expectancy and relatively greater sensitivity to radiation (the risk of radiation-induced leukemia is approximately twice as great in children as in adults). Because of their small body size, which results in increased exposure from internal scatter, the thyroid and gonadal doses are higher in children than in adults. The average entrance (skin) dose from a combined cardiac catheterization/angiocardiographic procedure is about 10 rad in a 5-year-old child and 30 rad in a 15-year-old adolescent. Although dose levels do not exceed permissible limits, every effort should be made to reduce radiation exposure, particularly in infants and young children.

Modern angiocardiographic suites incorporate "low-dose" fluoroscopy systems which significantly decrease radiation exposure to patient and staff when compared with conventional fluoroscopic equipment. It is possible to substantially decrease patient dose, with little if any loss of information, by using low pulse-rate fluoroscopy systems mated to videodisc recorders that can store a single image or dynamic sequence. Thyroid and gonadal exposure can be further reduced by placing the image intensifier as close as possible to the patient, by carefully collimating the beam, and by accurately calibrating the equipment. By using protective eyeglasses and lead shields, it is possible to reduce scattered radiation to the operator's eyes (lens) and thyroid to negligible levels.

PHYSIOLOGIC MONITORING AND RECORDING EQUIPMENT

In addition to imaging apparatus, the catheterization laboratory is equipped with a basic physiologic recording system, which is used to monitor, display, and record the patient's ECG and heart rate, intravascular and intracardiac pressures, and related hemodynamic data (Fig. 3.2). Transducers connected to fluid-filled catheters near the vascular access site are used to record intravascular and intracardiac pressures. Cardiac output is measured by the thermodilution method or, in certain situations, by the Fick method (see below). The availability of an oximeter in the catheterization laboratory permits more accurate measurements of cardiac output by the Fick method and facilitates the

CHAPTER LABELING KEY

RA	right atrium	LV	left ventricle
LA	left atrium	Ao	aorta
RV	right ventricle		

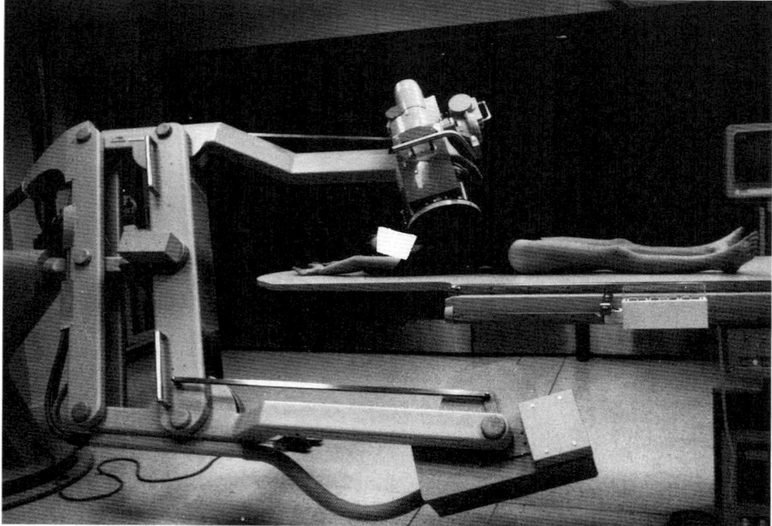

Fig. 3.1 X-ray equipment used for angiocardiography. Rotation and angulation of the X-ray tube and image intensifier system is simplified by this type of support. When combined with an additional X-ray tube and image intensifier for the horizontal plane, it is possible to perform biplane 35-mm cine angiography in multiple projections.

evaluation of shunts; by using fluoroscopy and transcatheter pressure monitoring to ascertain the position of the catheter tip, one can ascertain the location and magnitude (volume) of the shunt.

Recently, computerized systems for processing physiologic data have become popular. These sophisticated systems tabulate the catheterization data and generate a computerized report which includes automated wave-form and heart rate analysis and various calculated parameters (eg, transvalvular pressure gradients, calculated valve area of stenotic valves). On many of the more popular systems, left ventricular volume can be calculated by using a light pen or similar digitizing device to trace the outline of the chamber on the ventriculogram. (Applying the concept of quantitative ventriculography entails three-dimensional mathematical modeling. For accurate results, it is necessary to correct for magnification and "pincushion" distortion of the image. The correction factor is obtained by making an exposure with a grid or metal ball of known dimensions in the position of the left ventricle after the patient has been removed from the table.) Although these sophisticated systems have many useful features they are not necessary in small-volume laboratories that specialize in routine coronary arteriography.

EMERGENCY EQUIPMENT

In addition to systems for imaging and recording physiologic data, equipment and drugs needed to deal with medical emergencies should be available in the catheterization laboratory. Basic equipment and supplies consist of a defibrillator, oxygen, suction, ventilation devices, pacemakers, pericardiocentesis instruments, and appropriate medications. Many laboratories also stock an intra-aortic balloon assist device. Some laboratories with high patient volumes have ready access to an anesthesia machine and portable cardiopulmonary bypass equipment. Although the sophistication of the equipment may vary, it is

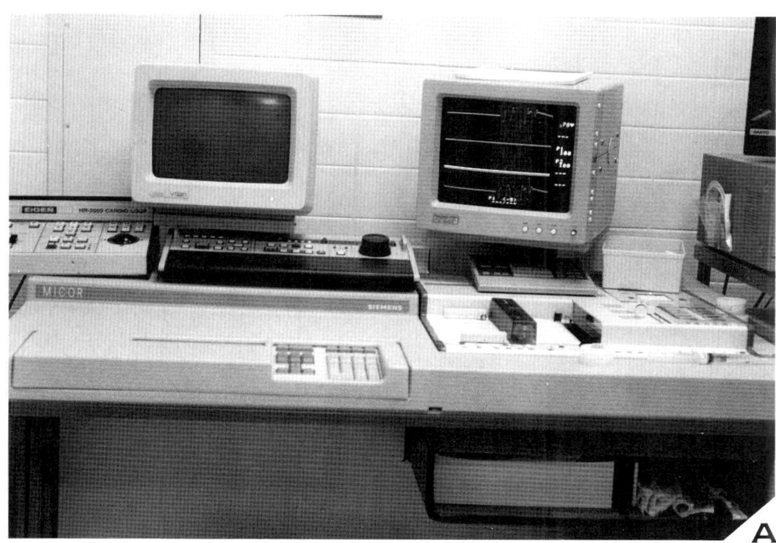

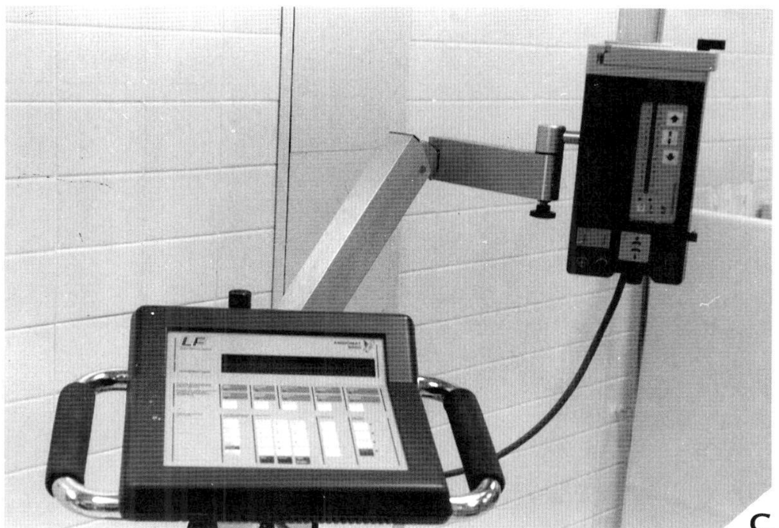

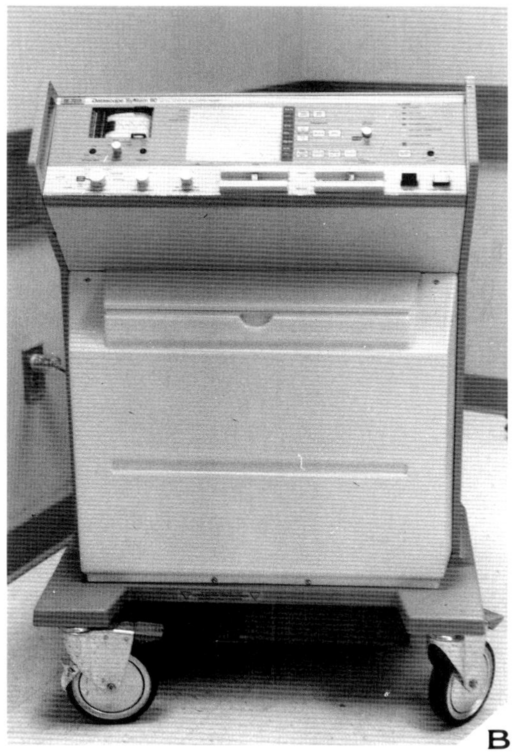

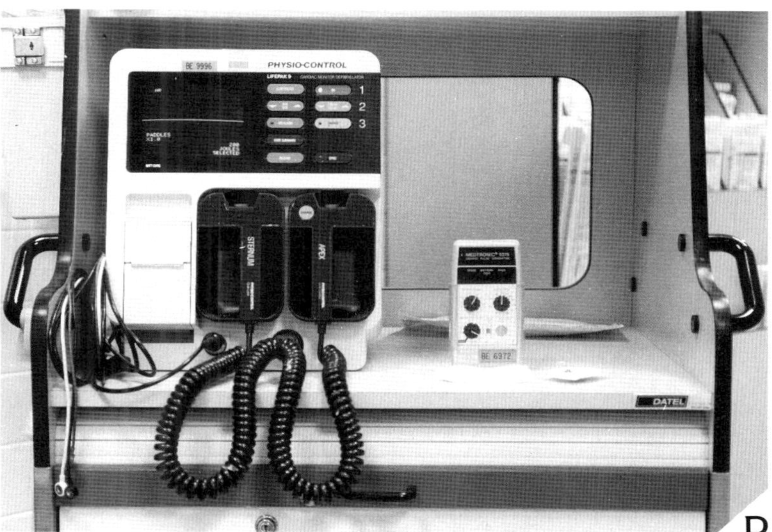

Fig. 3.2 Equipment used for cardiac catheterization and angiocardiography. (A) Equipment for recording pressures during catheterization; (B) intra-aortic balloon monitor; (C) power injector for contrast media; (D) ECG monitor and defibrillator.

axiomatic that laboratory personnel must be proficient in its use, so that emergency measures can be carried out quickly and effectively.

STAFF

The composition of the catheterization laboratory team has evolved over the years; in many respects it resembles its surgical counterpart. In addition to the cardiologist and assistant (if there is one), who may be a cardiology fellow or resident, the team commonly includes a scrub technician, a circulating nurse, a radiology technologist, and a technologist to record the physiologic data. Some laboratories utilize one person for more than one function.

PRINCIPLES OF CARDIAC CATHETERIZATION

In this technique, one or more catheters are introduced through a peripheral vein or artery and positioned under fluoroscopic guidance in the cardiac chambers and/or great vessels. (An abnormal course taken by the catheter is often a clue to the presence of cardiac malformation.) Pressures and oxygen content (saturation) are measured at various sites. By carefully analyzing the data, the cardiologist can obtain a wealth of anatomic, physiologic, and functional data (Fig. 3.3).

To catheterize the right side of the heart, the catheter is introduced into a systemic vein and advanced successively into the right atrium, right ventricle, and pulmonary trunk (Fig. 3.4). Left heart catheterization can be performed by either a retrograde or an antegrade approach. Retrograde catheterization is accomplished by introducing the catheter into a systemic artery and passing it retrogradely into the aorta and left ventricle; if necessary, the catheter can be passed retrogradely through the mitral valve into the left atrium (Fig. 3.5). In the antegrade approach, the catheter is introduced into a systemic vein and advanced into the right atrium; it is then passed into the left atrium via the foramen ovale (which generally remains "probe patent" throughout life) or an existing atrial septal defect. Once the catheter has entered the left atrium it can be manipulated across the aortic valve into the left ventricle and aorta. An alternative method of antegrade left heart catheterization is to perforate the atrial septum (transseptal catheterization) (Fig. 3.6).

The design of the catheter varies according to the use for which it is intended. Catheters employed exclusively for pressure measurements usually have an end hole. (This is always the case for catheters introduced into peripheral branches of the pulmonary arteries to measure wedge pressure.) Catheters used for angiocardiography, which is usually performed after the physiologic data have been collected, have an end hole and multiple side holes. A variety of specialized catheters have been developed for coronary arteriography (see Chapter 21). Swan–Ganz catheters, which are used to measure pressure in pulmonary arteries, have an inflatable balloon at the tip. When the catheter tip is positioned in a main pulmonary artery, the balloon is swept by the flowing blood into a peripheral branch. Specially designed balloon angioplasty catheters are used to treat congenital and acquired valvular stenoses, aortic coarctation, and coronary artery stenoses (see Chapters 16, 30 and 31).

Pressures are recorded by means of a transducer, a device that transforms mechanical into electrical energy. The data are displayed on a video monitor and inscribed on a continuous roll

FIG. 3.3 ANATOMIC, PHYSIOLOGIC, AND FUNCTIONAL DATA PROVIDED BY CARDIAC CATHETERIZATION

Anatomic Data	Physiologic Data*	Functional data*
Catheter position	Pressures	Calculated parameters
Septal defects	Cardiac chambers	Cardiac output
Patent ductus arteriosus	Aorta	Cardiac index
Anomalies of great veins	Pulmonary arterial tree	Left ventricular end diastolic volume
Anomalies of great arteries	Pulmonary capillary bed (wedge pressure)	Cardiac ejection fraction
	Gradient across a stenotic valve or coarctation	Left ventricular mass
	Oxygen saturation	Right ventricular mass
	Cardiac chambers	Oxygen consumption
	Great arteries	
	Great veins	
	Pulmonary arterial tree	
	Calculated parameters	
	Pulmonary resistance	
	Systemic resistance	
	Ratio between pulmonary and systemic resistance	

**At rest and in response to exercise or administration of drugs or oxygen.*

Fig. 3.3 Anatomic, physiologic, and functional data provided by cardiac catheterization.

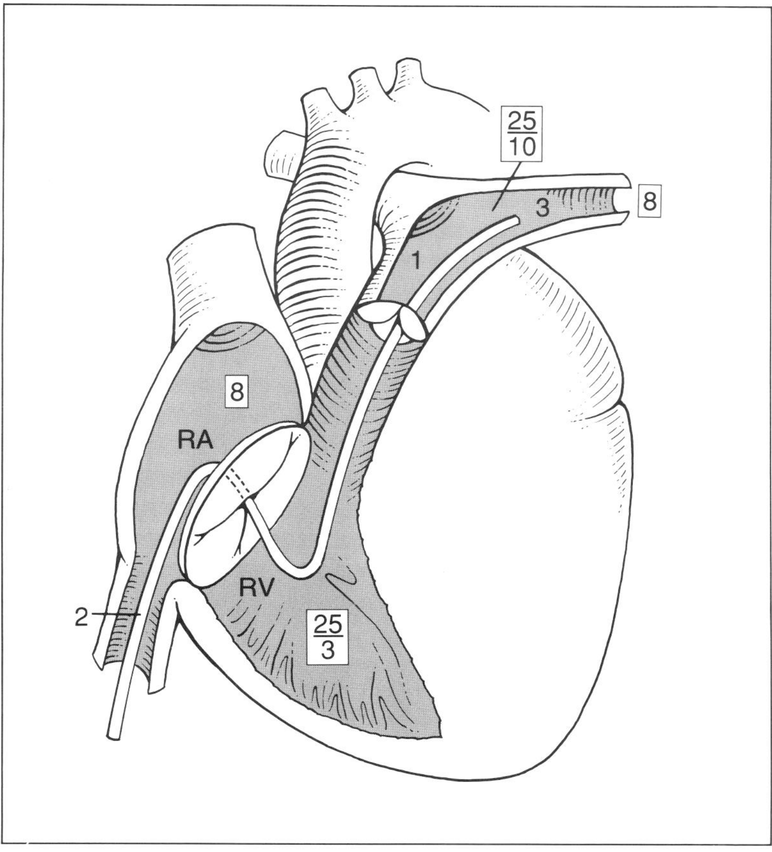

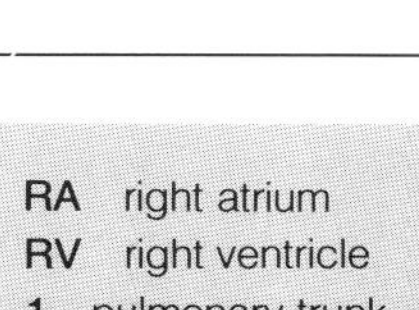

2 catheter (in inferior vena cava)
3 catheter position for pulmonary wedge pressure

Fig. 3.4 Right-sided catheterization via the inferior vena cava. Right ventricular pressure normally increases with exercise.

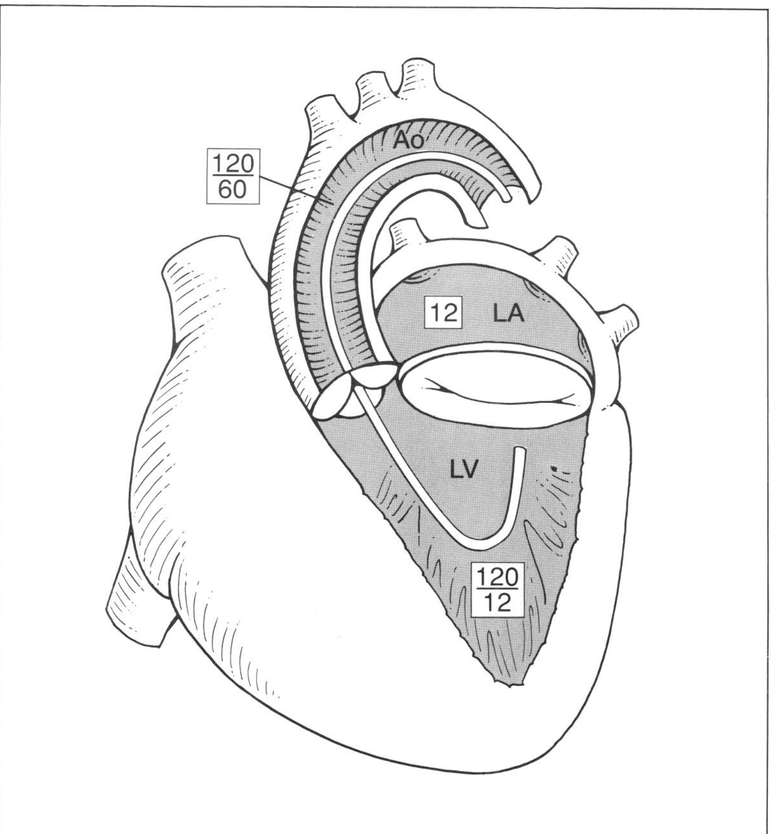

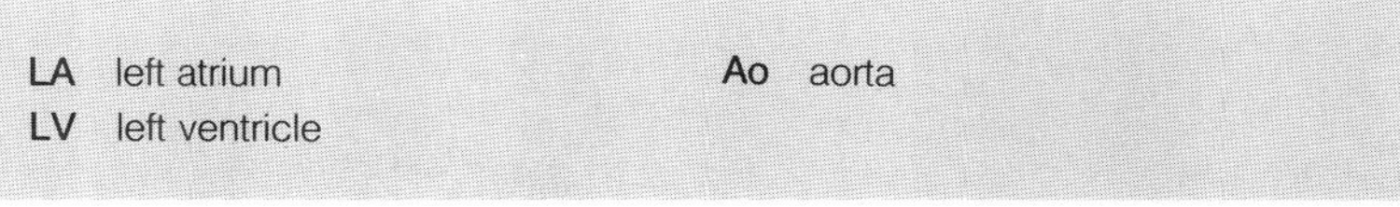

Fig. 3.5 Antegrade catheterization of left side of heart in the evaluation of congenital heart disease. The left heart can also be approached from the right atrium via the foramen ovale, which generally remains "probe patent" throughout life, or via a natural or surgically created atrial septal defect [eg, following a Rashkind procedure (balloon atrial septosomy)].

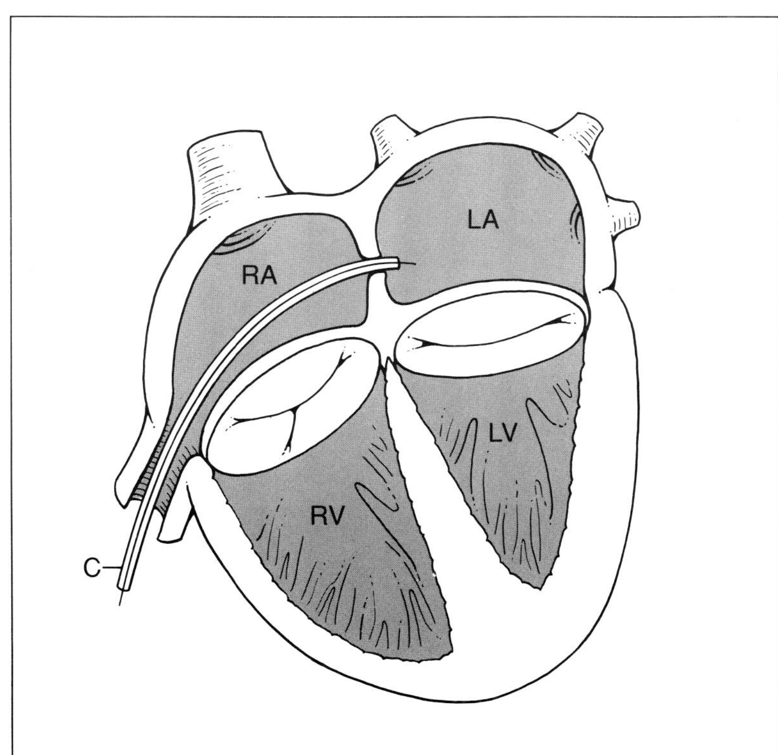

Fig. 3.6 Transseptal catheterization. The catheter (C) has been advanced from the inferior vena cava into the right atrium, and via the iatrogenic septal perforation into the left atrium. The catheter tip is positioned in the midportion of the left atrium. The catheter can be exchanged for larger catheters or a balloon catheter to create an atrial septal defect, or it can be advanced into the left ventricle. Applications include balloon valvotomy for mitral stenosis, left ventriculography following aortic valve replacement, percutaneous insertion of left ventricular assist devices, and left heart catheterization in patients with aortic stenosis when retrograde catheterization is not feasible.

of paper. Blood oxygen content at various sites is measured by oximetry; the data are used to calculate the magnitude of intra- and extracardiac shunts and other functional parameters.

The normal pressures on the left and right sides of the heart are shown in Figs. 3.4 and 3.5; (see also Fig. 3.9). By wedging an end-hole catheter into a peripheral pulmonary arterial branch, it is possible to measure the pulmonary wedge (capillary) pressure; the latter value, which reflects the pulmonary venous pressure, serves as an indirect measurement of left atrial pressure. The normal left atrial pressure is 12 mm Hg or less. The left ventricular diastolic pressure is normally equal to the main left atrial pressure (ie, 12 mm Hg or less). The normal left ventricular systolic pressure is 110 to 120 mm Hg. The normal aortic systolic pressure is the same as left ventricular systolic pressure. Aortic diastolic pressure is normally 80 mm Hg or less.

The catheterization data can be used to calculate the volume of blood in the systemic and pulmonary circulations, as well as the magnitude (volume) of any left to right or right to left shunt that may be present. The amount of blood pumped per minute equals the *cardiac output;* by normalizing this value to body surface, it is possible to calculate the *cardiac index* (blood flow per minute per square meter of body surface). The *ejection fraction,* the percentage of the ventricular content ejected during systole, is a useful parameter of ventricular function; it equals the end diastolic volume minus end systolic volume, divided by the end diastolic volume × 100). The normal left ventricular ejection fraction is above 50 percent. The left ventricular ejection fraction can also be estimated by echocardiography or MRI.

Cardiac output is most commonly measured by the thermodilution method, with computer analysis of the temperature curve; data analysis can be performed by a computer incorporated into the physiologic recording system or by a free-standing microcomputer. In the thermodilution technique, cold saline solution is injected through the proximal (right atrial) port of a balloon-tipped right heart catheter which has a thermistor at the distal (pulmonary artery) end. Although useful for routine studies, the thermodilution technique is inaccurate in a number of situations (eg, intra- and extracardiac shunts, tricuspid insufficiency, extremely low cardiac output). In such cases, cardiac output is usually measured by techniques based on the Fick principle (cardiac output equals oxygen consumption divided by the arterial–venous oxygen difference). If a metabolic analyzer is available, oxygen consumption can be measured directly; otherwise, a normal value (90 to 120 mL/min/M^2 body surface area) must be assumed.

To evaluate intra- or extracardiac shunts, O_2 saturation is measured at appropriate sites (determined by fluoroscopy or transcatheter pressure monitoring). Using the Fick principle, it is possible to calculate the magnitude (volume) of the shunt by measuring the difference between the arterial and venous oxygen content in each circuit. Using the Fick principle, it is also possible to estimate the pulmonary blood flow per unit time. [The volume of blood traversing the pulmonary circulation per minute is proportional to the amount of oxygen consumed during a given period of time; the latter value is calculated by subtracting the oxygen content of expired air from the oxygen content of room air (21 percent).] In a normal subject, the ratio of pulmonary to systemic blood flow is 1:1. If a shunt is present, the volume of blood flowing from the systemic circuit to the pulmonary circuit, or vice versa, can be calculated. The magnitude (volume) of the shunt, expressed in liters/minute, is expressed as the ratio between pulmonary and systemic blood flow; it may be 3:1 or greater in a patient with a large ventricular septal defect.

Blood flowing through the pulmonary vascular bed must overcome a certain resistance. Pulmonary vascular resistance, expressed mathematically as the pressure drop across the pulmonary vascular bed divided by the pulmonary blood flow, is another important parameter that can be determined from the catheterization data (Fig. 3.7). In both children and adults, pulmonary resistance is normally 1 to 6 units/M^2 (that is, corrected for body surface area). (To express pulmonary resistance as dyne–sec/cm^2, multiply units by 80.) In an infant with a large left to right shunt, pulmonary resistance typically begins to rise immediately after birth, progressively increasing until it reaches systemic or suprasystemic levels. A value greater than 8 units/M^2 suggests fixed, increased pulmonary resistance. Pa-

FIG. 3.7 FORMULA FOR CALCULATING PULMONARY VASCULAR RESISTANCE*

$$\text{Pulmonary resistance} = \frac{P_{PA}\,(\text{mean}) - P_{PV}\,(\text{mean})}{Q_P}$$

*P_{PA} (mean) = mean pulmonary arterial pressure (mm Hg);
PPV (mean) = mean pulmonary venous pressure (mm Hg);
QP = pulmonary blood flow (L/min).

Fig. 3.7 Formula for calculating pulmonary vascular resistance.

FIG. 3.8 FORMULA FOR CALCULATING SYSTEMIC VASULAR RESISTANCE*

$$\text{Systemic resistance} = \frac{P_{AO}\,(\text{mean}) - P_{RA}\,(\text{mean})}{S_f}$$

*For example, in a patient with a (normal) mean aortic pressure of 83 mm Hg, a (normal) mean right atrial pressure of 4 mm Hg, and a body surface of 4.4 square meters, the calculated systemic resistance is 18 units/square meter of body surface.
P_{AO} (mean) = mean aortic pressure (mm Hg);
P_{PV} (mean) = mean right atrial pressure (mm Hg);
S_F = systemic blood flow (liters/min).

Fig. 3.8 Formula for calculating systemic vascular resistance.

tients with levels above 40 units/M^2 have a very poor prognosis. Pulmonary resistance is decreased in patients with pulmonary arteriovenous fistulas, an anomaly in which a portion of the pulmonary blood flow bypasses the pulmonary capillary bed.

Systemic (peripheral) vascular resistance is calculated in the same manner as pulmonary vascular resistance (Fig. 3.8). Systemic resistance is normally 15 to 40 units/M^2 (to express resistance as dyne-sec/cm^2, multiply by 80). Increased peripheral resistance is characteristic of systemic hypertension, whereas decreased peripheral resistance is seen in patients with systemic arteriovenous fistulas (see Chapter 14), severe aortic insufficiency, and other disorders with similar hemodynamic features.

To sum up, cardiac catheterization accurately depicts the pathophysiology as well as the functional status of the heart in patients with congenital or acquired heart disease. In some instances the position of the catheter may also provide important anatomic information (see Fig. 3.3). Normal cardiac catheterization values are shown in Fig. 3.9.

PERFORMING THE STUDY

INDICATIONS AND RISKS

Invasive diagnostic procedures are performed to precisely define the pathophysiology and pathologic anatomy in patients whose clinical findings suggest a cardiac abnormality. In general, an invasive study is indicated when quantitative data needed to guide therapy or indicate prognosis cannot be obtained by noninvasive techniques such as echocardiography or MRI. Examples include symptomatic structural defects (congenital or acquired) and angina with a positive exercise stress test. Many physicians believe that any clinical findings compatible with coronary artery disease warrant coronary arteriography, even when the symptoms and/or objective evidence are minimal. This concept is based on data suggesting that the pathologic anatomy is a more accurate predictor of prognosis than the patient's symptoms.

Other candidates for invasive diagnostic studies include patients with a known diagnosis in whom it necessary to quantify the results of an intervention or to assess changes occurring over a period of time. Examples include patients with recurrent angina after coronary angioplasty for single-vessel disease and patients with recurrent symptoms after valve surgery.

Invasive diagnostic procedures are not always necessary or appropriate. For example, catheterization and angiocardiography can be omitted in an elderly patient with well-tolerated aortic incompetence which appears mild on echocardiography, or in a symptomatic patient with echocardiographically demonstrated mitral valve prolapse and a normal exercise stress test. In other words, an invasive diagnostic procedure is indicated only when it is clearly justified by the benefit-to-risk ratio. In each instance, the clinician must weigh both the medical risk and the cost and inconvenience to the patient, and then ask, "How will these data affect the management of this patient?"

In a relatively healthy patient, routine catheterization/angiography is associated with a relatively small risk. Advanced age, heart failure, peripheral vascular disease, renal or pulmonary insufficiency, and a history of asthma or severe allergy are

FIG. 3.9 NORMAL HEMODYNAMIC PARAMETERS OBTAINED FROM CARDIAC CATHETERIZATION

Normal values and pressures	
O_2 consumption (VO_2)	110–150/ml/min/M^2
Pulmonary A-V O_2 difference	3.5–4.7 vol.%
Systemic A-V O_2 difference	3.5–4.7 vol.%
Systemic O_2 saturation	>94%
Cardiac index (C.I.)	2.5–4.0 L/min/M^2
Systemic vascular resistance (SVR)	8.0–15.0 units
Pulmonary vascular resistance (PVR)	0.2–1.2 units
Total pulmonary resistance (TPR)	1.0–3.0 units
Aortic valve area (AVA)	2.6–3.5 cm^2
Mitral valve area (MVA)	4.0–6.0 cm^2
LV end diastolic volume	<90 ml/M^2
Ejection fraction	55–70%

Normal pressures (mm Hg)	
Right atrium (RA), mean	1–8
Right ventricle (RV), systolic	15–28
End diastolic (RVEDP)	0–8
Pulmonary artery (PA)	
Systolic	15–28
Diastolic	5–16
Mean	10–22
Pulmonary artery wedge (PAW)	
Mean	4–12
Left atrium (LA)	
Mean	4–12
Left ventricle (LV)	
Systolic	85–150
End diastolic (LVEDP)	4–12
Aortic (AO)	
Systolic	85–150
Diastolic	60–90
Mean	70–105

Fig. 3.9 Normal hemodynamic parameters obtained from cardiac catheterization.

important risk factors. In general, the sicker the patient—whether from cardiac or noncardiac disease—the greater the risk. Extreme examples include a patient in cardiogenic shock undergoing preoperative coronary angiography with an intra-aortic balloon pump in place, or an elderly patient with suspected severe aortic stenosis who presents with angina, congestive heart failure, and hypotension.

To minimize the risk, the patient should be in the best possible physiologic condition, with at least partial compensation of both the cardiac and the noncardiac disease. Associated conditions such as hypertension, hypotension, arrthythmias, heart failure, clotting abnormalities, and renal dysfunction should be corrected to the extent feasible, because this will not only increase the safety of the procedure but make the data more meaningful. The presence of an overt infection or unexplained fever may justify delaying the procedure. However, when the urgency of the situation warrants, the patient's physician and the invasive cardiology team may elect to perform the invasive study under less than ideal conditions after carefully considering the risks and benefits.

PREPARATION OF THE PATIENT

Once the decision has been made to recommend an invasive study and the patient appears to be in optimal condition, the risks and benefits should be discussed with the patient and family, and written permission obtained. (Because contrast material will be administered, an allergy history should also be elicited.)

The entry site is shaved the night before or on the day of the study. The patient is kept fasting on the day of the study to prevent vomiting and possible aspiration during the procedure. Routine premedication includes an antihistamine (to prevent contrast-induced vomiting) and possibly a mild sedative. We usually administer atropine intravenously just before injecting contrast material, to counter a pain-related vagal reaction that might cause hypotension and bradycardia. Premedication should be individualized. For example, an elderly patient may become agitated after administration of atropine; a patient with chronic obstructive pulmonary disease may deteriorate after sedation; or a patient with unstable angina may exhibit cardiac ischemia with tachycardia after antihistamine premedication.

For reasons of safety, intravenous access is established before the catheterization procedure is begun. The choice of intravenous fluids should reflect the underlying disease. For example, salt-containing fluids should not be given to any patient in congestive heart failure. On the other hand, salt-containing fluids may be warranted in a patient with renal insufficiency, since infusion of a liter of saline overnight may lower the serum creatinine. In such cases, we adminster saline the night before if the patient's cardiac status permits. Pretreatment with low ("renal") doses of dopamine may improve renal function in some patients with congestive heart failure, thereby increasing their tolerance for contrast media.

In infants and children, catheterization is performed under general anesthesia with endotracheal intubation. Sedation and other details of patient preparation are the responsibility of the anesthesiologist, and are therefore beyond the scope of this book.

PLANNING THE PROCEDURE

The invasive cardiologist should plan a suitable strategy beforehand and discuss it with other members of the team. Although elementary preparations usually suffice in a patient of average size who is being evaluated for angina, elaborate planning may be necessary for a patient with a complex congenital defect,

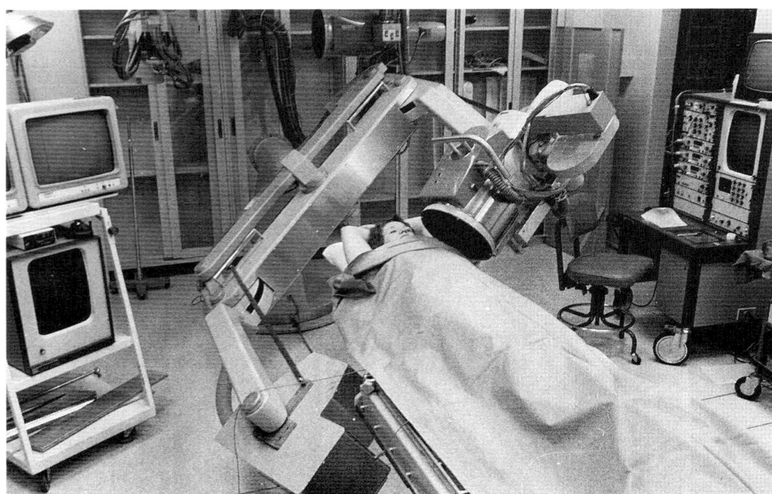

Fig. 3.10 The patient prior to catheterization.

limited vascular access, large body size, hemodynamic instability, or a need for ventilatory support. Hypothermia is a potential hazard in small infants.

In general, it is wise to insert all the vascular lines, make the necessary physiologic and hemodynamic measurements, and adjust the medication and/or mechanical support to optimize the patient's circulatory and respiratory status before performing the angiographic procedure. In planning the latter, the region of greatest clinical importance should be studied first (eg, the coronary arteries, left ventricle, aorta, or other region, depending on the clinical problem). In performing coronary arteriography with the Judkins (transfemoral) technique, the invasive cardiologist must decide which coronary artery to examine first. Because it is usually possible to pass a catheter with a right coronary artery curve across the aortic valve, it is possible to obtain a precontrast left ventricular pressure by introducing the right coronary catheter first. On the other hand, performing the left coronary arteriogram as the initial procedure can identify patients with a left dominant coronary artery pattern (see Chapter 21). Since the small right coronary artery is likely to be temporarily occluded by the catheter, appropriate precautions can be taken when performing the right coronary arteriogram.

CATHETERIZATION

Depending on the study to be performed, a suitable artery (femoral, brachial, or axillary) or vein (jugular, subclavian, femoral, or brachial) is used for vascular access. After sterile preparation of the entry site, local anesthetic is injected (Fig. 3.10).

Most invasive cardiac studies are performed with the Seldinger technique. After percutaneous puncture of the vessel to be catheterized, a guidewire is introduced. A dilator is passed over the guidewire and a sheath is inserted over the dilator. The guidewire and dilator are then removed, leaving the sheath in place. The catheter is introduced through the sheath and advanced into the region to be studied. Some invasive cardiologists prefer to heparinize the patient briefly with 2000 to 5000 units once the sheath is in place. For the Sones method of coronary arteriography, a cut-down is made over the left or right brachial artery, after which the catheter is introduced through a small arteriotomy.

Once vascular access is obtained, a wide variety of catheters are available. Most invasive cardiologists prefer to use the balloon-tipped 7F "Swan–Ganz" model for right heart catheterization and measurements of cardiac output by the thermal dilution technique in adults. (Smaller Swan–Ganz catheters are used in infants and children.) Not only does inflating the balloon facilitate passage of the catheter into the right ventricle, it also enables one to intermittently measure the pulmonary artery "wedge" pressure, which provides an indirect measurement of left atrial pressure. Swan–Ganz catheters can be safely left in place for several days to monitor the hemodynamic status of patients in the intensive care unit.

Arterial and left heart catheters are available in a variety of preshaped configurations. The most popular catheters for conventional coronary arteriography are Judkins catheters with left and right coronary curves, which are available in sizes from 6F to 8F. The smaller size is suitable for most noncomplex situations and can be used in patients whose body size is not too large. The advantage of the 6F catheter is that it allows the patient to ambulate as early as 6 hours after the procedure, whereas patients studied with an 8F catheter must remain in bed overnight. Angled "pigtail" catheters with side holes are favored for ventriculography. Using a catheter with side holes makes it possible to deliver larger volumes of contrast material (eg, 12 to 20 mL/second for 3 seconds) more safely, and with fewer ectopic beats, than is possible with an end-hole catheter of comparable size. Pigtail catheters are ideally suited for aortography, as well as for demonstrating regurgitant flow through an incompetent aortic or mitral valve. (A more detailed discussion of the great variety of preshaped catheter configurations designed for specific situations is beyond the scope of this book.)

ANGIOGRAPHY

After the catheters have been placed in the desired location and the hemodynamic data have been recorded, angiography is performed. Extreme care must be taken to avoid introducing air bubbles and to prevent thrombus formation in the oxygenated circulation proximal to the carotid arteries. After the study is complete and the catheters withdrawn, the injection site is compressed for up to 15 minutes. The patient is then returned to his room and observed for bleeding from the puncture site and other complications (eg, chest pain, ECG changes).

ANGIOCARDIOGRAPHY

Angiocardiography is used to evaluate both congenital malformations and acquired cardiac disorders. In addition, angiocardiography provides important functional data, including ventricular volume and mass, abnormal wall motion, and functional parameters such as myocardial and mechanical compliance.

Angiocardiographic diagnosis of cardiac malformations depends on a rigorous, systematic assessment of the various cardiac segments and connections and of the great vessels. Like other radiographic images, angiocardiograms project complex three-dimensional structures onto a two-dimensional plane; therefore, overlapping structures may not be adequately visualized. In addition, certain structures (eg, the ventricular septum, bifurcation of the pulmonary arteries) are not optimally displayed on standard frontal, lateral, and oblique projections. Special axial projections, obtained by angling the X-ray tube with respect to the coronal and sagittal planes, can usually overcome these difficulties (Figs. 3.10 to 3.12).

Conventional angiocardiography employs relatively large volumes of contrast material, which may be hazardous to infants or unstable patients, as well as to patients with impaired renal function. The risk is increased in complex cases that require multiple projections and large volumes of contrast material. To decrease the risk, which appears to be at least in part related to the total osmolar load, many cardiac catheterization laboratories have switched to low-osmolality contrast media. The disturbance of left ventricular function associated with left ventriculography (manfested by elevation of end diastolic left ventricular pressure and end diastolic left ventricular pressure) is not as severe when low-osmolality contrast agents are employed.

Digital angiography utilizes digital images processed through the video system, which can be manipulated electronically (eg, electronic subtraction significantly enhances subject contrast). Digital intravenous angiocardiography (DIVA) requires considerably less contrast material than conventional cineangiocardiography. In the least invasive technique, contrast material is injected into a peripheral vein and, after a timed delay, images are recorded when the region of interest is maximally opacified (Fig. 3.13). Although DIVA theoretically eliminates

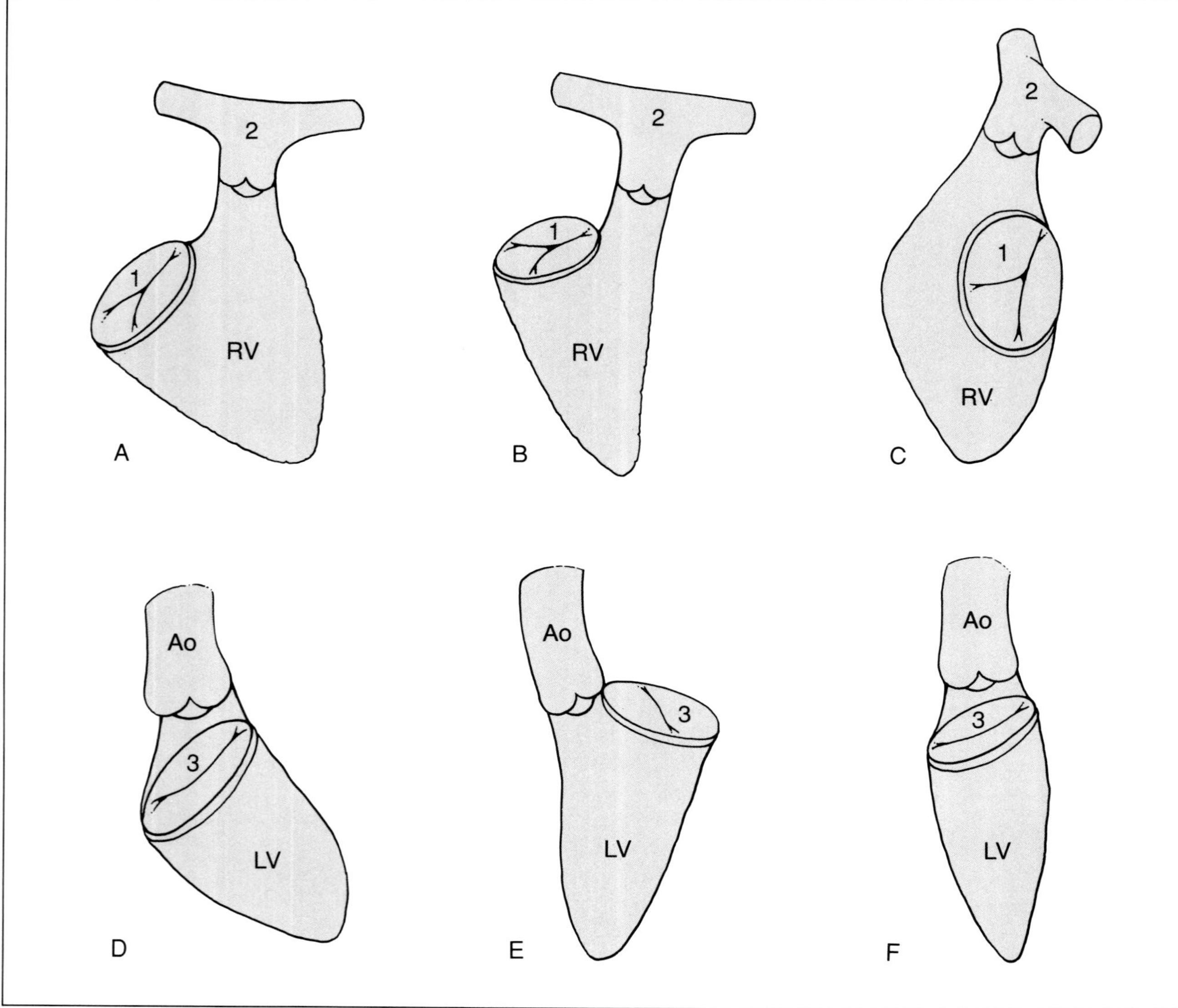

Fig. 3.11 Frontal and axial projections or normal ventricles. (A–C) Right ventriculogram. (A) Frontal projection. (B) Long axial projection. (C) Four-chamber projection. (D–F) Left ventriculogram. (D) Frontal projection. (E) Long axial projection. (F) Four-chamber projection. Muscular ventricular septal defects are best localized in the long axial projection. Atrioventricular septal defects are well seen in the four-chamber view of the left ventriculogram. Axial projections profile the ventricular and atrial septum, allowing a better assessment of their morphology than standard frontal and lateral projections. Ventricular septal defects of the muscular, trabecular, and outlet portions of the ventricular septum are best demonstrated in the long axial projection, whereas atrioventricular septal defects (which involve the inlet position of the ventricular septum) are best seen in the four-chamber projection.

1 tricuspid valve
RV right ventricle
2 pulmonary trunk
LV left ventricle
3 mitral valve
Ao aorta

the need for cardiac catheterization, the images are frequently degraded by motion artifacts and usually lack the resolution needed for intracardiac diagnosis. For this reason, DIVA is largely restricted to extracardiac diagnosis (eg, aortic arch anomalies, coarctation of the aorta, peripheral arterial stenosis). To adequately visualize intracardiac structures, it is necessary to inject the contrast material as close to the area of interest as possible (ie, through a catheter). Although the catheter technique is invasive, it requires much less contrast material than conventional cineangiocardiography and is useful in selected cases.

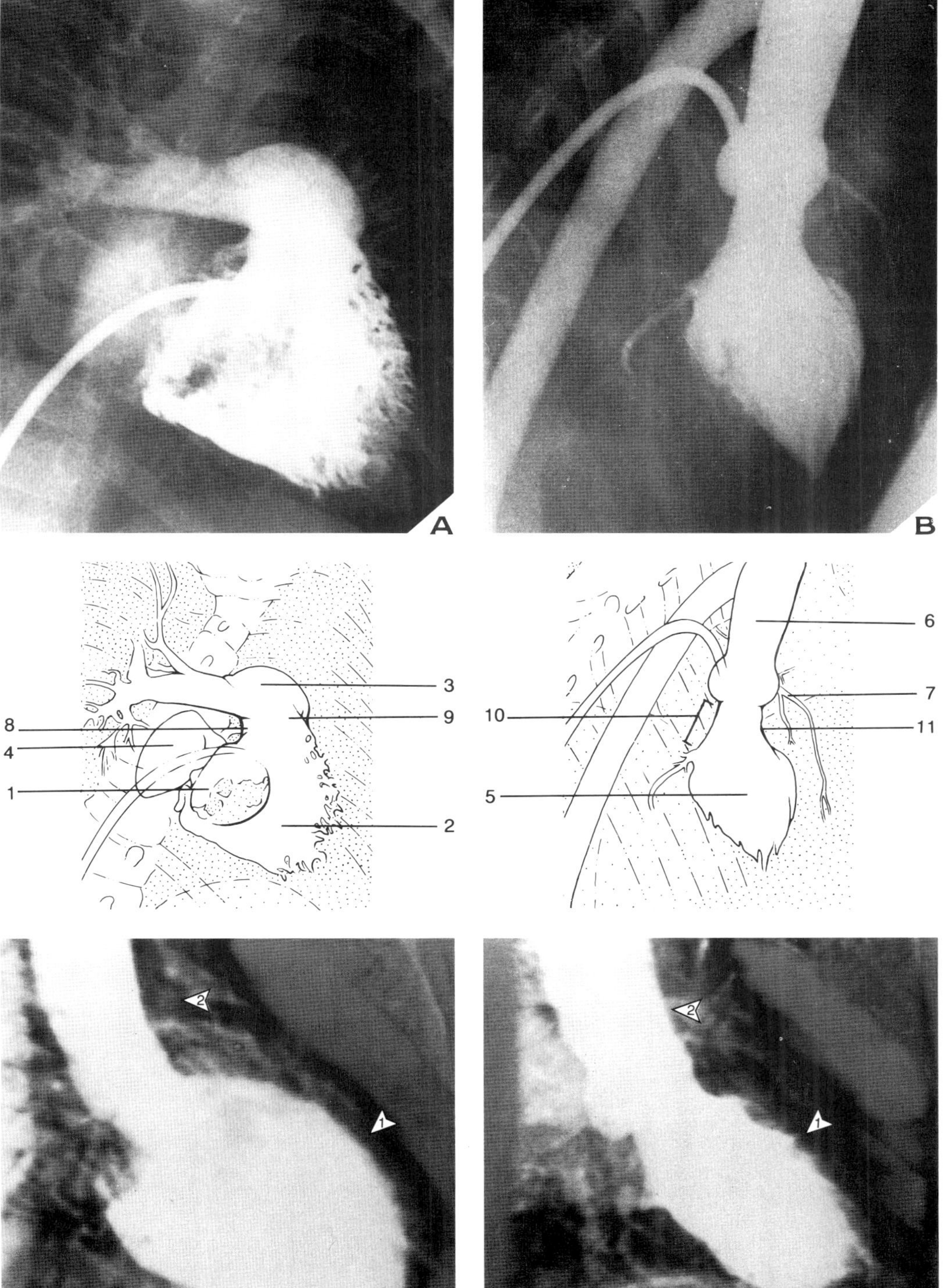

Fig. 3.12 Right and left ventriculography in the elongated right anterior oblique projection. (A) Normal right ventriculogram. The catheter has been advanced from the inferior vena cava into the right atrium and across the tricuspid valve. The opacification of the right atrium is due to catheter-induced tricuspid insufficiency. (B) Normal left ventriculogram. The catheter has been advanced across the foramen ovale and mitral valve into the left ventricle. The outflow tracts of the right and left ventricles are better demonstrated in the elongated right anterior oblique projection than in the standard frontal and lateral views. The crista supraventricularis appears as a discrete structure between the tricuspid and pulmonic valves, and is demarcated posteriorly by the right coronary cusp of the aortic valve. The atrioventricular septum forms the posteroinferior aspect of the left ventricular border and the conal (outlet) portion of the septum forms its left anterior border.

1	tricuspid valve
2	right ventricle
3	pulmonary trunk
4	right atrium
5	left ventricle
6	ascending aorta
7	coronary arteries
8	crista supraventricularis
9	pulmonic valve
10	atrioventricular septum
11	outlet septum

Fig. 3.13 Digital angiocardiography (catheter technique). Elongated right anterior projection of normal left ventricle in diastole (A) and systole (B). The contrast material has been injected via a catheter that was passed retrogradely into the left ventricle.

arrow 1	left ventricle	arrow 2	aorta

CORONARY ARTERIOGRAPHY

Coronary arteriography usually requires 3 to 10 mL of contrast material, which is injected manually over a period of 1 to 3 seconds (the size of the patient, the heart, and the coronary arteries, together with the run-off, dictate the volume and injection rate). After the initial run, the images are reviewed on videotape to see if additional projections or injections are required.

The newer low-osmolality contrast agents are cleared more rapidly from the coronary circulation and produce less myocardial hyperemia than conventional ionic contrast agents. However, it is not clear whether these agents, which are much more expensive than conventional ionic agents, significantly decrease the morbidity and mortality associated with this procedure. Although we do not routinely use low-osmolality agents for coronary arteriography, we believe that they are indicated in hemodynamically unstable patients, diabetics, and patients with severe renal failure.

Coronary arteriography is discussed more extensively in Chapter 21.

THERAPEUTIC CATHETER PROCEDURES

Since the introduction of balloon septostomy by Rashkind in 1968, the therapeutic use of percutaneously introduced vascular catheters has steadily increased. Current applications include balloon angioplasty of stenotic vessels (including the coronary arteries) and cardiac valves; embolotherapy to occlude arteriovenous fistulas, aortopulmonary collaterals, and patent ductus arteriosus; and palliative systemic–pulmonary shunts. The use of transvascular techniques in the treatment of congenital and acquired heart disease is discussed in Chapters 16 and 30.

SPECIAL SITUATIONS, PROBLEMS, AND TECHNIQUES

TRANSSEPTAL CATHETERIZATION

This technique allows percutaneous access to the left atrium from the right atrium, after which the catheter can be advanced across the mitral valve into the left ventricle (see Fig. 3.6). Although not as frequently employed as in the past, the transseptal approach is indicated in selected situations [eg, balloon valvotomy for mitral stenosis, left ventriculography following aortic valve replacement (Fig. 3.14), and percutaneous insertion of left ventricular assist devices], and remains an alternative in patients with aortic stenosis for whom retrograde catheterization of the left ventricle is not feasible (see Fig. 3.20).

The procedure utilizes a specially designed curved, thin-needle obturator which is sheathed in a pointed dilator and a long outer sheath (Fig. 3.15). Vascular access is gained via the right femoral vein. Under careful fluoroscopic guidance, the coaxial system is advanced until it abuts the atrial septum. The needle is then advanced, puncturing the septum; if pressure measurements do not clearly indicate that the needle tip is in the left atrium, it is withdrawn into the dilator and the coaxial system is repositioned for another attempt. If the needle position is satisfactory, the catheter is advanced over the needle and the coaxial system is withdrawn. Potential complications include pericardial tamponade (due to perforation of the atrial wall by the dilator) and hemodynamic collapse (due to perforation of the aorta). Successful application of this demanding technique requires a thorough assessment of the patient's anatomy and considerable experience on the part of the operator.

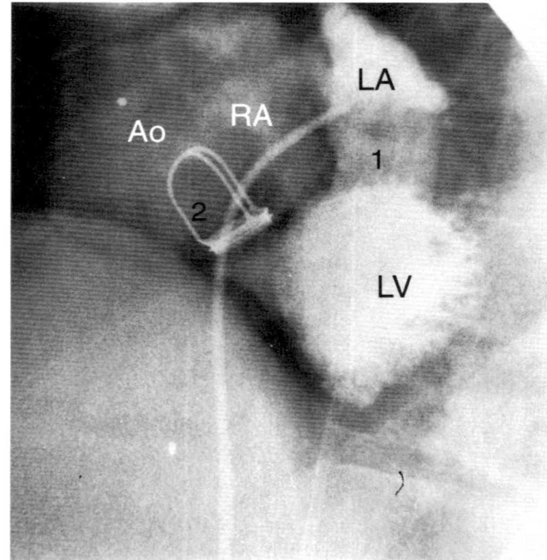

RA right atrium
LA left atrium
1 mitral valve
LV left ventricle
2 aortic valve prosthesis
Ao aorta

Fig. 3.14 Angiocardiography after transseptal catheterization. The angiographic catheter has been passed from the right atrium into the left atrium via the atrial septum. A four-chamber projection demonstrates opacification of the left atrium and left ventricle. There is a small amount of contrast material in the right atrium. If a selective left ventriculogram is desired, the catheter can be advanced across the mitral valve into the left ventricular cavity. The study was performed to evaluate left ventricular function in a patient with a mechanical aortic valve prosthesis.

PROSTHETIC VALVES

The invasive cardiologist is frequently called on to evaluate patients with prosthetic valves. Whereas patients with tissue valves (eg, commercially available stent-mounted heterografts) can be studied with standard techniques, provided that care is taken not to injure the valve, mechanical valves present special problems. Most invasive cardiologists believe that mechanical valves should not be crossed with a catheter because of the risk that the catheter may become entrapped, causing the valve to become incompetent. Therefore, if it is necessary to enter the left heart in a patient with a mechanical aortic valve prosthesis, transseptal catheterization (see above) is the procedure of choice. For patients with mitral and aortic valve prostheses, direct transthoracic needle puncture of the left ventricle via the

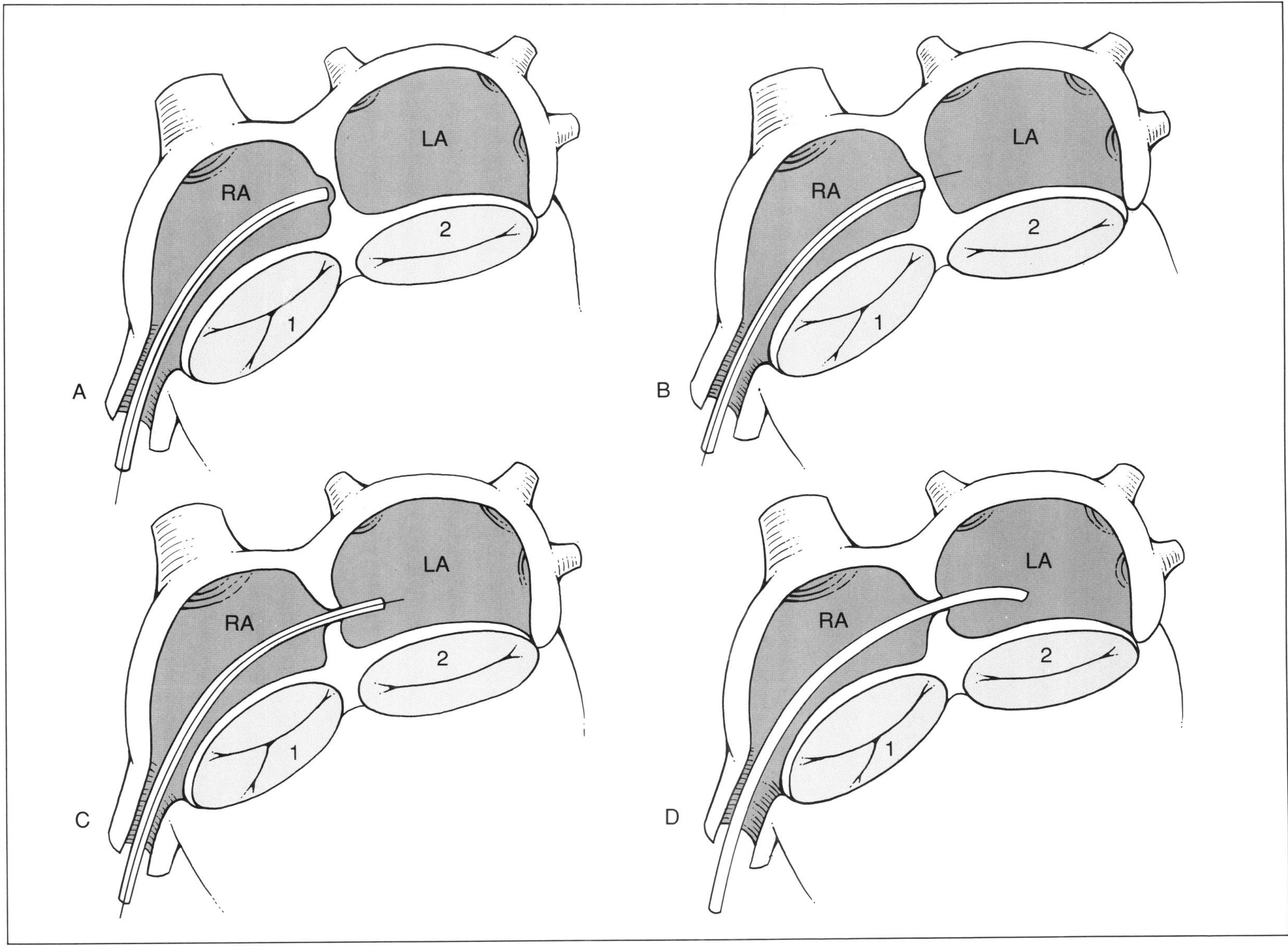

RA right atrium	**1** tricuspid valve
LA left atrium	**2** mitral valve

Fig. 3.15 Transseptal catheterization. Schematic representation of atrial septal puncture and catheter exchange. (A) The catheter is passed from the inferior vena cava into the right atrium and its tip is positioned in the fossa ovalis. (B) A guidewire with a hard core and a sharp tip is passed through the catheter and punctures the atrial septum. (C) The catheter–guidewire assembly is advanced a short distance into the left atrium and the guidewire is removed. (D) The catheter is then advanced into the left atrium.

LV apex should be considered (Figs. 3.16 and 3.17). This demanding technique is best employed in centers with considerable experience with complex interventions.

In general, standard techniques can be used in patients with mechanical mitral valve prostheses, provided that the catheter is kept clear of the valve to minimize the risk of dislodging a thrombus or entrapment of the catheter. Rarely, it is necessary to pass a catheter across a mechanical tricuspid or pulmonic valve prosthesis. A small balloon catheter can be used in such cases; although ball-cage prostheses usually present no problem, entrapment of the catheter is a potential risk in patients with flap valves. Whereas valvular incompetence secondary to catheter entrapment on the left side of the heart may have serious consequences, temporary valvular incompetence on the right side of the heart is usually well tolerated, even in patients who are quite ill.

AORTIC STENOSIS

Most invasive cardiologists have developed their own repertory of "tricks" for passing catheters retrogradely through stenotic aortic valves. The small valve orifice, dilated aortic root, turbulent blood flow, and the often ragged surface of the cusps contribute to the difficulty of the procedure. Nevertheless, it is necessary to persevere, since in many clinical settings (eg, elderly patients, poor ventricular function, associated coronary artery or noncardiac disease) the surgeon relies heavily on the pressure gradient and the calculated valve area in assessing the need for corrective surgery.

One technique that we have found to be reliable employs an Amplatz-configuration (S-shaped) coronary artery catheter containing a straight guidewire (Fig. 3.18). Using biplane or multiview fluoroscopy for guidance, the catheter tip is "aimed" at the valve from a distance of 1 or 2 cm, and repeated attempts are made to pass the guidewire across the valve. Once the guidewire has crossed the valve, it is usually possible to feed the catheter into the left ventricle. If this results in an excessive number of ventricular ectopic beats, or if a ventriculogram is desired, the Amplatz catheter can be replaced with a pigtail catheter (Fig. 3.19). The catheter exchange is done cautiously over a long J-shaped guidewire to minimize the risk of perforating the ventricular wall.

An alternative approach that can be employed when the retrograde technique is unsuccessful is to enter the left atrium via the transseptal approach, after which the catheter is passed through the mitral valve into the left ventricle (Fig. 3.20).

PROBLEMS OF VASCULAR ACCESS AND CATHETER PLACEMENT

Because of its ease and the low radiation dose to the operator, most angiographers prefer the femoral approach for aortography and coronary arteriography. Occasionally it may be very difficult—rarely, impossible—to position the catheter tip in the aortic root for these procedures. A number of special maneuvers can be employed in such cases. (The side with the strongest femoral pulse should be used.) A J-tip guidewire (or one with a soft tip and "torqueable" curve) can be employed if the iliac vessels or aorta are tortuous or stenotic, or both. Another frequently successful technique is to use a Judkins-shape right coronary artery catheter, making frequent test injections of contrast material to find a passage through which the catheter

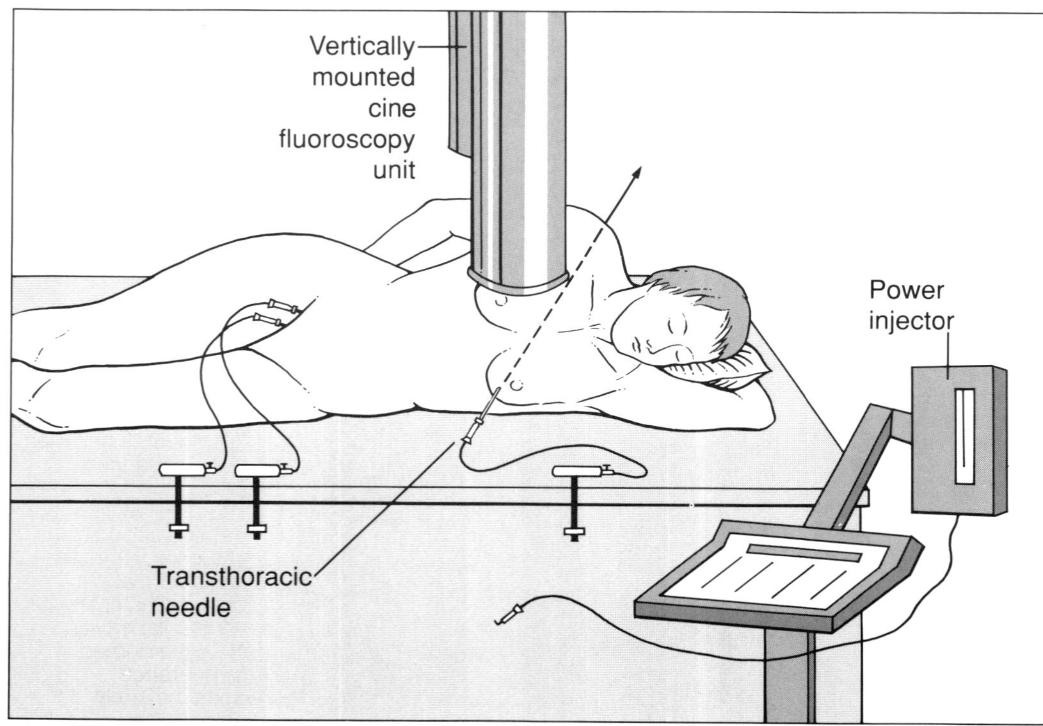

Fig. 3.16 Direct transthoracic transapical needle puncture of the left ventricle. The patient lies comfortably with his or her left side down. The patient's right side is slightly elevated so that the mitral prosthesis is in profile when viewed through the vertically mounted cine fluoroscopy unit. The shortest route between the skin surface and the cardiac apex is identified and the puncture site is prepared and anethetized. Under fluoroscopic control, the transthoracic needle is introduced and advanced in the direction of the right scapula until it enters the left ventricle. Contrast is then injected through a power injector (shown at patient's left). Systemic and pulmonary arterial "wedge" pressures are continuosly monitored during the procedure.

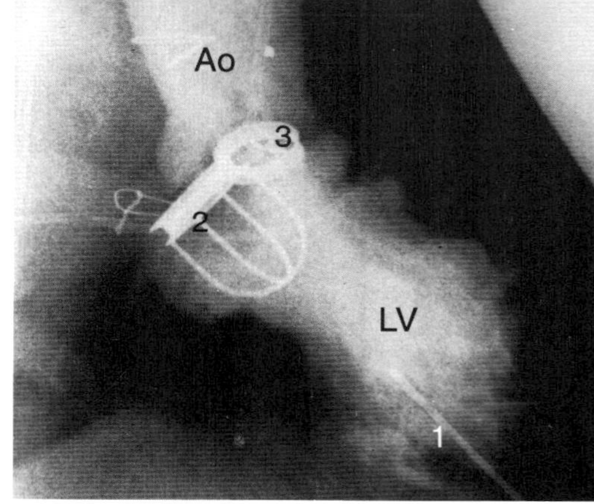

1 transapical catheter
LV left ventricle
2 prosthetic mitral valve
3 prosthetic aortic valve
Ao aorta

Fig. 3.17 Left ventriculography after transthoracic needle puncture of the left ventricle. Right anterior oblique projection of left ventriculogram in a patient with aortic and mitral valve prostheses. The tip of the catheter has been positioned in the midportion of the left ventricular cavity (the absence of contrast material in the left atrium rules out mitral incompetence). To complete the evaluation of a patient with mitral and aortic valve prostheses, the transthoracic transapical study is followed with a conventional thoracic aortogram to rule out aortic valvular incompetence.

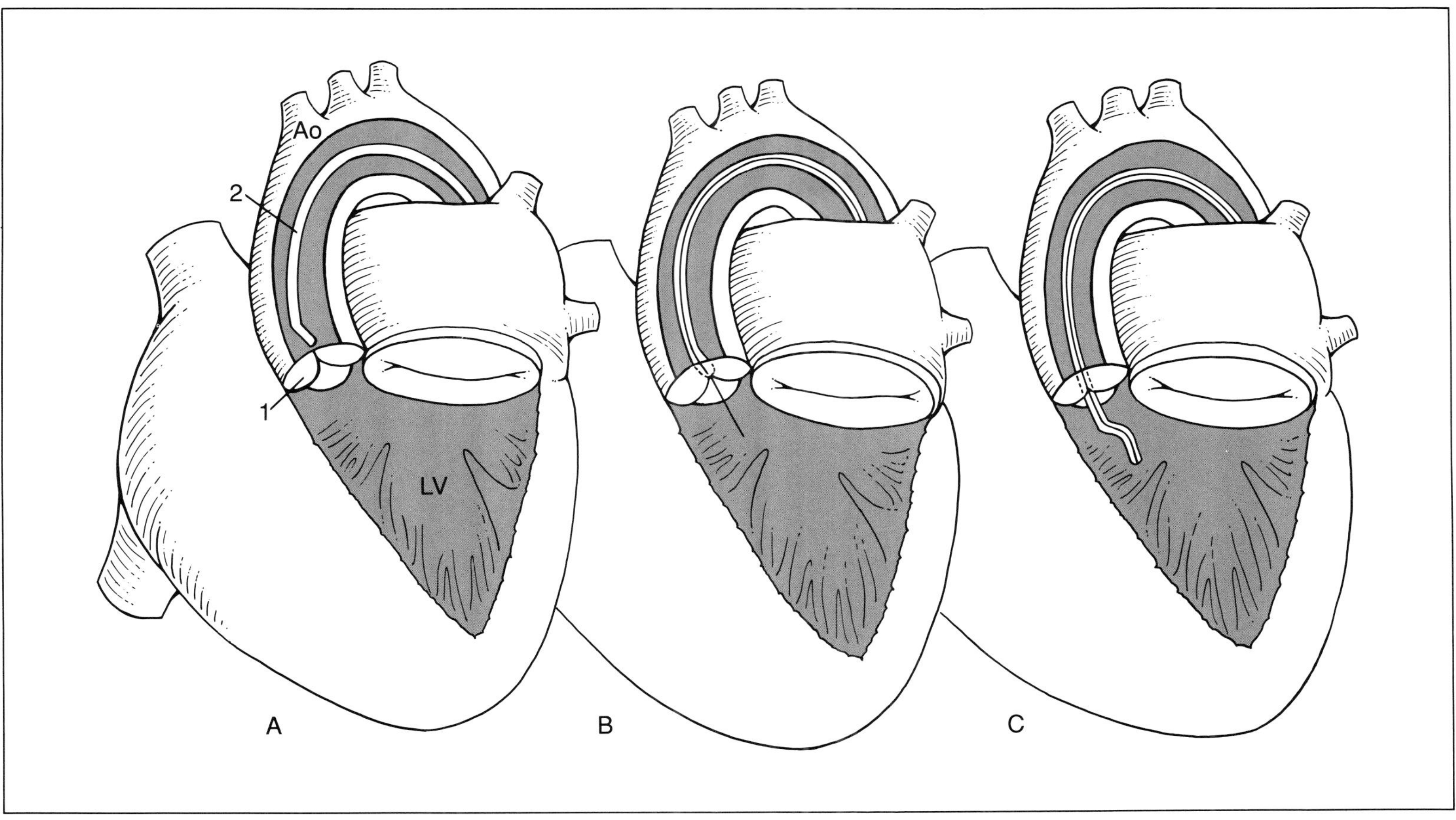

1 aortic valve
2 Amplatz catheter
Ao aorta
LV left ventricle

Fig. 3.18 Retrograde catheterization of left ventricle in patient with aortic stenosis using an Amplatz coronary artery catheter. (A) The Amplatz catheter, which has an angulated tip, is positioned with the end hole just above the aperture of the aortic valve. (B) The guidewire is advanced through the catheter tip, passing easily through the aortic valve into the left ventricle. (C) The catheter–guidewire assembly is then passed into the left ventricular cavity and the guidewire is withdrawn.

Fig. 3.19 Left ventriculogram in a patient with severe aortic stenosis (retrograde technique). The angiographic catheter has been passed from the aortic root across the stenotic aortic valve into the left ventricle. Note the domed appearance (*arrows*) of the aortic valve, indicating severe aortic stenosis.

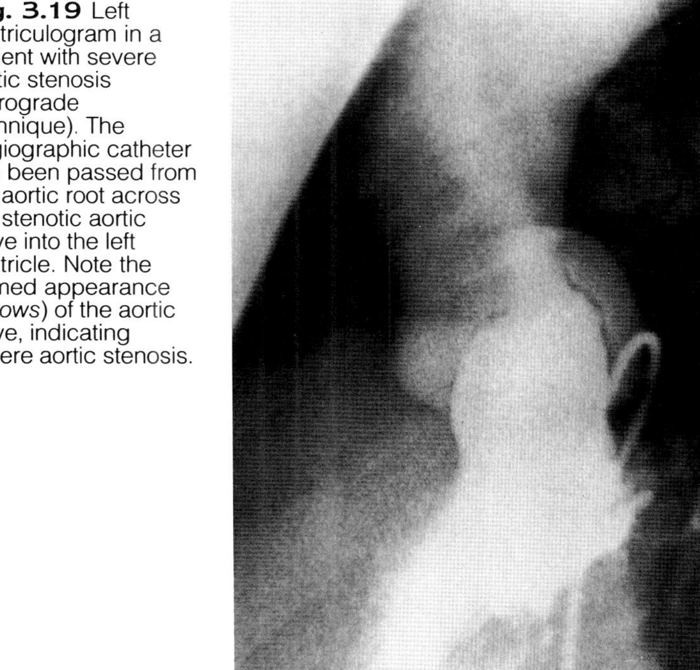

Fig. 3.20 Left ventriculogram in patient with aortic stenosis (transseptal technique). Left anterior oblique projection of left ventriculogram. The catheter has been passed from the inferior vena cava into the right atrum, through the atrial septum, and into the left atrium. It has then been advanced across the mitral valve into the inflow tract or trabecular portion of the left ventricle. Contrast material outlines the entire left ventricular cavity. Note the domed appearance of the severely stenotic aortic valve. The transseptal technique is employed in patients with severe aortic stenosis in whom it is not possible to pass a guidewire retrogradely through the valve orifice.

can be guided. The use of an extra-long (15 cm) sheath improves torque control in patients with very tortuous iliac arteries. Extreme care should be taken in patients with abdominal aortic aneurysms, particularly symptomatic ones, to avoid traumatizing the aorta during passage of the guidewire or catheter.

Femoral puncture is contraindicated in patients with a graft or scar from previous vascular surgery; entry into the vessel is likely to be difficult owing to the hard, noncompliant tissue, and hemostasis may be difficult or impossible to achieve when the catheter is removed. Alternatives include percutaneous puncture of the brachial or axillary artery or a brachial artery cutdown. (Heparin should be administered intra-arterially in such cases.) In patients undergoing coronary arteriography, the right arm is preferred for multipurpose and Sones catheters, whereas Judkins catheters can be used in either arm (Fig. 3.21). Percutaneously placed 6F sheaths are commonly used when Judkins catheters are employed. Excessive radiation exposure to the operator is a potential problem when the upper extremities are used for access. Technical aspects of coronary arteriography are discussed further in Chapter 21.

STUDY OF PATIENTS WITH COMPLEX CONGENITAL HEART DISEASE

These investigations, which may be technically very difficult, are best performed in larger centers. As much detailed information as possible should be available to help the invasive cardiologist plan the procedure. In planning the study of an adult patient with a complex defect, consultation with the pediatric cardiologist, radiologist, and surgeon may be helpful. Because many teenagers and adult patients are emotionally labile, general anesthesia may be necessary if the study is to progress in satisfactory fashion.

Polycythemia is a common problem in cyanotic patients. It predisposes to clotting of catheters and yet, paradoxically, impedes hemostasis after the catheter is removed. However, a preliminary phlebotomy is likely to have adverse hemodynamic effects and should be avoided. Great care should be taken to avoid air bubbles in the venous circulation in patients with right to left shunts. Arrthymias are common and usually transient. The most frequently encountered arrhythmias are transient ectopic beats of atrial or ventricular origin. Patients with Ebstein's malformation and congenital defects associated

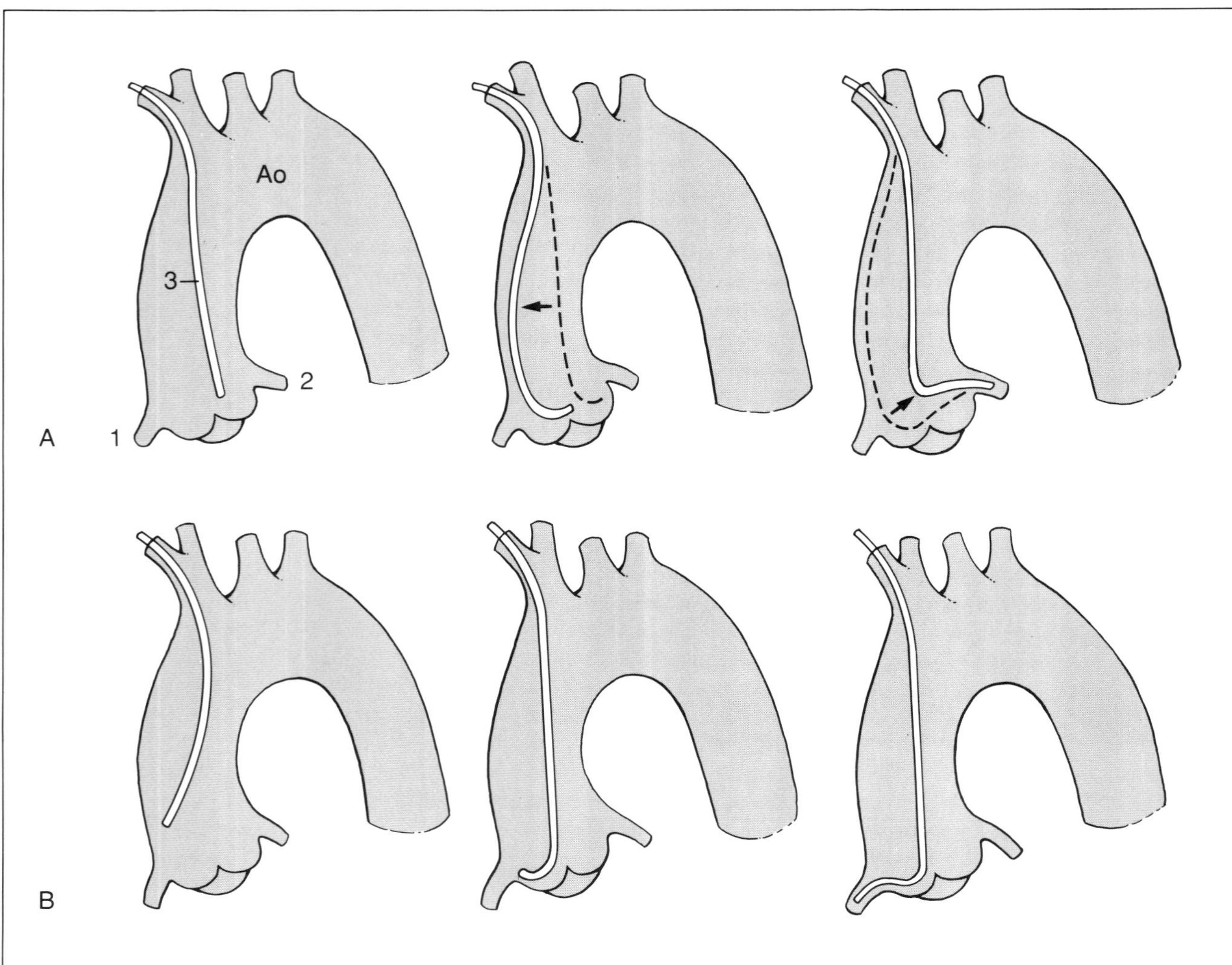

Fig. 3.21 Catheter course for coronary arteriography performed via right brachial artery. (A) Selective catheterization of left coronary artery. (B) Selective catheterization of right coronary artery.

Ao	aorta
1	right coronary artery
2	left coronary artery
3	catheter

with left axis deviation or right bundle branch block (eg, atrioventricular septal defect, discordant atrioventricular connection) are prone to develop arrhythmias during catheterization. Although most arrhythmias resolve spontaneously, a DC countershock may sometimes be necessary to restore a sinus rhythm.

When dealing with a complex defect, it may be necessary to deviate from the "physiological data first, angiography last" rule, since it is sometimes desirable to perform angiography early in the procedure to guide the operator in catheterizing a markedly disordered cardiovascular system (Fig. 3.22).

POSTPROCEDURAL HEMOSTASIS

Hemostasis at the entry site is seldom a problem after routine studies performed with the Seldinger technique via a femoral arterial puncture; manual compression just proximal to the entry site, maintained for 15 minutes and followed by 6 to 18 hours of bed rest, usually results in an uneventful recovery with minimal scarring. The steady increase in the number of interventional procedures which take longer than diagnostic procedures and entail a greater number of catheter and guidewire exchanges has led to increased concern about postprocedural bleeding.

Complications associated with inadequate hemostasis, which may occasionally require surgical intervention, include perivascular hematoma, arteriovenous fistula, arterial occlusion, and false aneurysm. Complications of this type can usually be avoided by making the arterial puncture well below the groin crease, so that when the catheter is withdrawn sufficient compressive force can be applied proximal to the puncture site to transiently occlude the artery. This is especially important in formerly obese patients who have recently lost a great deal of weight, resulting in an abnormally low interstitial tissue pressure.

Patients on anticoagulant therapy present a special problem. Simple compression may be insufficient in these patients, in which case it may be necessary to use a vascular clamp or pressure girdle to stop the bleeding. Hypertensive patients also present a special problem; lowering the blood pressure to normal with nitrates or sublingual liquid nifedipine may be effective in preventing or controlling bleeding at the entry site. The risk of postprocedural bleeding is particularly great in patients with aortic incompetence, owing to the elevated systolic pressure.

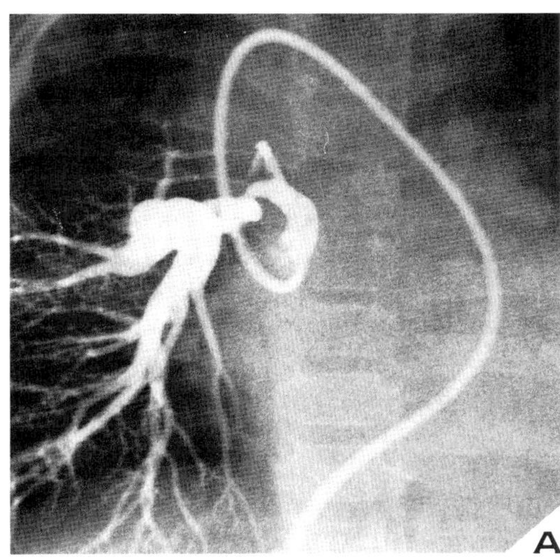

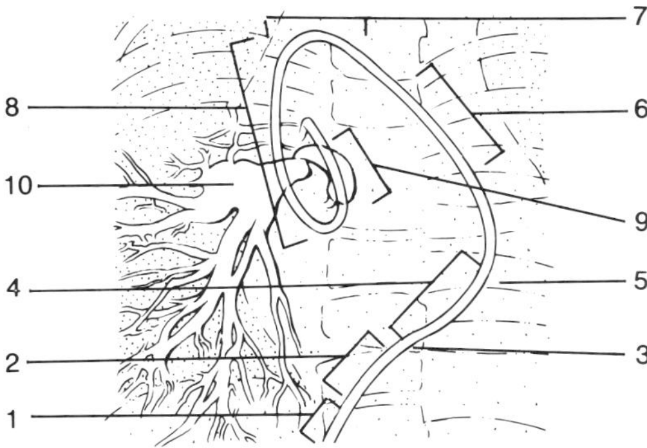

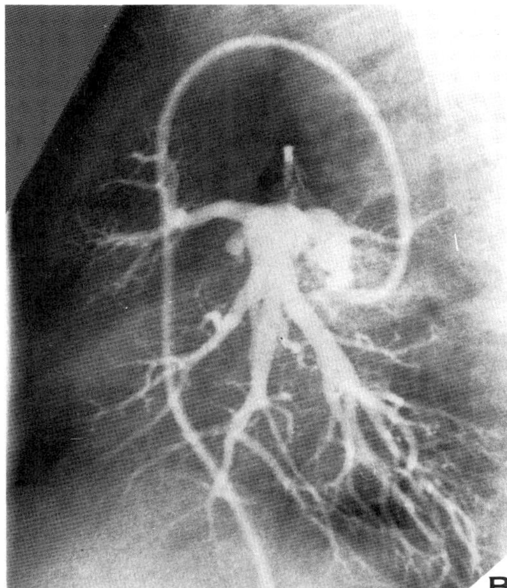

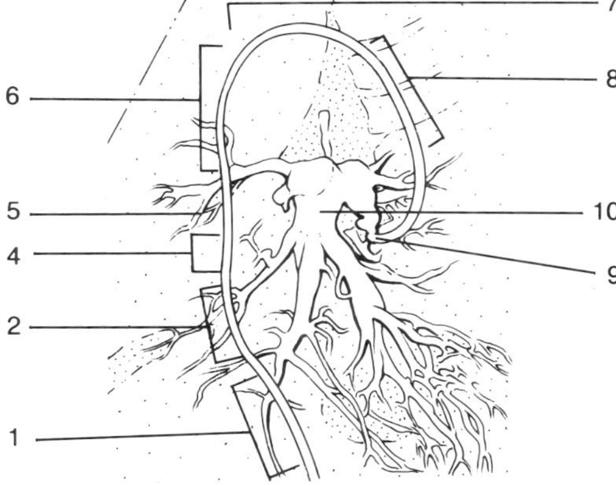

Fig. 3.22 Course of catheter in patient with complex congenital heart disease. (A) Frontal and (B) lateral projections of subselective right pulmonary arteriogram in a patient with pulmonary atresia with ventricular septal defect. The catheter was introduced into a femoral vein, advanced into the inferior vena cava, and passed into the right atrium. It then passed through the tricuspid valve to enter the right ventricle, crossed the ventriclar septal defect, and passed throgh the aortic valve into the ascending aorta. The upward course of the catheter indicates that it is in a right aortic arch. The catheter then courses downward to the right of the spine, indicating that the descending thoracic aorta is on the right. The catheter tip is in an aortopulmonary collateral that arises from the descending thoracic aorta and connects with lobar arteries supplying the right lower lobe. A preliminary arteriogram may be helpful when the course of the catheter is confusing.

1	inferior vena cava right atrium	7	right aortic arch
2	tricuspid valve	8	descending thoracic aorta
3	ventricular septal defect	9	aortopulmonary collateral (catheter tip)
4	right ventricle	10	lower lobe pulmonary artery
6	ascending aorta		

CHAPTER 4

Nuclear Magnetic Resonance Imaging

VERA A. BITTNER, M.D.
GEORGE B. CRANNEY, M.D.

Proton nuclear magnetic resonance (NMR) imaging, also known as magnetic resonance imaging (MRI), has been applied clinically to many areas of the body. It is noninvasive, yields excellent anatomic resolution, is intrinsically three dimensional, provides inherent contrast between tissues and flowing blood, and can often distinguish between normal and abnormal tissue on the basis of tissue relaxation properties. This chapter reviews basic principles of NMR physics and spectroscopy, discusses some common imaging sequences, and briefly outlines present and potential cardiovascular applications. The role of MRI in specific disease states will be addressed in later chapters.

BASIC PRINCIPLES

NMR PHYSICS

Certain atomic nuclei (usually those possessing odd numbers of nucleons) possess a net spin and an electric charge, and thus generate a small magnetic field. They can be thought of as small bar magnets. These nuclei exhibit nuclear magnetic resonance. Those with actual or potential medical relevance include ^{1}H (proton), ^{31}P (phosphorus), ^{23}Na (sodium), ^{13}C (carbon), and ^{19}F (fluorine).

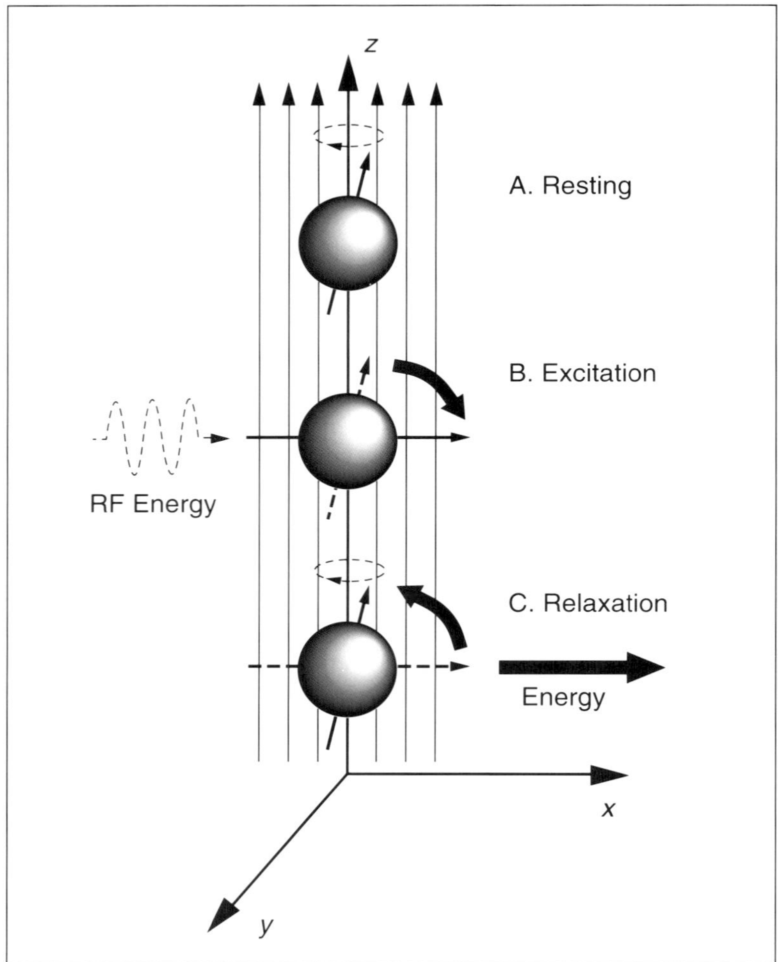

Fig. 4.1 Behavior of spins in a magnetic field. (A) Nuclei are aligned with the external magnetic field (vertical arrows) and precess around its axis (z-axis). (B) Radiofrequency (RF) energy at the Larmor frequency tips the nuclei away from the z-axis into the xy-plane, a process called excitation. (C) The nuclei gradually realign with the external magnetic field. During this process of relaxation, energy is released and a signal (the so-called FID or free induction decay) can be measured.

In the absence of an external magnetic field, the magnetic fields associated with these nuclei are randomly oriented, and there is no net magnetic moment. When placed in a magnetic field, the nuclei become aligned parallel or antiparallel to the extrinsic field and precess around its axis. Individual magnetic fields generated by the spinning charges no longer cancel each other, and a net magnetic moment in the direction of the external magnetic field is generated. The strength of this magnetic moment depends on the external field strength and on the concentration and the intrinsic magnetic sensitivity of the nuclei.

Nuclear magnetic resonance is exhibited because sensitive nuclei can absorb radiofrequency (RF) energy at a characteristic resonance frequency (or Larmor frequency). Absorption of the RF energy causes the nuclei to be tipped away from their alignment with the external magnetic field (Fig. 4.1). The degree of displacement is proportional to the duration and the power of the RF pulse. RF pulses strong enough to rotate the vector by 90 degrees ("90-degree pulses") and 180 degrees ("180-degree pulses") are frequently used in standard MRI (see below).

After cessation of the RF pulse, the nuclei realign with the external magnetic field through a process called relaxation (Fig. 4.2). During relaxation, a characteristic RF signal is released from these nuclei and can be measured as the so-called *free in-*

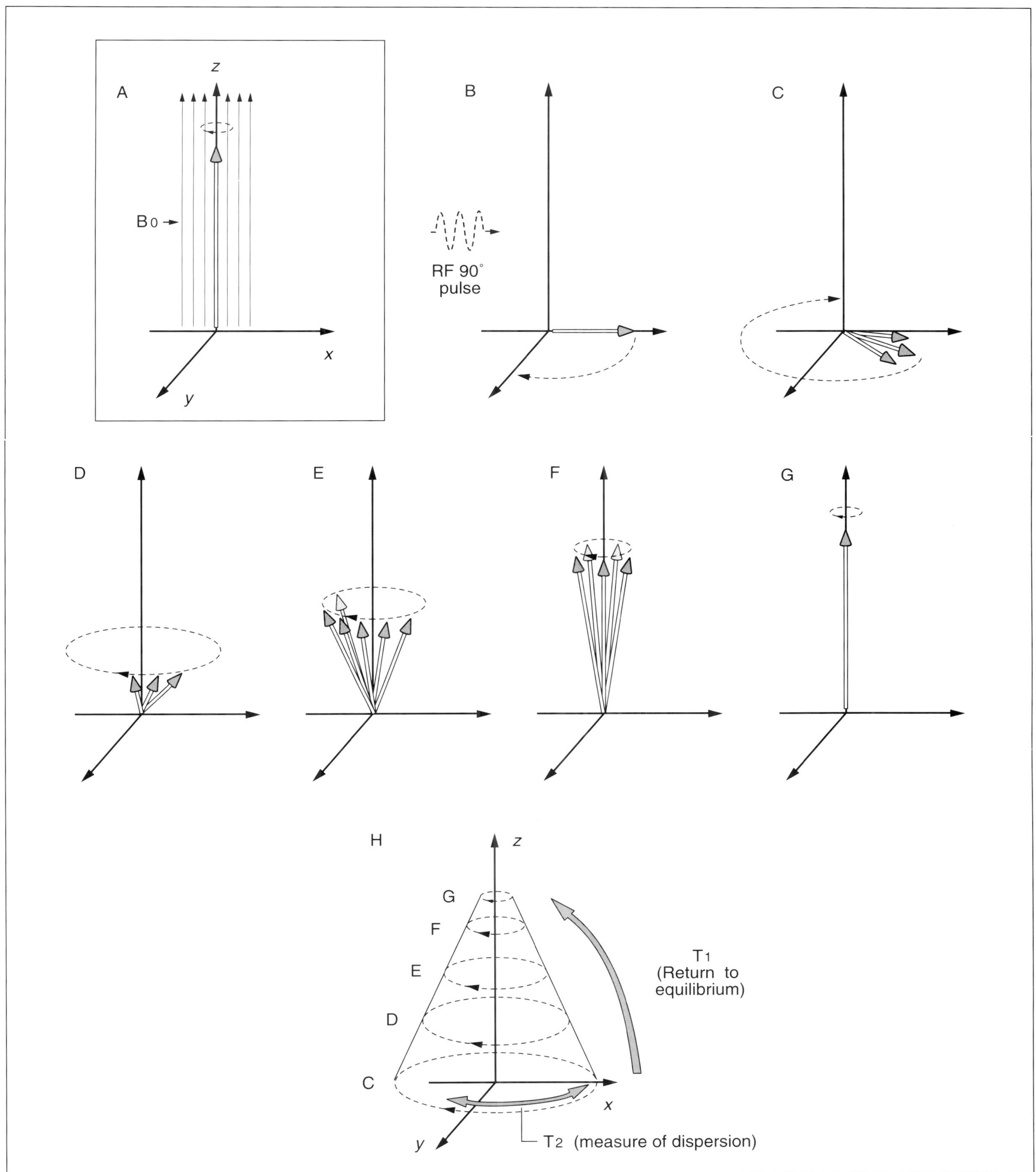

Fig. 4.2 Relaxation. (A) Spin magnetization (vertical arrow) is aligned with the external magnetic field (B_0) along the z-axis. (B) After experiencing a 90-degree RF pulse spins are now precessing around B_0 in the xy-plane. (C) Spins rotate around B_0 with slightly different speeds, resulting in dispersion of spins. The time constant of this relaxation process is called T2 (see H). (D–G) Nuclei gradually realign along the z-axis until spin magnetization is again aligned with B_0. The time constant of this portion of relaxation is called T1 (see H). (H) Summary diagram. T1 is the time constant that describes regrowth of magnetization along the z-axis. T2 describes the dispersion of spins in the xy-plane.

duction decay (FID). The relaxation process is characterized by two time constants, the *longitudinal* or spin–lattice relaxation time (T1) and the *transverse* or spin–spin relaxation time (T2). T1 relaxation is determined by the rate of growth of the magnetization vector along the direction of the extrinsic magnetic field (the "z-axis") from zero immediately after the RF pulse to a maximum value. After an RF pulse, all nuclei initially precess in phase. T2 describes the rate of dephasing of these nuclei that results in cancellation of the magnetization vector in the "xy-plane" perpendicular to the z-axis. The factors that influence proton T1 and T2 in tissue are complex; they include temperature, concentration, and compartmentalization of tissue water, intercompartmental exchange, the presence of macromolecules and paramagnetic metal ions, and the concentration and distribution of lipid. Relaxation times greatly influence NMR signal intensities during spectroscopy and imaging.

As indicated above, each nucleus has a characteristic resonance or Larmor frequency, which is dependent on magnetic field strength. Nuclei are subject to the external magnetic field modified by the magnetic microenvironment of the lattice surrounding the nucleus. Thus, nuclei of a given species at different positions within a molecule or in different molecules are exposed to a slightly different magnetic field, and therefore precess at slightly different frequencies. Corresponding differences in the resonance frequencies are referred to as "chemical shift." On the basis of this chemical shift, molecular structures can be determined in high-resolution NMR spectroscopy, and the signals from water protons and lipid protons can be distinguished in proton NMR spectroscopy as well as in chemical shift imaging. The field dependence of the Larmor frequency can also be exploited for spatial encoding in imaging. Instead of a homogeneous magnetic field, a magnetic field gradient is applied to the tissue, causing the magnetic field to differ from point to point within the sample. Accordingly, resonance frequency differs from point to point, and the particular location of a nucleus within the sample can thus be determined.

SPECTROSCOPY

NMR spectroscopy is based on the chemical shift phenomenon described above. Because chemical shift increases with increasing field strength, high field magnet systems provide better spectral resolution than systems operating at lower field strengths. Clinical spectroscopy is feasible at 1.5 Tesla and above.

In a basic spectroscopic experiment, an RF pulse tailored to the Larmor frequency of the nuclear species under investigation is delivered to the tissue sample and the FID is recorded. Multiple scans are averaged to achieve a better signal-to-noise ratio. Fourier transformation converts the averaged FIDs (signal in the time domain) to a spectrum (signal in the frequency domain). The chemical microenvironments of the nuclear species under investigation generate separate peaks at distinct locations. The area underneath the peaks is proportional to the concentration of the nuclei in the respective environment. Figure 4.3 shows a sample ^{31}P spectrum from a perfused rat heart. Distinct peaks of inorganic phosphate, phosphocreatine, and the three phosphates of ATP are visible.

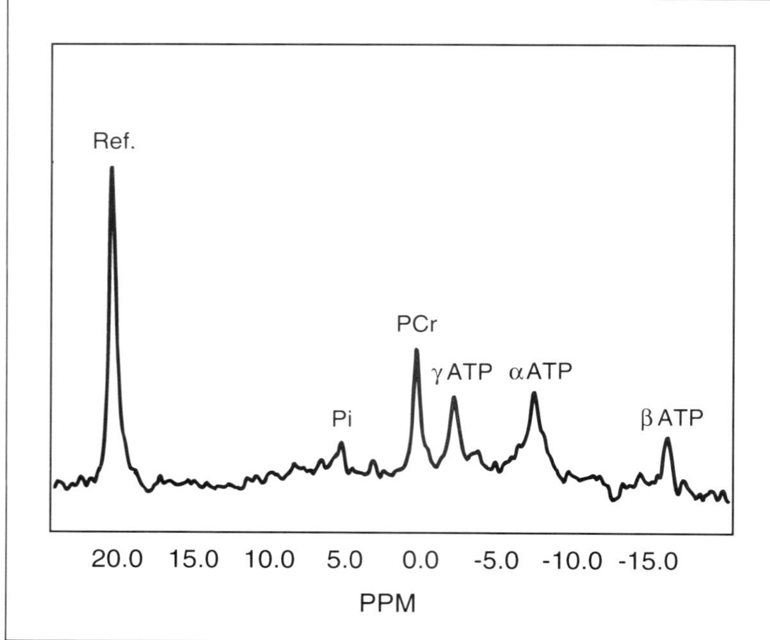

Fig. 4.3 ^{31}P spectrum of a perfused rat heart. The peaks for phosphocreatine (PCr) and ATP (gamma, alpha, and beta for the three phosphate groups) are well resolved. The inorganic phosphate peak is also visible upfield from phosphocreatine. Metabolite concentrations can be determined by normalizing peak areas to the MDP reference peak at 20 ppm (parts per million).

Proton, phosphorus, sodium, and carbon NMR spectroscopy have been widely applied to the study of myocardial metabolism in vitro, in perfused heart models, and in in vivo animal models of hypoxia, ischemia, and infarction, cardiomyopathy, and cardiac allograft rejection. In humans, ^{31}P spectroscopy has been successfully used to study skeletal muscle metabolism in normal volunteers, patients with myopathies, and those with peripheral vascular disease. Human cardiac ^{31}P spectroscopy is still in its infancy, although several recent reports describing localized spectroscopy in normal volunteers with surface coils at 1.5 T are encouraging. Further improvement in spectral quality can be expected at higher field strengths.

PRINCIPLES OF MRI IMAGING

As discussed above, the intensity of the signal generated during imaging of biological tissue depends on the species of nucleus being imaged, its concentration, the relaxation times (T1 and T2), and its motion. Protons have the highest NMR sensitivity and are the most abundant nuclei in biological tissue. Therefore, clinical applications of MRI have mainly utilized the proton. The appearance of tissue in MRI and the contrasts among various tissues in the same image can be manipulated to predominantly reflect proton concentration, T1, or T2, by varying the strength, duration, and timing of the perturbing RF pulses and the time at which the emitted RF signal is measured. Flowing blood provides natural contrast, appearing as either increased or decreased signal intensity depending on the flow velocity and the pulse sequence used. The RF signal emitted by the relaxing nuclei is detected by a receiver coil (analogous to an antenna). The coil is oriented such that only magnetization in the transverse plane (orthogonal to the axis of the external magnetic field) can be detected. To overcome motion artifact in cardiovascular imaging, imaging pulse sequences are triggered by successive R-waves of the electrocardiogram ("cardiac gating"). Respiratory gating may enhance image quality, but it markedly prolongs imaging time.

The pulse sequence most commonly used in imaging is the *spin–echo* sequence (Fig. 4.4A). An initial 90-degree pulse is followed after a short period by a 180-degree pulse. This 180-degree pulse rephases spins that had undergone transverse re-

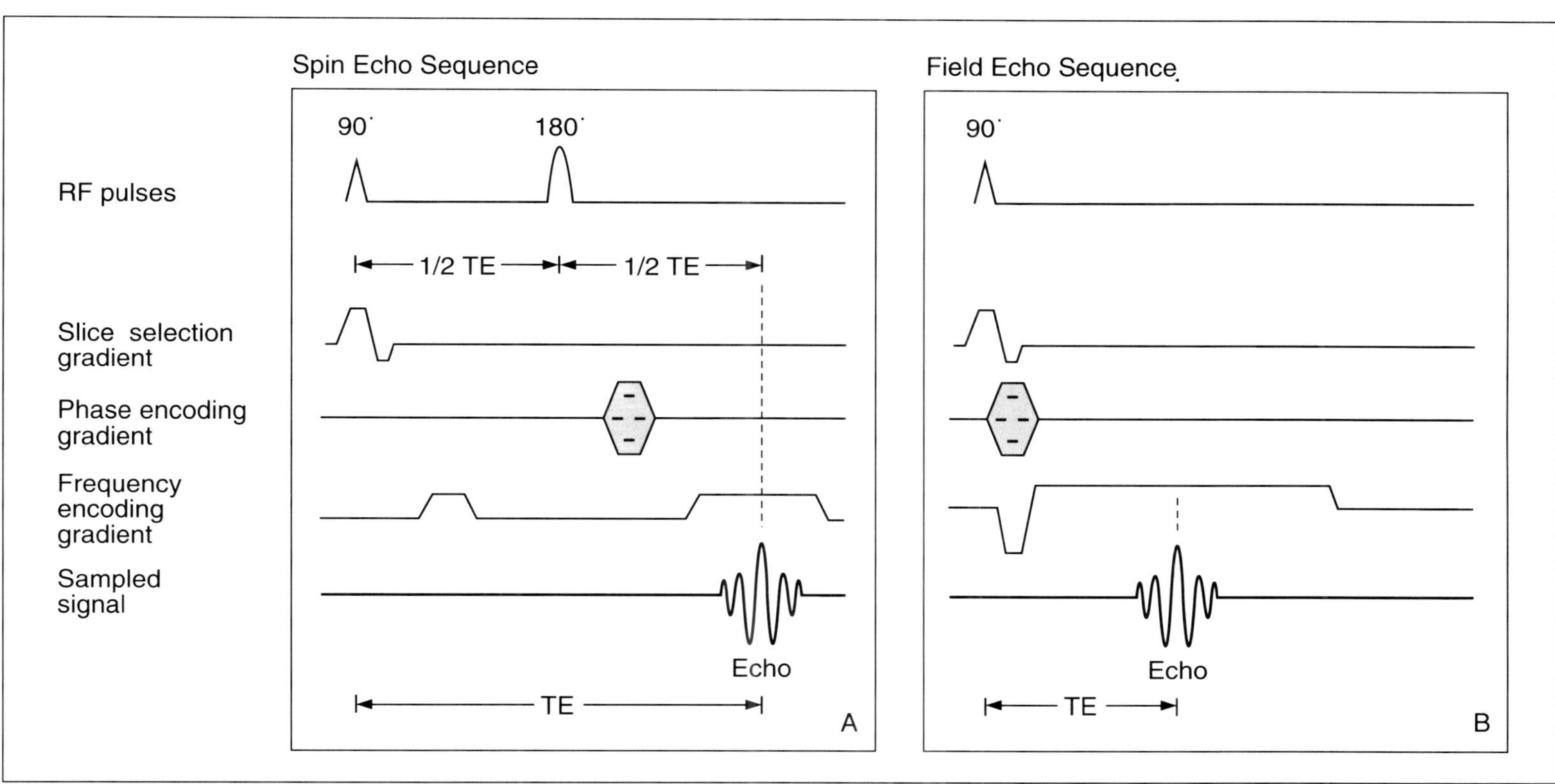

Fig. 4.4 Basic imaging sequences. (A) Spin–echo sequence. The basic spin–echo sequence consists of a 90-degree radiofrequency (RF) pulse followed after a time period of 1/2 TE (time to echo) by a 180-degree RF pulse. At time TE a free induction decay called an "echo" is generated and can be recorded. Slice selection, phase encoding, and frequency encoding gradients are applied for spin localization. During imaging this basic sequence is repeated many times to achieve an adequate signal-to-noise ratio. (B) Field echo sequence. This sequence forms the basis for gradient echo imaging sequences. Again a 90-degree pulse is applied at the beginning. In contrast to the spin– echo sequence, the echo is now generated by reversal of the frequency encoding gradient rather than by an additional RF pulse. Echo times are much shorter than with the spin–echo sequence and allow faster image acquisition.

laxation during the interpulse delay. When rephasing is complete after an echo time (TE), magnetization in the transverse plane is measured. The sequence can then be repeated. The repetition time between successive 90-degree pulses is called TR. This spin–echo sequence can be T2 weighted by using long TR and TE, or can be tailored to reflect primarily spin density (by using long TR and short TE) or to reflect T1 and spin density (by using short TR and TE). If T1 weighting is desired, a different sequence called "inversion recovery" (180-degree pulse followed by 90-degree pulse and a second 180-degree pulse) can be utilized. T1 and T2 are altered in many disease states, and MRI imaging can therefore be used to characterize tissue pathology. Paramagnetic substances, such as gadolinium, can be used to selectively alter intrinsic T1 and T2, and therefore have potential usefulness as contrast and perfusion agents.

During imaging, magnetic field gradients are superimposed on the homogeneous static magnetic field. Magnetic field strength therefore varies with position. As mentioned earlier, because the resonance frequency of a nucleus is proportional to the strength of the extrinsic magnetic field, protons at different locations in a graded magnetic field have unique resonance frequencies and can be selectively excited by tailored RF pulses. One or more parallel slices or a volume of tissue can thus be defined and imaged. Many systems not only allow imaging in the standard orthogonal planes (coronal, sagittal, transverse) but also allow definition of oblique imaging planes. Slice thickness can be varied by the operator. Images can be acquired either one slice at a time or by multi-slice imaging sequences. Slices may be contiguous, with or without a small interslice gap, or spatially remote. In traditional multi-slice imaging, each slice is imaged during a different phase of the cardiac cycle. Multi-slice, multi-phase spin–echo imaging is also feasible but very time consuming. Faster imaging techniques (see below) have made the latter technique more practical.

Several modifications of the spin–echo technique have been developed. A basic sequence called "field echo" is shown in Fig. 4.4B. After an initial 90-degree pulse, spins are rephased by application of a magnetic gradient. As in the spin–echo sequence, a signal can be recorded after an echo time TE. Faster imaging methods that generate echoes by application of magnetic field gradients, and which utilize excitation angles of less than 90 degrees and faster repetition times, are now widely applied in clinical imaging. These imaging methods are known as "gradient echo" MRI. Acquisition times are markedly reduced. With these methods, the flowing blood has a higher image intensity than the surrounding tissue. Up to 32 phases per slice can be obtained during a single acquisition, and the resultant images can be displayed in an endless-loop movie which resembles a conventional angiogram (thus the designation "cine MRI"). Echoplanar imaging and other rapid acquisition methods require specialized hardware and have only recently become available on whole-body imaging systems. These techniques generate single "shot" or multiple-shot images in 30 to 200 milliseconds. Image resolution is not yet equivalent to that of standard imaging methods, but is steadily improving.

ANGIOGRAPHY AND FLOW QUANTITATION

MRI has inherent flow sensitivity. In spin–echo MRI, flowing blood has lower signal intensity than stationary tissue because excited spins in flowing blood move out of the tissue slice selected for imaging before the spins can be refocused by the 180-degree pulse. In gradient–echo MRI, tissue signal intensity is lower owing to partial saturation of spins with rapid pulsing, whereas blood flowing into the slice being imaged contains fully magnetized spins and therefore appears bright. Flow not only affects signal amplitude by these wash-in/wash-out phenomena but also affects spin phase. Movement of spins along a magnetic gradient results in accumulation of a phase that is proportional to the spin velocity. Stationary spins do not acquire any phase shift. Images based on phase shift information can be reconstructed and used to differentiate flow from stationary tissue ("phase display imaging"). Quantitation of flow velocity based on phase shift information is also possible and, when combined with standard anatomic imaging to measure vessel cross-sectional area, allows determination of flow volume.

INSTRUMENTATION AND SAFETY

The external magnetic field of an MRI unit can be supplied by a permanent, a resistive, or a superconductive magnet. Only the latter is suitable for operation at the higher field strengths necessary to optimize in vivo NMR spectroscopy and imaging of nuclei other than protons. Most imaging units operate at a magnetic field strength of 0.15 to 2 Tesla; newer systems utilize 4 Tesla magnets. In comparison, the earth's magnetic field ranges from 0.0003 Tesla (3 gauss) at the equator to 0.0007 Tesla (7 gauss) at the north pole. Software for data acquisition and processing is continuously evolving. Even though MRI at current field strengths is believed to be safe, certain precautions must be taken (Fig. 4.5). A patient's predisposition to claustro-

FIGURE 5. CONTRAINDICATIONS TO MRI

Unstable, acutely ill patient
Claustrophobia
Ferromagnetic intracerebral surgical clips
Temporary or permanent pacemaker
Automatic internal defibrillator
Other implanted electronic devices
Ocular foreign bodies

Fig. 4.5 Contraindications to MRI.

phobia is at least a relative contraindication to MRI, because the internal diameter of current imaging systems is frequently reduced to approximately 60 cm when gradient and receiver coils are in place and the limited space may trigger a panic response. Imaging is contraindicated in patients with pacemakers or other implanted electronic devices because the magnetic field can interfere with the operation of these devices. Change to asynchronous mode, reed switch inhibition, and rapid pacing during RF pulsing have all been reported. MRI is similarly contraindicated in patients with ferromagnetic intracerebral surgical clips, although selected nonferromagnetic clips may be safe for imaging. Imaging of patients with weight-bearing prostheses or with prosthetic valves is safe, but image quality in the vicinity of the prosthetic material may be significantly degraded.

Loose ferromagnetic objects in the imaging room are attracted to the magnet and can become high-speed flying projectiles. Patients and employees must be carefully screened before entering the imaging room. Patient monitoring ability is limited during MRI, and access to the patient is cumbersome. MRI should therefore not be performed in clinically unstable patients. Even in patients considered to be stable, medical emergencies can arise. Procedures for patient evacuation from the immediate vicinity of the magnet and transport to an adjacent area where resuscitation can proceed without endangering the patient or members of the resuscitation team must be clearly defined and rehearsed at regular intervals.

CLINICAL APPLICATIONS

CARDIOVASCULAR ANATOMY

Spin–echo MRI provides high-resolution images of cardiovascular anatomy (Figs. 4.6 and 4.7). Cardiac chamber sizes, orientations, and wall thicknesses are well seen. Atrioventricular and ventriculoarterial connections are easily identified. Valve

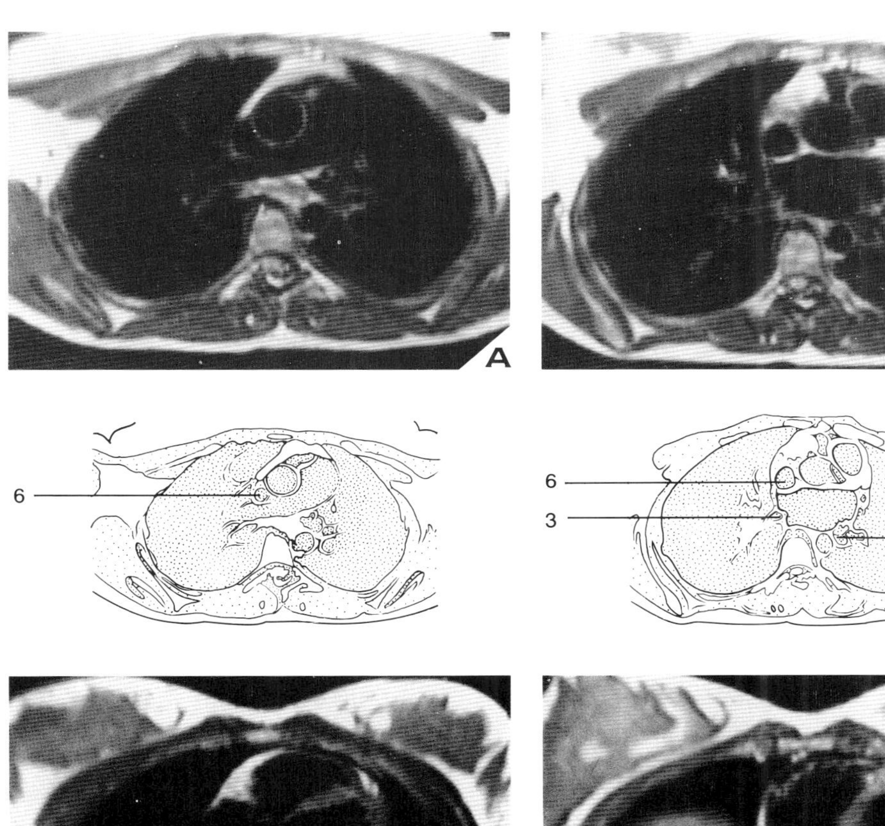

Fig. 4.6 Spin–echo imaging in the transverse plane in a normal volunteer. Four slices at different levels are shown. (A) Slice at the level of the pulmonary arteries. Ascending and descending thoracic aorta are also depicted. (B) Slice at the level of the left atrium and origin of the great vessels. Superior vena cava, ascending and descending aorta are easily distinguished. Pulmonary veins are seen to enter the left atrium. (C) Slightly lower than slice B. Right and left ventricles and portions of the left and right atrium are seen. (D) Slice just above the diaphragm. Both ventricles are again visualized.

1 left atrium; 2 left ventricle; 3 pulmonary veins; 4 right atrium; 5 right ventricle; 6 right superior vena cava.

leaflets, however, are not reliably imaged. The ventricular septum is well seen, and frequently the thinner atrial septum is also visualized. The pericardium appears as a thin, low signal intensity line between the bright signals originating from epicardial and pericardial fat. Systemic and pulmonary venous return can usually be seen. The central pulmonary arteries and the ascending and descending thoracic aorta are clearly depicted. Although most of the anatomic information can be derived from standard axial imaging planes, right and left ventricular wall thicknesses and chamber dimensions are more appropriately depicted with oblique imaging planes corresponding to the axes of the heart.

Clinically, cardiovascular spin–echo MRI has been applied in a variety of settings, including depiction of intra- and paracardiac masses, assessment of patients with congenital cardiac anomalies, demonstration of congenital and acquired anomalies of the great vessels (such as hypoplasia or dilatation of the central pulmonary arteries, aortic coarctation, aortic dissection, and aneurysmal dilatation of the thoracic and abdominal aorta), depiction of sequelae of myocardial infarction (such as wall thinning, ventricular aneurysm, and mural thrombus), and demonstration of the extent and distribution of hypertrophy in hypertensive heart disease and hypertrophic cardiomyopathy. Qualitative and quantitative diagnostic information derived from these MR images appears to correlate well with similar data obtained by traditional invasive and noninvasive imaging modalities.

GLOBAL AND REGIONAL VENTRICULAR FUNCTION

As discussed above, angulated spin–echo MRI can accurately assess ventricular wall thickness and chamber sizes. However, imaging times for multi-slice, multi-phase acquisitions with

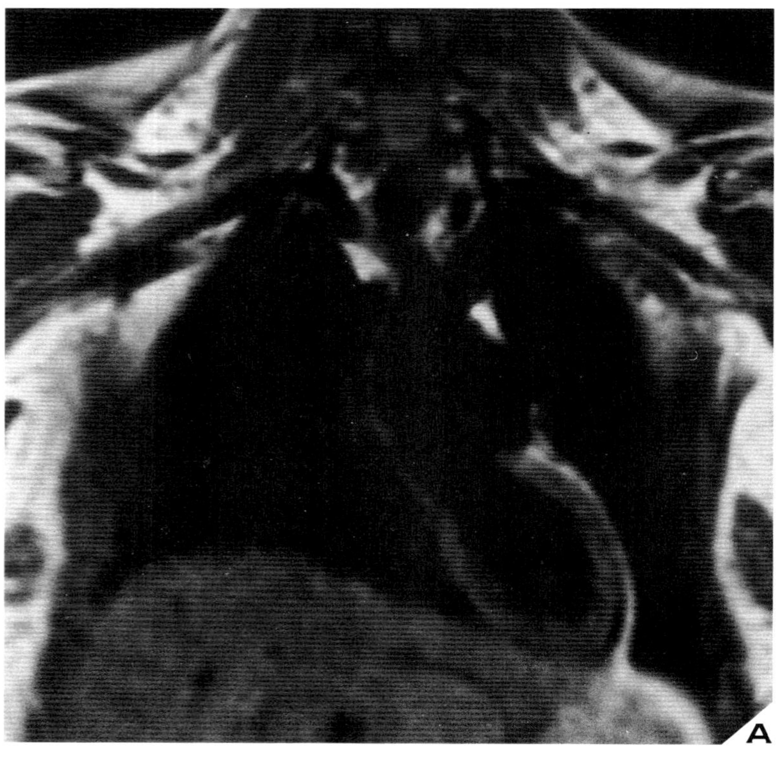

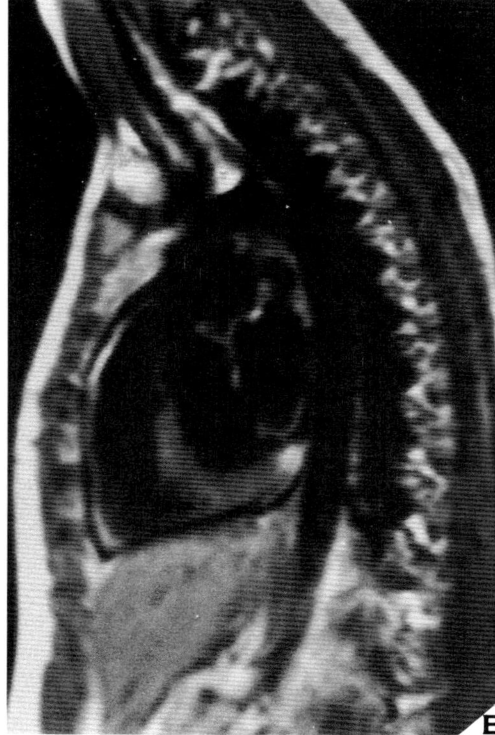

Fig. 4.7 Spin-echo imaging in the coronal and sagittal planes. (A) Coronal image at the level of the left ventricular outflow tract. The right atrium, the left ventricle, the ascending aorta, and the pulmonary trunk are clearly shown. (B) Sagittal image showing the right ventricular outflow tract. The aortic arch and descending aorta are well seen. A portion of the left ventricle and the left atrium are also depicted.

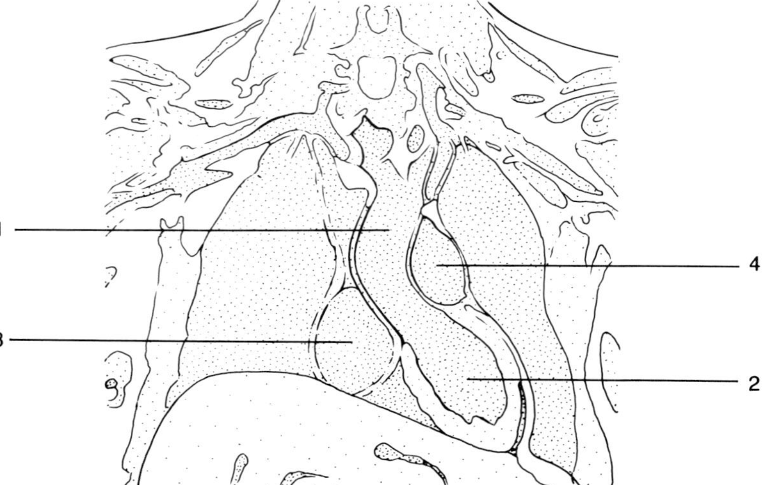

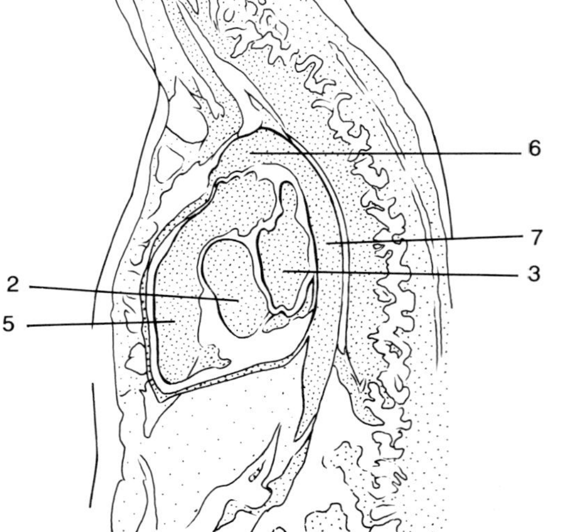

1 aorta
2 left ventricle
3 left atrium
4 pulmonary trunk
5 right ventricle
6 aortic arch
7 descending aorta
8 right atrium

standard spin–echo sequences are prohibitively long. Gradient–echo imaging allows clear depiction of anatomic detail and is considerably faster than spin–echo imaging. By applying standard formulas validated in the cardiac catheterization laboratory (Simpson's rule, Dodge–Sandler area length method, and others), parameters such as right and left ventricular end diastolic and end systolic volumes, ejection fraction, stroke volumes, cardiac output, and ventricular mass can be quantitated. Comparison of right and left ventricular stroke volumes allows calculation of shunts or regurgitant volumes in selected patients with congenital or acquired septal defects or univalvular regurgitation, respectively. Regional wall motion can be qualitatively assessed by cine loop display of multi-phase gradient echo images or quantitated by measuring regional shortening and wall thickening. Gradient–echo imaging is therefore the imaging sequence of choice at present for the evaluation of ventricular function by MRI (Figure 4.8). Even more precise analysis of regional wall motion may be possible in the future by radiofrequency tagging of selected myocardial segments. Off-line analysis of images with most current MRI processing software requires manual tracing of chamber outlines and is therefore cumbersome and time consuming. More sophisticated software for semiautomatic or automatic edge detection is under development and should markedly facilitate data analysis. The value of MRI for evaluation of ventricular function should improve even further when three-dimensional acquisition and processing strategies become available.

VISUALIZATION AND QUANTITATION OF FLOW

Cine MR images show laminar blood as a bright signal that contrasts well with the lower signal intensity of myocardium and vascular walls. Turbulent blood flow is seen as intraluminal loss of signal and has been observed distal to stenotic valves or vessels, at sites of intracardiac shunting, and proximal to regurgitant valves. Aortic regurgitation, for example, is seen as a low signal area in the left ventricle during diastole, and mitral regurgitation as a low signal area in the left atrium during systole. Sensitivity for the detection of regurgitation appears to be excellent, and qualitative estimates of its severity can be obtained by measuring the area of signal loss. Visualization of flow by cine MRI has also been used to identify coronary artery bypass graft patency. Because stenoses of grafts can not be assessed with this method, MRI is at best a screening device for graft patency and does not replace angiography at this time.

Imaging methods specifically geared towards detection of flow and depiction of vessel anatomy are based either on wash-

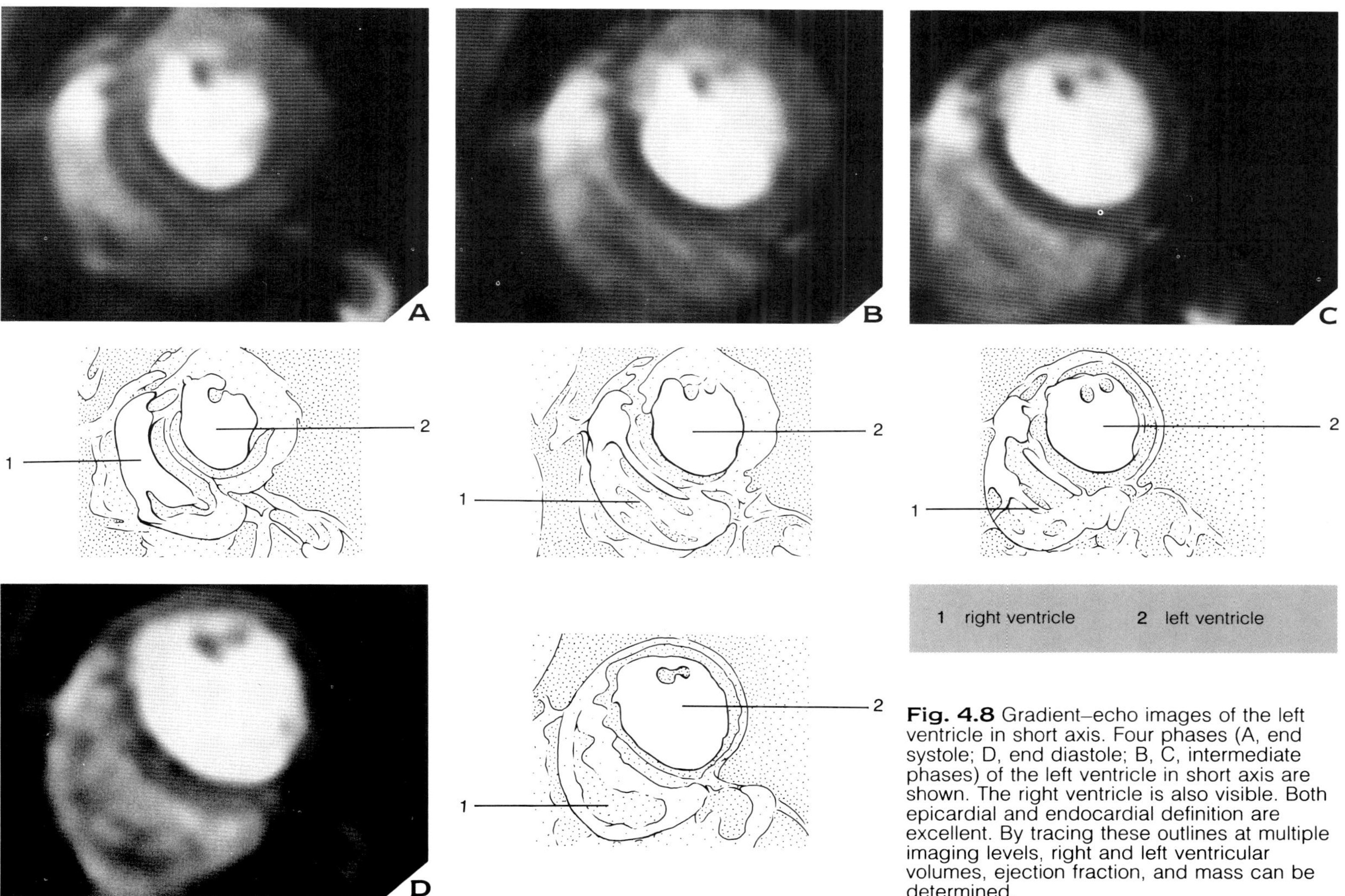

Fig. 4.8 Gradient–echo images of the left ventricle in short axis. Four phases (A, end systole; D, end diastole; B, C, intermediate phases) of the left ventricle in short axis are shown. The right ventricle is also visible. Both epicardial and endocardial definition are excellent. By tracing these outlines at multiple imaging levels, right and left ventricular volumes, ejection fraction, and mass can be determined.

in/wash-out phenomena or on velocity induced phase shifts. Excellent quality images of peripheral vessels have been obtained in healthy volunteers by either approach (Figure 4.9), and preliminary data in patients are encouraging. Coronary vessels cannot be reliably imaged with current technology. Bulk flows in the main pulmonary artery and in the ascending aorta have been quantitated and used to estimate shunt volume in patients with congenital heart disease. Pixel-by-pixel flow velocities can be determined in cross-sections of large vessels and have, for example, been used to construct detailed three-dimensional velocity profiles across the aorta throughout the cardiac cycle. Angiography and flow quantitation remain research tools at present but show great promise for future clinical application.

MYOCARDIAL TISSUE CHARACTERIZATION

Myocardial tissue characterization based on the relaxation parameters T1 and T2 has been applied to the evaluation of myocardial ischemia and infarction. Some investigators have seen increased signal intensity on T2 weighted images in areas of myocardial infarction (Figure 4.10), but the sensitivity and specificity of this signal enhancement appear to be limited. Paramagnetic contrast agents are compounds that possess unpaired electrons and can therefore alter T1 and T2 of surrounding protons by changing the local magnetic field. After intravenous infusion, these contrast agents are distributed in the myocardium according to regional blood flow, regional differences in cellular uptake by the myocardium, and diffusion of the contrast agent into and out of the interstitium. Differences in regional concentration of the contrast agent have been shown to induce differences in relaxation parameters between normal myocardium and infarcted tissue, and may thus allow detection of infarcts and quantitation of infarct size. Although these preliminary studies are encouraging, a clinical role for MRI contrast agents has not yet been defined.

Tissue characterization has also been suggested as a method to detect cardiac allograft rejection by MRI, but the results obtained by different investigators have been highly variable. Detection of abnormal metabolism by in vivo ^{31}P spectroscopy has greater potential as an eventual replacement for the more hazardous technique of serial endomyocardial biopsy as a means for diagnosing rejection.

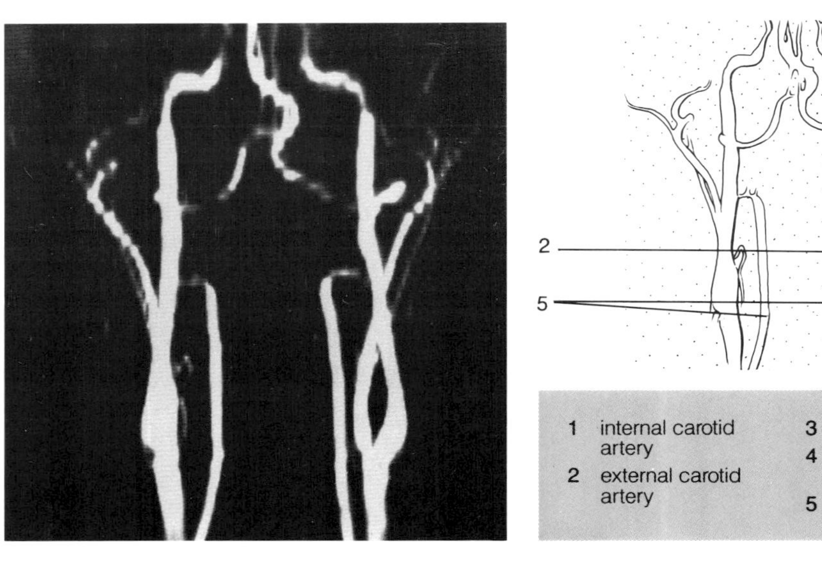

Fig. 4.9 MRI angiogram of the carotid circulation in a normal volunteer. Both common carotids and both internal and external carotids are well outlined. The carotid bifurcation, a frequent site of stenosis, is well visualized. The vertebral arteries are seen medial to the carotid vessels.

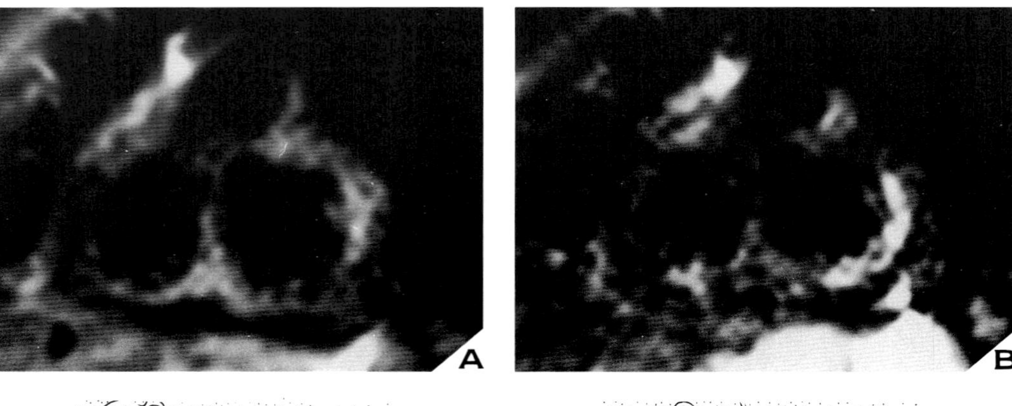

Fig. 4.10 T2 signal enhancement of myocardial infarction (A) Spin–echo image of the left ventricle with TE of 30 msec and repetition time TR of 1 sec. There is some signal inhomogeneity but the area of myocardial infarction is not clearly visible. (B) Spin–echo image of the left ventricle in the same projection and with the same TR as in A but obtained with a longer TE of 100 msec. Increased signal is seen in the region of infarction.

1 pulmonary trunk
2 right ventricle
3 left ventricle
4 increased signal in area of infarction

CHAPTER 4A

Nuclear Cardiology

MILENA HENZLOVA, M.D.
ROBERT C. BOURGE, M.D.

All radionuclide methods have in common the use of intravascularly introduced radiopharmaceuticals, which decay with the emission of gamma rays (originating from the nucleus), characteristic X-rays (originating from the orbital electrons), and/or positrons. Emitted radiation interacts with matter; the most important interactions include the Compton effect and the photoelectric effect. Before the emitted energy is detected externally, usually in a thin sodium iodine (NaI) crystal, some attenuation and scatter of the electromagnetic energy occurs owing to the interaction with the surrounding tissue. In addition, absorption of a small amount of the emitted energy represents the radiation exposure of the body, estimated to be equivalent to a standard chest X-ray for some nuclear medicine procedures.

RADIOACTIVE DECAY

The nucleus of an atom is composed of positively charged protons and neutral neutrons. Nonradioactive atoms have a stable neutron-to-proton ratio. Radioisotopes or radionuclides can achieve stability by emission of particles, which is usually accompanied by emission of electromagnetic energy. The nucleus is surrounded by negatively charged electrons arranged in orbits or shells. Electrons belonging to the same shell have the same energy. Movement of the electrons from one shell to another (caused by forces within or outside of the atom) is also accompanied by emission of electromagnetic energy.

The types of decay of the radionuclides utilized for cardiac imaging include beta (β-) decay, electron capture, internal conversion, and positron (β+) decay. *Beta (β-) decay* (examples: ^{3}H, ^{14}C, ^{32}P, ^{131}I) is characterized by the transformation of a neutron into a proton and an electron, accompanied by gamma ray emission. *Electron capture* (examples: ^{67}Ga, ^{111}In, ^{123}I, ^{125}I) is characterized by the "capture" of an orbital electron by the nucleus. The captured electron combines with a proton to form a neutron, and the process is accompanied by the emission of a characteristic X-ray. *Internal conversion* (example: ^{99m}Tc) is characterized by the transfer of the nuclear energy of an unstable radionuclide to an orbital electron; gamma rays are emitted. *Positron decay* (examples: ^{11}C, ^{13}N, ^{15}O) is characterized by the emission of a positively charged electron (e+) from the nucleus. The ejected positron ultimately comes to rest and interacts with an electron (e-). Both particles are annihilated in the process and mass is converted into energy. During the interaction, a pair of equally energetic photons (0.511 MeV) is released, traveling in opposite directions. Two opposing detectors, connected in coincidence to record simultaneous events, make positron emission tomography (PET) imaging possible.

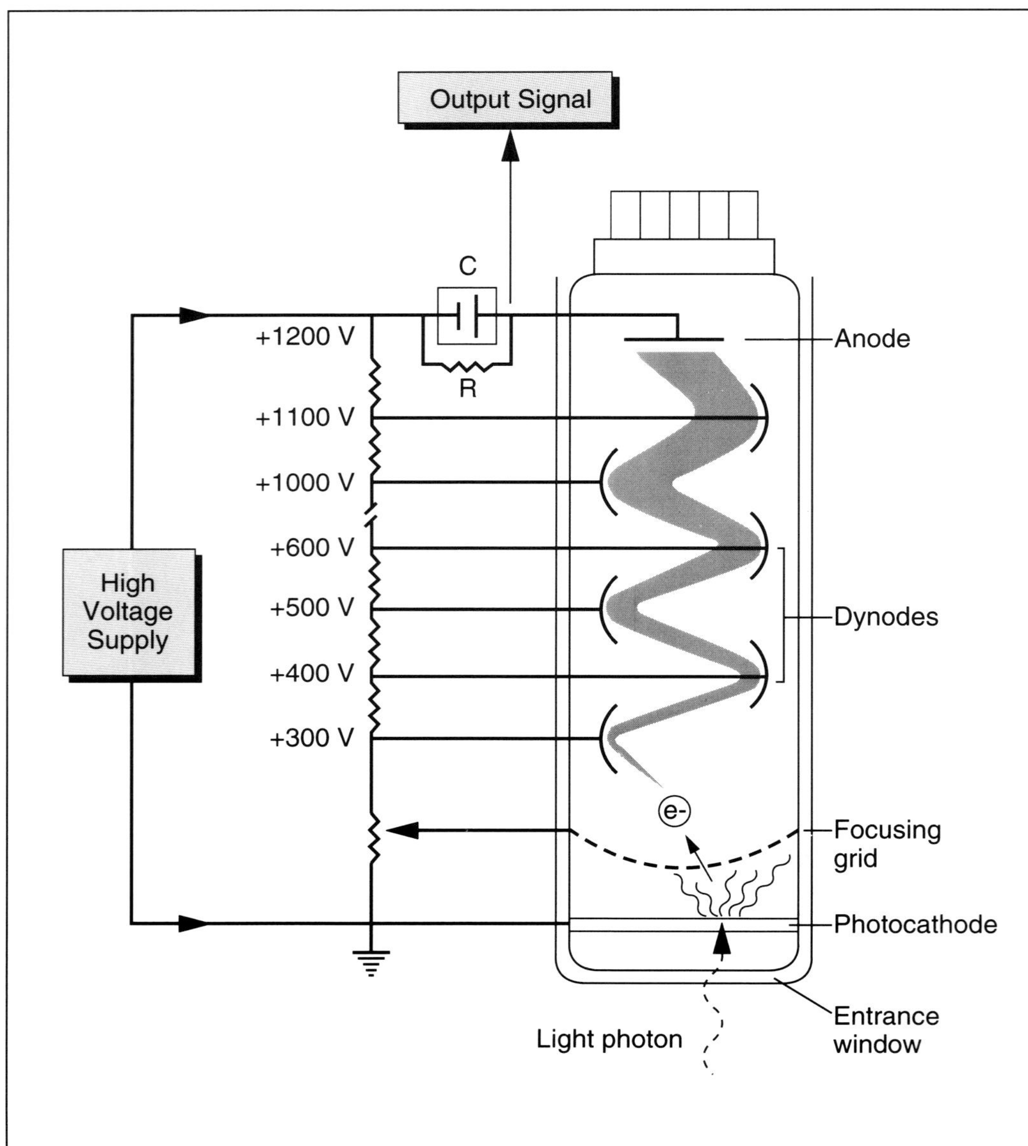

Fig. 4A.1 Components and principles of a photomultiplier tube.

Gamma and/or X-ray photons of different energies interact with the surrounding matter. A medium-energy photon can dislodge an outer (orbital) shell electron and continue to travel in a different direction and with lower energy (Compton scatter). A low-energy photon transfers all its energy to an inner shell electron and dislodges it from its orbital shell.

RADIATION DETECTION AND DETECTION DEVICES

When the described interactions occur in a sodium crystal, a flow of high-speed electrons is created. This leads to formation of ion pairs, which are subsequently trapped in the detection crystal by intentionally introduced impurities (such as thallium) and give rise to a visible light or scintillation (photoelectric effect). Visible light is converted to an electrical impulse, which is augmented in a photomultiplier tube (Fig. 4A.1). The signal is then analyzed by a pulse height analyzer to discriminate the radionuclides of different energies and to eliminate scattered gama rays, which degrade the nuclear images.

Since the late 1950s, the *Anger camera* (Fig. 4A.2) has been the instrument used most often for nuclear imaging. Components of this device include a collimator (to select desirable photons and "focus" the image information on the crystal), a sodium iodine crystal (0.25–0.5 inch thick, 300–500 mm in diameter), an array of photomultiplier tubes to detect and strengthen the energy detected in the crystal, position logic

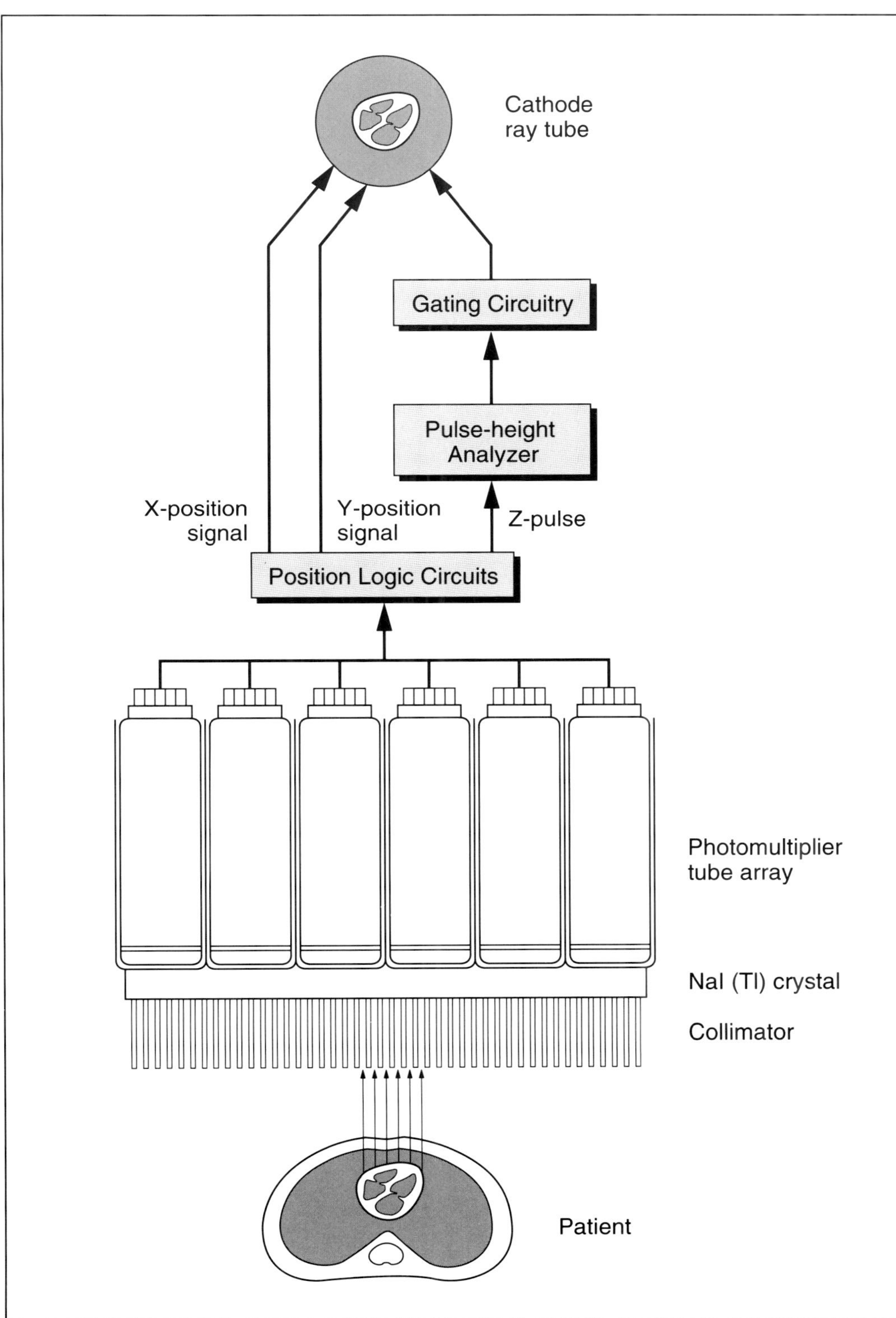

Fig. 4A.2 Components of the Anger camera.

circuits (for spatial orientation of the received signals), a pulse height analyzer (to analyze the energy of the individual detected photons), and a cathode ray tube (to display the localization and intensity of the energy detected in the crystal). Anger cameras can be stationary or mobile, and planar or rotational (Fig. 4A.3, Appendix).

The *multicrystal camera* consists of an array of up to 294 NaI crystals (1 cm × 1 cm × 1 inch), each coupled to two photomultiplier tubes. Fast counting is possible (>400,000 counts/sec), and dead time (time to process occurring events before responding to a new event) is shortened with these cameras. This device is particularly suitable for first-pass studies (see below).

The *PET camera* consists of two opposing crystals with appropriate electronics so that only simultaneously occurring events (release of a pair of equi-energetic annihilation photons traveling in opposite directions) are recorded and spatially oriented.

CARDIOPULMONARY RADIONUCLIDE IMAGING

Despite some limitations, radionuclide pulmonary arterial perfusion imaging (with or without ventilation imaging) remains the screening test of choice for most patients with suspected pulmonary thromboembolism. The radiopharmaceuticals most often used for perfusion imaging are ^{99m}Tc-labeled macroaggregated albumin or human albumin microspheres. Planar imaging is usually done with a single crystal gamma camera. Ventilation studies are optimally performed utilizing ^{133}Xe or ^{127}Xe gas techniques. Recently, ^{99m}Tc DTPA aerosol ventilation studies have become more widely used owing to the lack of need for very specialized equipment used in gas ventilation studies and lower cost. The clinical applications of pulmonary scanning techniques are outlined in Chapter 24.

CLINICAL APPLICATION OF CARDIAC RADIONUCLIDE IMAGING

Radionuclide imaging is unique in its ability to provide quantitative physiologic information. It can not compete with other invasive and noninvasive imaging methods in morphologic assessment, because radionuclide image resolution is low.

Clinically used cardiac radionuclide imaging methods include:

1. Assessment of global and regional ventricular function.
2. Imaging of myocardial perfusion.
3. Detection of myocardial viability, myocardial necrosis, and myocardial substrate utilization.

ASSESSMENT OF GLOBAL AND REGIONAL VENTRICULAR FUNCTION

Radionuclide angiography has been used for more than a decade to evaluate ventricular function. Left and right ventricular function can be assessed using the first-pass (or initial transit) technique or multigated equilibrium radionuclide angiography.

The *first-pass technique* follows the passage of the bolus of the tracer through the cardiac chambers during rapid serial imaging. A single-crystal Anger camera or, preferably, a multicrystal camera, is employed to acquire 400,000 to one million counts per second. Images are acquired at 25-millisecond intervals. Cardiac chambers are visualized in one view per injection of 25–30 mCi of ^{99m}Tc pertechnate, ^{99m}Tc sulfur colloid, or ^{99m}Tc DTPA. After the acquisition, a time–activity curve of the region of interest is generated. Three to six cycles are usually available for analysis. Good separation of the right and left ventricle in the 30° right anterior oblique (RAO) position allows evaluation of right and left ventricular function and visualization of intracardiac shunts. After injection of another bolus of the isotope, usually minutes after the previous bolus, a different projection of the heart or function during a different physiologic state (exercise, drug effect) can be imaged. However, repeated imaging is limited by increased background radiation after each injection.

Red blood cells labeled with ^{99m}Tc make *blood pool imaging* possible. Three methods are available for labeling: the in vivo method, the modified in vivo method, and the in vitro method. All three methods employ stannous pyrophosphate, a bone-scanning agent that sensitizes the red blood cell membrane and makes it permeable to ^{99m}Tc pertechnate, which binds irreversibly to the globin portion of the hemoglobin molecule.

For the *in vivo method*, the patient receives 50 mg of pyrophosphate intravenously; 20 minutes later 15–30 mCi of ^{99m}Tc pertechnate are injected intravenously. Labeling efficiency is approximately 85 percent.

The *in vitro method*, which is used least often, requires withdrawal of 20 mL of the patient's blood, which is incubated for 20 minutes with pyrophosphate, is then mixed with 30 mCi of ^{99m}Tc pertechnate, and is reinjected into the patient. Tagging efficiency approaches 95 percent. The *modified in vitro method* combines features of the other two methods. The patient is injected with pyrophosphate to sensitize the red blood cells. However, the ^{99m}Tc erythrocyte labeling is done in vitro, in a syringe of withdrawn blood, which is reinjected after 15 minutes of equilibration. Tagging efficiency is again close to 95 percent. Some pharmaceuticals, such as heparin and sulfa drugs, may interfere with erythrocyte labeling.

The labeled blood pool can be imaged a number of times over a 6-hr period. When the scintillation Anger camera is used, image acquisition requires 2 to 10 minutes. The left anterior oblique (LAO) view, which best delineates the intraventricular septum, is usually obtained first. Subsequent views are standardized in relation to the optimal LAO angulation. Data acquisition is computerized. Electronic gating permits accumulation of data from specified portions of multiple cardiac cycles. The R-R interval is usually divided into 16–24 sections, and image frames are acquired for a preselected number of cycles or a desired number of counts. Most cameras are equipped with an arrhythmia beat rejection system. Frame-mode acquisition rejects all abnormally long or abnormally short cycles. When too many cycles are rejected, a longer acquisition time is needed to compensate. List-mode acquisition, which requires more computer memory, stores all data for each cycle.

An R-R histogram is plotted after completion of the acquisition. To create the histogram, the operator selects the acceptable cycle length for image reconstruction. For each part of the cardiac cycle, a sufficient number of frames are summated to create a cycle of sufficient length to permit computerized calculation of the ejection fraction and an image adequate for visual analysis (Fig. 4A.4). Processed data are displayed in a cine loop mode for qualitative analysis. Ventricular size, motion, and shape can be assessed by observing the endless loop movie on a computer console or on a videotape. Global ventricular function, expressed most often as an ejection fraction value, can be derived from end diastolic and end systolic counts, independent of ventricular geometry. Regional ventricular function can be assessed semiquantitatively by dividing each left ventricular projection into three to five segments and grading the wall motion as normal, hypokinetic, akinetic, or dyskinetic. Quantitative analysis of wall motion is also possible. Right ventricular ejection fraction can also be calculated from both the first-pass and the blood pool study. However, the accuracy and validation of right ventricular ejection fraction remain elusive owing to variability of right ventricular shape and the overlay with other cardiac structures.

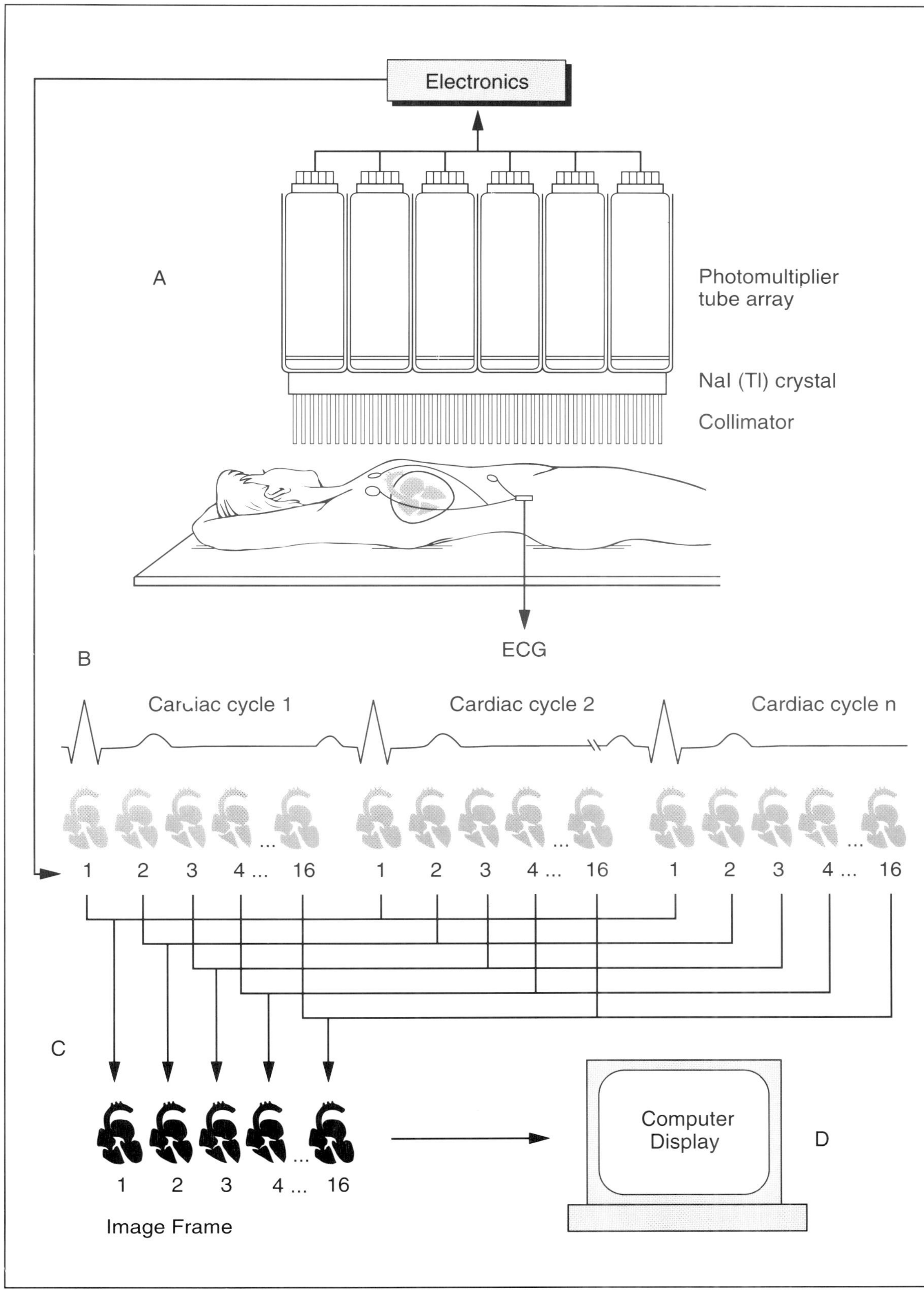

Fig. 4A.4 Principles of gated radionuclide angiography. After labeling of the blood pool (see text): (A) the patient is positioned under an Anger camera with ECG signal from the patient routed to the computer controlling acquisition of data. (B) Each cardiac cycle is divided into 16 or more frames, which represent specific portions of the cardiac cycle referenced to the R-wave of the ECG. Individual frames are stored in the computer memory. (C) The frames are then summed to allow enough image information representing each portion of the cardiac cycle to be used for ejection fraction processing and display. (D) The computer allows display of the cardiac cycle via an "endless loop" display of the summed frames for visual analysis.

MYOCARDIAL PERFUSION TECHNIQUES

THALLIUM (^{201}Tl)

^{201}Tl is a cyclotron-produced isotope with a physical half-life of 73.5 hours. The most abundant photon emission has an energy of 69–83 keV, which is somewhat less than the optimal energy for Anger camera imaging (greater than 100 keV). ^{201}Tl is a monovalent cation with biologic characteristics similar to potassium. After intravenous injection of 2–3 mCi of ^{201}Tl, distribution of the tracer in the myocardium is proportional to the regional blood flow, with a first-pass extraction of 80 percent. Myocyte uptake of ^{201}Tl is an active process, requiring energy to activate the sodium–potassium ATPase mechanism. Therefore, only viable myocytes can accumulate ^{201}Tl. After initial uptake, ^{201}Tl clears from the myocardium with a biologic half-life of 4 to 6 hours. The clearance rate is known to depend on the extent of regional ischemia (washout is slower in ischemic segments), level of exercise (washout is faster after a higher level of exercise), and plasma insulin level (washout is faster with a higher insulin level).

Initial ^{201}Tl images, usually obtained after exercise minutes after radionuclide injection, depict initial myocardial perfusion distribution. Areas with decreased flow (eg, supplied by stenosed coronary arteries) appear as defects on the initial image. Late images are obtained 3 to 4 hours after tracer injection. The phenomenon of ^{201}Tl "redistribution" enables one to distinguish between a "fixed" defect, usually representing nonviable myocardium, and a "reversible" defect, probably representing hypoperfused but viable myocardium. Two mechanisms contribute to the "redistribution" or "fill-in" of the initial defect. First, tracer clearance from the ischemic segments is slow. Therefore, the initial activity persists longer in the hypoperfused segments, decreasing the regional disparity on late images. In addition, ^{201}Tl continues to be taken up from the circulating blood, making the initial disparity less pronounced on late images. The utility of thallium imaging in patients with chronic coronary artery disease is described in Chapter 20. Imaging can be done in planar or tomographic modes (see Figs. 20.13–20.16).

Intraobserver variability is a significant factor in the interpretation of ^{201}Tl scans. For this reason, computerized programs have been devised to quantify initial and delayed abnormalities, thus decreasing the subjectivity of the interpretation. A program developed at our institution realigns early and late images, subtracts left ventricular background activity, and generates circumferential activity profiles for each view acquired. Early and delayed ventricular activity profiles are then superimposed, and the ratio between early and delayed activity is expressed as a percentage. The hottest myocardial pixel, which is considered to represent normal myocardium, is assigned a value of 100 percent. With the data displayed in this fashion it is easy to appreciate both segmental activity differences and temporal changes (Fig. 4A.5).

Additional information which can be derived from the planar images includes: assessment of left ventricular cavity size and of stress-induced changes in cavity size; demonstration of exercise-induced increase in lung ^{201}Tl activity, expressed as a "heart: lung ratio," which has been observed in patients with exercise-induced left ventricular dysfunction (seen most often in patients with diffuse three-vessel coronary artery disease) and transient pulmonary hypertension; and delayed segmental ^{201}Tl clearance, which corresponds to regional hypoperfusion and ischemia.

Like the planar images, the tomographic slices are arranged side by side to facilitate qualitative assessment. Circumferential profiles can be generated for quantitative analysis. Another type of display uses short-axis circumferential profiles to construct a myocardial map (see Chapter 20).

TECHNETIUM-99m (^{99m}Tc) IMAGING

The use of ^{99m}Tc radiopharmaceuticals for myocardial perfusion studies results in improved image resolution and decreased soft-tissue attenuation. ^{99m}Tc, which is usually produced on site from a molybdenum generator, emits photons with an energy of 140 keV—optimal for Anger camera imaging—and has a physical half-life of 6 hours. Two classes of ^{99m}Tc-labeled agents are being clinically tested for myocardial perfusion studies: ^{99m}Tc-labeled isonitriles (MIBI agents; Sestamibi or Cardiolite), and ^{99m}Tc-labeled boronic acid derivatives (BATO agents; Teboroxime or Cardiotec). Isonitriles are efficiently extracted by the myocardium by passive diffusion; because they bind to intracellular protein, they do not significantly redistribute. Therefore, stress imaging requires a separate study. However, since no significant redistribution occurs, initial imaging can be delayed by several hours.

Teboroxime is extracted by the myocardium at slightly higher rate than isonitriles; however, myocardial retention is much shorter, lasting only minutes. Initial imaging must therefore be done immediately after injection; repeat studies or stress studies can be done shortly afterward.

POSITRON EMISSION IMAGING

The positron-emitting nuclide most often used for cardiac perfusion studies is rubidium-82 (^{82}Rb), produced in a strontium-82 (^{82}Sr) generator. ^{82}Rb distributes in the myocardium in a manner similar to potassium and ^{201}Tl. Because it has a half-life of 75 seconds it must be continuously infused for imaging studies. N-13 (^{13}N) ammonia, which is cyclotron produced, is also taken up by the myocardium proportionally to the regional blood flow; it has a half-life of 10 minutes. Both ^{82}Rb and ^{13}N-ammonia are used to assess myocardial blood flow distribution at rest or with stress (dipyridamole infusion or hand-grip exercise.)

DETECTION OF VIABILITY, MYOCARDIAL NECROSIS, AND SUBSTRATE UTILIZATION

Many patients with persistent thallium defects on 3- or 4-hour scans have no history or other evidence of previous myocardial infarction. Up to 40 percent of these persistent defects do not represent "scar." Three methods are presently available to study persistent defects, which were until recently considered to represent nonviable myocardium. The first technique uses late imaging: a third set of scans is obtained 18 to 72 hours after the ^{201}Tl injection. The disadvantages of this approach are that it requires a second visit by the patient to the nuclear cardiology laboratory and that late images are of poor quality owing to a decreased concentration of the tracer in the myocardium.

Another recently described technique uses ^{201}Tl "reinjection." A second smaller dose of ^{201}Tl (1–2 mCi) is injected 2 to 4 hours after the initial scan; the scan is then repeated 15 to 20 minutes later. The third method uses dual positron-emitting isotope imaging (PET). ^{13}N-labeled ammonia is used as a perfusion agent and F-18 fluorodextrose is used as a tracer of glucose metabolism. Ischemic myocardium preferentially utilizes glucose as opposed to preferential lipid utilization in nonischemic myocardium (see also Chapter 20). PET perfusion defects that accumulate labeled glucose are considered to be underperfused but viable.

Infarct-avid tracers (eg, the bone imaging agent ^{99}Tc-labeled stannous pyrophosphate) bind to the intracellular calcium, which crystallizes within the necrotic myocyte. Delivery of the tracer depends on residual regional coronary blood flow. Planar or gated SPECT images are acquired 1 to 2 hours after administration of the tracer. Pyrophosphate uptake in necrotic myocardium begins 6 to 12 hours after the onset of injury, peaks at 24 to 72 hours, and often becomes undetectable in 10 to 14 days. Qualitative interpretation is based on a relative scale (0–4+) which relates myocardial activity to the adjacent bone activity. Pyrophosphate imaging is useful in patients with difficult to interpret ECG and enzyme changes, eg, patients who present late (>18 to 24 hours after symptom onset) or patients who have recently undergone cardiac surgery. An obvious drawback of the technique is the long interval before the scan becomes positive. In addition, the specificity of a positive scan is low. Recent chest contusion, cardioversion, myocarditis, amyloidosis, radiation therapy, chemotherapy, and remote myocardial infarction are known causes of a false-positive pyrophosphate scan.

The newest method of myocardial necrosis imaging uses labeled antimyosin antibodies. Antimyosin (Myoscint) is an F(ab) fragment of a monoclonal antibody which binds to the exposed myosin of an irreversibly damaged myocyte. The antibody, which is tagged with indium-111 (^{111}In) and injected intravenously, is taken up by the necrotic myocardium; images are obtained 24 to 48 hours later. Antimyosin imaging has also been used for detection of necrosis in patients with chest trauma or cardiomyopathy, and for detection of rejection in patients who have undergone cardiac transplantation.

PERSPECTIVES IN NUCLEAR CARDIOLOGY

The first-pass and blood pool studies provide both an accurate assessment of the global and regional ventricular function and an estimate of ventricular volumes. Particularly in patients with chronic coronary artery disease, data obtained at rest and during exercise have been proven to be of significant prognostic value and of use for patient risk stratification. The ejection fraction at peak exercise, rather than the difference between the resting and the exercise value, appears to be the most powerful predictor of future cardiac mortality and is comparable to cardiac catheterization data in its predictive power.

The newest technetium-labeled myocardial perfusion agents permit simultaneous assessment of ventricular function and of myocardial perfusion. With these agents, radionuclide ventriculography can be performed, using the first-pass technique, at the time of bolus injection of the radiopharmaceutical agent.

After almost a decade in which only a single radiopharmaceutical agent was available for myocardial perfusion studies, three agents will soon be available: ^{201}Tl, ^{99m}Tc Sestamibi, and ^{99m}Tc Teboroxime. The choice of the perfusion agent will

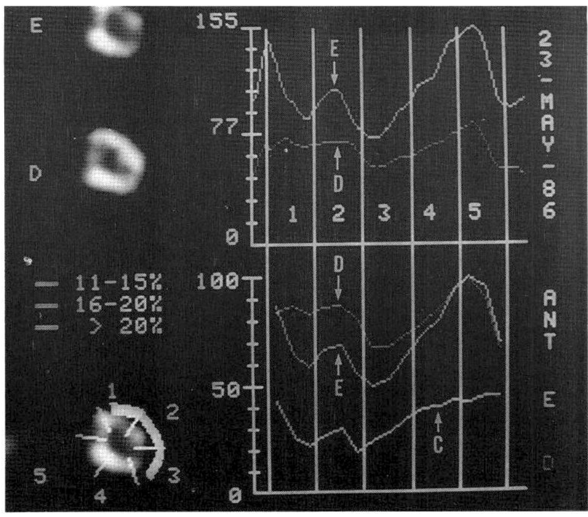

Fig. 4A.5 Quantitative computerized analysis of a ^{201}Tl myocardial perfusion image in the anterior view, depicting anterolateral wall redistribution (ischemia). The background-corrected images (early and delayed) are on the left (left upper panel). Circumferential myocardial activity in 5 myocardial segments (depicted in the left lower panel) is expressed in absolute counts (right upper panel) and in percent, normalized to the hottest pixel (right lower panel). Early images have higher absolute counts (upper line in the right upper panel) than the delayed images (lower line).

depend on the indication for the test performance and on the clinical circumstances. Some of the similarities and differences of the three agents are summarized in Fig. 4A.6.

In patients who are unable to exercise adequately (eg, because of orthopedic disability, leg claudication, pulmonary disease, or poor motivation), pharmacologic alternatives to exercise can be used for perfusion imaging. Two vasodilating agents will soon be available for intravenous infusion: dipyridamole (0.14 mg/kg/min for 4 minutes) and adenosine (140 μg/kg/min for 6 minutes). Dipyridamole induces coronary vasodilatation by inhibition of endogenous adenosine breakdown. Adenosine has a direct vasodilating effect on the precapillary arterioles. Because the hyperemic response to the increased adenosine concentration is reduced or absent in significantly stenosed coronary arteries, regional perfusion inhomogeneities are accentuated. Compared with adequate exercise, which increases resting coronary blood flow 2–2.5 times, intravenous dipyridamole or adenosine increases resting coronary blood flow four to five times. The diagnostic and prognostic agreement, as well as the safety of the pharmacological stress tests, has been confirmed in several recent comparative studies.

^{201}Tl and PET glucose imaging are used for detection of myocardial viability. Dual isotope imaging with ^{112}In-labeled antimyosin and ^{201}Tl has emerged as another method for assessing viability. Antimyosin, a "cold spot" agent, images necrotic myocardium with high sensitivity and specificity; ^{201}Tl a "hot spot" agent, is taken up only by viable myocardium. Antimyosin-thallium "match" (no overlap) indicates absence of viability in a hypoperfused myocardial segment; a "mismatch" (overlap of the territory avid for both agents) indicates the presence of viable myocardium in the hypoperfused segment.

Fig. 4A.7 depicts the spectrum of different states of the myocardium and imaging options. "Stunned" myocardium represents myocardial function altered by a recent insult. "Hibernating" myocardium represents myocardial function altered by chronic hypoperfusion.

Fig. 4A.6 Some comparisons of myocardial perfusion imaging agents

	201 Thallium	Isonitriles (MIBI)	BATO Agents (Teboroxine)
Radiopharmaceutical	201 Thallium Chloride	99m Technetium	99m Technetium
Charge	Cation	Cation	Neutral
Dose	2-3 mCi	15-30 mCi	15-30 mCi
Energy for imaging	68-83 keV	140 keV	140 keV
Myocardial extraction fraction	0.80	0.65	0.71
Myocardial T-½	3-4 hrs	6-7 hrs	10-15 minutes
Optimal time for imaging after injection	5-10 minutes	1-2 hours	1-2 minutes
First-pass imaging	No	Yes	Yes
Redistribution	Yes	No	Yes
Myocardial counts	Low	High	High
SPECT imaging	Yes	Yes	Possibly
Duration of the test	3-4 hours	3-4 hours	60-90 minutes

Fig. 4A.7 Imaging options for different states of myocardial function

Myocardium	Contractility	Viability	Tl-201 Stress	Tl-201 Delayed (up to 72 hrs)	Antimyosin Uptake	PET Viability
Normal	Normal	+	No defect	No change	No	+
"Stunned"	↓ - ↓ ↓	+	Defect	No change/Redist.	No	+
"Hibernating"	↓ - ↓ ↓	+	Defect	No change/Redist.	No	+
Acutely infarcted	↓ ↓ ↓	+/−	NA	NA	Yes	−
Chronically infarcted	↓ ↓ ↓	−	Defect +/−	No Change	No	−

NA = Nonapplicable, Redist. = Redistribution

CHAPTER 18

Acquired Valvular Disease

Dysfunction of the cardiac valves, which may manifest as stenosis, insufficiency, or a combination of the two, results from distortion of the leaflets or the supporting structures.

AORTIC VALVE

AORTIC VALVULAR STENOSIS

Aortic stenosis is defined as a condition in which opening of the aortic valve in systole is restricted. It may result from a variety of disorders that affect the cusps or annulus, the underlying cause varying with the age of the patient (Fig. 18.1).

Calcification of a bicuspid aortic valve, which is common in patients over 60 years of age, is the most frequent cause of aortic stenosis in the elderly (Fig. 18.2). In younger individuals, aortic valve calcification is usually a sequela of inflammation, affecting normally formed (ie, tricuspid) valves.

PATHOPHYSIOLOGY

In the normal subject the systolic pressure in the left ventricle is equal to that in the aorta. Patients with clinical manifestations of aortic stenosis with a valve orifice measuring less than 2 cm^2 per square meter of body surface have a significant gradient. Left ventricular outflow obstruction results in increased resistance to ejection. The pressure overload leads to left ventricular hypertrophy. The thick-walled left ventricle contracts poorly and eventually dilates; as left ventricular compliance decreases, the end diastolic pressure rises and the left atrium becomes enlarged.

In patients with severe, longstanding aortic stenosis, the left ventricle is markedly dilated and contracts poorly. The coronary arteries can no longer adequately perfuse the thickened myocardium, leading to myocardial ischemia. Coronary artery stenosis, which is present in about 20 percent of patients with aortic stenosis, is often an aggravating factor.

CLINICAL FEATURES

Patients with aortic stenosis typically present with chest pain, dizziness, and/or syncope. Sudden death, probably resulting from ischemic changes in the conducting system and/or exercised-induced hypotension, is not uncommon. On physical examination, the cardiac apex is displaced to the left and there is a palpable systolic thrill in the left second intercostal space, close to the sternum. The characteristic auscultatory findings are a single second sound and a systolic murmur, which is best heard at the base and radiates into the neck. Often, particularly in younger patients, there is a delayed upstroke of the arterial pulse.

Electrocardiograms show left ventricular hypertrophy. The latter is often associated with a ''strain'' pattern (ie, increased voltage in the left precordial leads with a T-wave vector opposite in direction to the QRS complex). The voltage may be normal, however, in patients with coexistent pulmonary disease.

Bacterial endocarditis is a relatively infrequent complication. In one large autopsy series, 7 percent of bicuspid aortic valves showed evidence of infection, which was similar to the frequency in normally formed valves. However, normal healing is less likely in patients with malformed valves. Factors predisposing to bacterial endocarditis include intravenous drug abuse, alcoholism, immune deficiency, and operative procedures.

An apparent association between aortic stenosis, cystic medial necrosis of the aorta, and aortic dissection has been suggested. In one study, which included 119 patients with fatal dissection associated with cystic medial necrosis, 9 percent had congenital bicuspid aortic valves (expected frequency 1 to 2 percent), and 5 percent had aortic stenosis. This may be a chance association, however, because the true frequency of bicuspid aortic valve (which is often asymptomatic) in the general population is unknown.

IMAGING AND INVASIVE DIAGNOSIS

Chest Films

The chest film may be normal early in the course of the disease, when there is left ventricular hypertrophy without left ventricular dilatation. Chest films of patients with significant longstanding aortic stenosis show cardiomegaly, with the characteristic findings of left ventricular enlargement (Fig. 18.3). On the frontal projection, the left lower heart border is unusually prominent and the apex is displaced laterally and inferiorly, depressing the diaphragm. On the lateral projection, the posterior border of the left ventricle is seen to project posterior to the

CHAPTER LABELING KEY

RA	right atrium	Ao	aorta
LA	left atrium	RVOT	right ventricular outflow tract
RV	right ventricle		
LV	left ventricle		

FIG. 18.1 ETIOLOGY OF AORTIC STENOSIS AT VARIOUS AGES

Age	Usual Etiology
Infant and child	Congenital malformation of valve cusps or annulus
Teenager and young adult	Inflammatory (usually rheumatic endocarditis)
60–75 years	Calcification of bicuspid aortic valve
Over 75 years	Degeneration of valve cusps or annulus

Fig. 18.1 Etiology of aortic stenosis at various ages

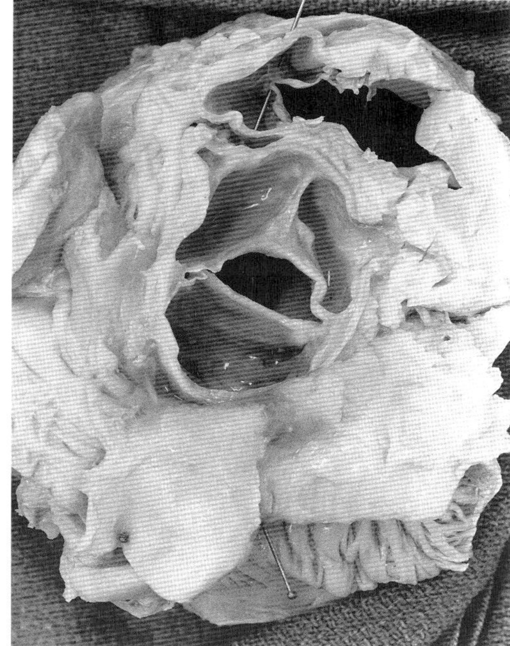

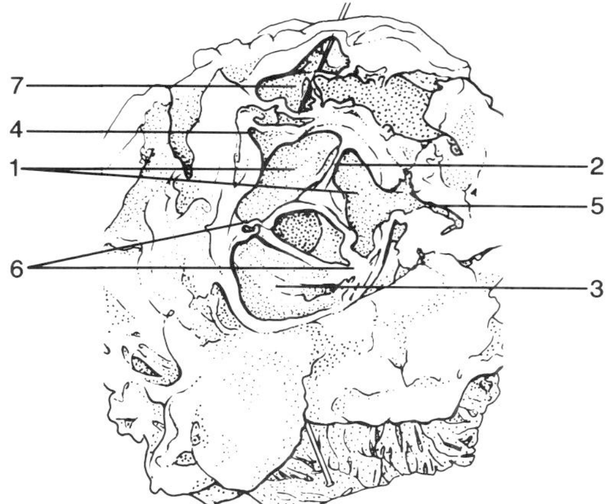

Fig. 18.2 Stenotic bicuspid aortic valve. As viewed from above, the right and left coronary cusps have joined to form a common anterior coronary cusp; the site of union is indicated by a raphe in the midportion of the common cusp. The ostia of the coronary arteries are located at each end of the common anterior cusp. The noncoronary cusp is posterior and to the right of the common anterior cusp. The commissures separating the common anterior and noncoronary cusps are partially fused. The free borders of the valve leaflets are slightly thickened.

1 common anterior coronary cusp
2 raphe (site of union of right and left coronary cusps)
3 noncoronary cusp
4 orifice of right coronary artery
5 orifice of left coronary artery
6 partial fusion of cusps
7 pulmonic valve

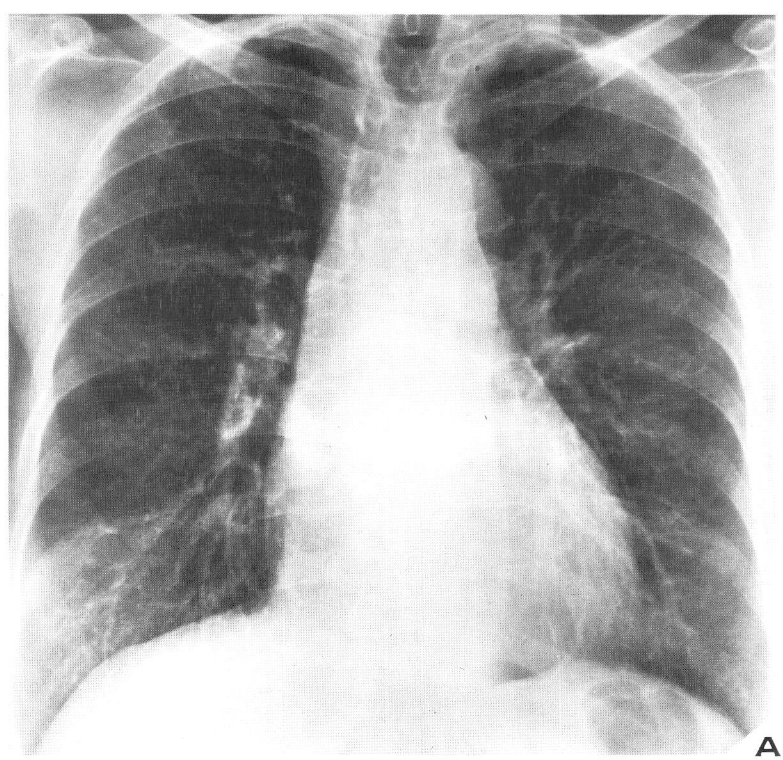

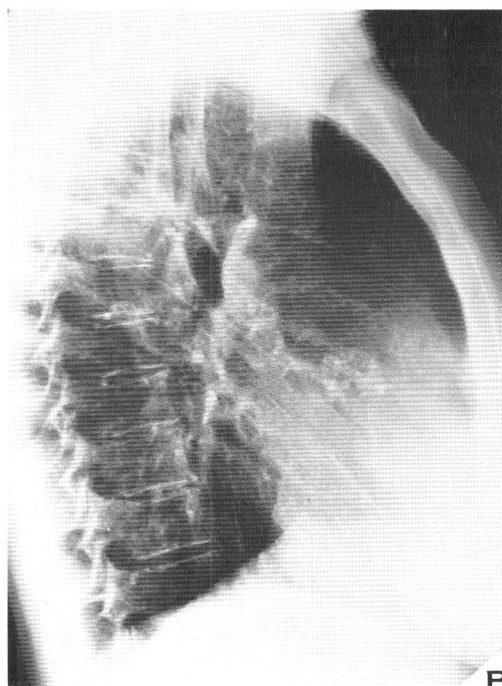

Fig. 18.3 Calcific aortic stenosis. (A) Frontal and (B) lateral chest films show slight cardiomegaly with prominence of the left ventricle. The pulmonary vasculature and mediastinum are unremarkable. Dense calcification with irregular contours is seen in the position of the aortic valve in B. Although the ascending aorta is not significantly enlarged, the left ventricular enlargement and aortic valve calcification make the diagnosis of calcific aortic stenosis almost certain.

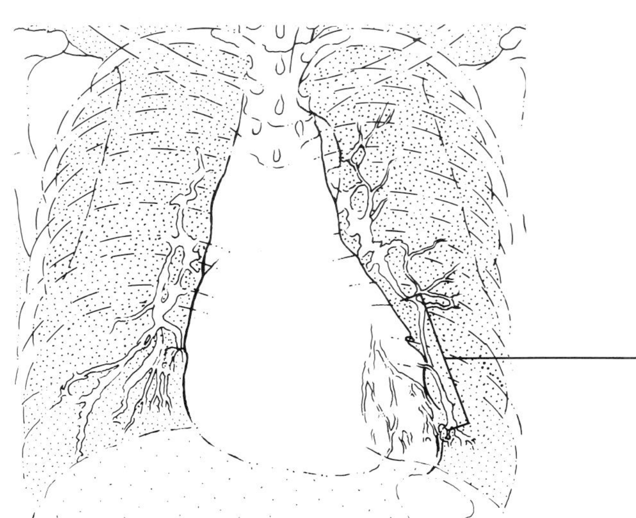

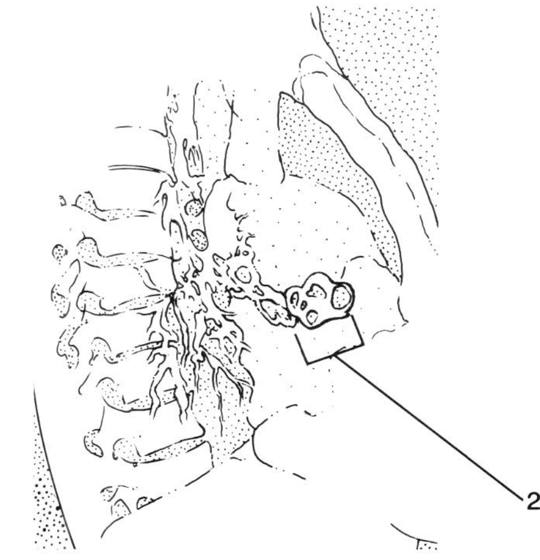

1 enlarged left ventricle
2 calcified aortic valve

inferior vena cava, and is often inferiorly displaced as well (Fig. 18.4B).

Enlargement of the ascending aorta secondary to poststenotic dilatation is relatively frequent. In these patients, frontal films show protrusion of the right border of the ascending aorta, and filling in of the retrosternal clear space is apparent on the lateral (Fig. 18.4). The poststenotic dilatation reflects the damage to the aortic wall produced by the turbulent flow (jet effect) that results when blood passes through a stenotic aortic valve. In most patients, the mural injury caused by the jet effect involves the anterior and right lateral wall of the aorta. In some patients the injury resulting from the jet effect is confined to the left lateral and/or posterior walls of the aorta, in which case widening of the ascending aorta is not apparent on chest films.

Calcification of the aortic valve can often be identified on lateral chest films. A heavily calcified valve appears as an irregularly marginated calcific density, often with a ring-like configuration, in the middle of the heart (Figs. 18.3B and 18.4B). Valve calcification that cannot be appreciated on chest films can often be detected by fluoroscopy or cineangiocardiography. Although clinically silent aortic valve calcification is not uncommon in autopsy series, its demonstration in a living subject almost always reflects functionally significant aortic stenosis.

Plain films in infants and children with congenital aortic stenosis typically show cardiomegaly with features of left ventricular and left atrial enlargement; valve calcification is not observed at this age (Fig. 18.5). Poststenotic dilatation of the ascending aorta is common; however, it is often obscured by the thymus on both frontal and lateral chest films. The radiologic findings in patients with congenital aortic stenosis are discussed further in Chapter 12.

Echocardiography

Echocardiography has proven a reliable technique for diagnosing and assessing the severity of aortic stenosis. On a complete study, with M-mode and two-dimensional images, it is possible to measure the aortic annulus, evaluate the morphology of the cusps and their displacement during the cardiac cycle, and assess various parameters of left ventricular function (eg, left ventricular volume, left ventricular mass, ejection fraction). The use of transesophageal probes increases diagnostic accuracy (Figs. 18.6 and 18.7). By employing various Doppler techniques (pulsed, continuous wave, color-flow), the cardiologist can assess the degree of aortic stenosis both qualitatively and quantitatively (Figs. 18.8 and 18.9; see Appendix). By measuring maximum Doppler velocity across the valve, one can calculate the instantaneous peak gradient (ie, the highest systolic pressure gradient during systole). This value is generally higher than the peak-to-peak gradient measured in the cardiac catheterization laboratory. The mean systolic gradient is determined by averaging multiple instantaneous gradients during a single systolic ejection period.

Because pressure gradients are flow dependent they do not accurately characterize the degree of stenosis. Echocardiographic measurements of aortic valve area enable more precise assessment of the severity of the stenosis. By combining two-dimensional and Doppler electrocardiography, one can measure the diameter of the left ventricular outflow tract, the velocity of blood flowing through the left ventricular outflow tract (ie, proximal to the aortic valve), and the maximum flow velocity across the aortic valve (Fig. 18.9). The simplified continuity equation permits calculation of the aortic valve area. Recent reports indicate a strong correlation between these parameters and cardiac catheterization data.

A

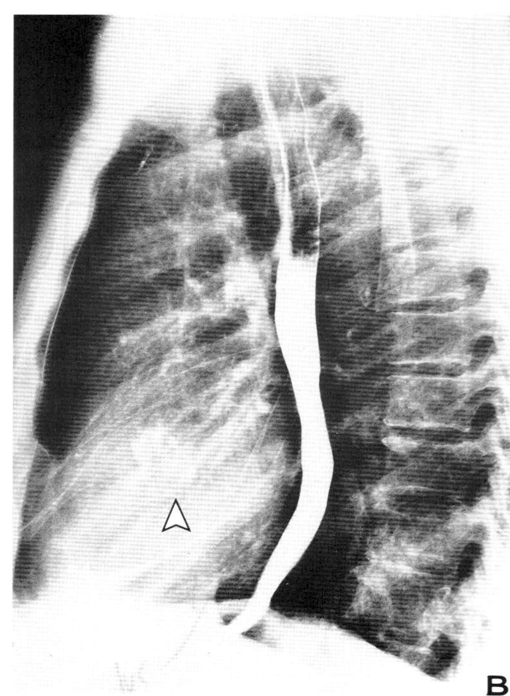

B

Fig. 18.4 Calcific aortic stenosis. (A) The cardiac silhouette is normal on the frontal projection. (B) On the lateral view the ascending aorta is prominent and abuts the anterior chest wall, indicating enlargement of this vessel in the sagittal plane. The left ventricle is enlarged posteriorly, projecting well behind the inferior vena cava. Note dense, irregular calcification of the aortic valve (*arrow*).

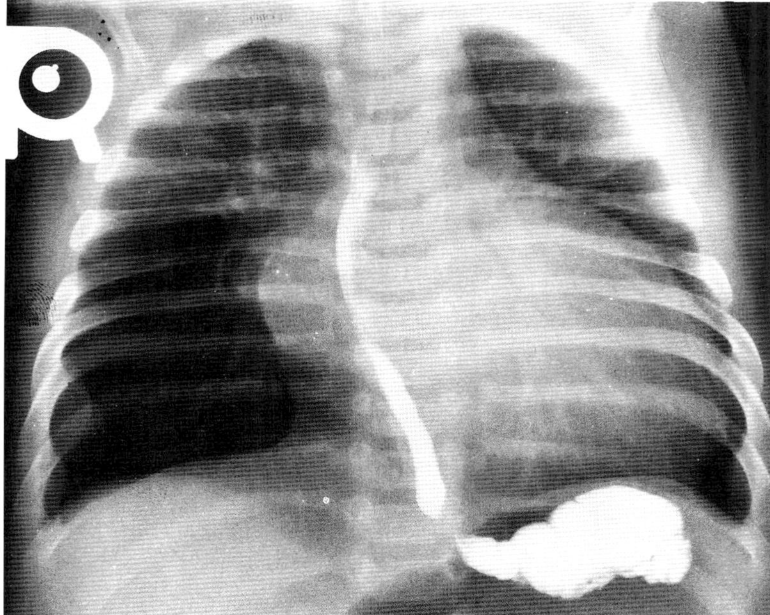

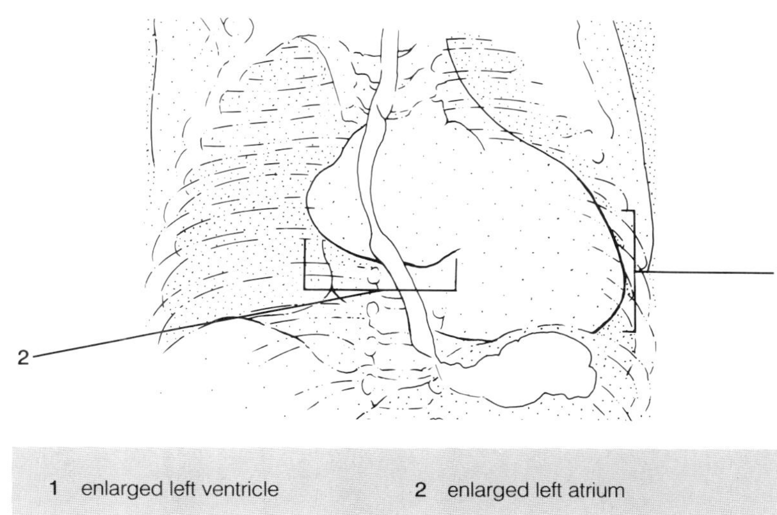

1 enlarged left ventricle	2 enlarged left atrium

Fig. 18.5 Congenital aortic stenosis. Supine chest film in an infant with congenital aortic stenosis shows cardiomegaly with left ventricular enlargement. Note enlargement of left atrium secondary to the decrease in left ventricular diastolic pressure. The pulmonary vasculature is normal. The overinflation of the right lower lobe is unrelated to the cardiac problem.

Fig. 18.6 Stenosis of trifoliate aortic valve. Transesophageal electrocardiogram of aortic root (basal short axis view); systole. The aortic leaflets are thick and do not separate widely.

1 right coronary cusp	3 noncoronary cusp
2 left coronary cusp	4 left atrium
	5 right ventricle

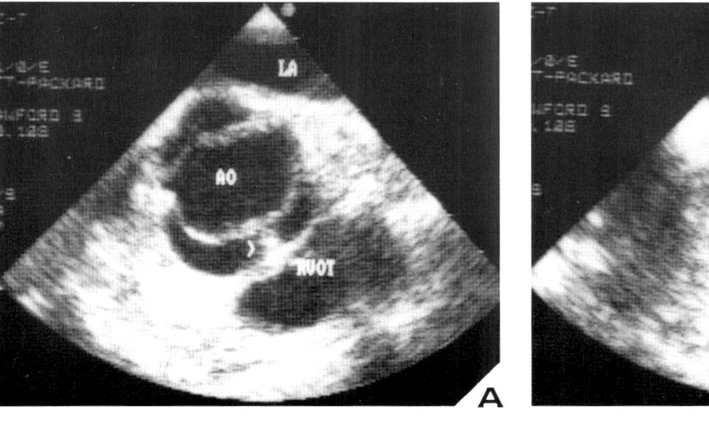

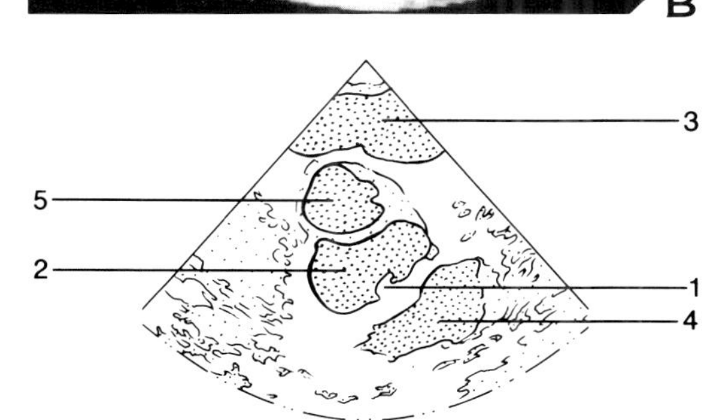

Fig. 18.7 Stenosis of bicuspid aortic valve. Transesophageal electrocardiogram of aortic root (basal short axis view). (A) Systole; (B) diastole. The midportion of the common anterior leaflet has a rough edge. The noncoronary cusp is related to the left atrium and the coronary cusp is related to the right ventricular outflow tract. Opening of the aortic valve is restricted.

1 raphe of common anterior leaflet	4 right ventricular outflow tract
2 aorta	5 noncoronary cusp
3 left atrium	

MRI

Moderate to severe aortic stenosis can be demonstrated by cine MRI, which combines excellent spatial resultion with an increased signal from flowing blood. The aortic valve is best evaluated on images obtained in the transverse sagittal plane. The morphology of the cusps can sometimes be demonstrated on spin-echo images. MRI is more sensitive for aortic insufficiency than for aortic stenosis (see below).

Cardiac Catheterization

With rare exceptions, aortic stenosis is strongly suggested by the history and physical examination and is confirmed by the plain film and echocardiographic findings. In practice, the assessment of aortic stenosis by noninvasive means is so precise that cardiac catheterization is seldom necessary. Catheterization data can be used to measure the pressure gradient across the aortic valve and the cross-sectional area of the valve. A

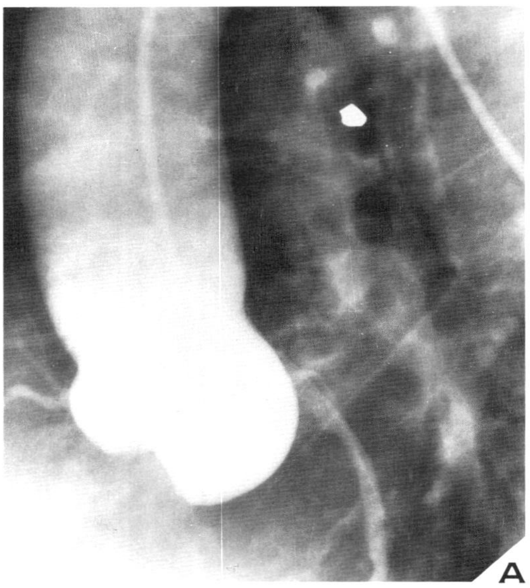

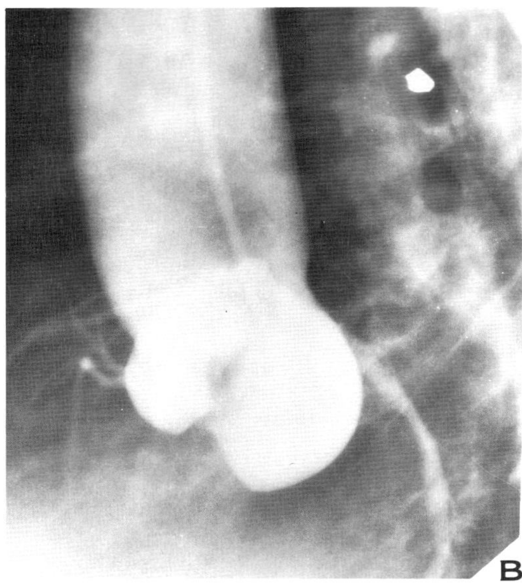

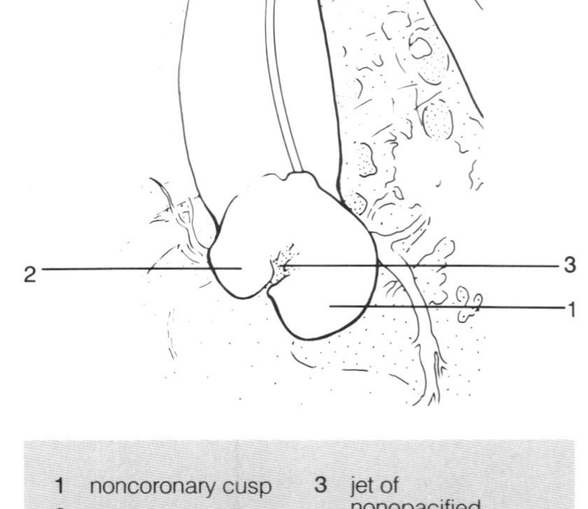

1	noncoronary cusp	3	jet of nonopacified blood
2	coronary cusp		

Fig. 18.10 Severe stenosis of bicuspid aortic valve. Lateral projections of thoracic aortogram in diastole (A) and systole (B). The posterior (noncoronary) cusp is larger than the anterior (coronary) cusp. The jet of nonopacified blood in B indicates the presence of a tight valvular stenosis.

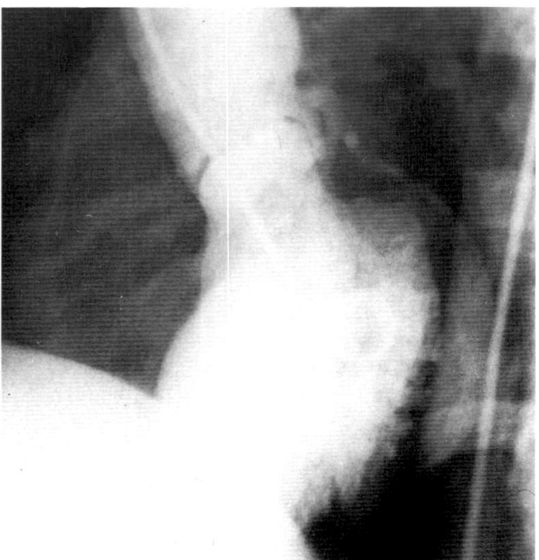

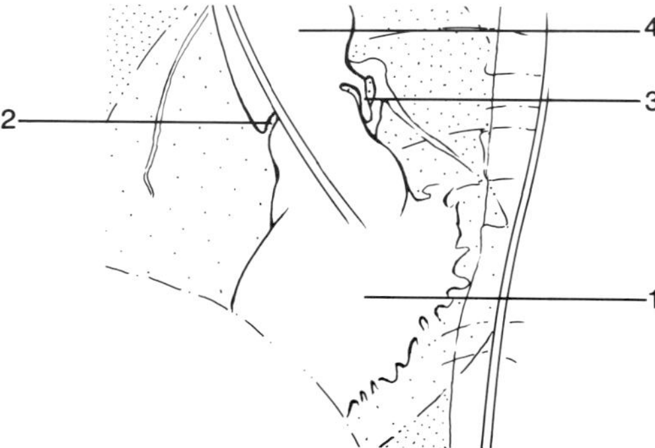

Fig. 18.11 Stenosis of trifoliate aortic valve. Long axis projection of left ventriculogram (in systole) shows "doming" of the left and right coronary cusps owing to restricted movement of the valve leaflets. The ascending aorta is only minimally dilated.

1	left ventricle	3	leaflet of left coronary cusp
2	leaflet of right coronary cusp	4	ascending aorta

cross-sectional area of 0.9 cm^2 per square meter of body surface denotes mild stenosis; 0.6 to 0.9 cm^2/M^2, moderate stenosis; and 0.4 to 0.6 cm^2/M^2, severe stenosis.

Cardiac catheterization is almost always performed in combination with coronary arteriography, owing to the frequent association of coronary artery disease with aortic stenosis. In our opinion, coronary arteriography is indicated in all patients over 40 years of age and in those with symptoms of ischemic heart disease.

Angiocardiography

Left ventriculography and thoracic aortography demonstrate the pertinent anatomy. In patients with a stenotic bicuspid aortic valve, which is usually calcified as well, angiography demonstrates a bicuspid (bifoliate) valve that does not open fully during systole (Fig. 18.10). In patients with a tricuspid (trifoliate) valve, it is possible to identify all three leaflets during diastole; owing to the restricted movement of the leaflets, the valve has a distinctive domed appearance during systole (Figs. 18.11 and 18.12).

CHRONIC AORTIC INSUFFICIENCY

PATHOLOGY

Aortic insufficiency (the inability of the aortic valve to seal off its orifice during diastole) can result from a variety of lesions affecting the cusps, the annulus, or both. In the Mayo Clinic surgical series, the most common cause of aortic insufficiency was dilatation of the aortic root, resulting in widening of the annulus (37 to 40 percent), followed by rheumatic heart disease (29 percent), and congenital malformation of the valve (24 percent). Less frequent causes of chronic aortic insufficiency include endocarditis involving a congenitally bicuspid valve and a prolapsed sinus of Valsalva with or without a VSD. [Acute aortic insufficiency (which may result from various causes, including bacterial or fungal endocarditis, aortic dissection, trauma, rupture of a congenital aneurysm of the sinuses of Valsalva) is discussed in the following section.]

The most frequent cause of aortic insufficiency is so-called medial degeneration of the aortic wall, which may be isolated (idiopathic aortic ectasia) or associated with Marfan syndrome;

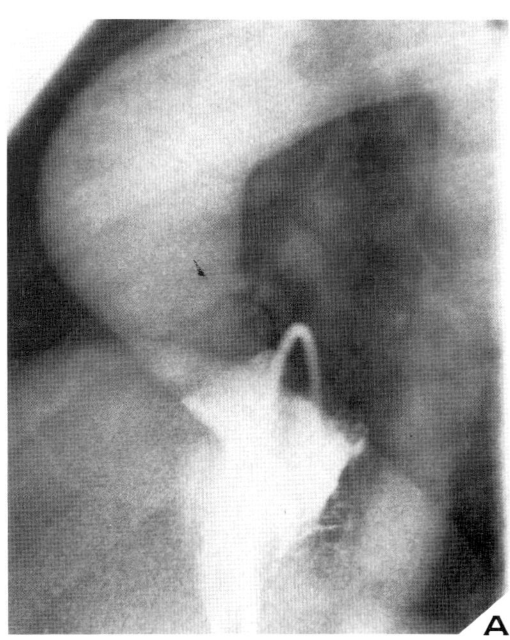

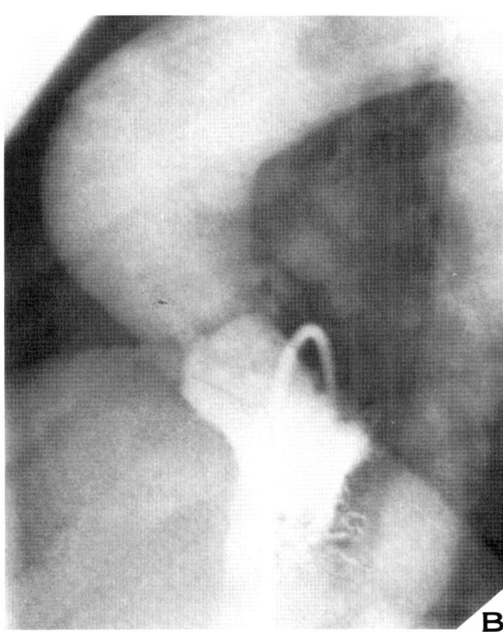

Fig. 18.12 Severe stenosis of trifoliate aortic valve. Long axis projection of left ventriculogram in diastole (A) and systole (B). There are three valve cusps (best seen in B); the right cusp is anterior, the left cusp is posterior, and the noncoronary cusp is in between and slightly lower. During systole the right and left coronary cusps form a continuous line with a very small jet in between, indicating severe aortic stenosis caused by fusion of the commissures. Note left ventricular hypertrophy and marked dilatation of the ascending aorta.

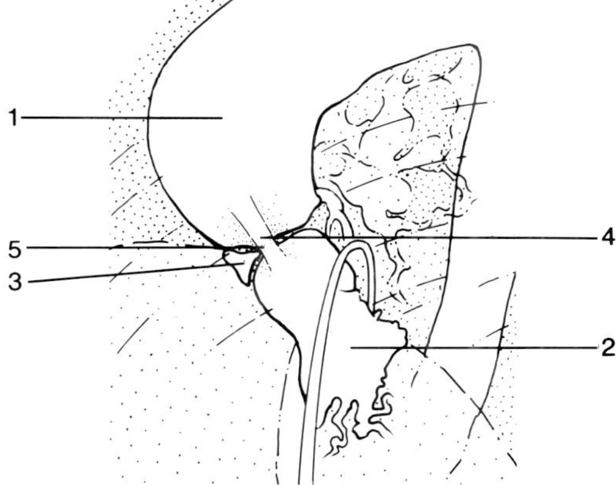

1 ascending aorta
2 left ventricle
3 right coronary cusp
4 left coronary cusp
5 jet of unopacified blood

less common causes are syphilitic aortitis and aortic root dilatation of unknown etiology. Microscopic examination in patients with medial degeneration of the aortic wall reveals cystic or mucoid degeneration of the media. These histologic changes are similar to those seen in the normal aging aorta. The medial changes result in weakness of the aortic annulus and dilatation of the aortic root (aortic–annular ectasia). In the Mayo Clinic series, only 8 percent of the patients with aortic root dilatation had Marfan syndrome, and only 2 percent had syphilitic aortitis. (Although chronic systemic hypertension is the most frequent cause of aortic root dilatation, it does not often lead to aortic insufficiency. Slight dilatation of the aortic root may also be seen in patients with aortic insufficiency secondary to rheumatic heart disease or a congenitally bicuspid aortic valve.)

The leaflets (cusps) are well formed in patients with congenital aortic insufficiency; however, they are too short to seal the orifice. In patients with rheumatic aortic insufficiency, the cusps are scarred and fibrotic; however, the commissures remain open, resulting in wide separation of the cusps (Fig. 18.13). In patients with aortic insufficiency secondary to bacterial endocarditis, the cusps are perforated or prolapsed; in extreme instances they may be destroyed. In such cases the destructive changes are usually most pronounced in the vicinity of the commissures (Fig. 18.14).

Aneurysmal dilatation of the ascending aorta, with inflammation and fibrosis of the sinuses of Valsalva and proximal aorta, may occur in patients with ankylosing spondylitis or rheumatic arthritis. The process may involve the aortic valve annulus, forming a subvalvular ridge, and may even extend into the anterior leaflet of the mitral valve.

CLINICAL FEATURES

Patients with mild aortic insufficiency are usually asymptomatic, whereas those with severe aortic insufficiency have symptoms of pulmonary venous hypertension; the latter range from exertional dyspnea to overt pulmonary edema. Angina pectoris is uncommon in patients with isolated aortic insufficiency. When it is present, it is usually secondary to associated coronary artery disease.

Palpation of the carotids and other peripheral arteries reveals bounding pulsations, with a striking diastolic collapse. There is lateral displacement of the cardiac apex, and auscultation reveals an early diastolic decrescendo murmur which radiates laterally. A systolic click and/or systolic ejection murmur may also be present.

Initially, the systolic pressure is elevated (200 to 250 mm Hg) and the diastolic pressure is markedly decreased (50 mm Hg or less). The wide pulse pressure, which reflects increased stroke volume, indicates that the left ventricle, although dilated, still has normal contractility. In time, with progressive left ventricular failure, the systolic pressure may fall to normal levels.

The electrocardiogram reveals evidence of left ventricular hypertrophy and enlargement, with increased voltage and T-wave inversion over the left precordium. The ECG may show P-wave prolongation in patients with longstanding "pure" aortic insufficiency.

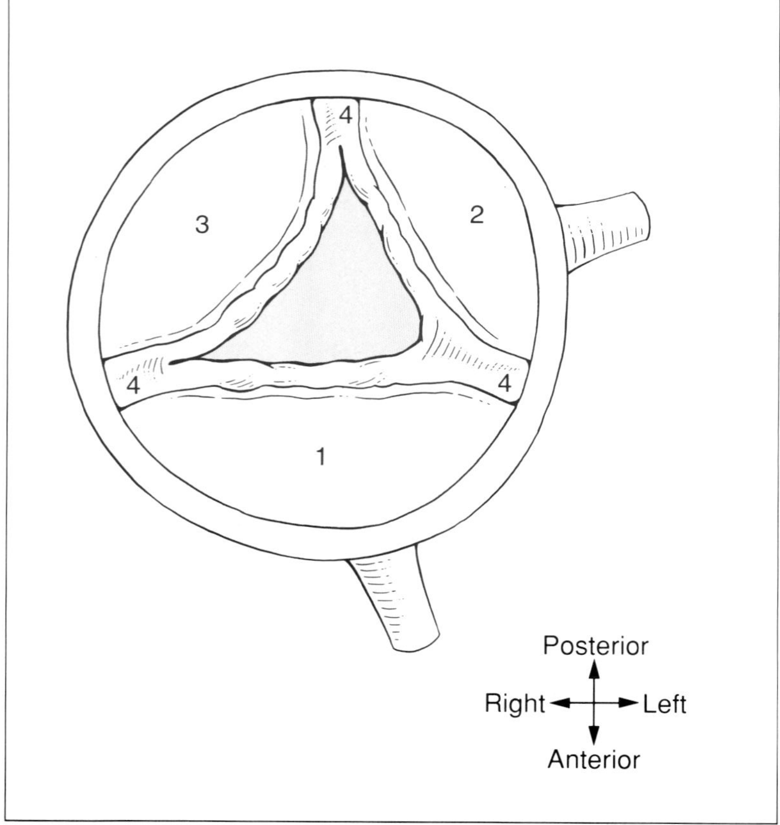

Fig. 18.13 Aortic insufficiency secondary to rheumatic heart disease. The aortic valve is viewed from above. The leaflets are short and thick, with nodular borders. The leaflets are fused at the commissures. Note the abnormally wide gap between the partially fused right and left cusps, indicating that the intercommissural ring is dilated.

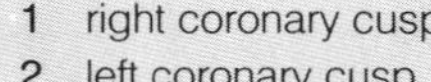

1	right coronary cusp	3	noncoronary cusp
2	left coronary cusp	4	fused commissures

IMAGING AND INVASIVE DIAGNOSIS

Plain Chest Films

Frontal and lateral projections typically show cardiomegaly with left ventricular enlargement. The left lower border of the heart is unusually prominent and is displaced to the left, the apex projecting below the dome of the diaphragm. On the lateral projection, the lower heart border projects behind the inferior vena cava (Fig. 18.15). Although the left atrium is usually normal in size, it may be enlarged in patients with longstanding aortic insufficiency. Aortic valve calcification is uncommon, although it is seen in some older patients.

When aortic insufficiency is secondary to isolated valve pathology, the ascending aorta is dilated in systole and normal (or small) during diastole; depending on the phase of the cardiac

Fig. 18.14 Aortic insufficiency secondary to bacterial endocarditis. The aortic valve is viewed from above. The right and noncoronary cusps are partially destroyed, with a perforation of the right coronary cusp. There are mass-like vegetations at the free margin of the noncoronary cusp.

1 right coronary cusp
2 left coronary cusp
3 noncoronary cusp
4 vegetations
5 perforation

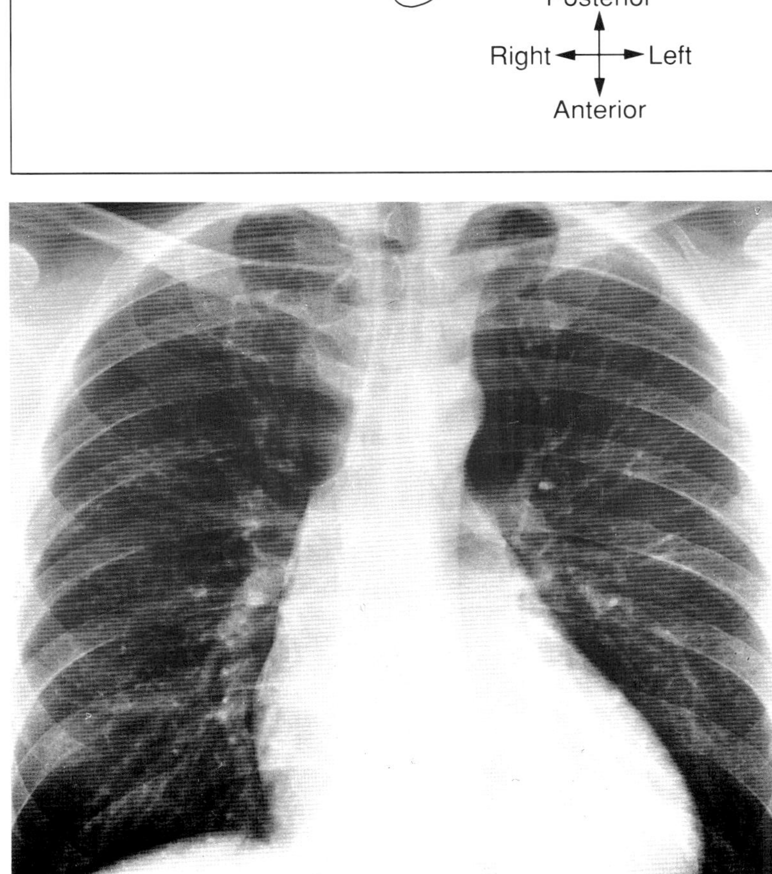

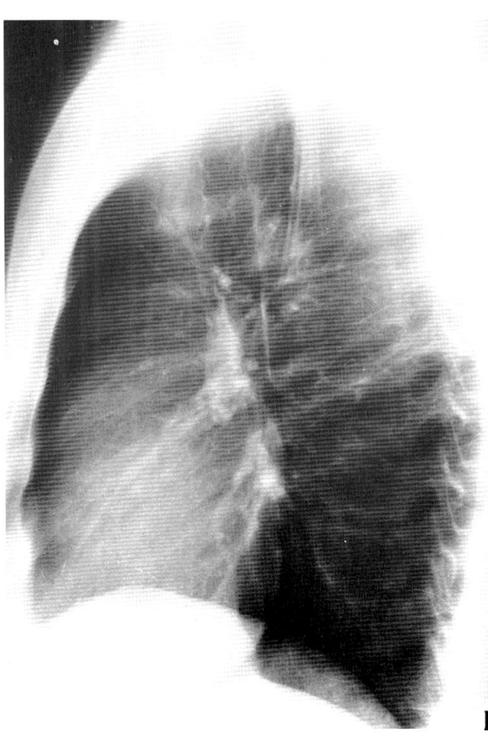

Fig. 18.15 Aortic insufficiency without left ventricular failure. (A) Posteroanterior and (B) lateral chest radiographs demonstrate moderate cardiomegaly with enlargement of the left ventricle, which projects posteriorly, inferiorly, and to the left. The cardiac apex projects beneath the diaphragm in A. The left atrium and aorta are normal. The pulmonary vascularity is normal, indicating that the pulmonary wedge pressure is normal or nearly normal, ie, that the left ventricle has not decompensated.

cycle at the time of the exposure, the right upper mediastinal contour may or may not appear prominent on the frontal projection. In patients with aortic insufficiency secondary to dilatation of the aortic root, the ascending aorta remains dilated throughout the cardiac cycle, filling in the retrosternal space on the lateral projection. In some individuals the markedly dilated aortic root may contribute to the left mediastinal border on the frontal projection.

When aortic insufficiency is due to an aneurysm of the aortic root (eg, in Marfan syndrome), the dilatation is limited to the annulus and the portion of the aorta or aortic arch; in such cases the aorta may project anteriorly or to the right or left. When it projects to the left, it may displace the pulmonary trunk to the left, the latter structure appearing as a localized bulge in the midportion of the cardiac silhouette on the frontal projection (Fig. 18.16).

The appearance of the pulmonary vasculature reflects left ventricular performance. When it is adequate, the pulmonary vasculature is normal, regardless of the duration of the disease. On the other hand, when left ventricular failure secondary to longstanding aortic insufficiency is present, there is radiographic evidence of pulmonary venous hypertension. The left atrium is usually enlarged in these patients (Fig. 18.17).

Echocardiography

Echocardiography accurately depicts the morphology of the aortic root and valve leaflets; measurement of end diastolic and end systolic volumes and the fractional shortening provide objective parameters of left ventricular size and function. Chronic aortic insufficiency leads to dilatation of the left ventricular cavity as well as "eccentric" hypertrophy of the left ventricular wall. Typically, left ventricular mass is markedly increased, whereas mural thickness is only slightly increased.

In patients with aortic insufficiency secondary to inflammatory disorders (eg, rheumatic endocarditis), M-mode, 2-D, and transesophageal echocardiography demonstrates thick, shortened leaflets which are widely separated at the commissures (Fig. 18.18). In patients with aortic insufficiency secondary to a dilated aortic root, echocardiograms show normal leaflets; however, the leaflets are too small to occlude the widened

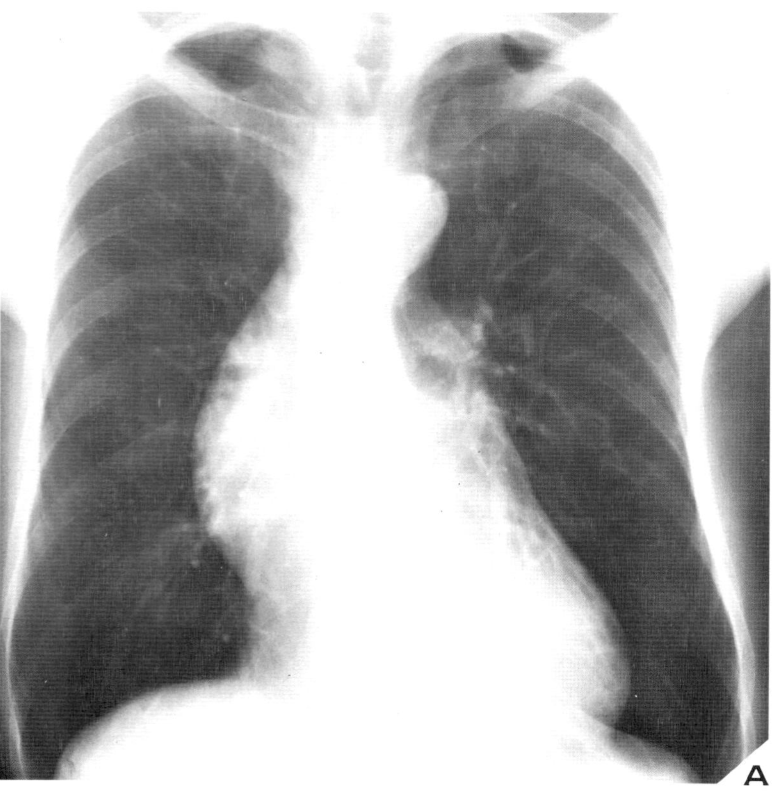

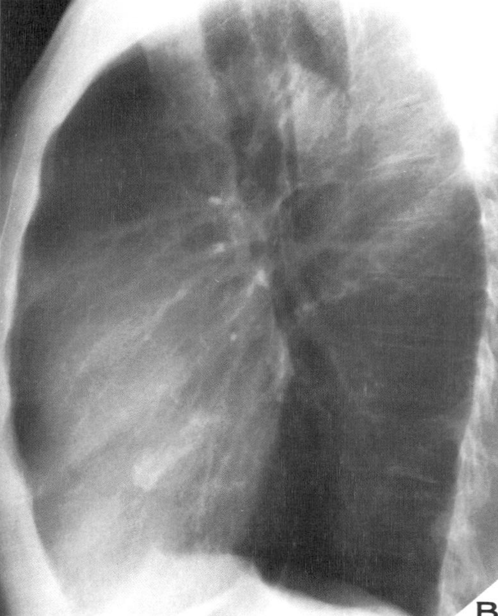

Fig. 18.16 Aortic insufficiency secondary to dilated aortic root (dilated annulus). (A) Posteroanterior and (B) lateral chest films show cardiomegaly with mild left ventricular enlargement. The dilated ascending aorta projects to the right on the frontal projection and fills in the retrosternal clear space on the lateral. The deformity of the midportion of the left heart border in A is produced by the pulmonary trunk, which has been displaced to the left by the dilated aortic root. The pulmonary vascularity is normal.

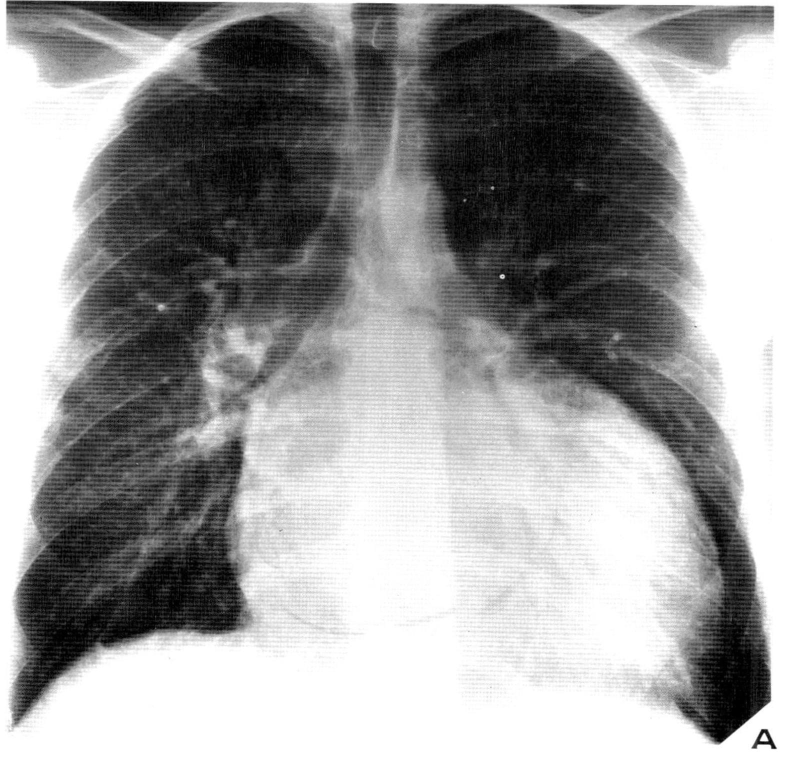

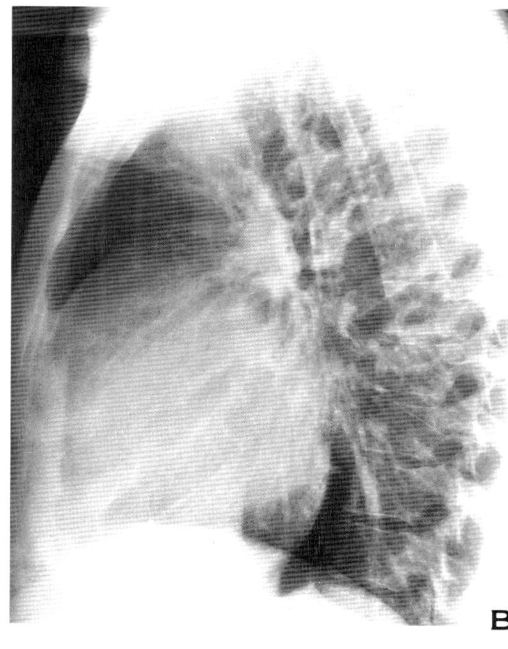

Fig. 18.17 Severe aortic insufficiency with congestive heart failure. (A) Posteroanterior and (B) lateral chest films show marked cardiomegaly with left ventricular and left atrial enlargement. Note interstitial edema, indicating the presence of pulmonary venous hypertension secondary to increased left atrial pressure (owing to left ventricular failure).

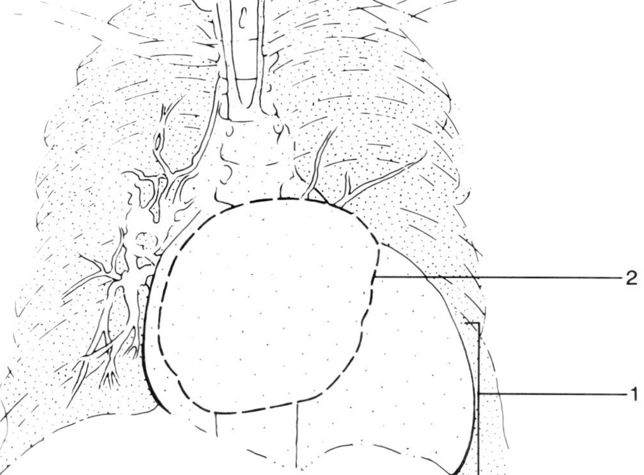

1 enlarged left ventricle
2 enlarged left atrium

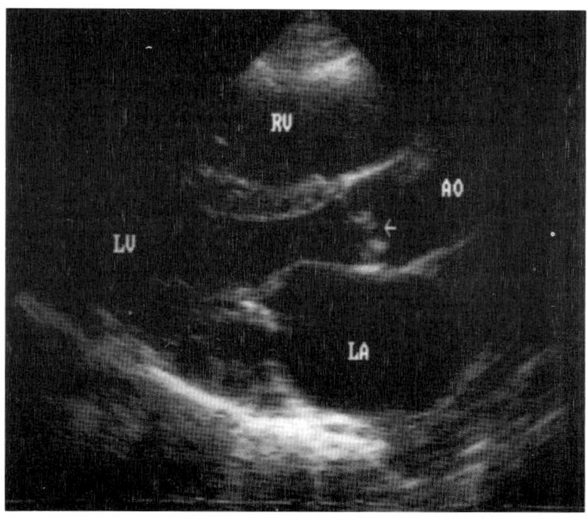

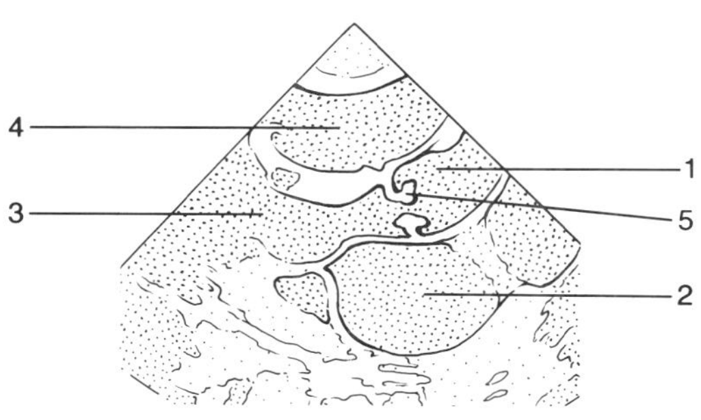

Fig. 18.18 Aortic insufficiency secondary to rheumatic heart disease. Parasternal long-axis view of 2-D echocardiogram in a patient with aortic and mitral valve disease shows thickening and distortion of the aortic valve leaflets. The left atrium is markedly enlarged owing to associated mitral stenosis.

1 aorta
2 left atrium
3 left ventricle
4 right ventricle
5 aortic valve

valve orifice (Fig. 18.19). When aortic insufficiency is caused by bacterial or fungal endocarditis, echocardiograms demonstrate vegetations as echogenic masses surrounding the leaflets; abscesses and/or fistula tracts can sometimes be appreciated as well (Fig. 18.20). Prolapse of the leaflets is clearly depicted on 2-D images (Fig. 18.21; see Appendix).

The degree of aortic incompetence can be evaluated by 2-D and Doppler (pulsed, continuous wave, and color) echocardiography. The size and dynamic changes in the left ventricular cavity, as seen on 2-D images, enable indirect assessment of the severity of the aortic insufficiency. On pulsed Doppler echocardiography, the severity is graded according to how far the regurgitant jet extends into the left ventricle. On continuous-flow Doppler images the wave form reflects the instantaneous pressure difference between the aorta and the left ventricle; the velocity profile contour derived from these data provides a valuable semiquantitative estimate of the severity of the aortic insufficiency. The area and width of the regurgitant jet can be measured on color Doppler images. The ratio of the area (or width) of the jet to the area (or width) of the left ventricular outflow tract correlates closely with the quantitative assessment of aortic insufficiency derived from cardiac catheterization data

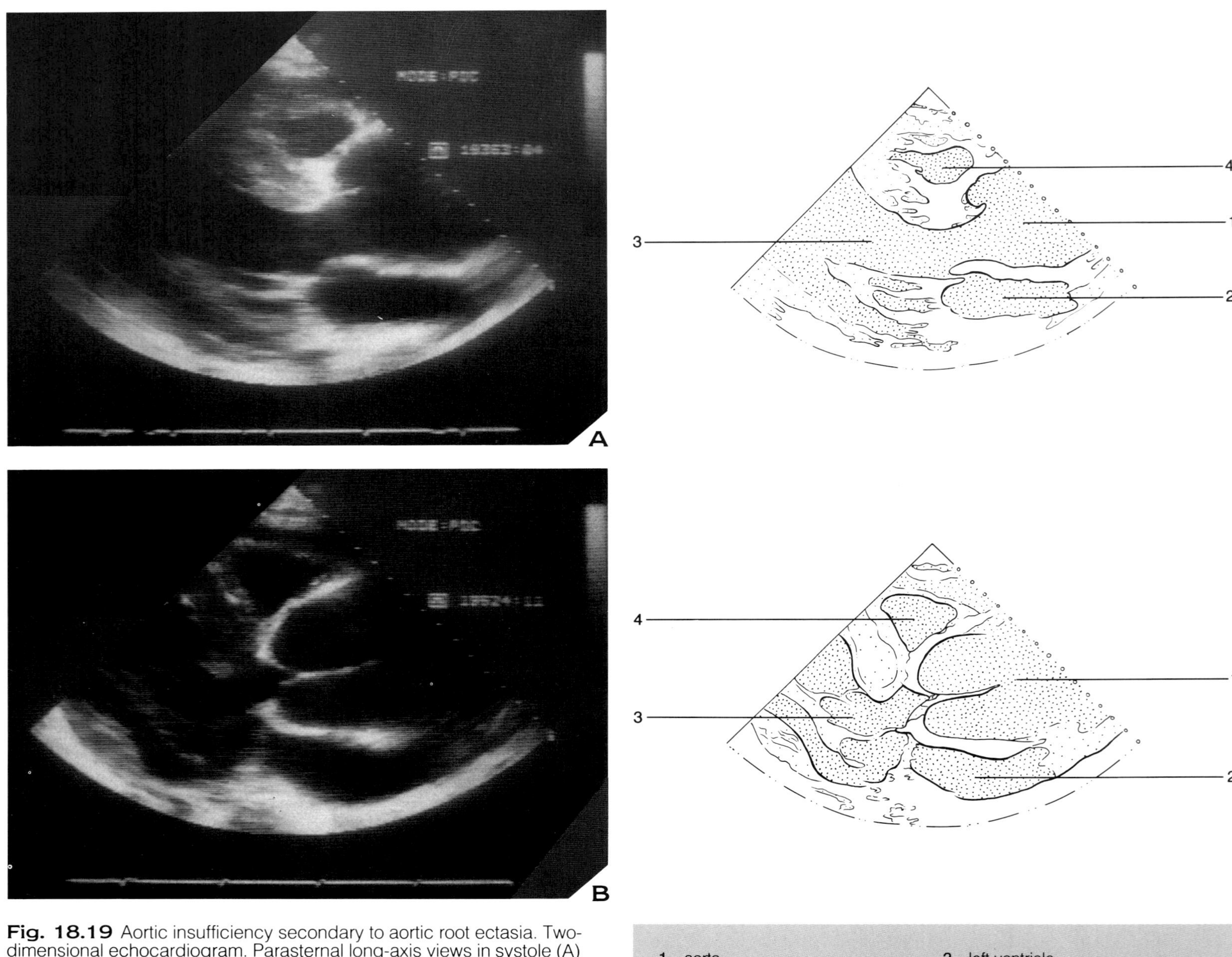

Fig. 18.19 Aortic insufficiency secondary to aortic root ectasia. Two-dimensional echocardiogram. Parasternal long-axis views in systole (A) and diastole (B) show marked dilatation of the aortic annulus and the aortic root. The transverse diameter of the aortic annulus is 60 mm (normal 40 to 45 mm).

(Fig. 18.22; see Appendix). The use of serial echocardiography is very important in the long-term follow-up of patients with aortic insufficiency, as these echocardiograms provide much of the information on which the timing of corrective surgery is based.

MRI

Aortic insufficiency is clearly depicted on cine MRI images, on which the regurgitant jet appears as a negative filling defect (Fig. 18.23). Measurements of the size and contractility of the left ventricle correlate well with echocardiographic data.

Cardiac Catheterization and Angiocardiography

Catheterization and angiocardiography are performed to assess the degree of aortic insufficiency and to ascertain the morphology of the coronary arteries and related structures. Typically, the left ventricular systolic pressure is markedly elevated and the left ventricular diastolic pressure is elevated as well.

To assess the severity of the aortic insufficiency, contrast material is injected into the aortic root, just above the sinuses of Valsalva. We employ the grading system devised by Hunt, which assigns grades of 1 (minimal) to 5 (severe) according to

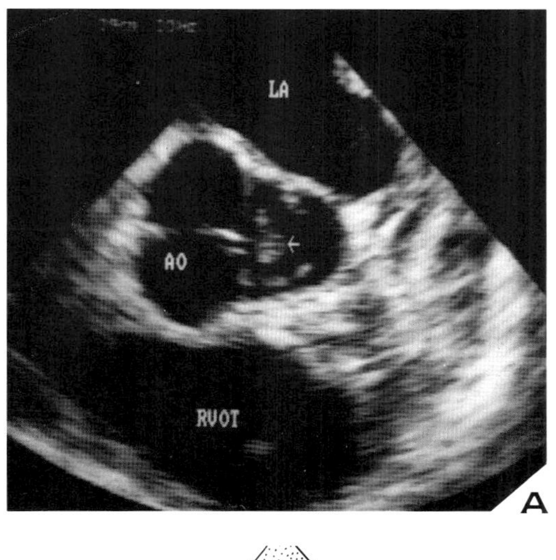

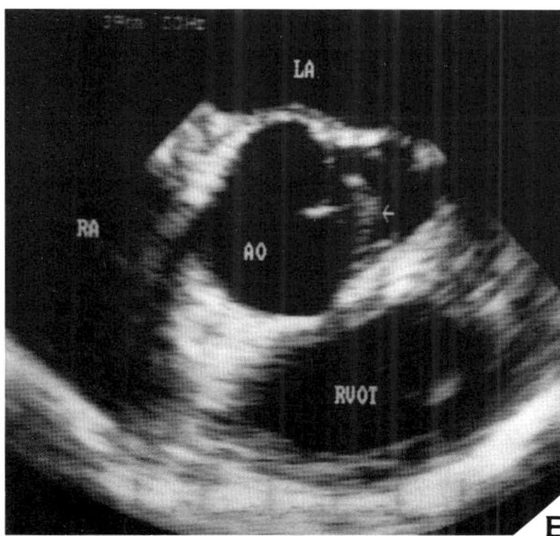

Fig. 18.20 Aortic insufficiency secondary to bacterial endocarditis. Transesophageal echocardiogram (basal short axis scan through aortic root). Two frames in diastole (A, B) demonstrate an echogenic mass on the left coronary cusp which represents a vegetation.

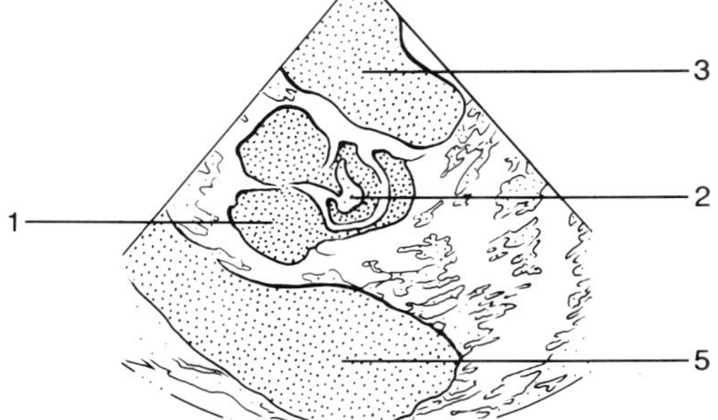

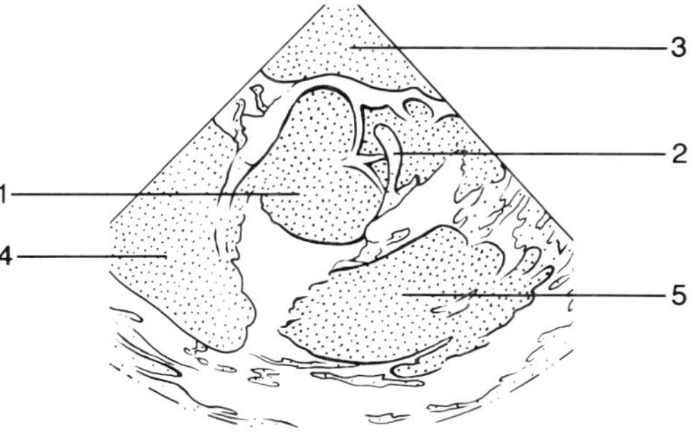

1	aorta	3	left atrium
2	vegetation on noncoronary cusp	4	left ventricle
		5	right ventricle

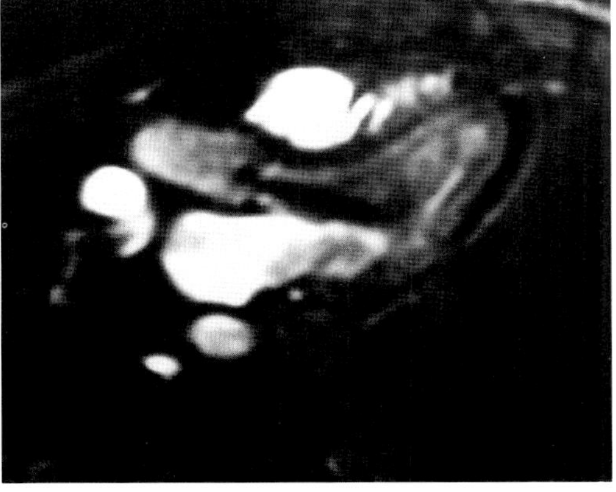

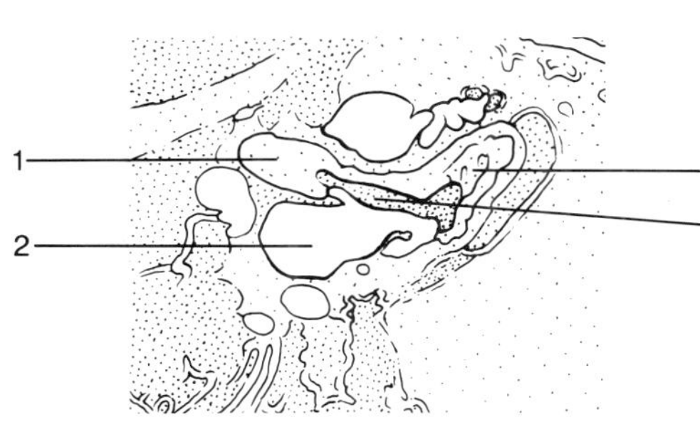

Fig. 18.23 Aortic insufficiency. Frame from cine MRI demonstrates turbulence in the left ventricular outflow tract during systole due to regurgitant flow through the incompetent aortic valve.

1	ascending aorta	4	regurgitant jet through incompetent aortic valve
2	left atrium		
3	left ventricle		

the density of the contrast material refluxing into the left ventricle and the rate at which the left ventricular cavity becomes opacified (Figs. 18.24 and 18.25). In patients with severe aortic insufficiency, the left ventricular chamber is densely opacified; its size, morphology, and contractility can thus be accurately assessed (Fig. 18.26). In patients with milder degrees of aortic regurgitation, a left ventriculogram is usually obtained to evaluate left ventricular morphology and contractility, although these parameters also can be accurately assessed by nonangiographic techniques (echocardiography and MRI).

The aortic root injection demonstrates the morphology of the aortic valve leaflets and the origin of the coronary arteries; however, selective coronary arteriography is necessary to exclude coincidental coronary artery stenosis, which is not uncommon in patients over 40 years of age with aortic insufficiency.

In patients with aortic insufficiency secondary to rheumatic heart disease, the mitral valve also may be incompetent secondary to inflammatory changes, or it may become incompetent due to left ventricular dilatation. A left ventricular injection, or an aortic root injection in patients with severe aortic insufficiency, will demonstrate the status of the left ventricle in such cases.

COMBINED AORTIC INSUFFICIENCY AND AORTIC STENOSIS

Some patients with aortic stenosis have minimal aortic insufficiency; conversely, some patients with aortic insufficiency have minimal aortic stenosis. In either instance the clinical manifestations are those of the dominant lesion. A minority of patients with combined lesions have hemodynamically significant degrees of stenosis and insufficiency (which may be balanced). Echocardiography or cardiac catheterization can identify patients with combined lesions, who require special management.

ACUTE AORTIC INSUFFICIENCY

ETIOLOGY AND PATHOGENESIS

Bacterial or fungal endocarditis, aortic dissection, and trauma are the most frequent causes of acute aortic insufficiency, a life-threatening condition which requires prompt treatment. Rupture of a congenital aneurysm of the sinuses of Valsalva is a relatively infrequent cause of acute aortic insufficiency.

Infective endocarditis of the aortic valve is most often caused by gram-positive cocci, alpha-streptococcus in particular. Risk factors include a previously abnormal valve, intravenous drug abuse, alcoholism, immune deficiency states, and manipulative procedures (eg, surgery, childbirth, dental extraction). The infection results in perforation and/or destruction of the cusps and aneurysm formation at or near the affected cusps, and predisposes to the formation of vegetations on the leaflets, which may interfere with their normal apposition during systole, resulting in varying degrees of insufficiency.

In aortic dissection, the false channel usually originates in or progresses to involve the middle segment of the ascending aorta. It may progress proximally to involve the aortic annulus, disrupting the supporting structures of the aortic valve. The resultant malalignment of the leaflets leads to aortic insufficiency of varying degree (see Fig. 18.29).

Traumatic aortic insufficiency is usually secondary to acute deceleration injuries (eg, falls, motor vehicle accidents) or to blunt trauma. In addition, direct injuries of the aortic valve can result from penetrating injuries, such as those caused by gunshot or knife wounds.

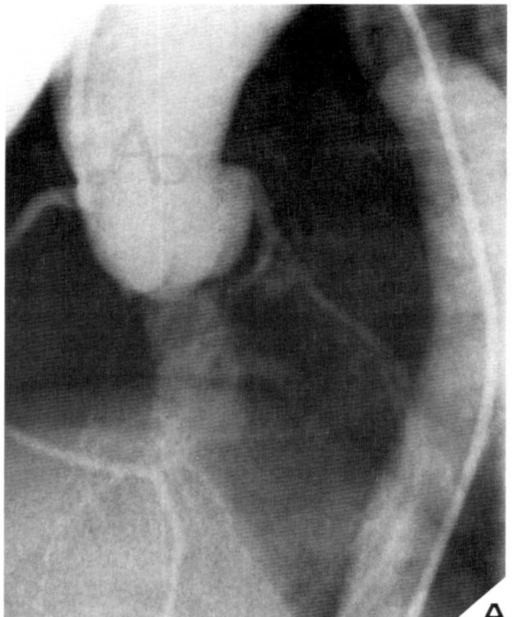

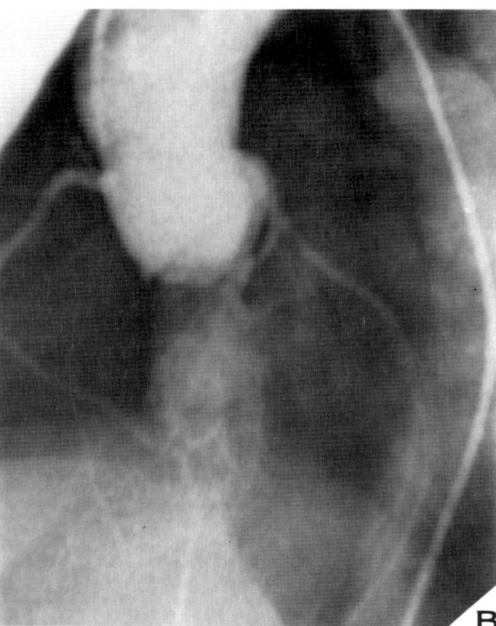

Fig. 18.24 Mild (Grade 1) aortic insufficiency. (A, B) Two diastolic frames of thoracic aortogram (left anterior oblique projection) show a trifoliate aortic valve with reflux limited to the left ventricular outflow tract.

HEMODYNAMICS AND CLINICAL FEATURES

Abrupt onset of congestive heart failure is the classic clinical presentation of acute aortic insufficiency. The acutely increased volume load on the left ventricle causes a marked elevation of the left ventricular end diastolic pressure, with a decrease in the effective (ie, forward) stroke volume and cardiac output. Left ventricular diameter, mass, and wall motion are usually normal in patients with acute aortic regurgitation. This is in sharp contrast to patients with chronic aortic insufficiency, in whom there has been time for compensatory left ventricular dilatation and hypertrophy to develop. The diagnosis of acute aortic insufficiency usually presents no difficulty, provided one suspects it and orders the appropriate studies.

IMAGING

Chest Films

Heart size is usually normal in patients with acute bacterial or fungal endocarditis; however, the lungs reveal evidence of pulmonary venous hypertension. The ascending aorta is usually normal.

In patients with acute aortic insufficiency secondary to aortic dissection, the ascending aorta may be dilated, with blurring of its borders secondary to local edema or mediastinal hemorrhage. In about one third of patients with aortic insufficiency secondary to aortic dissection, the mediastinum is unremarkable. Although heart size is usually normal, there is usually evidence of congestive heart failure (pulmonary venous hypertension or pulmonary edema) (Fig. 18.27).

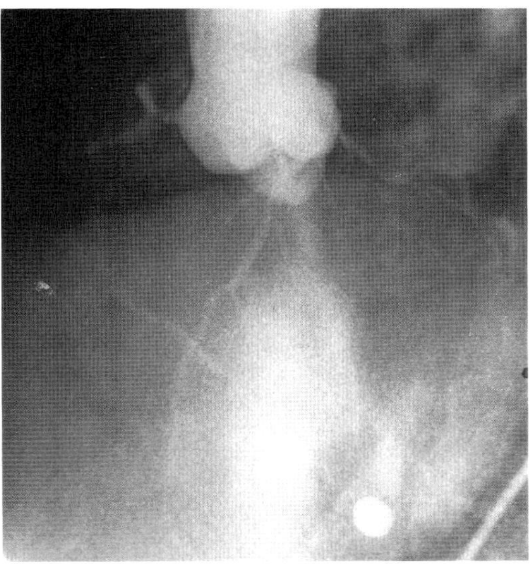

Fig. 18.25 Moderate (Grade 3) aortic insufficiency. Diastolic frame of thoracic aortogram (right anterior oblique projection) shows a trifoliate aortic valve with reflux into the left ventricle. Although the entire left ventricular cavity is opacified, the density is less than that of the ascending aorta.

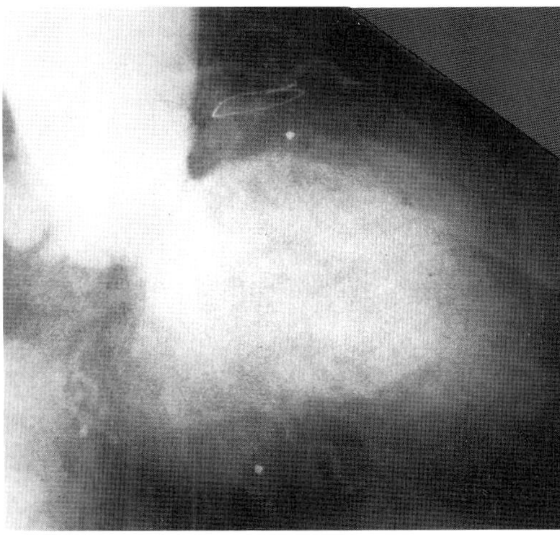

Fig. 18.26 Severe (Grade 5) aortic insufficiency. Right anterior oblique projection of thoracic aortogram demonstrates opacification of the entire left ventricle. The refluxed contrast material has the same density as the ascending aorta.

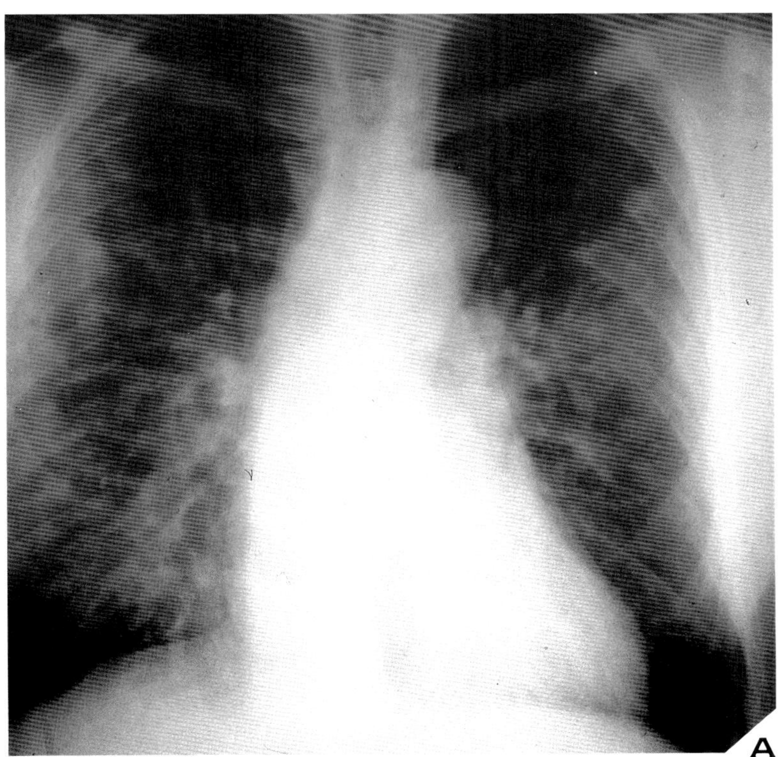

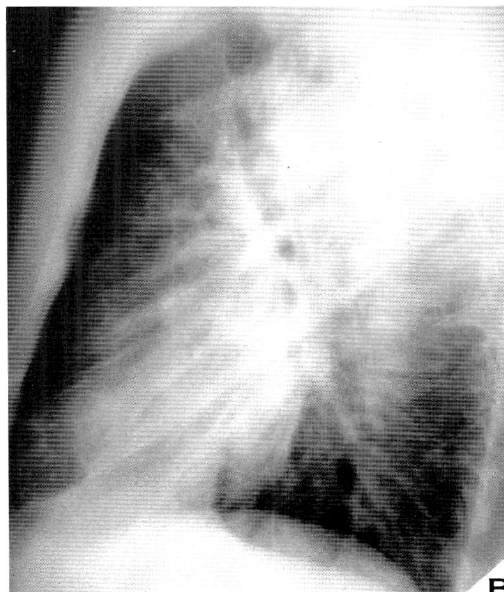

Fig. 18.27 Acute aortic insufficiency. (A) Posteroanterior and (B) lateral chest films in patient with aortic dissection show borderline cardiac enlargement with prominence of the left ventricle. There is severe pulmonary edema, particularly in the central portions of the lungs. Echocardiography demonstrated severe aortic regurgitation.

Echocardiography

As in the case of chronic aortic insufficiency (see above), conventional 2-D and color-flow Doppler echocardiography can be employed to confirm the diagnosis and assess the degree of functional abnormality. Echocardiography can detect vegetations greater than 2 to 3 mm in diameter and is the modality of choice in patients with suspected infective endocarditis. The presence of an abnormal linear echo paralleling the aortic lumen strongly suggests the diagnosis of aortic dissection; dilatation of the aorta and pericardial effusion are other suggestive findings (see Chapter 27). Conventional 2-D and color-flow Doppler images clearly depict aortic insufficiency secondary to a ruptured sinus of Valsalva aneurysm (Fig. 18.28; see Appendix).

MRI

Spin-echo images accurately depict the location and extent of the aortic dissection, as well as the involvement of surrounding structures (see Chapter 27). Aortic insufficiency is clearly seen on cine MRI (see Fig. 18.23).

Angiography

Thoracic aortography, preferably with 35 mm cine images, is the standard diagnostic procedure in patients with acute aortic insufficiency. A catheter is passed from a peripheral artery into the aortic root and contrast material is delivered at a high rate (30 mL/second) to adequately opacify the aortic root. At least two projections are essential to assess the severity of the aortic insufficiency; the left and right anterior oblique projections and the lateral projection are the most useful. As in patients with chronic aortic insufficiency, the severity is graded according to the rate at which contrast material refluxes from the aorta into the left ventricle during diastole and the degree of opacification of the left ventricular cavity. In patients with dissection involving the aortic root, aortography may demonstrate distortion of the sinuses of Valsalva (Fig. 18.29). In patients with aortic insufficiency caused by bacterial endocarditis, aortography may demonstrate a filling defect attached to one or more of the cusps, which represents vegetations, or a saccular dilatation of the aortic root.

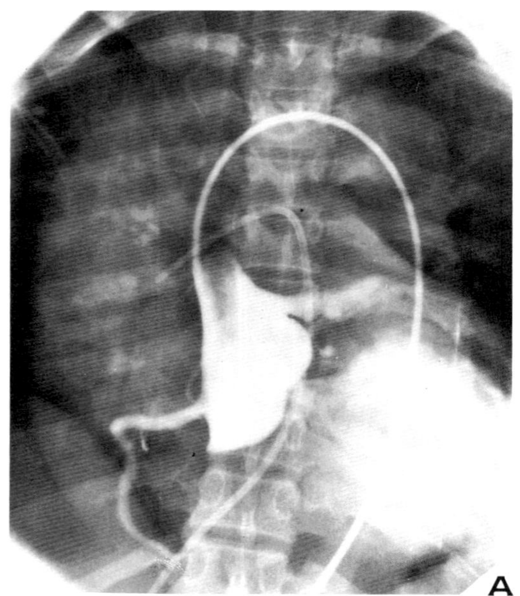

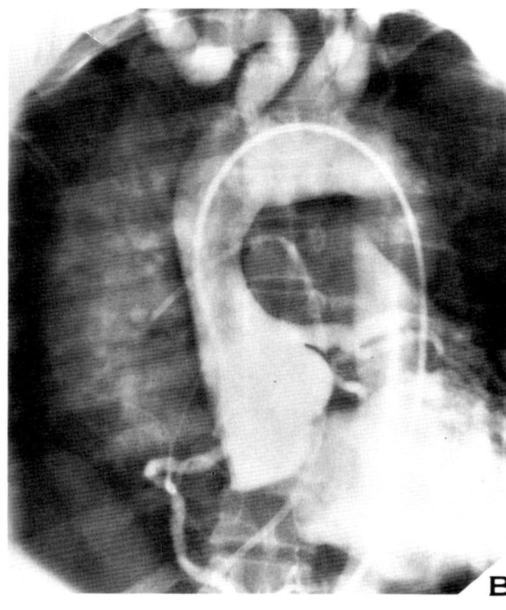

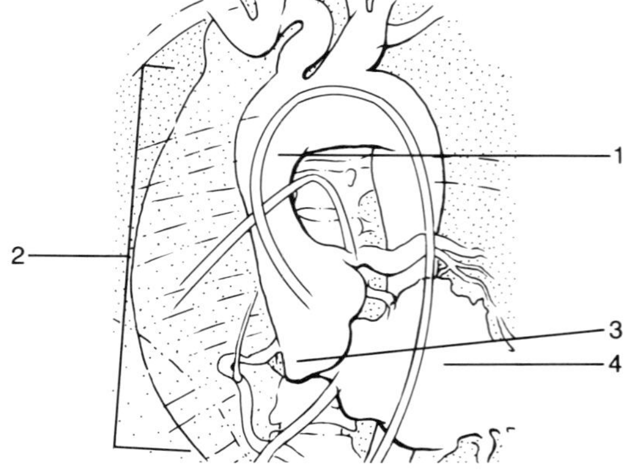

1	true lumen of ascending aorta	3	right coronary cusp
2	false lumen (dissected channel)	4	left ventricle

Fig. 18.29 Acute aortic insufficiency (Grade 5) secondary to dissection of the aortic root. (A) Early and (B) late phases of thoracic aortogram (frontal projection) show deformation of the ascending aorta by the false lumen (dissected channel). The deformation extends from the right coronary sinus to the aortic arch. There is dense opacification of the entire left ventricular cavity.

MITRAL VALVE

Malfunction of the mitral valve can lead to mitral stenosis, mitral insufficiency, or both. These functional abnormalities result from morphological changes in the leaflets, the annulus, or a combination of the two.

MITRAL STENOSIS

Restricted opening of the mitral valve during diastole (mitral stenosis) results in left ventricular inlet obstruction, with a diastolic pressure gradient between the left atrium and the left ventricle. Rheumatic heart disease is by far the most common cause of acquired mitral stenosis. Left atrial neoplasms, mainly myxomas, are a rare cause of inlet obstruction (see Chapter 26). Congenital malformations, such as a supravalvular mitral ring, can cause left ventricular inlet obstruction in both teenagers and adults (see Chapter 17).

PATHOLOGY

Rheumatic mitral stenosis results from fusion of the anterolateral and/or posteromedial commissures and thickening of the valve leaflets, particularly at their free margins. Although the structural changes may be limited to the leaflets, in most patients the chordae tendineae (subvalvular apparatus) are affected as well. The chordae tendineae are short and thick; often they are fused, forming a mass beneath the commissures (Fig. 18.30). Extensive fusion of the chordae tendineae may create the appearance of a second annulus closer to the apex. In these patients the deformed mitral valve resembles a funnel, with its

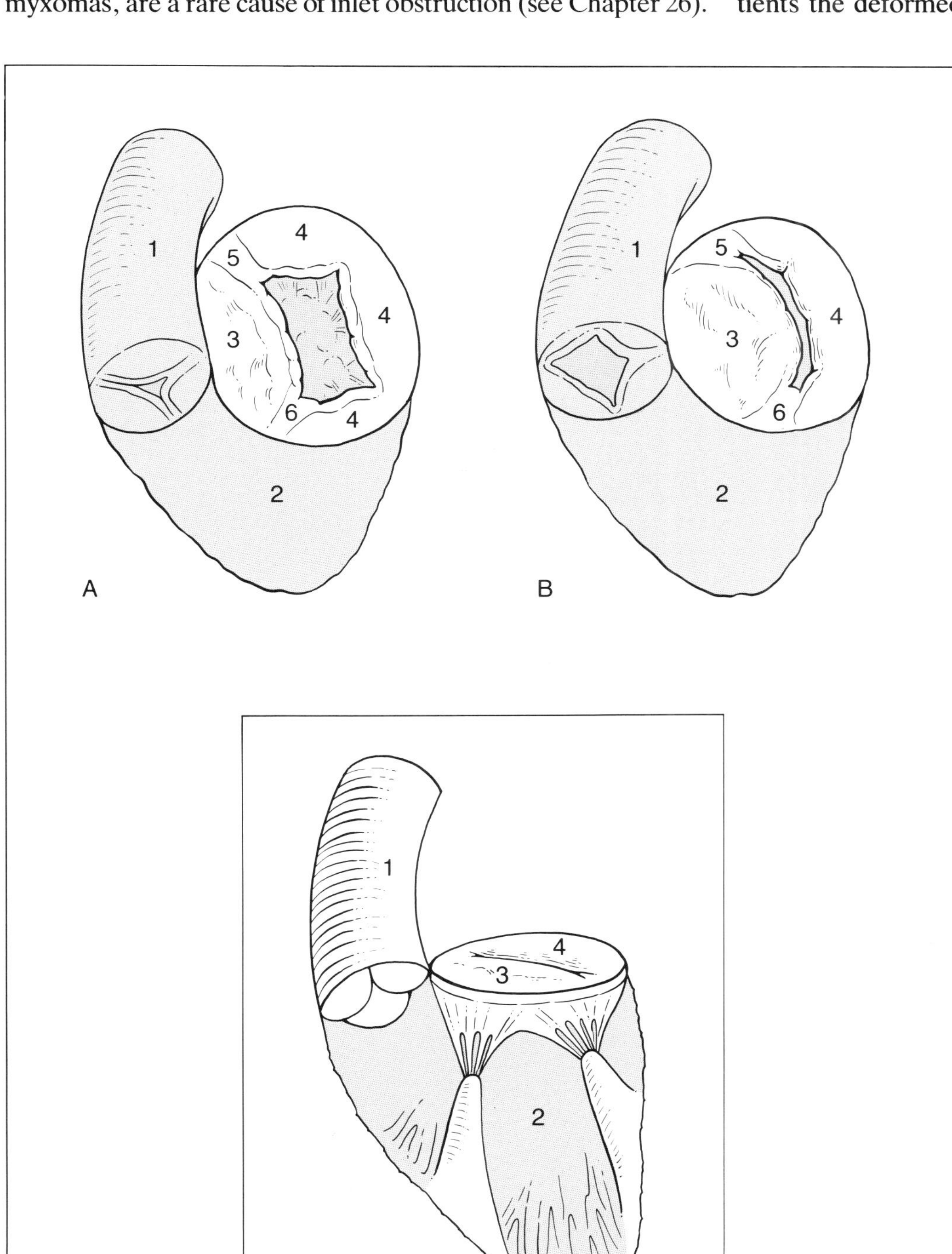

Fig. 18.30 Mitral stenosis secondary to rheumatic heart disease. Mitral valve (viewed from the left atrium) in diastole (A) and systole (B). The leaflets are thickened and fused at the level of the commissures. The chordae tendineae are short (C). The increased thickness of the leaflets and the fusion of the commissures restrict the opening of the valve during diastole.

1 aorta
2 left ventricle
3 anterior leaflet of mitral valve
4 posterior leaflet of the mitral valve (with its three scallops)
5 fused anterolateral commissure
6 fused posteromedial commissure

widest part of the level of the true annulus and its "spout" within the body of the left ventricle (Fig. 18.31). Calcification is very common in older patients with rheumatic mitral stenosis. The calcifications are located at the free borders or at the level of the commissures, and may extend for a variable distance into the annulus.

PATHOPHYSIOLOGY

Owing to the increased pressure load, the left atrium is markedly enlarged in most patients with hemodynamically significant mitral stenosis. The chronically elevated left atrial pressure results in pulmonary venous hypertension and pulmonary edema. Pulmonary venous hypertension, in turn, leads to pulmonary arterial hypertension, resulting in right ventricular dilatation and hypertrophy and ultimately leading to right ventricular failure. The left ventricle is usually morphologically normal; however, localized fibrosis secondary to rheumatic carditis may cause abnormal wall motion.

Longstanding pulmonary venous hypertension leads to increased pulmonary vascular resistance; the latter usually disappears after the stenosis is surgically corrected. Rarely, pul-

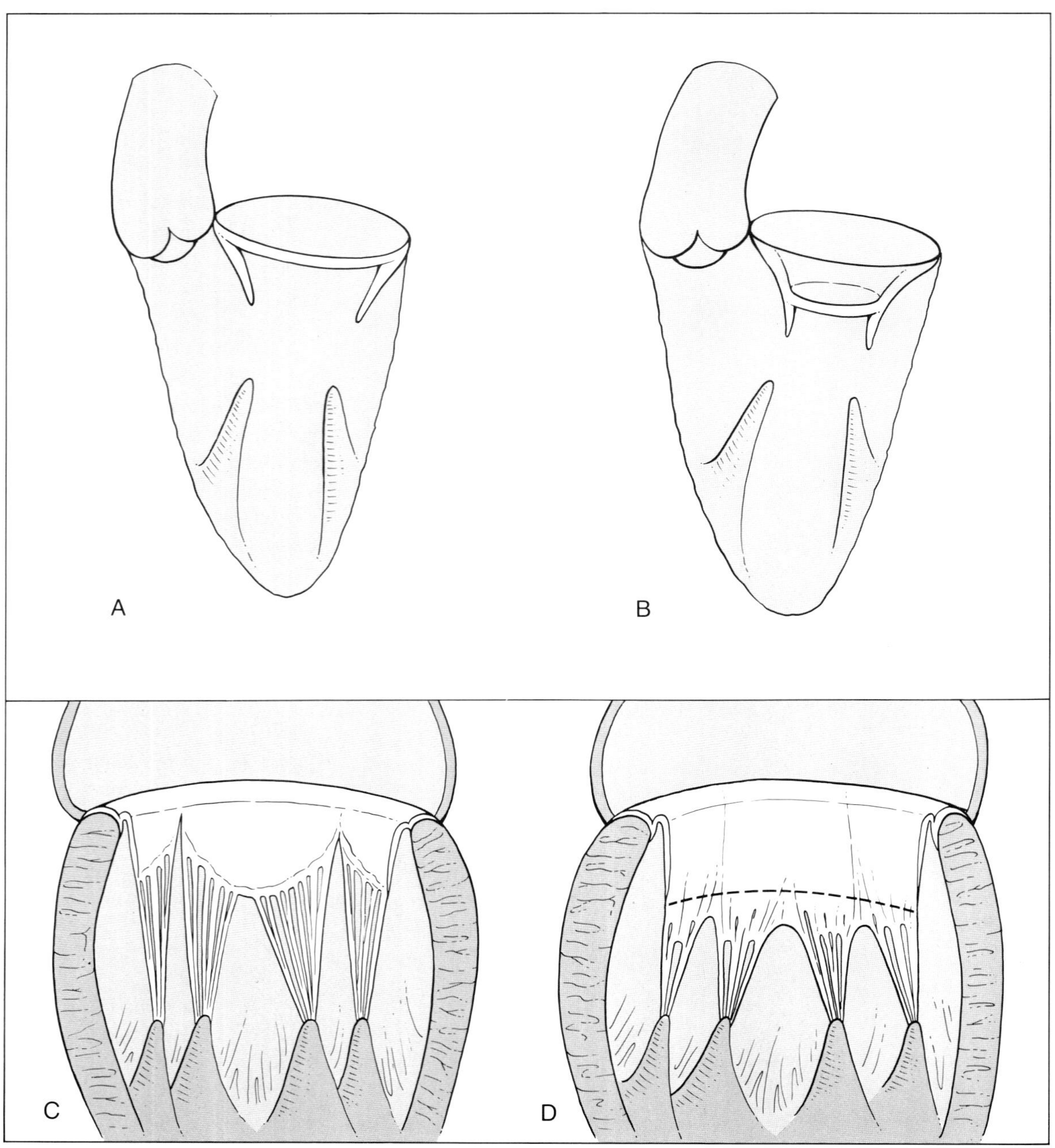

Fig. 18.31 Severe mitral stenosis: fusion of the chordae tendineae producing apparent displacement of the annulus. Ventriculographic appearance of the normal (A) and stenotic mitral valve (B) and the anatomic relations of the normal (C) and stenotic (D) mitral valve are shown schematically. Severe mitral stenosis is accompanied by fusion of the commissures and shortening of the chordae tendineae, creating a funnel-shaped deformity. The "mouth" of the funnel is at the level of the anatomic annulus; the "spout" projects into the left ventricle. The apparent mitral annulus (as seen on the ventriculogram) lies caudal to the true mitral annulus, ie, it is closer to the apex. The heads of the papillary muscles appear much closer to the annulus than normal.

monary vascular disease may progress to obliteration of small pulmonary arteries and arterioles (resistance vessels), leading to fixed pulmonary hypertension and further increasing the pressure load on the right ventricle. The tricuspid valve may become incompetent in patients with marked right ventricular enlargement.

CLINICAL FEATURES

Patients with mitral stenosis typically present with nonspecific respiratory symptoms (dyspnea, cough, or "chronic bronchitis"), orthopnea, or paroxysmal nocturnal dyspnea. The symptoms are aggravated by exercise and are often worse when the patient is recumbent. Symptoms related to chronic congestive right ventricular failure (eg, right upper quadrant pain and nausea caused by a large congested liver) are late manifestations. About 10 percent of patients with mitral stenosis complain of chest pain.

Auscultation reveals a loud first sound, an opening snap (not always present), and a characteristic diastolic rumble with a presystolic crescendo. A typical murmur may not be heard, however, in patients with atrial fibrillation.

Electrocardiograms typically show P-wave prolongation (characteristic of left atrial enlargement). Patients with severe, longstanding disease have ECG changes indicating right ventricular hypertrophy secondary to pulmonary hypertension. The frequency of atrial fibrillation varies with the severity of the obstruction, the size of the left atrium, and the age of the patient. Atrial fibrillation is present in about 50 percent of patients with severe, longstanding mitral stenosis. Atrial fibrillation is an important risk factor for early death in such patients.

Systemic embolization from an atrial thrombus is not uncommon in patients with tight mitral stenosis and may occur early in the course of the disease. The risk of embolization, which may affect the brain, kidneys, spleen, limbs or other peripheral arteries, is greatly increased in patients with atrial fibrillation.

Hemoptysis is a manifestation of severe, longstanding pulmonary venous hypertension. Once commonplace in patients with severe mitral stenosis, hemoptysis is seldom encountered in the present era of aggressive diuretic therapy and early surgical replacement of the mitral valve.

IMAGING AND INVASIVE DIAGNOSIS

Chest Films

Frontal and lateral projections almost always reveal left atrial enlargment, manifested by elevation and posterior displacement of the left mainstem bronchus and a "double density" on the frontal projection. The left atrial appendage appears as a bulge in the midportion of the left heart border. If barium is given, posterior displacement of the esophagus can be appreciated on the lateral and right anterior oblique projections (Figs. 18.32 to 18.34).

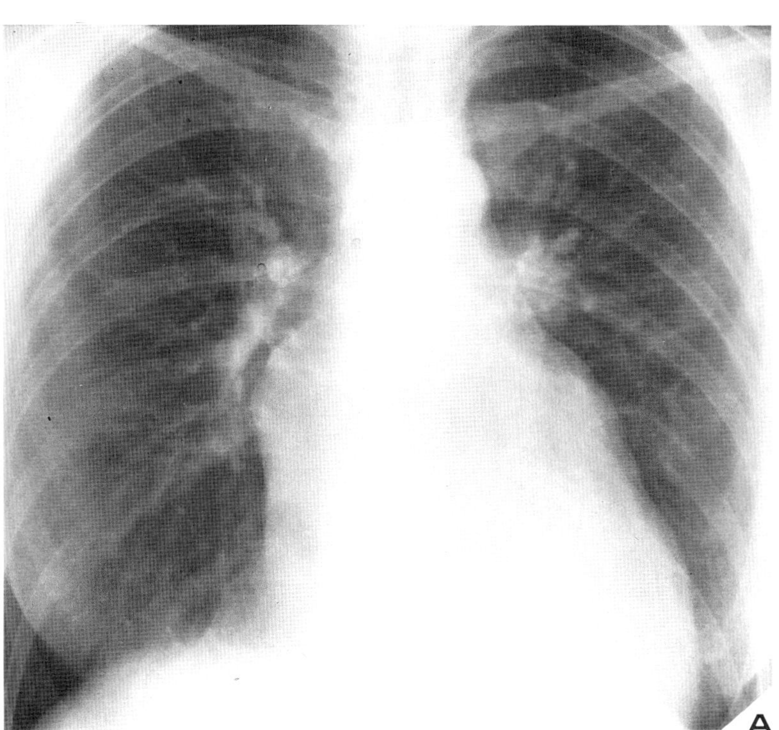

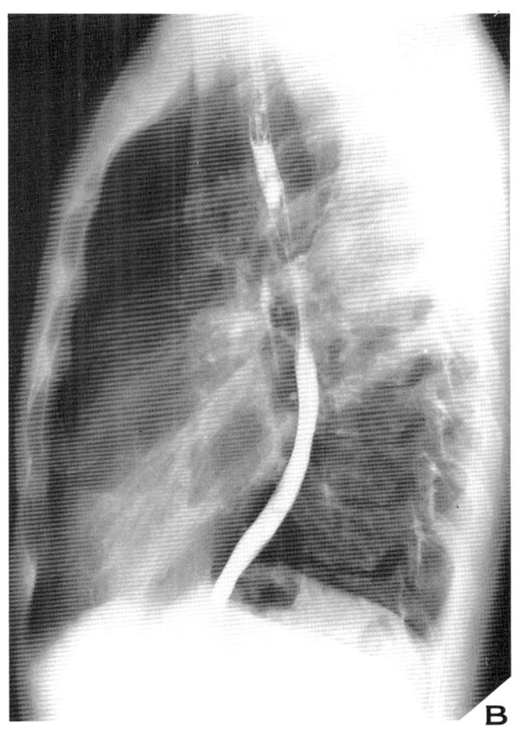

Fig. 18.32 Mitral stenosis. (A) Posteroanterior projection. There is moderate cardiomegaly with marked left atrial enlargement. The right border of the enlarged left atrium projects beyond the right atrial contour. The left atrial appendage is displaced to the left and forms a bulge in the midportion of the left heart border. The main portion of the left atrium elevates the left main bronchus and appears as a "double density" within the heart. The left ventricle is slightly smaller than average. There is evidence of both pulmonary venous hypertension [the arteries and veins are more prominent in the upper lung fields than in the lower zones ("cephalization")] and pulmonary arterial hypertension (the pulmonary trunk and the left and right main pulmonary arteries are enlarged). (B) Lateral projection. The opacified esophagus is displaced posteriorly by the large left atrium. There is moderately heavy calcification of the mitral valve.

Calcification of the mitral valve is not uncommon in patients with rheumatic mitral stenosis, although it is only infrequently evident on plain films (Figs. 18.32B and 18.34). It can be detected fluoroscopically in about 10 percent of patients with rheumatic mitral valve disease. Mitral valve calcification associated with rheumatic heart disease must be differentiated from "physiologic" calcification of the mitral annulus, which is common in the elderly and is part of the normal aging process. "Physiologic" calcification typically occurs on the ventricular side of the annulus, at the junction between the leaflet and the ventricular wall. [Although "physiologic" calcification usually does not interfere with the functioning of the leaflet, large calcium deposits that extend into the wall of the left ventricle or left atrium can cause mitral valvular dysfunction (insufficiency and/or stenosis).] "Physiologic" calcification typically appears on chest films as a dense C-shaped or ring-shaped opacity in the

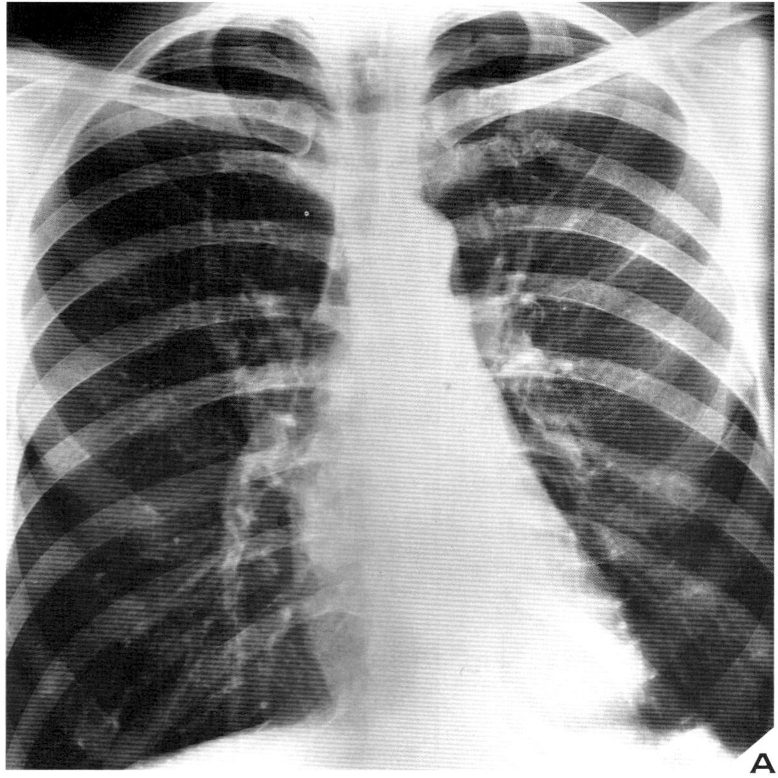

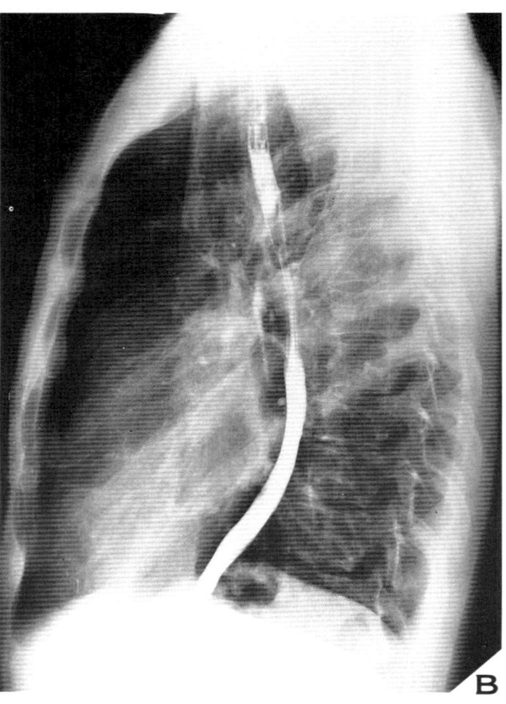

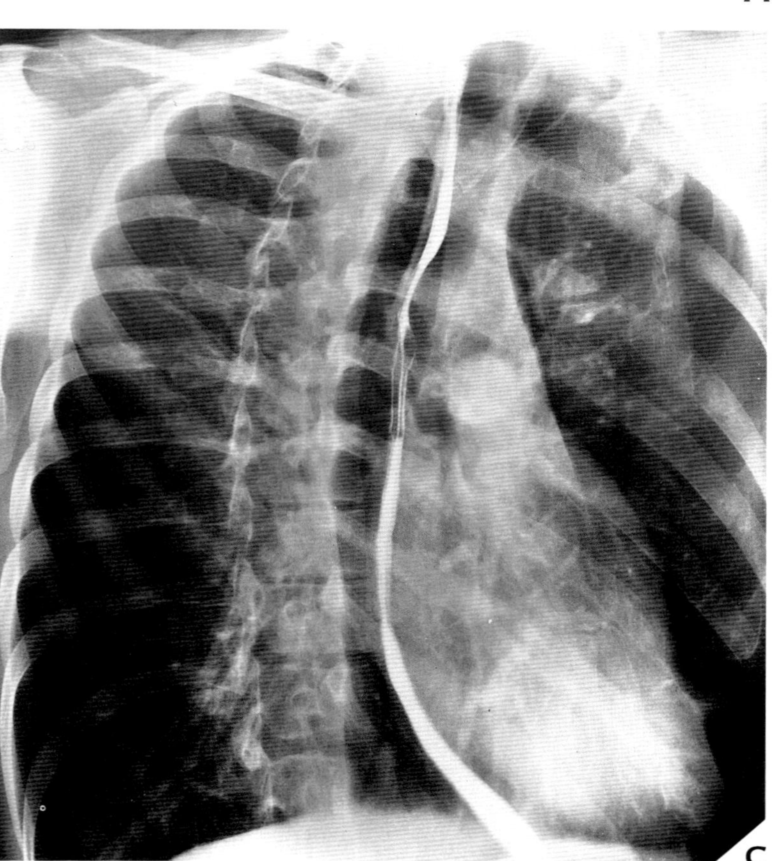

Fig. 18.33 Mitral stenosis. (A) Posteroanterior, (B) lateral, and (C) right anterior oblique projections show a normal-sized heart. Although the left atrium appears normal in A, posterior displacement of the esophagus (B, C) and left main bronchus (B) indicates the presence of left atrial enlargment. The left ventricle is smaller than average. There is "cephalization" of the pulmonary vasculature, indicating the presence of pulmonary venous hypertension.

position of the mitral annulus (Fig. 18.35). Calcifications associated with rheumatic mitral stenosis are usually limited to the leaflets, typically occurring at the level of the commissures. On chest films they appear as irregular, ill-defined high-density shadows within the mitral orifice. Fluoroscopy reveals wide excursion of the calcified leaflet (or leaflets), whereas a calcified annulus exhibits very little motion during the cardiac cycle. Occasionally, the calcification associated with rheumatic heart disease involves the mitral annulus as well as the mitral valve. In such cases, the presence of characteristic abnormalities of the heart and pulmonary vasculature will suggest the correct diagnosis. Heavy calcification, together with plain film findings of pulmonary venous hypertension, indicates severe mitral stenosis, even though the radiologic appearance of the calcification may be indistinguishable from that of "physiologic" calcification.

Radiologic evidence of pulmonary venous hypertension is invariably present in patients with rheumatic mitral stenosis. Mildly increased left atrial pressure is manifested by constriction of the arteries in the lower zones and dilatation of the arteries in the upper zones ("cephalization" of the pulmonary circulation) (Figs. 18.32 and 18.33). The redistribution of pulmonary blood flow results from the accumulation of interstitial fluid in the lower zones, which prevents the pulmonary vascular bed from expanding normally. When left atrial pressure exceeds 20 mm Hg, plain films begin to show evidence of interstitial pul-

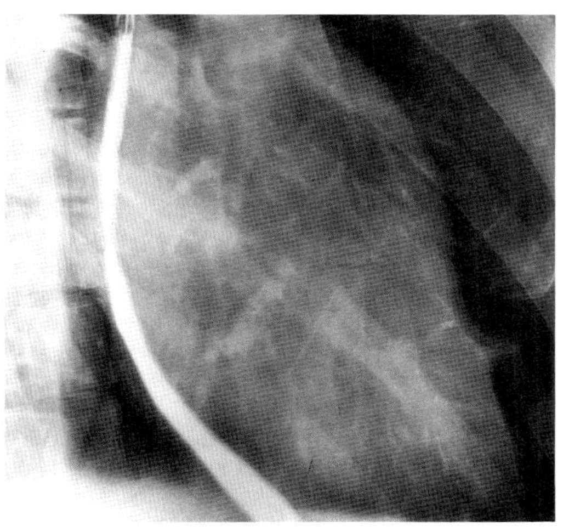

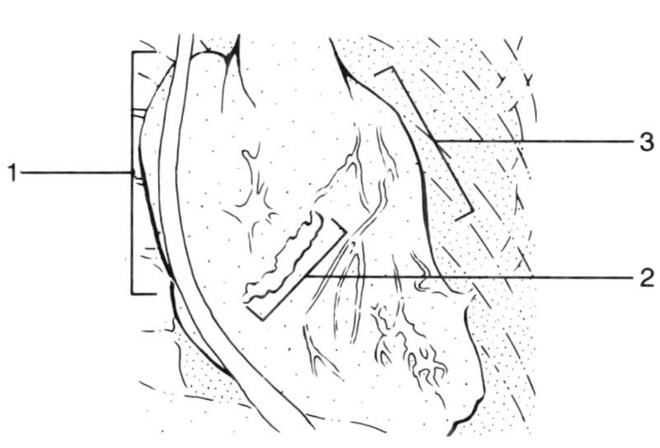

Fig. 18.34 Mitral stenosis. Right anterior oblique projection shows posterior displacement of the esophagus by the enlarged left atrium. The mitral valve is heavily calcified. Note prominence of right ventricular outflow tract and pulmonary trunk secondary to pulmonary arterial hypertension.

1	enlarged left atrium	3	dilated right ventricular outflow tract and pulmonary trunk
2	calcified mitral valve		

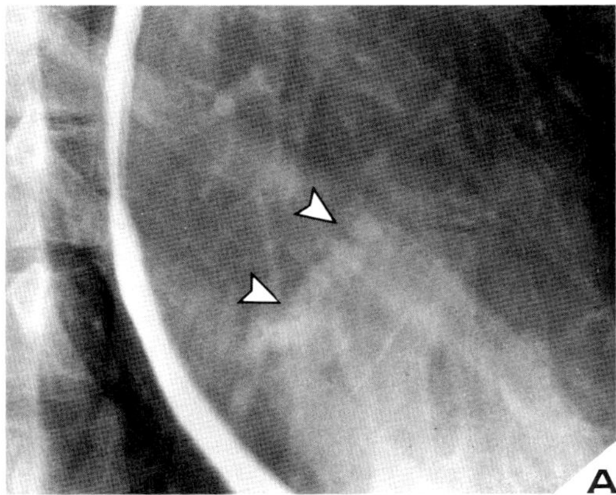

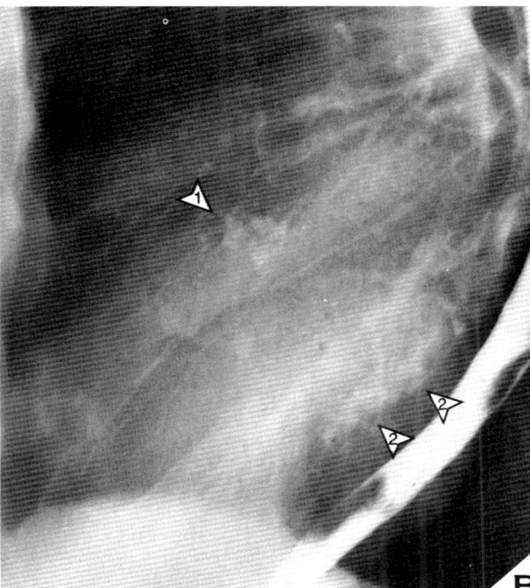

Fig. 18.35 "Physiologic" versus pathological calcification of the mitral valve. (A) Close-up of lateral chest film shows mottled calcification of the mitral leaflets *(arrows)* in a patient with mitral stenosis secondary to rheumatic heart disease. (B) Close-up of lateral chest film in another patient shows a C-shaped calcification (*arrow* 1) at the insertion of the posterior mitral leaflet. This appearance is typical of "physiologic" calcification of mitral annulus. This patient also has calcific aortic stenosis [note calcification of aortic valve (*arrows* 2)].

monary edema (Kerley A, B, and C lines) (Fig. 18.36). Further elevation of left atrial pressure leads to alveolar pulmonary edema, which manifests initially as perihilar densities (''butterfly'' pattern). Some patients with severe, longstanding mitral stenosis exhibit a prominent nodular–interstitial pattern reflecting hemosiderin deposition in the interlobular septa. (Owing to advances in therapy, hemosiderin deposition is seldom seen nowadays.) Right ventricular enlargement and dilatation of the pulmonary trunk and central pulmonary arteries are reliable plain film evidence of pulmonary arterial hypertension (Fig. 18.34). Right atrial enlargement usually indicates tricuspid insufficiency secondary to right ventricular overload.

Echocardiography

Transthoracic or transesophageal 2-D echocardiography clearly depicts the pathologic changes in the leaflets, annulus, and chordae tendineae characteristic of rheumatic mitral stenosis (Figs. 18.37 and 18.38). The ''funnel'' configuration associated with severely damaged valves is also well seen. In this acquired malformation, the functional annulus is interposed between the true annulus and the apex and papillary muscles; thus the latter, which are usually normal, are much closer to the valve orifice than normal (Fig. 18.39; see also Fig. 18.31). Conventional and color Doppler imaging demonstrates the stenotic mitral valve, as well as any coexistent mitral insufficiency, and provides data that can be used to quantitate the severity of the left ventricular inflow obstruction (Figs. 18.40 and 18.41; see Appendix). Either 2-D or M-mode echocardiography can be used to determine left atrial size. The former can also detect left atrial thrombi, especially those in the left atrial appendage, which are often difficult to demonstrate by angiography. Associated abnormalities of the aortic valve, commonly present in patients with rheumatic mitral stenosis, can be studied by various echocardiographic techniques. The clinical and plain film findings in patients with left atrial myxoma and patients with mitral stenosis are very similar; echocardiography readily differentiates the two (see Chapter 26).

MRI

Spin–echo and cine MRI have a limited ability to demonstrate the morphologic and functional abnormalities in patients with acquired mitral stenosis. At present, MRI has only a minor role in evaluation of patients with rheumatic mitral stenosis.

Cardiac Catheterization

In most instances the clinical history, physical examination, plain films, and echocardiography will establish the diagnosis of mitral stenosis and indicate its severity. Cardiac catheterization provides additional functional data. Measurements of left atrial pressure indicate the severity of the pulmonary venous hypertension. (The pulmonary capillary wedge pressure serves as an indirect measurement of left atrial pressure.) The gradient between the capillary wedge pressure and the left ventricular diastolic pressure indicates the severity of the left ventricular inlet obstruction. Although this parameter is flow dependent, a diastolic gradient of 10 mm Hg or greater at rest can be taken as

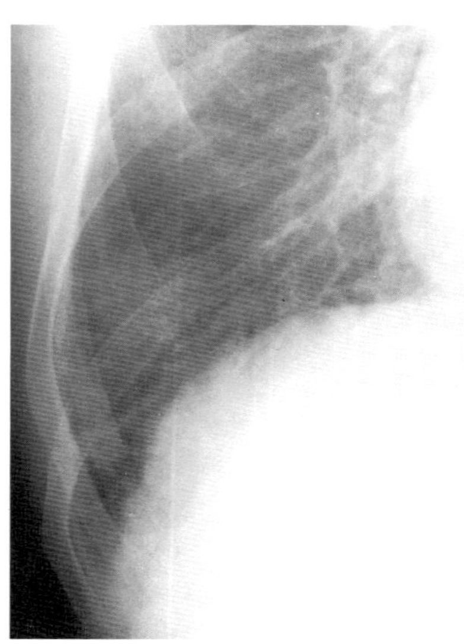

Fig. 18.36 Mitral stenosis with moderately severe pulmonary venous hypertension. Detail of chest film shows short, straight horizontal lines perpendicular to the pleural surface (Kerley B lines) at the right lung base and a small pleural effusion.

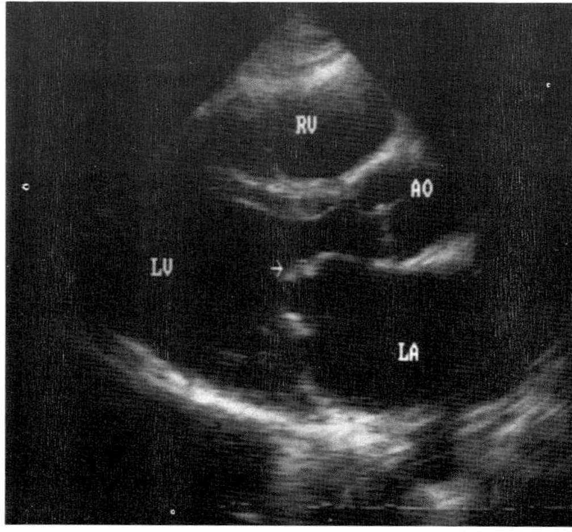

Fig. 18.37 Mitral stenosis. Two-dimensional echocardiography (parasternal long axial view, in diastole) in a patient with rheumatic heart disease. There is thickening of the free borders of the anterior and posterior leaflets of the mitral valve. The leaflets do not coapt normally and have a "domed" configuration. The left atrium is enlarged.

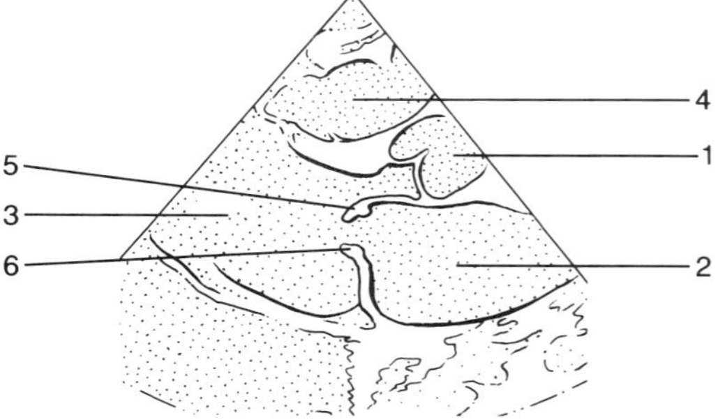

1 aorta
2 left atrium
3 left ventricle
4 right ventricle
5 thickened free border of anterior leaflet
6 thickened free border of posterior leaflet

evidence of severe mitral stenosis. Using the Gorlin modified orifice equation, one can calculate the cross-sectional area of the mitral valve. This value ranges from 0.5 to 0.8 cm^2 per square meter of body surface in most patients with symptomatic mitral stenosis. Estimates of severity derived from the catheterization data usually correlate closely with the clinical picture.

Angiocardiography

The morphologic and functional abnormalities associated with mitral stenosis can be demonstrated by selectively opacifying the left atrium and left ventricle. Coronary arteriography is performed in patients with suspected coronary artery disease and in all patients 40 years of age of older whether symptomatic or not.

Left Ventriculography. Selective left ventriculography is performed via a catheter introduced through a femoral artery puncture. The long axial projection (60° right anterior oblique with a 30° craniocaudal tube tilt) is the most useful for evaluating mitral valve pathology. The elongated right anterior oblique view is useful for demonstrating the papillary muscles and their relation to the annulus. In classical mitral stenosis, the shape of the mitral valve apparatus is best seen in diastole, as nonopacified blood passes from the left atrium into the left ventricle. The anterior and posterior leaflets are clearly seen, and the heads of the papillary muscles are close to the functional annulus. Filling defects are seen beneath the mitral valve apparatus, in the vicinity of the commissures. During systole the anterior and posterior leaflets come together, the thickened borders of the leaflets appearing as a filling defect in the midportion of the mitral

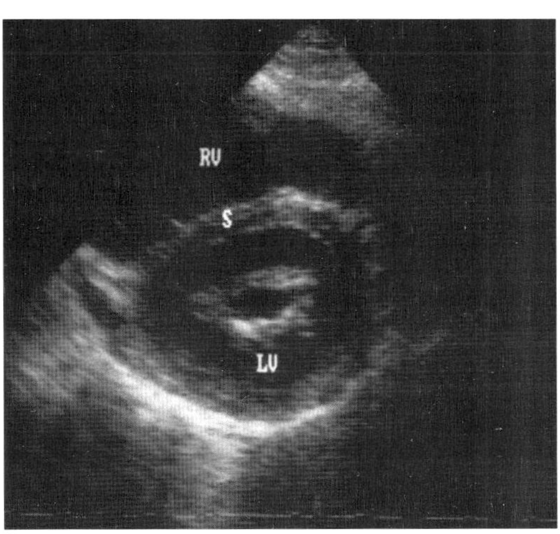

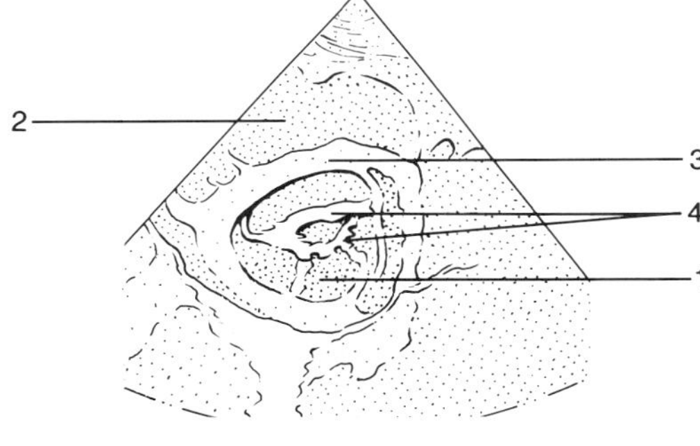

Fig. 18.38 Mitral stenosis. Two-dimensional echocardiogram (parasternal short-axis view, in diastole) in a patient with rheumatic heart disease shows a restricted mitral valve orifice and thickening of the leaflets, mainly at the commissures. The calculated mitral valve area was 1.4 cm^2 (normal, 3.0 to 3.5 cm^2).

1 left ventricle
2 right ventricle
3 ventricular septum
4 thickened mitral valve leaflets

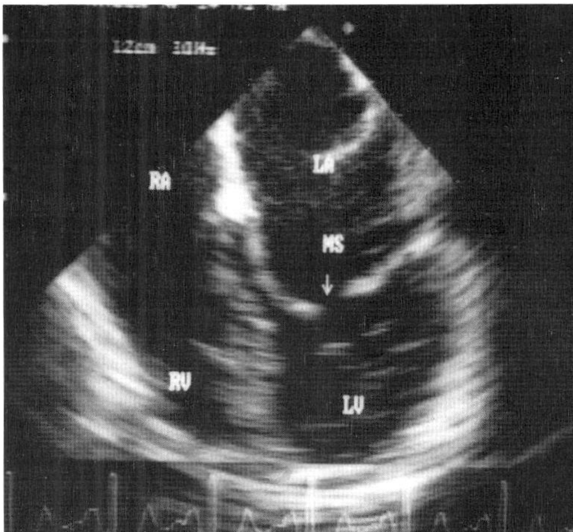

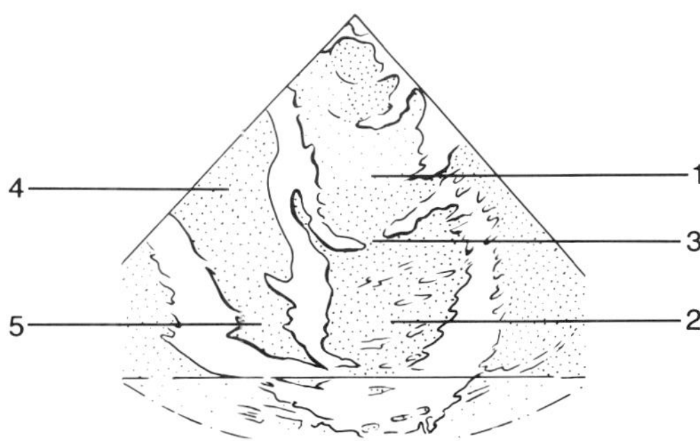

Fig. 18.39 Mitral stenosis. Transesophageal echocardiogram (4-chamber view, in diastole) demonstrates thickening and doming of the anterior and posterior leaflets of the mitral valve and narrowing of the mitral orifice. Note the apical displacement of the mitral orifice. In normal hearts the orifice of the mitral valve lies at the same level as the mural insertion of the leaflets (ie, the anatomic annulus).

1 left atrium
2 left ventricle
3 apically displaced orifice of stenotic mitral valve
4 right atrium
5 right ventricle

annulus (Fig. 18.42). A filling defect is sometimes seen caudal to the level of the commissures on the long axial projection, representing fibrosis of the subvalvular apparatus. The relations of the mitral annulus and the papillary muscles are more clearly seen on the elongated right anterior oblique projection; in patients with a "funnel" deformity of the mitral valve apparatus, the heads of the papillary muscles appear closer to the mitral annulus than normal (Fig. 18.43; see also Fig. 18.31).

Left Atriography. When the left atrium is adequately opacified, it is possible to measure the diameter of the mitral annulus, to assess the degree to which valve opening is restricted during diastole, and to detect atrial thrombi. The left atrium is opacified on the late phase of a right ventriculogram or pulmonary arteriogram; it is also opacified (by reflux) after a left ventricular injection in patients with coexistent mitral insufficiency. In each instance, the left atrium may not be opaci-

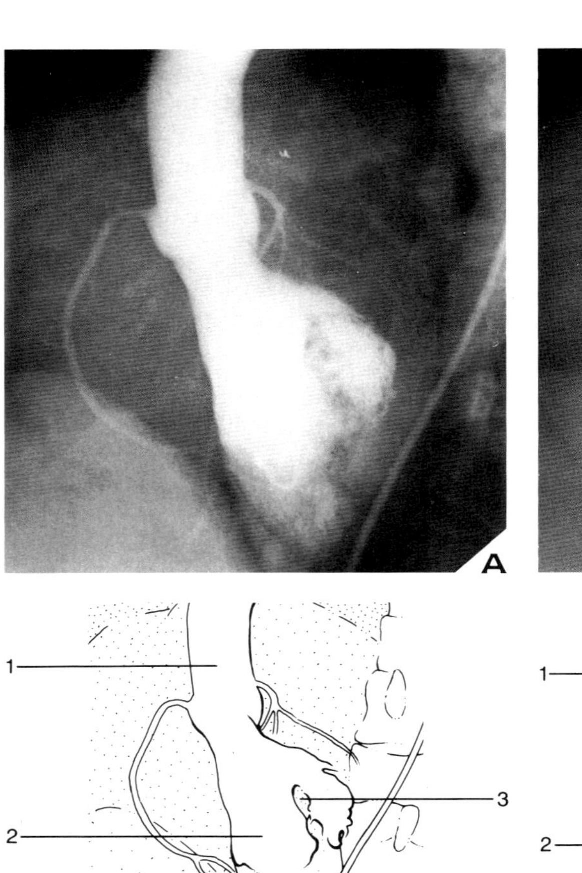

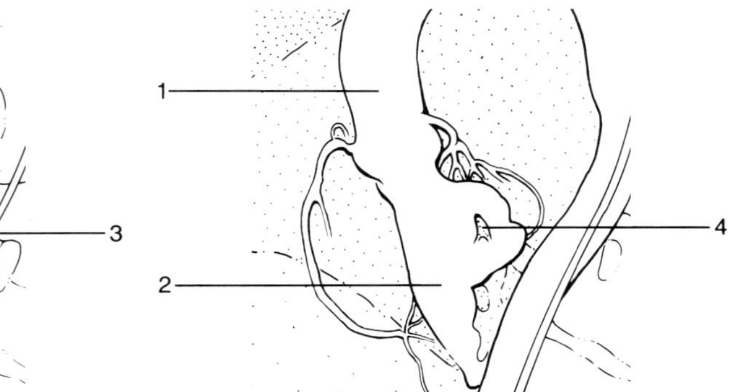

Fig. 18.42 Mitral stenosis. Selective left ventriculogram (long axis view). (A) Diastole. Mitral valve opening is markedly restricted. (B) Systole. There is a filling defect in the area normally occupied by the free borders of the mitral leaflets, presumably produced by fibrous tissue in the posteromedial commissure and thickening of the valve leaflets.

1	aorta	4	filling defect produced by thickened leaflets and fibrosis in the posteromedial commissure
2	left ventricle		
3	restricted opening of mitral valve		

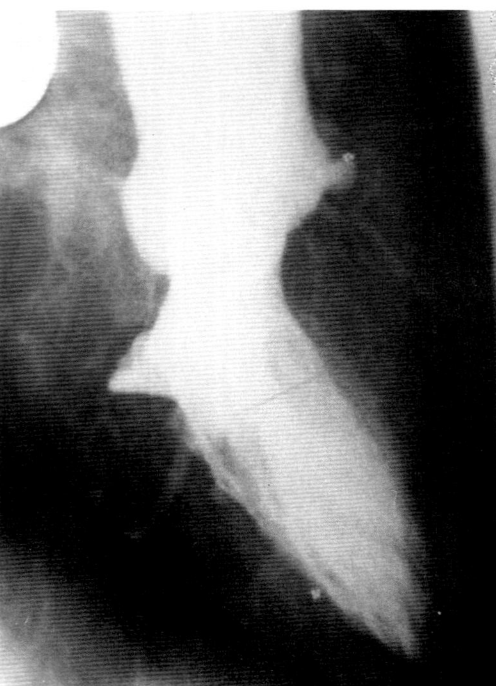

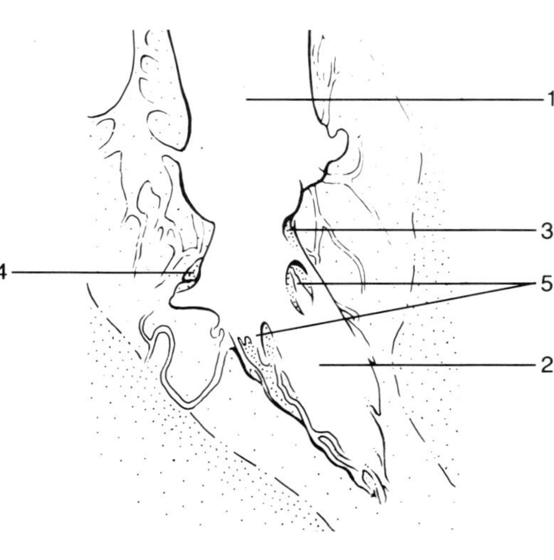

Fig. 18.43 Mitral stenosis. Left ventriculogram (elongated right anterior oblique view, in diastole). The mitral valve is well seen in diastole, which is not the case for normal mitral valves. The functional (false) annulus is displaced apically. The heads of the papillary muscles are unusually close to the dynamic annulus owing to the shortness of the chordae tendineae and fusion of the posteromedial commissure of the mitral valve.

1	aorta	4	posterolateral commissure
2	left ventricle	5	heads of papillary muscles
3	anterolateral commissure		

fied densely enough to demonstrate structural detail or exclude a left atrial thrombus. If necessary, the left atrium can be selectively opacified by puncturing the atrial septum and passing a catheter from the right atrium into the left atrium (Fig. 18.44).

MITRAL INSUFFICIENCY

Mitral insufficiency is defined as the inability of the mitral valve apparatus to completely seal the mitral orifice during ventricular systole. It can result from abnormalities of the leaflets, subvalvular apparatus, and/or annulus. The most frequent cause of isolated mitral insufficiency in Europe and the Western Hemisphere is prolapse of the mitral valve ("floppy" mitral valve), which accounts for 38 percent of all cases. Rheumatic heart disease (31 percent) is the second most frequent cause. Less common causes include rupture of the chordae tendineae, infective endocarditis, papillary muscle ischemia secondary to coronary artery disease, and distortion of the subvalvular apparatus secondary to left ventricular dilatation.

PATHOGENESIS

Prolapsed ("Floppy") Mitral Valve

This disorder, which results in moderate to severe mitral insufficiency, is believed to be caused by age-related changes engrafted on a congenitally malformed valve. Pathologically, all three components of the mitral valve apparatus are affected (Fig. 18.45). The mitral annulus is dilated and sometimes calcified. The leafets are thickened and redundant. The chordae tendineae are thick and elongated, and often are fused or ruptured. Usually there is prolapse of both leaflets or only of the posterior leaflet; isolated prolapse of the anterior leaflet is unusual. Complications include infective endocarditis and systemic embolization of noninfected thrombotic vegetations, which frequently form on the valve leaflets. Prolapse of the mitral valve must be differentiated from midsystolic click syndrome, a common (and relatively innocuous) condition in which mitral valve function is only minimally affected.

Prolapse of the mitral valve is sometimes seen in patients with dysautonomia, a disorder of the autonomic nervous sys-

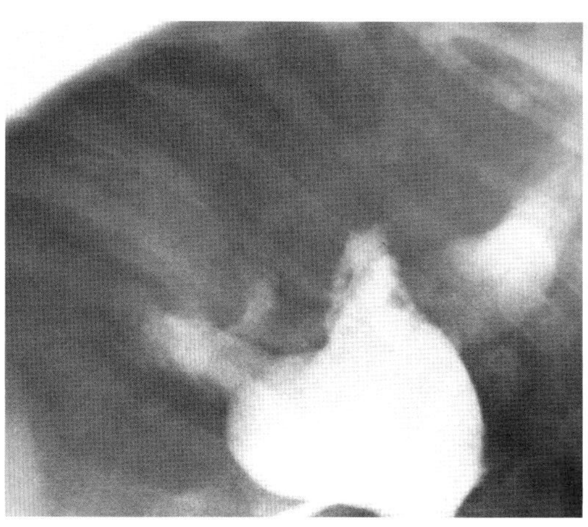

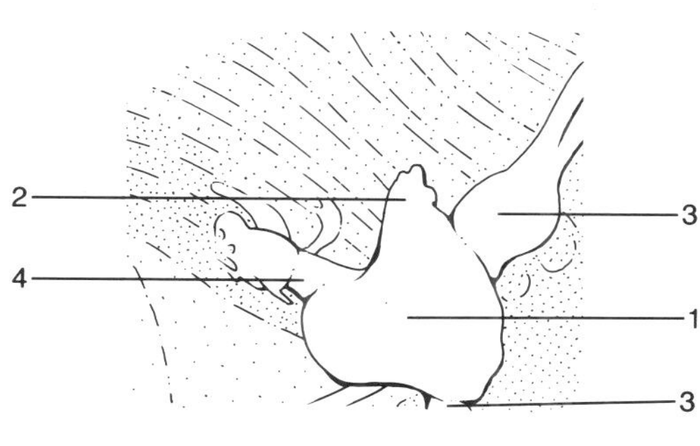

Fig. 18.44 Mitral stenosis. Transseptal selective left atriogram (elongated right anterior oblique projection) demonstrates moderate left atrial enlargement. The mitral valve is narrow and has a funnel-shaped appearance.

1	left atrium	3	pulmonary veins
2	left atrial appendage	4	stenotic mitral valve

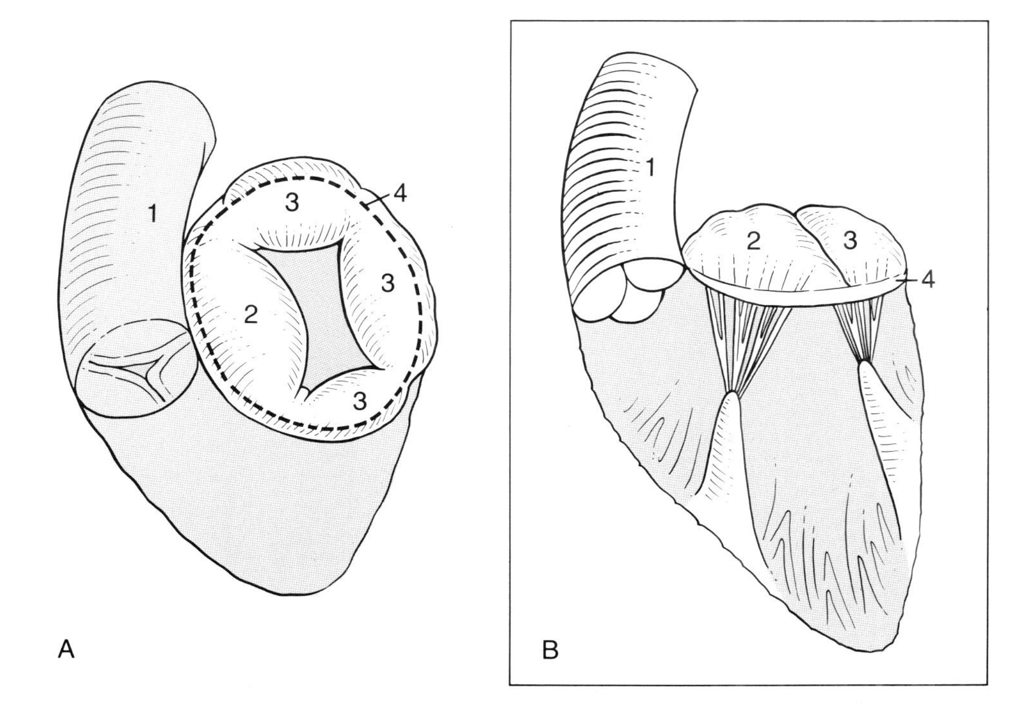

Fig. 18.45 Prolapse of both mitral leaflets. (A) Superior view; (B) Lateral view. Both leaflets are redundant and protrude into the left atrium. The chordae tendineae are elongated.

1	aorta	3	prolapsed posterior mitral leaflet
2	prolapsed anterior mitral leaflet	4	mitral annulus

tem characterized by defective lacrimation, blotchy skin lesions (secondary to vasomotor instability), emotional lability, motor incoordination, and hyporeflexia.

Coronary Artery Disease

Papillary muscle dysfunction secondary to fibrosis can lead to severe mitral insufficiency in patients with ischemic heart disease. Rupture of a papillary muscle, resulting in severe mitral insufficiency of abrupt onset, can also occur, although it is less common.

Infective Endocarditis

Infection results in perforation or partial destruction of the mitral leaflets. Involvement of the aortic and/tricuspid valves, leading to aortic and/or tricuspid insufficiency, may also be present, particularly in intravenous drug abusers.

CLINICAL FEATURES

Chronic Mitral Insufficiency

Early in the course of the disease, before the onset of significant left ventricular failure, there are no symptoms; at this stage, a cardiac murmur may be the only evidence of mitral insufficiency. Later, when left ventricular function deteriorates, symptoms of left ventricular failure (eg, shortness of breath) appear.

The classical murmur of mitral insufficiency is a pansystolic murmur which is loudest at the apex and radiates towards the left axilla and left lung base. There may be an associated diastolic rumble. In patients whose mitral insufficiency is mainly due to prolapse of the posterior leaflet, the murmur radiates anteriorly toward the aortic root and is maximal parasternally. In such patients the murmur may radiate into the neck along the course of the carotid arteries. Patients with severe mitral in-

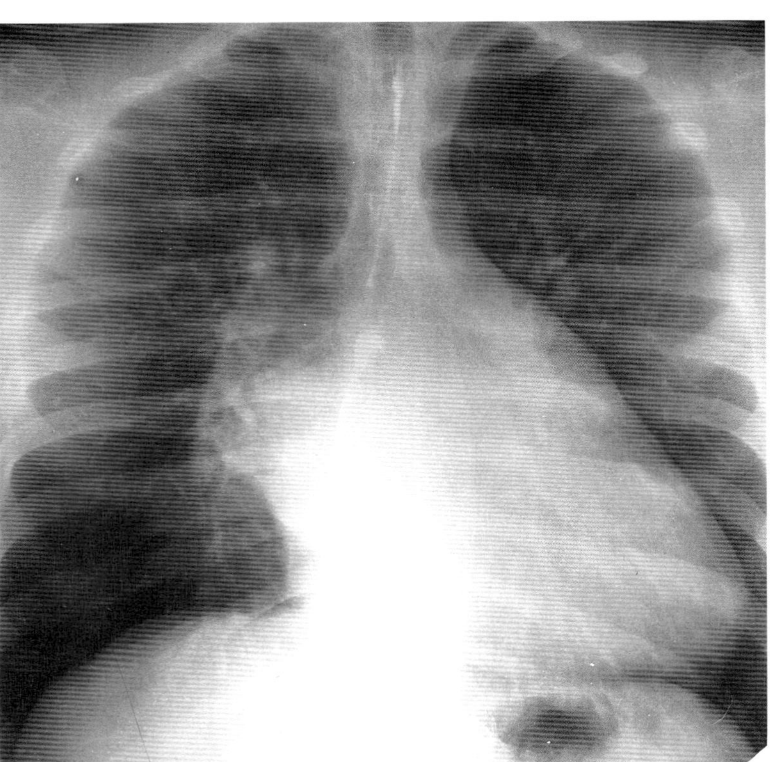

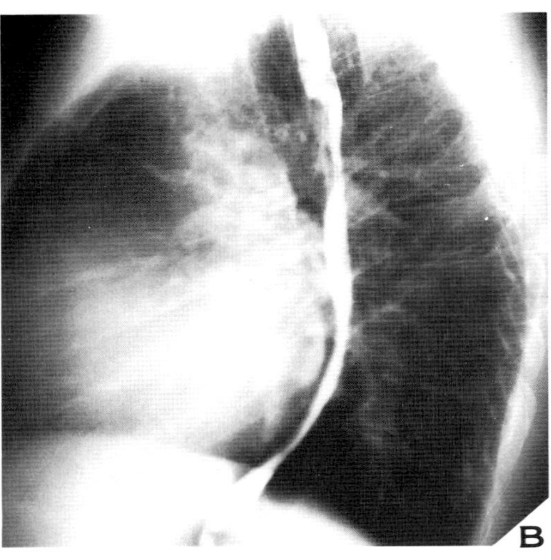

Fig. 18.46 Moderately severe mitral insufficiency. (A) Posteroanterior and (B) lateral chest views show marked cardiomegaly with prominence of the left ventricle, which projects inferiorly, posteriorly, and to the left. The left atrium is markedly enlarged, forming a double density within the heart and extending to the right of the right atrial contour. The bulge of the left upper heart border represents the left atrial appendage. On the lateral, the enlarged left atrium displaces the esophagus posteriorly. The pulmonary vasculature is normal. The absence of pulmonary venous hypertension in a patient with an enlarged left atrium is characteristic of isolated mitral insufficiency.

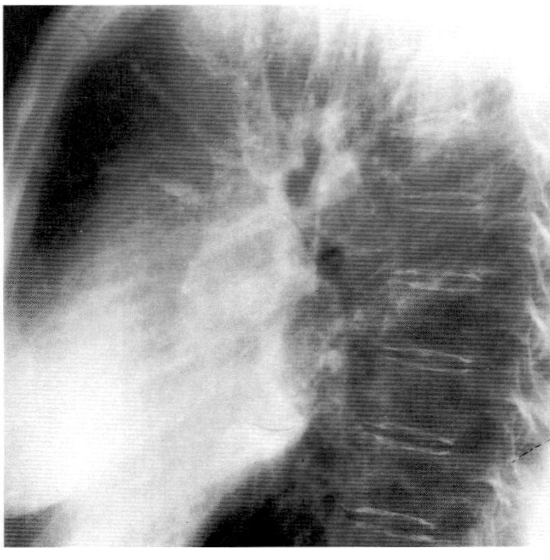

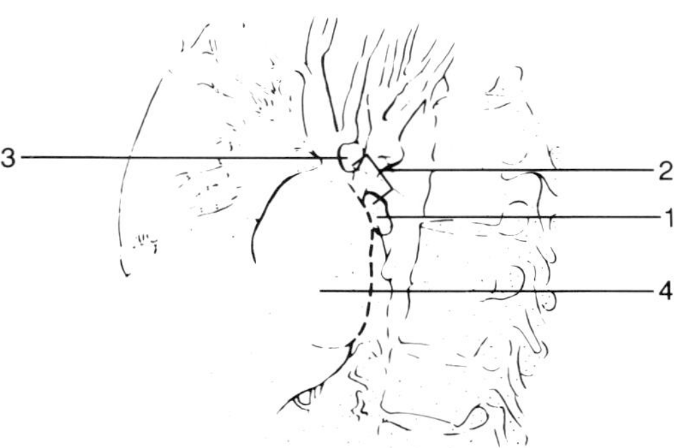

Fig. 18.47 Left atrial enlargement due to mitral insufficiency. The enlarged left atrium bulges posteriorly above the left atrium. The left mainstem bronchus is displaced posteriorly. (The carina lies midway between the right upper lobe bronchus and the left upper lobe bronchus, both of which appear as circular images on the lateral projection.)

1	left upper lobe bronchus	3	right upper lobe bronchus
2	left main bronchus	4	enlarged left atrium

competence associated with marked left atrial enlargement may have a pulsatile precordial lift.

Electrocardiograms typically reveal left ventricular enlargement and P-wave abnormalities characteristic of left atrial enlargement ("P-mitrale"). Atrial fibrillation is very common. Patients with pulmonary hypertension secondary to left ventricular failure have ECG findings of right ventricular hypertrophy.

Acute Mitral Insufficiency

Patients with acute mitral insufficiency (eg, secondary to infective endocarditis or rupture of the chordae tendineae or a papillary muscle) present with clinical signs of congestive heart failure and pulmonary edema, the severity varying with the degree of valvular incompetence. Auscultation reveals an apical systolic murmur which varies in intensity and timing.

IMAGING AND INVASIVE DIAGNOSIS

Plain Films

In patients with moderate to severe mitral insufficiency, frontal and lateral films show left atrial and left ventricular enlargement. On the frontal projection, left atrial enlargement is manifested by a double density within the cardiac silhouette and straightening or convexity of the left heart border owing to enlargement of the left atrial appendage (Fig. 18.46). The lateral projection reveals posterior displacement of the left main bronchus and esophagus (Figs. 18.46B and 18.47). If the left ventricular end diastolic pressure is not elevated, the pulmonary vasculature is usually normal. (Although measurements of lung water indicate that subclinical pulmonary edema is present in some asymptomatic patients with mitral insufficiency, this is usually not evident radiographically.) When the left ventricle decompensates, plain films show the typical findings of pulmonary venous hypertension [cephalization and interstitial edema (Kerley A, B, and C lines)] and/or alveolar edema (Fig. 18.48).

In patients with longstanding mitral insufficiency and chronically increased pulmonary vascular resistance, chest films demonstrate the typical findings of pulmonary arterial hypertension: enlargement of the right ventricle and dilatation of the pulmonary trunk and central pulmonary vessels. The right atrium is often enlarged secondary to tricuspid insufficiency (Fig. 18.48). In some instances, right ventricular enlargement may be difficult to appreciate owing to the superimposed left ventricular enlargement.

Chest films of patients with acute mitral insufficiency (eg, secondary to infective endocarditis or rupture of the chordae tendineae or a papillary muscle) typically show a normal-sized heart and central pulmonary edema.

Echocardiography

Echocardiography demonstrates the morphology of the mitral annulus, leaflets, chordae tendineae, and papillary muscles, as well as the degree of mitral insufficiency and the presence of complications (eg, endocarditis). The leaflets and subvalvular apparatus are seen to best advantage on four-chamber and long axial sections, on which the leaflets appear as a strand-like

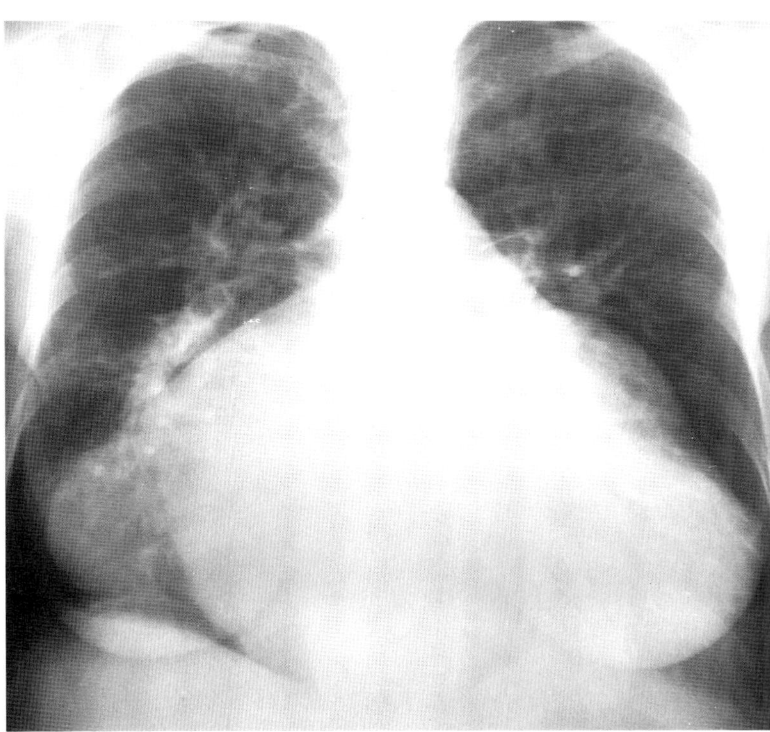

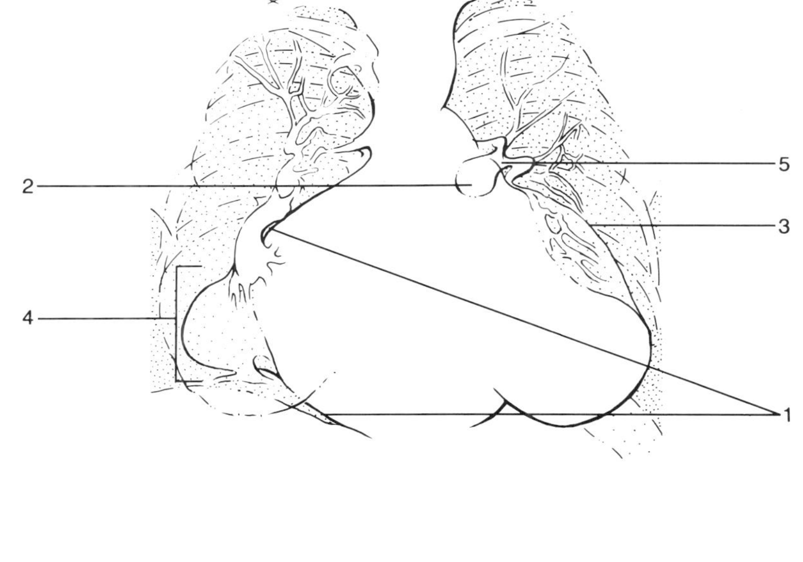

1 right border of left atrium
2 elevated left main bronchus
3 prominent left atrial appendage
4 lateral border of right atrium
5 pulmonary trunk

Fig. 18.48 Severe mitral insufficiency. Posteroanterior chest film in a patient with severe mitral insufficiency, pulmonary arterial hypertension, and tricuspid insufficiency demonstrates a huge left atrium, which appears as a double density within the heart; the left and right inferior borders of the left atrium reach the diaphragm and the left main bronchus is markedly elevated. Both the left ventricle and the right atrium are markedly enlarged, the latter structure forming a bulge along the right lower heart border. The pulmonary trunk is prominent. There is mild interstitial pulmonary edema. The combination of pulmonary hypertension (manifested by the dilated pulmonary trunk) and interstitial pulmonary edema indicates the presence of significant left ventricular failure.

complex (Figs. 18.49 to 18.51). In patients with mitral insufficiency the leaflets are usually larger and thicker than normal. The leaflets do not coapt normally and protrude into the left atrium during systole. Doppler images demonstrate a regurgitant jet extending from the valve into the left atrium; the larger the jet, the more severe the insufficiency (Figs. 18.52 and 18.53; see Appendix).

In patients with longstanding disease, the size of the left atrium correlates well with the degree of mitral insufficiency. Whereas the left atrium is invariably enlarged in patients with longstanding severe mitral insufficiency, it is usually *not* enlarged in patients with acute mitral incompetence, no matter how severe.

Two-dimensional echocardiography usually allows a definitive diagnosis of acute mitral insufficiency. Transesophageal echocardiography is particularly sensitive in this regard. Perforation of a leaflet in a patient with infective endocarditis is clearly shown with this modality (echo-dense images representing vegetations along the borders of the leaflets also may be seen in such cases). Loosened support of the affected leaflet indicates rupture of the chordae tendinae or a papillary muscle; the displaced leaflet appears as an echo-dense image which is displaced into the left atrium during systole. Color Doppler imaging can be used to document the severity of the mitral insufficiency and to confirm the diagnosis of perforated leaflet.

MRI

Spin–echo images with electrocardiographic gating demonstrate enlargement of the left ventricle and increased mitral valve area, indirectly indicating the presence of mitral insufficiency (Fig. 18.54). Displacement of the leaflets may be apparent in patients with prolapse of the posterior and/or anterior leaflets. Enlargement of a mitral leaflet is a common finding, particularly in patients with prolapse of one or both leaflets or end-stage cardiomyopathy; it is uncommon in those with infective endocarditis or rheumatic mitral valve disease. Abnormal left ventricular wall motion and abnormal systolic motion of the mitral leaflets may be evident in patients with mitral insufficiency secondary to myocardial ischemia.

Cine MRI demonstrates a low-intensity signal in the left atrium, which represents turbulent regurgitant flow through the relatively narrow mitral orifice (Fig. 18.55). Although cine MRI is very sensitive in detecting mitral insufficiency, false positives sometimes occur. Nor does cine MRI accurately indicate the

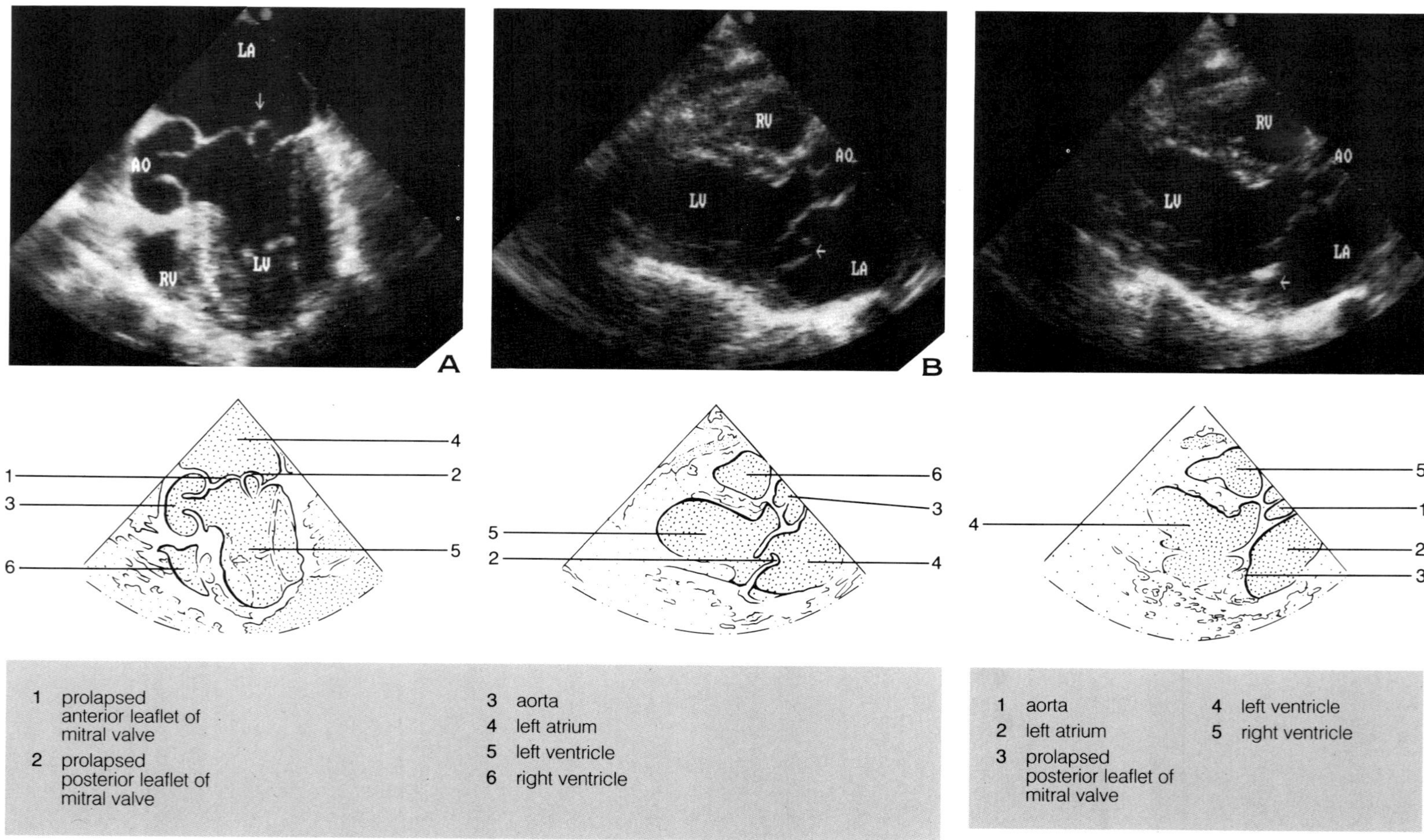

1 prolapsed anterior leaflet of mitral valve
2 prolapsed posterior leaflet of mitral valve
3 aorta
4 left atrium
5 left ventricle
6 right ventricle

Fig. 18.49 Mitral valve prolapse. Transesophageal echocardiogram. (A) Frontal long axial view through left ventricular outflow tract (systole) shows the anterior leaflet of the mitral valve protruding into the left atrium (it projects above the level of the anatomic mitral annulus). (B) Parasternal long axial scan in systole shows the posterior leaflet of the mitral valve protruding into the left atrium. The two leaflets fail to coapt, indicating mitral insufficiency.

1 aorta
2 left atrium
3 prolapsed posterior leaflet of mitral valve
4 left ventricle
5 right ventricle

Fig. 18.50 Mitral insufficiency with prolapse of the posterior leaflet and calcification of the mitral annulus. Two-dimensional echocardiogram (parasternal long-axis view, in systole) demonstrates a high-intensity echo characteristic of a calcification within the posterior portion of the mitral annulus. There is slight protrusion of the posterior leaflet of the mitral valve into the left atrium.

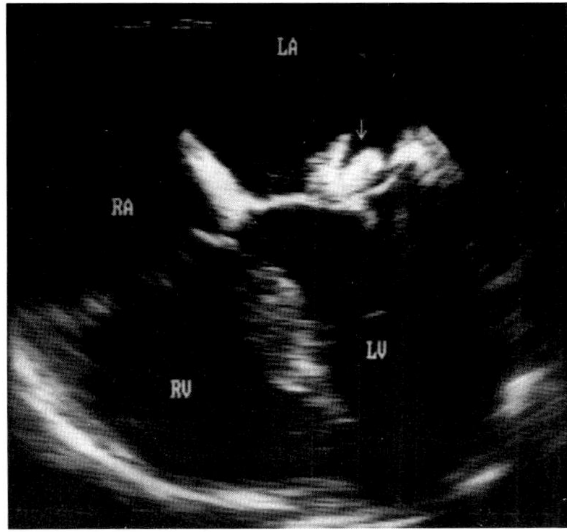

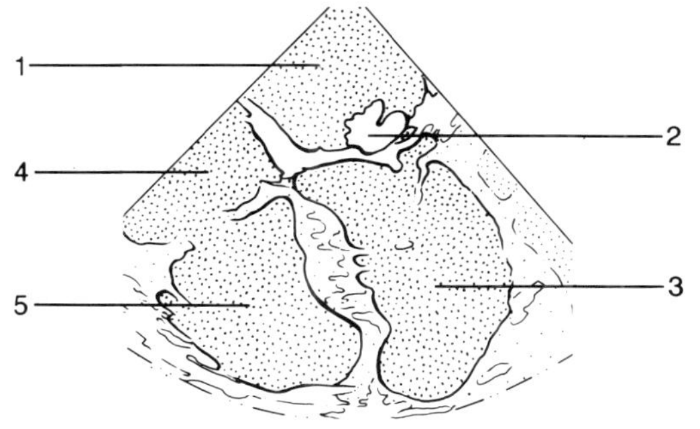

Fig. 18.51 Mitral insufficiency secondary to valvular endocarditis. Transesophageal echocardiogram (four-chamber view, in systole) demonstrates an echogenic structure immediately above the mitral valve. On the real-time study it was attached to the atrial surface of the anterior leaflet. The vegetation prevents the leaflets from coapting normally, resulting in mitral insufficiency.

1 left atrium
2 vegetation on anterior leaflet of mitral valve
3 left ventricle
4 right atrium
5 right ventricle

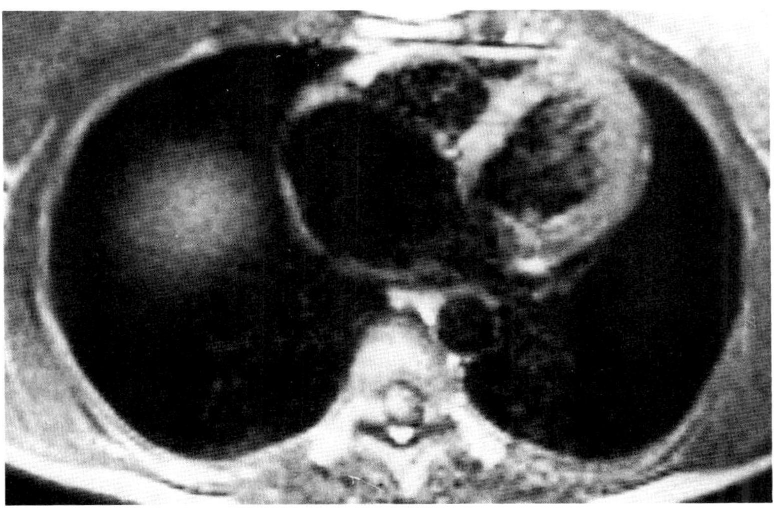

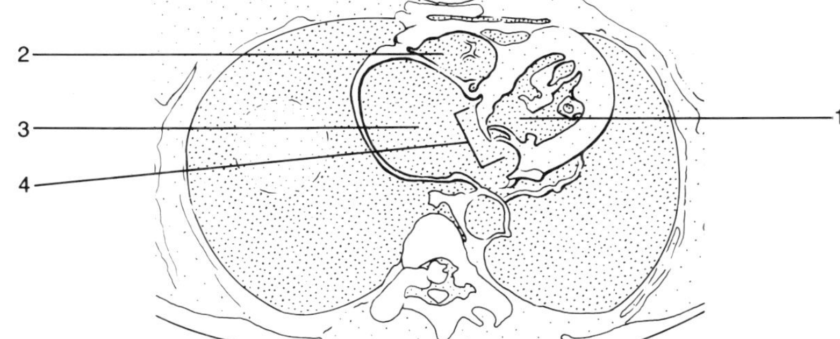

1 left ventricle
2 right ventricle
3 left atrium
4 mitral valve

Fig. 18.54 Mitral insufficiency. Axial spin–echo MR image at the level of the atrioventricular valves shows mild enlargement of the mitral annulus.

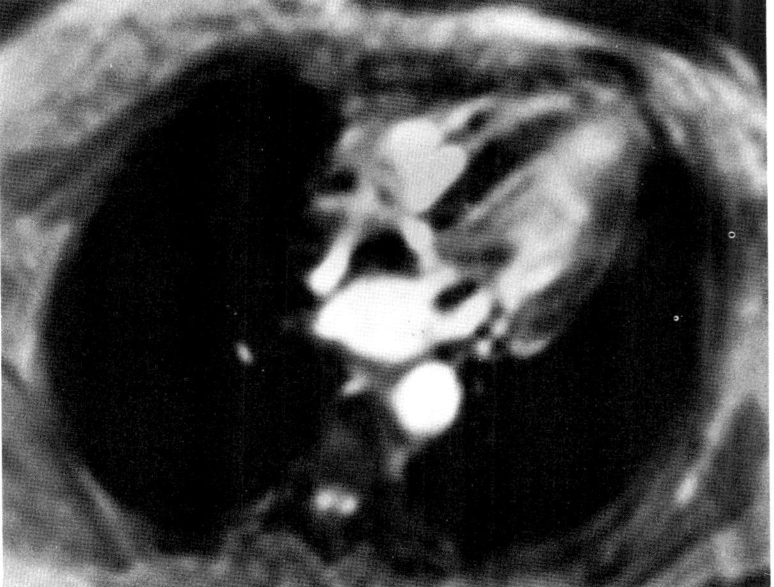

1 left ventricle
2 left atrium
3 right ventricle
4 regurgitant jet through mitral valve

Fig. 18.55 Mitral insufficiency. Frame of cine MRI (during systole). Axial projection at the level of the mitral valve. Note area of low signal intensity in the left atrium (just above the mitral valve) which represents regurgitant flow through the incompetent mitral valve.

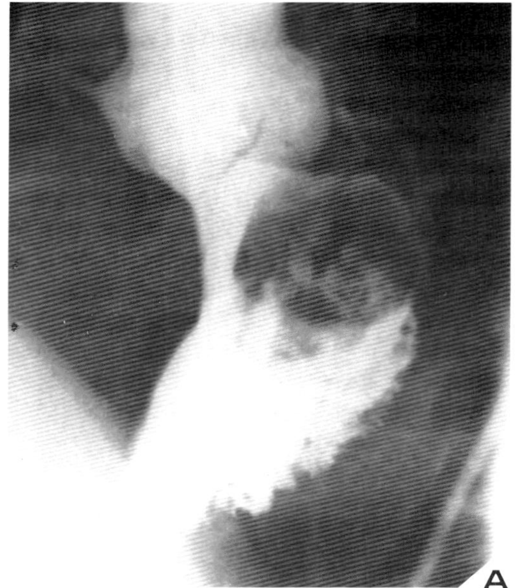

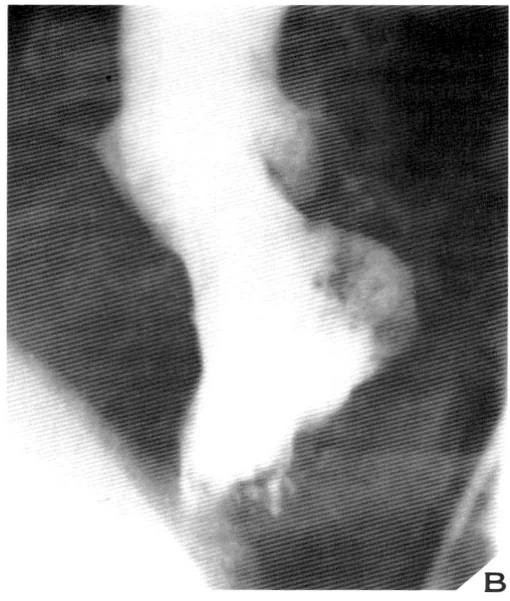

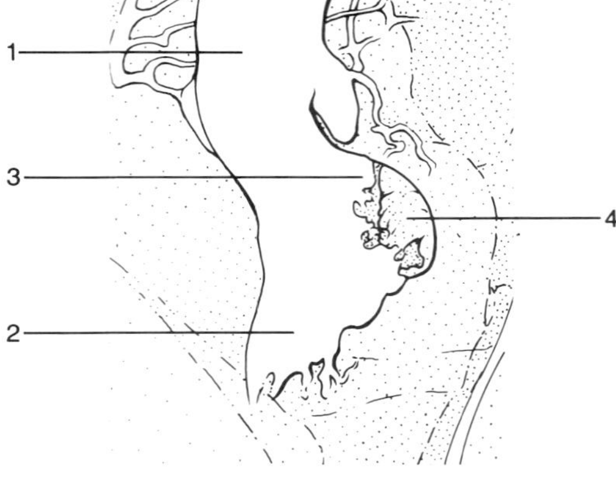

Fig. 18.56 Mild prolapse of posterior leaflet. Long axial projection of left ventriculogram in diastole (A) and systole (B). Note accumulation of contrast material beneath the posterior leaflet of the mitral valve. The posterior leaflet protrudes above the level of the mitral annulus during systole, indicating a mild degree of prolapse. The anterior leaflet is normal.

1 aorta
2 left ventricle
3 anterior leaflet of mitral valve
4 prolapsed posterior leaflet of mitral valve

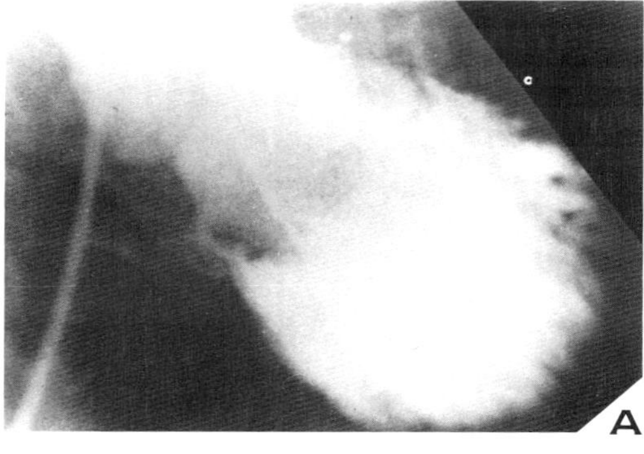

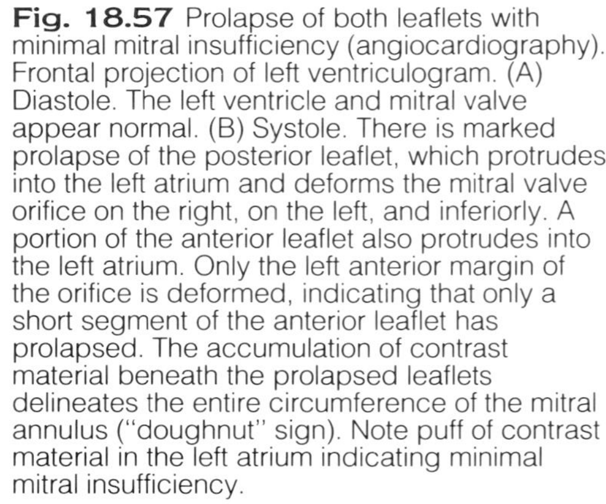

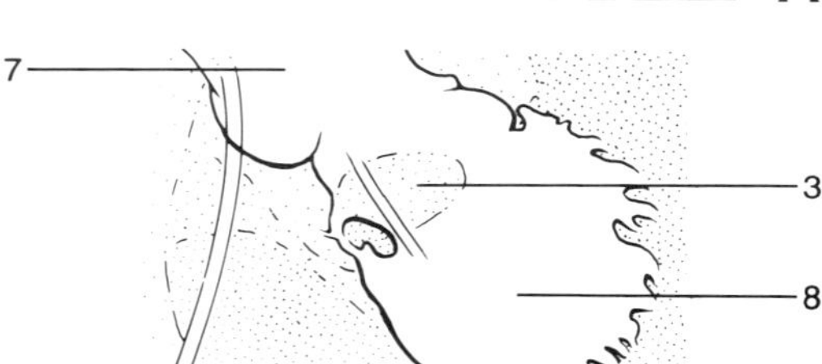

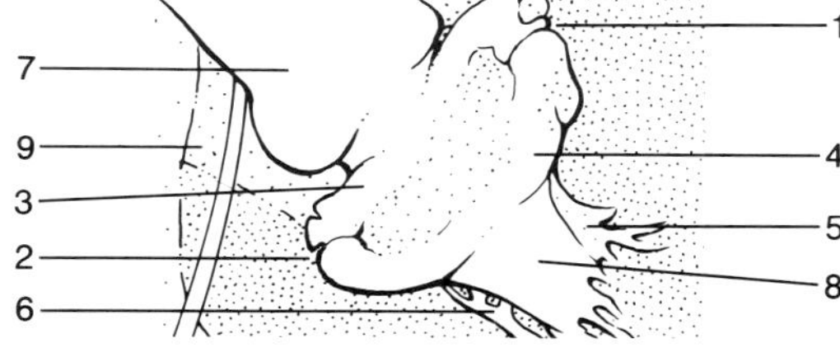

1 anterolateral commissure
2 posterolateral commissure
3 prolapsed anterior mitral leaflet
4 prolapsed posterior mitral leaflet
5 anterior papillary muscle
6 posterior papillary muscle
7 aorta
8 left ventricle
9 left atrium

Fig. 18.57 Prolapse of both leaflets with minimal mitral insufficiency (angiocardiography). Frontal projection of left ventriculogram. (A) Diastole. The left ventricle and mitral valve appear normal. (B) Systole. There is marked prolapse of the posterior leaflet, which protrudes into the left atrium and deforms the mitral valve orifice on the right, on the left, and inferiorly. A portion of the anterior leaflet also protrudes into the left atrium. Only the left anterior margin of the orifice is deformed, indicating that only a short segment of the anterior leaflet has prolapsed. The accumulation of contrast material beneath the prolapsed leaflets delineates the entire circumference of the mitral annulus ("doughnut" sign). Note puff of contrast material in the left atrium indicating minimal mitral insufficiency.

severity of the insufficiency, because the appearance of the regurgitant jet and the depth to which it penetrates the left atrial cavity depend on the imaging plane and other technical factors.

Cardiac Catheterization

The main role of cardiac catheterization is to measure the left ventricular pressure, particularly the end diastolic pressure, and left atrial pressure, which can be measured directly or indirectly (pulmonary wedge pressure). Right ventricular catheterization, which is needed to verify pulmonary arterial pressure and to assess pulmonary resistance, is routinely performed.

Angiocardiography

Mitral insufficiency is best demonstrated on left ventriculograms obtained in the left and right anterior oblique projections with cranial angulation of the tube, which show abnormal movement of the valve leaflets and reflux into the left atrium during systole (Figs. 18.56 and 18.57). (In patients with an irritable left ventricle, the injection of contrast material may induce premature ventricular contractions. Because dense opacification of the left ventricle is necessary to demonstrate left atrial reflux, an injection made during a ventricular ectopic beat may fail to detect mitral insufficiency or may not accurately indicate its severity. An injection made during a premature ventricular beat may also produce artifactual mitral insufficiency. These pitfalls can be avoided by limiting the analysis to contractions that occur during periods of regular cardiac rhythm.)

The appearance of the regurgitant jet often indicates the nature of the underlying abnormality: A wide jet usually indicates malfunction of both leaflets. An anterior jet, just behind the aortic valve, usually indicates prolapse of the posterior leaflet (Fig. 18.58A). Conversely, a posterior jet (ie, one directed towards

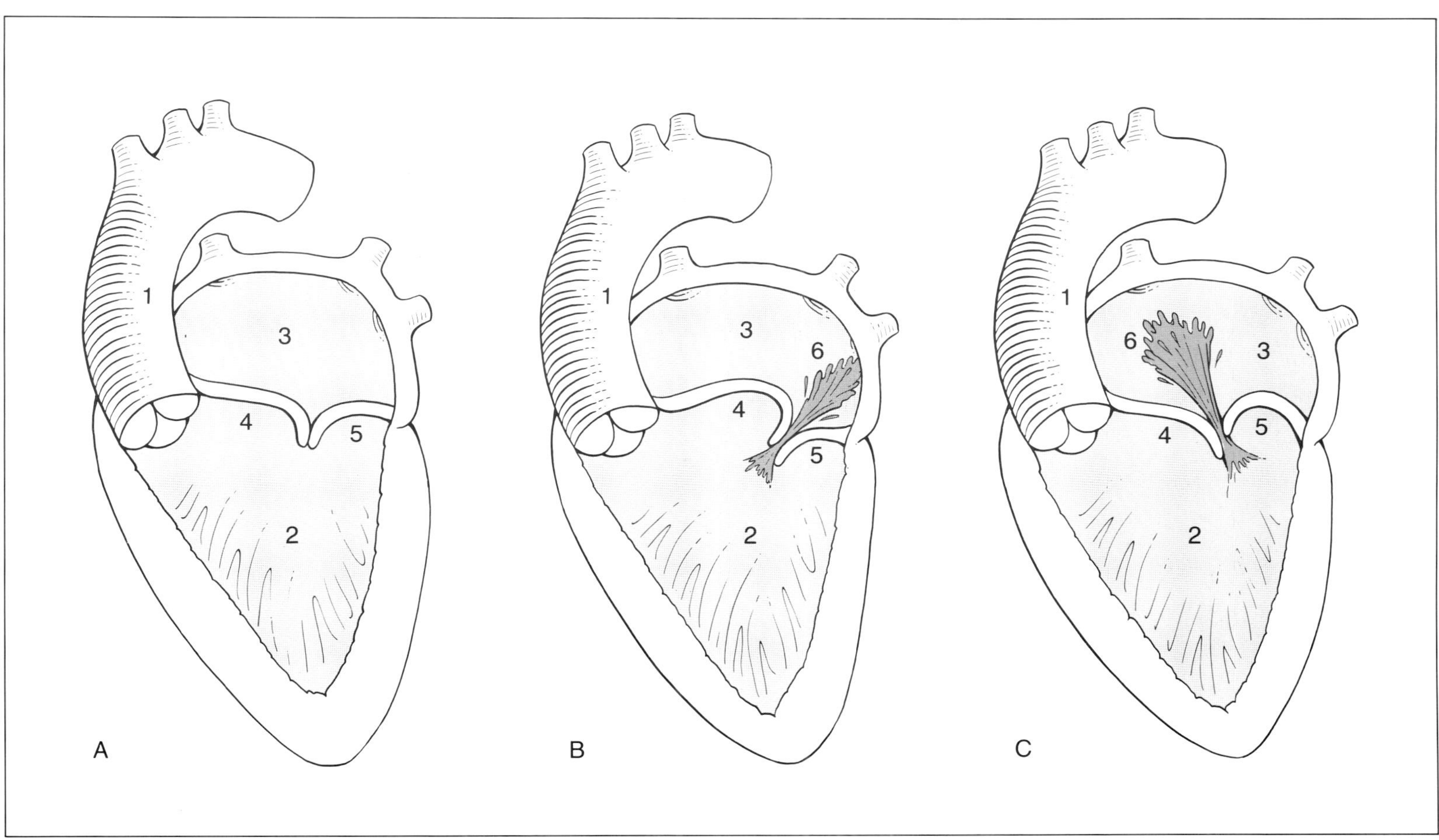

Fig. 18.58 Direction of regurgitant jet in prolapse of the mitral valve leaflets. (A) Normal mitral valve; (B) prolapsed anterior leaflet; (C) prolapsed posterior leaflet.

1 aorta
2 left ventricle
3 left atrium
4 anterior mitral leaflet
5 posterior mitral leaflet
6 regurgitant jet

the posterior wall of the left atrium) usually indicates malfunction of the anterior leaflet (Figs. 18.58B and 18.59). When the regurgitant jet is located close to the posterior medial commissure, it is best seen in the right anterior oblique projection. On the other hand, jets in the vicinity of the anterolateral commissure are more clearly depicted in the long axial projection. In patients with a malfunctioning posterior leaflet, the regurgitant jet is directed anteriorly, towards the aorta.

The severity of mitral insufficiency is graded according to the size of the left atrium and the rate at which it becomes opacified after contrast material is injected into the left ventricle. In minimal (Grade I) mitral insufficiency the left atrium is not enlarged and is only slightly opacified (ie, its margins are only partially outlined by refluxed contrast material). In moderate (Grade II) mitral insufficiency the left atrium is not enlarged; although its margins are clearly outlined by contrast material, the lumen remains less densely opacified than the left ventricle throughout the cardiac cycle (Fig. 18.60). In severe (Grade III) mitral insufficiency the left atrium is large and densely opacified throughout the cardiac cycle (Fig. 18.61). Although opacification of the

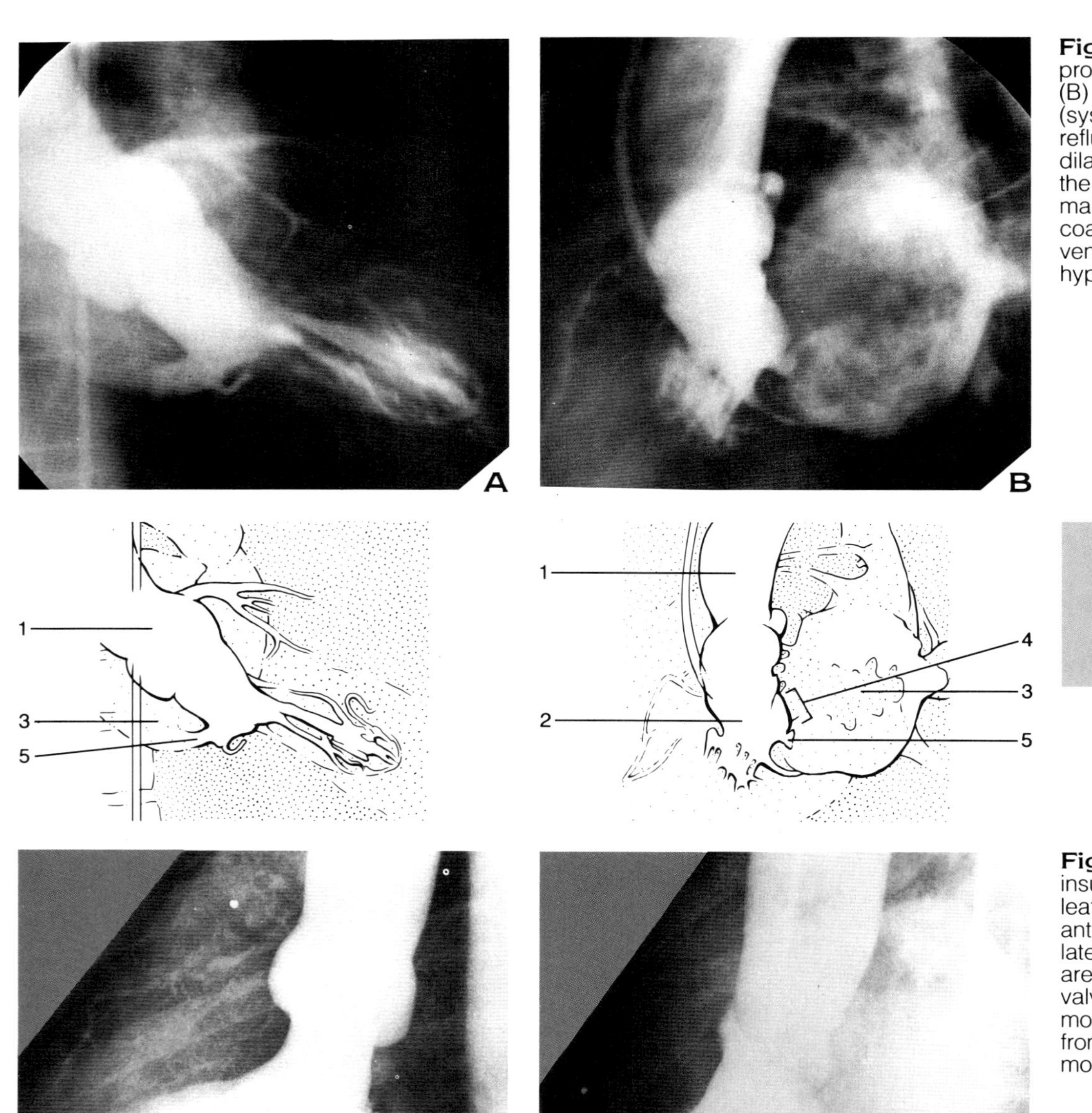

Fig. 18.59 Mitral insufficiency secondary to prolapse of the anterior leaflet. (A) Frontal and (B) lateral projections of left ventriculogram (systole) demonstrate a jet of contrast material refluxing into the left atrium, which is massively dilated. The regurgitant jet is directed towards the posterior wall of the left atrium, indicating a malfunctioning anterior leaflet which does not coapt properly with the posterior leaflet. The left ventricle contracts normally, although its wall is hypertrophied.

1 aorta
2 left ventricle
3 left atrium
4 anterior leaflet of mitral valve
5 regurgitant jet (directed posteriorly)

Fig. 18.60 Severe (Grade III) mitral insufficiency secondary to prolapse of posterior leaflet. Left ventriculogram (elongated right anterior oblique projection). (A) Early systole; (B) late systole. Left ventricular size and contractility are normal. The posterior leaflet of the mitral valve protrudes posteriorly into the left atrium. A moderate amount of contrast material refluxes from the left ventricle into the left atrium, which is moderately enlarged.

1 aorta
2 left ventricle
3 posterior leaflet of mitral valve
4 left atrium

pulmonary veins indicates abnormal stiffness of the left atrial wall, it does not reliably indicate the severity of the mitral insufficiency.

For many years cardiac catheterization and cine angiocardiography have been the standard modalities for confirming the diagnosis of mitral insufficiency and assessing its severity. However, because angiographic estimates of severity are imprecise, many clinicians now rely on echocardiography for both diagnosis and functional analysis.

TRICUSPID VALVE

TRICUSPID STENOSIS AND INSUFFICIENCY

The tricuspid valve is affected by several conditions that cause stenosis, insufficiency, or a combination of the two. Infective endocarditis, most often the result of intravenous drug abuse, is the most common cause of tricuspid insufficiency; less frequent causes include trauma, carcinoid syndrome, rheumatic heart disease, and idiopathic prolapse of the tricuspid leaflets.

PATHOGENESIS

Infective endocarditis leads to rapid destruction of the leaflets. Trauma causes flaring of the affected leaflet (usually the anterior leaflet), resulting in tricuspid insufficiency; the clinical manifestations may not appear for many years after the traumatic event. In patients with the carcinoid syndrome, which may develop after serotonin-secreting tumors of the gastrointestinal tract have metastasized to the liver, the tricuspid valve becomes shrunken and deformed, resulting in both tricuspid stenosis and tricuspid insufficiency. The pulmonic valve may be similarly affected. Rheumatic heart disease can result in tricuspid stenosis or tricuspid insufficiency. Another cause of tricuspid insufficiency in patients with rheumatic heart disease is right ventricular dilatation secondary to lesions of the mitral or aortic valve. Masses in the right ventricle or right atrium obstructing the tricuspid orifice must also be considered in the differential diagnosis of tricuspid stenosis (see Chapter 26).

CLINICAL FEATURES

Tricuspid Insufficiency

Patients with tricuspid insufficiency of rapid onset (usually secondary to infectious endocarditis) typically present with pulmonary symptoms. In patients with chronic tricuspid insufficiency the physical examination reveals jugular venous distension and characteristic abnormalities of the jugular venous pulse (dominant, fused "c" and "v" waves followed by a sharp, deep "y" descent). Typically, there is a systolic murmur along the left sternal border. The murmur is often high pitched and its intensity tends to increase on inspiration. The liver is enlarged and demonstrates systolic pulsations. Patients with severe, longstanding tricuspid insufficiency have signs and symptoms of right heart failure (eg, peripheral edema, ascites).

Tricuspid Stenosis

In patients with tricuspid stenosis and a sinus rhythm, the jugular pulse demonstrates a prominent "a" wave. This finding is absent in patients with atrial fibrillation. Typically there is a

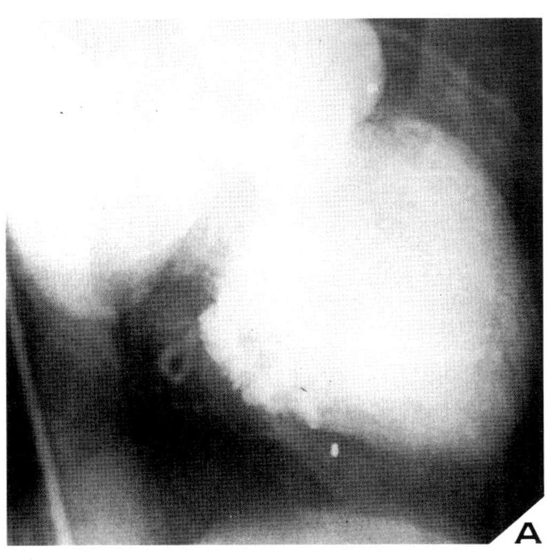

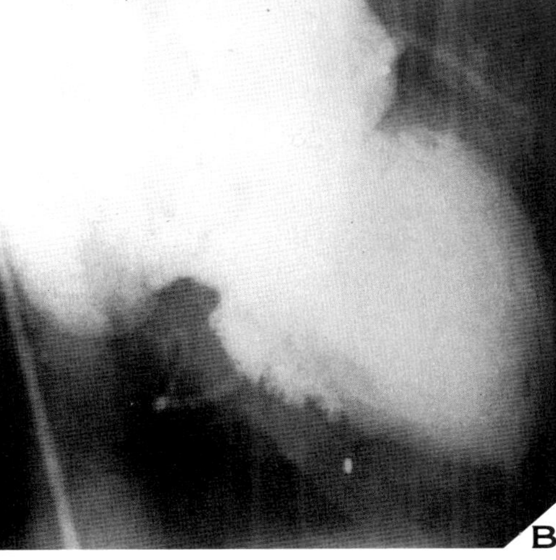

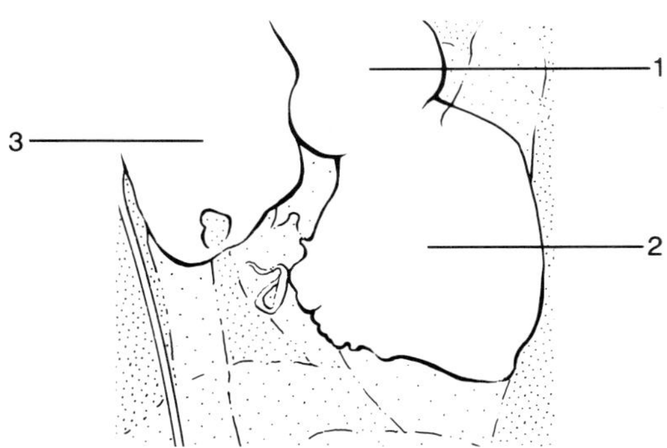

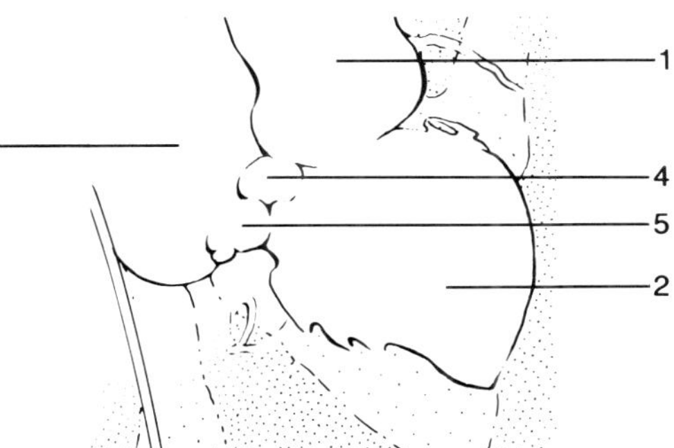

Fig. 18.61 Severe (Grade III) mitral insufficiency. Elongated right anterior oblique projection of left ventriculogram in diastole (A) and systole (B) shows a normal-sized left ventricle and an enlarged left atrium, which is completely opacified. The density of the left atrium is equal to that of the left ventricle and aorta, indicating severe mitral insufficiency.

1 aorta
2 left ventricle
3 left atrium
4 prolapsed anterior mitral leaflet
5 prolapsed posterior mitral leaflet

mid-diastolic murmur along the lower left sternal border, which increases in intensity during inspiration. The liver is usually large but not pulsatile.

IMAGING

Plain Films

Chest films show right atrial enlargement, prominence of the superior vena cava, and dilatation of the azygos vein (Fig. 18.62). The plain film findings in tricuspid insufficiency and tricuspid stenosis are similar.

Echocardiography

A reduced diastolic slope, characteristic of tricuspid stenosis, can be demonstrated by transthoracic or transesophageal echocardiography. Echocardiography will also exclude cardiac tumor, a rare cause of clinical tricuspid stenosis. Two-dimensional echocardiography accurately depicts the morphologic abnormalities in patients with tricuspid insufficiency secondary to infective endocarditis, carcinoid syndrome, traumatic lesions, and prolapse of the valve leaflets. Color Doppler demonstrates turbulence in the right atrium during systole, and is the method of choice for assessing the severity of tricuspid insufficiency (Fig. 18.63; see Appendix).

Cardiac Catheterization and Angiocardiography

Tricuspid Insufficiency. Cardiac catheterization demonstrates increased pressure in the right atrium during systole. The pressure curve is characterized by fused "c" and "v" waves followed by a sharp, deep "y" descent. Because true tricuspid insufficiency cannot be differentiated from artifactual (catheter-induced) tricuspid insufficiency, right ventriculography is of little value in detecting mild to moderate degrees of tricuspid insufficiency.

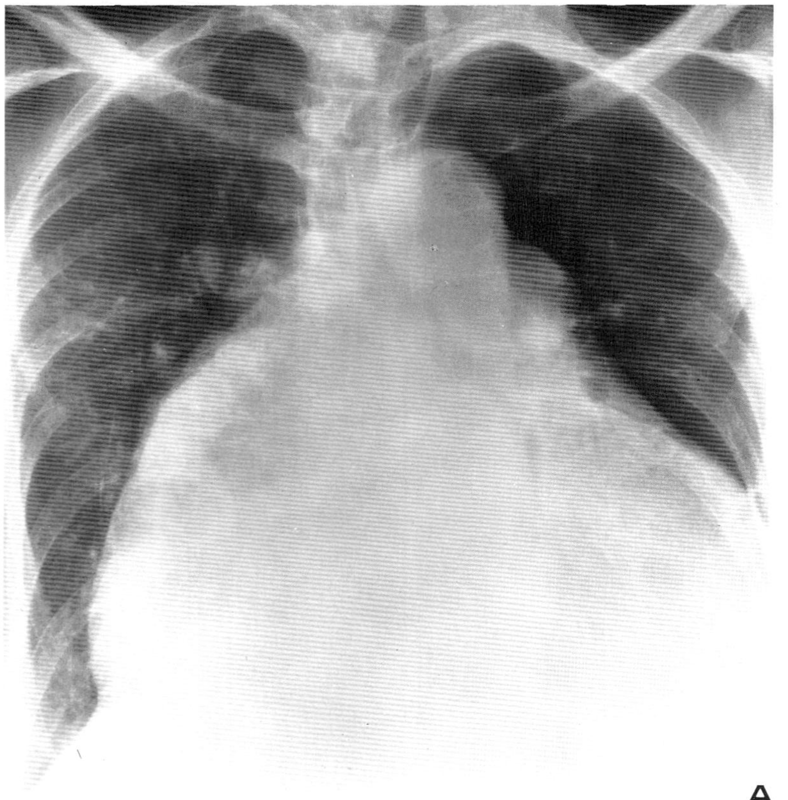

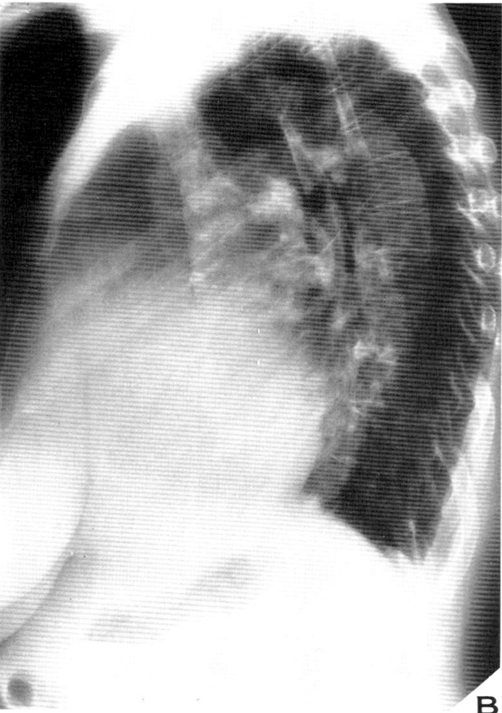

Fig. 18.62 Severe tricuspid insufficiency. (A) Frontal and (B) lateral projections show massive cardiomegaly, predominantly due to right ventricular and right atrial enlargement, with dilatation of the azygos vein. The pulmonary vasculature is normal.

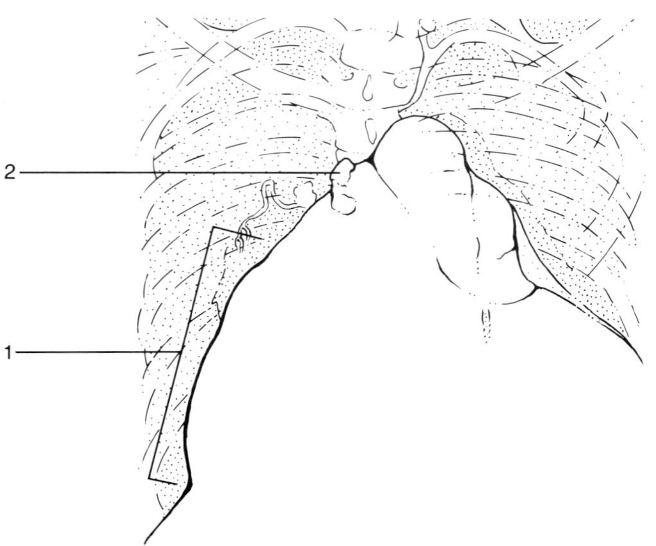

1 enlarged right atrium　　2 dilated azygos vein

Tricuspid Stenosis. During cardiac catheterization, obstruction can be demonstrated at the level of the tricuspid valve by measuring the diastolic pressure in the right atrium and right ventricle. A gradient of 4 mm Hg or more across the tricuspid valve is considered evidence of tricuspid stenosis.

PULMONIC VALVE

PULMONIC STENOSIS

Acquired pulmonic stenosis is rare. The most common cause is rheumatic endocarditis, which leads to fusion of the commissures. A less frequent cause is the carcinoid syndrome, which results in constriction of the pulmonic valve ring and retraction and fusion of the valve cusps; the intense fibrotic reaction associated with this disorder may extend into the right ventricular outflow tract.

Imaging

The radiographic and echocardiographic findings in acquired pulmonic stenosis are similar to those of the congenital disorder (see Chapter 12).

PULMONIC INSUFFICIENCY

The most common cause of acquired pulmonic insufficiency is dilatation of the valve ring secondary to pulmonary hypertension (see Chapter 24). Other causes include idiopathic dilatation of the pulmonic valve and connective tissue disorders. The pulmonic valve may also become incompetent after surgical treatment of tetralogy of Fallot or VSD (see Chapter 17).

IMAGING AND INVASIVE DIAGNOSIS

Plain Films

Chest films show right ventricular enlargement and dilatation of the pulmonary trunk similar to the findings in congenital absence of the pulmonic valve leaflets.

Echocardiography

Short-axis views through the plane of the pulmonic valve, augmented with color Doppler imaging, are highly accurate in detecting pulmonic insufficiency. Dilatation of the right ventricular outflow tract and the pulmonary trunk are clearly demonstrated, and the pulmonic valve leaflets are seen to flutter in the right ventricular outflow tract. Color Doppler imaging demonstrates a regurgitant jet during diastole; the size of the jet correlates with the severity of the insufficiency.

Angiocardiography

Angiocardiography is much less sensitive than echocardiography and is seldom used to evaluate pulmonic insufficiency.

CHAPTER 19

Myocardial Disorders

This chapter will consider a number of disorders in which the myocardium is primarily affected. In most of these conditions, known as cardiomyopathies, the etiology is unknown. The myocardium may also be affected by a number of systemic disorders of known or unknown etiology.

CARDIOMYOPATHIES

Cardiomyopathy, defined as a primary myocardial disease of undetermined cause, can take one of three forms: dilated, hypertrophic, or restricted.

DILATED CARDIOMYOPATHIES

This group of conditions is characterized by dilatation of one or both ventricles. The diagnosis of cardiomyopathy is made only when other conditions that cause ventricular dilatation have been excluded.

PATHOLOGIC FEATURES

In most instances, both ventricles undergo hypertrophy and dilatation; one or both atria are commonly dilated as well. Although the ventricular wall is usually of normal thickness, its weight is increased by 25 to 50 percent (Fig. 19.1). Subendocardial and transmural scarring and mural thrombus are frequently present. Endocardial fibrosis may be a prominent feature, particularly in children with the dilated form of endocardial fibroelastosis (see Chapter 29). When the right ventricle is involved, the tricuspid annulus enlarges, resulting in tricuspid insufficiency. In patients with left ventricular involvement, the altered geometry of the left ventricular cavity and the malalignment of the papillary muscles commonly lead to mitral insufficiency.

Microscopically, there is myocardial hypertrophy and interstitial infiltration of inflammatory cells (myositis), with sarcoplasmic degeneration and drop-out of myocytes. Interstitial and subendocardial fibrosis are present to a variable degree. It should be emphasized, however, that the histologic picture is nonspecific, and the diagnosis of dilated cardiomyopathy cannot therefore be made solely on the basis of the pathologic findings.

CLINICAL FEATURES

Most patients with dilated cardiomyopathy are between 20 and 50 years of age. Men are more often affected than women, in a ratio of 1.6 to 1. Most patients present with signs and symptoms of chronic, progressive congestive heart failure resulting from the marked reduction in the left ventricular ejection fraction. In a few patients the onset of the disorder is heralded by chest pain, arrhythmia, or systemic thromboembolism.

Physical examination typically reveals cardiomegaly with a poor-quality cardiac impulse and atrial and filling gallop rhythms. Patients with a significant decrease in cardiac output exhibit poor peripheral perfusion, pale extremities (often with a tinge of cyanosis), and low-amplitude arterial pulses. In patients with tricuspid insufficiency secondary to right ventricular failure, physical examination reveals pulsatile jugular distension and a pulsatile liver. The ECG findings are nonspecific (low-voltage QRS complex, flat or inverted T-wave). Conduction disturbances are very common, left bundle branch block and atrial fibrillation each occurring in about 20 percent of patients with this disorder. The clinical and radiologic findings in infants with endocardial fibroelastosis are discussed in Chapter 29.

IMAGING AND INVASIVE DIAGNOSIS

Plain Films

The radiographic findings are often nonspecific. Typically, there is generalized cardiac enlargement involving both sides of the heart to about the same degree (Fig. 19.2), although occasionally one side or the other may predominate. (Often, however, accurate assessment of individual chamber enlargement is difficult.) The degree of cardiomegaly is quite variable, depending on the severity of the disease, its chronicity, and the extent of myocardial damage. In patients with left ventricular failure, chest films show evidence of pulmonary venous and pulmonary arterial hypertension (Fig. 19.2). Dilatation of the superior vena cava and the azygos vein secondary to systemic venous hypertension indicates the presence of right ventricular failure.

In patients with massive cardiomegaly, the differential diagnosis includes massive pericardial effusion, multiple valvular disease (eg, rheumatic heart disease affecting the mitral, tricuspid, and aortic valves), and Ebstein's anomaly. Massive

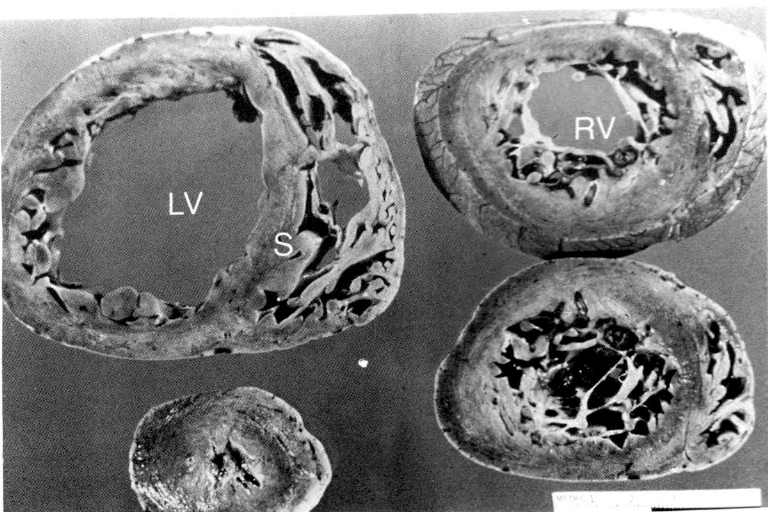

Fig. 19.1 Dilated cardiomyopathy. Cross-sections of the ventricular segment of the heart (beginning clockwise from the right): immediately beneath the atrioventricular valves; through the midportion of the ventricles; slightly cephalad to the apex; through the apex of the left ventricle. The total muscle mass of the left ventricle is increased and its cavity is enlarged. The right ventricle is also dilated but its wall is not thickened. Note that these changes involve the ventricles from the base to the apex. (LV = left ventricle; RV = right ventricle; S = ventricular septum

pericardial effusion typically produces a deformity of the left heart border which extends upward to include the pulmonary trunk but spares the aortic arch; posterior displacement of the epicardial fat is seen on the lateral projection. The pulmonary vasculature is usually normal (see Chapter 22). Patients with multivalvular disease typically have dilatation of the ascending aorta, calcification of the aortic and/or mitral valve, and a history of valvular disease (see Chapter 18). Adults with Ebstein's anomaly typically have right atrial and right ventricular enlargement without enlargement of the left atrium and left ventricle (which may be difficult to appreciate in patients with massive right-sided enlargement); the pulmonary vascularity is usually decreased owing to the presence of a right to left shunt at the atrial level (see Chapter 17). Thus, dilated cardiomyopathy is the most likely diagnosis in a patient with massive cardiomegaly and pulmonary venous hypertension who has no history of valvular disease or evidence of a pericardial effusion on imaging studies.

Echocardiography

Two-dimensional echocardiography demonstrates the size of the ventricular chambers and their contractility and confirms the absence of pericardial effusion. Mural thrombus can also be identified. In a typical case, both ventricles appear dilated and contract poorly (Fig. 19.3; see Appendix). By calculating ventricular volume, ejection fraction, and fractional shortness (a parameter indicating velocity of contractility), it is possible to quantify the degree of ventricular dysfunction; using color flow Doppler, one can assess the severity of the tricuspid or mitral insufficiency that is commonly present.

CT and MRI

Cine CT accurately depicts the size, configuration, and contractility of the ventricles. Although cine CT can be used to calculate the ventricular ejection fraction, the degree of tricuspid or mitral insufficiency cannot be assessed with this technique. Either conventional or cine CT will exclude a pericardial effu-

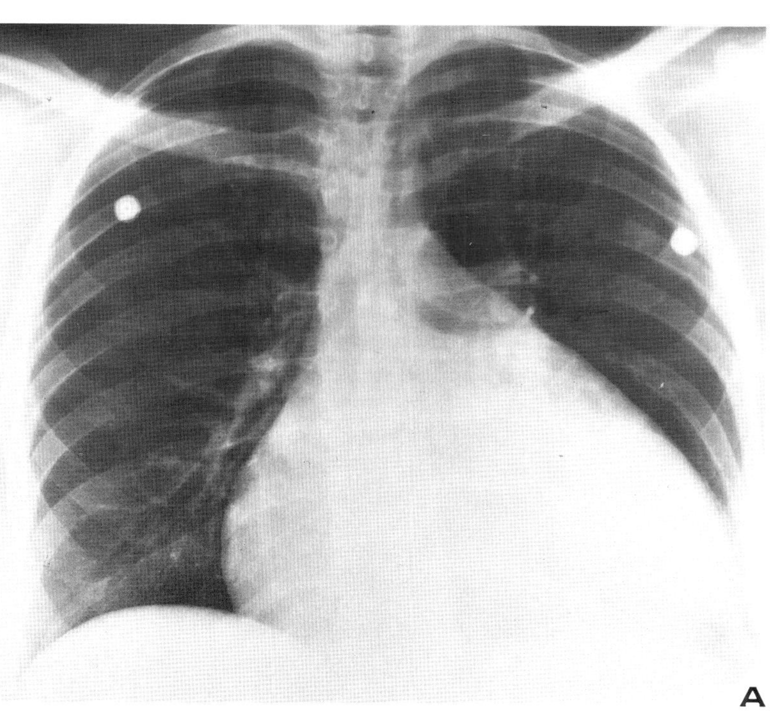

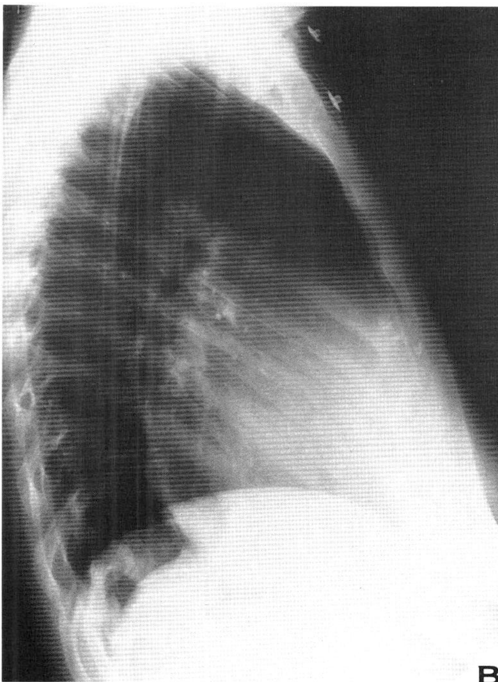

Fig. 19.2 Dilated cardiomyopathy. (A) Posteroanterior and (B) lateral chest films show massive cardiomegaly with enlargement of all four chambers. The vascular pedicle is normal; however, the pulmonary trunk is prominent, reflecting the increased pulmonary arterial pressure. The pulmonary vasculature shows evidence of pulmonary venous hypertension.

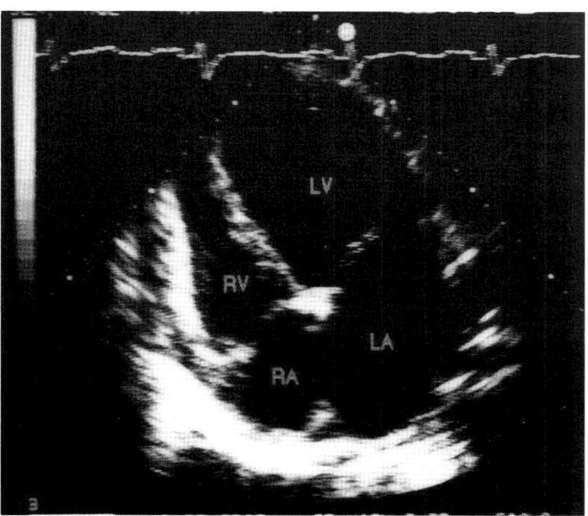

Fig. 19.3 Dilated cardiomyopathy. Apical four-chamber view of 2-D echocardiogram shows marked enlargement of the left ventricle. Note that the mitral and tricuspid valves are in normal position, separated from each other by the atrioventricular septum.

sion or extracardiac condition (eg, mediastinal tumor) that may cause enlargement of the cardiac silhouette.

Spin–echo MR images accurately depict the morphology and contractility of the affected ventricle (Fig. 19.4). Cine MRI demonstrates abnormal ventricular contractions and can be used to calculate the ejection fraction and other parameters of left ventricular function. Cine MRI clearly demonstrates mitral or tricuspid insufficiency and can be used to assess its severity (see Chapter 18).

Cardiac Catheterization

Cardiac catheterization demonstrates low cardiac output, decreased stroke volume, and elevated left ventricular diastolic pressure; pulmonary arterial pressure is usually only moderately elevated. In some instances the pulmonary arterial pressure may rise to almost systemic levels secondary to the reactive pulmonary hypertension associated with left ventricular failure. In patients with tricuspid insufficiency, right atrial pressure is increased.

Angiography

Left ventriculography demonstrates a large, globular left ventricle with severely diminished contractility; all segments of the left ventricle are affected (Fig. 19.5). Some patients exhibit focal dyskinesis or akinesis, which reflects the interstitial fibrosis commonly present. The mitral annulus is dilated, with variable degrees of insufficiency. The left atrium is usually enlarged and contracts poorly (Fig. 19.6). The left ventricular outflow tract is usually not obstructed, and the aortic valve is normal.

In patients with right ventricular involvement, the right ventricle appears enlarged and globular. Opacification of the right atrium and caval veins is commonly observed after a right ventricular injection, indicating the presence of tricuspid insufficiency (Fig. 19.7).

Mural thrombi in the right atrium, right ventricle, and/or left ventricle are quite common. They appear as eccentric filling defects, usually adjacent to an area of severe hypokinesis. Mural thrombi typically have smooth contours, which serves to distinguish them from the surrounding endocardium.

Selective coronary arteriography is routinely performed to exclude obstructive coronary artery disease. Although the coronary arteries are usually normal, some patients (mainly those over 50 years of age) exhibit atherosclerotic changes. Only 5 percent of patients with dilated cardiomyopathy have significant stenosis of the coronary arteries, in which case differentiation from ischemic cardiomyopathy may be difficult.

Because of the frequent occurrence of pulmonary thromboembolism in patients with dilated cardiomyopathy, pulmon-

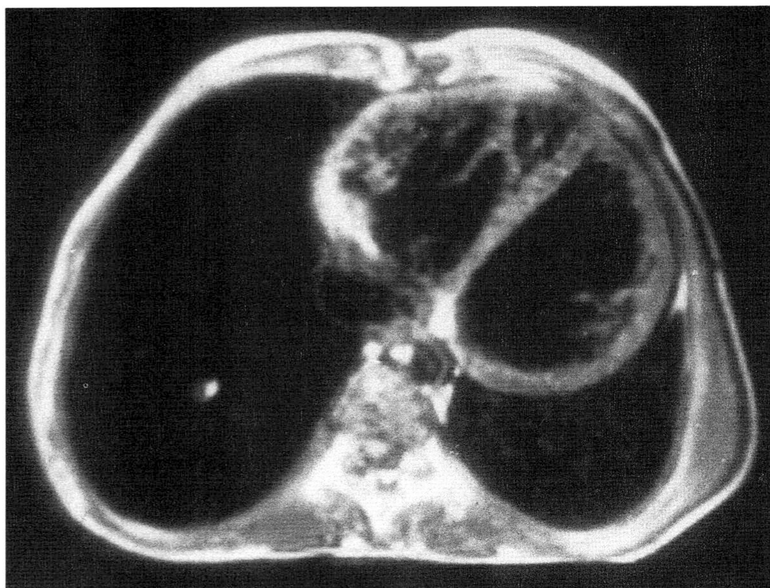

Fig. 19.4 Dilated cardiomyopathy. On axial spin–echo MR image, the right and left ventricles are dilated to approximately the same degree. The myocardium of both ventricles is abnormally thin relative to the size of the ventricular cavity. The right atrium is also dilated. The pericardium is normal.

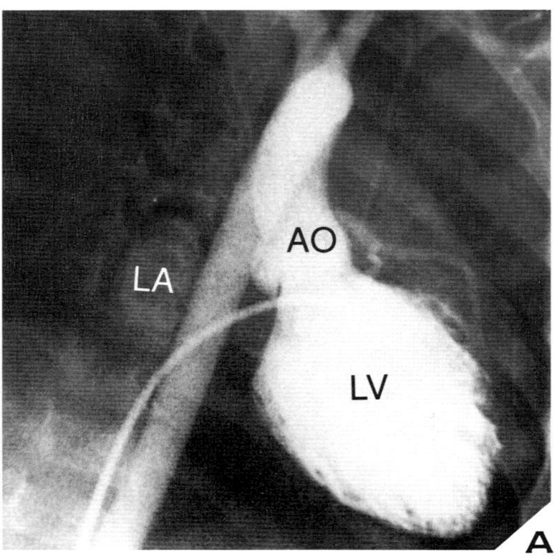

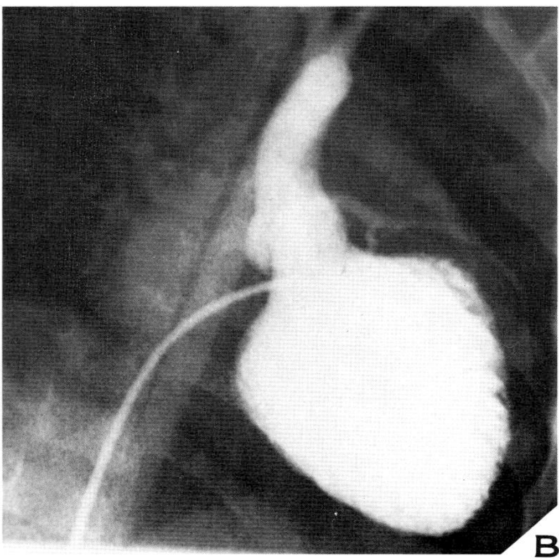

Fig. 19.5 Dilated cardiomyopathy. Elongated right anterior oblique projection of cine left ventriculogram in (A) systole and (B) diastole. The catheter has been passed from the inferior vena cava into the left ventricle (LV) via a patent foramen ovale. The left ventricle is markedly dilated and its contractility is uniformly reduced. A small amount of contrast refluxes across the mitral valve during systole, faintly opacifying the left atrium (LA). The free wall of the left ventricle, delineated by the left anterior descending coronary artery, is only minimally thickened. (Ao = Aorta)

ary arteriography is often indicated. This complication should be suspected in any patient with dilated cardiomyopathy who has a lung infiltrate associated with cough, pleuritic pain, or other suggestive clinical findings (see Chapter 24).

HYPERTROPHIC CARDIOMYOPATHY

Hypertrophic cardiomyopathy is a primary disorder of heart muscle which is characterized by symmetric or asymmetric hypertrophy of one or both ventricles; occasionally the hypertrophy is concentric. Systolic and diastolic function, as well as cardiac rhythm, are affected.

PATHOLOGY

Hypertrophic cardiomyopathy is classified as *symmetric* or *asymmetric* according to the location and extent of the hypertrophy. In the more common asymmetric form, the hypertrophy primarily affects the ventricular septum, typically involving the entire trabecular septum or its middle or apical portion. Occasionally, the posterior or lateral portions of the septum are predominantly involved.

On gross examination, the ventricular mass is markedly increased, the heart weight being two to three times greater than normal. The hypertrophy typically extends for a variable distance into the anterior and free wall of the left ventricle. In

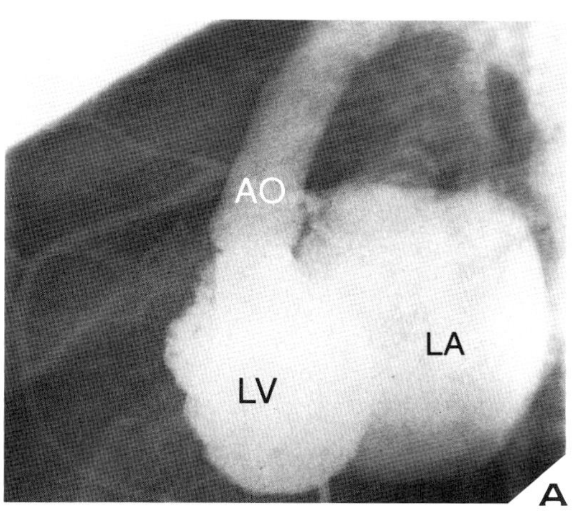

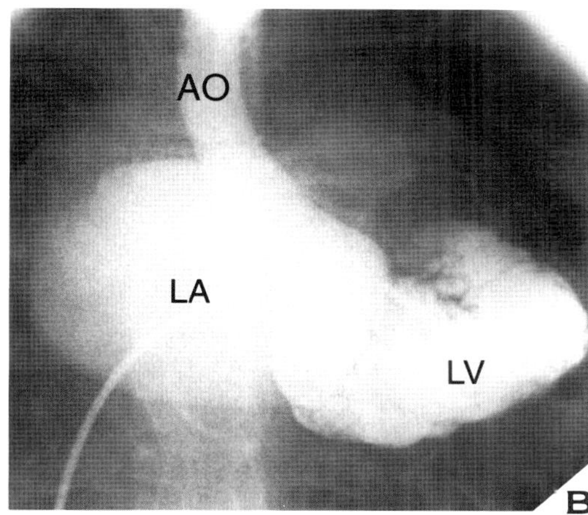

Fig. 19.6 Dilated cardiomyopathy. (A) Frontal and (B) lateral projections of left ventriculogram show moderate dilation of the left ventricle (LV). The entire left atrium (LA) is opacified, indicating severe mitral insufficiency. The ascending aorta (Ao) and coronary arteries are normal.

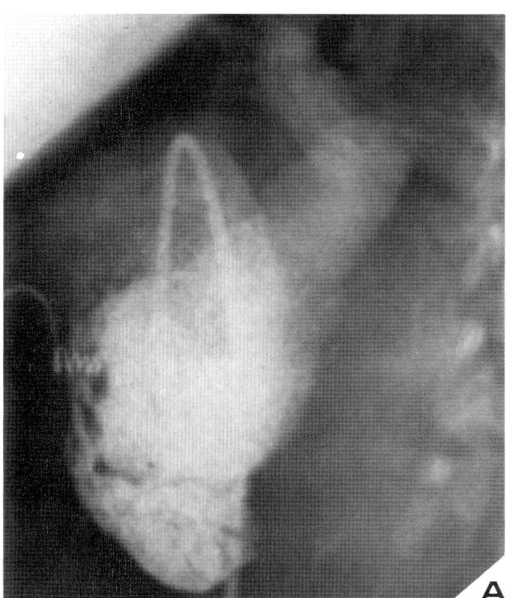

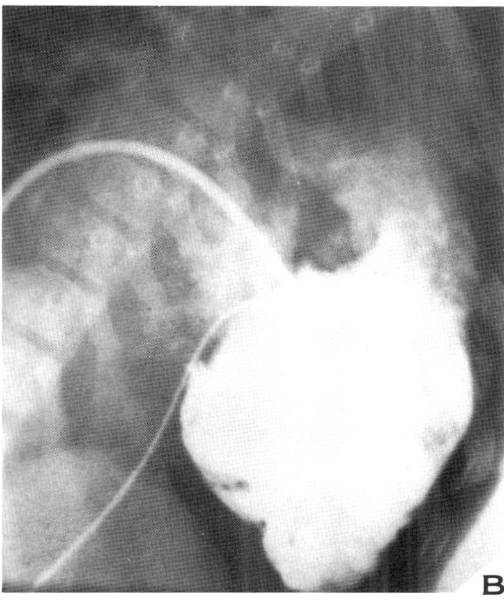

Fig. 19.7 Dilated cardiomyopathy. (A) Right anterior oblique and (B) left anterior oblique projections of cine right ventriculogram demonstrate moderate enlargement and decreased contractility of the right ventricle. Note opacification of right atrium, indicating the presence of tricuspid insufficiency, a common finding in patients with dilated cardiomyopathy affecting the right ventricle. (The degree of tricuspid insufficiency cannot be assessed owing to the presence of the catheter.)

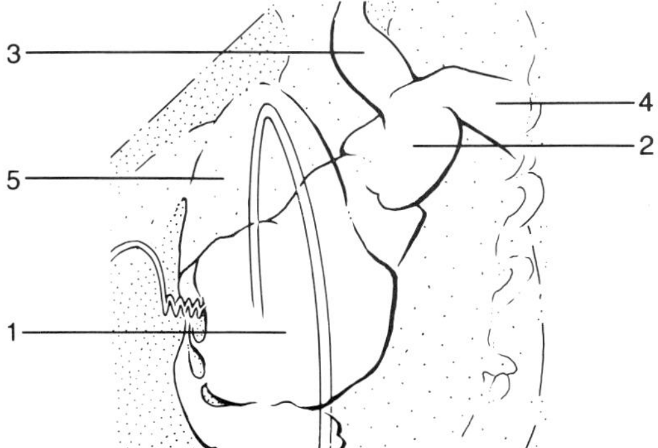

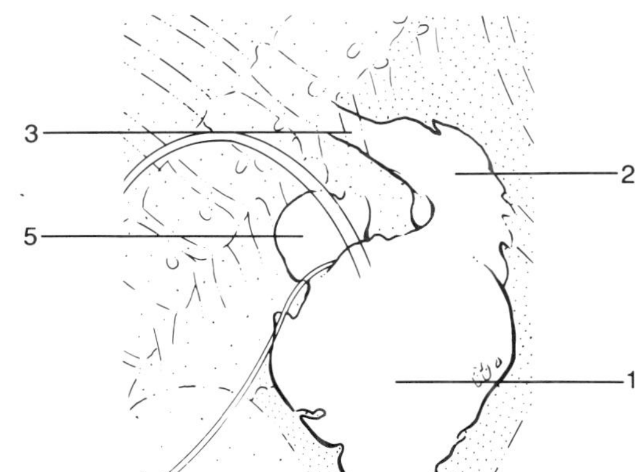

1 right ventricle
2 pulmonary trunk
3 right pulmonary artery
4 left pulmonary artery
5 right atrium

most cases the ventricular septum is thicker than the lateral (free) wall of the left ventricle (Fig. 19.8). In some instances the septum and lateral wall are hypertrophied to the same degree (Fig. 19.9). When the hypertrophy is limited to the septum, it typically involves the trabecular portion at its junction with the outlet portion [idiopathic hypertrophic subaortic stenosis (IHSS)], although on occasion it may extend into the middle or apical portions. The ventricular chambers are usually not dilated. Both atria are usually dilated, reflecting the elevated end diastolic pressure in the ventricles (secondary to decreased compliance) and, in patients with advanced disease, the presence of mitral and tricuspid insufficiency. Chronic contact between the anterior mitral leaflet and the hypertrophied septum results in thickening of the anterior mitral leaflet and endocardial fibrosis in the subaortic segment of the septum.

Microscopically, there is disarray of cellular organization, characterized by a whorled, intertwined cluster of myocytes and loss of the normal parallel arrangement of the contractile elements of the cytoplasm. Although this pattern is typical of hypertrophic cardiomyopathy, it can also be seen in patients with left ventricular outlet obstruction (eg, aortic stenosis) and in some normal hearts. Other common histologic features include subendocardial fibrosis, particularly in the subaortic region, and patchy interstitial fibrosis. Narrowing of the lumen of the intramyocardial branches of the coronary arteries has also been described in this condition.

CLINICAL FEATURES

IHSS, the best known but probably not the most common variety of hypertrophic cardiomyopathy, typically occurs in middle-aged women. It is occasionally familial. The usual presenting complaints are angina pectoris and palpitations. Syncopal or presyncopal episodes are very common. An occasional patient may present with orthopnea or paradoxical nocturnal dysnea, in which case confusion with congestive heart failure may occur.

Physical examination may be normal when left ventricular outlet obstruction is minimal or absent. In patients with significant left ventricular outlet obstruction the apical precordial impulse is displaced laterally and is unusually forceful and prominent; a systolic thrill can frequently be palpated at the apex or along the lower sternal border. In patients with diminished right ventricular compliance secondary to massive septal hypertrophy, the jugular venous pulse usually demonstrates a prominent "a" wave.

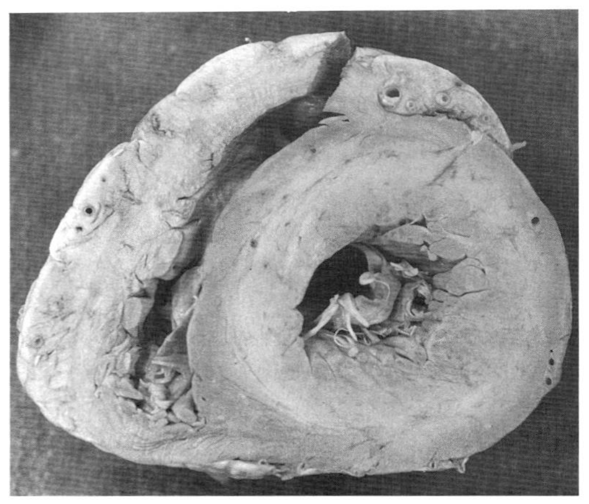

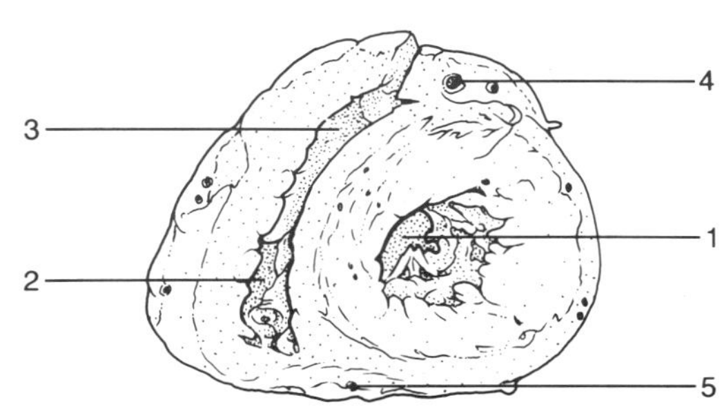

Fig. 19.8 Hypertrophic cardiomyopathy. Transverse section of heart specimen shows hypertrophy of the septum and free wall of the left ventricle; the septal hypertrophy is greater than that of the free wall. Right ventricular hypertrophy is also present.

1 left ventricle
2 right ventricle
3 right ventricular outflow tract
4 left anterior descending coronary artery
5 posterior descending coronary artery

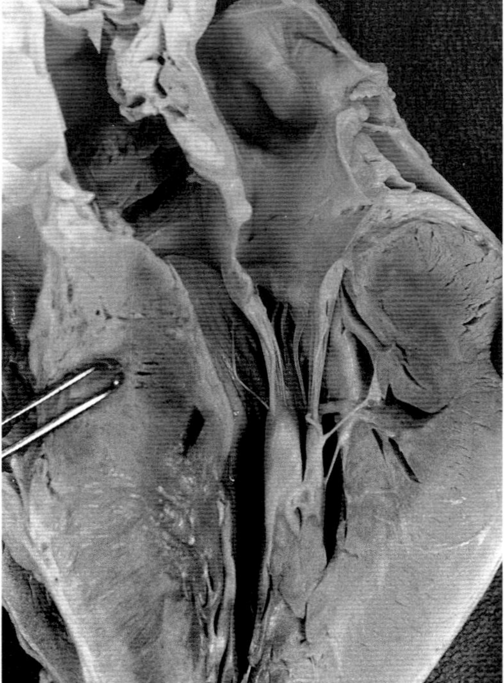

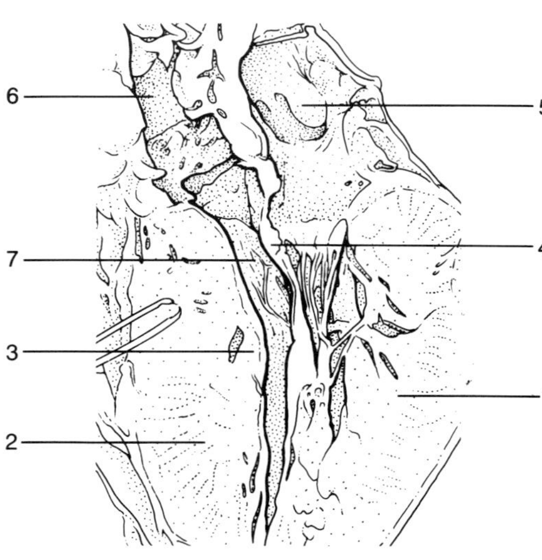

Fig. 19.9 Hypertrophic cardiomyopathy. Coronal section through the ventricular septum shows marked hypertrophy of the septum and free wall of the left ventricle, which are enlarged to approximately the same degree. Note marked narrowing of left ventricular outflow tract (subaortic segment), which is mainly due to the hypertrophied septum. The anterior leaflet of the mitral valve is well formed; however, there is fibrosis of its free border. Note endocardial fibrosis opposite the anterior mitral leaflet resulting from repetitive trauma.

1 free wall of left ventricle
2 hypertrophied ventricular septum
3 endocardial thickening (on ventricular septum)
4 anterior leaflet of mitral valve
5 left atrium
6 aorta
7 left ventricular outflow tract

The classic murmur of IHSS is a harsh, crescendo–decrescendo systolic murmur, which is produced by turbulent blood flow through the narrow left ventricular outflow tract and mitral regurgitation. The murmur typically begins well after the first heart sound and is best heard along the left sternal border and at the apex, where it is often more holosystolic and has a blowing quality. The carotid pulse is of low amplitude and slow (pulsus parvus et tardus).

The ECG is frequently normal in asymptomatic patients without left ventricular outflow obstruction. Symptomatic patients typically have ST-segment and T-wave abnormalities, with evidence of left ventricular hypertrophy (increased QRS voltage, particularly in the midprecordial leads). Other ECG findings include Q-wave abnormalities in the inferior leads and prominent P-waves indicating left atrial enlargement. Atrial fibrillation is present in 5 to 10 percent of symptomatic patients. Exercise testing may provoke a ventricular arrhythmia.

IMAGING AND INVASIVE DIAGNOSIS

Plain Films

The plain film findings depend on the degree of muscular hypertrophy and on the presence or absence of left or right ventricular outflow tract obstruction. Patients without significant obstruction have no radiographic abnormalities. Most symptomatic patients exhibit moderate cardiomegaly with prominence of the left lower segment of the cardiac silhouette on the frontal projection, which gives the heart a globular configuration. On the lateral projection, increased density can be appreciated in the area beneath the aortic valve (Fig. 19.10). Left atrial enlargement secondary to mitral insufficiency is a common finding in patients with severe IHSS. Although the pulmonary vasculature is usually normal, patients with left ventricular failure may have radiographic evidence of pulmonary venous hypertension (Fig. 19.11). Dilatation of the central pulmonary arteries may be seen in patients with pulmonary

A

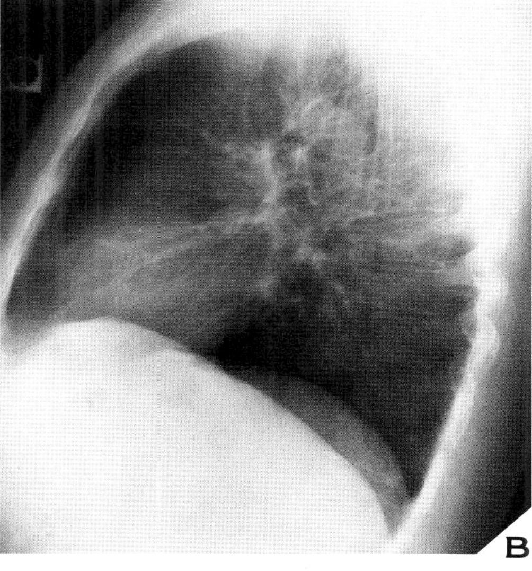

B

Fig. 19.10 Hypertrophic cardiomyopathy. (IHSS). (A) Frontal chest film shows a normal-sized heart with mild left ventricular hypertrophy (note prominence of left lower heart border). The ascending aorta, aortic arch, and pulmonary vascularity are normal. (B) The lateral projection demonstrates increased density in the region just inferior to the aortic valve, further evidence of left ventricular hypertrophy.

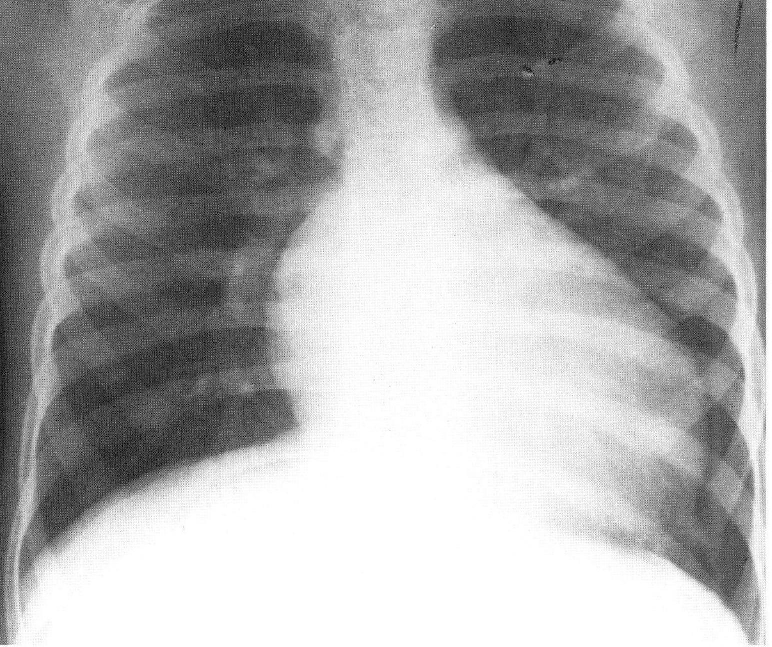

Fig. 19.11 Hypertrophic cardiomyopathy (IHSS). Posteroanterior chest film shows marked cardiomegaly with left ventricular and left atrial enlargement. The aorta and main pulmonary arteries are normal. The pulmonary vasculature shows a cephalization pattern, indicating the presence of pulmonary venous hypertension secondary to left ventricular failure.

arterial hypertension, reflecting long-standing pulmonary venous hypertension.

Although the findings described are suggestive of hypertrophic cardiomyopathy, an unequivocal diagnosis cannot be made on the basis of the plain film findings alone. For example, patients with aortic valvular disease or long-standing severe systemic hypertension may have left ventricular hypertrophy with similar plain film findings. (The presence of a dilated ascending aorta and marked tortuosity of the descending aorta favors the diagnosis of hypertension.) It may be impossible to differentiate hypertrophic cardiomyopathy from mitral valvular disease in patients whose plain films demonstrate various combinations of left ventricular enlargement, left atrial enlargement, and pulmonary venous hypertension.

Echocardiography

Echocardiography remains the most useful imaging technique for the diagnosis and assessment of hypertrophic cardiomyopathy. Either the transthoracic or the transesophageal approach can be used to evaluate the size of the ventricular cavities and the thickness of the ventricular wall. The standard examination consists of short axis views obtained at the subvalvular level and at the midportion of the septum, and long axis views obtained via a parasternal or axial window; an apical or parasternal four-chamber view also may be helpful. Extension of the hypertrophic process into the free wall of the right or left ventricle is best seen in the four-chamber view.

The diagnosis of septal and ventricular hypertrophy is based on measurements at various points. Left ventricular hypertrophy is diagnosed when the thickness of the ventricular wall is >15 mm (>17 mm at the junction of the septum and the free wall). In a normal heart, the mean thickness of the septum and free wall of the left ventricle is 8 ± 0.2 mm (range 7 to 10 mm), and the ratio of the septum to the free wall is 1:1. Hypertrophy may be limited to the septum or the free wall, or both may be involved to a greater or lesser extent (Figs. 19.12 and 19.13). In the most severe form, which results in obstruction of the left ventricular outflow tract, both the septum and the free wall are hypertrophied. When the hypertrophy is limited to the septum, there is a discrepancy between the thickness of the septum and that of the free wall; in such cases the septum to free wall ratio is greater than 1.5:1.

Abnormal displacement of the anterior mitral leaflet during systole—the hallmark of IHSS—is well seen on two-dimensional echocardiography. Normally, the anterior leaflet is displaced posteriorly and superiorly throughout systole. In IHSS, the leaflet moves into an anterior position during the latter part of systole, resulting in mitral regurgitation and left ventricular outflow tract obstruction (Fig. 19.14). With color flow Doppler, it is possible to document the presence of mitral insufficiency and to evaluate its severity.

It should be emphasized that abnormal anterior systolic motion of the septal leaflet is not pathognomic of hypertrophic cardiomyopathy. It can also be seen in patients with concentric

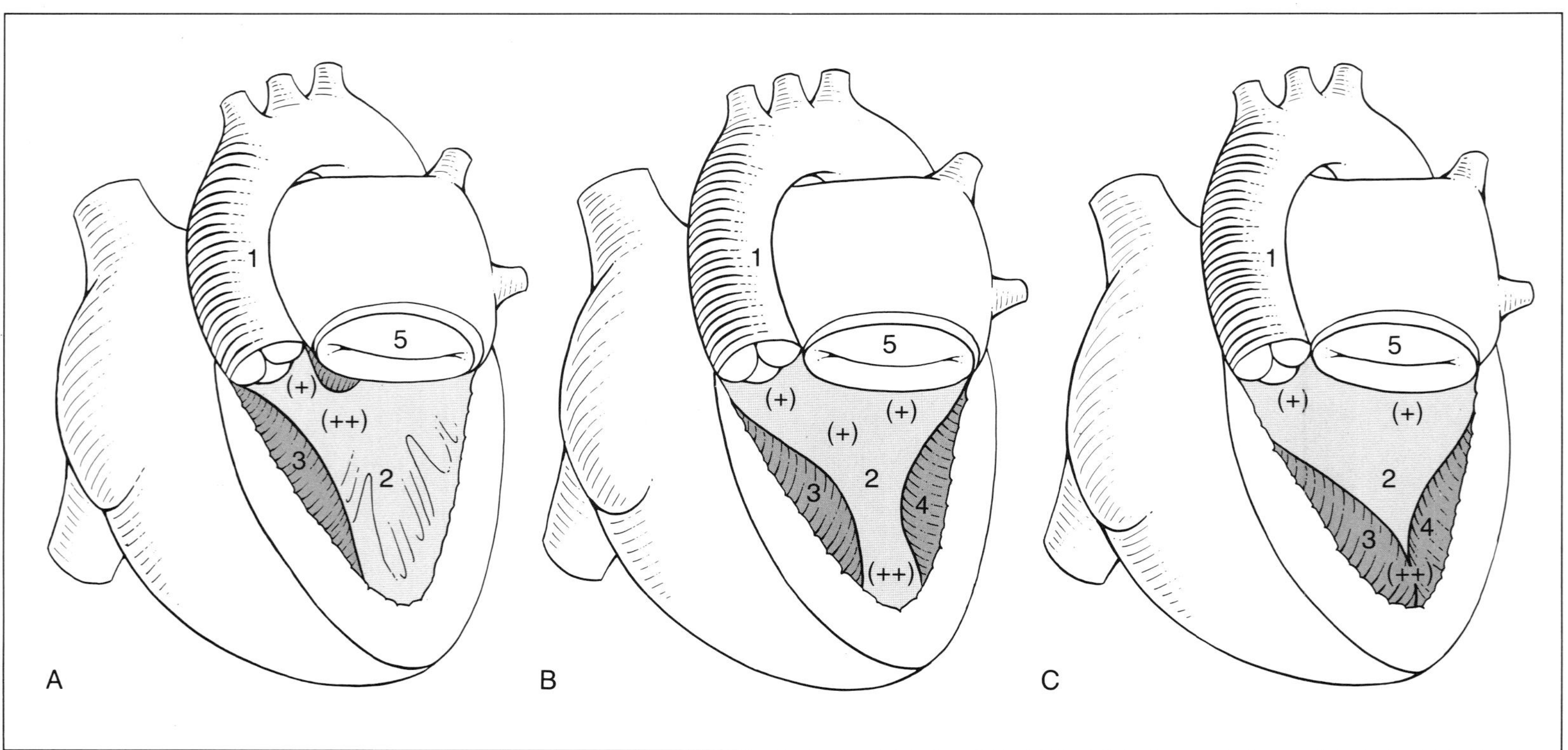

Fig. 19.12 Patterns of left ventricular obstruction in hypertrophic cardiomyopathy. The sites of obstruction in the three most common varieties of hypertrophic cardiomyopathy are shown schematically. (A) Subaortic (left ventricular outflow tract) form. (B) Midventricular form. (C) Apical form.

1 aorta
2 left ventricular cavity
3 hypertrophy of ventricular septum
4 hypertrophy of free wall
5 mitral valve
\+ region of normal systolic pressure
\+ + region of increased systolic pressure

hypertrophy secondary to aortic stenosis or to longstanding systemic hypertension.

Cine CT and MRI

Cine CT and gated spin–echo MR images provide information similar to that obtained from two-dimensional echocardiography. Both CT and MRI demonstrate the hypertrophy of the ventricular wall and septum and indicate the relative thickness of each (ie, the septum to free wall ratio). Either modality can be used to calculate the end diastolic and end systolic volumes and the ejection fraction.

Cine MRI demonstrates the morphology of the mitral leaflets and the abnormal motion of the anterior mitral leaflet. It is also possible to detect mitral insufficiency, which results in a signal void in the left atrium during systole. However, cine MRI offers no advantage over echocardiography; the latter remains the modality of choice for noninvasive evaluation of hypertrophic cardiomyopathy.

Cardiac Catheterization

The major hemodynamic aberrations associated with hypertrophic cardiomyopathy affect the left ventricle. Left heart catheterization demonstrates diminished diastolic compliance and a pressure gradient between the inlet and outlet portions of the left ventricle. Four types of systolic pressure gradient are encountered in hypertrophic cardiomyopathy, depending on the site of obstruction:

1. A small early systolic gradient across the aortic valve. Although this is a normal phenomenon, resulting from early systolic flow acceleration, the gradient is often greater than normal owing to the rapid ejection in early systole. It does not extend beyond midsystole.

2. A systolic intraventricular gradient at the level of the papillary muscles (see Figs. 19.12 and 19.16). This type of gradient, which is seen in patients with midventricular obstruction, occurs in the midportion of the left ventricle between the inlet and outlet segments, and lasts throughout systole.

3. A systolic gradient at the subaortic level, caused by contact between the anterior mitral leaflet and the septum (see Figs. 19.12 and 19.17). This type of gradient, which is seen in patients with IHSS, occurs during the second part of systole when the anterior leaflet of the mitral valve is displaced anteriorly. The gradient is between the inlet and outlet segments of the left ventricle and is associated with increased pressure in the inlet and trabecular segments.

4. A systolic gradient due to cavity obliteration (see Figs. 19.12 and 19.18). In this type of gradient, seen in patients with the apical form of IHSS, the catheter is usually entrapped in the apical segment, where a high systolic pressure is recorded. There is no gradient between the inlet and outlet segments of the left ventricle.

In patients with a subaortic pressure gradient, all of the intraventricular pressures proximal to the obstruction are elevated, including that of the inflow segment. Some patients with hypertrophic cardiomyopathy do not exhibit a systolic gradient at rest; in such cases a gradient may be demonstrated during exercise or by provoking premature ventricular contractions.

Approximately 25 percent of patients with hypertrophic cardiomyopathy have mild pulmonary hypertension secondary to the elevated left atrial pressure. Approximately 15 percent have elevated right ventricular and right atrial pressures, which are believed to result from abnormal muscular contraction of the infundibular segment.

ANGIOCARDIOGRAPHY

Hypertrophy of the septum and free wall of the left ventricle is best seen on left ventriculograms in the long axial and elongated right anterior oblique projections. Representative examples of

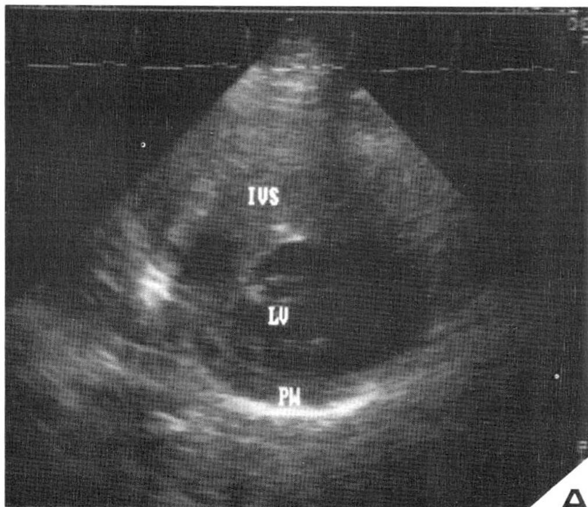

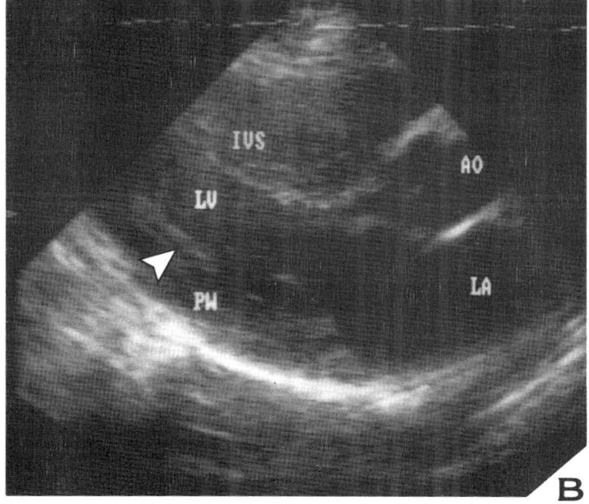

Fig. 19.13 Hypertrophic cardiomyopathy (IHSS) (echocardiographic findings). (A) Short axis view. The thickness of the ventricular septum (IVS) is markedly increased when compared with that of the posterior wall (PW) of the left ventricle (LV); the septum-to-free wall ratio is 2:1. (B) Long axis view (in diastole). The ventricular septum (IVS) is markedly thickened. The left ventricular chamber (LV) is of normal size. The anterior mitral leaflet (arrow) makes contact with the ventricular septum (IVS) during diastole. (AO = aorta; LA = left atrium)

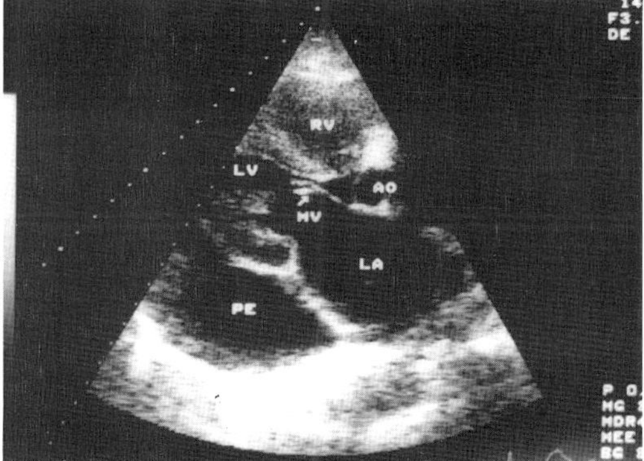

Fig. 19.14 Hypertrophic cardiomyopathy (IHSS) (echocardiographic findings). Long axial view in systole shows contact between the anterior mitral leaflet and the hypertrophied ventricular septum, resulting in obstruction of the left ventricular outflow tract. Note the small pericardial effusion (PE) posterior to the heart.

RV right ventricle
LV left ventricle
arrow hypertrophied septum
AO aorta
MV anterior leaflet of mitral valve
PE pericardial effusion

obstructive and nonobstructive hypertrophic cardiomyopathy are shown in Figs. 19.15 to 19.20. Hypertrophy of the free wall is manifested by an abnormally wide separation between the inferior border of the ventricular cavity and the posterior descending coronary artery; a corrected measurement of 1.5 cm or more (in diastole) indicates severe hypertrophy (Fig. 19.19). Septal hypertrophy is suggested by deformity of the septal aspect of the left ventricle, which appears as a shelf immediately

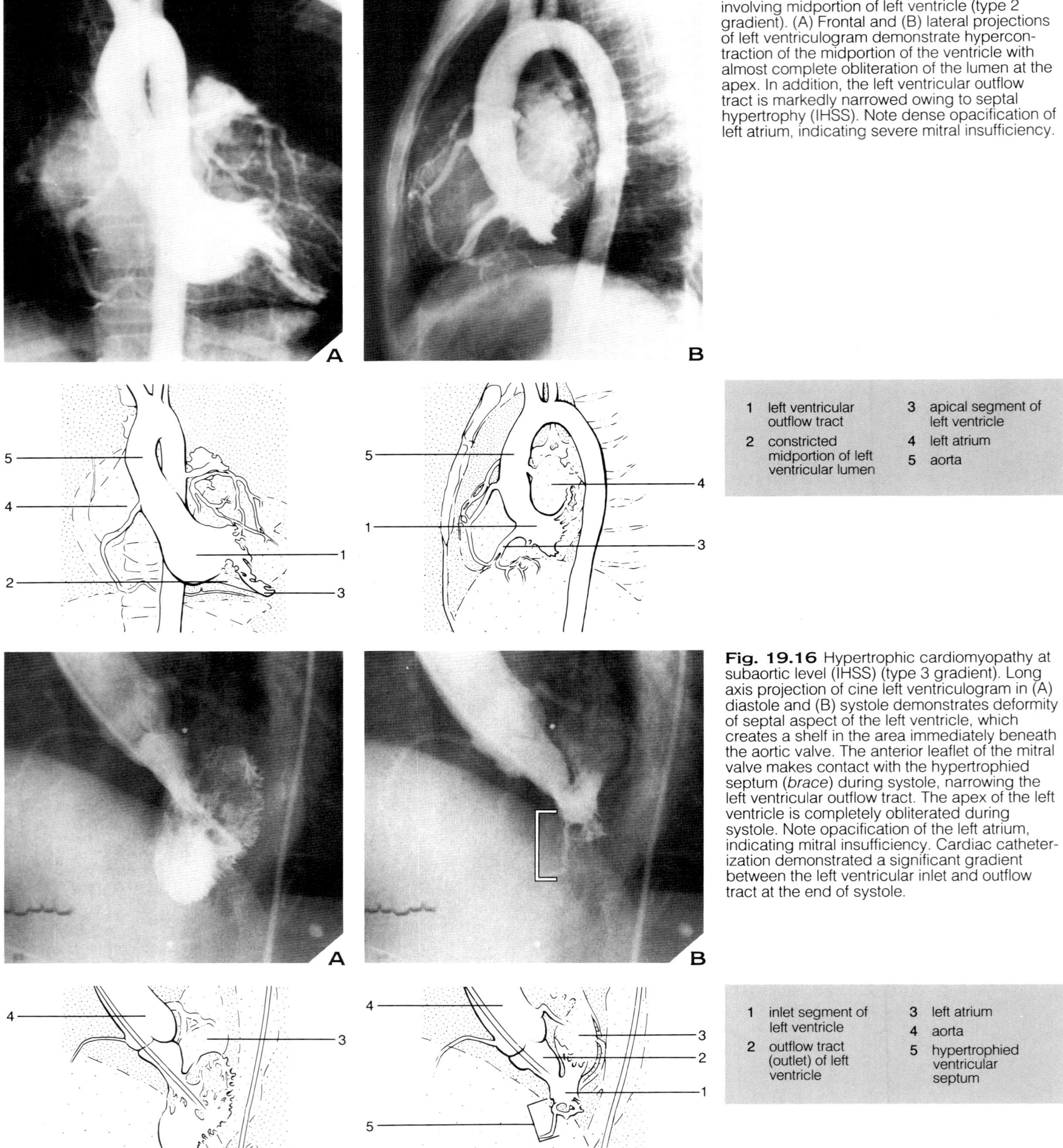

Fig. 19.15 Hypertrophic cardiomyopathy involving midportion of left ventricle (type 2 gradient). (A) Frontal and (B) lateral projections of left ventriculogram demonstrate hypercontraction of the midportion of the ventricle with almost complete obliteration of the lumen at the apex. In addition, the left ventricular outflow tract is markedly narrowed owing to septal hypertrophy (IHSS). Note dense opacification of left atrium, indicating severe mitral insufficiency.

1 left ventricular outflow tract
2 constricted midportion of left ventricular lumen
3 apical segment of left ventricle
4 left atrium
5 aorta

Fig. 19.16 Hypertrophic cardiomyopathy at subaortic level (IHSS) (type 3 gradient). Long axis projection of cine left ventriculogram in (A) diastole and (B) systole demonstrates deformity of septal aspect of the left ventricle, which creates a shelf in the area immediately beneath the aortic valve. The anterior leaflet of the mitral valve makes contact with the hypertrophied septum (*brace*) during systole, narrowing the left ventricular outflow tract. The apex of the left ventricle is completely obliterated during systole. Note opacification of the left atrium, indicating mitral insufficiency. Cardiac catheterization demonstrated a significant gradient between the left ventricular inlet and outflow tract at the end of systole.

1 inlet segment of left ventricle
2 outflow tract (outlet) of left ventricle
3 left atrium
4 aorta
5 hypertrophied ventricular septum

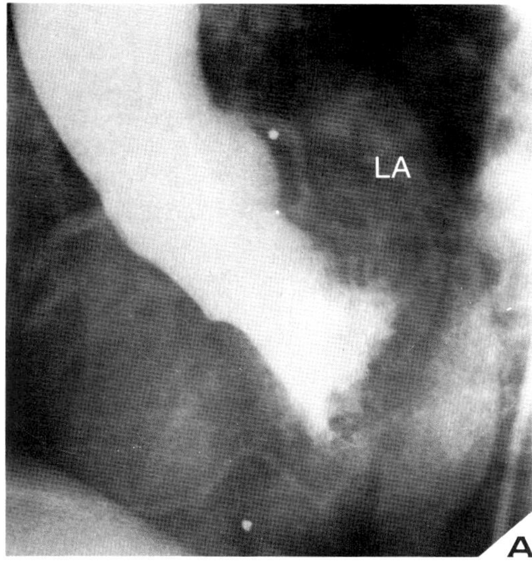

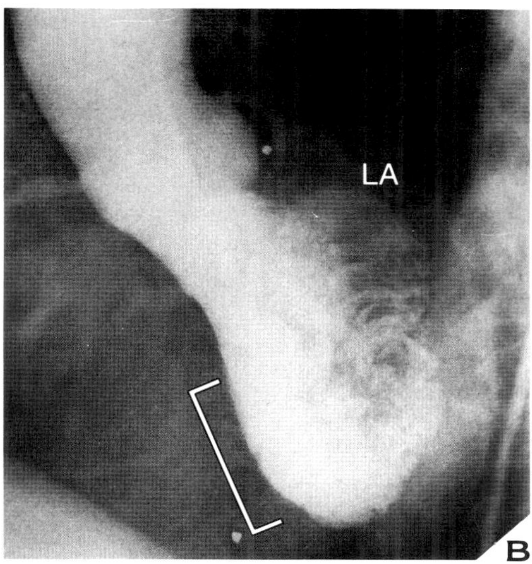

Fig. 19.17 Apical form of hypertrophic cardiomyopathy (type 4 gradient). Left anterior oblique projection of cine left ventriculogram in (A) systole and (B) diastole. The left ventricle contracts vigorously in systole, obliterating the lumen in the trabecular portion of the chamber; only the inlet and outlet portions of the left ventricle remain open. The trabecular portion of the septum (*brace*) is well demonstrated in diastole. (LA = left atrium)

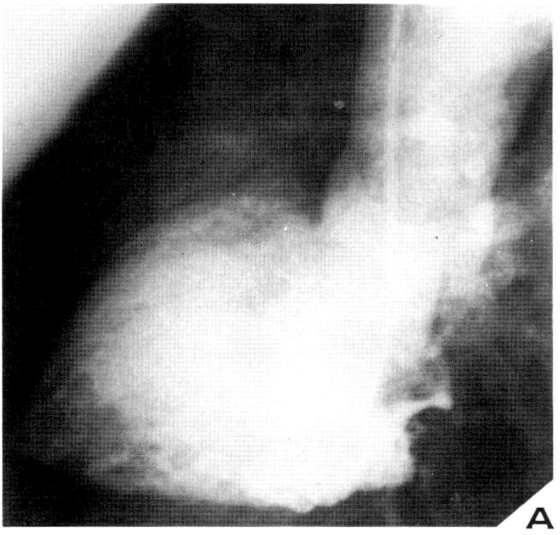

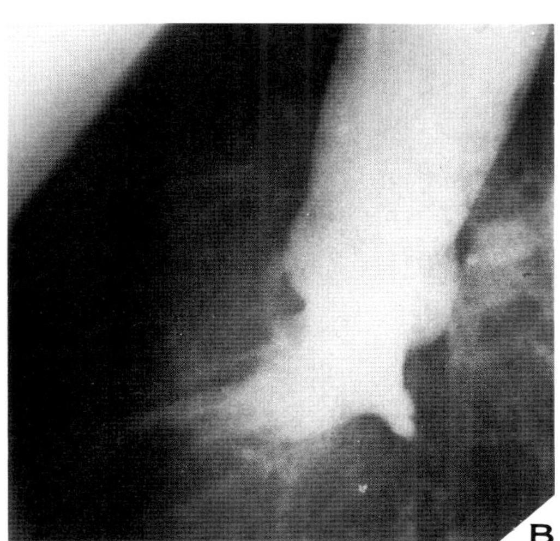

Fig. 19.18 Apical (nonobstructive) form of hypertrophic cardiomyopathy. Long axial view of cine left ventriculogram in (A) diastole and (B) systole. The entire left ventricle is well demonstrated in diastole but the middle and distal (apical) portions are obliterated during systole. There is no mitral insufficiency.

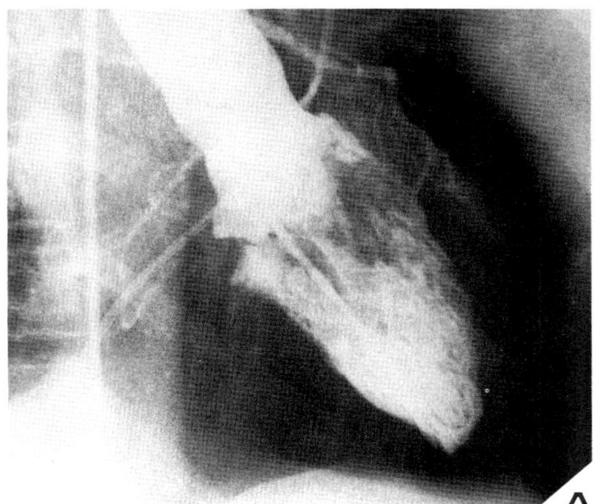

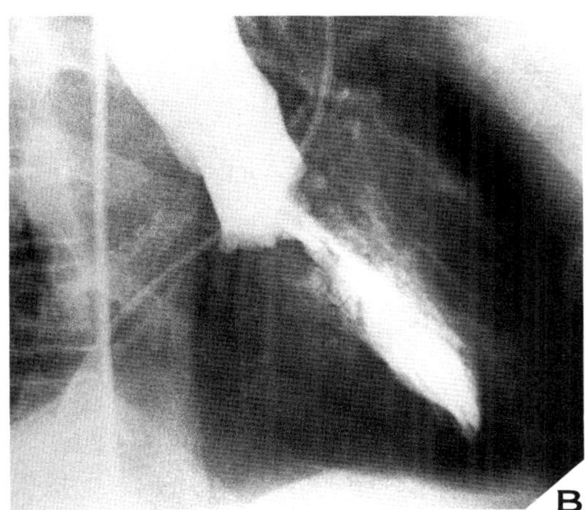

Fig. 19.19 Hypertrophic cardiomyopathy involving midportion of left ventricle. Frames of cine left ventriculogram in (A) diastole and (B) systole (right anterior oblique projection) demonstrate marked narrowing of midportion of the left ventricle, ie, at the junction of its outlet and trabecular portions; the distal (apical) and subaortic (outlet) portions of the left ventricle are normal. The left anterior descending coronary artery is widely separated from the border of the left ventricular lumen, indicating hypertrophy of the free wall. No mitral insufficiency was demonstrated.

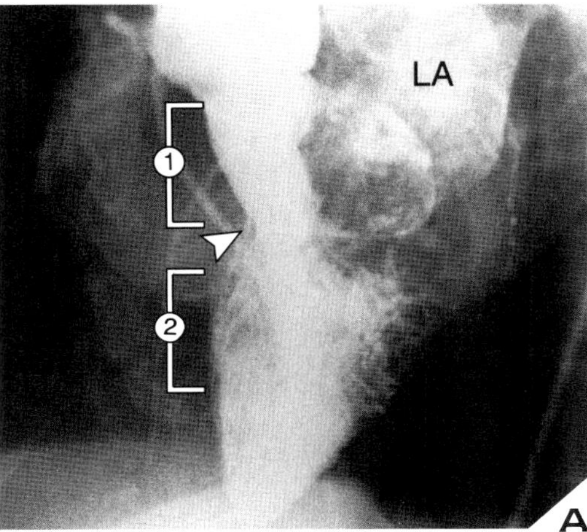

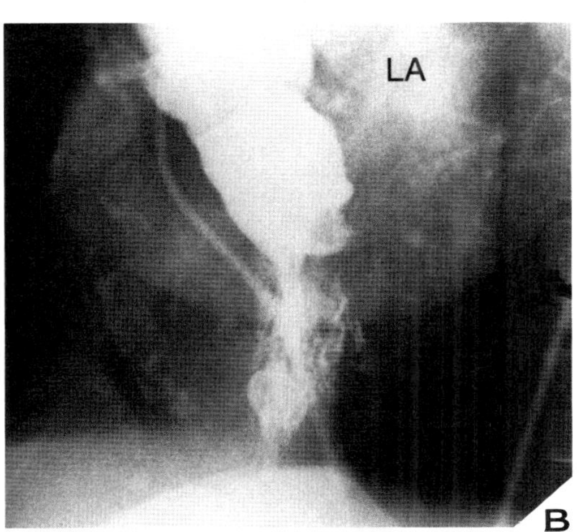

Fig. 19.20 Hypertrophic cardiomyopathy (IHSS). Long axial view of cine left ventriculogram in (A) diastole and (B) systole. There is significant narrowing of the left ventricular outflow tract (*brace* 1) during systole; the hypertrophied ventricular septum (*brace* 2) produces a distinct shelf-like impression (*arrow*). Note reflux of contrast material into the left atrium (LA), indicating mitral insufficiency.

beneath the aortic valve in the long axial view (Fig. 19.20). Biventricular angiocardiography is needed to measure the thickness of the septum; however, this is not necessary in most cases.

In patients with hypertrophy of the apical segment, the left ventricle is of normal size during diastole, and its inlet, trabecular, and outlet portions are well outlined. During systole, the apical portion disappears, and only the inlet and outlet portions remain opacified (Figs. 19.16 and 19.17).

Right ventricular hypertrophy is demonstrated by right ventriculography in the long axial and elongated right anterior oblique projections. Hypertrophy of the septum and crista supraventricularis results in narrowing of the right ventricular outflow tract in late systole (Fig. 19.21). In some patients the hypertrophy is mainly at the level of the moderator band.

The abnormal motion of the anterior (septal) leaflet and the insufficiency of the mitral valve are best demonstrated by left ventriculography in the long axial projection (see Fig. 21.13). In early systole the anterior leaflet is in normal position. In midsystole the anterior leaflet assumes an anterior position, sometimes touching the septum, resulting in narrowing of the outflow portion of the left ventricle. The leaflets are abnormally apposed during systole, so that the rough surface of the posterior leaflet makes contact with the smooth surface of the anterior leaflet (Fig. 19.22). At the same time, a jet of contrast material can be seen escaping from the left ventricle into the left atrium, indicating mitral insufficiency (the jet is usually directed towards the posterior wall of the left atrium).

The great majority of patients with obstructive hypertrophic cardiomyopathy have mitral insufficiency. (Those with the nonobstructive form may have mitral insufficiency secondary to primary mitral valve disease.) Prolapse of the posterior mitral leaflet (see Chapter 18) has been reported in patients with hypertrophic cardiomyopathy.

Coronary arteriography is usually performed in conjunction with angiocardiography to exclude obstructive coronary artery disease, which occurs in 10 to 15 percent of cases.

RESTRICTED CARDIOMYOPATHY

Restricted cardiomyopathy is defined as a condition in which ventricular compliance is abnormal in the presence of normal systolic function. The underlying pathologic process is myocardial fibrosis or hypertrophy, or infiltration of the myocardium by abnormal substances (eg, amyloid). Involvement of the inlet portion of the ventricles causes obstruction during diastole, resulting in mitral and/or tricuspid stenosis. The resulting hemodynamic disturbance is similar to that seen in constrictive pericarditis (see Chapter 22). The thickness of the ventricular wall is usually normal. Restricted cardiomyopathy occurs in a number of systemic and primary cardiac disorders, including amyloidosis, hemochromatosis, glycogen storage disease, endocardial fibrosis, and eosinophilic cardiomyopathy.

CLINICAL FEATURES

Patients with restricted cardiomyopathy typically present with exercise intolerance, weakness, and dyspnea; a small percentage complain of chest pain. Patients with advanced disease present with peripheral edema, hepatomegaly, ascites, or anasarca. Physical examination usually reveals a systolic murmur reflecting mitral or tricuspid regurgitation. Jugular venous distension may be present in advanced cases.

Differentiation from constrictive pericarditis and certain other conditions may be not be possible even after a thorough evaluation, including echocardiography and cardiac catheterization. In such cases a myocardial biopsy may be needed for definitive diagnosis.

IMAGING AND INVASIVE DIAGNOSIS

Plain Films

The plain film findings are nonspecific. The heart is usually of normal size or is minimally to moderately enlarged. Cardiomegaly, when present, is mainly the result of left atrial dilatation. The involved ventricle (or ventricles) is usually of normal

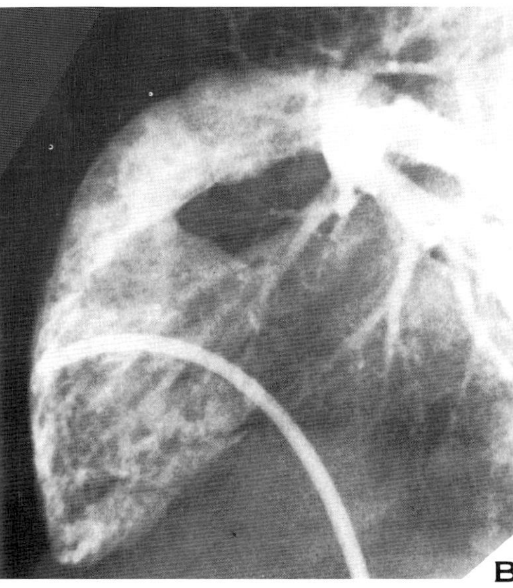

Fig. 19.21 Hypertrophic cardiomyopathy involving right ventricle. (A) Frontal and (B) lateral projections of cine right ventriculogram (in systole). The walls of the right ventricle are thick and trabeculated, particularly along the septal border, where the septal parietal (moderator) bands are identified. The infundibulum is narrowed owing to hypertrophy of the crista supraventricularis. The pulmonary arteries are normal.

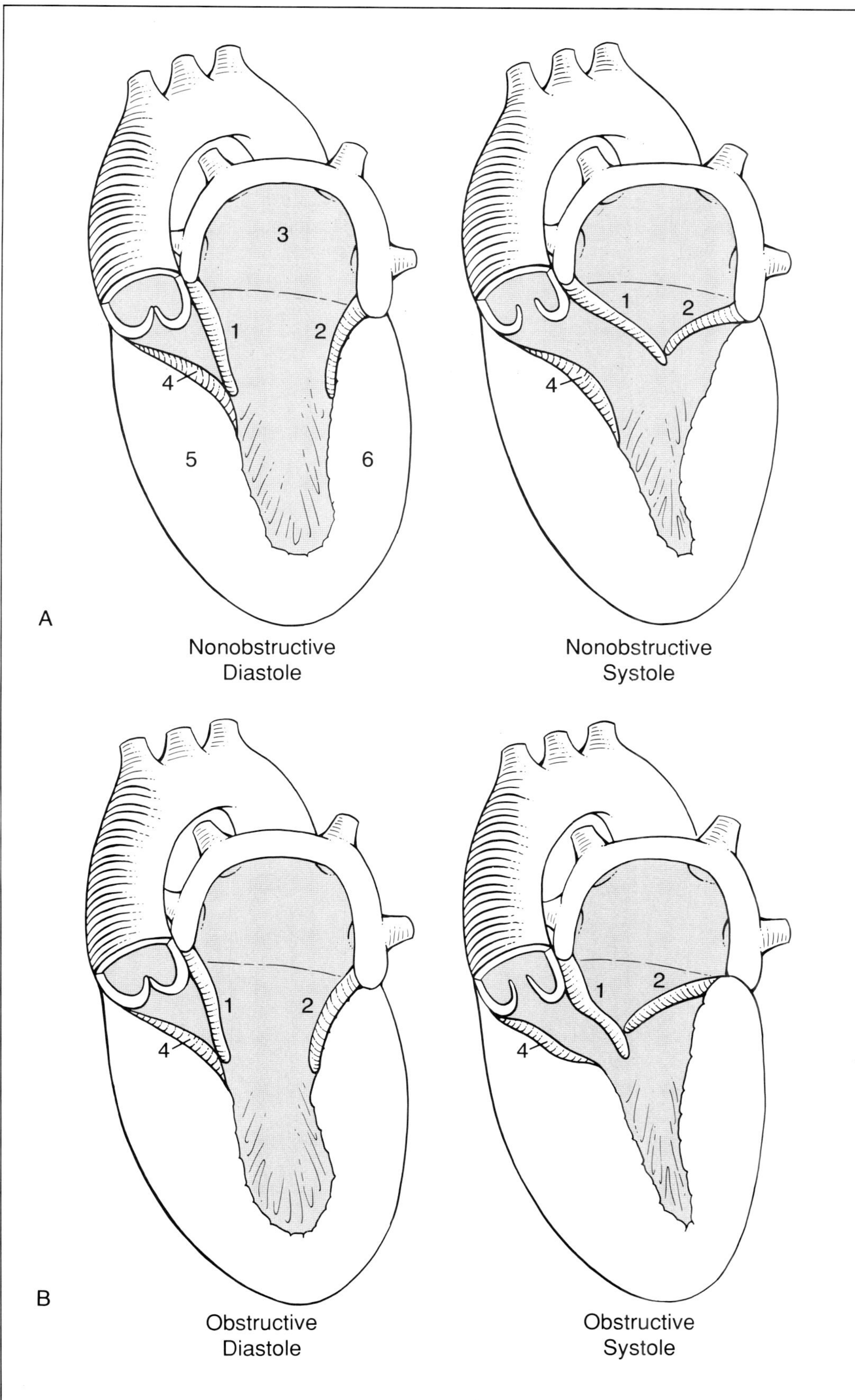

Fig. 19.22 Abnormal motion of anterior leaflet of mitral valve in hypertrophic cardiomyopathy (schematic). (A) Nonobstructive; (B) Obstructive. Abnormal apposition of the anterior and posterior leaflets in systole is a common finding in the obstructive form of hypertrophic cardiomyopathy.

1 anterior (septal) leaflet of mitral valve
2 posterior leaflet of mitral valve
3 left atrium
4 endocardial thickening of septum (due to repetitive trauma by anterior leaflet)
5 hypertrophied septum
6 hypertrophied free wall of left ventricle

size. The vascular pedicle commonly appears normal. Pulmonary venous hypertension, reflecting increased left ventricular end diastolic pressure, is often seen in symptomatic patients (Fig. 19.23).

Differentiation from such disorders as constrictive pericarditis, mediastinal fibrosis, and mitral insuffiency is seldom possible on the basis of the plain film findings alone. The presence of pericardial calcification strongly favors the diagnosis of restrictive pericarditis; however, calcification is present in only 50 percent of patients with this condition.

Echocardiography

Echocardiography in various projections is useful for diagnosis of restricted cardiomyopathy and assessment of the severity of the hemodynamic disturbance. With conventional two-dimensional echocardiography it is possible to accurately assess the thickness of the ventricular wall and the size of the ventricular chambers and to detect left atrial enlargement (which is commonly present). With color flow Doppler, it is possible to detect the presence of mitral and/or tricuspid insufficiency.

Abnormalities of the diastolic function of the left ventricle

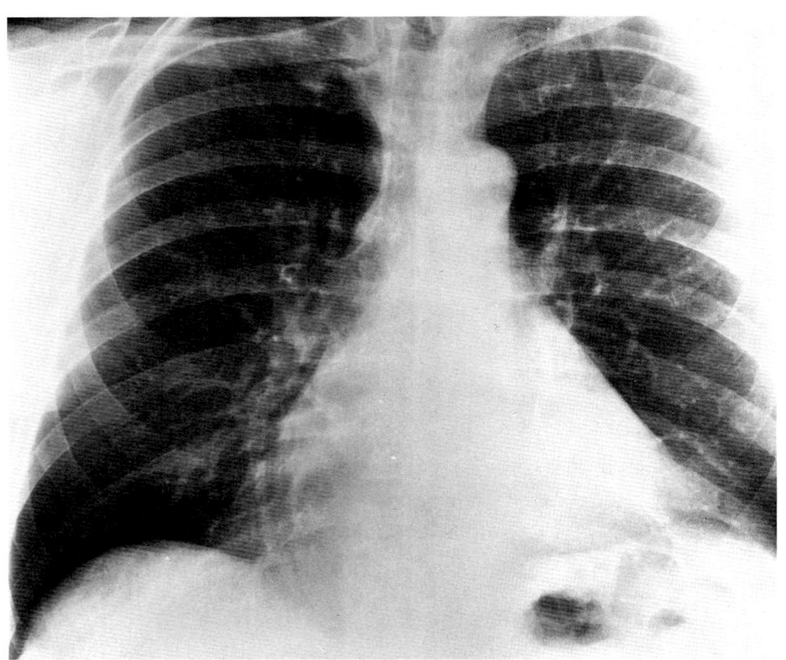

Fig. 19.23 Restricted cardiomyopathy. Frontal chest film shows a slightly enlarged heart with a prominent left ventricle. The left atrium is only minimally enlarged. The pulmonary vasculature shows signs of pulmonary venous hypertension (cephalization pattern). Although the radiographic findings suggest mitral insufficiency, the clinical data did not support this diagnosis. In a patient with no clinical or echocardiographic evidence of mitral valve disease, this radiographic appearance should raise the question of restricted cardiomyopathy or constrictive pericarditis. The diagnosis of restricted cardiomyopathy was confirmed by open biopsy in this patient.

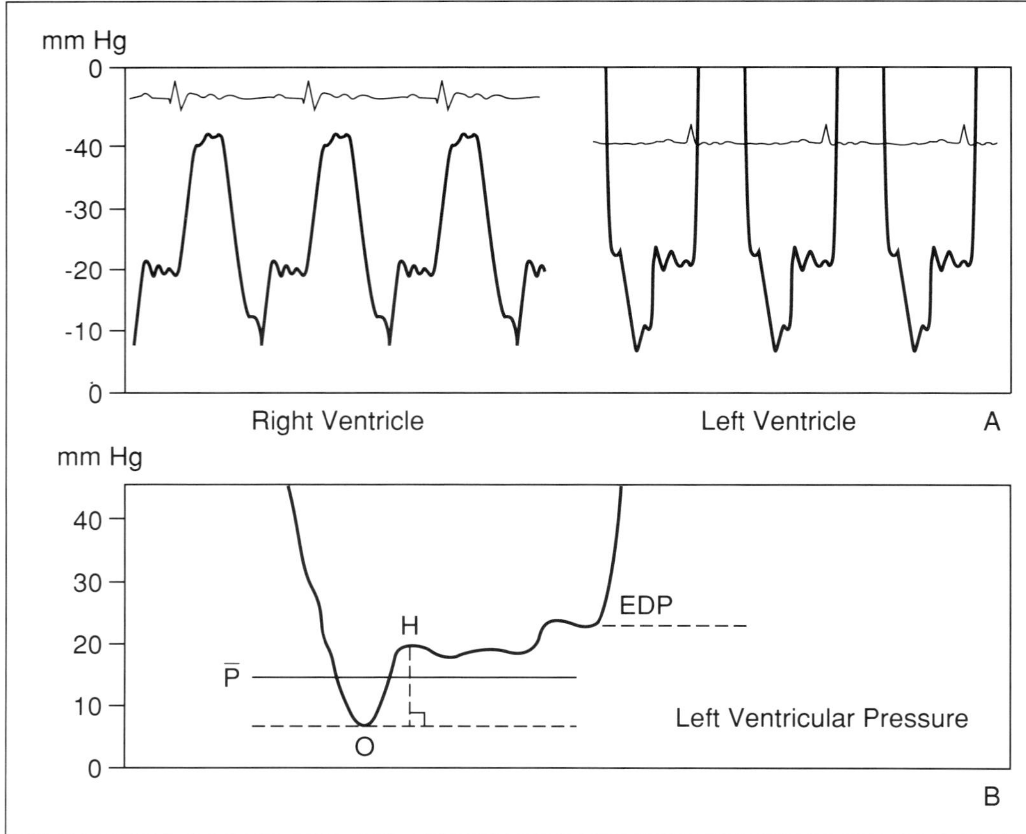

Fig. 19.24 Ventricular pressure in restricted cardiomyopathy. (A) Tracing of right and left ventricular pressure curves. Both tracings show an early diastolic dip followed by a plateau of stable pressure: the "square root sign." The end diastolic pressure is similar in both ventricles. (B) Left ventricular diastolic pressure tracing (scale 0–40 mm Hg).

H	diastolic plateau	EDP	end of diastole (onset of systole)
O	lowest diastolic pressure		

can be detected early in the course of the disease by Doppler flow analysis. Diastolic impairment is characterized by a decrease in diastolic filling and an increase in velocity during atrial contractions. Abnormal reflection of the ultrasonic beam can be detected by high-resolution ultrasonography when the myocardium has been infiltrated by abnormal substances (amyloid, hemochromatin) or tissue elements (endocardial fibroelastosis, eosinophils). The clinical efficacy of high-resolution ultrasonography has not yet been validated in large series.

Cardiac Catheterization

Cardiac catheterization demonstrates characteristic hemodynamic aberrations in patients with restricted cardiomyopathy. However, these changes are not pathognomonic, since they may also occur in constrictive pericarditis, mediastinal fibrosis, and other disorders associated with impaired diastolic function (eg, myocardial infarction with biventricular involvement, right ventricular enlargement with compression of the left ventricle posteriorly against the normal pericardium, neoplastic infiltration of the pericardium). The ventricular pressure tracing demonstrates a deep and rapid early decline in ventricular pressure at the onset of diastole, followed by a rapid rise to a plateau in early diastole; this distinctive configuration has been termed the "square root sign." The atrial pressure tracing reveals a prominent "Y" descent, followed by a rapid rise to a plateau. The "X" descent may also be rapid, resulting in a characteristic "M" or "W" wave form. The "A" wave is prominent and is often of the same amplitude as the "V" wave (Fig. 19.24). Systemic and pulmonary venous pressure, as well as left and right end diastolic pressure, are elevated. The pressure elevations are exacerbated by exercise. Pulmonary artery pressure is elevated, reflecting the left atrial hypertension.

Angiocardiography

Angiocardiography is seldom indicated when the diagnosis of restricted cardiomyopathy has been established by other means. Left and right ventriculography demonstrate normal-sized chambers with relatively normal contractility. However, it is difficult to evaluate diastolic function with this technique. Absence of the normal effect of left atrial contraction during ventricular diastole can often be appreciated on cine studies. (Normally, left ventricular filling is rapid during the first part of diastole and slows progressively until the end of diastole. Late in diastole, the left atrium contracts, increasing left ventricular volume—a phenomenon known as the "atrial kick." Owing to the impaired relaxation of the left ventricle in patients with restricted cardiomyopathy, left atrial contraction is not effective in increasing left ventricular volume at the end of diastole.) Left ventriculography frequently demonstrates mitral insufficiency, a common sequela of this disorder.

Coronary arteriography is indicated in any patient over 40 years of age to rule out associated obstructive coronary artery disease. Coronary arteriography typically demonstrates decreased excursion of the epicardial and septal arteries during the cardiac cycle, an observation that may be helpful in differentiating restricted cardiomyopathy from constrictive pericarditis (the septal arteries tend to show increased mobility in the latter condition) (see Chapter 21).

SPECIFIC MYOCARDIAL DISEASES

The myocardium may be involved in a variety of systemic disorders (Fig. 19.25). These disorders may manifest with the morphologic and hemodynamic features of a dilated cardiomyopathy (eg, alcoholic heart disease), hypertrophic cardiomyopathy (eg, glycogen storage disease, Niemann–Pick disease, Friedreich's ataxia), or restricted cardiomyopathy (eg, amyloidosis, hemochromatosis). In addition, some systemic disorders may also affect the endocardium and cardiac valves (eg, carcinoid syndrome, methysergide toxicity).

TABLE 19.25 SYSTEMIC DISORDERS ASSOCIATED WITH MYOCARDIAL DYSFUNCTION.

Category	Examples
Infectious (myocarditis)	Viral, rickettsial, bacterial, trepanosomal (Chagas disease)
Granulomatous disorders	Sarcoidosis
Neoplastic disorders	Leukemia
Endocrine disorders	Thyrotoxicosis, hypothyroidism, adrenocortical insufficiency, pheochromocytoma, acromegaly
Metabolic and nutritional disorders	Hypokalemia, hyperkalemia, hypomagnesemia, kwashiorkor, beri-beri
Storage and infiltrative disorders	Hemochromatosis, glycogen storage disease, mucopolysaccharidoses (Hurler, Hunter, Morquio–Ullrich), Niemann–Pick disease, histiocytosis X (Langerhans type)
Amyloid deposition	Primary, secondary, and familial forms
Connective tissue disorders	Systemic lupus erythematosus, polyarteritis nodosa, scleroderma, rheumatoid arthritis
Muscular and neuromuscular disorders	Muscular dystrophy (Duchenne, myotonic dystrophy), Friedreich's ataxia
Hypersensitivity and toxicity	Alcohol, sulfonamide, penicillin, antimony, cobalt, isoprenaline, anthracene
Therapeutic irradiation	Postirradiation cardiomyopathy

Fig. 19.25 Systemic disorders associated with myocardial dysfunction.

CHAPTER 20

Ischemic Heart Disease: Clinical Features and Noninvasive Diagnosis

GENERAL CONSIDERATIONS

PATHOPHYSIOLOGY

Ischemic heart disease is the consequence of an inadequate supply of oxygenated blood to the myocardium. It can be caused by decreased myocardial blood flow resulting from obstructive disease, spasm or thrombosis of the coronary arteries, by increased myocardial oxygen demand, or by a combination of the two. The resulting myocardial hypoxemia leads to metabolic disturbances at the cellular level, which are manifested clinically by metabolic, electrophysiologic, and hemodynamic aberrations of variable severity.

METABOLIC DISTURBANCES

The metabolic changes associated with myocardial ischemia are complex. The various clinical manifestations of ischemic heart disease reflect the locally decreased oxygen saturation, as well as the accumulation of toxic metabolites such as lactic acid and

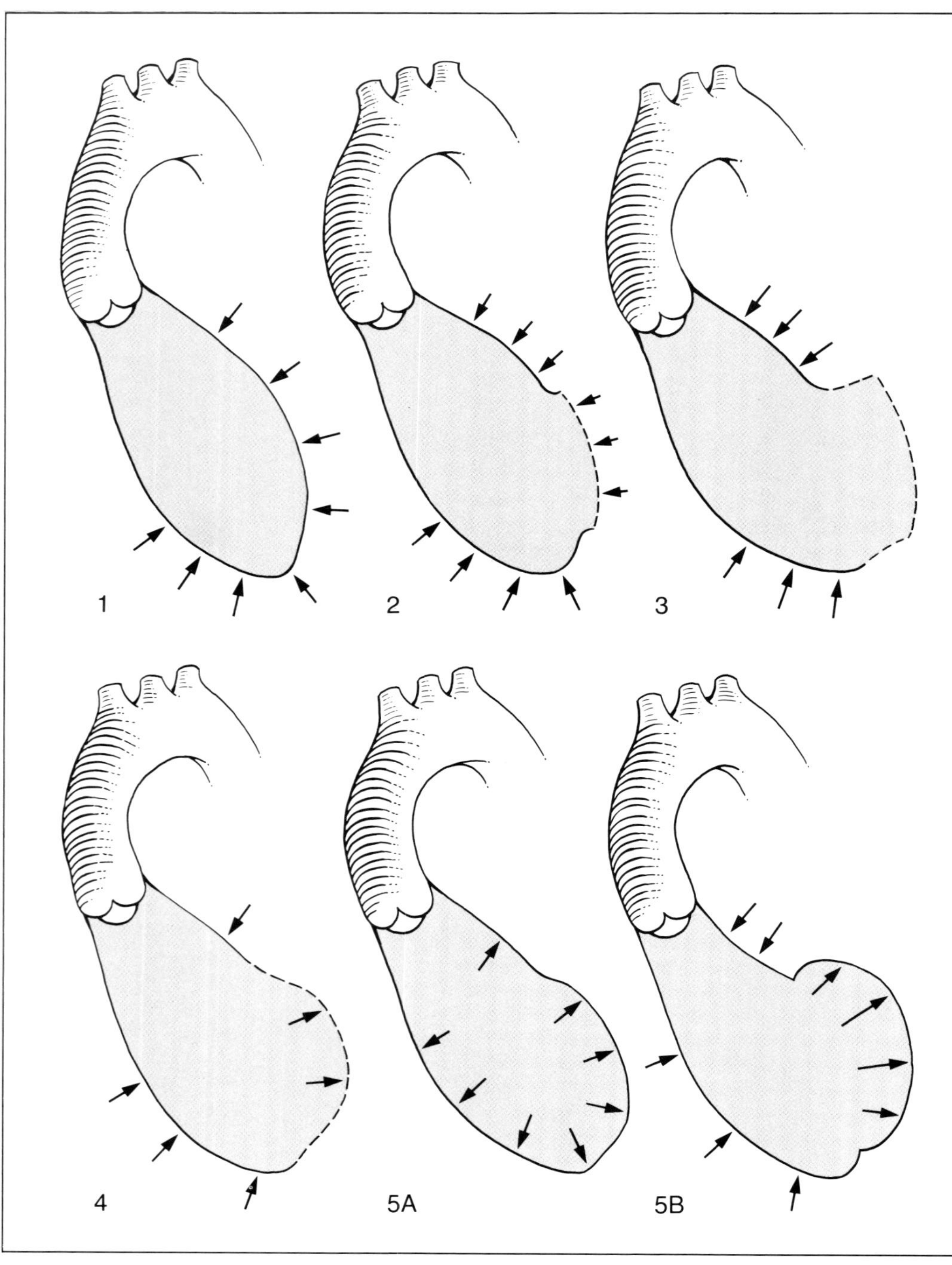

Fig. 20.1 Patterns of myocardial dysfunction observed on imaging studies. In the following examples, the dysfunction involves the anterolateral wall of the left ventricle. (1) Normal systole. Concentric inward displacements of all segments of the left ventricle. (2) Hypokinesis. There is diminished inward displacement of the anterolateral wall of the left ventricle during systole. The involved segment is displaced inward, but the displacement is less than that of the normal surrounding myocardium. (3) Akinesis. There is no inward displacement of the anterolateral wall of the left ventricle during systole. (4) Dyskinesis. The anterolateral wall of the left expands during systole while the remainder of the left ventricular wall is displaced inward. (5A and 5B) Left ventricular aneurysm. (A) End diastole. The anterolateral wall of the left ventricle is deformed (B) Systole. The abnormal segment expands, while the normal surrounding myocardium is displaced inward.

ammonia. Myocardial ischemia results in significant aberrations of calcium metabolism. (The tendency for calcium to accumulate in areas of myocardial necrosis has led to the use of ^{99m}Tc-tagged calcium salts in scintigraphic tests used for diagnosis of myocardial infarction.) Elevated serum levels of creatine phosphokinase (CPK) and lactic dehydrogenase (LDH) are sensitive indicators of myocardial necrosis and subendocardial ischemia, forming the basis of the most widely used clinical tests for myocardial infarction.

ELECTROPHYSIOLOGIC DISTURBANCES

Although myocardial ischemia is associated with significant and constant changes in the ECG, the underlying mechanisms are not well understood. Abnormalities of the ST-segment are commonly seen in patients with ischemic heart disease. Elevation of the ST-segment implies severe ischemia or necrosis, whereas depression is associated with subendocardial ischemia without transmural necrosis. The leads in which these changes occur indicate the site of the ischemia. Thus, ST-segment changes in leads V1 and V6 indicate ischemia in the anteroapical segment of the left ventricle, whereas ST-segment changes in leads II, III, and aVF reflect ischemia in the inferior wall of the left ventricle. However, it should be emphasized that the absence of ST-segment changes does not exclude the possibility of clinically significant myocardial ischemia. Indeed, 5 to 10 percent of patients with angina pectoris have a normal resting ECG. Conversely, some individuals without signs or symptoms of ischemic heart disease exhibit significant ST-segment changes both at rest and with exercise.

HEMODYNAMIC DISTURBANCES

A significant reduction (or interruption) of the blood supply to a portion of the myocardium leads to a decrease in the ability of the affected ventricle to contract and relax. The degree of ventricular dysfunction depends on the severity and extent of the myocardial ischemia. Both the systolic and diastolic function of the ventricle are affected; however, systolic function may be normal in the early stages of ischemic heart disease.

Several patterns of myocardial dysfunction are observed on imaging studies in patients with ischemic heart disease (Fig. 20.1):

1. Hypokinesis. The affected segment contracts and relaxes poorly.
2. Dyskinesis. The affected segment expands during systole.
3. Akinesis. A portion of the myocardium does not contract or relax during the cardiac cycle (any apparent motion of the affected segment is due to displacement of the adjacent normal myocardium).
4. Ventricular aneurysm. When an extensive segment of the myocardium dies and is replaced by fibrous tissue, the affected portion of the ventricular wall protrudes beyond the normal ventricular contour during diastole and expands during systole, resulting in a significant deformity of the cardiac silhouette throughout the cardiac cycle.

To compensate for the localized dysfunction, the normal myocardium surrounding the ischemic region undergoes hypertrophy and remodeling. These adaptations may allow the affected ventricle to function normally (or almost normally). However, when myocardial damage is very extensive these compensatory mechanisms are insufficient to prevent ventricular failure.

ISCHEMIC HEART DISEASE SECONDARY TO CORONARY ATHEROSCLEROSIS

CLINICAL MANIFESTATIONS

In the Framingham study, approximately 1 percent of men 30 to 60 years of age developed symptoms of ischemic heart disease per year. The initial manifestation was angina pectoris in 45 percent, myocardial infarction in 42 percent, and sudden death in 13 percent. Many of these patients had premature ventricular contractions at the time of presentation. Although congestive heart failure is rarely the initial manifestation of ischemic heart disease in young adults, it is the initial manifestation in 58 percent of patients who are 70 years of age or older at the time of diagnosis.

CHRONIC ISCHEMIC HEART DISEASE

ANGINA PECTORIS

Although chest pain is the hallmark of myocardial ischemia, it occurs in many nonischemic cardiac conditions and in a variety of gastrointestinal, neuromuscular, and respiratory disorders (Fig. 20.2). The term *angina pectoris* ("angina") is used to describe the chest pain associated with myocardial ischemia. *Classical angina* is a transient precordial or substernal discomfort which is typically provoked by exertion, emotion, stress, ingestion of a meal, heat, cold, or excessive humidity, and is

FIGURE 20.2 CARDIAC AND NONCARDIAC DISORDERS ASSOCIATED WITH CHEST PAIN MIMICKING ANGINA PECTORIS

Nonischemic cardiac conditions

Aortic valvular stenosis and insufficiency
Cardiomyopathy (dilated, hypertrophic)
Mitral valve prolapse
Pericarditis
Aortic dissection
Pulmonary embolism
Pulmonary hypertension

Noncardiac conditions

Digestive tract
- Esophagitis
- Peptic ulcer
- Gastritis

Musculoskeletal
- Shoulder arthropathy
- Chest wall pain

Lung and mediastinum
- Pneumothorax
- Pleuritis
- Mediastinitis

Fig. 20.2 Cardiac and noncardiac disorders associated with chest pain mimicking angina pectoris.

promptly relieved by rest or nitrates (eg, nitroglycerine). *Atypical angina* is characterized by chest pain similar to classical angina; however, one or more of the additional features that typify classical angina are lacking. *Angina equivalent* is characterized by dyspnea or pain in the left shoulder or arm; like classical angina, it is provoked by exertion and relieved by rest or nitrates. In *variant (Prinzmetal's) angina,* pain is present at rest or awakens the patient from sleep, and is not precipitated by physical exertion.

Angina pectoris is caused by obstructive disease of the large coronary arteries; one, two, or three coronary arteries may be involved. The location, quality, duration, severity, and frequen-

FIGURE 20.3 CLINICAL GRADING OF ANGINA PECTORIS

Grade I	Angina occurs with usual activity but does not result in functional impairment
Grade II	Angina occurs with prolonged activity and results in minimal functional impairment
Grade III	Angina occurs with usual activity and results in functional impairment
Grade IV	Angina occurs at rest and the patient is incapacitated for usual activities

Fig. 20.3 Clinical grading of angina pectoris.

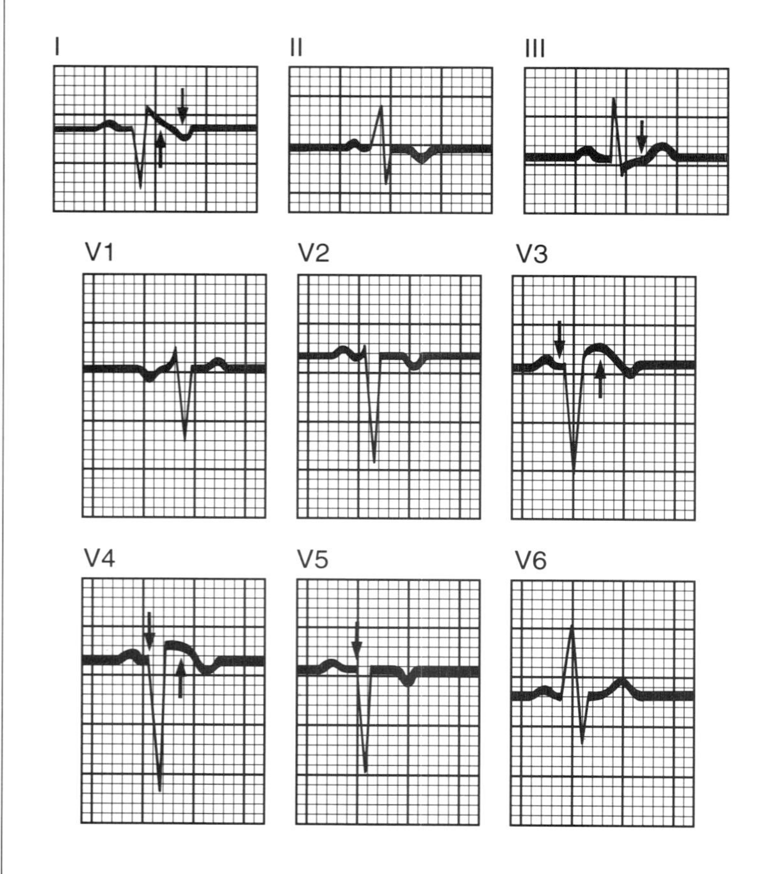

Fig. 20.4 Anterior myocardial infarction (ECG findings). In I, the ST-segment is elevated and the T-wave is inverted. In III, the ST-segment is depressed. The ST-segment is elevated in leads V3 and V4. Note absence of R-waves and prominence of Q-waves in V3, V4, and V5. This pattern is typical of an old anterior myocardial infarct secondary to occlusion of the left anterior descending coronary artery.

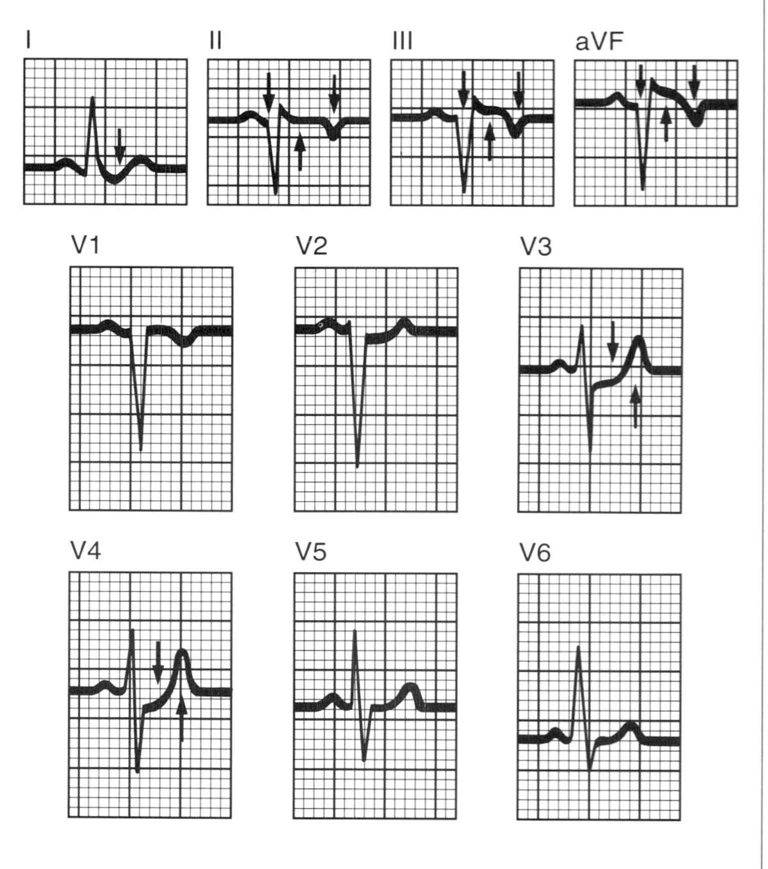

Fig. 20.5 Posteroinferior myocardial infarction. In I, there is significant depression of the ST-segment. In II and III, the R-wave is absent, the ST-segment is elevated, and the T-waves are inverted. In V3, the ST-segment is markedly depressed but the ST-segment is elevated. In V4, the T-wave is still higher and the ST-segment is markedly depressed. This pattern is typical of an old posteroinferior infarct secondary to occlusion of the circumflex artery.

cy of the pain, as well as the provoking factors, have considerable prognostic importance. Angina pectoris is graded according to the pattern of pain occurrence and the degree of functional impairment (Fig. 20.3).

PHYSICAL FINDINGS

The physical examination is usually unremarkable in patients with chronic ischemic heart disease. Occasionally there is a widened or diffuse apical impulse secondary to left ventricular enlargement. PVCs are quite common; although ventricular ectopic beats may indicate the presence of a left ventricular aneurysm, they can also occur in normal individuals. Auscultatory findings indicating left ventricular dysfunction (eg, muffled S1, paradoxically split second heart sound) are sometimes present. An apical systolic murmur of mitral insufficiency (due to papillary muscle dysfunction or a dilated mitral annulus) can be heart in an occasional patient.

ELECTROCARDIOGRAPHIC FINDINGS

The resting ECG is the initial diagnostic test in patients with suspected ischemic heart disease. The most common abnormalities are pathologic Q-waves (which usually indicate previous myocardial infarction), abnormal repolarization (ST-segment and T-wave abnormalities) (Figs. 20.4 and 20.5), disturbances of atrioventricular and intraventricular conduction, and signs of left atrial enlargement. These findings may be seen in a number of cardiac disorders other than ischemic heart disease and therefore are not pathognomonic of the latter.

The correlation between certain ECG findings and coronary artery disease is well established. For example, in patients with previous myocardial infarction the nature of the Q-wave changes usually indicates the location and extent of coronary artery involvement; however, both false negatives and false positives may occur. In one study, single-vessel disease was more likely to be encountered in patients with a normal QRS-complex than in patients with ECG evidence of infarction; almost two thirds of the patients with double- or triple-vessel disease had a normal QRS-complex (Hamby, 1977).

The *electrocardiographic exercise stress test* ("ECG stress test") is commonly used in patients with suspected ischemic heart disease. Its goal is to induce a controlled, temporary ischemic state during a period of continuous clinical and ECG observation. The patient is then classified as being at high, intermediate, or low risk for coronary artery disease. The interpretation is based on the ST-segment, R-wave, T-wave, and Q-wave changes elicited by exercise (walking on a treadmill or riding a bicycle). The duration of the test, the work performed by the patient ("load"), and changes in hemodynamic status (reflected by systemic blood pressure and heart rate) must also be taken into account. ST-segment depression greater than 1 mm, usually seen in leads V5 and aVf, is interpreted as a positive ECG stress test (Fig. 20.6). The predictive value of this finding is increased when the ST-segment depression occurs soon after exercise is begun or is associated with a decrease in systemic blood pressure. The exercise stress test has a sensitivity of 62 to 80 percent (mean 65 percent) and a specificity of 83 to 96 percent (mean 85 percent) for coronary artery disease. Its sensitivity and specificity are lower in women than in men.

IMAGING AND INVASIVE DIAGNOSIS

Plain Films

The radiographic findings associated with ischemic heart disease vary with the nature and duration of the symptoms. Most patients who present with chest pain have a normal chest film (Fig. 20.7). Patients in whom congestive heart failure is the initial manifestation typically exhibit radiographic evidence of

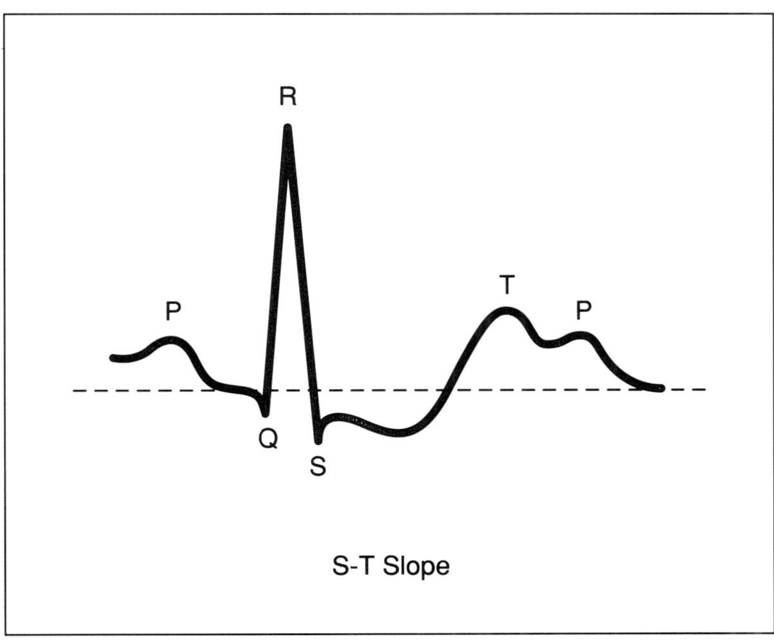

Fig. 20.6 Abnormal electrocardiographic exercise stress test. Depression of the ST-segment during exercise, usually seen in V5, indicates myocardial ischemia (ie, a "positive" stress test).

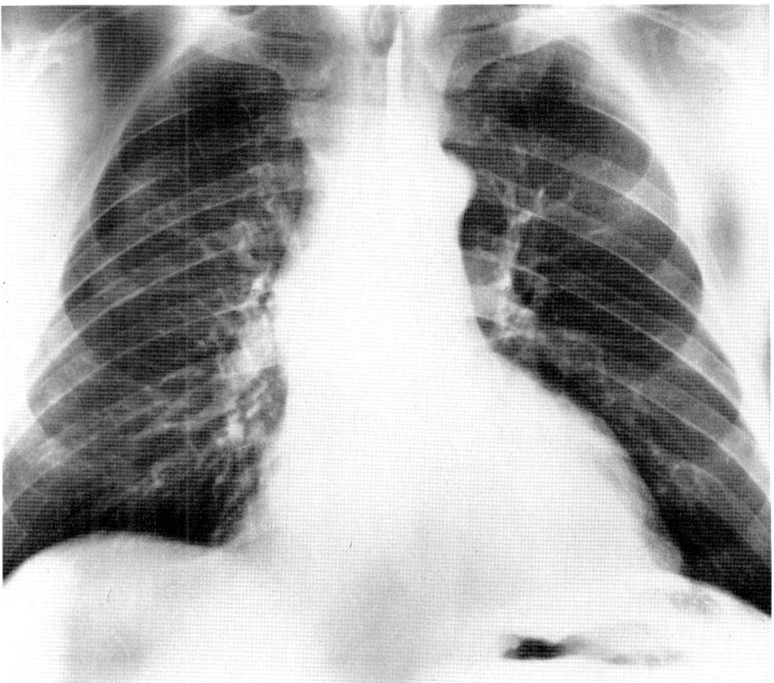

Fig. 20.7 Ischemic heart disease. Posteroanterior chest film of a patient with three-vessel obstructive coronary artery disease shows a normal-sized heart with left ventricular enlargement. The pulmonary vasculature is normal.

pulmonary venous hypertension, left ventricular enlargement, and moderate left atrial dilatation (Fig. 20.8). About 50 percent of patients who present with an arrhythmia have a normal chest film; however, cardiomegaly with left ventricular and left atrial enlargement is not uncommon in this setting. The presence of cardiomegaly and/or pulmonary venous hypertension usually indicates a decrease in the left ventricular ejection fraction secondary to a previous myocardial infarction (Fig. 20.8); both radiographic findings have an adverse prognostic significance. It should be emphasized that a normal chest film does not exclude significant left ventricular enlargement.

Calcification of the coronary arteries—which is much more likely to be detected by fluoroscopy than on chest films—is a good indicator of coronary atherosclerosis (Fig. 20.9). Although calcification of the coronary arteries can be appreciated fluoroscopically in about 75 percent of patients with coronary artery disease, it is seen in only 25 percent of those with severe obstructive disease. Coronary artery calcification in symptomatic patients between 40 and 50 years of age almost always indicates severe ischemic heart disease. (Coronary artery calcification are very common after 70 years of age and therefore correlate poorly with ischemic heart disease in the elderly.) The extent of the calcification does not correlate with the severity of the obstructive disease; this is especially true in elderly patients.

Although the presence or absence of coronary artery calcification is of little consequence in symptomatic patients, its presence is of great significance in asymptomatic individuals. In one study, 20 percent of asymptomatic individuals between 40 and 50 years of age with coronary artery calcification detected during routine chest fluoroscopy were subsequently shown to have significant coronary artery disease. It is therefore important for the radiologist to routinely look for coronary artery calcification when performing an esophagram, barium enema, or upper gastrointestinal series.

Echocardiography

Echocardiography, particularly when the transesophageal approach is employed, can consistently detect stenosis of the proximal segments of the right and left main coronary arteries. However, the efficacy of echocardiography in detecting coronary artery disease has yet to be validated in large clinical studies. At present, its main role is to assess left ventricular function and morphology. Echocardiography accurately detects abnormal wall motion, left ventricular dilatation, and congestive heart failure, all of which have considerable prognostic significance (Fig. 20.10; see Appendix). The cardiac valves, pericardium, and the presence or absence of left ventricular thrombus can also be assessed.

The echocardiographic exercise stress test has been proposed as an alternative to the ECG stress test. In the absence of ischemic heart disease, all segments of the ventricular wall exhibit normal motion at rest and with exercise (stress). In a normal subject, the left ventricular ejection fraction increases with exercise. Abnormal wall motion is defined as segmental hypokinesis, akinesis, or dyskinesis. The development of additional abnormalities of wall motion in conjunction with an abnormal resting study (or the development of any abnormality in conjunction with a normal resting study) is indicative of myocardial ischemia. A decreased ejection fraction with exercise in the absence of abnormal wall motion indicates global left ventricular dysfunction. In various published series, the mean

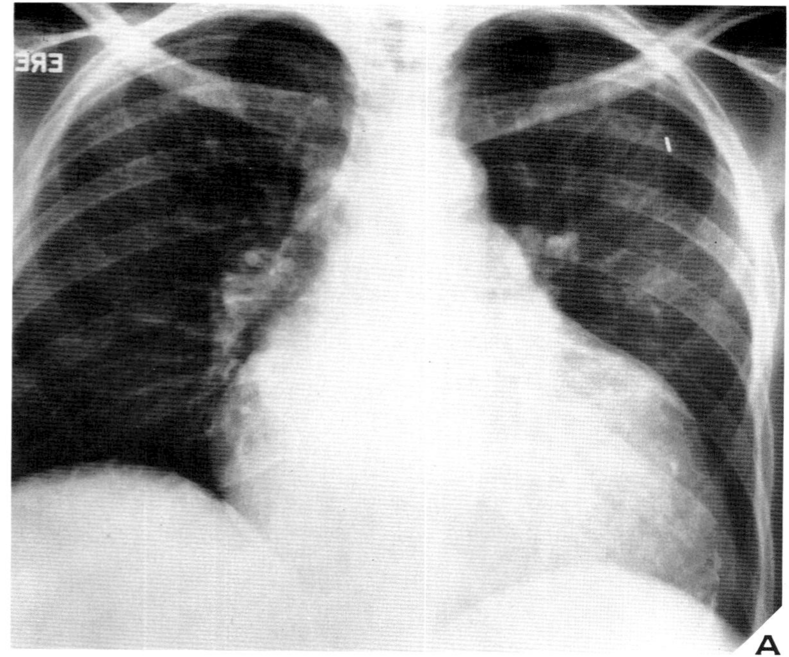

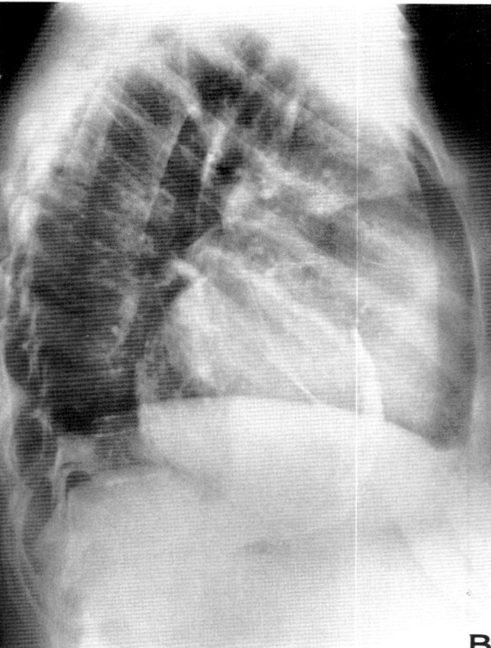

Fig. 20.8 Congestive failure secondary to ischemic heart disease. (A) Frontal and (B) lateral chest films in a patient with angina pectoris show marked enlargement of the left ventricle, which projects to the left, inferiorly, and posteriorly. Note the curvilinear calcification in the anterolateral wall of the left ventricle, the site of a previous myocardial infarction. There is evidence of left ventricular failure (note left atrial enlargement and cephalization pattern indicating pulmonary venous hypertension).

sensitivity of the echocardiographic exercise stress test in detecting ischemic heart disease is 65 percent (range, 62 to 80 percent), with a mean specificity of 87 percent (range 83 to 96 percent). There is a strong correlation between the segmental distribution of the abnormal wall motion and the territory of the stenotic coronary artery (sensitivity, 80 percent; specificity, 87 percent).

Nuclear Medicine

Chronic ischemic heart disease and its sequelae can be evaluated by a number of scintigraphic tests. Various blood pool tests delineate the morphology of the cardiac chambers and can be used to assess myocardial contractility. By using radiopharmaceuticals whose distribution corresponds to myocardial blood flow, one can assess myocardial perfusion. Other radiopharmaceuticals are used to assess metabolic function and viability.

Blood Pool Studies (Radionuclide Angiography). This technique, which employs ^{99m}Tc-labeled erythrocytes, ^{99m}Tc-labeled human albumin, or the recently introduced ^{99m}Tc-labeled methoxyisobutyl isonitrile (MiBi), is based on the principle that the substance labeled with the tracer is distributed uniformly in the circulating blood. In the most popular technique, known as multiple gated acquisition scanning (MUGA), activity in the cardiac chambers is recorded in multiple projections during systole and diastole over a 5- to 10-minute period. By limiting the acquisition of counts to the period of the R-wave (ECG gating), it is possible to obtain a series of images that delineate ventricular morphology and contractility. Thus, regional and global function of each ventricle can be assessed during rest and exercise. With this noninvasive technique, it is possible to calculate global and regional ventricular ejection fractions and relative and absolute ventricular volumes, which provide useful information about the dynamic changes associated with ischemic heart disease (Figs. 20.11 and 20.12, Appendix). By means of blood pool studies it is possible to measure the regional ejection fraction and assess changes in regional wall motion.

Injecting the tracer during exercise increases the sensitivity of the test. Certain functional and dynamic abnormalities indicating myocardial ischemia that are not evident on the resting study (eg, abnormal global or segmental contraction) may be seen only on the exercise study. By assessing wall motion, ejection fraction, and ventricular volume at rest and during exercise, 75 to 90 percent of patients with ischemic heart disease can be identified.

The first-pass technique is used to exclude an intracardiac shunt, which can occur as a complication of ischemic heart disease (eg, perforation of the ventricular septum). In this technique, the radiopharmaceutical is injected into a peripheral vein and its course through the right heart, pulmonary circulation, left heart, and aorta is recorded on sequential scintigrams. Increased activity in the pulmonary circulation on the levophase indicates a left to right shunt.

Tests of Myocardial Perfusion. Radioisotopes that concentrate in the myocardium are useful to study myocardial perfusion. The most widely used agent is ^{201}Tl (thallium), which is taken up by viable myocytes via the sodium–potassium pump.

Thallium can be administered at rest or at peak exercise. Approximately 88 percent of an intravenously administered dose of thallium is cleared by the myocardium during the first pass; its myocardial distribution is proportional to coronary blood flow. Although the factors that affect myocardial thallium uptake are not completely understood, the most important appear to be local ischemia, the exercise level at the time of administration, and the serum insulin level. After initial uptake, thallium is progressively "washed out" from the myocardium into the circulating blood. Fifty percent of an administered dose of thallium, which has a physical half-life of 72 hours, disappears from the myocardium in 4 to 7 hours and is

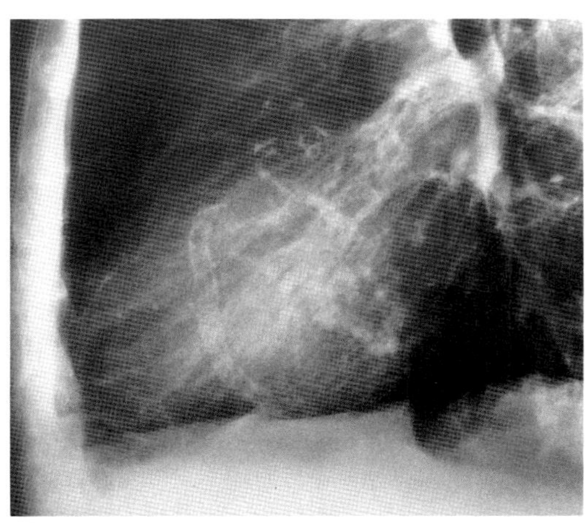

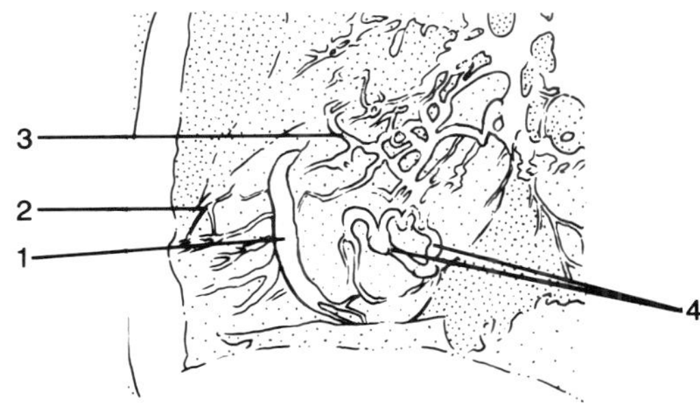

Fig. 20.9 Coronary artery calcification. Lateral chest film of a patient with ischemic heart disease shows extensive calcification of the right coronary artery and of the left anterior descending and circumflex branches of the left coronary artery. There is also calcification of the mitral valve.

1 right coronary artery
2 left anterior descending coronary artery
3 circumflex artery
4 calcified mitral valve

rapidly cleared by the kidneys; once cleared from the myocardium, the half-life of thallium in the circulating blood is 30 seconds.

In a normal individual, the rate of thallium uptake and wash-out is uniform throughout the myocardium (Fig. 20.13). Segmentally diminished uptake indicates poor myocardial perfusion (ie, ischemic heart disease).

Nonviable myocardium appears as a region of abnormally decreased uptake which persists for the duration of the study (4 to 24 hours) (Fig. 20.14). Abnormally slow uptake of tracer with prolonged retention (delayed wash-out) indicates that the myocardium is viable but underperfused (Fig. 20.15).

The scintigraphic images can be recorded by either the planar or the tomographic method. In the latter technique, known as single photon emission tomography (SPECT), sections of the heart at different planes are displayed separately (Figs. 20.13 to 20.15) or as concentric rings ("bulls-eye") using a polar-coordinate mapping technique (Fig. 20.16; see Appendix). It is much easier to detect underperfused segments on SPECT images than on planar images.

Thallium scintigraphy is highly accurate for diagnosis of coronary artery disease, with a sensitivity of 90 to 95 percent and a specificity of 85 to 90 percent. Even more important than its accuracy is its ability to localize the myocardial damage to specific vascular territories (ie, the distribution of specific coronary arteries). Thallium scintigraphy is particularly useful in patients with an abnormal resting ECG and clinical manifestations of myocardial ischemia, in patients on drug therapy, and in patients with impaired exercise tolerance. Patients unable to perform the standard exercise test, which employs a treadmill or bicycle, can be studied after a dose of dipyridamole, a drug that enables the examiner to stress the heart under controlled conditions.

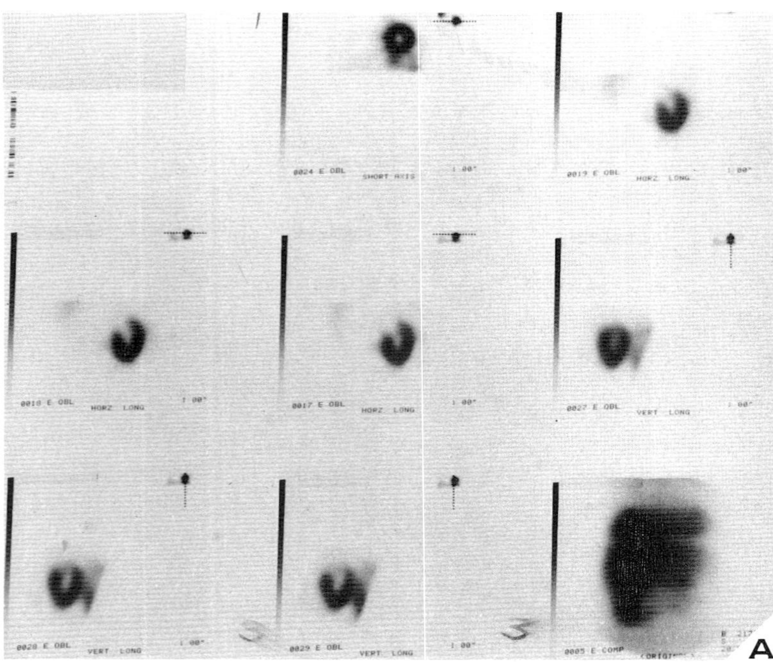

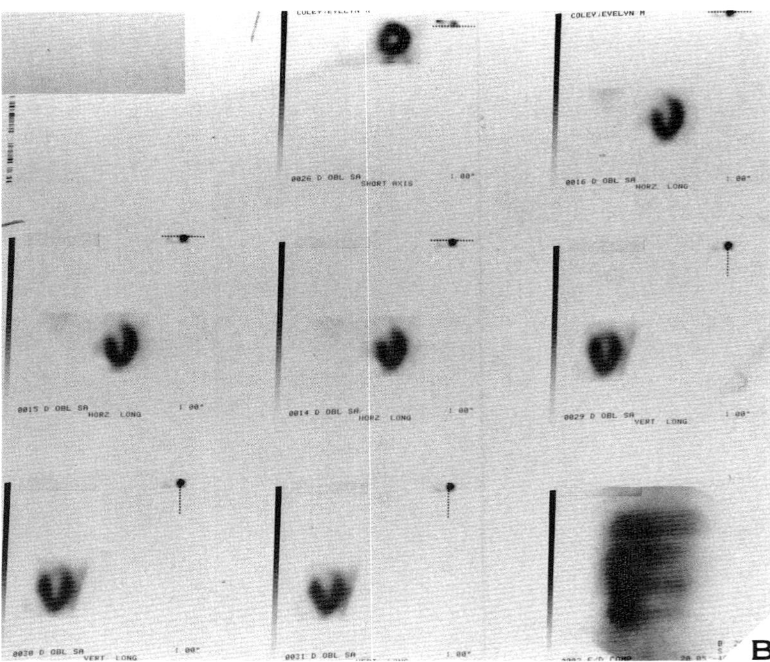

Fig. 20.13 Normal myocardial perfusion (thallium) exercise test. SPECT images in multiple projections following intravenous administration of 3 mCi of thallium-201 (A) Early phase. (B) Three hours after injection. All segments of the left ventricular myocardium show uniform uptake and wash-out of the radiopharmaceutical. The radiopharmaceutical was injected during maximal exertion, during which time the systolic blood pressure rose 5 mm Hg from the baseline level. The simultaneous ECG tracing was normal and the patient did not complain of chest pain. (1 = short axis projection; 2 = left anterior oblique projection; 3 = vertical longitudinal projection.)

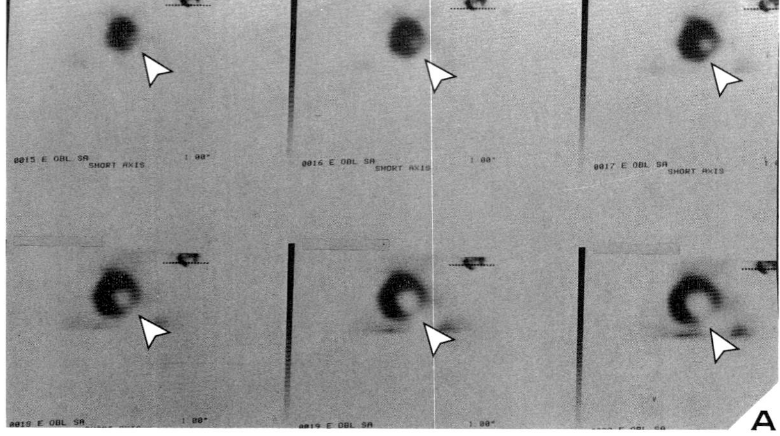

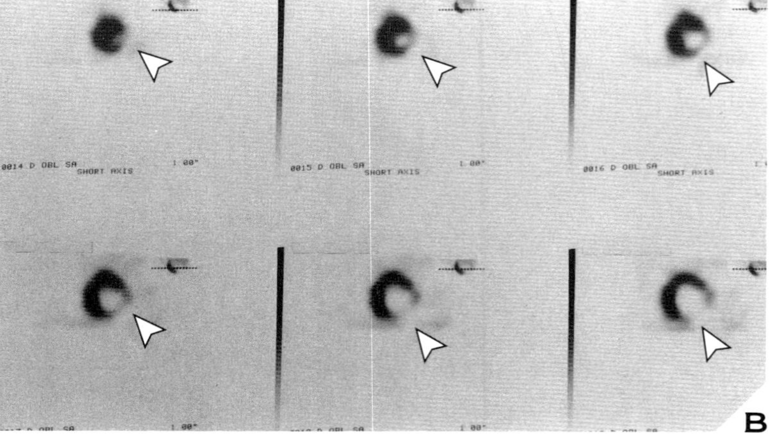

Fig. 20.14 Abnormal myocardial perfusion on resting thallium study. (A) Early and (B) delayed (3 hour) tomographic (SPECT) images in short axis projection following administration of 3 mCi of ^{201}T1. Note the area of decreased uptake (*arrows*) in the posterolateral segment of the left ventricle which persists on the delayed images.

Myocardial perfusion can also be assessed by positron emission tomography (PET) employing ^{13}N-labeled ammonia, ^{3} ^{8}K, or generator-produced ^{82}Rb. (^{13}N and ^{38}K are cyclotron byproducts; ^{38}Rb is generator-produced.) These radionuclides decay by producing a positron, a particle having the same mass as an electron but an opposite charge; when the positron encounters an electron outside the nucleus, the electron–positron pair undergoes annihilation, converting the masses of the two particles into two 0.511 meV photons which travel away from the annihilation site in opposite directions. The PET scanner consists of an array of detector elements coupled to electronics and a computer; in most devices the detector elements (which consist of a single crystal coupled to a single photomultiplier tube) are arranged in a circular ring (Fig. 20.17). Two protons that arrive simultaneously at a pair of detectors at opposite sides of the ring are recorded as a single annihilation event. With this technique, it is possible to precisely localize the annihilation events, yielding scintigraphic images with excellent spatial resolution.

Tests of Cardiac Metabolism. Several scintigraphic tests assess the metabolic status of the myocardium. Most of these measure the rate of uptake of substrates such as fatty acids and glucose or its analogue 2-deoxyglucose. The uptake of amino acids into myosin, the contractile protein of cardiac muscle, has not been extensively studied with scintigraphic techniques. Scintigraphic studies of cardiac metabolism are limited by technical problems in labeling the substrate and the rate at which the substrate is metabolized.

The radiopharmaceuticals most commonly used for studies of cardiac metabolism are glucose or 2-deoxyglucose labeled with the positron emitters ^{11}C or ^{16}F. Both glucose and 2-deoxyglucose are phosophorylated by glucokinase to form glucose-6-phosphate. Whereas most cells utilize glucose as their main energy source, normal myocardial cells preferentially utilize fatty acids for this purpose. On the other hand, ischemic but viable myocardial cells preferentially utilize glucose. Ischemic myocardium, as well as myocardium that is recovering from a recent ischemic event,

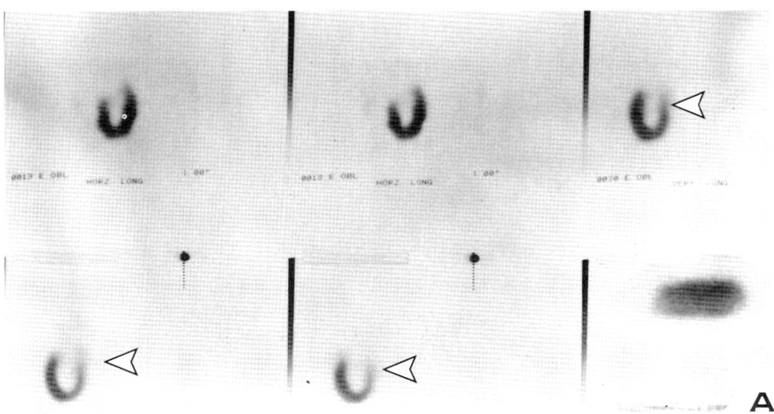

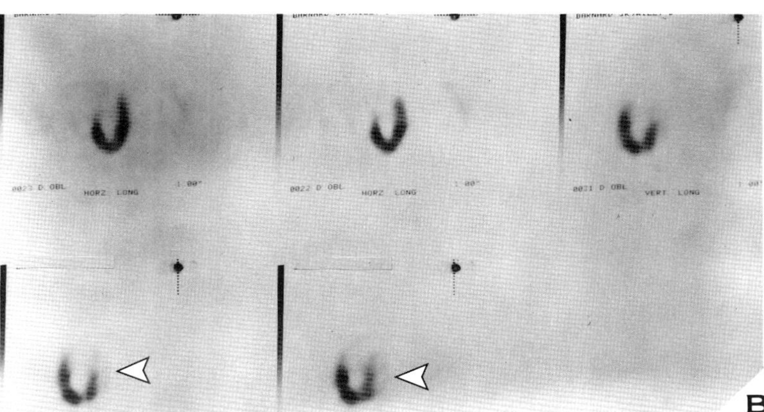

Fig. 20.15 Abnormal thallium exercise study in a patient with angina pectoris. Tomographic (SPECT) study following administration of 3 mCi of ^{201}T1. The radiopharmaceutical was administered during exercise, which was terminated prematurely when the patient complained of chest pain; the ECG revealed 2-mm elevation of the ST-segment. (A) Early and (B) delayed (3 hour) images in the left anterior oblique projection in the horizontal long axis (1-2) and vertical long axis (3-5) planes. Note diminished uptake (*arrows*) in the posterolateral segment of the left ventricle (4 and 5) on the early images. The delayed images show further accumulation of the radiopharmaceutical, with better delineation of the wall of the affected segment. The redistribution of the tracer indicates that the myocardium in the affected segment is viable but underperfused.

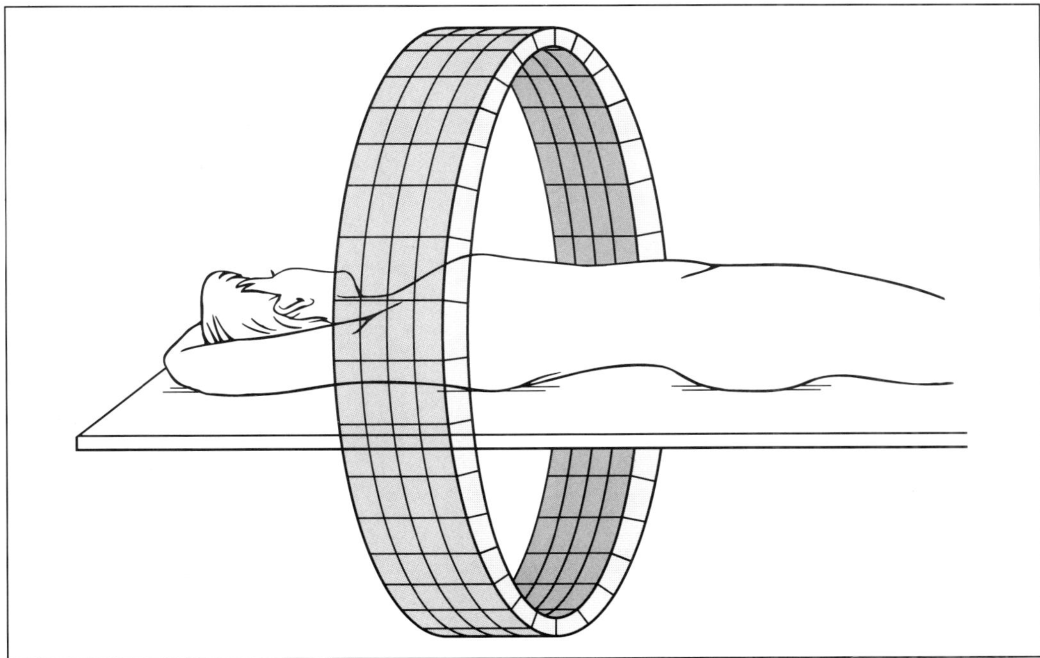

Fig. 20.17 PET scanner. The detectors are stacked in circular array. Each detector consists of a single crystal coupled to a single photomultiplier tube.

exhibits increased uptake of the tracer when compared with normal myocardium.

Long-chain fatty acids provide more than 90 percent of the myocardial energy requirement under aerobic conditions. Long-chain nonesterified fatty acids (NEFAs) are rapidly cleared from the blood (half-time less than 2 minutes) and are taken up by the myocardium during the first pass, with an extraction rate of 50 to 60 percent. Scintigraphic studies utilizing labeled fatty acids provide valuable insight into the efficiency of myocardial energy production in patients with ischemic heart disease, cardiomyopathy, and myocardial hypertrophy, and after myocardial infarction. Radiopharmaceuticals currently available for such studies include intrinsically ^{11}C-labeled palmitate and a series of analogues labeled with positron or single-photon emitters. Both unmodified palmitate and its phenyl- and phenylmethyl-substituted analogues are rapidly concentrated in the myocardium and rapidly catabolized. The clearance rate and the total uptake and oxidation are significantly decreased in ischemic myocardium. Studies have shown that the contribution of NEFAs to total myocardial energy production drops to about 30 percent (normal, 50 to 60 percent) in ischemic myocardium. This decrease is probably due to a shift to an alternate oxidation pathway which catabolizes NEFAs one carbon atom at a time.

Other Invasive Modalities

Obstruction of the coronary arteries by atherosclerotic plaques can be demonstrated angiographically in approximately 90 percent of patients with signs and symptoms of ischemic heart disease. In the remainder, the obstruction is secondary to dissection, coronary artery emboli, or vasculitis (eg, periarteritis nodosa).

Ventricular dysfunction, which can be demonstrated by various imaging modalities, is a common sequela of ischemic heart disease. In patients with stable angina, myocardial damage is minimal; although there may be some destruction of myocardial cells in the subendocardial region, most of the myocardium is unaffected. In patients with severe, longstanding angina the damage may be more extensive, with replacement of a portion of the myocardium by fibrous tissue which lacks the ability to contract and relax. Extensive myocardial damage (eg, after a transmural myocardial infarction) may lead to formation of a ventricular aneurysm. Right ventricular infarction (resulting in right ventricular dysfunction) is much less common than left ventricular infarction, and is almost always associated with the latter.

Cine coronary arteriography is the standard technique for evaluating the morphology of the coronary arteries. Although the role of other imaging methods (eg, echocardiography, MRI, cine CT) continues to evolve, angiocardiography (left ventriculography) remains the method of choice for assessing changes in the left ventricular wall produced by ischemic heart disease. Coronary arteriography and angiocardiography are further discussed in the following chapter.

ACUTE MYOCARDIAL INFARCTION

PATHOLOGY

Acute myocardial infarction is defined as necrosis of a significant portion of the myocardium caused by an abrupt interruption of the blood supply. Histologically, an acute myocardial infarct consists of an area of tissue necrosis surrounded by a region of patchy cell death and edema. Microscopically, dead muscle fibers exhibit loss of striations, eosinophilia, fragmentation, and gradual disappearance of the nuclei. The infarcted region is initially invaded by polymorphonuclear leukocytes and later by macrophages; in the final stage of repair the infarcted muscle is replaced by fibrous tissue.

Myocardial infarcts are described according to the anatomic region affected. For example, an anteroseptal infarct involves the anterior portion of the myocardium and the adjacent ventricular septum; a posteroseptal infarct involves the posterior ventricular wall and the adjacent septum; and a lateral infarct involves the free wall, sparing the septum. These patterns, which correspond to the territories of the major coronary arterial branches (Fig. 20.18), are discussed further in the following chapter.

The artery supplying the affected myocardial segment is occluded or markedly narrowed in 90 percent of patients who die of acute myocardial infarction. In one patient study, 85 percent of the coronary arteriograms obtained within 4 hours

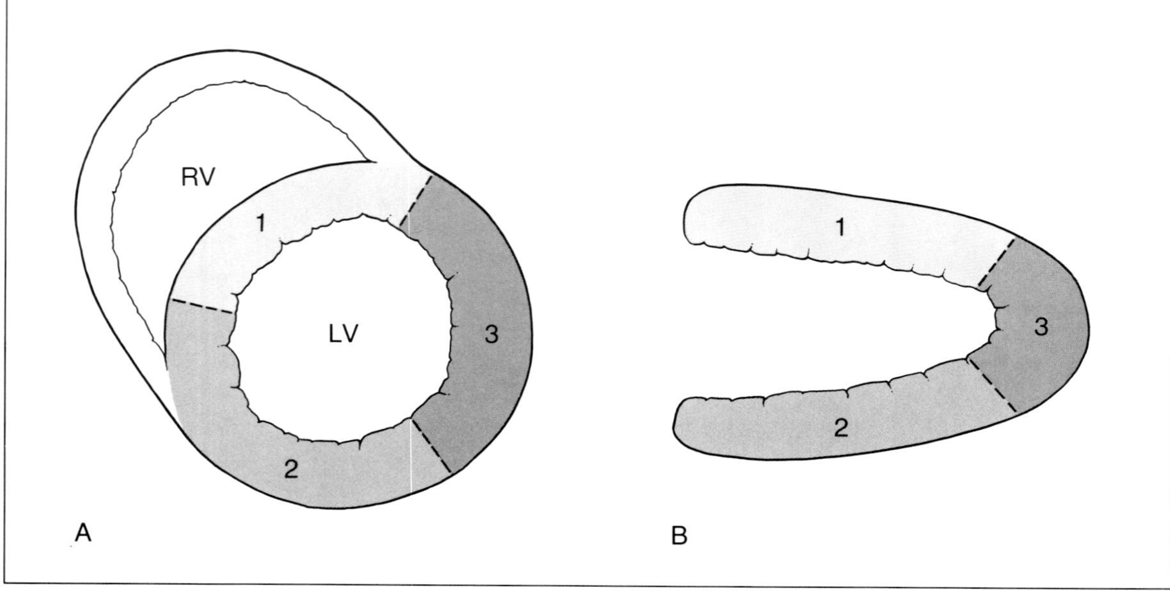

Fig. 20.18 Anatomic patterns of acute myocardial infarction. Schematic representation showing how the usual patterns of myocardial infarction correspond to the territories supplied by the major coronary arteries. (A) Short axis projection. (B) Left anterior oblique projection.

1 anteroseptal infarct (territory normally supplied by left anterior descending artery)
2 posteroseptal infarct (territory normally supplied by distal right coronary artery and its posterior descending branch)
3 posterolateral infarct (territory normally supplied by the circumflex artery)

after onset of symptoms demonstrated coronary artery occlusion. Angiograms performed at a greater interval after onset of symptoms demonstrate a lower rate of occlusion (Fig. 20.19), suggesting that some acutely occluded arteries subsequently reopen. In a small percentage of cases the coronary artery supplying the infarcted region is entirely normal. In such cases one can speculate that the infarction was caused by a transient interruption of myocardial blood flow caused by spasm.

The recanalization process, which usually proceeds at a relatively slow rate, can be accelerated by thrombolytic therapy and other therapeutic measures (see Chapters 30 and 31). It has been shown that the extent of myocardial damage can be decreased by early reperfusion of the ischemic region.

In young adults in whom myocardial infarction is the first manifestation of ischemic heart disease, the artery supplying the infarcted region is usually occluded very close to its origin; in such cases few or no collaterals are demonstrated by coronary arteriography or autopsy.

CLINICAL MANIFESTATIONS

The diagnosis of acute myocardial infarction is based on three criteria: clinical history, characteristic ECG changes, and elevated serum cardiac enzyme levels. At least two of these criteria (one of which must be elevation of cardiac enzyme levels) are required for unequivocal diagnosis of acute myocardial infarction. Because cardiac enzyme levels are not elevated until 2 to 15 hours after the onset of symptoms, unequivocal diagnosis is usually not possible at the time of admission, when only the clinical history and abnormal ECG findings are usually available.

Chest pain, typically accompanied by nausea, anxiety, and sweating, is the classical presenting symptom of acute myocardial infarction. Initially, the ECG demonstrates elevation or depression of the ST-segment, inversion of the T-wave, and absence of the R-wave; deep Q-waves are usually a late manifestation (Fig. 20.20). In approximately 75 percent of cases, acute myocardial infarction is strongly suggested by the clinical history and the ECG findings.

Ventricular function is affected to a variable degree, depending on the extent of myocardial damage; some patients exhibit no evidence of ventricular malfunction, whereas others present with severe congestive heart failure or cardiogenic shock secondary to profound ventricular failure. On the basis of the hemodynamic changes, patients with acute myocardial infarction can be classified into four categories (Kembal et al, 1967).

Category 1. No congestive heart failure.
Category 2. Mild congestive heart failure.
Category 3. Pulmonary edema.
Category 4. Cardiogenic shock.

Cardiogenic shock is the acute inability of the left ventricle to perfuse the vital organs: death is imminent without effective

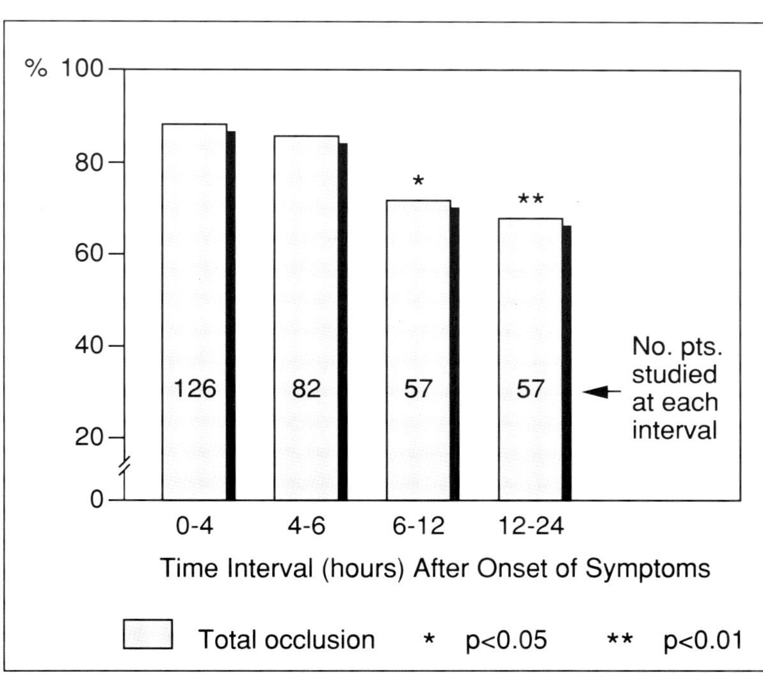

Fig. 20.19 Frequency of total occlusion of infarct-related artery in patients with acute myocardial infarction at discrete time intervals after onset of symptoms (Adapted from DeWood MA, et al: Prevalence of total occlusion during the early hours of transmural myocardial infarction. (*N Engl J Med* 1980; 303:897.)

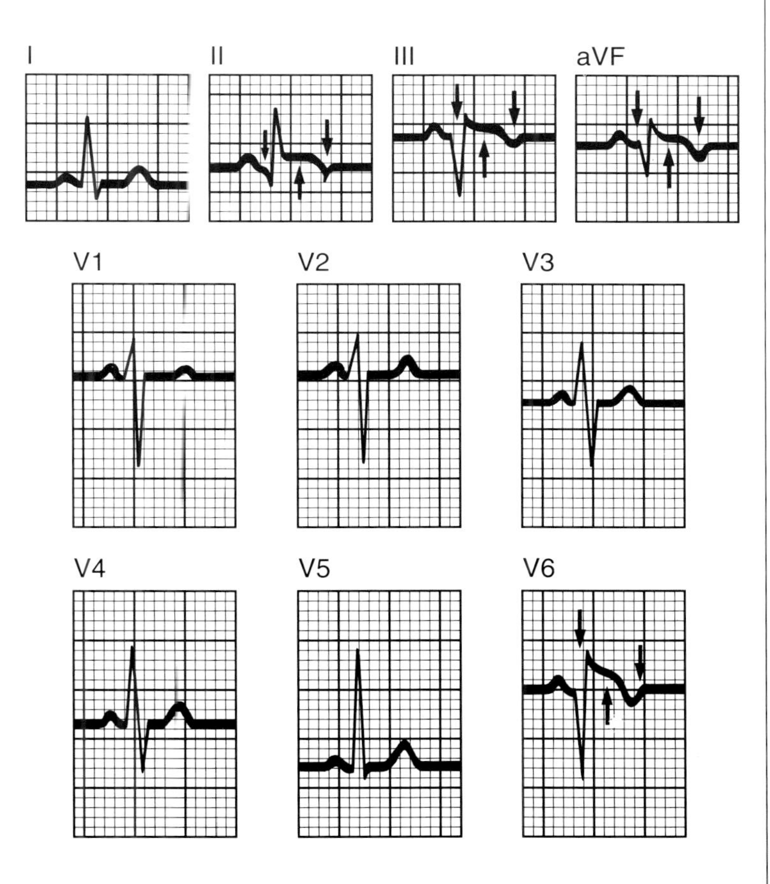

Fig. 20.20 Acute posterolateral myocardial infarction secondary to occlusion of a large marginal artery. Note 2-mm ST-segment elevation and T-wave inversion in II. Deep Q-waves, ST-segment elevation, and T-wave inversion are seen in II, V6, and aVf.

cardiovascular support. A systolic blood pressure of 70 mm Hg or less usually indicates the presence of cardiogenic shock. The Kembal classification has considerable prognostic value. Whereas the mortality in Categories 1, 2, and 3 is 7, 29, and 26 percent, respectively, the mortality in Category 4 is 90 percent (ie, only 10 percent of patients who present in cardiogenic shock survive the acute episode).

Acute complications of myocardial infarction include perforation of the ventricular septum, perforation of the free wall of the affected ventricle (cardiac rupture), and papillary muscle rupture resulting in acute mitral insufficiency. Subacute and late complications include the postmyocardial infarction (Dressler) syndrome (see Chapter 22), left ventricular aneurysm, and chronic left ventricular failure.

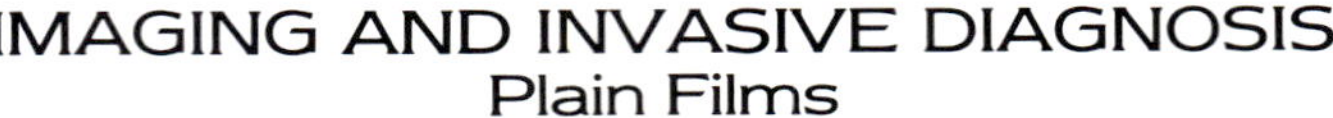

IMAGING AND INVASIVE DIAGNOSIS

Plain Films

In most patients with acute myocardial infarction left ventricular output is only slightly decreased, in which case the chest film is usually normal. Patients with more extensive myocardial damage may exhibit radiographic signs of left ventricular failure (Fig. 20.21). Acute pulmonary edema signals massive left ventricular involvement (Fig. 20.22).

Echocardiography

Echocardiography can be performed to verify the extent of left and right ventricular myocardial damage. The extent of the lesion correlates with the extent of abnormal wall motion. Patients with involvement of more than 50 percent of the left

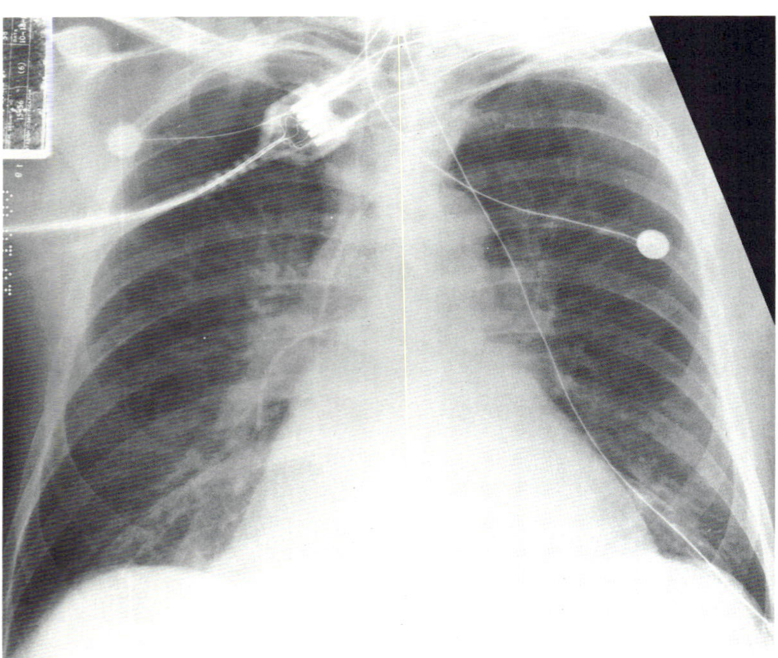

Fig. 20.21 Acute myocardial infarction. Supine portable chest film demonstrates mild left ventricular enlargement and moderate pulmonary edema (note perihilar haze). A Swan–Ganz catheter has been inserted; its tip is in the right lower lobe artery. Other studies confirmed the presence of a large myocardial infarct secondary to occlusion of the left anterior descending coronary artery.

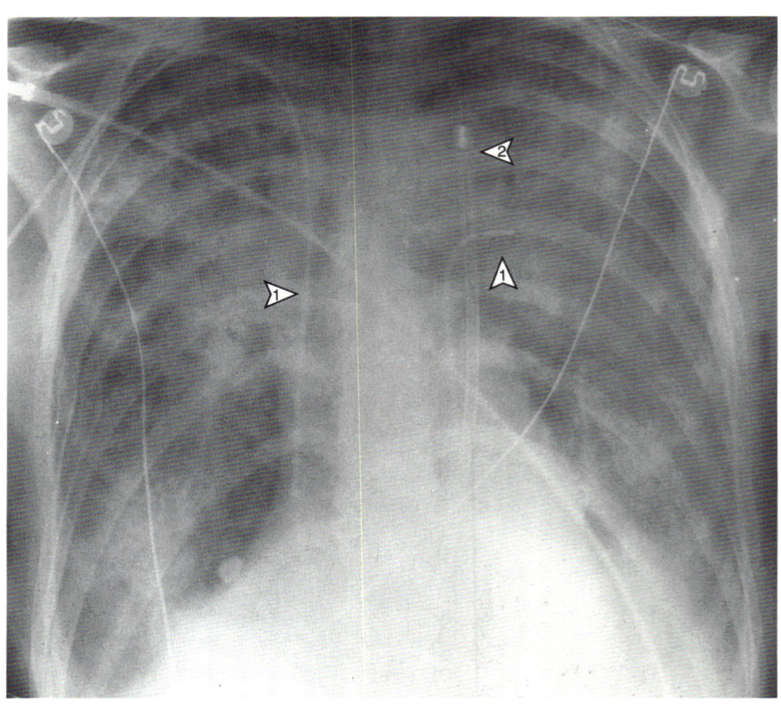

Fig. 20.22 Acute myocardial infarction with left ventricular failure and mitral insufficiency. Supine portable chest film in a patient with extensive myocardial damage with papillary muscle dysfunction shows bilateral alveolar pulmonary edema. The heart is not significantly enlarged. There is no left atrial enlargement. A Swan–Ganz catheter (*arrows* 1) is in place, with its tip in a branch of the left pulmonary artery. An intra-aortic counterpulsion balloon catheter (*arrow* 2) is also present, with its tip at the level of the aortic arch.

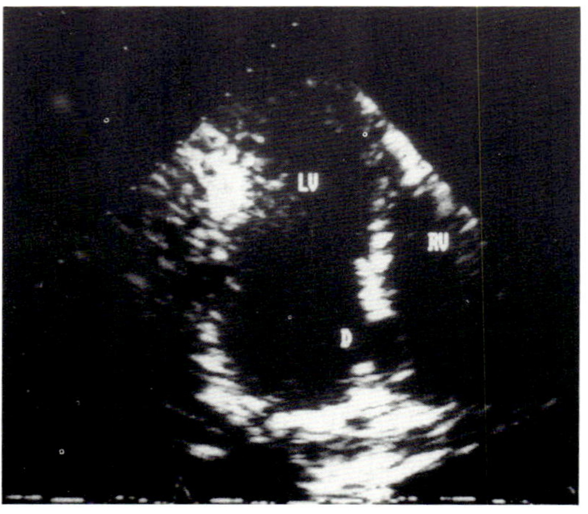

Fig. 20.23 Acute myocardial infarction with rupture of the ventricular septum. Apical four-chamber projection demonstrates an echo-free region (D) in the position of the inlet portion of the ventricular septum, which represents the ruptured segment. The left ventricle (LV) is enlarged. (RV = right ventricle)

ventricular myocardium are at increased risk for death during the acute stage. The early development (within 24 hours of the onset of symptoms) of a "functional aneurysm" is also associated with increased mortality. (A "functional aneurysm" is defined as a ventricular segment that behaves like an aneurysm but whose wall consists of viable myocardium.)

Various complications of acute myocardial infarction, such as acute mitral insufficiency secondary to rupture of a papillary muscle, hemopericardium secondary to rupture of the free wall of the left ventricle, and rupture of the ventricular septum (Fig. 20.23), can be demonstrated by echocardiography.

Nuclear Medicine

Cardiac scintigraphy with ^{99m}Tc-pyrophosphate ("pyrophosphate") can confirm the presence of myocardial necrosis. The principle of the test is that the cell membrane of necrotic myocardial cells loses its normal permeability, leading to excessive intracellular accumulation of calcium. Thus, an intravenously administered dose of the radiopharmaceutical accumulates in the infarcted segment (Fig. 20.24). Persistent abnormal pyrophosphate accumulation has been associated with an increased incidence of recurrent infarction and sudden death.

The disadvantage of pyrophosphate scintigraphy is that the abnormal accumulation of pyrophosphate in necrotic myocardium is a late event, and is seldom detected scintigraphically less than 3 days after the acute episode. (In animal studies pyrophosphate accumulation may occur as early as 12 hours, or as late as 10 days, after coronary artery ligation.) For this reason, this test is no longer widely used.

During acute myocardial infarction the soluble light chain of cardiac myosin leaks from myocardial cells into the blood, whereas the insoluble heavy chain remains inside the cells until it is digested by leukocytes (liquefactive necrosis). Studies in experimental animals and man have shown that ^{99m}Tc- or ^{111}In-labeled antibodies directed against the heavy chain of cardiac myosin (papain-digested fragment of antimyosin Fab) accumulate in necrotic myocardium; in the animal model, abnormal uptake of the radiopharmaceutical in the region of the infarct can be detected as early as 6 hours after coronary artery ligation. Although early results are encouraging, this test has not yet been approved for general clinical use. At present there are no clinically available nuclear medicine techniques capable of detecting the early stage of myocardial infarction.

Invasive Diagnosis

Coronary arteriography is used to localize the obstruction, verify catheter placement, and monitor the therapeutic response in patients undergoing thrombolytic therapy for acute myocardial infarction (see Chapters 21 and 31). Left ventriculography demonstrates the extent of the myocardial damage and can be used to assess the function of the surrounding myocardium. It also demonstrates the presence of mitral insufficiency secondary to papillary muscle dysfunction or dilatation of the mitral annulus. Complications such as perforation of the ventricular septum and papillary muscle rupture are clearly depicted by left ventriculography (see Chapter 21). Because comparable information can be obtained by noninvasive techniques, and because it is potentially hazardous in the presence of acute myocardial infarction, left ventriculography is rarely indicated.

Cardiac catheterization is seldom performed in patients with acute myocardial infarction. Right heart catheterization demonstrates increased oxygen saturation in the right ventricle and pulmonary artery in patients with a left to right shunt secondary to rupture of the ventricular septum.

VENTRICULAR ANEURYSM

A ventricular aneurysm is defined as a large segment of nonviable myocardium which is deformed during diastole and expands (dilates) during systole. Left ventricular aneurysm is a relatively

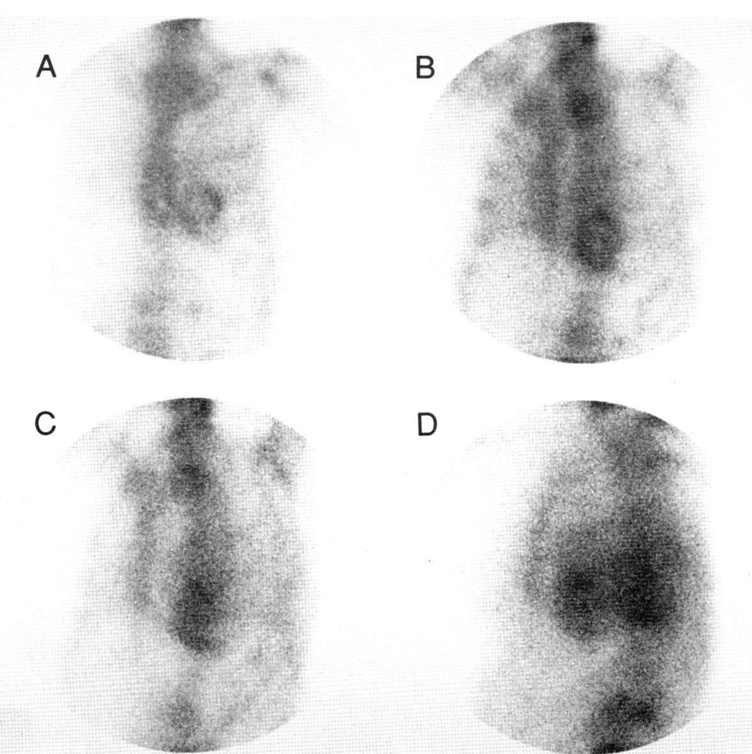

Fig. 20.24 Acute myocardial infarction demonstrated by pyrophosphate scintigraphy. This 36-year-old woman presented with acute cardiogenic shock. The ECG showed evidence of extensive anterior wall infarction, consistent with occlusion of the left anterior descending artery. (A–D) Pyrophosphate scan obtained 24 hours after the onset of symptoms in (A) anterior, (B) 30° LAO, (C) 60° LAO, and (D) left lateral projections shows 4+ uptake (significantly greater than bone uptake in the ribs and sternum) in a large "doughnut"-shaped lesion. The lesion migrates with the sternum, indicating its anterior location. The doughnut configuration indicates absence of flow in the center of the infarcted region, with abnormal uptake by the compromised myocardium at the periphery of the lesion. This scintigraphic pattern connotes a poor prognosis. (Courtesy of Arnold Strashun, MD, Brooklyn, New York.)

frequent late complication of acute myocardial infarction, occurring in 15 to 20 percent of patients with transmural involvement. In one study, 47 percent of patients with left ventricular aneurysms were still alive 5 years after the acute episode; only 18 percent were alive at 10 years (Grondin et al, 1979). Mural thrombus is a frequent sequela of left ventricular aneurysms (see below).

Left ventricular aneurysms usually involve the anterolateral and apical regions; the posterolateral and diaphragmatic regions are less frequently affected (Fig. 20.25). About 5 percent of all ventricular aneurysms involve the inferior wall of the right ventricle. Left ventricular aneurysms are most commonly associated with combined lesions of the left anterior descending, circumflex, and right coronary arteries ("triple vessel disease"), with isolated stenosis of the left anterior descending artery next in order of frequency. The latter is the most common underlying coronary artery lesion in patients 40 to 50 years of age.

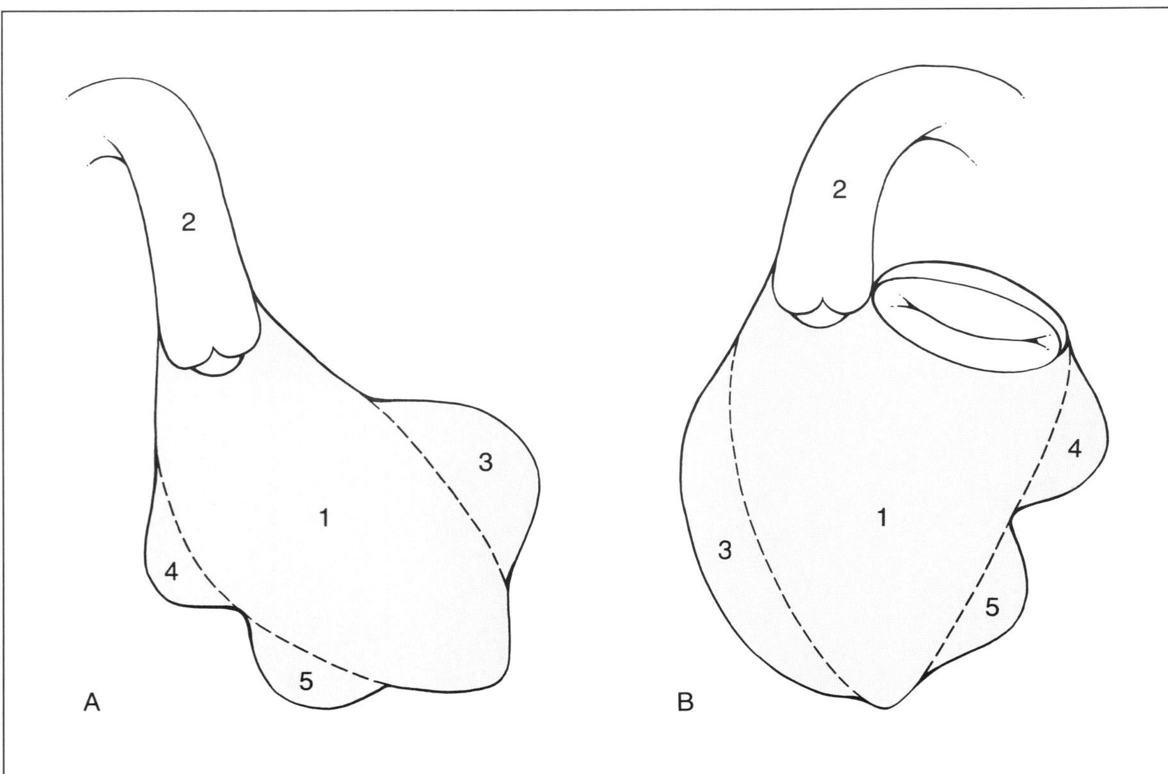

Fig. 20.25 Location of left ventricular aneurysms. The most common locations are shown schematically in the (A) right anterior oblique and (B) left anterior oblique projections. The most common site is the anterolateral wall of the left ventricle, corresponding to the territory normally supplied by the left anterior descending coronary artery. Aneurysms of the diaphragmatic and posterobasal segments (the territories of the right coronary and circumflex arteries, respectively) are less common.

1 left ventricle
2 aorta
3 aneurysm of anterolateral and septal segment of left ventricle
4 aneurysm of posterobasal and superlateral segments of left ventricle
5 aneurysm of diaphragmatic and inferolateral segments of left ventricle

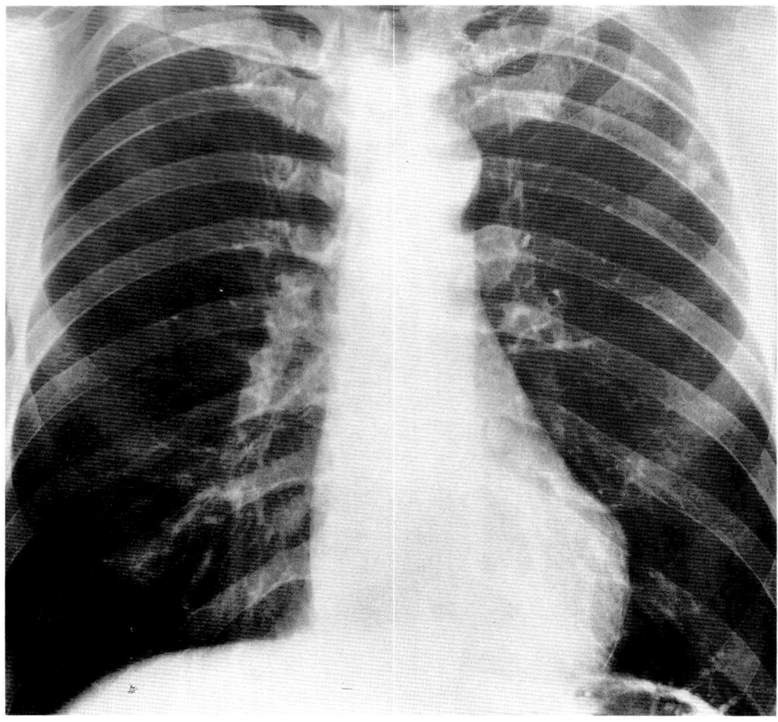

Fig. 20.26 Left ventricular aneurysm. Posteroanterior chest film of a patient with a history of a previous myocardial infarction shows a subtle deformity of the left interior border of the cardiac silhouette, suggesting localized left ventricular enlargement. However, the presence of a linear calcification in this region indicates that the deformity represents a left ventricular aneurysm.

CLINICAL MANIFESTATIONS

There is usually a history of a previous acute myocardial infarction. The usual complaints are (in order of frequency) dyspnea on exertion, easy fatigability, and angina; less frequent symptoms include palpitations, dyspnea at rest, and syncope. Physical examination may reveal expansion and leftward displacement of the apical impulse. Not uncommonly there is a murmur of mitral insufficiency, a frequent sequela of left ventricular aneurysms. Systemic embolic phenomena strongly suggest the presence of mural thrombus in the left ventricle.

IMAGING AND INVASIVE DIAGNOSIS

Plain Films

Frontal and lateral chest films typically show cardiomegaly with left ventricular enlargement and a localized deformity of the left ventricular contour (Figs. 20.26 and 20.27). Only 5 percent of patients with left ventricular aneurysm have normal plain films. ["Radiologically silent" aneurysms usually arise from the inferior (diaphragmatic) aspect of the left ventricle.] The lateral chest film often shows a characteristic double density in the area beneath the aortic valve (Fig. 20.27B). Aneurysms located in the posteroinferior portion of the left ventricle typically deform the diaphragm (the posterioinferior contour of the left ventricle is often deformed as well). Calcification of the wall of the aneurysm can be detected radiographically or fluoroscopically in 20 to 30 percent of patients with left ventricular aneurysms (Fig. 20.26). Although often difficult to appreciate on plain films, the calcification is easily detected fluoroscopically.

Left atrial enlargement usually indicates mitral insufficiency. Congestive failure, a frequent sequela of left ventricular aneurysm, is manifested radiographically by pulmonary venous hypertension (cephalization pattern) and pulmonary edema.

Echocardiography

Echocardiography is a highly sensitive and specific method for detecting left ventricular aneurysms, and provides a noninvasive way to assess the severity of the resulting functional disturbance (Fig. 20.28). Although most aneurysms are clearly shown on long axial two-chamber and four-chamber views, the precise location and extent of the aneurysm are most clearly seen on transesophageal images.

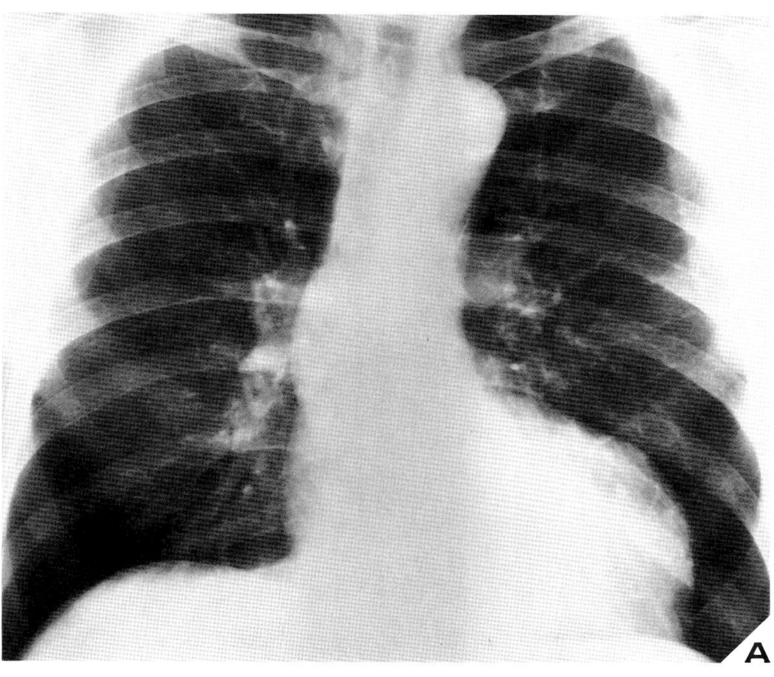

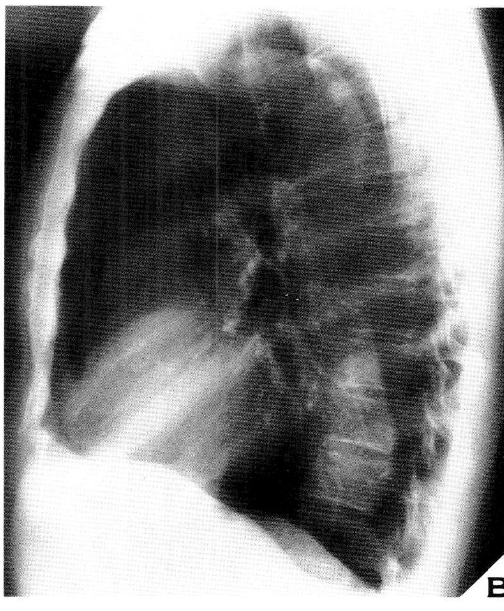

Fig. 20.27 Left ventricular aneurysm. (A) Posteroanterior chest film shows left ventricular enlargement, with a localized deformity just above the apex. (B) Lateral projection shows increased radiopacity in the area beneath the aortic valve, which represents an aneurysm of the anterolateral segment of the left ventricle. The patient had a history and ECG evidence of a previous myocardial infarction.

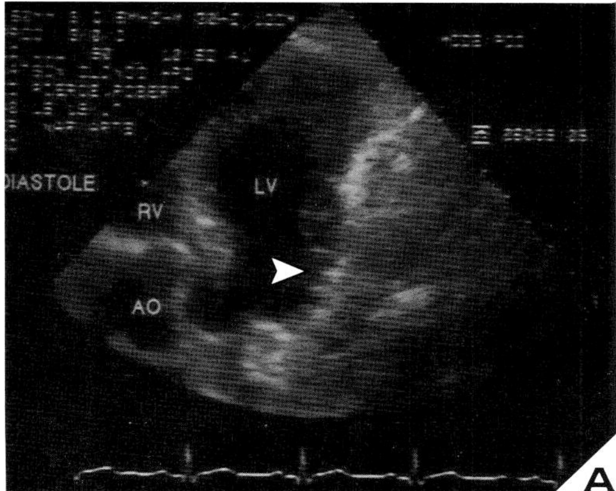

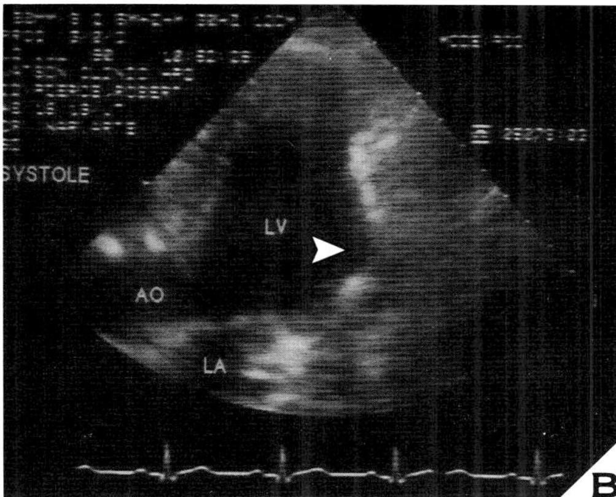

Fig. 20.28 Left ventricular aneurysm (echocardiographic findings). Apical long-axis views in (A) diastole and (B) systole demonstrate a deformity of the posteroinferior aspect of the left ventricle (LV) with thinning (*arrows*) of the ventricular wall in this region. A portion of the thinned wall protrudes beyond the ventricular wall during systole, confirming that it represents an aneurysm; the other portions of the left ventricle contract normally. The calculated ejection fraction was 55 percent. Coronary arteriography revealed occlusion of the right coronary artery. (AO = aorta; LA = left atrium)

(This is particularly true of aneurysms located in the posteroinferior portion of the left ventricle.) Color Doppler images demonstrate the abnormal flow pattern characteristic of a ventricular aneurysm (Fig. 20.29; see Appendix), as well as the mitral insufficiency that is commonly present.

Computed Tomography

Left ventricular aneurysms are clearly demonstrated on contrast-enhanced images. "Fast" or cine CT images obtained in the transverse or oblique plane accurately depict the location and extent of the aneurysm (Fig. 20.30).

MRI

MRI has the same sensitivity and specificity as "fast" or cine CT in detecting left ventricular aneurysms. Static and cine MR images demonstrate the size and location of the aneurysm and the status of the surrounding myocardium (Fig. 20.31). Cine MRI is particularly useful in detecting both mitral insufficiency and the mural thrombus that is present in approximately 50 percent of patients with left ventricular aneurysms.

Angiography

Left ventricular aneurysm and its sequelae (eg, mitral insufficiency, mural thrombus) are clearly depicted by left ventriculography (see following chapter).

MURAL THROMBUS

Mural thrombus is a frequent sequela of both acute myocardial infarction and left ventricular aneurysm, and occasionally occurs in patients with dilated cardiomyopathy. (Mural thrombus is so common in patients with left ventricular aneurysm that some authors include it in the definition of the latter.) In one study, mural thrombus was present in 32 percent of patients with acute myocardial infarction and in 50 percent of those with left ventricular aneurysms (Keating et al, 1983).

PATHOGENESIS

The thrombotic process is initiated by aggregation of platelets in the immobile segment of the ventricular wall, which leads to deposition of variable amounts of fibrin and blood clot. This results in enlargement of the thrombus, which is eventually replaced by organized fibrous tissue. Longstanding mural thrombi may undergo calcification, although this is uncommon. Grossly, mural thrombi are usually broadly attached to the ventricular wall; only rarely are they pedunculated.

CLINICAL MANIFESTATIONS

The presence of mural thrombus in the left ventricle is rarely suspected on clinical grounds. Peripheral embolic phenomena suggest the diagnosis; however, this complication is very unusual.

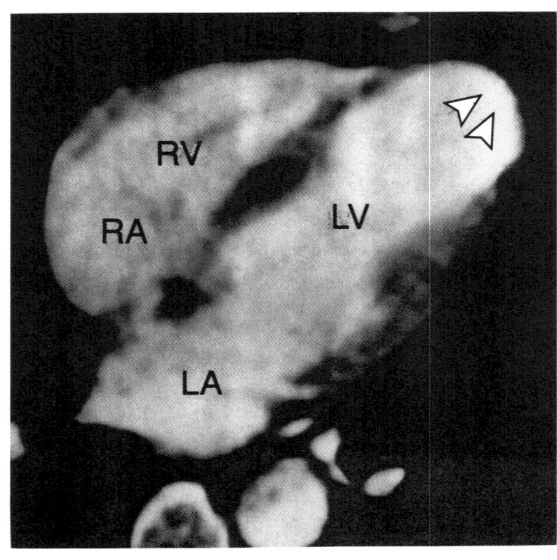

Fig. 20.30 Left ventricular aneurysm (CT findings). ECG-gated CT scan following bolus injection of contrast material (scan time, 4.5 seconds). Section through the left ventricle shows a localized dilation (*arrows*) of the left ventricular cavity (LV) with thinning of the overlying myocardium. The ventricular cavity protrudes beyond the contour of the heart during systole. ECG showed evidence of an old anterior myocardial infarct. (Courtesy of Klaus Lackner, MD, Bonn, Federal Republic of Germany.)

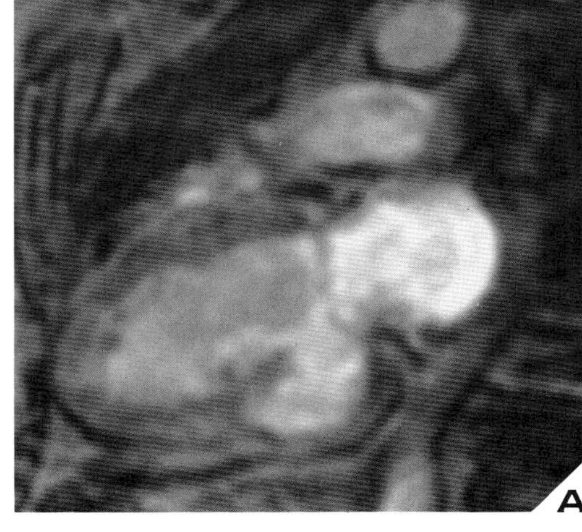

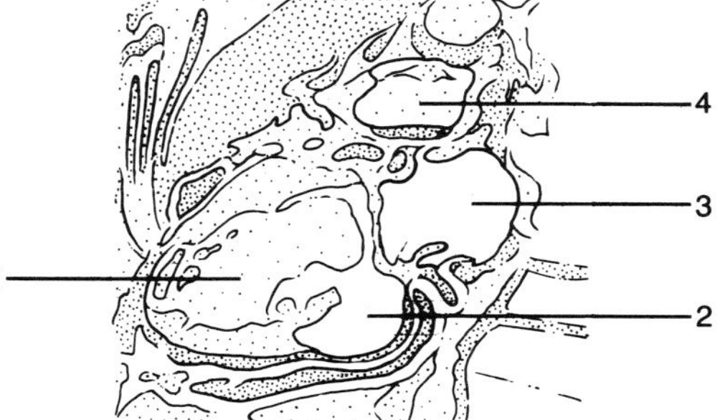

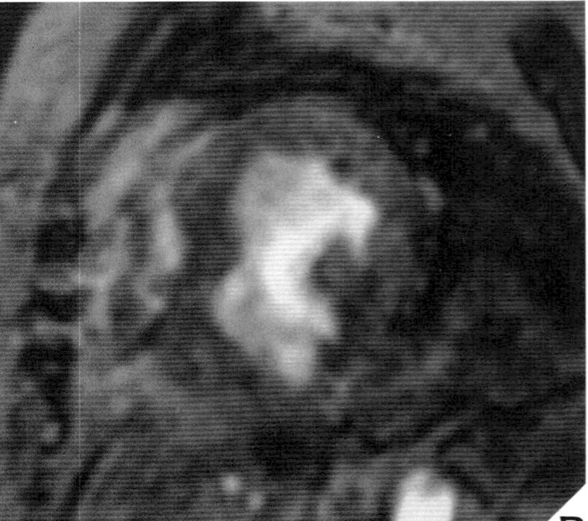

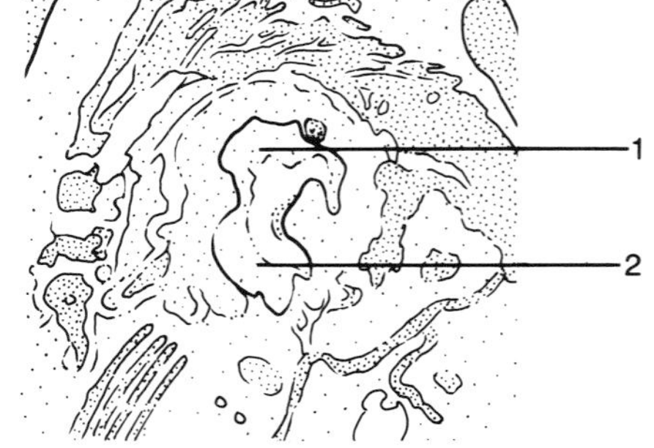

Fig. 20.31 Left ventricular aneurysm (MRI findings). Gradient–echo study (cine MRI). (A) Long-axis and (B) short-axis sections through the left ventricle demonstrate an aneurysm of the posterolateral segment. The aneurysm communicates widely with the left ventricular cavity, which is only minimally enlarged.

1	left ventricle	3	left atrium
2	aneurysm	4	pulmonary trunk

IMAGING AND INVASIVE DIAGNOSIS

Mural thrombi are usually detected by echocardiography and confirmed by cine angiocardiography. On echocardiography, a mural thrombus appears as an echo-dense image adjacent to the wall of the left ventricle; it is usually surrounded by an aneurysm or a markedly hypokinetic segment (Fig. 20.32). On "fast" or cine CT or cine MRI, the thrombus appears as a negative image which is adjacent to the ventricular wall and moves with it. Cine angiocardiography (see Chapter 21) appears to be slightly more accurate than other imaging modalities in the diagnosis of mural thrombi.

PSEUDOANEURYSM (FALSE ANEURYSM) OF THE LEFT VENTRICLE

A pseudoaneurysm (false aneurysm) represents a cavity that communicates with the ventricular lumen but whose wall is not formed by myocardium (Fig. 20.33). Pseudoaneurysms result from rupture of the left ventricle. After rupture of the ventricular wall, the extravasated blood clots and becomes organized by fibrous tissue; the mass of clot and fibrous tissue is then remodeled by the pulsating blood, resulting in the formation of a

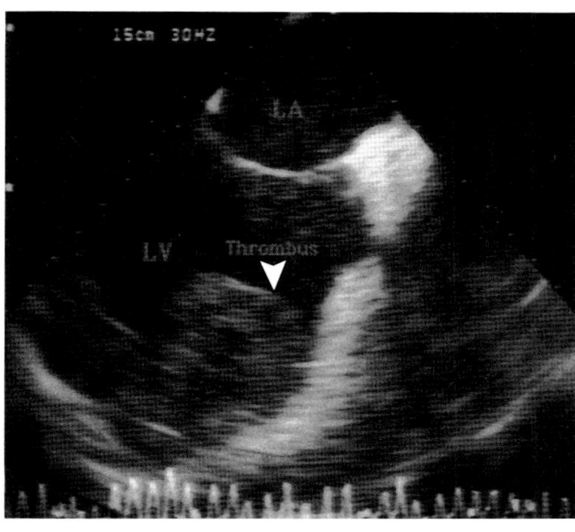

Fig. 20.32 Left ventricular aneurysm with mural thrombus (echocardiographic findings) Transesophageal four-chamber projection demonstrates a markedly dilated left ventricle (LV) with an aneurysm involving the posterolateral wall and apex. The large echo-dense image (*arrow*) within the aneurysm represents a mural thrombus. (LA = left atrium)

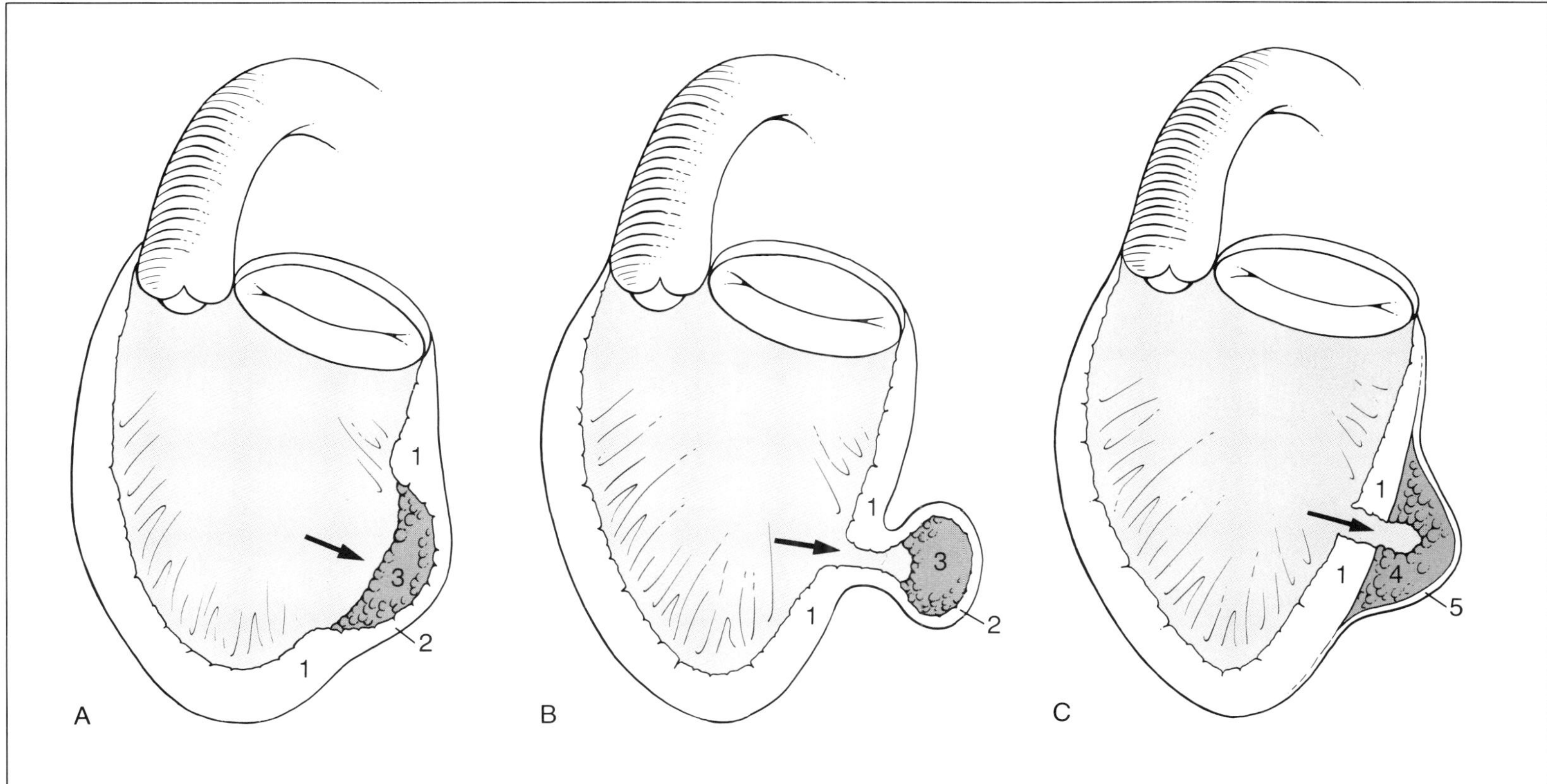

Fig. 20.33 Morphology of true and false aneurysms of the left ventricle. Schematic representation of various types of left ventricular aneurysm. (A) Typical wide-mouthed aneurysm with mural thrombus. (B) Saccular aneurysm with mural thrombus. (C) False aneurysm (pseudoaneurysm). Pseudoaneurysms result from rupture of the ventricular wall. Unlike true aneurysms (A and B), the wall of a pseudoaneurysm is not formed by myocardium; rather, it consists of thrombus which is contained by the pericardium. Recanalization of the thrombus leads to progressive enlargement of the pseudoaneurysm, which may eventually rupture. Although differentiation from typical aneurysms, which communicate widely with the ventricular lumen, usually presents no difficulty on imaging studies, differention from a saccular aneurysm with a narrow neck may be difficult.

1 wall of left ventricle
2 wall of ventricular aneurysm
3 mural thrombus
4 thrombus in false aneurysm
5 pericardium

sac of variable thickness. Pseudoaneurysms tend to enlarge progressively and are prone to rupture, a catastrophe that almost always leads to sudden death.

CLINICAL MANIFESTATIONS

The clinical manifestations of left ventricular pseudoaneurysms are similar to those of left ventricular aneurysms.

IMAGING AND INVASIVE DIAGNOSIS

Plain Films

In general, the plain film findings are similar to those of true aneurysms. A left ventricular pseudoaneurysm typically appears as a discrete extracardiac mass (Fig. 20.34). The mass is usually anterolateral, but may occasionally occur along the diaphragmatic aspect of the heart. Congestive heart failure, manifested radiographically by pulmonary venous hypertension or pulmonary edema, is not uncommon.

Echocardiography

In general, the echocardiographic features of left ventricular pseudoaneurysms resemble those of true aneurysms (ie, deformity of the left ventricular contour with paradoxical expansion during systole). The presence of a narrow neck between the ventricular cavity and the lumen of the aneurysmal sac favors the diagnosis of pseudoaneurysm.

Computer Tomography and Magnetic Resonance Imaging

Both CT and MRI clearly depict the pseudoaneurysm, which appears as a sac connected to the ventricular lumen via a narrow neck (Fig. 20.35).

Coronary Arteriography and Angiocardiography

The characteristic morphologic features of the lesion are clearly shown by left ventriculography. False aneurysms are easily distinguished from true aneurysms by coronary arteriography, which is usually performed in conjunction with left ventriculography (see Chapter 21).

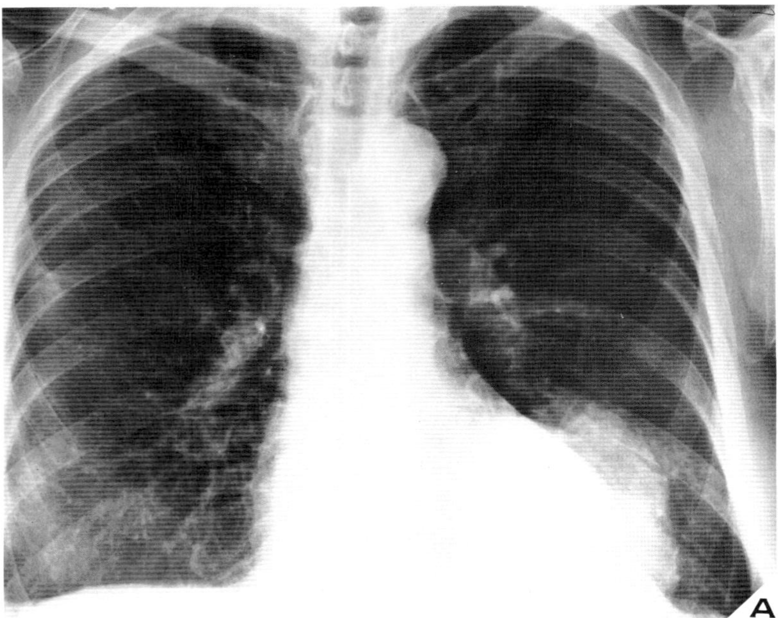

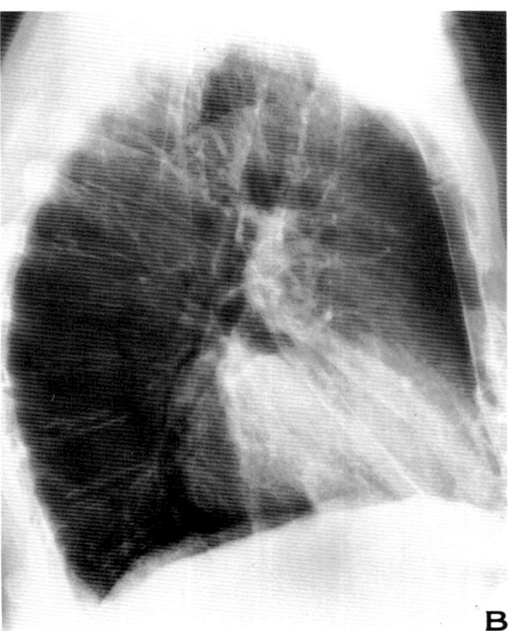

Fig. 20.34 Pseudoaneurysm of the left ventricle. (A) Posteroanterior chest film shows a mass adjacent to the left heart border. The left ventricle is only minimally enlarged. (B) On the lateral projection the mass, which represents a large pseudoaneurysm, projects posteriorly. The patient had a history of a previous myocardial infarction and presented with symptoms of congestive heart failure.

TREATMENT OF ISCHEMIC HEART DISEASE CAUSED BY CORONARY ATHEROSCLEROSIS

The various procedures used to treat ischemic heart disease caused by coronary atherosclerosis (including coronary artery angioplasty, thrombolytic therapy, and surgical revascularization) are discussed in Chapters 30 and 31.

ISCHEMIC HEART DISEASE SECONDARY TO CONGENITAL MALFORMATIONS OF THE CORONARY ARTERIES

ANATOMY AND PATHOPHYSIOLOGY

A great many anomalies of the coronary arteries have been documented, most of which are of no clinical significance.

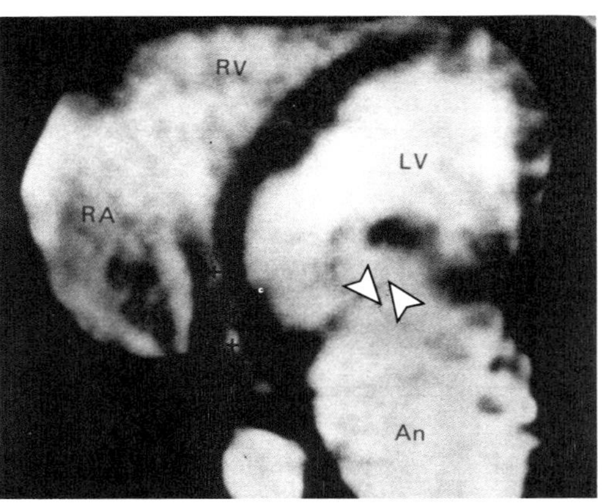

Fig. 20.35 Pseudoaneurysm of the left ventricle (CT findings). ECG-gated CT after administration of a bolus of contrast material (scan time, 4.5 seconds). Axial section through the left ventricle shows a large pseudoaneurysm (An) arising from the left posterior aspect of the left ventricle (LV). Note the narrow neck (*arrows*) at the site of the ventricular rupture. The filling defects within the pseudoaneurysm and along its margin represent thrombus. (RV = right ventricle; RA = right atrium) (Reproduced by permission from Lackner K, Thurn P: Computed tomography of the heart: ECG-gated and continuous scans. *Radiology* 1981; 140:413.)

Of the various aberrant branching patterns that have been described, only one is unequivocally associated with myocardial ischemia: interposition of the left main coronary artery between the aorta and pulmonary trunk. Although the precise mechanism is not clear, the observation that the origin of the left coronary artery takes an unusually oblique course in individuals with this anomaly (it is usually perpendicular) has led to speculation that it may be compressed in patients with a dilated aortic root. Indeed, a slit-like left coronary ostium may be responsible for the symptoms in some individuals with this anomaly.

Anomalous origin of the left coronary artery from the pulmonary trunk results in a coronary artery to pulmonary artery fistula, which in turn leads to diminished perfusion of the myocardium. The decreased myocardial perfusion can lead to myocardial infarction or dilated ischemic cardiomyopathy of the affected ventricle. Anomalous origin of the left anterior descending coronary from the pulmonary trunk is less likely to cause symptoms than anomalous origin of the left coronary artery; occasionally, however, it has been associated with clinically significant myocardial ischemia. (Anomalous origin of the right coronary artery from the pulmonary trunk, which is usually detected incidentally in patients undergoing coronary arteriography, is only rarely responsible for significant myocardial ischemia.)

Abnormal communications (fistulas) between the coronary arteries and the cardiac chambers, either directly or via the cardiac veins, may accompany certain congenital cardiac defects (eg, pulmonary atresia with intact ventricular septum) or may occur as an isolated malformation. In the latter case, the abnormal connection is (in decreasing order of frequency) to the right ventricle, right atrium, pulmonary trunk, left atrium, or to more than one cardiac chamber.

CLINICAL MANIFESTATIONS

Individuals with anomalous origin of the left coronary artery from the pulmonary trunk typically present with signs and symptoms of congestive heart failure in early infancy; occasionally, the condition may go unrecognized until 4 to 6 months of age, when signs and symptoms of left ventricular failure appear. (There are isolated case reports in which the anomaly was first diagnosed in old age.) The ECG findings in young infants are nonspecific; however, in infants with extensive ischemic lesions the ECG shows ST-segment depression and Q-waves in leads III and aVf (Fig. 20.36).

Individuals with anomalous origin of the right coronary artery

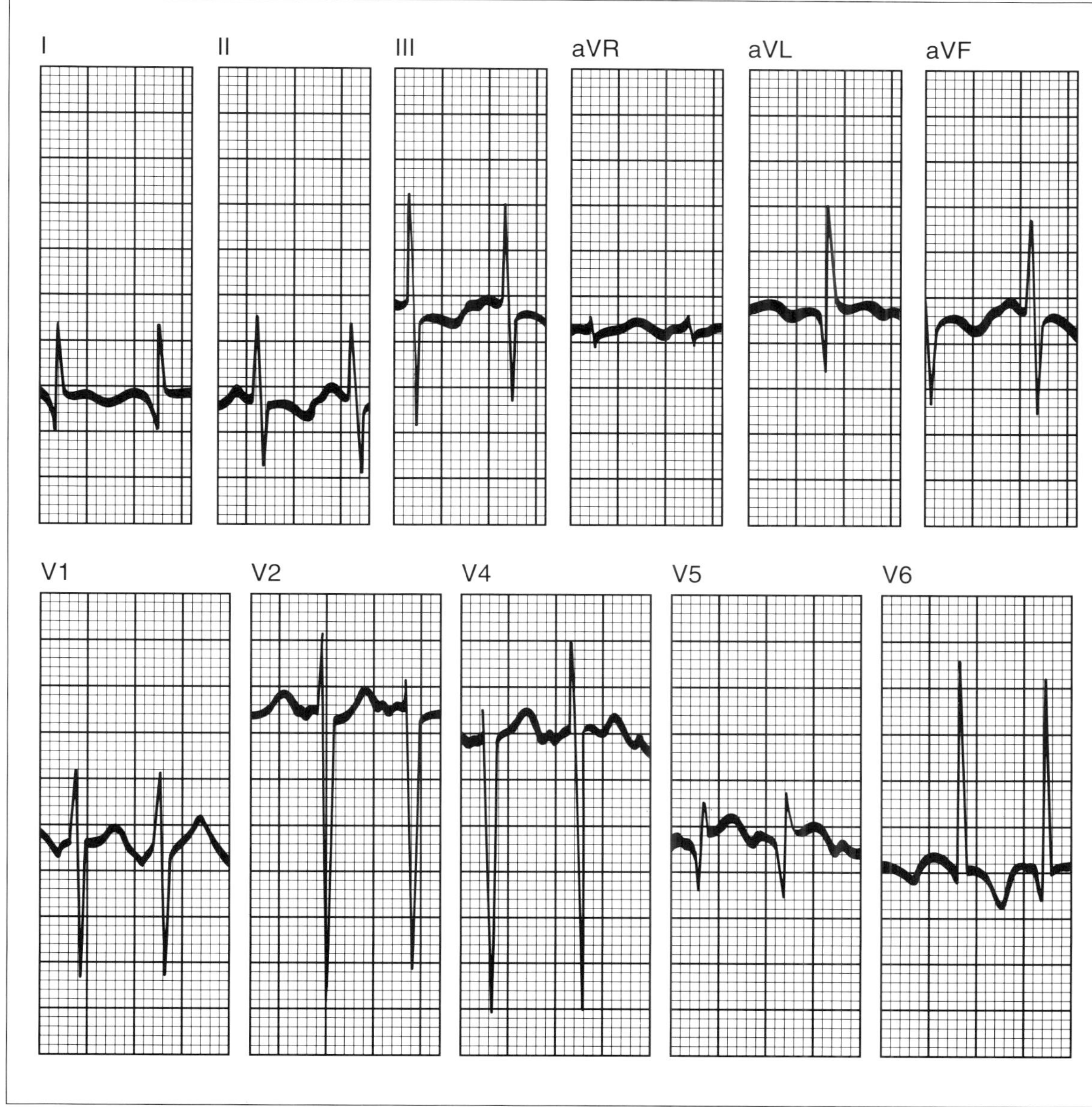

Fig. 20.36 Anomalous origin of the left coronary artery from the pulmonary trunk. ECG of a 3-month-old infant who presented in congestive heart failure shows T-wave inversion in II, III, aVf, and V6; elevation of the ST-segment in V5; and Q-waves in V1, V5, and aV1. These findings are consistent with infarction of the posterolateral portion of the left ventricle.

from the pulmonary trunk are usually asymptomatic. Only rarely is the left to right shunt associated with this anomaly large enough to cause clinically significant right ventricular overload. Patients with coronary artery fistulas to the various cardiac chambers or to the venous system are usually asymptomatic; auscultation occasionally reveals a continuous murmur. Neither of these anomalies is associated with clinical or ECG evidence of myocardial ischemia.

IMAGING AND INVASIVE DIAGNOSIS

Plain Films

Chest films of young infants with anomalous origin of the left coronary artery from the pulmonary trunk typically reveal massive cardiomegaly, with left ventricular or predominance and evidence of pulmonary venous hypertension (Fig. 20.37). Although this pattern is suggestive of dilated cardiomyopathy in an older child, anomalous origin of the left coronary artery is the presumptive diagnosis in an infant with this pattern.

Chest films are normal in patients with a coronary–cavitary or coronary–venous fistula unless the left to right shunt is very large, in which case there may be evidence of right-sided enlargement (Fig. 20.38).

Echocardiography

The anomalous left or right coronary artery is easily identified as an anomalous vessel arising from the pulmonary trunk on sections that show this structure to advantage. Typically, the anomalous coronary artery is seen during systole, when pulmonary artery pressure is high, and disappears during diastole, when the direction of blood flow is reversed. The anomaly is particularly well seen on color Doppler images (Fig. 20.39; see Appendix). The anomalous left coronary artery usually arises from the right posterior aspect of the pulmonary trunk, just anterior to the left sinus of Valsalva. The anomalous right coronary artery usually originates from the right anterior aspect of the pulmonary trunk, just anterior to the right sinus of Valsalva. Occasionally the anomalous coronary artery originates high in the pulmonary trunk. In an exceptional case it may arise from the right or left pulmonary artery.

Angiography

The various congenital anomalies of the coronary arteries associated with myocardial ischemia are clearly depicted by angiography (see Chapter 21).

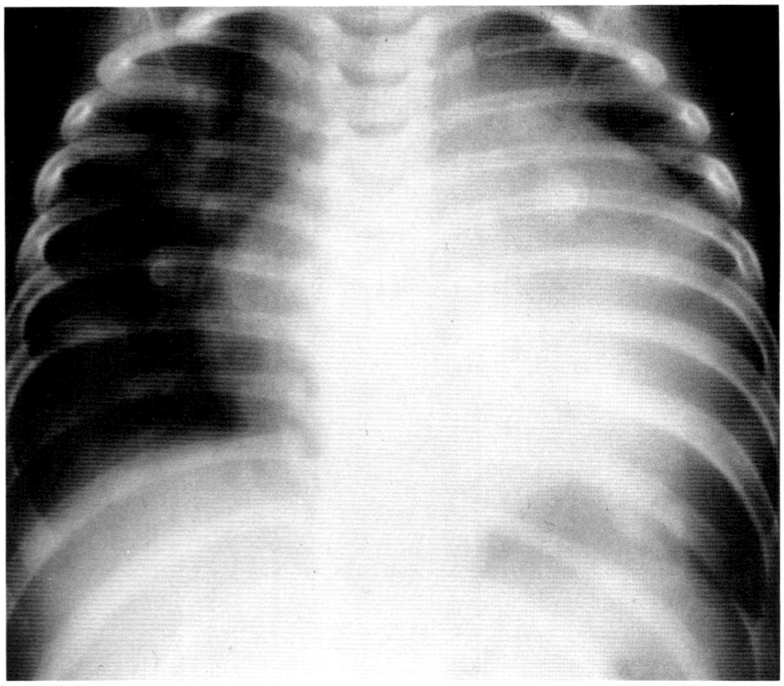

Fig. 20.37 Anomalous origin of the left coronary artery from the pulmonary trunk. Chest film of a 6-month-old infant demonstrates massive cardiomegaly with left ventricular enlargement. The pulmonary trunk is prominent and there is evidence of pulmonary hyptertension. Anomalous origin of the left coronary artery and cardiomyopathy should be considered in the differential diagnosis in an infant with these radiographic findings.

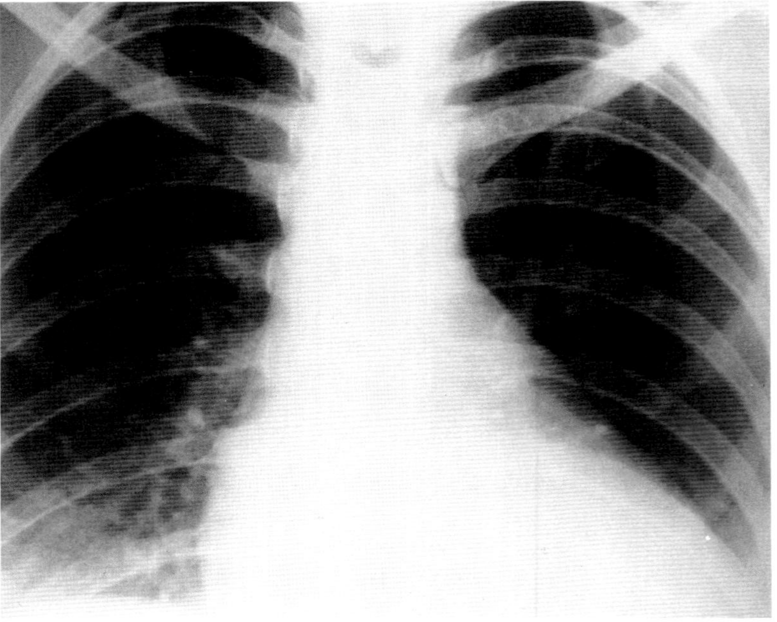

Fig. 20.38 Right coronary artery–right ventricular fistula. Posteroanterior chest film shows moderate cardiomegaly with right ventricular enlargement. The pulmonary vasculature is normal. Unless the left to right shunt is very large, the plain films are usually normal or nearly normal in patients with coronary–venous and coronary–cavitary fistulas.

CHAPTER 21

Ischemic Heart Disease: Invasive Diagnosis

This chapter will discuss the angiographic techniques used to identify abnormalities of the coronary arteries responsible for ischemic heart disease and to evaluate the sequelae of myocardial infarction.

CORONARY ARTERIOGRAPHY AND LEFT VENTRICULOGRAPHY

The coronary arteries are best visualized by selective injection of contrast material at the level of the coronary ostia. By using selective techniques it is possible to avoid interference from the opacified aorta, a common problem when the coronary arteries are studied by injecting contrast material into the aortic root. In addition, selective techniques require a relatively small volume of contrast material, so that multiple projections can be obtained with little increased risk to the patient.

Left ventriculography is usually performed in conjunction with selective coronary arteriography to assess left ventricular function and morphology. For left ventriculography, the angiographic catheter is passed retrogradely through the aortic valve into the left ventricle.

EQUIPMENT

The angiographic suite should be equipped for biplane ventriculography and single-plane coronary arteriography with cinefluorographic recording (see Chapter 3). Cinefluorography, which provides a readily accessible anatomic and dynamic display of the coronary arterial tree, is essential for accurate evaluation of left ventricular function. A 35-mm camera with framing rates of 30–60 frames/second provides a permanent record of the images viewed on the image intensifier. A recording system that allows rapid retrieval and manipulation of the images is regarded as indispensable by many angiographers. With such equipment the angiographer can analyze each run immediately, "fine-tune" the radiographic technique, and obtain any additional projections that may be needed to optimally display the entire coronary arterial tree.

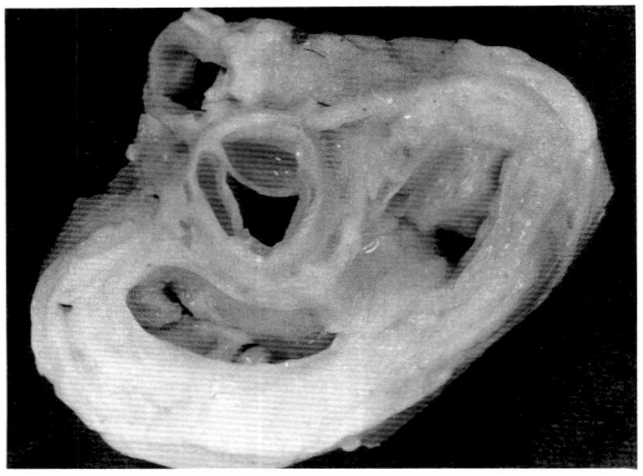

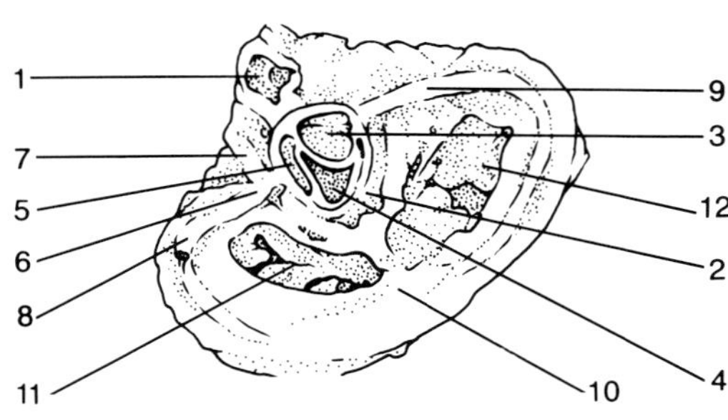

Fig. 21.1 Origin of the coronary arteries. Anatomic specimen of the base of the heart at the level of the arterial and atrioventricular valves (viewed from above). The aorta is wedged between the mitral and tricuspid valves. The right coronary artery arises from the right (anterior) coronary cusp. The left coronary artery arises from the left (posterior) coronary cusp and quickly bifurcates into the left anterior descending and circumflex arteries.

1	pulmonary trunk	7	left anterior descending artery
2	aorta	8	circumflex artery
3	right (anterior) coronary cusp	9	right coronary artery
4	noncoronary cusp	10	crux cordis
5	left (posterior) coronary cusp	11	mitral valve
6	left main coronary artery	12	tricuspid valve

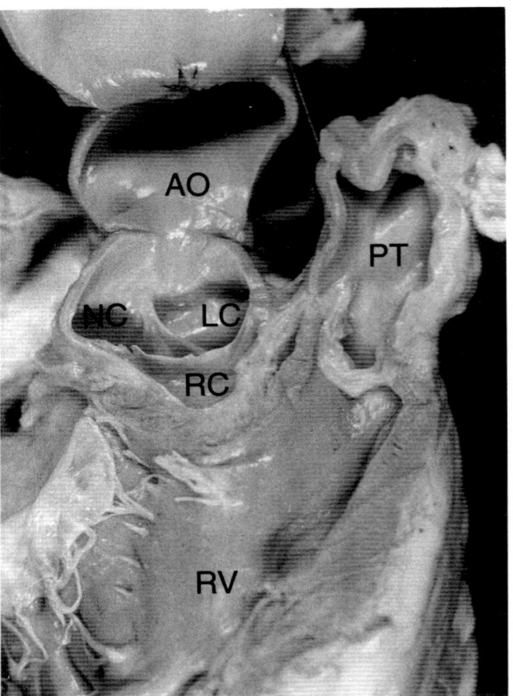

Fig. 21.2 Relations of the aortic valve and right ventricular outflow tract. Anatomic preparation [as viewed from the right ventricle (RV)]. The crista supraventricularis has been removed to display the aortic valve and the three sinuses of Valsalva. The right coronary cusp (RC), the site of the right coronary artery orifice (ostium), is posterior to the crista supraventricularis. The left coronary cusp (LC), the site of the left coronary artery orifice (ostium), is posterior and to the left of the right coronary cusp. (AO = aorta; PT = pulmonary trunk; NC = noncoronary cusp)

TECHNIQUE

To optimally visualize the entire coronary arterial tree, it is necessary to selectively catheterize both main coronary arteries. This can be accomplished by either the Judkins or the Sones method. In the Judkins method, the catheter is introduced over a guidewire (Seldinger technique) via a percutaneous femoral artery puncture (see Chapter 3); a separate preshaped catheter is used for each coronary artery. The Sones technique employs a single end-hole catheter which is inserted via a brachial artery cut-down; by modifying its shape in the aortic root, one can use the same catheter to selectively cannulate the right and left coronary arteries.

The contrast material is injected at a rate sufficient to completely displace nonopacified blood from the coronary arteries for a period of 3 to 4 seconds, during which time high-resolution cine images are obtained. The catheter is then passed across the aortic valve for biplanar cine left ventriculography. Left ventricular function is best assessed on images obtained during a period of sinus rhythm. Premature ventricular contractions can usually be avoided by the use of a multiple-sidehole catheter, which is positioned with its tip in the trabecular segment, and a moderate flow rate (10–14 mL/second for 4 to 5 seconds). Nitroglycerine administration or postextrasystolic potentiation is useful in evaluating contractile reserve.

The choice of contrast material for coronary arteriography and left ventriculography should be individualized. We continue to employ conventional ionic contrast agents for clinically stable patients who are being studied on an elective basis. However, we have switched to the newer low-osmolality (nonionic) contrast agents for severely ill, hemodynamically unstable patients and for patients with diabetes or renal failure. The choice of contrast media for angiography is discussed further in Chapter 3.

MORPHOLOGY OF THE CORONARY ARTERIES

The right and left coronary arteries usually originate from the aorta as separate channels (rarely, from a single trunk). The right coronary artery arises from the anterior (right) coronary cusp and the left coronary artery arises from the posterior (left) coronary cusp (Figs. 21.1 and 21.2). Not infrequently, however, the orifice (ostium) of either or both coronary arteries may be at a distance from the cusp, in the tubular portion of the aorta.

The course of the major coronary arteries is shown schematically in Fig. 21.3. The right coronary artery is a large vessel which runs within the right atrioventricular groove to the crux cordis, where it bifurcates into the posterior descending

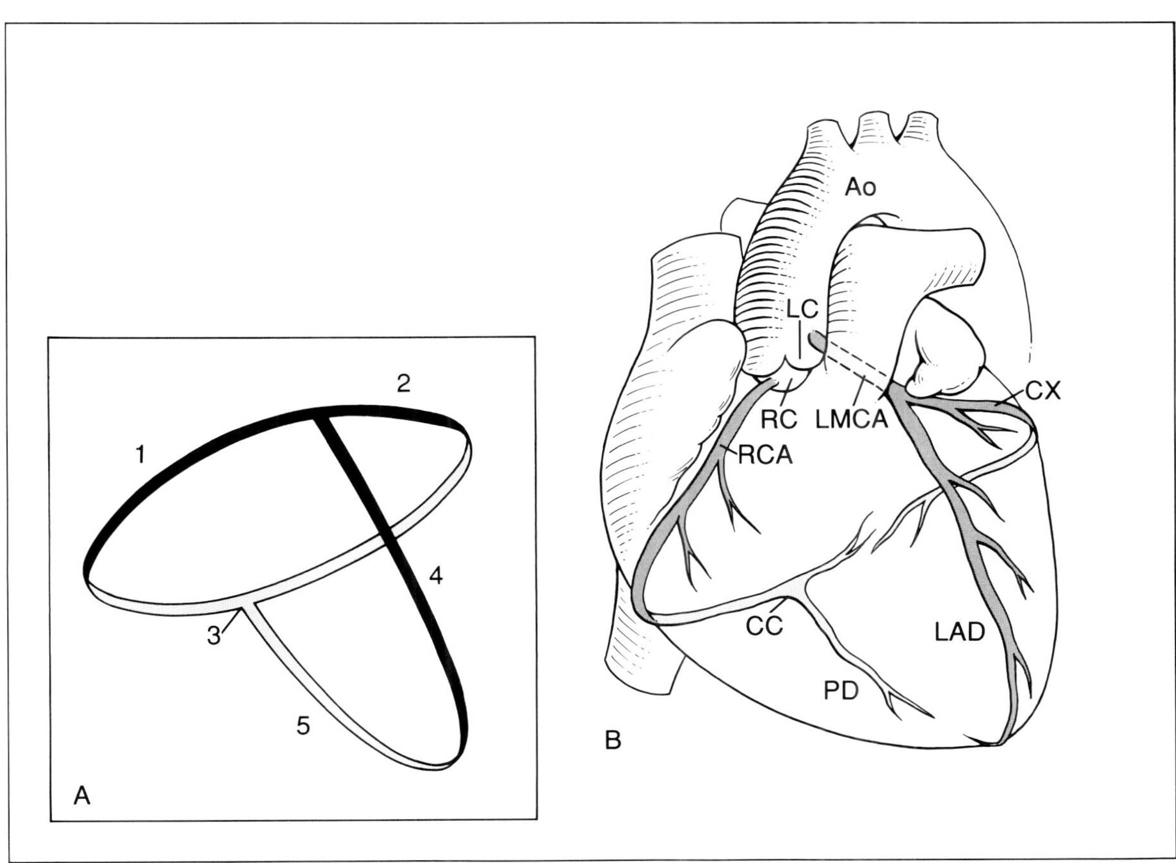

Fig. 21.3 Course of the coronary arteries around the heart. (A) In this schematic representation, the cardiac apex is oriented anteriorly, inferiorly, and to the left, following the usual anatomic arrangement. The atrioventricular groove is represented by a circle and the anterior and posterior interventricular sulci by a loop (the right ventricle is on the right and the left ventricle is on the left). The right part of the circle represents the right atrioventricular groove and marks the course of the right coronary artery. The left part of the circle represents the left atrioventricular groove and marks the course of the circumflex artery. The anterior part of the loop is formed by the anterior interventricular sulcus and marks the course of the left anterior descending artery. The inferior part of the loop is formed by the posterior interventricular sulcus and marks the course of the posterior descending artery. The crux cordis marks the take-off of the posterior descending artery from the right coronary artery. (B) The course of the coronary arteries and their major branches is shown schematically.

1 right atrioventricular groove
2 left atrioventricular groove
3 crux cordis
4 anterior interventricular sulcus
5 posterior interventricular sulcus

AO aorta
RC right coronary cusp
LC left coronary cusp
LMCA left main coronary artery
LAD left anterior descending coronary artery

CX circumflex artery
RCA right coronary artery
CC crux cordis
PD posterior descending coronary artery

and posterolateral arteries. The posterior descending artery runs in the posterior interventricular sulcus towards the cardiac apex. The left coronary artery is a short vessel, 10 to 15 mm in length, which runs for a short distance just posterior to the pulmonary trunk. It bifurcates into two branches before reaching the atrioventricular groove. The left anterior descending artery runs along the anterior interventricular sulcus from the base of the heart to the apex. The left anterior descending artery gives rise to septal perforating branches (septal arteries) and branches to the free wall of the left ventricle (diagonal branches). The circumflex artery runs along the left atrioventricular groove to the obtuse margin of the heart (Fig. 21.4). The circumflex artery gives rise to branches to the free wall of the left ventricle (marginal branches) and to the left atrium (atrial branches).

It is evident from the above description that the four main branches of the coronary arterial tree have a distinctive arrangement: the right coronary and circumflex arteries form a circle within the atrioventricular groove, while the left anterior descending branch of the left coronary artery and the posterior descending branch of the right coronary artery form a loop within the anterior and posterior interventricular sulci, respectively (Fig. 21.3). (It is noteworthy that the right and left coronary arteries usually conform to the position of the corresponding ventricles; therefore, in patients with ventricular inversion the right coronary artery is usually on the left side of the ventricular septum and the left coronary artery is usually on the right side of the ventricular septum.)

Variations of the coronary arterial pattern are common, occurring in about 10 percent of the population. The most common variant is a hypoplastic (nondominant) right coronary artery. In such cases the circumflex artery is dominant, providing circulation to the posterior septum via the posterior descending artery, and to the inferior left ventricular wall via the left posterolateral arteries.

There are many possible collateral routes between the territories of the three main coronary arteries. However, most patients with ischemic heart disease exhibit one of four angiographic patterns (Fig. 21.5):

1. In a right coronary dominant system, connection between the distal circumflex artery and the left posterolateral artery at the level of the left atrioventricular groove.
2. Connection between the left anterior descending artery and the posterior descending artery in the region of the apex.
3. Connection between the proximal segment of the right coronary artery and the proximal segment of the left anterior descending artery.

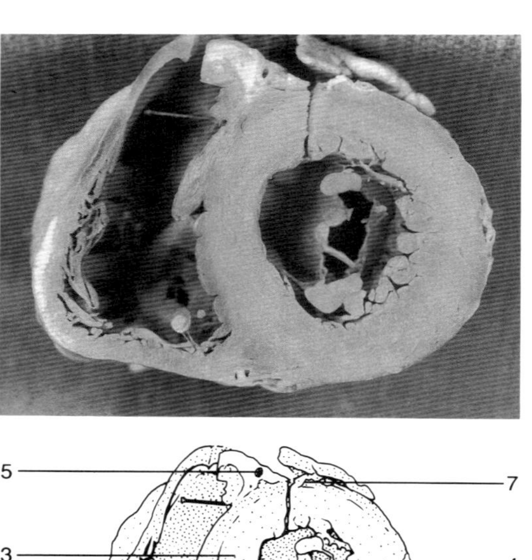

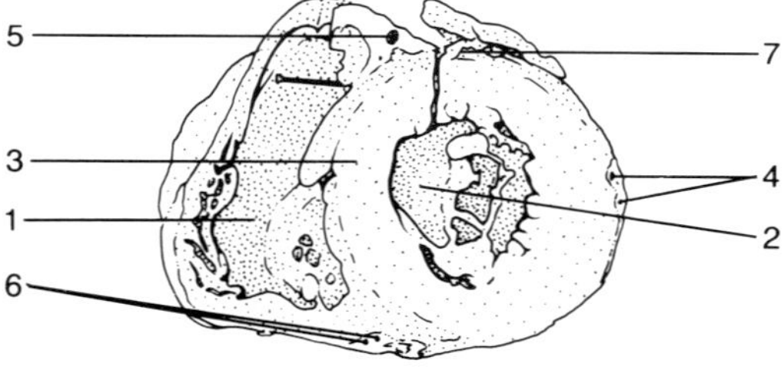

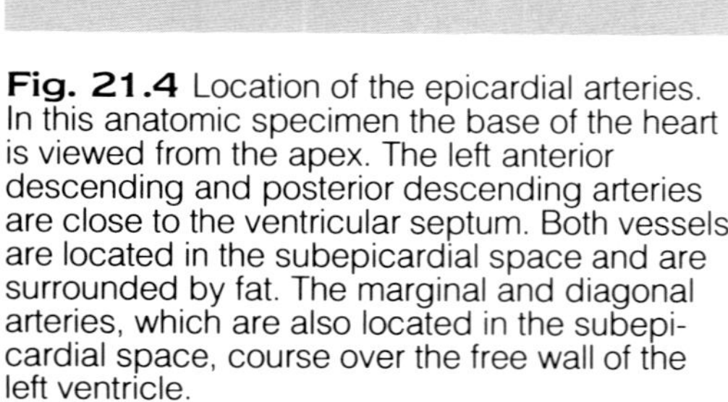

Fig. 21.4 Location of the epicardial arteries. In this anatomic specimen the base of the heart is viewed from the apex. The left anterior descending and posterior descending arteries are close to the ventricular septum. Both vessels are located in the subepicardial space and are surrounded by fat. The marginal and diagonal arteries, which are also located in the subepicardial space, course over the free wall of the left ventricle.

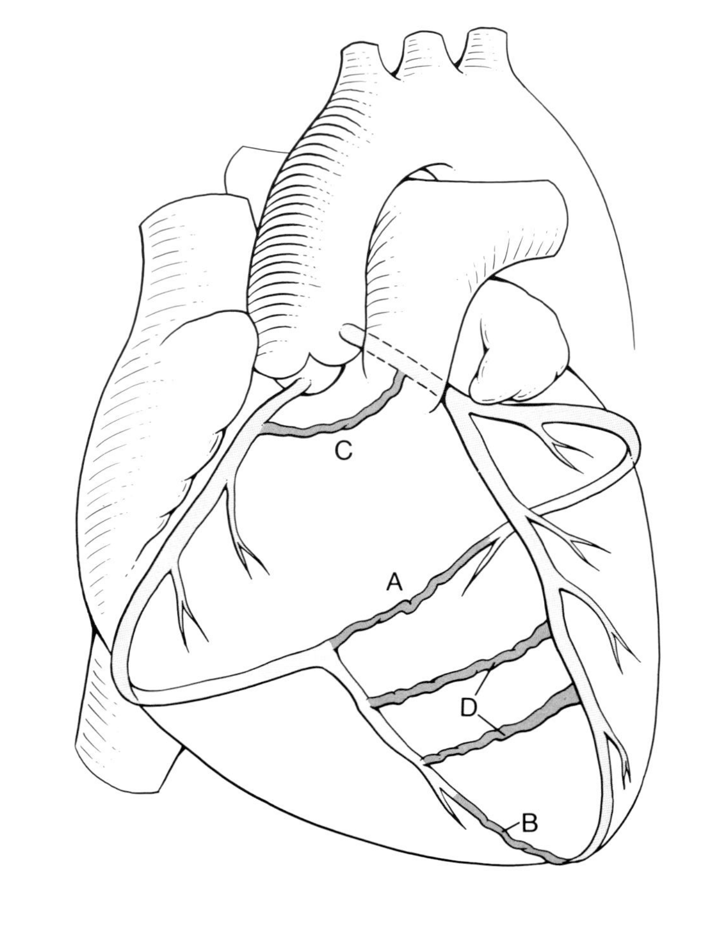

Fig. 21.5 Collateral circulation. The most common collateral pathways between the right and left coronary arteries are shown schematically. (A) Connection between posterolateral and distal circumflex arteries. (B) Connection between distal left anterior descending and posterior descending arteries. (C) Connection between right coronary and left anterior descending arteries via the conus artery. (D) Connection between left anterior descending and posterior descending arteries via septal arteries.

4. Connection (via septal arteries) between the left anterior descending and inferior septal arteries, permitting collateral flow between the left anterior descending and the posterior descending arteries.

The collateral circulation is described in greater detail in the section on coronary artery stenosis (see below).

The vascular territories of the left ventricle are shown in Fig. 21.6. In general, significant stenosis of the left anterior descending artery produces ischemia in the anterior and anterolateral segments of the left ventricular myocardium, as well as in the anterior portion of the septum. Significant narrowing of the right coronary artery produces ischemia in the inferior segment and posterior septum, as well as the right ventricle. Partial or complete obstruction of the circumflex artery produces ischemia in the posterolateral and posterior segments of the left ventricle.

ANGIOGRAPHIC ANATOMY OF THE CORONARY ARTERIES

The *right coronary artery* is divided into three segments: proximal, middle, and distal. The boundaries between these segments are arbitrary; it is customary to divide the entire right coronary artery into three segments, beginning at the ostium and ending at the bifurcation at the level of the crux cordis (Fig. 21.7). In most individuals the *posterior descending artery*

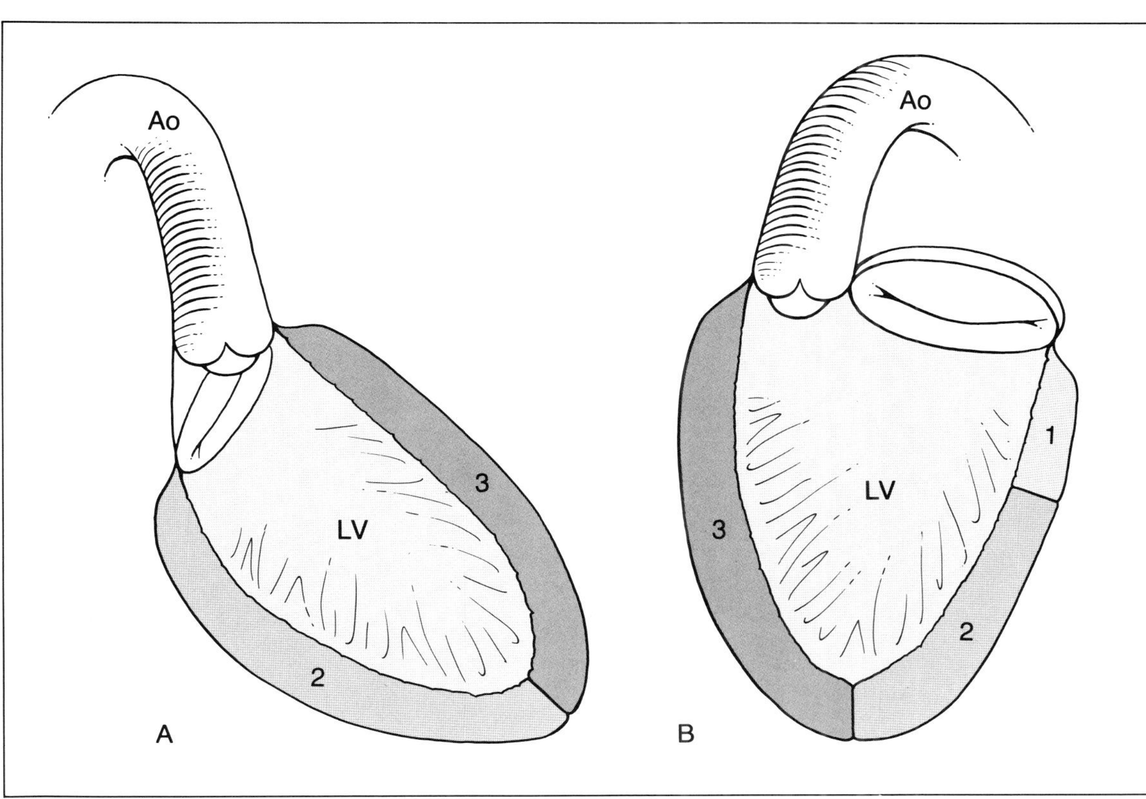

Fig. 21.6 Vascular territories of the left ventricle. (A) Right anterior oblique projection of left ventriculogram. (B) Left anterior oblique projection of left ventriculogram. The cardiac apex is an area of overlapping circulation, supplied by both the left anterior descending and circumflex arteries.

1 territory of right coronary artery
2 territory of circumflex artery (overlaps territory of right coronary, artery)
3 territory of left anterior descending artery
LV left ventricle
AO aorta

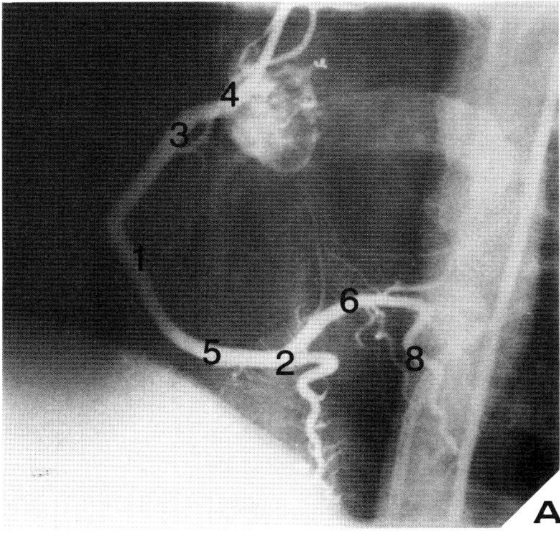

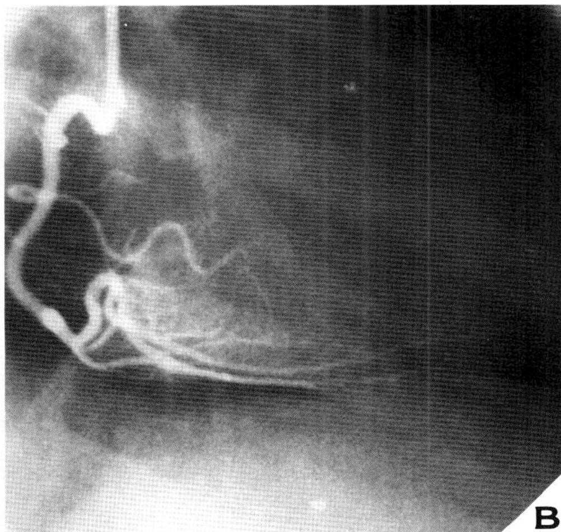

Fig. 21.7 Right coronary artery. Selective right coronary arteriograms (A) in the left anterior oblique projection with craniocaudal angulation and (B) in the right anterior oblique projection without craniocaudal angulation. The right coronary artery is a large vessel originating in the right coronary cusp and terminating at the crux cordis; its entire course is within the right atrioventricular groove. The right coronary artery is divided by convention into the proximal, middle, and distal segments. At the level of the crux cordis it bifurcates into the posterior descending and posterolateral arteries. The latter vessel runs in the left atrioventricular groove, where it gives off branches to the inferior wall of the left ventricle. In the right anterior oblique projection, the posterior descending artery is overlapped by branches of the posterolateral artery (the latter can be identified by their characteristic displacement during the cardiac cycle).

1 ostium of right coronary artery
2 crux cordis
3 proximal segment of right coronary artery
4 middle segment of right coronary artery
5 distal segment of right coronary artery
6 posterolateral artery
7 posterior descending artery
8 branch of posterolateral artery

originates from the right coronary artery; it runs in the posterior interventricular sulcus, where it gives off a number of septal branches. The *posterolateral artery* runs in the distal portion of the left atrioventricular groove. The proximal connection of the posterolateral artery varies. Most often the posterolateral artery originates from the right coronary artery, in which case it is called the "right posterolateral branch of the right coronary artery." Occasionally it arises from the distal portion of the circumflex artery, in which case it is called the "left posterolateral segmental artery."

The *left main coronary artery* (Fig. 21.8) is a short vessel (1 to 2 cm in length) which arises from the left coronary cusp. It courses posteriorly and to the left of the right ventricular outflow tract, where it bifurcates into the left anterior descending and circumflex arteries. (Rarely, the left main coronary artery is absent, in which event the left anterior descending and circumflex arteries arise directly from the aorta.)

The *left anterior descending artery* (Fig. 21.8) courses along the anterior interventricular sulcus. It is divided into three segments. The proximal segment extends from the origin of the vessel to the origin of the first septal branch. The middle and distal segments are arbitrarily divided at a point midway between the origin of the first septal branch and the apex. The epicardial branches of the left anterior descending artery *(diagonal arteries)* are designated diagonal arteries one, two, three, and so forth (diagonal artery one is the most proximal).

The *circumflex artery* (Fig. 21.8) courses in the left atrioventricular sulcus. It has two segments: the proximal segment extends from the origin to the take-off of the first marginal artery, and the distal segment extends from the origin of the first marginal artery to the left posterolateral segmental artery. The *marginal arteries* are distributed over the lateral free wall of the left ventricle; they are designated marginal arteries one, two, and three, and so forth, one being the most proximal.

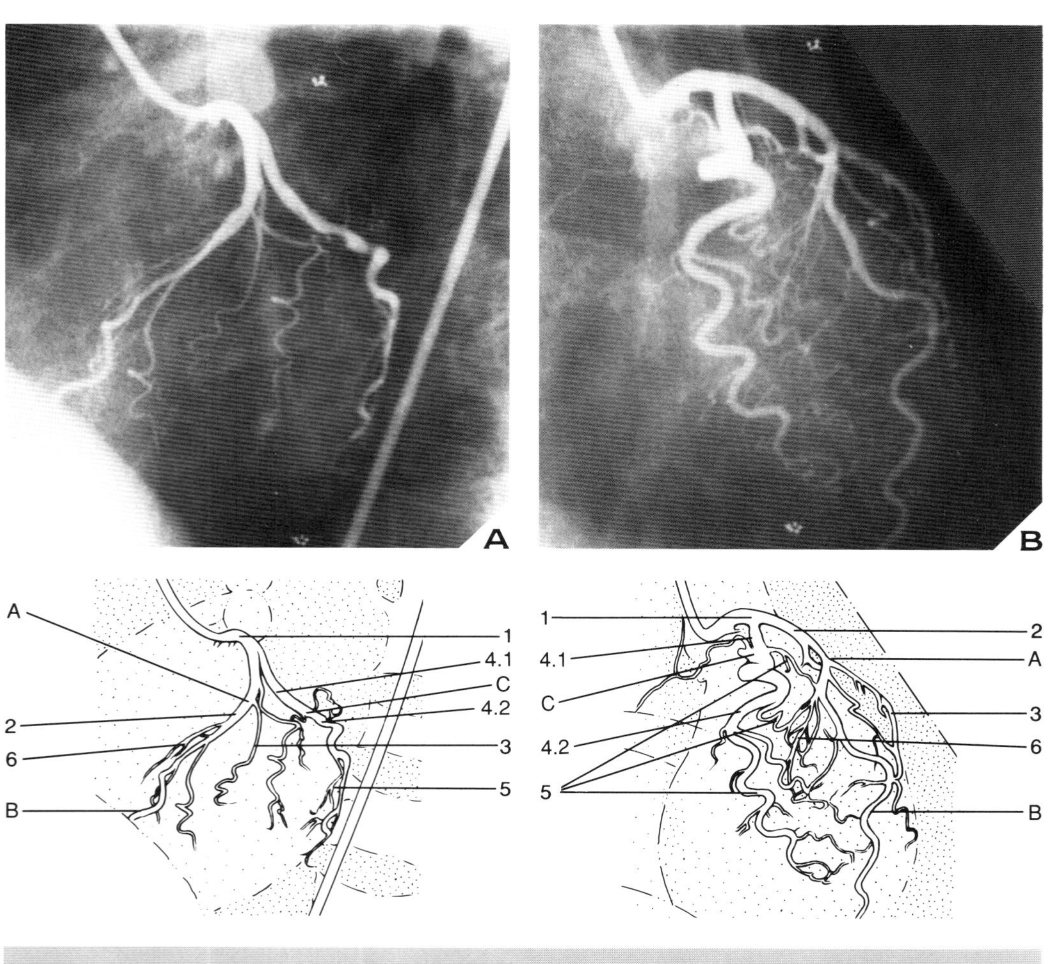

Fig. 21.8 Left coronary artery. (A) Left anterior oblique and (B) right anterior oblique projections of selective left coronary arteriogram. The left coronary artery is a short (1 to 2 cm) vessel which divides into two large branches: the left anterior descending and circumflex arteries. The left anterior descending artery courses in the anterior interventricular sulcus, where it gives off diagonal and septal branches. The diagonal arteries are distributed to the free wall of the left ventricle; the septal arteries penetrate into the muscular ventricular septum and supply this structure. The circumflex artery, which courses in the left atrioventricular groove, supplies the lateral portion of the left ventricle. It gives off a variable number of marginal arteries, which are distributed to the free wall of the left ventricle, and several posterosuperior branches, which are distributed to the left atrium. By convention, the left anterior descending coronary artery is divided into three segments: the proximal segment extends from the ostium to the origin of the first septal artery; the middle segment extends from the first septal artery to the midpoint of the remaining artery. The circumflex artery is divided into two segments: the proximal segment extends from its origin to the take-off of the first important marginal artery; the distal segment represents the remainder of this vessel.

The arteries that are distributed over the free wall of the left ventricle undergo significant displacement during the cardiac cycle (they are short in systole and elongated in diastole), whereas the arteries that course within the interventricular sulcus exhibit little displacement during the cardiac cycle.

- 1 left main coronary artery
- 2 left anterior descending coronary artery
- 3 diagonal arteries
- 4.1 proximal segment of circumflex artery
- 4.2 distal segment of circumflex artery
- 5 marginal branches
- 6 septal arteries
- A division between promimal and middle segments of left anterior descending artery
- B division between middle and distal segments of left anterior descending artery
- C division between proximal and distal segments of circumflex artery

In most individuals the posterior descending artery originates from the right coronary artery, a pattern known as *right coronary dominance* (Fig. 21.7). In some individuals the posterior coronary artery arises from the distal portion of the circumflex artery (left posterolateral segmental artery), a pattern known as *left coronary dominance* (Figs. 21.9 and 21.10).

The *sinus node artery* originates from the right coronary artery in 60 percent of the population and from the proximal segment of the circumflex artery in the rest. The sinus node artery, which is usually the largest of the atrial branches, courses

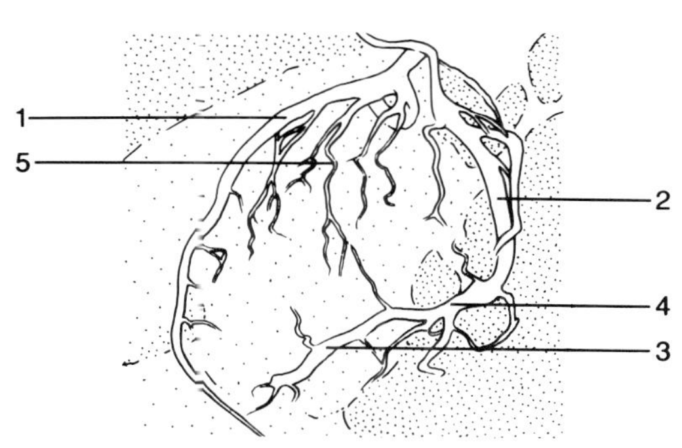

Fig. 21.9 Dominant left coronary pattern. Lateral projection of selective left coronary arteriogram shows the posterior descending coronary artery arising from the distal portion of the circumflex artery.

1	left anterior descending coronary artery	4	left posterolateral artery
2	circumflex artery	5	diagonal branches
3	posterior descending coronary artery		

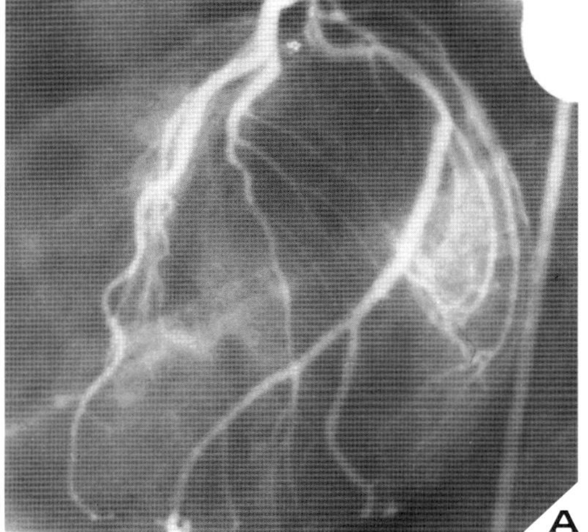

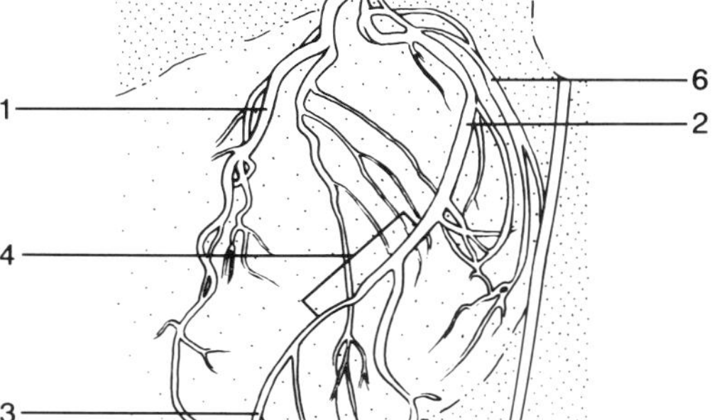

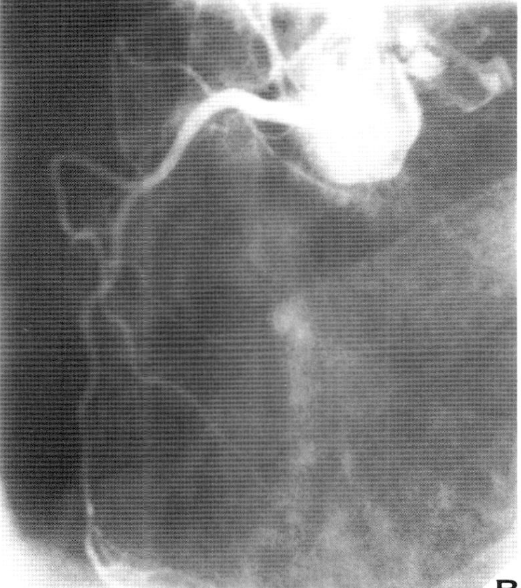

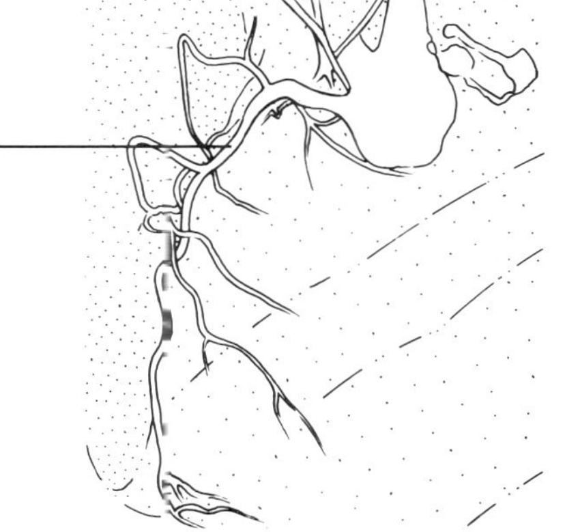

Fig. 21.10 Left dominant coronary pattern. Selective (A) left and (B) right coronary arteriograms (left anterior oblique projection) show a small right coronary artery which is distributed only to the free wall of the right ventricle and does not extend into the right atrioventricular groove. The right coronary artery does not give rise to the posterior descending artery. The left anterior descending artery is normal and gives rise to several diagonal branches. The circumflex artery is unusually large; it continues into the posterior aspect of the left atrioventricular groove, where it connects with the posterior descending coronary artery.

1	left anterior descending coronary artery	4	left posterolateral artery
2	circumflex artery	5	small (hypoplastic) nondominant right coronary artery
3	posterior descending coronary artery	6	marginal arteries

in a posterosuperior direction until it reaches the junction of the superior vena cava and right atrium. Its distal branches have a circular configuration (Fig. 21.11).

The *atrioventricular node artery* originates from the right coronary artery at the level of the crux cordis in 90 percent of the population and from the left posterolateral artery in 10 percent. It appears angiographically as a straight, vertically oriented channel which terminates at the apex in a right angle (Fig. 21.12).

PROJECTIONS USED FOR CORONARY ARTERIOGRAPHY

A complete angiographic evaluation of the coronary arteries consists of a series of projections which, taken together, allow a thorough evaluation of the entire coronary arterial tree. Because specific portions of the coronary arterial tree are clearly depicted in each projection, while others are obscured, a series of projections is needed to completely evaluate the coronary

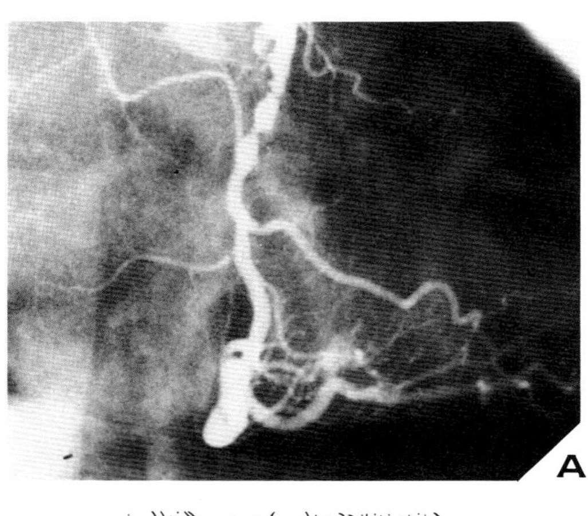

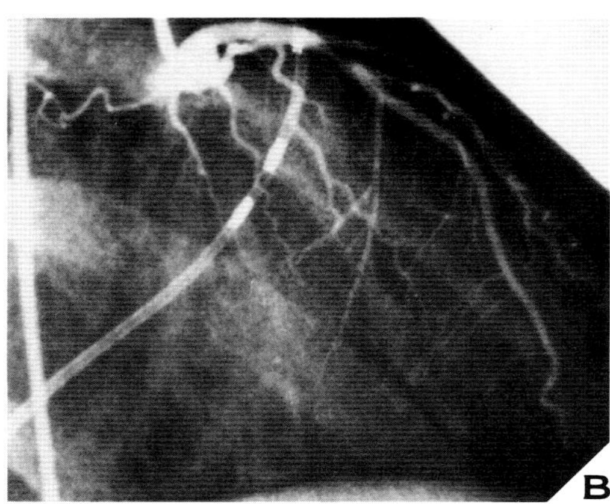

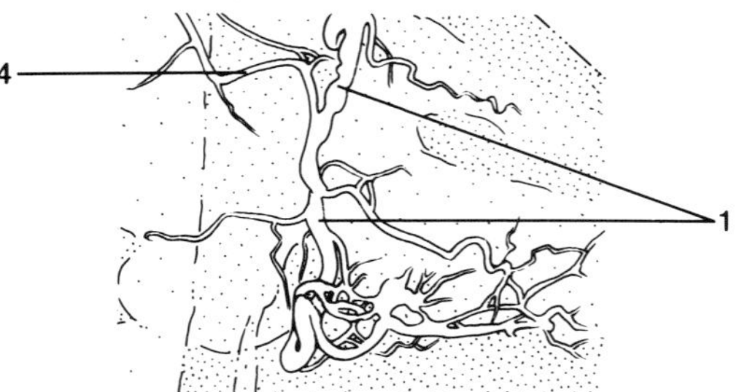

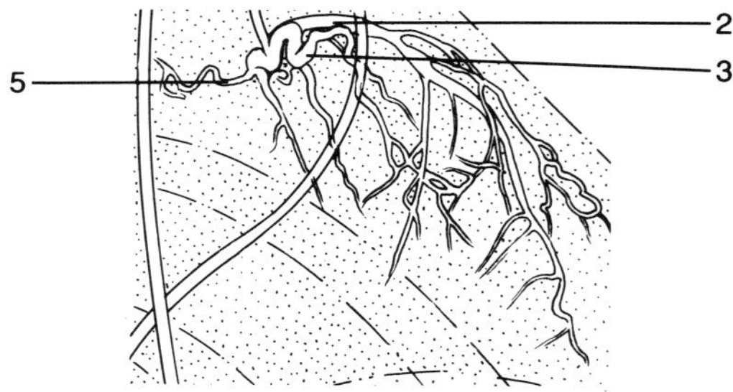

Fig. 21.11 Sinus node artery. (A) Right and (B) left selective coronary arteriograms in two different patients (right anterior oblique projection). The sinus node artery originates from the proximal segment of the right coronary artery and courses posteriorly and superiorly to the area of the junction of the superior vena cava and right atrium. At this point the sinus node artery divides into an anterior and a posterior branch, which typically encircle the caval–atrial junction. In about 40 percent of normal subjects the sinus node artery originates from the circumflex artery (B) and courses from left to right to reach the caval–atrial junction, where it divides into anterior and posterior branches as described above.

1 right coronary artery
2 left anterior descending coronary artery
3 marginal branches
4 sinus node artery originating from right coronary artery
5 sinus node artery originating from circumflex artery

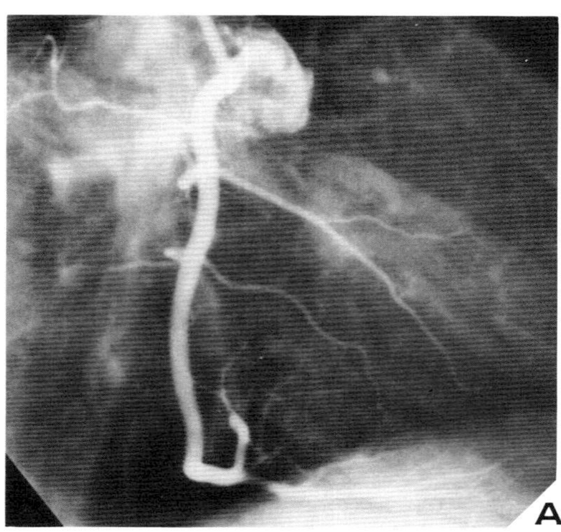

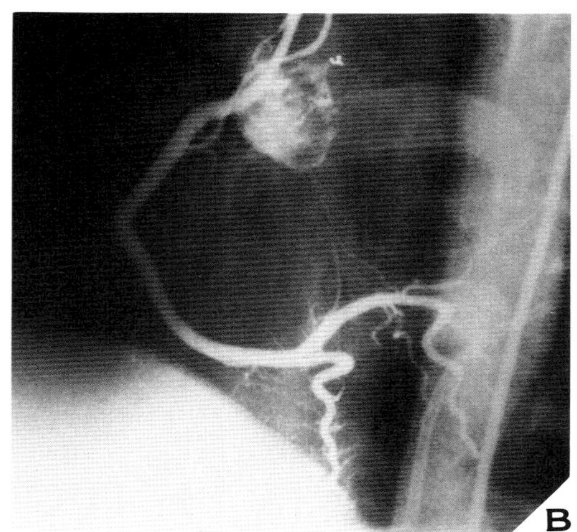

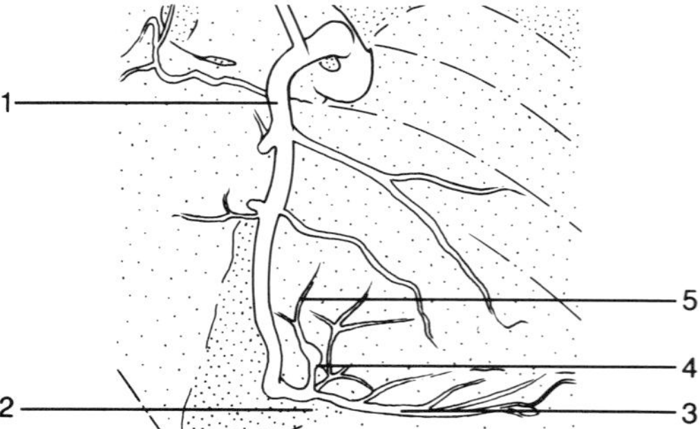

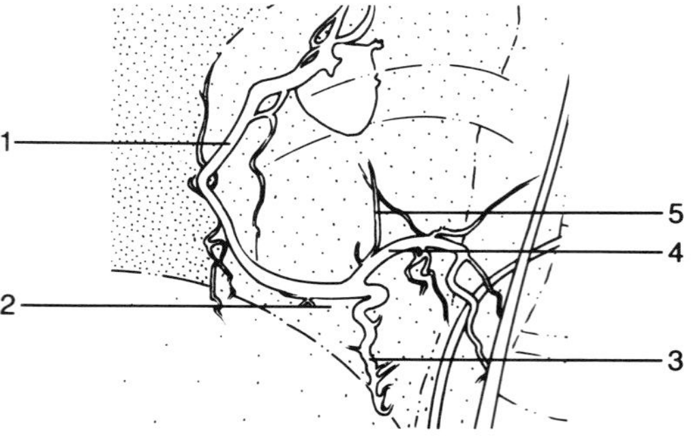

Fig. 21.12 Artery to the atrioventricular node. (A) Right anterior oblique and (B) left anterior oblique projections of selective right coronary arteriogram demonstrate the atrioventricular node artery arising as a branch of the distal segment of the right coronary artery at the level of the crux cordis. The atrioventricular node is supplied by a branch arising from the artery that reaches the crux cordis; in 90 percent of cases it arises from the right coronary artery. The atrioventricular node artery is a very small, straight vessel which courses superiorly and anteriorly to reach the apex of the triangle of Kock, where it ends in a right angle.

1 right coronary artery
2 crux cordis
3 posterior descending coronary artery
4 posterolateral artery
5 artery to the atrioventricular node

arterial tree. In addition, individual anatomic variations often make it necessary to modify the examination. Other factors governing the choice of projection are the size of the patient and his or her ability to inspire deeply during the filming sequence. Portions of the coronary arterial tree may be obscured by the diaphragm and dense upper abdominal organs in some patients and in certain projections.

The terminology used to describe angiographic projections varies from author to author. The terminology used in the following discussion relates to the angiographic equipment used in our laboratory, which allows isocentric rotation of the image intensifier and X-ray tube in the axial and sagittal planes. However, these terms can be employed with any type of equipment.

In our laboratory, as in most angiographic laboratories, the image intensifier (II) is located above the radiographic table and the X-ray tube is located below the table. Thus, with the patient lying supine, the II is anterior (superior) to the patient and the X-ray tube is posterior (inferior) to the patient. If the II–X-ray tube system is perpendicular to the patient ("zero position"), the resulting view is described as a *posteroanterior (PA) or frontal projection* (Fig. 21.13A). If the II–X-ray tube system is partially rotated in the axial plane so that the II is to the left of the patient and the X-ray tube is to the right, the resulting view is described as a *left anterior oblique (LAO) projection* (ie, the X-ray beam is traveling from the right posterior aspect to the left anterior aspect of the patient) (Fig. 21.13B). Conversely, if the II–X-ray tube system is partially rotated to the right, so that the II is to the patient's right, the resulting view is described as a *right anterior oblique projection* (Fig. 21.13C).

When the II is angulated towards the patient's head and the X-ray tube is angulated in the opposite direction (ie, towards the patient's feet), the resulting projection is described as

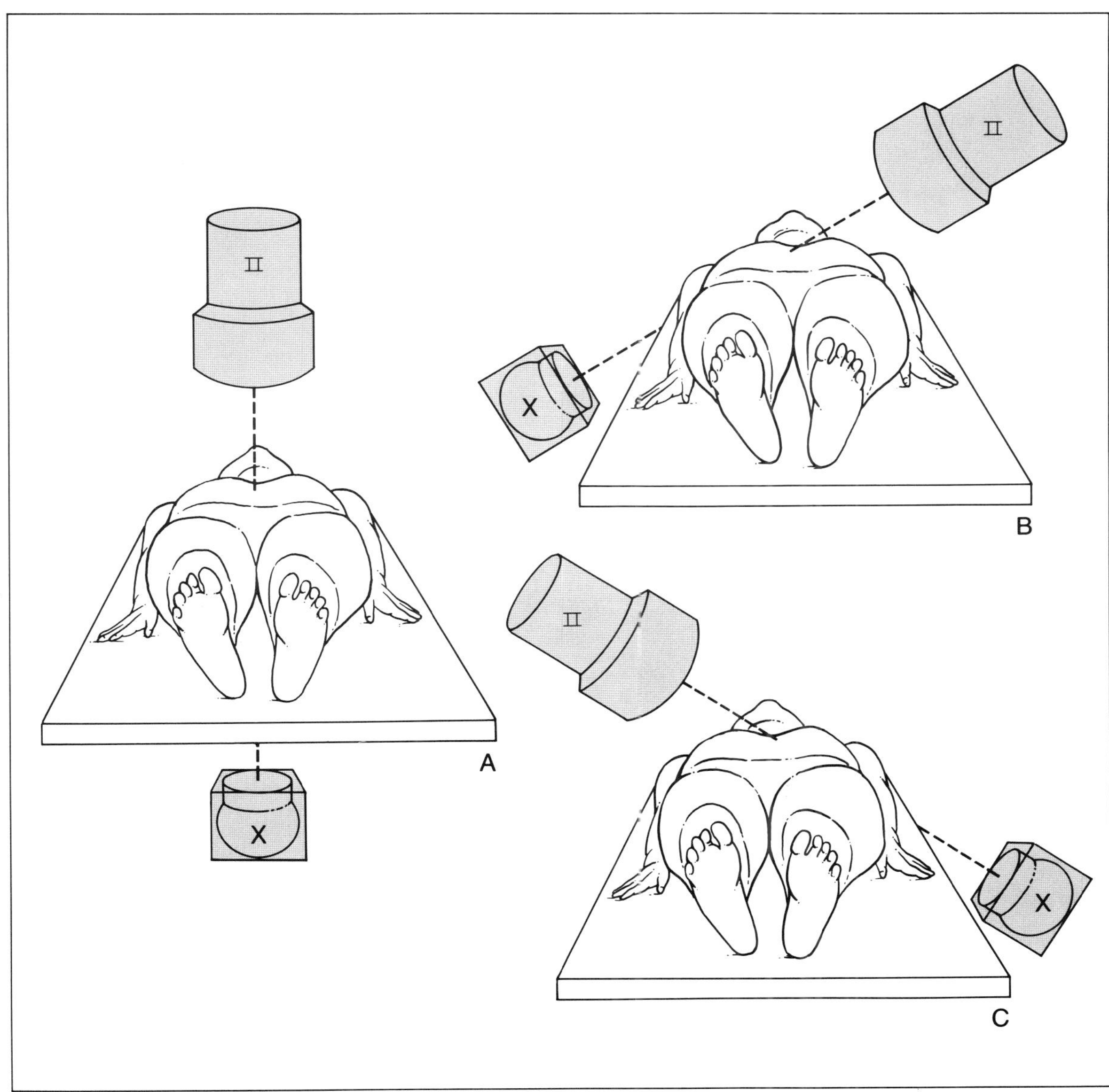

Fig. 21.13 Radiographic projections used for coronary angiography. In most equipment used for coronary angiography the image intensifier (II) is above the radiographic table and the X-ray tube (X) is below it. (A) To obtain a posteroanterior (frontal) projection the II–X-ray tube system is perpendicular to the patient. (B) Left anterior oblique projection is obtained by rotating the II to the patient's left and rotating the X-ray tube to the patient's right. (C) Right anterior oblique projection is obtained by rotating the II to the patient's right and rotating the X-ray tube to the patient's left. (Right and left anterior oblique projections can also be obtained by turning the patient without shifting the II–X-ray tube system.) This terminology is now standard in all cardiac laboratories.

cranially or craniocaudally (Cr) angulated (Fig. 21.14A,B). (With angiographic equipment that allows isocentric rotation of the II–X-ray tube system in the sagittal plane, the II will be displaced towards the patient's feet and the X-ray tube will be displaced by an equivalent distance towards the patient's head.) If the angulation is in the opposite direction, the resulting view is described as *caudally or caudocranially (Cd) angulated* (Fig. 21.14C).

Rotation of the II–X-ray tube system to the right or left can be combined with cranial or caudal angulation. The resulting projection can be described as "left anterior oblique with craniocaudal angulation (LAO-Cr)" or "right anterior oblique with caudocranial angulation (RAO-Cd)," and so forth. Each of these angles can be varied over a considerable range, creating a wide variety of possible projections. It should be kept in mind that the necessary angulation or rotation can be obtained by moving the II–X-ray tube system while the patient remains supine, or by moving the patient while the II–X-ray tube system remains vertically oriented ("zero position"), or by moving both the patient and the II–X-ray tube system.

The various projections used for coronary arteriography are listed in Fig. 21.15. The following projections, or variations thereof, are usually considered essential for a complete evaluation of the coronary arterial tree.

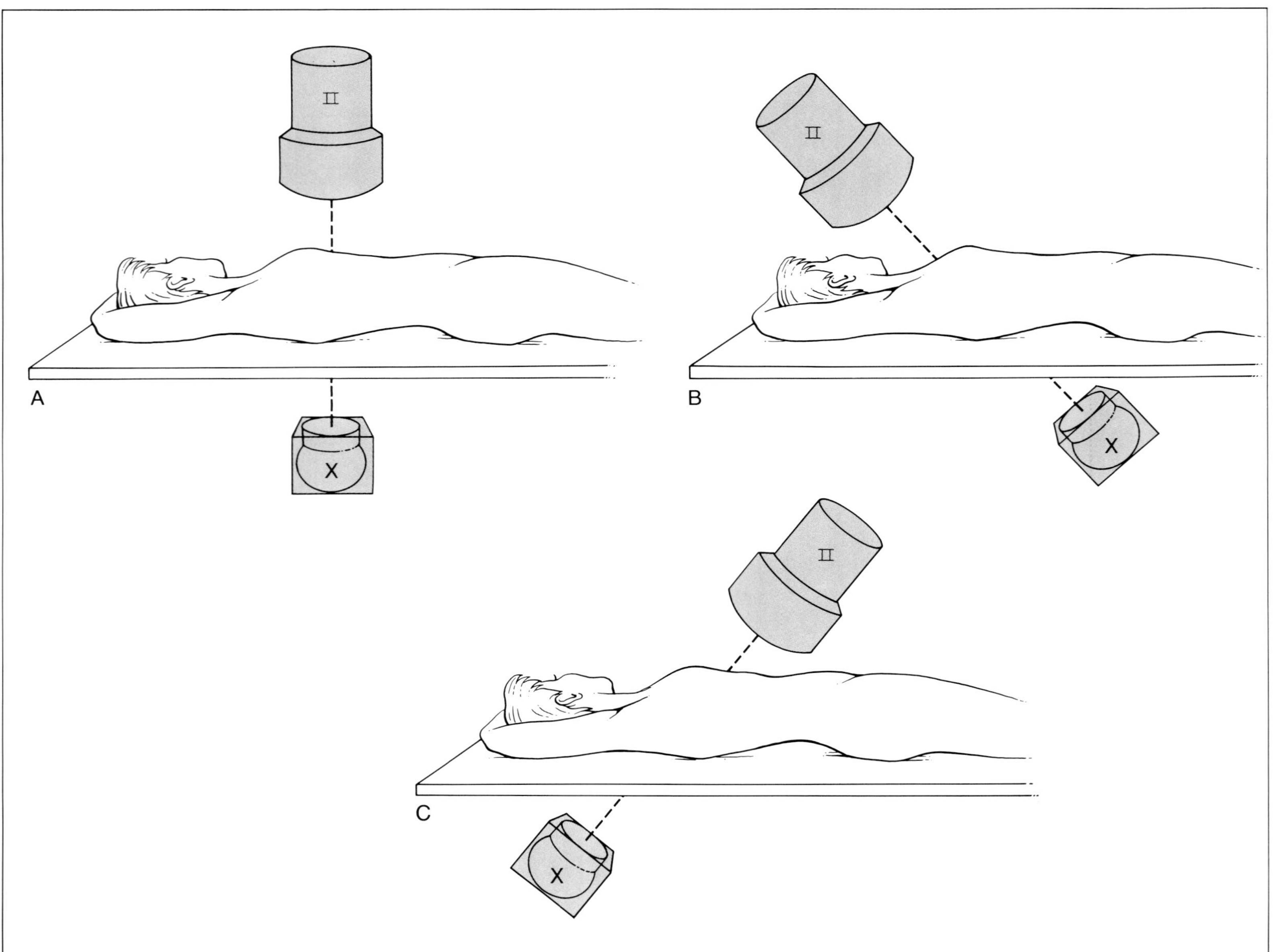

Fig. 21.14 Craniocaudal and caudocranial angulation. (A) Vertical orientation ("zero position"). (B) Craniocaudal angulation. In an isocentric system (ie, one with the patient or the radiographic table at the center of rotation). The II is shifted closer to the patient's head and the X-ray tube is shifted closer to the patient's feet. (C) Caudocranial angulation. The II is shifted closer to the patient's feet and the X-ray tube is shifted closer to the patient's head. Craniocaudal and caudocranial angulation can be combined with axial rotation of the II–X-ray tube system to obtain right or left anterior oblique projections with craniocaudal or caudocranial angulation.

TABLE 21.15 PROJECTIONS USED FOR CORONARY ARTERIOGRAPHY

Projection	Comment
Left anterior oblique (LAO)	
A. Without angulation (standard LAO)	Seldom used
B. With craniocaudal angulation (LAO-Cr)	Useful for 1. Right coronary artery, particularly bifurcation and posterolateral branch 2. Proximal segment of circumflex artery 3. Middle segment of left anterior descending artery and diagonal branches
C. With caudocranial angulation (LAO-Cd)	Useful for 1. Left main coronary artery 2. Proximal segment of circumflex artery 3. Proximal segment of left anterior descending artery 4. The "ramus medianus"
Right anterior oblique	
A. Without angulation (standard RAO)	Useful for 1. Middle and distal segments of right coronary artery 2. Posterior descending artery
B. With craniocaudal angulation (RAO-Cr)	Useful for 1. Middle segment of right coronary artery and posterior descending artery 2. Left anterior descending artery and diagonal branches
C. With caudocranial angulation (RAO-Cd)	Useful for 1. Posterior descending artery 2. Left main coronary artery 3. Circumflex artery and marginal branches
Lateral	Useful for 1. Middle segment of right coronary artery 2. Middle and distal segments of left anterior descending artery
Projections for special problems	
A. Visualizing left main coronary artery and LAD	Combination of frontal or LAO projections with 15° RAO/30° craniocaudal angulation (Timi projection)
B. Visualizing coronary ostia	Frontal and LAO projections with craniocaudal and caudocranial angulation

LEFT CORONARY ARTERIOGRAPHY
60° Left Anterior Oblique With 30° Craniocaudal Angulation (LAO-Cr) (Fig. 21.16)

In this projection the origin of the left main coronary artery from the left (posterior) coronary cusp is clearly seen. The left main coronary artery courses posteriorly and inferiorly towards its bifurcation; it length is variable (mean, approximately 1.5 cm). Although the bifurcation is usually clearly seen, it is sometimes overlapped by the proximal segments of the left anterior descending and circumflex arteries, a problem that can usually be solved by rotating the II to the patient's left. Although the proximal segment of the left anterior descending artery is foreshortened, its middle and distal portions are well visualized in this projection.

The LAO-Cr projection is especially useful for visualizing the diagonal arteries as they arise from the proximal and middle

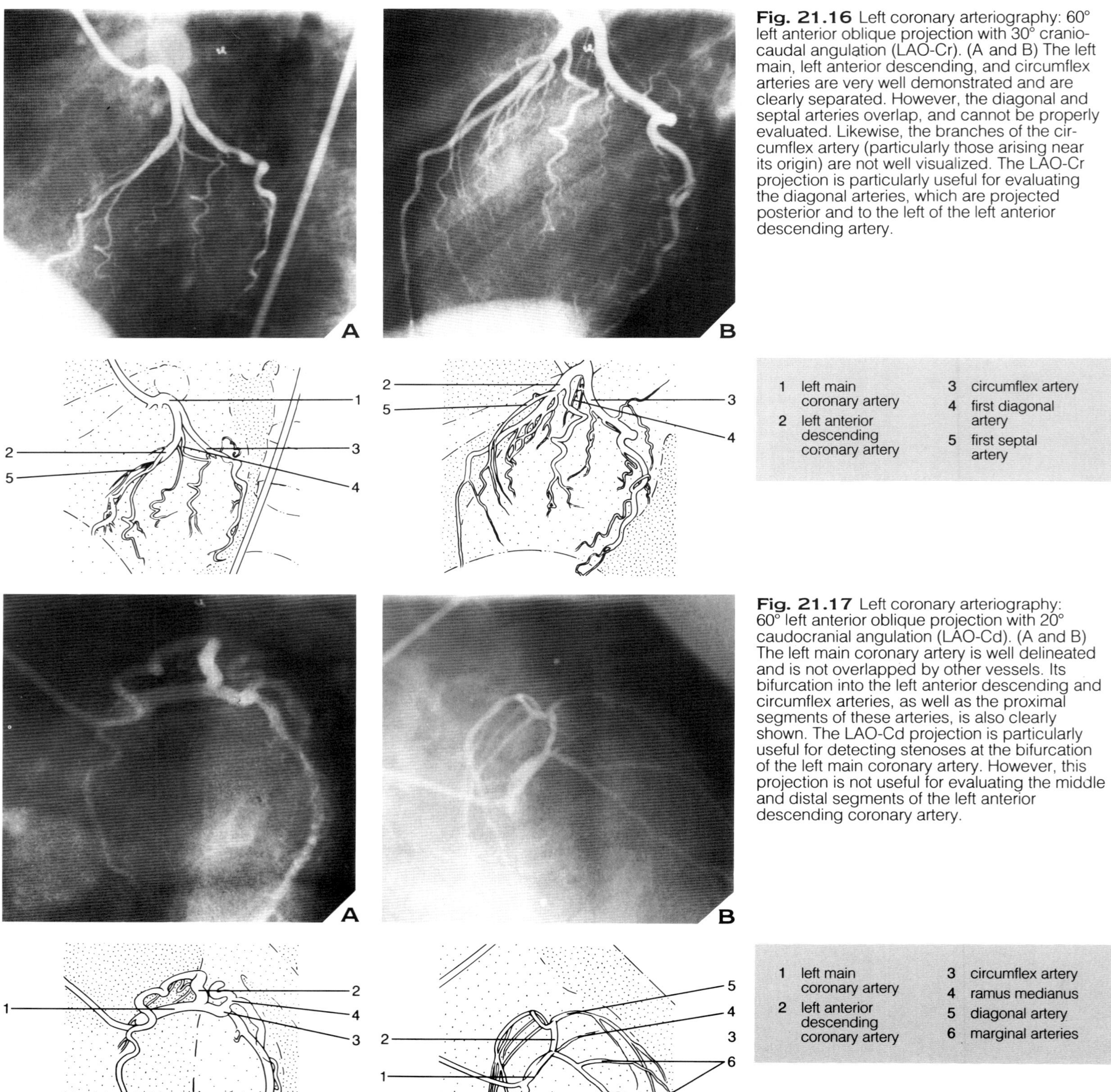

Fig. 21.16 Left coronary arteriography: 60° left anterior oblique projection with 30° craniocaudal angulation (LAO-Cr). (A and B) The left main, left anterior descending, and circumflex arteries are very well demonstrated and are clearly separated. However, the diagonal and septal arteries overlap, and cannot be properly evaluated. Likewise, the branches of the circumflex artery (particularly those arising near its origin) are not well visualized. The LAO-Cr projection is particularly useful for evaluating the diagonal arteries, which are projected posterior and to the left of the left anterior descending artery.

Fig. 21.17 Left coronary arteriography: 60° left anterior oblique projection with 20° caudocranial angulation (LAO-Cd). (A and B) The left main coronary artery is well delineated and is not overlapped by other vessels. Its bifurcation into the left anterior descending and circumflex arteries, as well as the proximal segments of these arteries, is also clearly shown. The LAO-Cd projection is particularly useful for detecting stenoses at the bifurcation of the left main coronary artery. However, this projection is not useful for evaluating the middle and distal segments of the left anterior descending coronary artery.

segments of the left anterior descending artery. The septal branches overlie the left anterior descending artery in this projection; their identification is facilitated by observing their characteristic displacement during the cardiac cycle.

The proximal segment of the circumflex artery courses posteriorly and inferiorly over the posterior aspect of the heart. The proximal and distal segments of the circumflex artery are not well seen in this projection because they are obscured by the marginal branches, which run in the same direction. When the circumflex artery supplies the inferior wall of the left ventricle through its left posterolateral branch, both the circumflex artery and its branches are well visualized as they course over the inferior aspect of the heart. In individuals with a left dominant coronary arterial system, the posterior descending artery can be seen as a vertically oriented channel arising from the distal portion of the circumflex artery and extending from the level of the crux cordis towards the apex (see Fig. 21.10).

60° Left Anterior Oblique with 20° Caudocranial Angulation (Fig. 21.17)

This projection is mainly used to identify the left main coronary artery and its bifurcation into the left anterior descending and circumflex arteries. The proximal segment of the circumflex arteries and the branches that arise from it are particularly well visualized in this projection. The proximal segment of the left anterior descending artery and its first diagonal branch are also well seen; however, the middle and distal segments of the left anterior descending artery are poorly visualized. This projection is particularly useful for identifying the artery that occasionally originates at the bifurcation of the left main coronary artery, the so-called ramus medianus.

The LAO-Cd projection is recommended for patients whose heart is horizontally oriented owing to a high position of the left hemidiaphragm, and in those who cannot perform a deep inspiration. In such patients it is difficult to adequately visualize the left main coronary artery in the LAO-Cr projection.

Left Lateral (Fig. 21.18)

The left main coronary artery overlies the proximal segments of the circumflex and left anterior descending arteries in the left lateral projection; therefore, this projection is not useful for evaluating the left main coronary artery. The middle and distal segments of the left anterior descending artery are seen in profile, and are clearly separated from the diagonal branches all the way to the apex. Although the proximal segment of the circumflex artery is not well seen, its distal segment is clearly visualized in the lateral projection.

30° Right Anterior Oblique Without Angulation (RAO) (Fig. 21.19)

In this projection the left main coronary artery appears as a short channel which arises from the left coronary cusp and courses towards the left atrioventricular groove. The left anterior descending artery appears to arise as a continuation of the

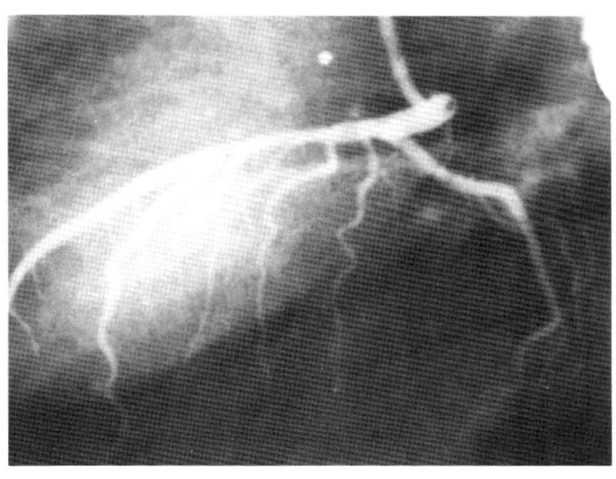

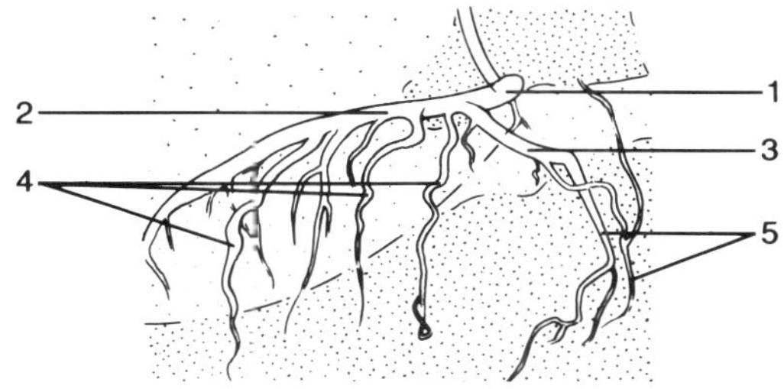

Fig. 21.18 Left coronary arteriography: lateral projection. The middle and distal segments of the left anterior descending artery are clearly visualized; however the bifurcation and the distal part of the left main coronary artery are not well seen. The lateral projection is particularly useful for identifying the distal portions of the diagonal arteries.

1 left main coronary artery	3 circumflex artery
2 left anterior descending coronary artery	4 diagonal branches
	5 marginal branches

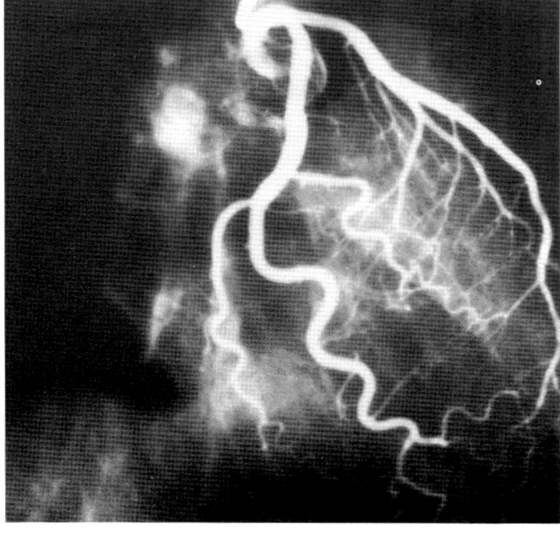

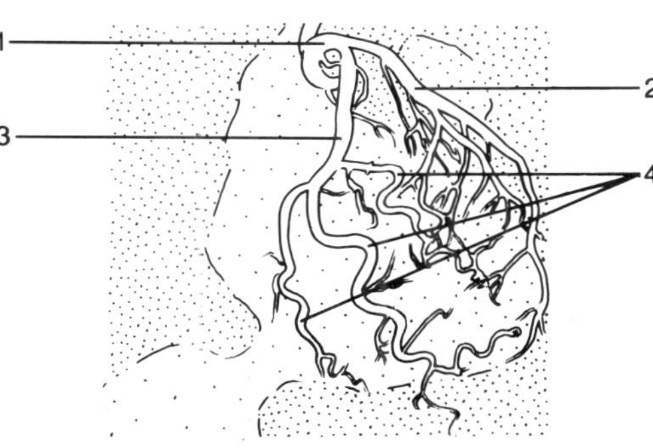

Fig. 21.19 Left coronary arteriography: right anterior oblique projection without angulation (RAO). The left main coronary artery is clearly visualized and separated from the other vessels. The circumflex artery is also nicely demonstrated as it courses within the left atrioventricular groove. The tortuosity of the marginal arteries indicates that this frame was exposed in systole.

1 left main coronary artery	3 circumflex artery
2 left anterior descending coronary artery	4 marginal branches of circumflex artery

left main coronary artery. The diagonal branches overlap the proximal and middle segments of the left anterior descending artery, so that neither can be properly evaluated in this projection. The distal segment of the left anterior descending artery (which lies in the interventricular groove) and the distal portions of the large diagonal branches (which course over the free wall of the left ventricle) are clearly separated. Although the proximal segment of the circumflex artery is not well visualized, its distal segment and branches are clearly seen in this projection.

30° Right Anterior Oblique With 30° Caudocranial Angulation (RAO-Cd) (Fig. 21.20)

The RAO-Cd projection is particularly useful for visualizing the circumflex artery, which appears as a channel separate from the left main coronary artery; it runs inferiorly and posteriorly in the left atrioventricular groove before terminating at the midportion of this anatomic landmark. The circumflex artery, which appears foreshortened on the standard RAO projection, is "stretched out" on the RAO-Cd projection, so that the origin and course of the marginal branches are clearly seen. The left anterior descending artery and its branches are not adequately visualized on the RAO-Cd projection owing to the superimposition of the diagonal arteries.

30° Right Anterior Oblique With 30° Craniocaudal Angulation (RAO-Cr) (Fig. 21.21)

The RAO-Cr projection provides excellent visualization of the left main coronary artery and its continuation into the left anterior descending artery. The proximal, middle, and distal segments of the left anterior descending artery are projected clear of the diagonal and marginal branches, which obscure it on the standard RAO projection. Although the marginal and diagonal arteries overlap, they can be distinguished by their different patterns of movement during the cardiac cycle. The circumflex artery is poorly visualized in this projection.

A modification of the standard RAO-Cr projection which combines 15° RAO with 30° craniocaudal angulation provides excellent visualization of the left anterior descending artery and its diagonal branches (Fig. 21.22).

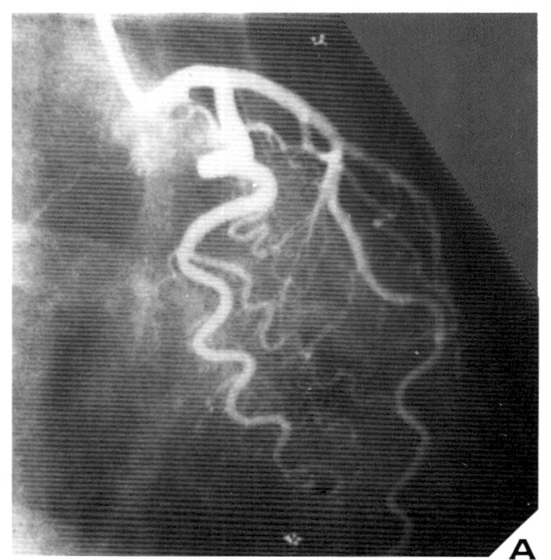

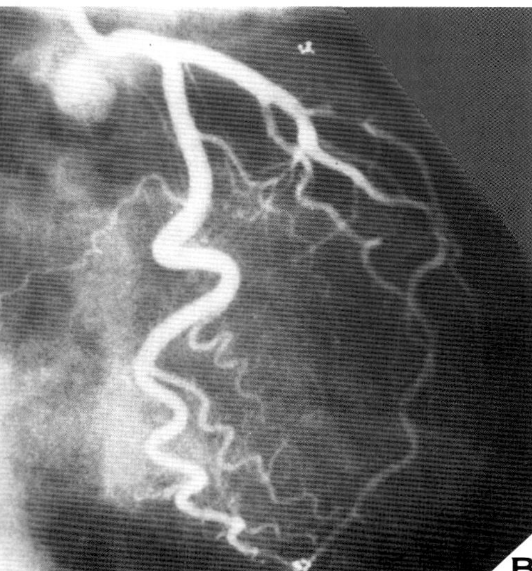

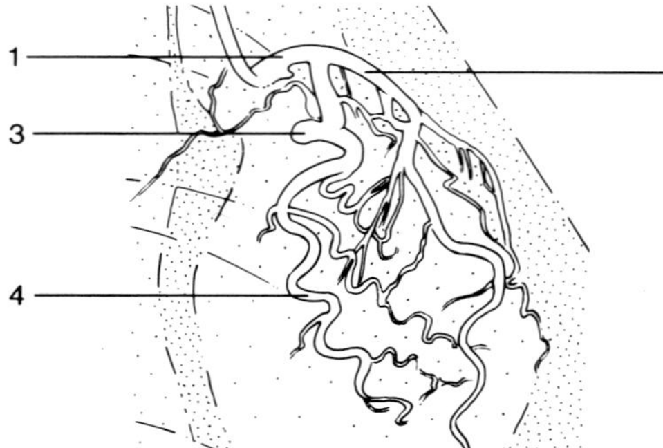

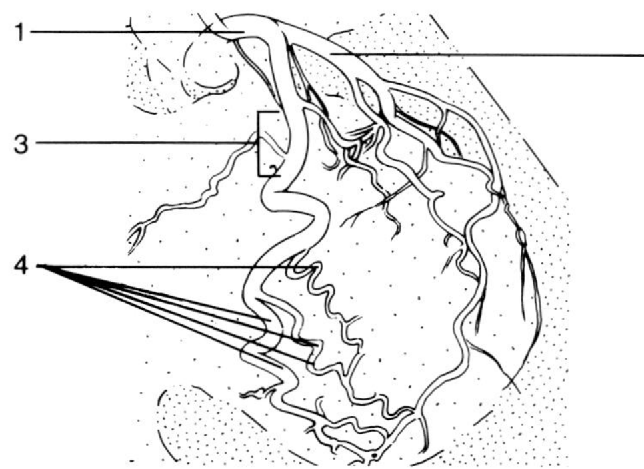

Fig. 21.20 Left coronary arteriography: right anterior oblique projection without (RAO) and with caudal angulation (RAO-Cd). (A) Without caudal (caudocranial) angulation (RAO). The left anterior descending and diagonal arteries are well demonstrated. However, a portion of the circumflex artery within the left atrioventricular groove is not well seen. (B) With caudal angulation the portion of the circumflex artery obscured on the unangled view is now clearly seen. (Note its straight course.)

1 left main coronary artery
2 left anterior descending coronary artery
3 circumflex artery
4 marginal branches of circumflex artery

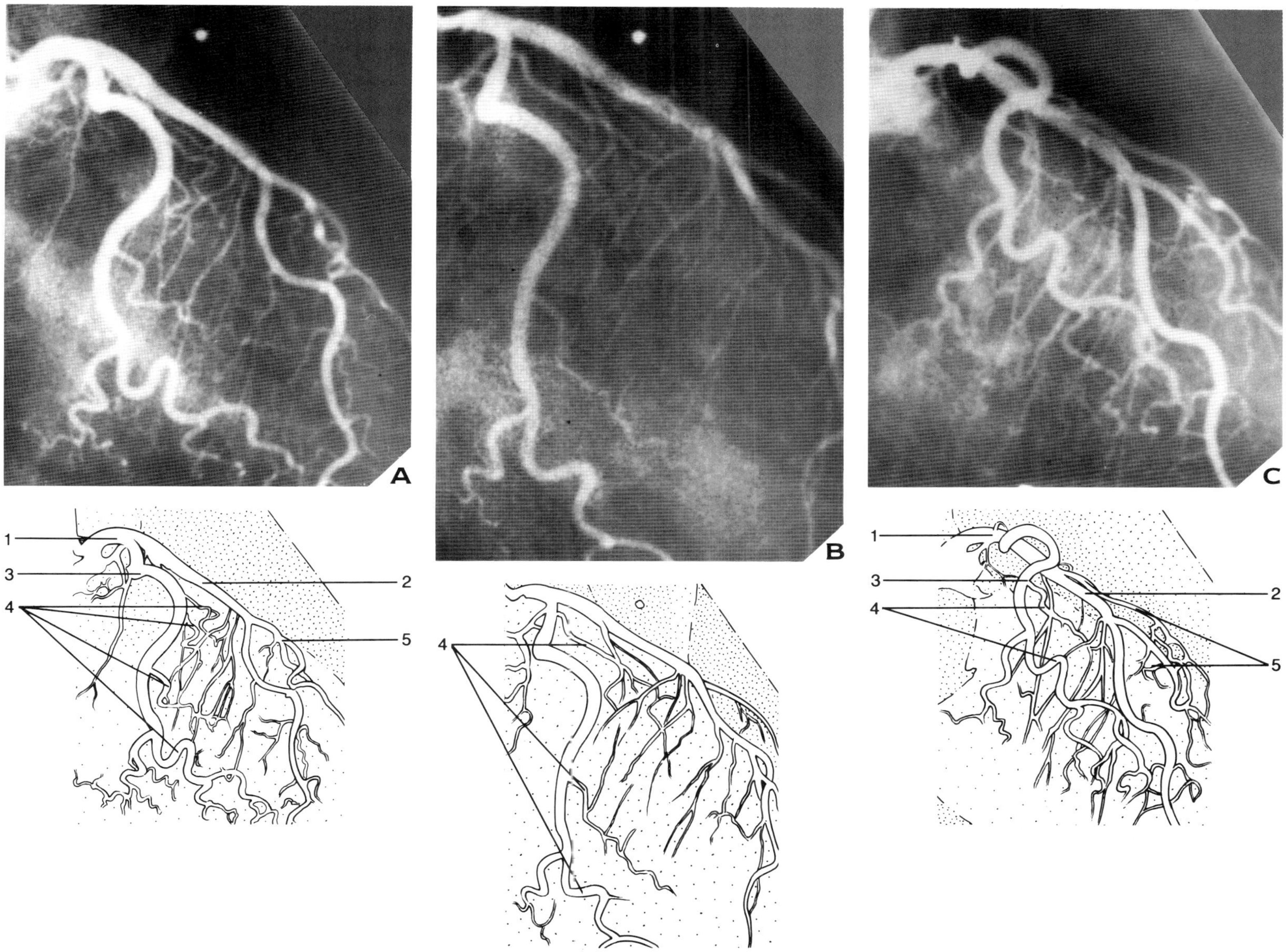

1	left main coronary artery	4	marginal branches of circumflex artery
2	left anterior descending coronary artery	5	diagonal branches of left anterior descending artery
3	circumflex artery		

Fig. 21.21 Left coronary arteriography: right anterior oblique projection: RAO, RAO-Cd, RAO-Cr projections. (A) Without angulation (RAO). (B) RAO with caudal (caudocranial) angulation (RAO-Cd). The circumflex artery and its marginal branches are clearly seen. (C) RAO with cranial (craniocaudal) angulation (RAO-Cr). The left anterior descending artery and its diagonal branches are well visualized.

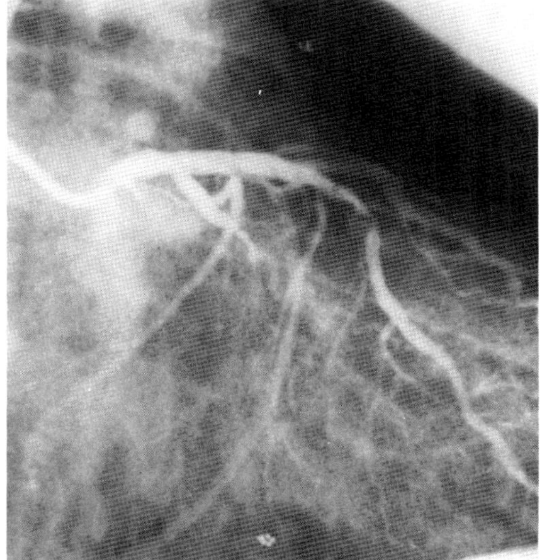

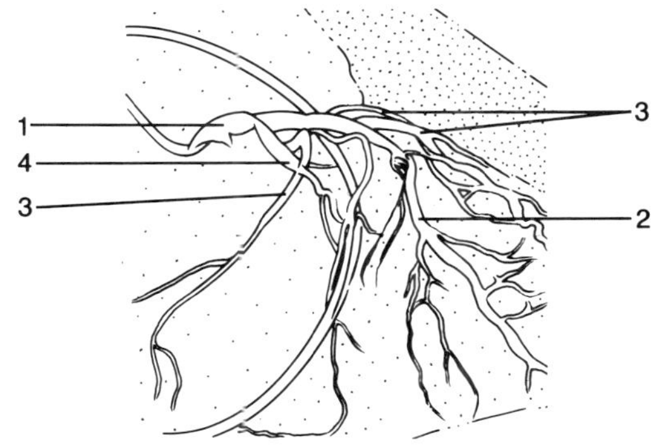

Fig. 21.22 Left coronary arteriography: 15° right anterior oblique projection with 30° craniocaudal angulation (Timi projection). This projection is designed to display the entire course (ie, all three segments) of the left anterior descending artery. The left main coronary artery and its continuation as the left anterior descending coronary artery, as well as the origins of the diagonal arteries, are well seen. However, the circumflex artery and its marginal branches are poorly visualized in this view. There is a severe stenosis in the middle segment of the left anterior descending coronary artery, just beyond the origin of the first septal artery.

1	left main coronary artery	2	left anterior descending coronary artery	3	diagonal arteries	4	circumflex and marginal arteries

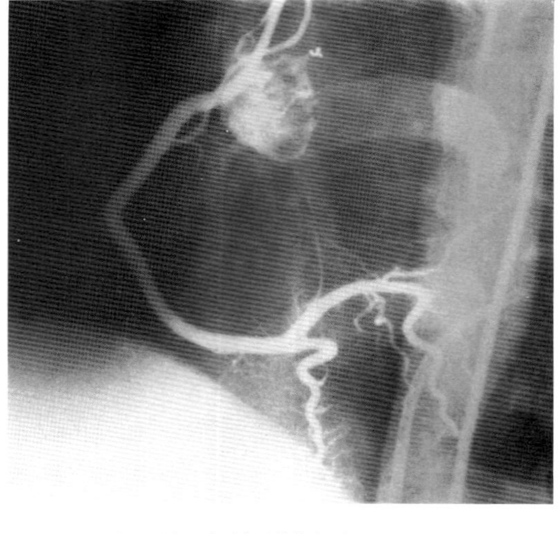

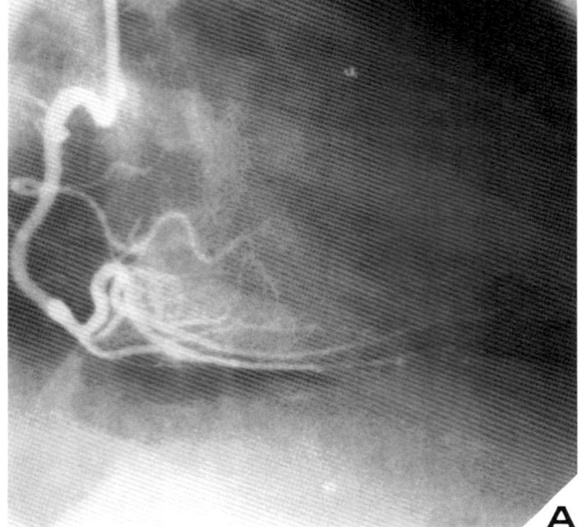

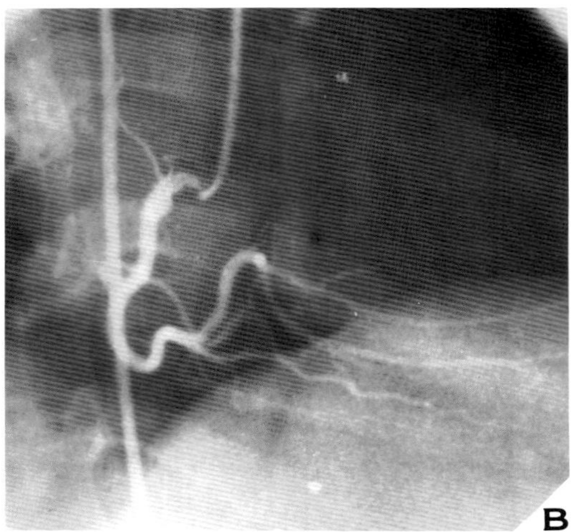

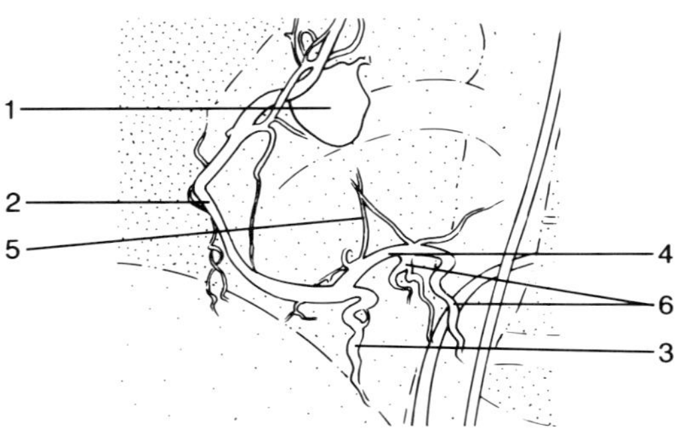

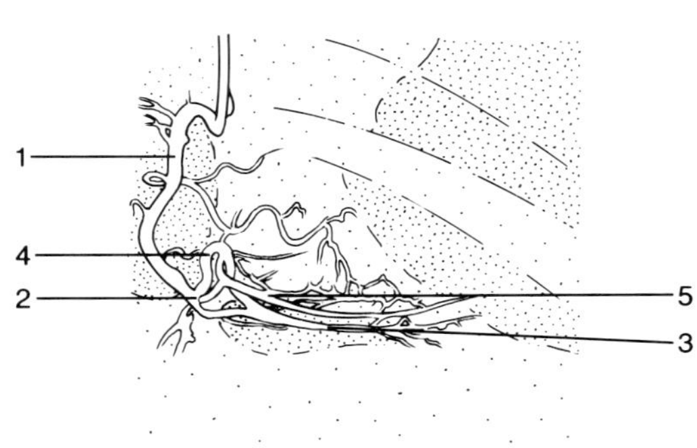

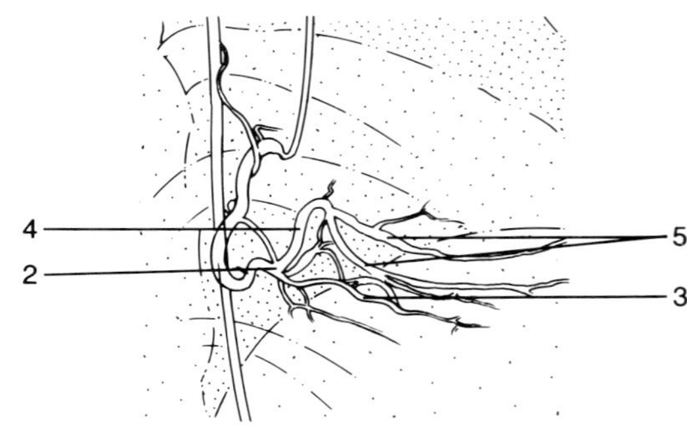

1	right coronary cusp	4	posterolateral artery
2	right coronary artery	5	artery of the atrioventricular node
3	posterior descending coronary artery	6	branches of the posterolateral artery

Fig. 21.23 Right coronary arteriography: left anterior oblique projection with 30° craniocaudal angulation (LAO-Cr). In this projection the entire right coronary artery and its branches are visualized (note reflux of contrast material into the right coronary cusp). The right coronary artery arises at the right coronary cusp and courses within the right atrioventricular groove. At the level of the crux cordis it bifurcates into the posterior descending and posterolateral arteries. The posterolateral artery gives off many branches which supply the inferior wall of the left ventricle; they are numbered one, two, or three, and so forth according to their relation to the origin of the posterolateral artery. The artery supplying the atrioventricular node is a straight branch of the posterolateral artery which runs superiorly in the direction of the right coronary cusp.

1	right coronary artery	3	posterior descending coronary artery	5	branches of the posterolateral artery
2	bifurcation of right coronary artery (at level of crux cordis)	4	posterolateral artery		

Fig. 21.24 Right coronary arteriography: right anterior oblique projection without (RAO) and with cranial angulation (RAO-Cr). The RAO projection demonstrates the middle segment of the right coronary artery as well as the posterior descending artery and the branches of the posterolateral artery. (A) On the unangled RAO projection the bifurcation of the right coronary artery and the proximal and distal segments of the posterior descending and posterolateral arteries overlap each other and are difficult to identify. (B) With cranial angulation (RAO-Cr) these branches are separated.

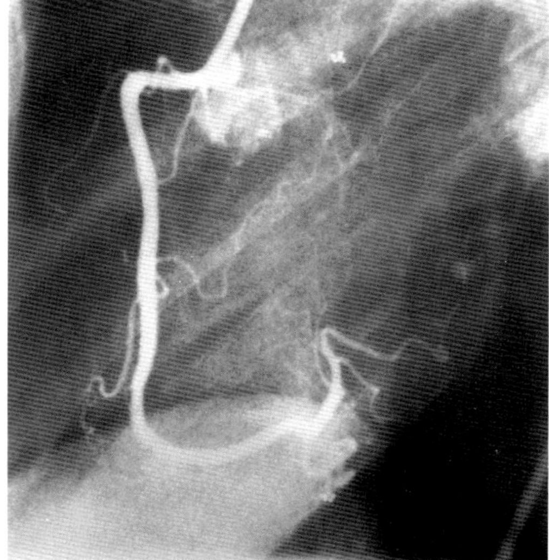

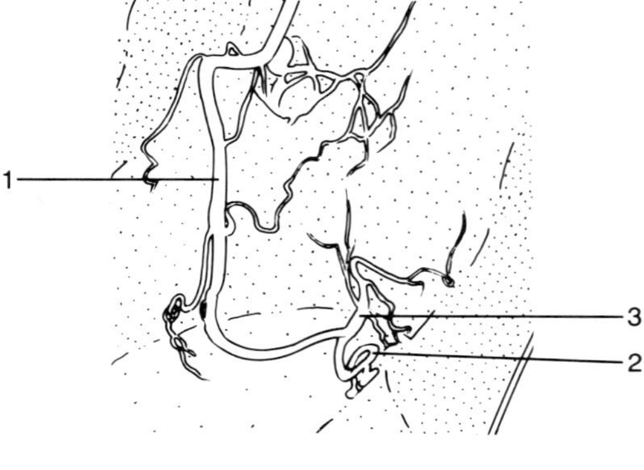

Fig. 21.25 Right coronary arteriography: left lateral projection. This projection is useful for demonstrating the origin of the right coronary artery from the right coronary cusp. The proximal and middle segments of the right coronary artery are also clearly seen. However, its distal segment, bifurcation, and major branches (posterolateral and posterior descending arteries) are not well visualized in this projection.

1	right coronary artery	3	posterolateral artery
2	posterior descending coronary artery		

RIGHT CORONARY ARTERIOGRAPHY

60° Left Anterior Oblique With 30° Craniocaudal Angulation (LAO-Cr) (Fig. 21.23)

This projection displays the entire length of the right coronary artery as it courses within the right atrioventricular sulcus. Its origin from the right (anterior) coronary cusp is seen in profile. The right coronary artery itself appears as a semicircle which is open posteriorly, superiorly, and to the left. Its right marginal branches of the right coronary artery are seen end-on in this projection.

In individuals with right coronary dominance, the distal portion of the right coronary artery can be seen to bifurcate into the posterior descending and right posterolateral arteries at the crux cordis. The right posterolateral artery then continues in the left atrioventricular groove. Its branches, which vary in number from one to four, are seen in profile as they course from the left atrioventricular groove towards the apex. The posterior descending artery appears as a vertically oriented channel extending from the right coronary artery bifurcation towards the cardiac apex. The middle and distal segments of the posterior descending artery and the branches of the right posterolateral artery are seen end-on in this projection.

30° Right Anterior Oblique Without Craniocaudal Angulation (30° RAO) (Fig. 21.24)

In this projection the middle and distal segments of the right coronary artery are visualized almost up to the bifurcation. The origin and proximal segment of the right coronary artery are seen end-on. The posterior descending artery is projected onto the inferior surface of the heart, and appears as a straight channel with the septal arteries oriented upward. For this reason, the 30° RAO projection is particularly useful for studying this vessel and its branches. The posterolateral artery is seen end-on; because its branches run parallel to the posterior descending artery, they can be identified throughout their entire course.

In some individuals the right posterolateral artery overlies the distal segment of the right coronary artery, making it difficult to evaluate either vessel. Increasing the angulation by 15°, either cranially or caudally, usually solves the problem.

The right marginal and atrial arteries are also well seen in the RAO projection. The most important atrial branch of the right coronary artery is the sinus node artery, which can be clearly seen as it courses superiorly and posteriorly towards the junction of the superior vena cava and right atrium.

Left Lateral (Fig. 21.25)

In the left lateral projection the right coronary artery courses inferiorly and posteriorly until the level of the crux cordis, where it bifurcates into the posterior descending and right posterolateral arteries. The former courses anteriorly and inferiorly, while the latter courses posteriorly into the left portion of the atrioventricular groove. Because the left lateral projection offers no advantage over the RAO and LAO projections, it is infrequently used.

SPECIAL SITUATIONS

Inadequate Visualization of the Left Main Coronary Artery

Adequate visualization of the left main coronary artery may be difficult owing to its orientation, short length, or the presence of disease. However, because of the lethal nature of high-grade obstructing lesions of this artery, accurate diagnosis is essential. A combination of a frontal projection and a shallow (15°) right anterior oblique projection with 30° craniocaudal angulation will demonstrate the entire course of the left main coronary artery in most patients (Fig. 21.26). The LAO-Cd and LAO-Cr projections may be helpful in problem cases.

Stenosis of the Coronary Ostia

Stenosis at the ostium of the right or left coronary artery may be difficult to demonstrate. Ostial stenosis should suspected if an arteriogram obtained with the catheter tip beyond the ostium fails to demonstrate reflux into the aorta. (The arteriogram may not actually demonstrate the stenosis in such cases.) Another suggestive sign is dampening of the arterial pressure when the catheter tip is positioned in the main coronary artery. In such cases it may be possible to demonstrate the stenotic ostium by injecting contrast material while slowly withdrawing the catheter from the main coronary artery into the aorta, or by injecting contrast material into the cusp.

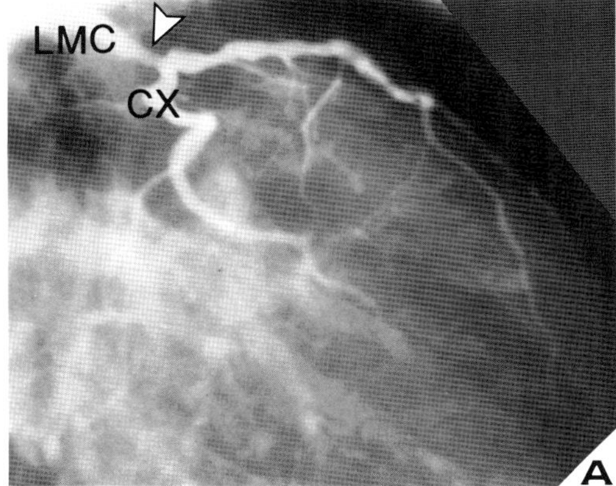

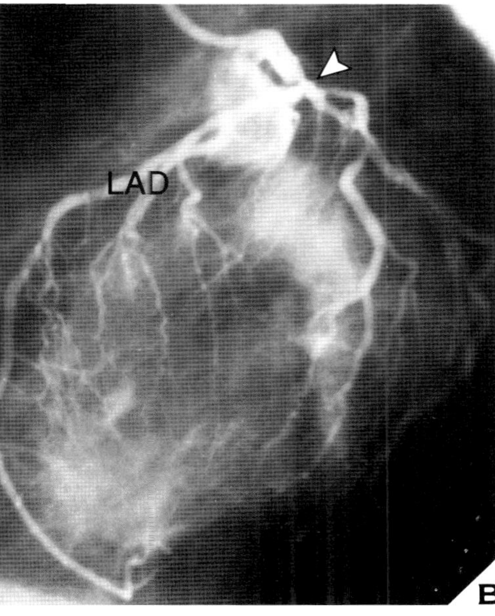

Fig. 21.26 Special projections for visualizing left main coronary artery. Selective left coronary arteriography in two different patients. (A) Frontal projection demonstrates stenosis (*arrow*) of the middle portion of the left main coronary artery. The ostium is widely patent. The distal portion of the left main coronary artery (LMC) is not visualized in this projection. (B) Left anterior oblique projection with craniocaudal angulation (LAO-Cr) demonstrates a severe stenosis (*arrow*) of the distal portion of the left main coronary artery, just proximal to the bifurcation. (CX = circumflex artery; LAD = left anterior descending artery).

CORONARY ARTERY STENOSIS

PATHOGENESIS

Coronary artery stenosis is almost always caused by atheromatous plaque, which consists of an accumulation of fat and other material in the subintimal space. Progressive enlargement of the plaque may lead to endothelial injury. Increased endothelial permeability results in an influx of plasma proteins into the arterial wall. (In severe cases, erythrocytes may penetrate into the media.) The atheromatous plaque may undergo erosion, resulting in ulceration and fissuring, which may extend into the media. Endothelial injury predisposes to platelet aggregation, which may occur at any stage of the process and may progress to thrombosis and occlusion of the arterial lumen. The pathogenesis of coronary artery atherosclerosis and its sequelae is discussed further in Chapter 30.

ANGIOGRAPHIC FINDINGS

Accurate assessment of the degree of coronary artery stenosis is critical for determining its functional significance. Obstructing atherosclerotic lesions may affect one, two, three, or all four of the major coronary arteries. The most common sites of stenosis are the left main coronary artery, the proximal segment of the left anterior descending artery, the circumflex artery, and the right coronary artery.

Coronary artery stenosis is graded according to the percentage of narrowing (decrease in diameter) when compared with an adjacent nonstenotic segment of the affected artery: *Grade 1,* less than 50%; *Grade 2,* 50 to 75 percent; *Grade 3,* over 75 percent; and *Grade 4,* complete occlusion (Figs. 21.27 to 21.32). Correlative studies have shown that stenosis of 50 percent or greater is associated with a significant decrease in myocardial perfusion.

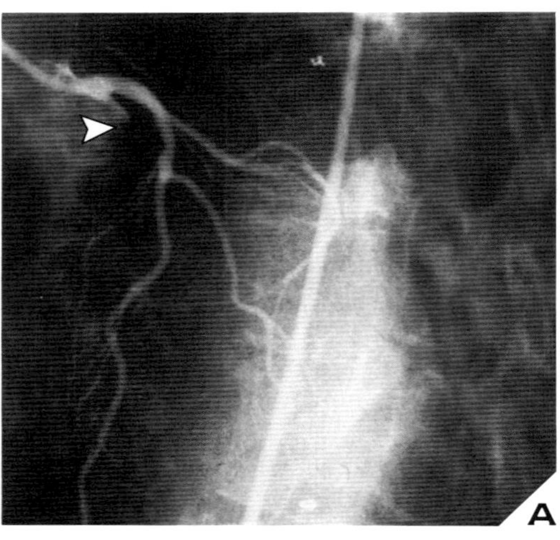

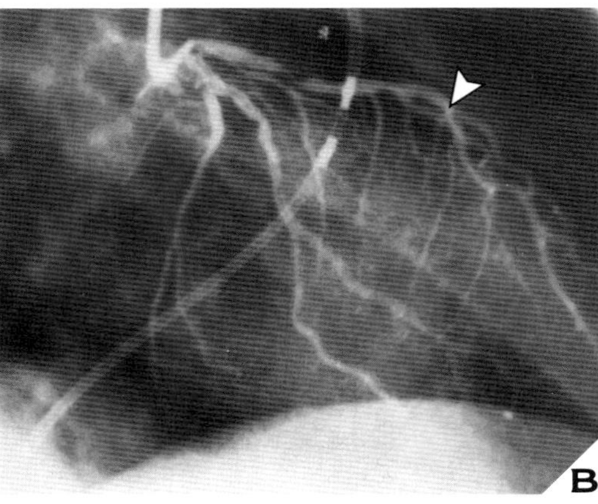

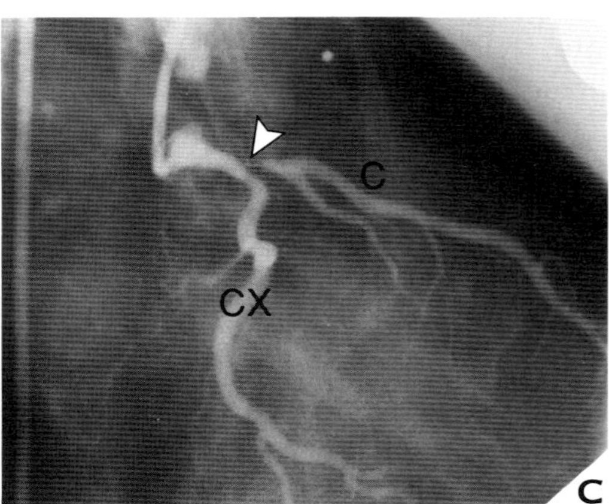

Fig. 21.27 Coronary artery stenosis (single artery stenosis). (A–C) Selective coronary arteriograms in three different patients. (A) 30 percent (nonsignificant) stenosis (*arrow*) of the proximal segment of the left anterior descending artery(LAO-Cr projection). (B) 70 percent (significant) stenosis (*arrow*) of the middle segment of the left anterior descending artery (RAO projection). (C) 90 percent stenosis of left anterior descending artery (RAO-Cd projection). (CX = circumflex artery)

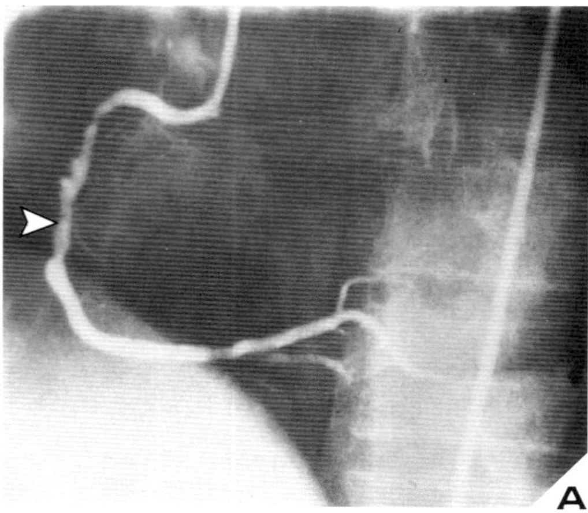

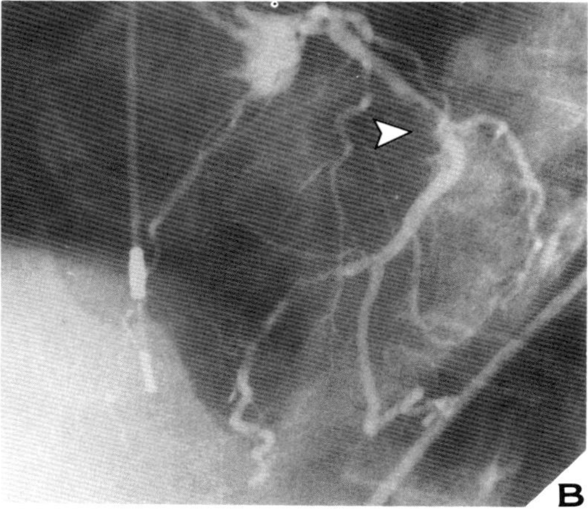

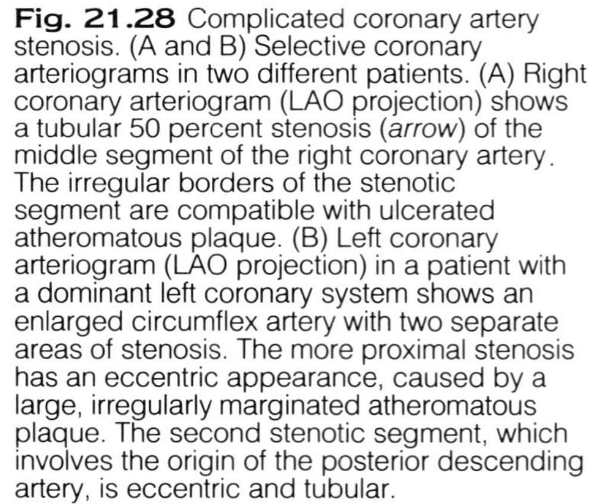

Fig. 21.28 Complicated coronary artery stenosis. (A and B) Selective coronary arteriograms in two different patients. (A) Right coronary arteriogram (LAO projection) shows a tubular 50 percent stenosis (*arrow*) of the middle segment of the right coronary artery. The irregular borders of the stenotic segment are compatible with ulcerated atheromatous plaque. (B) Left coronary arteriogram (LAO projection) in a patient with a dominant left coronary system shows an enlarged circumflex artery with two separate areas of stenosis. The more proximal stenosis has an eccentric appearance, caused by a large, irregularly marginated atheromatous plaque. The second stenotic segment, which involves the origin of the posterior descending artery, is eccentric and tubular.

1 left anterior descending artery
2 enlarged circumflex artery
3 eccentric stenosis of circumflex artery caused by ulcerated atheromatous plaque
4 eccentric tubular stenosis of circumflex artery
5 posterior descending artery

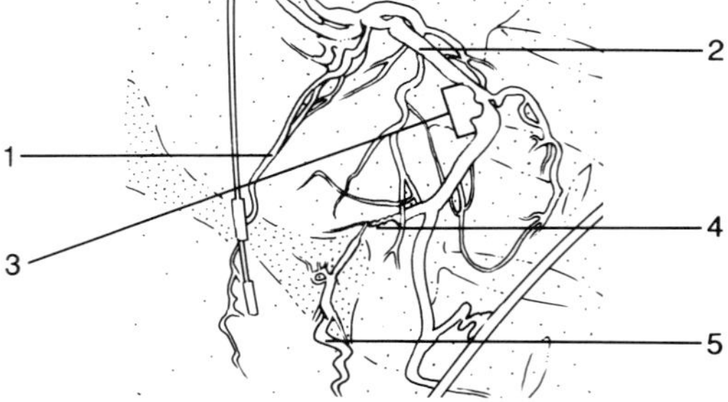

The various pathologic lesions associated with coronary atherosclerosis are clearly depicted on selective coronary arteriograms. The most common lesions are chronic stenoses, which have smooth borders, usually with a triangular configuration (Fig. 21.27A). The lesions may be isolated or multiple, affecting two or more vessels (Fig. 21.29). In stenoses associated with ulcerated atheromatous plaque, the stenosis is usually eccentric and the ulcer can be identified by its irregular borders (Fig. 21.28); the mural irregularity may not correspond to the site of the maximal luminal narrowing. Chronic stenoses typically have a triangular configuration (Fig. 21.29). Acute occlusions typically have irregular borders (Fig. 21.30). Intraluminal filling defects representing thrombus are commonly seen in acute occlusions. They are typically elongated, with their long axis parallel to that of the artery, and may severely compromise the arterial lumen.

The stenotic lesions of coronary atherosclerosis typically occur at the origin of the affected artery. The stenotic segment may measure 1 cm or more in length (Fig. 21.28B). Multiple projections may be required to accurately assess the extent and morphology of the obstructing lesion.

CLINICAL CORRELATION

In general, the angiographic findings correlate with the clinical manifestations, as well as with the waxing and waning nature of the symptoms that is typical of ischemic heart disease. Patients with stable atheromata (Fig. 21.27B) usually have stable angina, whereas those with ulcerated plaques (Fig. 21.28A,B) commonly have accelerated angina; in the latter, platelet aggregation may lead to thrombotic occlusion and sudden death. Healing of the ulcerated plaque results in progressive stenosis of the affected artery, which is usually associated with stable angina; recurrent ulceration initiates a new cycle. Thrombosis is usually associated with unstable angina; progression of the thrombus may lead to complete occlusion, resulting in acute myocardial infarction (Fig. 21.30). Alternatively, the thrombus may undergo organization and become incorporated into the atheromatous plaque, resulting in the formation of a stable atheroma; this process, which causes progressive stenosis, is usually associated with stable angina (Fig. 21.31).

The most common sites of involvement in patients with angina pectoris are (in order of frequency) the proximal seg-

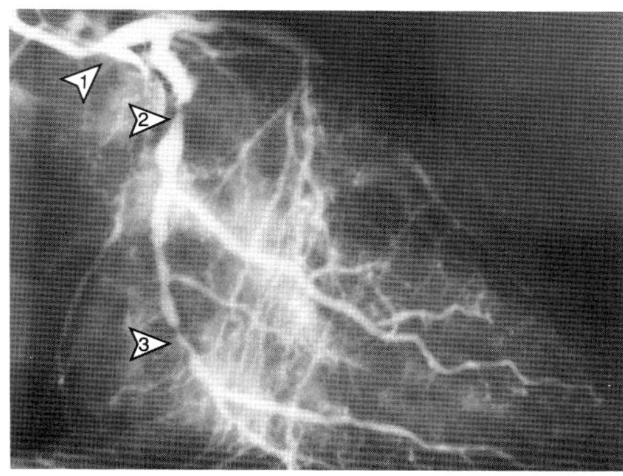

Fig. 21.29 Occlusion of right coronary artery with severe stenosis of circumflex artery. Left coronary arteriogram (RAO projection) shows occlusion (*arrow* 1) of the left anterior descending artery just beyond the origin of the first septal artery. Note the triangular configuration of the proximal margin of the occluded segment, indicating that the preexisting stenosis was of long duration. [This interpretation is supported by the observation that the segment distal to the occlusion (LAD) has been opacified via collaterals.] In addition, there is a significant (80 percent) circumscribed stenosis (*arrow* 2) of the circumflex artery, and another (*arrow* 3) in the proximal segment of its third marginal branch.

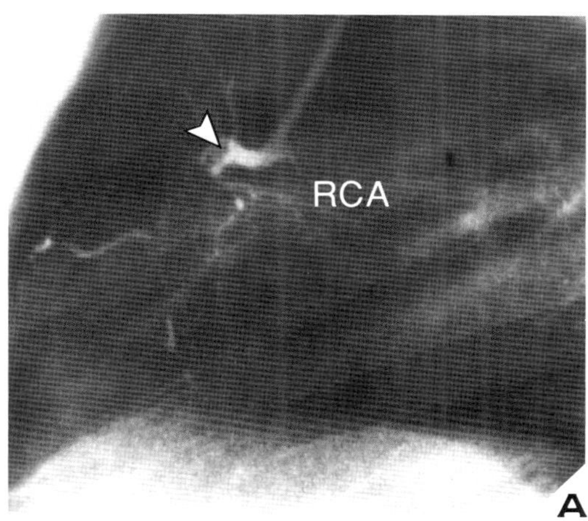

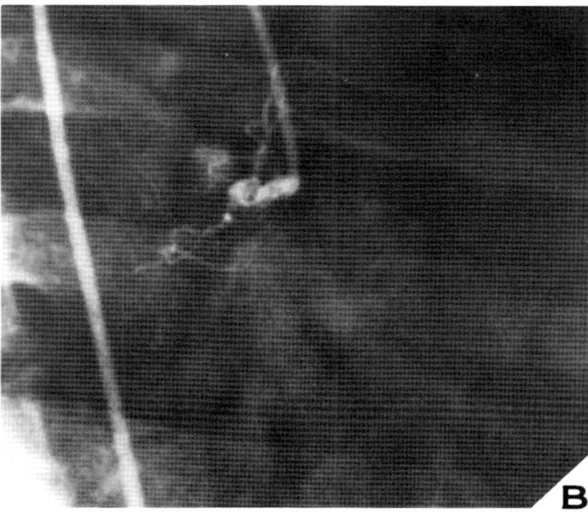

Fig. 21.30 Acute occlusion of right coronary artery. (A) Lateral and (B) RAO projections of right coronary arteriogram demonstrate occlusion of the proximal segment of the right coronary artery (RCA). Note the straight border of the occluded segment, which is typical of an acute myocardial infarction. The oval intraluminal filling defect (*arrow*) just proximal to the obstruction represents thrombus, a common finding in acute coronary artery occlusions.

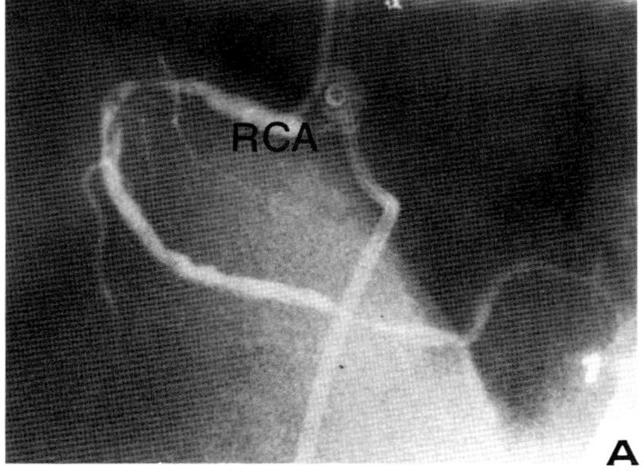

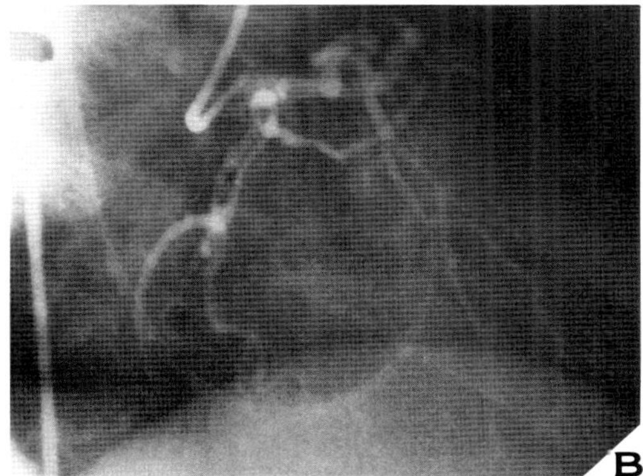

Fig. 21.31 Organized thrombus. Selective coronary arteriograms in two different patients. (A) Right coronary arteriogram (LAO-Cr projection) shows an 80 percent stenosis of the middle segment of the right coronary artery (RCA). The segment distal to the stenosis is patent but contains a filling defect (organized thrombus) which extends for an additional 1.5 cm. (B) Left coronary arteriogram (RAO-Cd projection) demonstrates severe stenosis of the circumflex artery caused by a large organized thrombus, which appears as an elongated filling defect.

ment of the left anterior descending artery, the right coronary artery, and the circumflex artery. Often, however, more than one artery is affected. Left anterior descending/circumflex and left anterior descending/right coronary are the most frequent combinations; however, other patterns of two- or three-vessel disease are not uncommon (Fig. 21.32).

Although coronary atherosclerosis is by far the most common cause of angina pectoris, other conditions that must be considered in the differential diagnosis include coronary artery spasm (Fig. 21.33); various acquired disorders of the coronary arteries, including embolism, aortic dissection, syphilitic aortitis, mediastinal irradiation, tumor infiltration, and periarteritis nodosa (Fig. 21.34); hereditary connective tissue disorders such as homocystinuria, Hurler syndrome (gargoylism), Marfan syndrome, and cystic degeneration of the aortic wall; and aortic stenosis.

COLLATERAL CIRCULATION

Severe stenosis or occlusion of a large coronary artery generates the hemodynamic conditions that lead to the formation of collateral channels which supply the territory normally supplied by the obstructed artery. Branches proximal to the obstruction enlarge and develop connections (via the capillary network) with arteries that have been deprived of their blood supply or are being perfused at low pressure. The arterial segment dis-

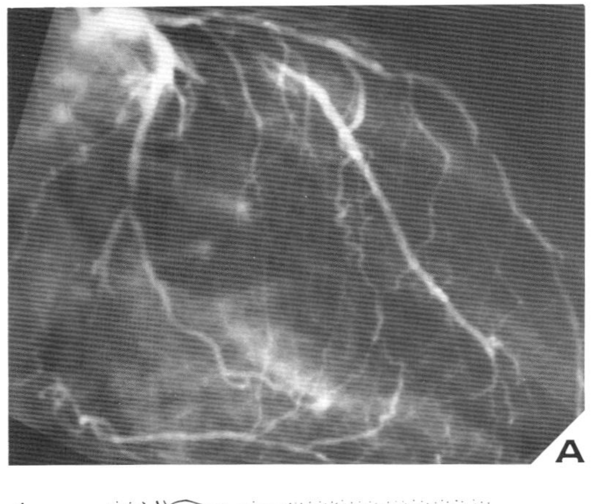

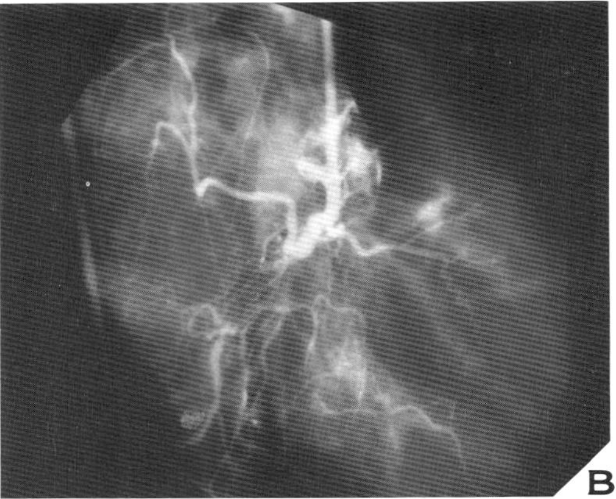

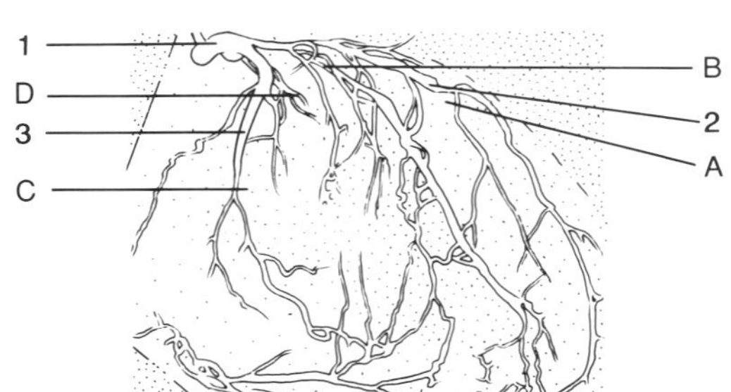

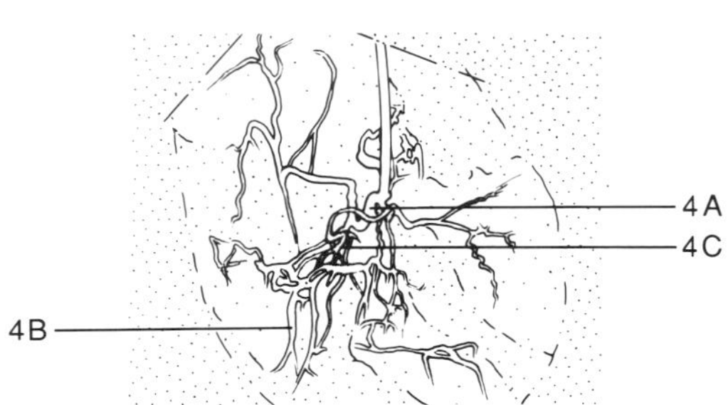

Fig. 21.32 Three-vessel disease. (A) Left and (B) right selective coronary arteriograms (RAO projection) in a patient with severe angina pectoris demonstrate severe stenosis or occlusion of all three major vessels. There is mild (50 percent) stenosis of the middle segment of the left anterior descending artery; severe (90 percent) stenosis of the first large diagonal artery, which supplies most of the free wall of the left ventricle; and moderately severe (70 percent) stenosis of the distal third of the circumflex artery. The first marginal artery is occluded. The proximal segment of the right coronary artery is also occluded; its distal portion is supplied by collaterals arising from the diagonal arteries and via the septal branch.

1 left main coronary artery
2 left anterior descending artery
3 circumflex artery
4 right coronary artery
A mild (50 percent) stenosis of middle segment of left anterior descending artery
B severe (90 percent) stenosis of largest diagonal artery
C significant (70 percent) stenosis of distal circumflex artery
D occlusion of first marginal artery

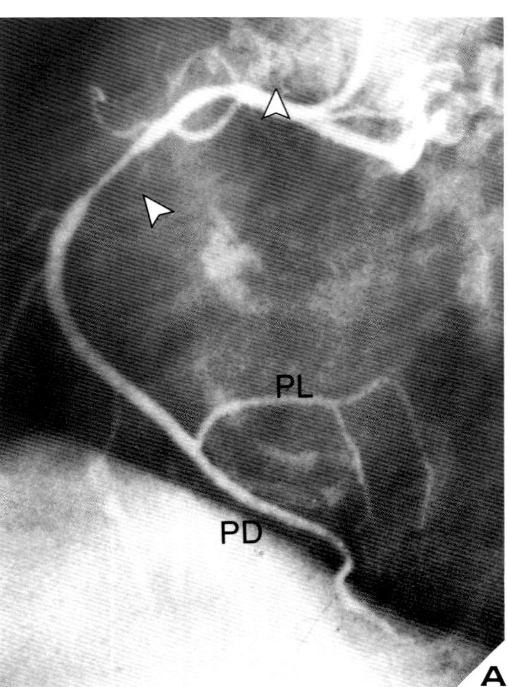

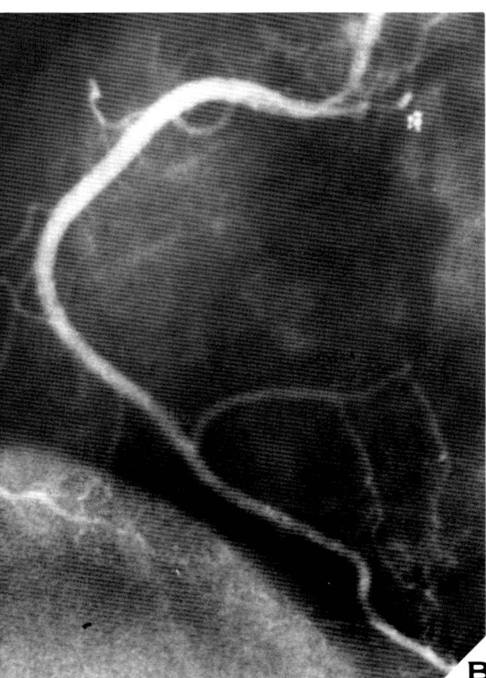

Fig. 21.33 Spasm resulting in ischemia in territory of right coronary artery. Right coronary arteriogram (LAO projection) before (A) and immediately after (B) administration of nitroglycerine. The narrowing (*arrow*) in the middle segment of the right coronary artery seen in A has completely disappeared in B. The patient complained of chest discomfort which was relieved by nitroglycerine; this sequence was replicated during the angiographic procedure. The angiographic findings confirm the ischemic nature of the chest pain. (PL = posterolateral artery; PD = posterior descending artery)

tal to the obstruction may be perfused via this collateral pathway, which has been called the *intraarterial collateral circulation.* Alternatively, the distal portion of the obstructed artery may be supplied through natural connections with neighboring territories, which, collectively, are known as the *interarterial collateral circulation.* The most common collateral pathways are the connection between the posterolateral artery and the distal segment of the circumflex artery; the connection between the distal part of the left anterior descending coronary artery and the distal, portion of the posterior descending artery; and the connection between the right coronary artery with the left anterior descending artery via the conus branch (Fig. 21.35; see also

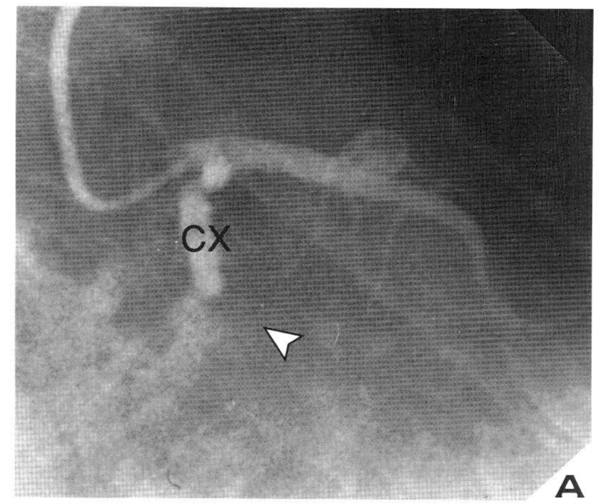

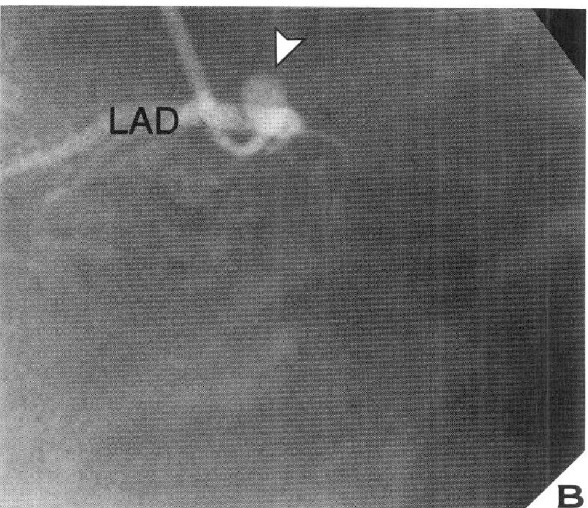

Fig. 21.34 Periarteritis nodosa (Kawasaki's disease). This 6-year-old child presented with mucocutaneous erythema and vague chest pain. Left coronary arteriogram in (A) RAO and (B) lateral projections demonstrate occlusion (*arrow*) of the middle segment of the circumflex artery (CX) just proximal to the origin of the first marginal branch. There is a saccular aneurysm (*arrow*) of the proximal segment of the left anterior descending artery (LAD); the filling defect within the aneurysm represents thrombus.

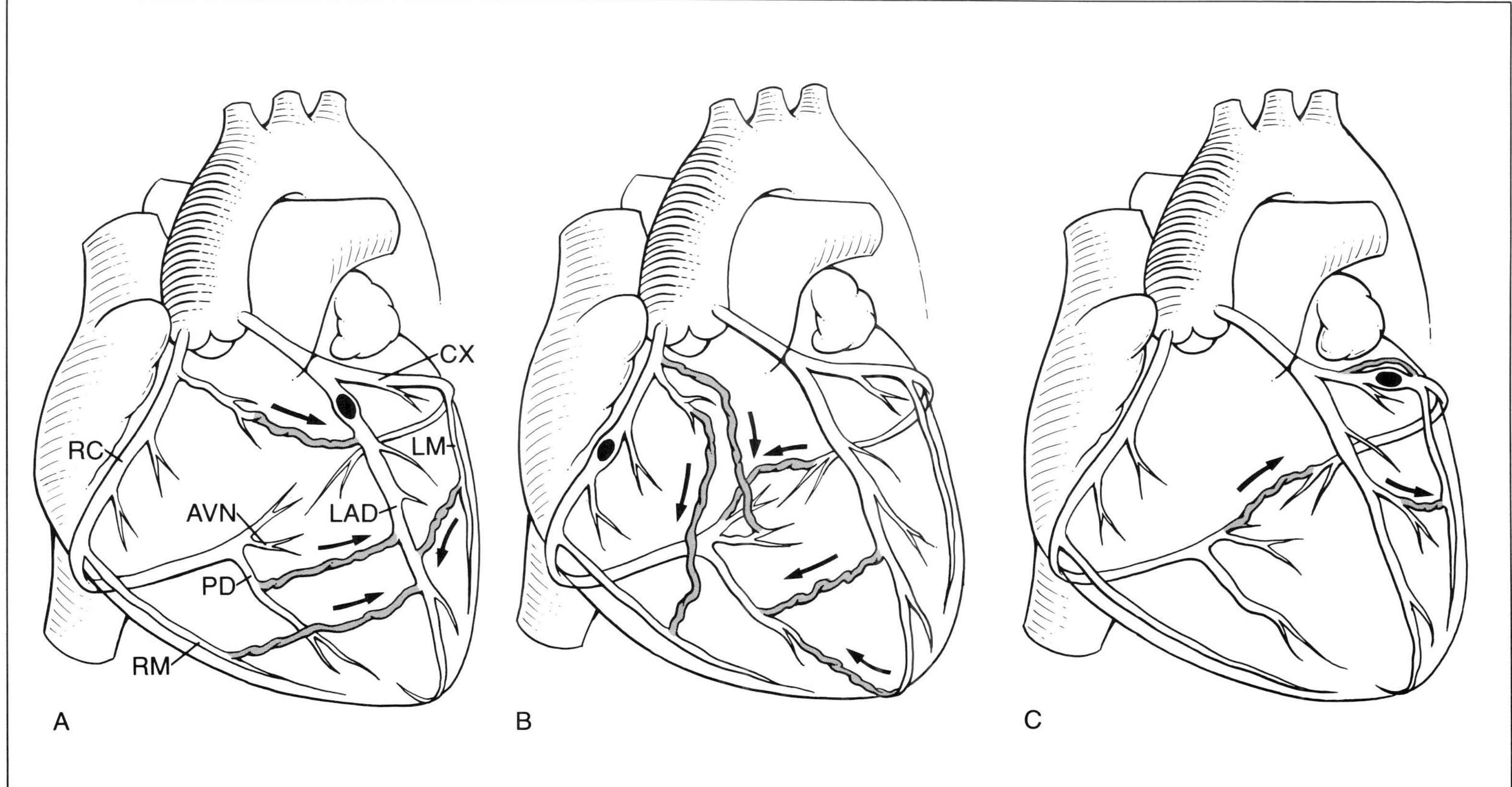

CX	circumflex artery	**RM**	right marginal artery
LM	left marginal artery	**AVN**	atrioventricular node artery
PD	posterior descending artery	**LAD**	left anterior descending artery
RC	right coronary artery		

Fig. 21.35 Collateral pathways of the coronary circulation. (A) After occlusion of the left anterior descending artery, its territory may be supplied by collaterals originating from right coronary artery via the conus artery; via septal arteries originating from the posterior descending artery; and via the right marginal arteries, and/or marginal branches of the circumflex artery over the free wall and apex of the left ventricle. (B) After occlusion of the right coronary artery, its territory may be supplied by septal branches of the left anterior descending artery, epicardial branches of the left anterior descending artery at the level of the apex, branches of the circumflex artery with the posterolateral artery over the posterior aspect of the heart, and/or intra-arterial collaterals to the right main coronary trunk. (C) After occlusion of the circumflex artery its territory may be supplied by the left diagonal arteries (branches of the left anterior descending artery); connections between the distal segment of the posterolateral artery and the distal segment of the circumflex artery; and or intra-arterial collaterals to the middle segment of the circumflex artery.

Fig. 21.5). Other interarterial collateral pathways connect minor branches (eg, connections between the diagonal and marginal branches; between the right marginal and left anterior descending arteries; and between the marginal arteries and branches of the posterolateral artery). A collateral pathway also may be established between the left anterior descending and posterior descending arteries via septal branches (Fig. 21.36).

ISCHEMIC HEART DISEASE

LEFT VENTRICULAR DYSFUNCTION

The left ventricle has been divided into ten angiographic segments to facilitate analysis of abnormal wall motion caused by ischemic heart disease (Fig. 21.37). This scheme roughly corresponds to the territories of the three main coronary arteries (left anterior descending, circumflex, and right coronary arteries), although there is some overlap. The territory of the right coronary artery is represented by the posterobasal and diaphragmatic segments; the territory of the circumflex artery is represented by the inferolateral and posterolateral segments; and the territory of the left anterior descending artery is represented by the septal, anterolateral, and apical segments (Fig. 21.38; see also Fig. 21.6).

LEFT VENTRICULOGRAPHY

Left ventriculography is performed by injecting 40 to 60 mL of contrast material through a pigtail catheter. Right and left anterior oblique projections with cranial and caudal angulation are routinely obtained. These projections clearly depict all ten left ventricular segments, facilitating analysis of wall motion, and demonstrate mitral insufficiency (if present). As noted earlier, left ventriculography is hazardous in patients with left ventricular failure, and can usually be omitted in such cases, since similar information can be obtained by echocardiography or nuclear angiography (blood pool imaging).

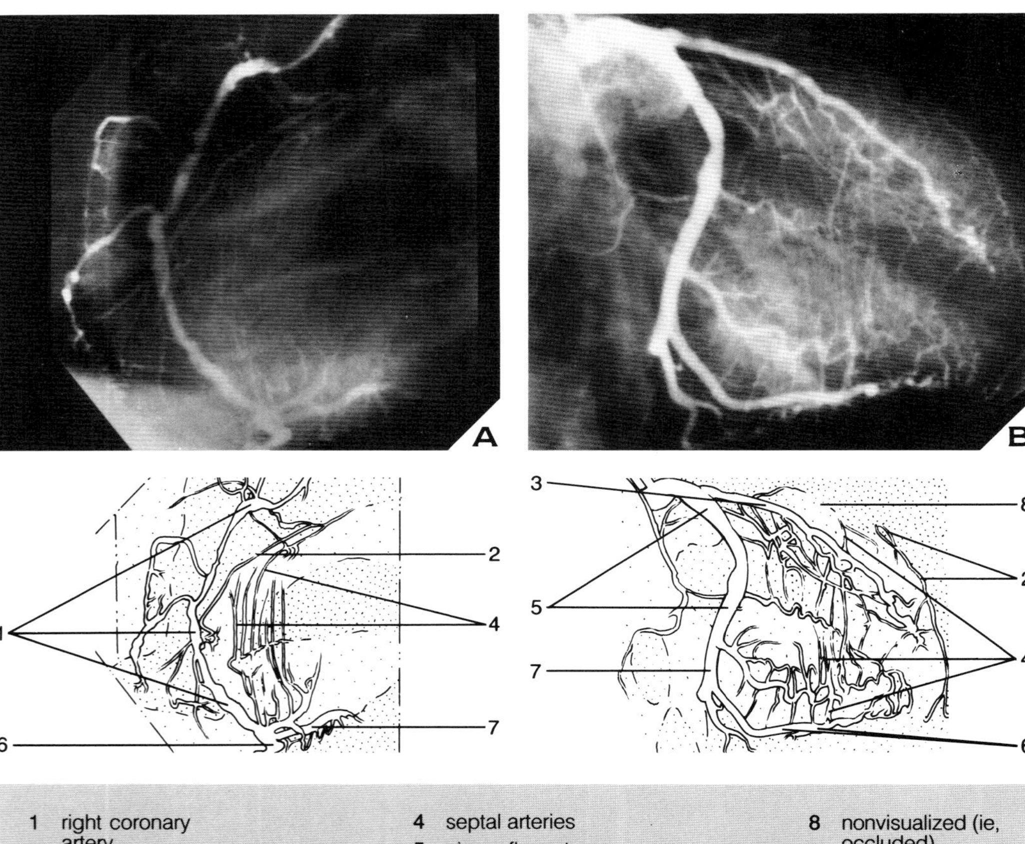

1 right coronary artery
2 left anterior descending artery
3 large first diagonal artery
4 septal arteries
5 circumflex artery
6 posterior descending artery
7 posterolateral artery
8 nonvisualized (ie, occluded) proximal and middle segments of left anterior descending artery

Fig. 21.36 Patterns of collateral circulation. Selective coronary arteriograms in two different patients. (A) Right coronary arteriogram (lateral projection) in a patient with complete occlusion of the left anterior descending coronary artery demonstrates severe stenosis of the middle segment of the right coronary artery. The territory of the left anterior descending artery is supplied by the right posterior descending artery via septal branches which connect with the septal branches of the left anterior descending artery. The entire left anterior descending artery is well opacified. (B) Left coronary arteriogram (RAO projection) in a patient with a dominant left coronary system and occlusion of the left anterior descending artery. (The first branch beyond the bifurcation of the left main coronary artery is a large first diagonal branch.) Although the proximal and middle segments of the left anterior descending artery are not visualized, its distal segment is opacified by septal arteries arising from the posterior descending artery. Additional collateral circulation to the distal left anterior descending artery is provided by the large diagonal artery and marginal branches.

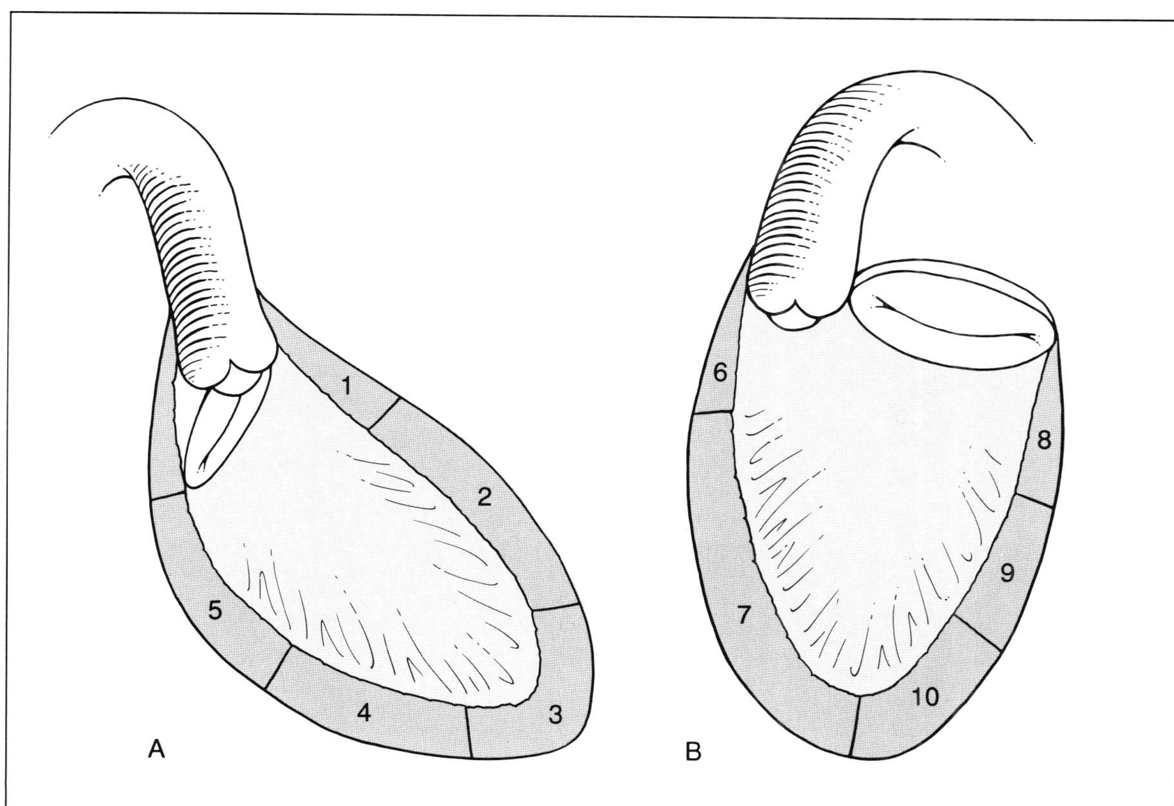

Fig. 21.37 Segments of the left ventricle. (A) Right anterior oblique projection. (B) Left anterior oblique projection. The artery that supplies each segment is shown in parentheses: LAD = left anterior descending artery; CX = circumflex artery; RCA = right coronary artery.

1 anterobasal segment (RCA or LAD, or both)
2 anterolateral segment (LAD)
3 apical segment (LAD)
4 diaphragmatic segment (RCA or CX)
5 posterobasal segment (RCA)
6 basal septal segment (RCA + LAD)
7 distal septal segment (LAD)
8 superolateral segment (RCA or XC, or both)
9 inferolateral segment (CX)
10 posterolateral segment (CX + RCA)

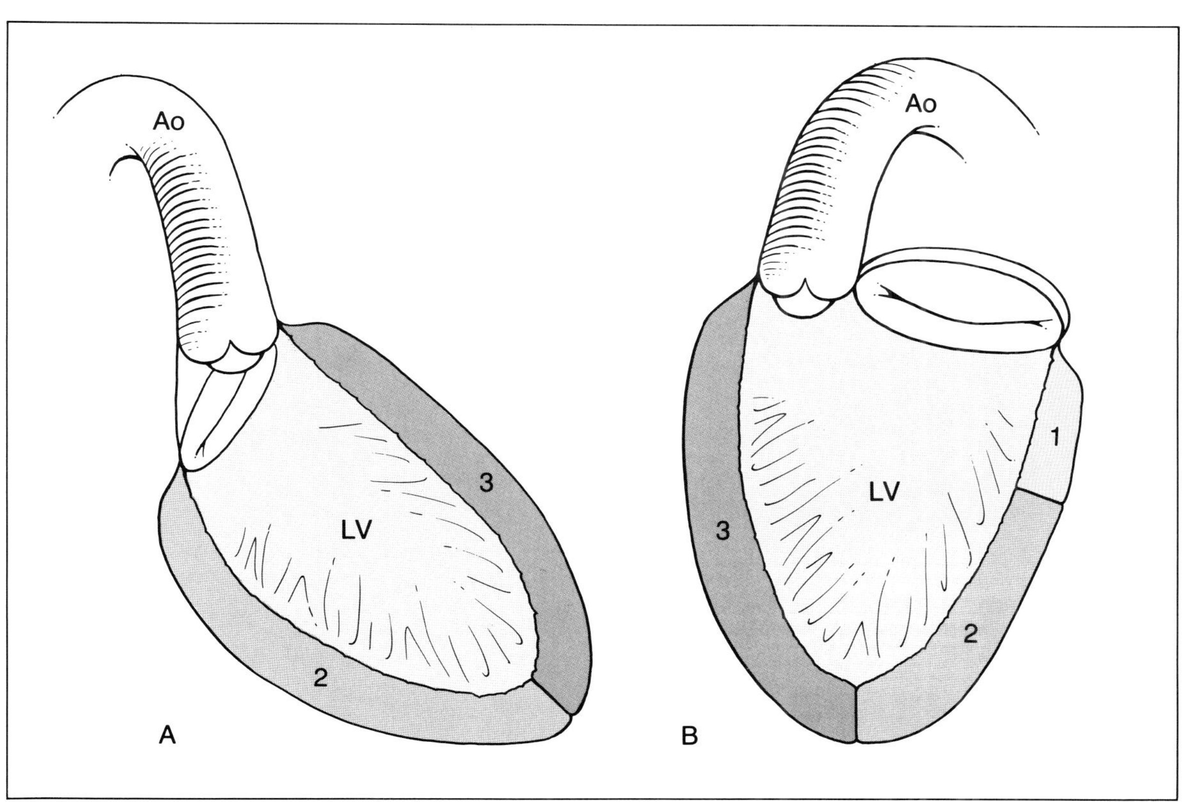

Fig. 21.38 Territories of the major coronary arteries as seen on left ventriculography. (A) Left anterior oblique projection. (B) Right anterior oblique projection.

1 territory of right coronary artery
2 territory of circumflex artery (overlaps territory of right coronary, artery)
3 territory of left anterior descending artery
LV left ventricle
AO aorta

Abnormal motion of the left ventricular wall is classified as hypokinesis (diminished contractility) (Fig. 21.39); akinesis (absence of motion during systole with relaxation during diastole); or dyskinesis (systolic expansion of the involved segment, which may appear normal during diastole) (Fig. 21.40). (Absence of wall motion in an akinetic segment can sometimes be difficult to appreciate owing to displacement by normally contracting neighboring segments.) One or more contiguous segments may exhibit abnormal wall motion; involvement of multiple segments is the rule when more than one coronary artery is involved. Although abnormal wall motion does not necessary indicate nonviability of the affected segment, particularly during the early stage of myocardial infarction, there is an approximate correlation between the number of dysfunctional segments and the extent of myocardial damage caused by chronic ischemic heart disease and/or myocardial infarction. Mitral insufficiency is a common finding in patients with ischemic heart disease (see Chapter 18) (Fig. 21.41).

ACUTE MYOCARDIAL INFARCTION

CORONARY ARTERIOGRAPHY

In acute myocardial infarction the artery supplying the infarcted region ("infarct-related artery") is usually markedly narrowed or occluded. The margins of the occluded or stenotic segment ("occlusion") have a variable appearance. In a minority of cases the margins of the occlusion are smooth (see Fig. 21.29). More often, however, the margins are irregular (Fig. 21.42). Irregularly shaped intraluminal filling defects, which represent thrombus, can often be identified just proximal to the occlusion (Figs.

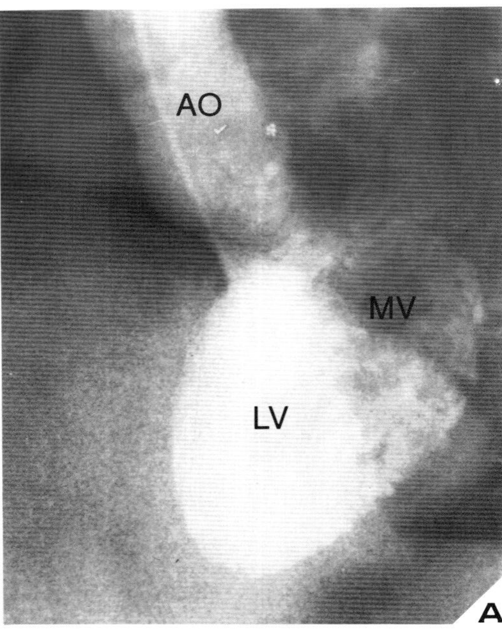

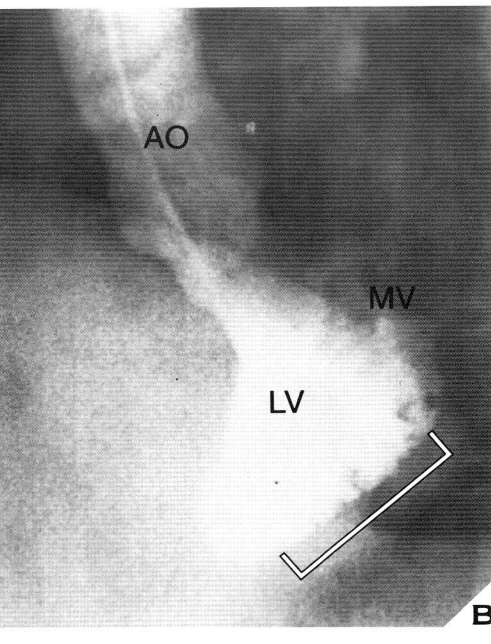

Fig. 21.39 Hypokinesis of superlateral and inferolateral segments of the left ventricle. (A and B) LAO projection of left ventriculogram. (A) Diastole. The profile of the left ventricle (LV) is normal. (B) Systole. The affected segments (*brace*), which are supplied by the circumflex artery and its branches, exhibit very little motion. The rest of the left ventricle contracts normally. (Ao = aorta; MV = mitral valve)

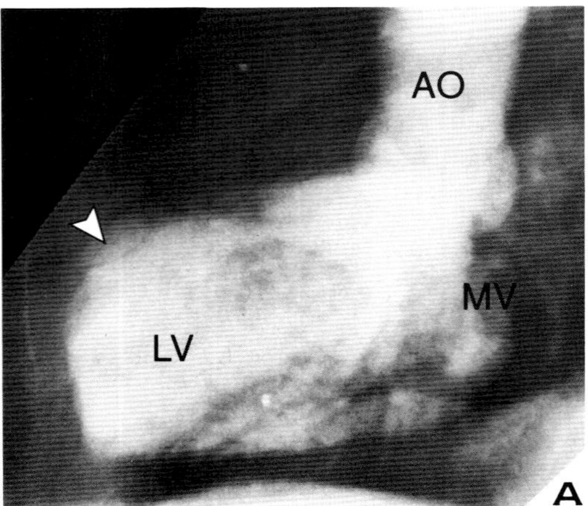

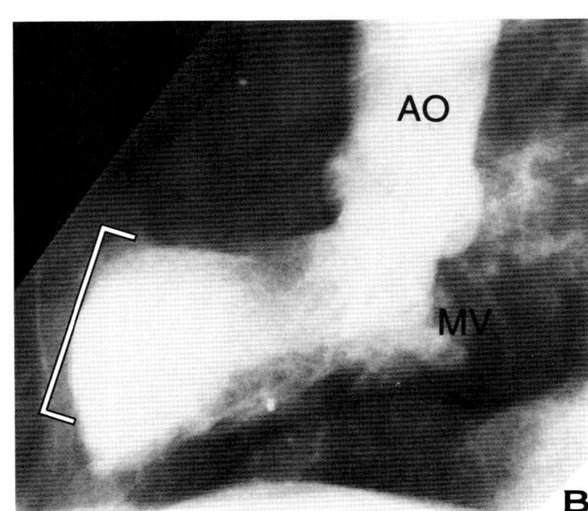

Fig. 21.40 Dyskinesis of anterolateral wall of left ventricle. RAO projection of left ventriculogram. (A) Diastole. The anterolateral wall (*arrow*) of the enlarged left ventricle (LV) is minimally deformed. (B) Systole. The affected segments (*brace*), which are supplied by the left anterior descending artery and its branches, protrude beyond the normal contour of the left ventricular cavity. The other segments contract normally. (Ao = aorta; MV = mitral valve)

21.42 and 21.43; see also Fig. 21.30). The portion of the infarct-related artery distal to the occlusion is usually opacified in retrograde fashion by collaterals. Although contrast material does not clear as rapidly from the distal segment of the infarct-related artery as it does from normal coronary arteries of comparable size, this is due to lack of flow rather than thrombus formation. Occasionally, however, intraluminal thrombi are seen distal to the occlusion.

In patients in whom myocardial infarction has occurred without occlusion of the infarct-related artery, the latter usually exhibits significant stenosis (75 percent or more). In some instances, however, the infarct-related artery is normal or only minimally narrowed. Such infarcts are presumably due to prolonged spasm of the infarct-related artery.

Coronary arteriograms obtained 1 week after the acute episode demonstrate significant stenosis of the infarct-related artery; however, the number of occluded branches is less than that observed on angiograms obtained within hours after the onset of symptoms (see Chapter 20).

LEFT VENTRICULOGRAPHY

Left ventriculography demonstrates the extent of myocardial damage, the function of the surrounding myocardium, and the status of the mitral valve, which is compromised in a high

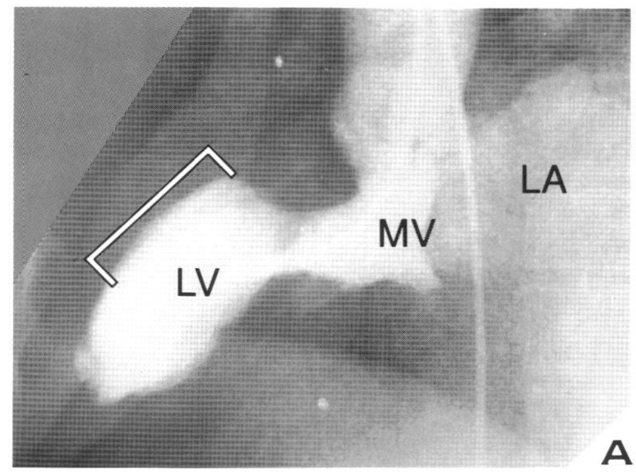

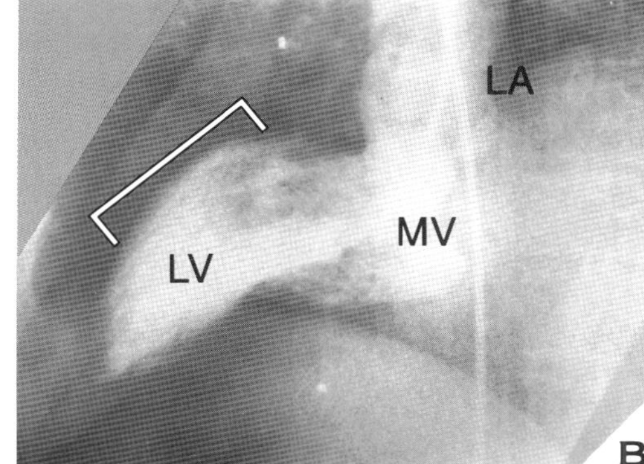

Fig. 21.41 Dyskinesis associated with mitral insufficiency and mural thrombus. RAO projection of left ventriculogram. (A) Diastole. Note localized deformity (*brace*) of anterolateral wall of left ventricle (LV). (B) Systole. The abnormal segment (*brace*) is displaced beyond the normal left ventricular contour. The filling defect at the apex (*arrows* in A and B) represents a mural thrombus. Note opacification of left atrium (LA) in B indicating mitral insufficiency. Coronary arteriography demonstrated occlusion of the left anterior descending artery. (MV = mitral valve)

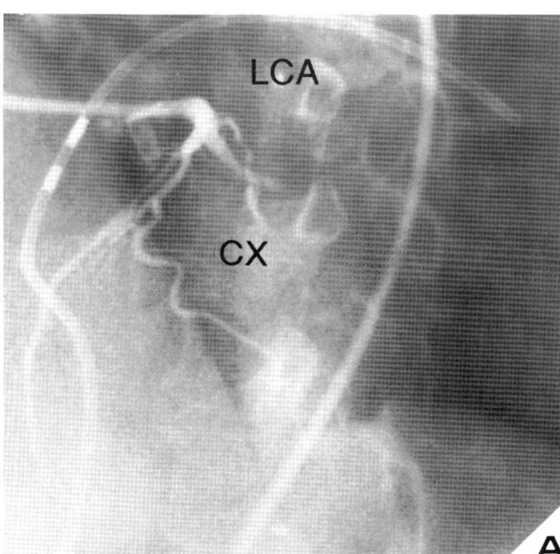

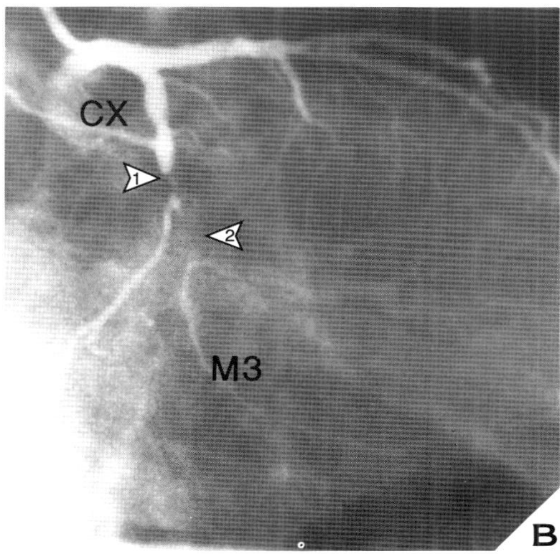

Fig. 21.42 Acute myocardial infarction. (A) LAO and (B) RAO projections of selective left coronary arteriogram in a patient with an acute posterolateral myocardial infarction demonstrate occlusion (*arrow* 1) of the circumflex artery (CX) just beyond the origin of the small second marginal artery. The distal segment of the circumflex artery is very small. The third marginal artery is occluded (*arrow* 2) just beyond its origin; however, its distal portion (M3), which is supplied by collaterals from the left anterior descending artery, is patent. Note the irregular outline of the circumflex artery just proximal to the occlusion, which suggests the presence of thrombus. (LCA = left main coronary artery)

Fig. 21.43 Acute myocardial infarction secondary to multiple vessel involvement. Left coronary arteriogram (shallow LAO projection) demonstrates a large, irregularly marginated filling defect attached to the superior wall of the left main coronary artery; this appearance is typical of mural thrombus. In addition, there is severe stenosis (*arrow*) of the proximal segment of the circumflex artery caused by atheromatous plaque (note irregular margins). Severe (70 percent) stenosis of the first diagonal artery is also demonstrated.

percentage of cases (Figs. 21.44 and 21.45). Complications such as perforation of the ventricular septum (Fig. 21.46) or papillary muscle rupture (Fig. 21.47) are also clearly shown by left ventriculography. (Rupture of the ventricular septum is confirmed by demonstrating increased saturation in the right ventricle and pulmonary trunk.)

Because of its invasiveness and potential side effects, which can lead to clinical deterioration, left ventriculography is seldom indicated in severely ill patients with acute myocardial infarction, as left ventricular function can be accurately assessed by noninvasive means in this setting (see Chapter 20).

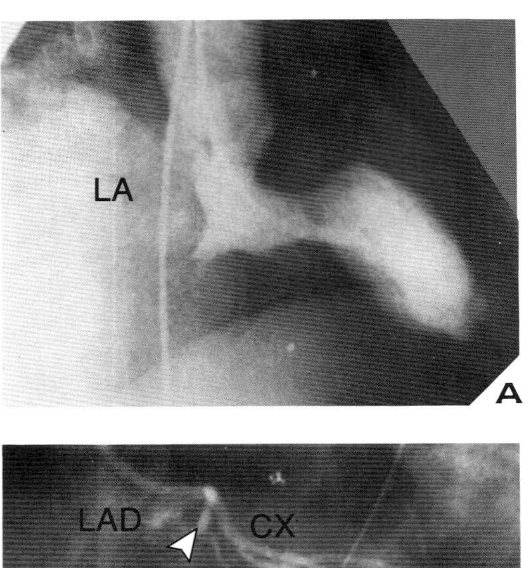

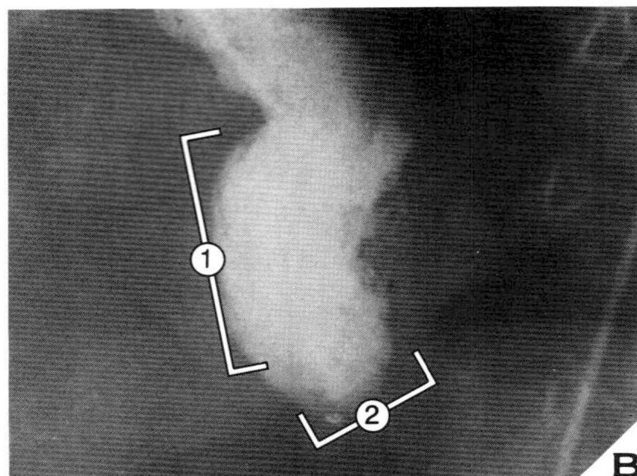

Fig. 21.44 Acute myocardial infarction. (A) RAO and (B) LAO projections of left ventriculogram (in systole) demonstrate a large akinetic segment involving the anterolateral wall distal septum (*brace* 1), and apex (*brace* 2) of the left ventricle. A small amount of contrast material is refluxing into the left atrium (LA), indicating mild mitral insufficiency.

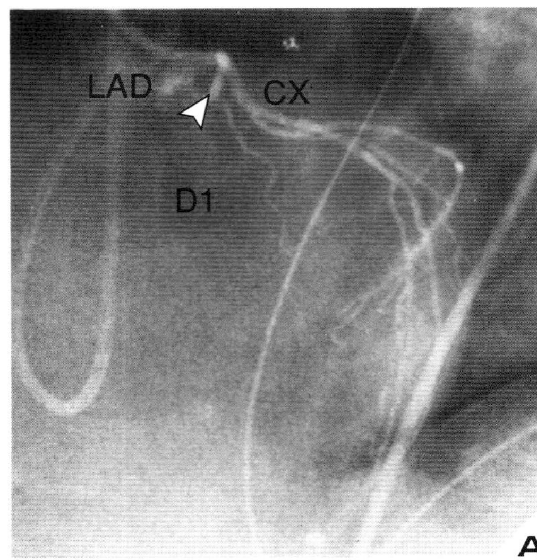

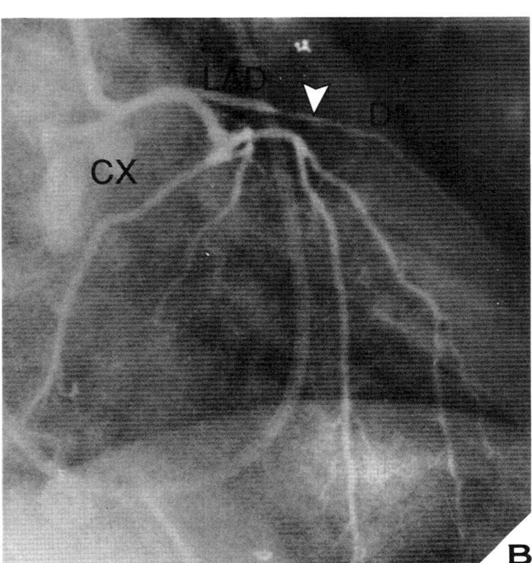

Fig. 21.45 Acute myocardial infarction. Same patient as shown in previous figure. Left coronary arteriogram in (A) LAO and (B) RAO projections demonstrate occlusion (*arrow*) of the proximal segment of the left anterior descending artery (LAD) just beyond the origin of the first diagonal branch (DI). The proximal margin of the occlusion has a smooth, triangular configuration. The distal segment of the left anterior descending artery is not opacified (the absence of collaterals suggests that the occlusion is acute). The circumflex artery (CX) is patent.

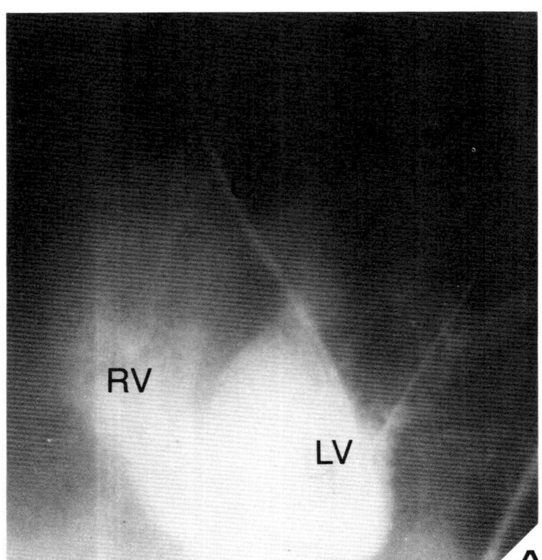

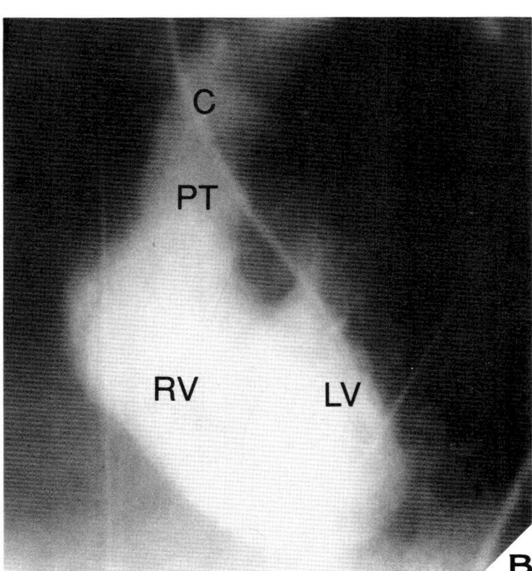

Fig. 21.46 Septal perforation secondary to acute myocardial infarction. (A) Early and (B) late phases of left ventriculogram (long-axial projection) shows dense opacification of the right ventricle (RV) and pulmonary trunk (PT). The left ventricle (LV) is not enlarged. (C = catheter)

LEFT VENTRICULAR ANEURYSM

LEFT VENTRICULOGRAPHY

Cine left ventriculography depicts the extent of the aneurysm and the functional status of the surrounding myocardium, and provides a means of assessing total and regional ventricular function. Mitral insufficiency, mural thrombus, and other sequelae of myocardial infarction are also demonstrated with this technique. Most aneurysms are clearly shown in the elongated right anterior oblique and long-axial projections. The aneurysm appears as a focal deformity during diastole which paradoxically expands during systole (Fig. 21.48).

Although noninvasive techniques (echocardiography, MRI, CT) can suggest the presence of mural thrombus, the definitive diagnosis is usually made by cine left ventriculography, on which it appears as a filling defect attached to the left ventricular

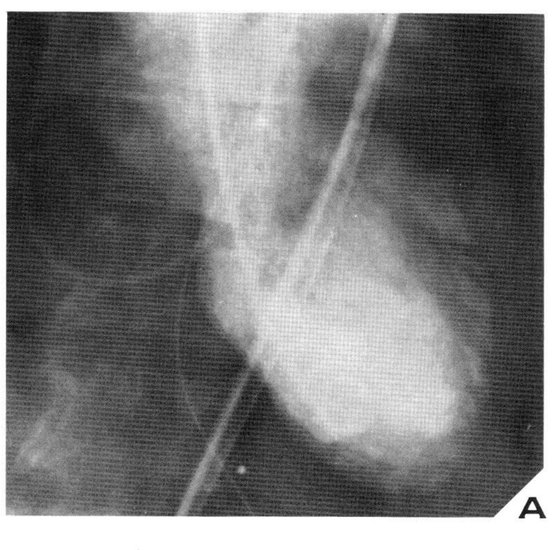

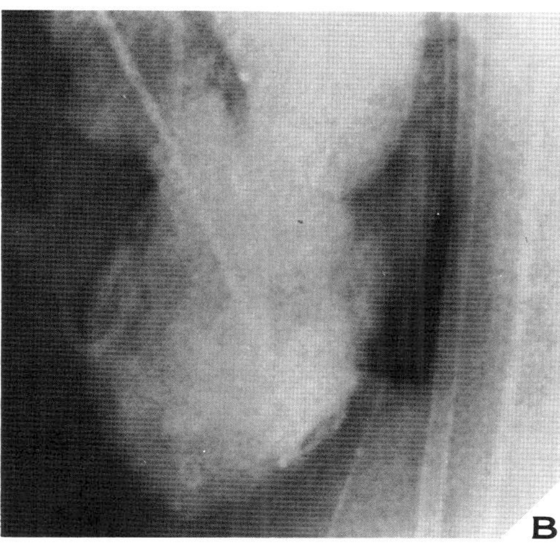

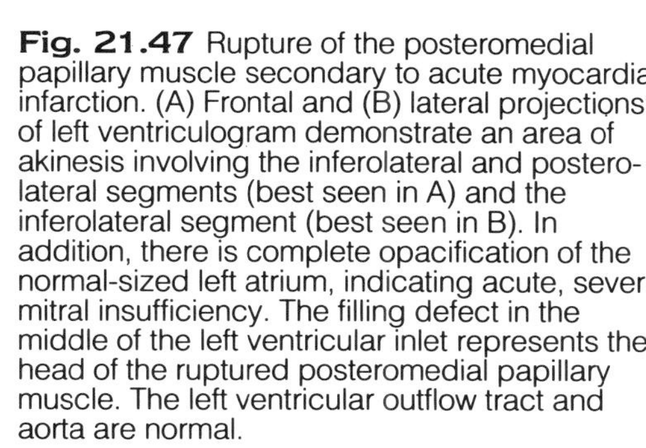

Fig. 21.47 Rupture of the posteromedial papillary muscle secondary to acute myocardial infarction. (A) Frontal and (B) lateral projections of left ventriculogram demonstrate an area of akinesis involving the inferolateral and posterolateral segments (best seen in A) and the inferolateral segment (best seen in B). In addition, there is complete opacification of the normal-sized left atrium, indicating acute, severe mitral insufficiency. The filling defect in the middle of the left ventricular inlet represents the head of the ruptured posteromedial papillary muscle. The left ventricular outflow tract and aorta are normal.

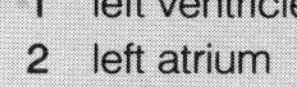

1 left ventricle
2 left atrium
3 aorta
4 ruptured posteromedial papillary muscle

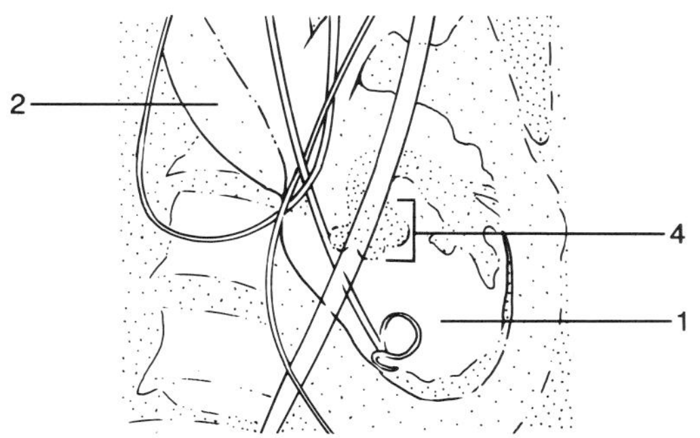

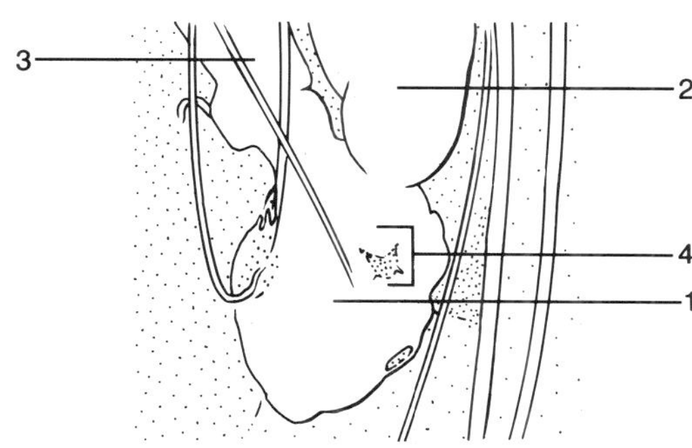

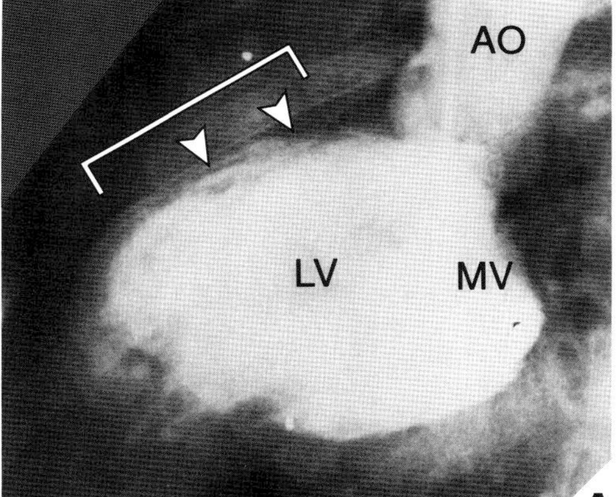

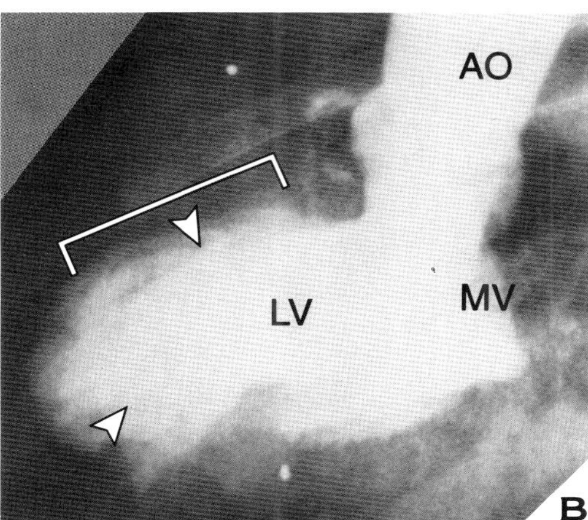

Fig. 21.48 Left ventricular aneurysm. RAO projection of left ventriculogram in (A) diastole and (B) systole. Note deformity (*brace*) of the anterosuperior aspect of the left ventricle (LV) in A, which exands further in B. The posterobasal, diaphragmatic, superolateral, and inferolateral segments of the left ventricle contract normally. The filling defect (*arrows*) adjacent to the inferior wall represents a mural thrombus. The patient had previously sustained an acute myocardial infarction secondary to occlusion of the left anterior descending artery. (Ao = aorta; MV = mitral valve)

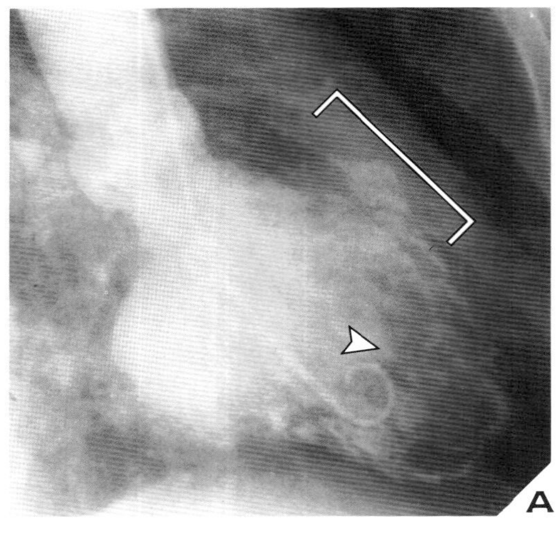

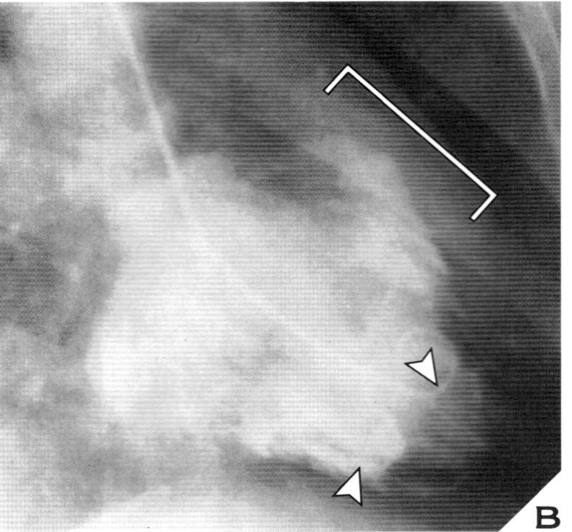

Fig. 21.49 Left ventricular aneurysm with mural thrombus. RAO projection of left ventriculogram in (A) systole and (B) diastole demonstrates an area of dyskinesis (*brace*) in the anterolateral aspect of the left ventricle. The large filling defect (*arrows*) at the apex represents a mural thrombus. The patient had recently sustained an acute anterolateral myocardial infarction secondary to occlusion of the left anterior descending artery.

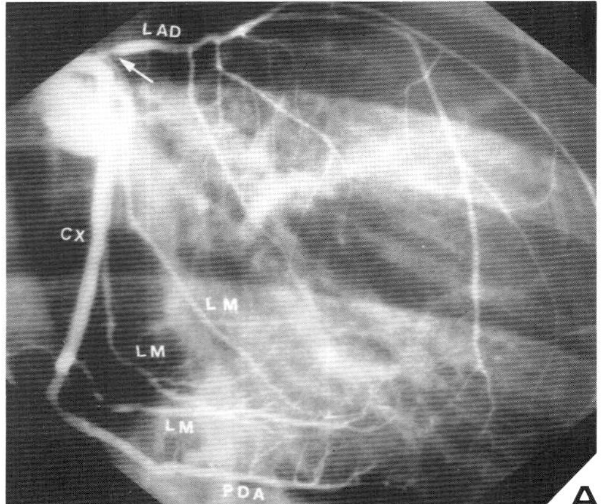

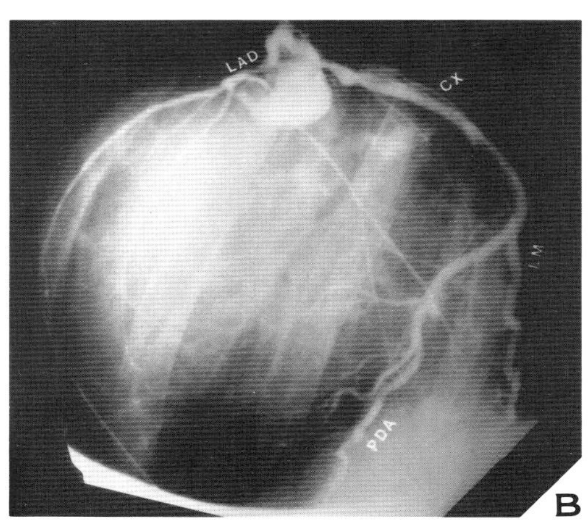

Fig. 21.50 Left ventricular aneurysm. (A) RAO and (B) LAO projections of left coronary arteriogram in a patient with an anterolateral wall aneurysm demonstrate significant stenosis (*arrow*) of the proximal segment of the left anterior descending artery (LAD); its branches are displaced anteriorly and to the left by the aneurysm. There is a paucity of branches arising from the middle and distal segments of the LAD [compare with the branches of the normal circumflex (CX) and left marginal (LM) arteries]. These angiographic findings suggest that the myocardium in the territory of the LAD is nonviable. (PDA = posterior descending artery)

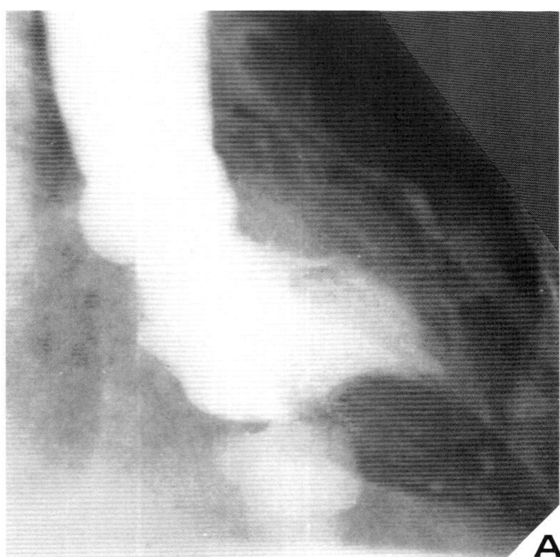

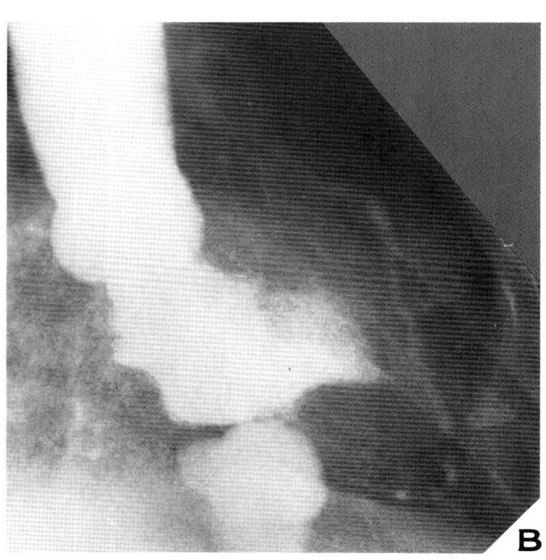

Fig. 21.51 Pseudoaneurysm of left ventricle. (A) Early and (B) late phases of left ventriculogram (RAO projection) in a patient with a recent acute myocardial infarction involving the inferior wall. The false aneurysm appears as a sac connected to the ventricular cavity by a narrow tract. The coronary arteries are related to the neck of the aneurysm and do not course over the surface (compare with previous figure). The filling defects within the pseudoaneurysm represent thrombus.

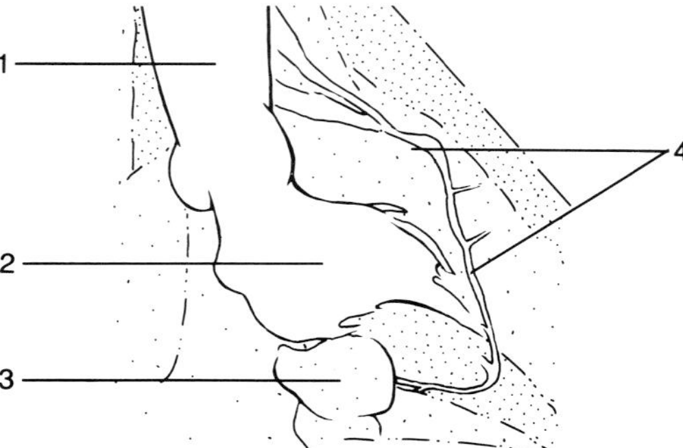

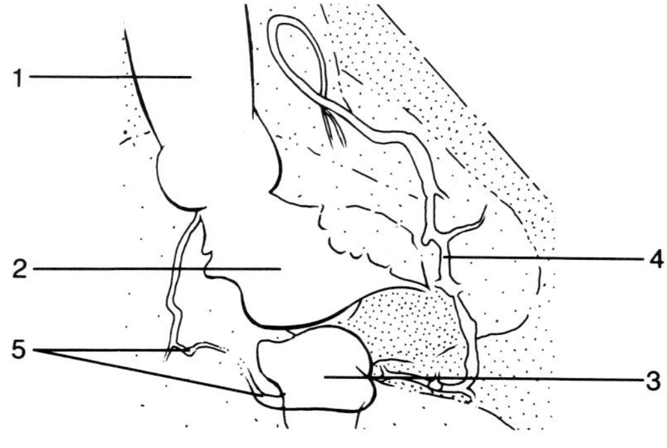

1 aorta
2 left ventricle
3 pseudoaneurysm
4 left anterior descending artery reaching neck of pseudoaneurysm
5 branches of posterior descending artery reaching neck of pseudoaneurysm thrombus

wall (Fig. 21.49). Because of the smooth luminal surface and the absence of trabeculation, it is usually possible to differentiate mural thrombus from normal or infarcted myocardium.

CORONARY ARTERIOGRAPHY

The coronary artery supplying the region of the ventricular aneurysm, if patent, is of small caliber and has a paucity of branches owing to the occlusion of the small intramyocardial and epicardial branches (Fig. 21.50).

LEFT VENTRICULAR PSEUDOANEURYSM (FALSE ANEURYSM)

On left ventriculography a pseudoaneurysm typically appears as a sac that communicates with the left ventricular cavity through a narrow channel (Fig. 21.51). Although a narrow neck is typical of left ventricular pseudoaneurysms, it is also seen in some true aneurysms (see Fig. 21.50A). Coronary arteriography, usually performed in conjunction with left ventriculography in such cases, will usually differentiate the two: Since coronary arteries lie within the epicardial fat, they course over the surface of a true aneurysm and around the neck of a pseudoaneurysm (Fig. 21.52). This distinction can also be made on the aortic phase of the left ventriculogram when the coronary arteries are adequately opacified (Fig. 21.51).

ISCHEMIC HEART DISEASE SECONDARY TO CONGENITAL ANOMALIES OF THE CORONARY ARTERIES

There is considerable variation in the origin, branching pattern, and course of the coronary arteries. The great majority of these variants are of no clinical significance; however, certain anomalies are associated with myocardial ischemia.

ANOMALOUS ORIGIN OF A CORONARY ARTERY FROM THE PULMONARY TRUNK

As noted in the previous chapter, myocardial ischemia may result when the left coronary artery originates from the pulmonary trunk (less often from the right or left pulmonary artery),

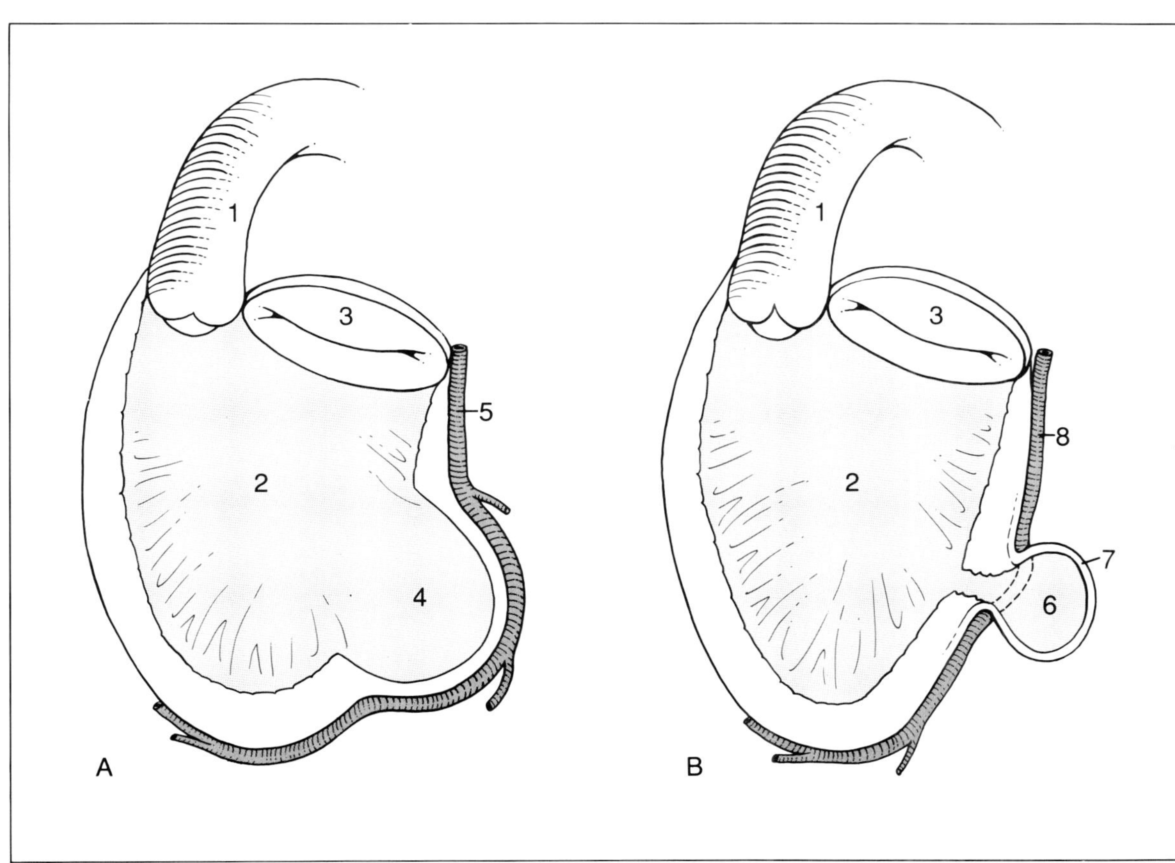

Fig. 21.52 Relations of coronary arteries to true and false left ventricular aneurysms. (A and B) Schematic representation of left ventriculogram in long axial projection. (A) True aneurysms are covered by myocardium; thus, the coronary arteries course over the outer wall of the aneurysm. True aneurysms usually have a wide connection with the ventricular cavity. (B) The wall of a false aneurysm (pseudoaneurysm) is formed by organized thrombus and pericardium; hence the coronary arteries do not course over its outer wall. Pseudoaneurysms typically have a narrow neck, an appearance that can be mimicked by a saccular aneurysm.

1 aorta
2 left ventricle
3 mitral valve
4 true aneurysm of left ventricle
5 coronary artery surrounding true aneurysm
6 false aneurysm (pseudoaneurysm) of the left ventricle
7 pericardium forming part of wall of pseudoaneurysm
8 coronary artery coursing around neck of pseudoaneurysm

resulting in a coronary–pulmonary fistula (Fig. 21.53). Anomalous origin of the left anterior descending artery from the pulmonary trunk is a less common anomaly which can sometimes cause clinically significant myocardial ischemia. Anomalous origin of the right coronary artery from the pulmonary trunk (Fig. 21.54) is a rare anomaly, usually discovered incidentally during coronary arteriography; it is of no importance unless the left coronary artery is stenotic, in which case it may aggravate the myocardial ischemia.

Anomalous origin of either coronary artery from the pulmonary trunk is best demonstrated by thoracic aortography, which demonstrates absence of the anomalous coronary artery and enlargement of its normal counterpart; if the study is carried out far enough into the venous phase, opacification of the anomalous coronary artery and its connection with the pulmonary trunk will be demonstrated (Figs. 21.55A and 21.56A). It can also be demonstrated more clearly by selectively injecting the normal coronary artery (Figs. 21.55B and 21.56B). The anomalous connection can be verified by passing a catheter into the pulmonary trunk and selectively opacifying the anomalous coronary artery; however, this is rarely necessary. In some instances an injection into the pulmonary trunk will opacify the

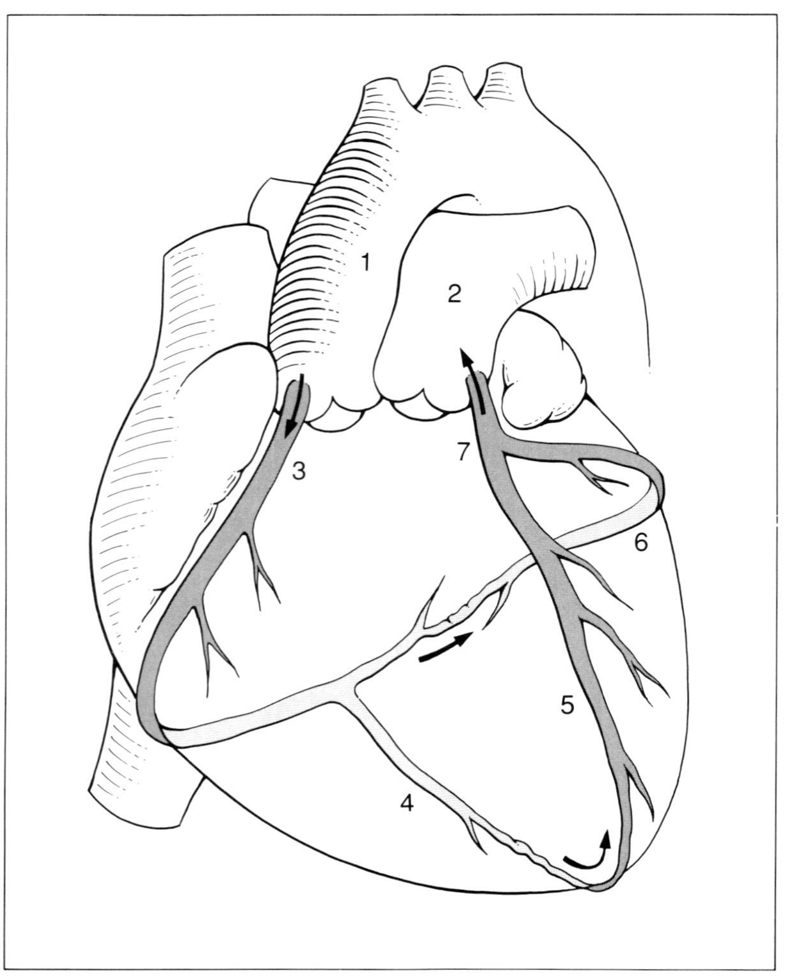

1 aorta
2 pulmonary trunk
3 right coronary artery
4 posterior descending artery
5 left anterior descending artery
6 circumflex artery
7 left main coronary artery

Fig. 21.53 Anomalous origin of the left coronary artery from the pulmonary trunk (schematic). The relatively low pressure in the branches of the anomalous left coronary artery results in a shunt between the right coronary artery (which originates normally) and peripheral branches of the left anterior descending and circumflex arteries; blood then flows into the low-pressure pulmonary trunk. As a result of the coronary–coronary shunt, the myocardium is underperfused. The right coronary artery is usually enlarged, and the connection between its posterolateral branch and the circumflex artery is easily demonstrated angiographically.

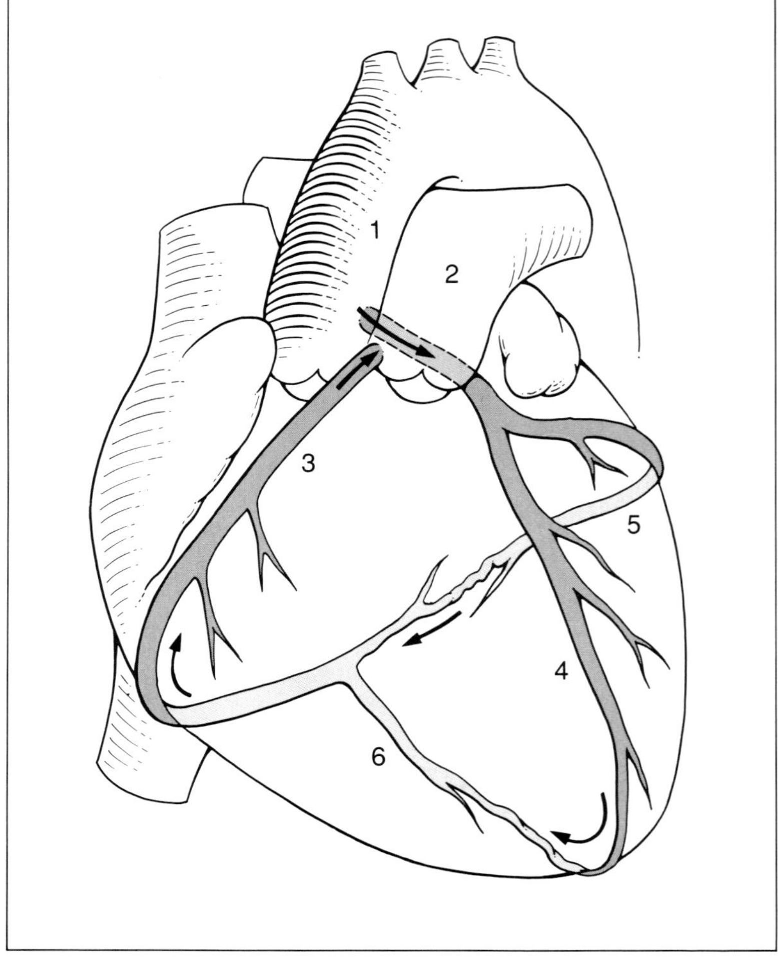

1 aorta
2 pulmonary trunk
3 right coronary artery
4 left anterior descending artery
5 circumflex artery
6 posterior descending artery

Fig. 21.54 Anomalous origin of the right coronary artery from the pulmonary trunk. In this anomaly, a shunt is established between the left coronary artery and the right coronary artery, from which blood flows into the low-pressure pulmonary trunk. The coronary–coronary shunt results in underperfusion of the right ventricular or myocardium, which is well tolerated.

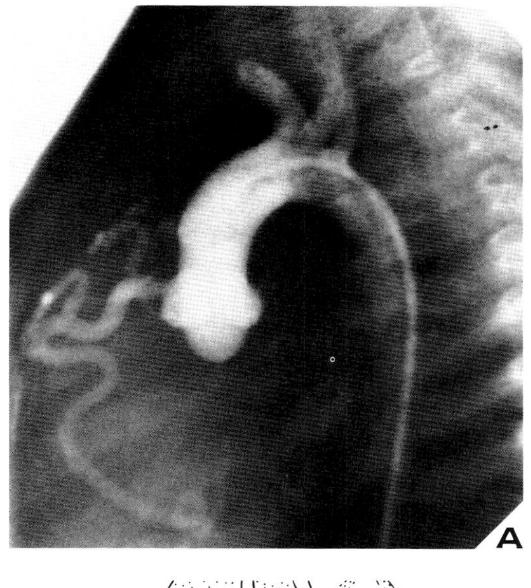

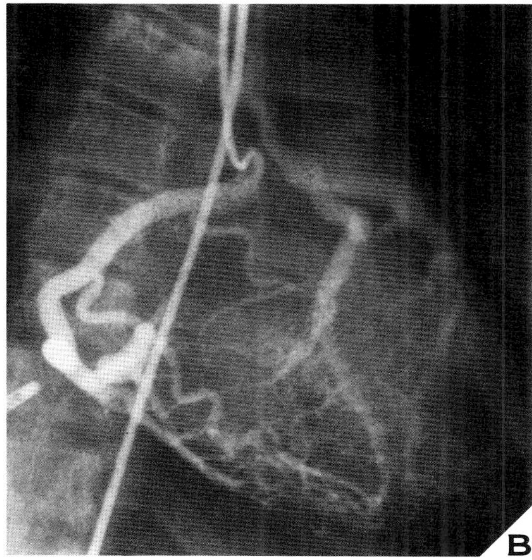

Fig. 21.55 Anomalous origin of the left coronary artery from the pulmonary trunk. (A) Lateral projection of thoracic aortogram demonstrates absence of the left coronary artery. The right coronary artery is enlarged and its branches are dilated. (B) Selective right coronary anteriogram (RAO projection) demonstrates enlargement of the right coronary artery and its posterior descending and posterolateral branches. Many collateral channels connect branches of the right coronary artery to the left anterior descending, circumflex, and marginal arteries, all of which are well opacified. Contrast material then flows in retrograde fashion into the left main coronary artery and thence into the pulmonary trunk, which is faintly opacified.

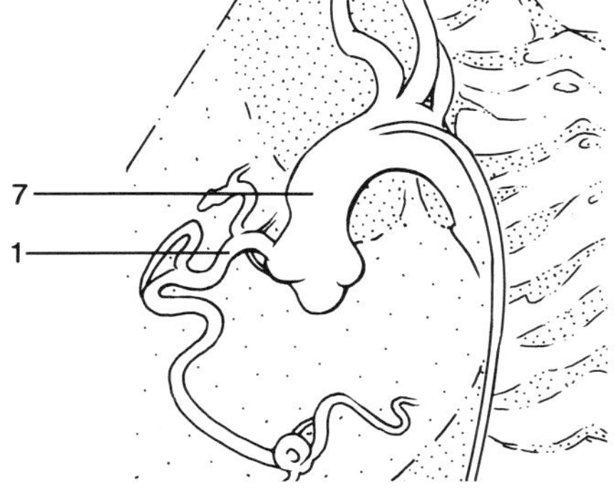

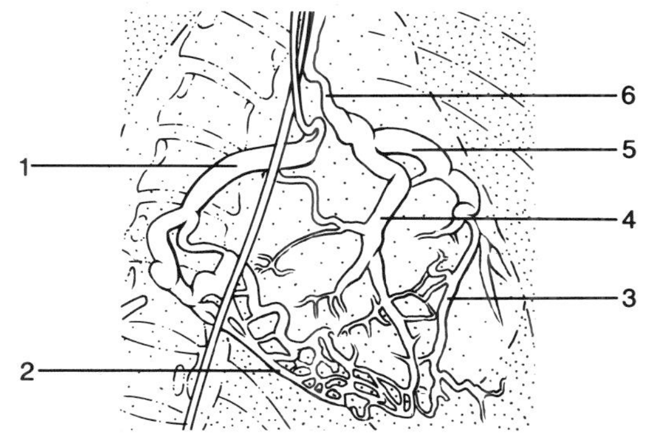

1 right coronary artery
2 posterior descending artery
3 left anterior descending artery
4 circumflex artery
5 left main coronary artery
6 pulmonary trunk
7 aorta

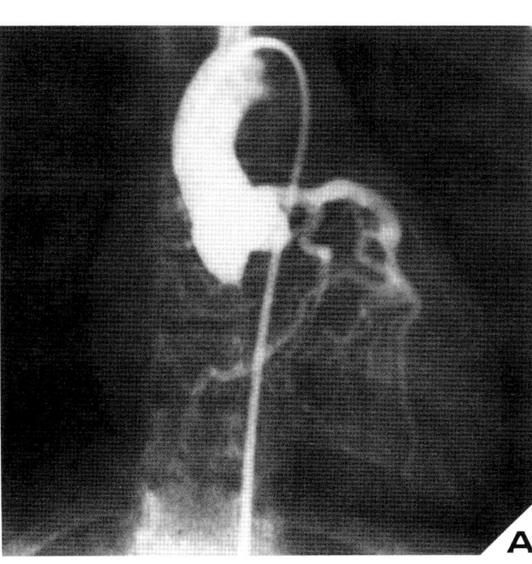

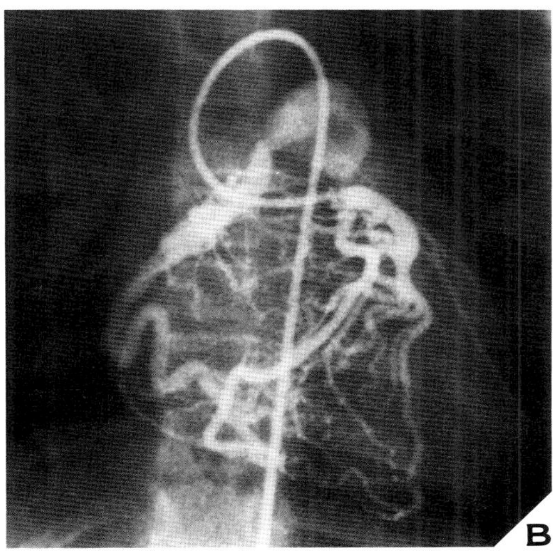

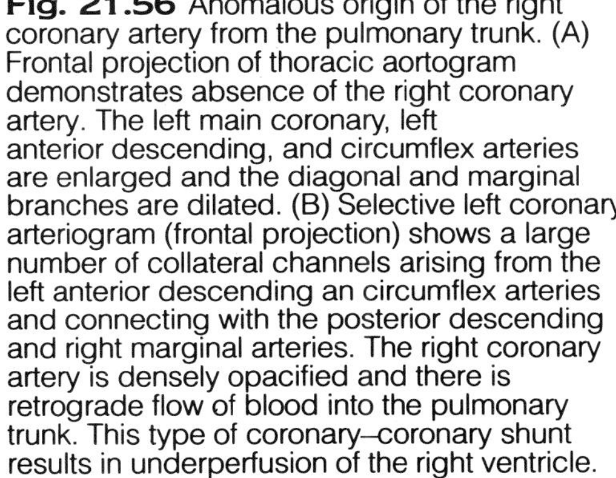

Fig. 21.56 Anomalous origin of the right coronary artery from the pulmonary trunk. (A) Frontal projection of thoracic aortogram demonstrates absence of the right coronary artery. The left main coronary, left anterior descending, and circumflex arteries are enlarged and the diagonal and marginal branches are dilated. (B) Selective left coronary arteriogram (frontal projection) shows a large number of collateral channels arising from the left anterior descending an circumflex arteries and connecting with the posterior descending and right marginal arteries. The right coronary artery is densely opacified and there is retrograde flow of blood into the pulmonary trunk. This type of coronary–coronary shunt results in underperfusion of the right ventricle.

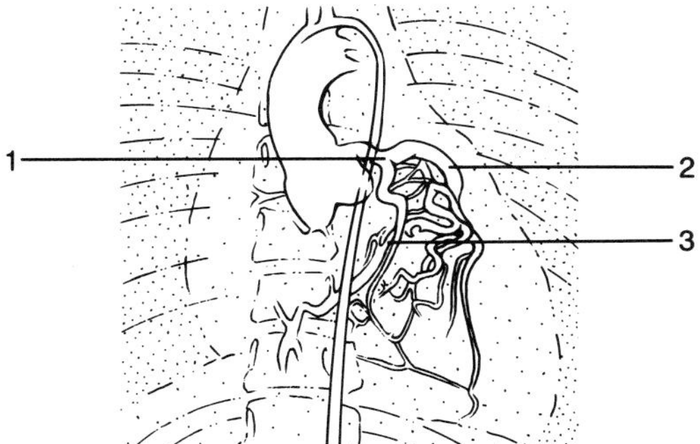

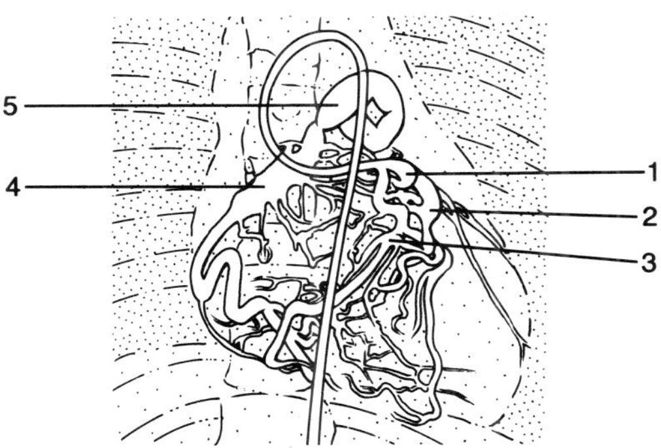

1 left main coronary artery
2 left anterior descending artery
3 circumflex artery
4 right coronary artery
5 pulmonary trunk

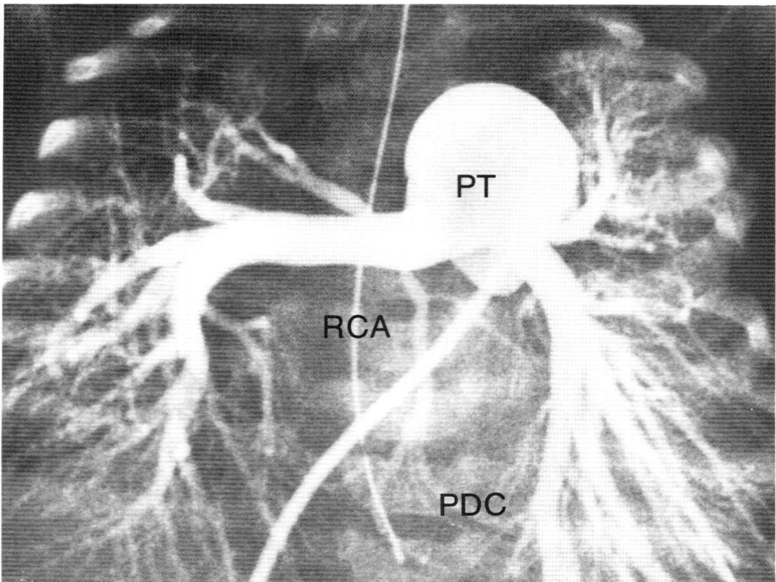

Fig. 21.57 Anomalous origin of the right coronary artery from the right pulmonary artery. Frontal projection of pulmonary arteriogram shows dilation of the pulmonary trunk (PT). The right and left pulmonary arteries are distributed normally. The right coronary artery (RCA) arises from the proximal segment of the right pulmonary artery and is distributed over the right ventricle. The anomalous right coronary artery and its branches are well opacified owing to the low right ventricular pressure. (During diastole, right ventricular pressure is lower than pulmonary artery pressure, thus increasing flow through coronary artery branches which course over the right ventricle.) (PDC = posterior descending coronary artery)

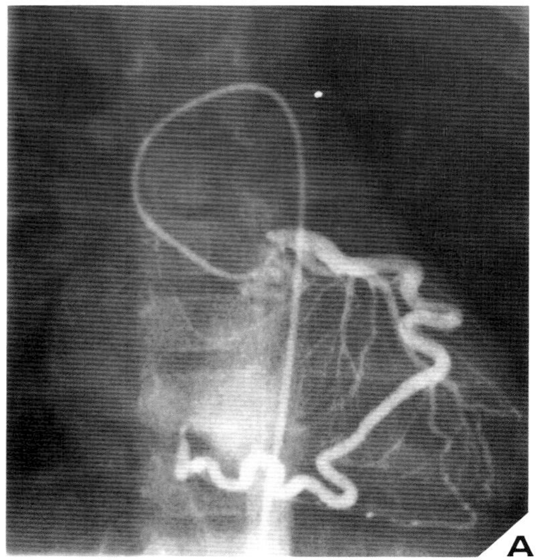

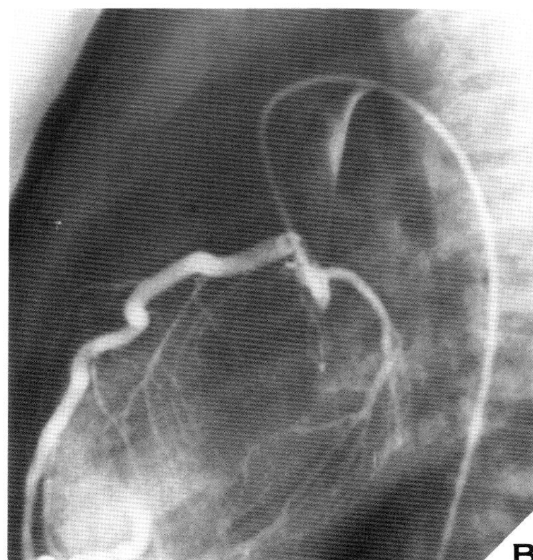

Fig. 21.58 Left coronary artery–right ventricular fistula. (A) Frontal and (B) lateral projections of selective left coronary arteriogram demonstrates marked dilation of the left anterior descending artery. A large right diagonal artery arises from the middle segment of the left anterior descending artery, courses over the right ventricle, and enters the inlet portion of the right ventricle through a narrow channel. The right ventricle is incompletely opacified. The course of the circumflex artery is normal.

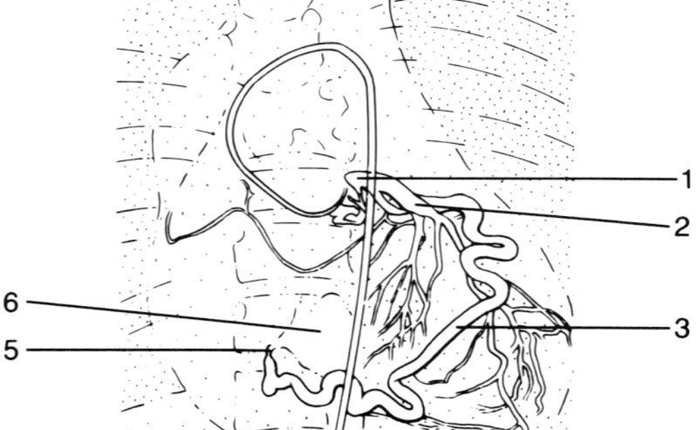

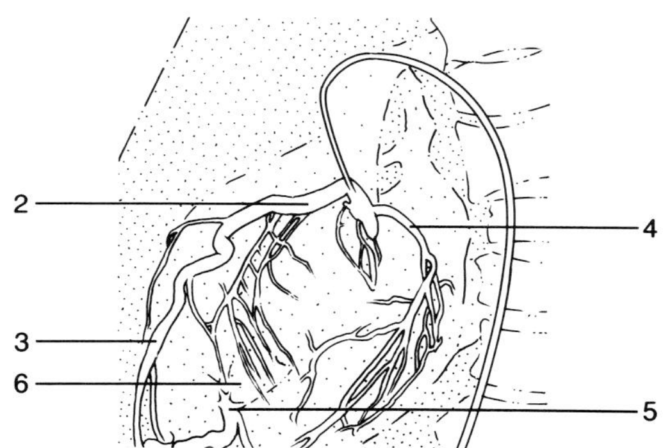

1 left main coronary artery
2 left anterior descending artery
3 right diagonal artery
4 circumflex artery
5 connection between diagonal artery and right ventricle
6 right ventricle

anomalous coronary artery; this is most likely to occur in the presence of pulmonary arterial hypertension, or if the anomalous coronary artery originates from the right or left pulmonary artery (Fig. 21.57).

CORONARY–CAVITARY FISTULA

Coronary–cavitary fistulas, which represent large, anomalous connections between the coronary circulation and a heart chamber or systemic vein, are sometimes associated with myocardial ischemia. Depending on the size of the fistula and its site of drainage, the patient may remain asymptomatic for a long time; eventually, however, signs and symptoms of myocardial ischemia may appear (see Chapter 20).

The fistula is demonstrated by selective coronary arteriography, which shows the enlarged feeding artery as well as its connection with the recipient chamber (Figs. 21.58 to 21.60). Flow of contrast material occurs during diastole and ceases during systole. Multiple projections may be required to demonstrate the precise location of the fistula, which must be known before corrective surgery can be undertaken. Occasionally it is not possible to demonstrate a large fistula with conventional angiographic techniques; the problem can usually be solved by using a large-bore catheter and a high-pressure injector (Fig. 21.60).

Coronary–left ventricular fistulas are rare. As with other coronary–cavitary fistulas, the connection between the feeding artery and the recipient chamber is seen during diastole (in systole, the fistula is occluded as a result of myocardial contraction and because left ventricular pressure exceeds the pressure in the feeding artery). Systolic opacification of the left ventricle occurs during coronary arteriography in some normal individuals and as an incidental finding in some patients with coronary

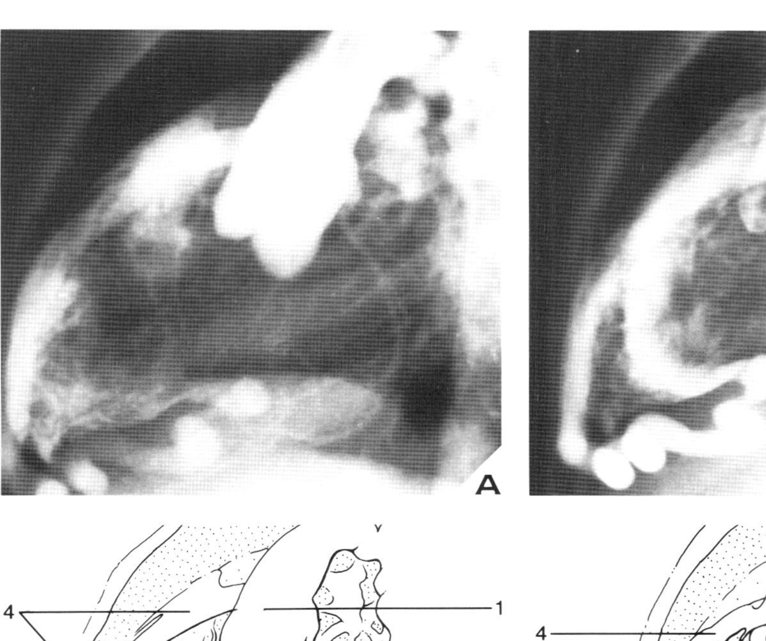

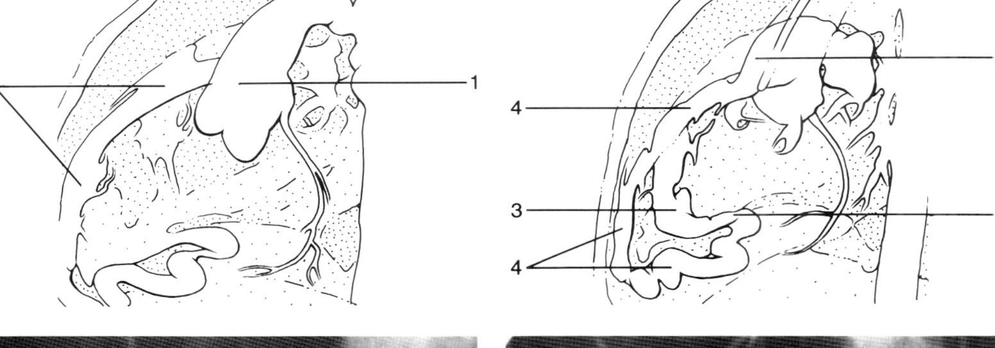

Fig. 21.59 Large right coronary artery-right ventricular fistula. (A) Early and (B) late phases of thoracic aortogram (lateral projection) show massive dilation of right coronary artery, which continues as a large channel that communicates with the inlet portion of the right ventricle through a wide opening. The right ventricle and pulmonary trunk are well opacified.

1 aorta
2 pulmonary trunk
3 right ventricle
4 right coronary artery
5 connection between right coronary artery and right ventricle

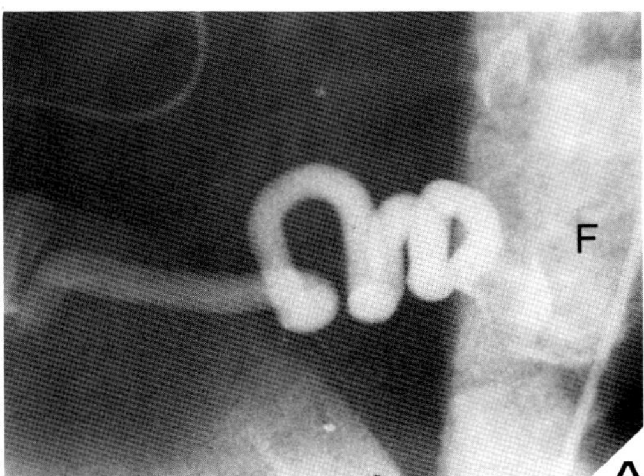

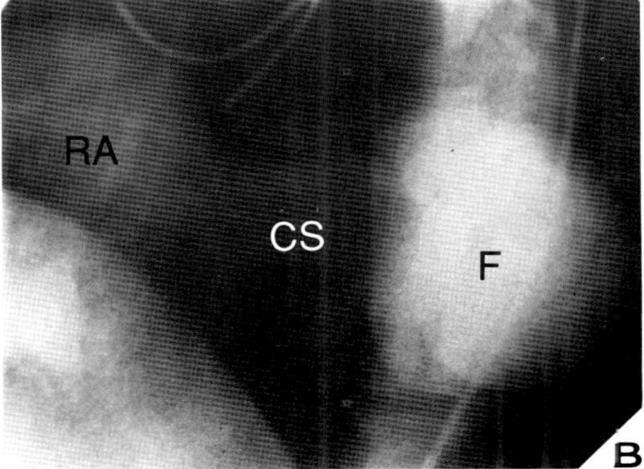

Fig. 21.60 Right coronary artery–coronary sinus fistula. The right coronary artery was selectively opacified by injecting a bolus of 20 mL of contrast material with a high-pressure injector. (A) Early and (B) late phases of right coronary arteriogram show marked enlargement of the right coronary artery, which terminates in an aneurysm-like fistula (F) that connects with the distal portion of the coronary sinus (CS). The patient had a moderately large (1:1.5) left to right shunt. (RA = right atrium)

artery disease (Fig. 21.61). This phenomenon, which has no clinical significance, is believed to result from the persistence of embryonic tissue in the left ventricular myocardium which communicates with the left ventricular cavity through defects in the endocardium. Blood fills this tissue during diastole, during which time the endocardial defects are occluded by a valve-like mechanism; during systole, this blood is expressed into the ventricular cavity.

Coronary–right ventricular fistula has been reported as an iatrogenic complication of endocardial biopsy, which is commonly performed after cardiac transplantation (Fig. 21.62). Published reports from a number of centers performing these procedures indicate that this complication, which results from injury to subendocardial branches of the coronary arteries by the biopsy instrument, is quite common.

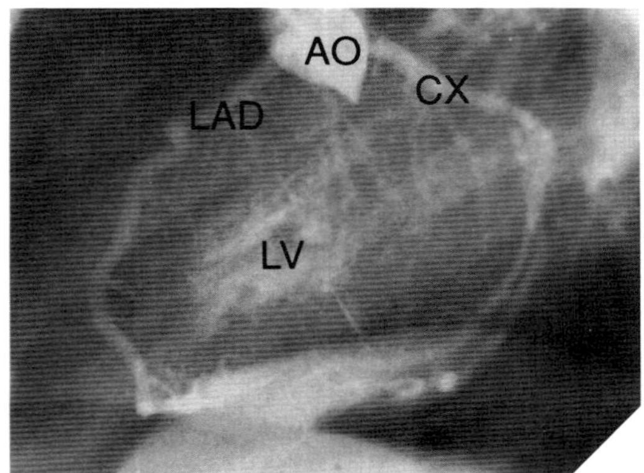

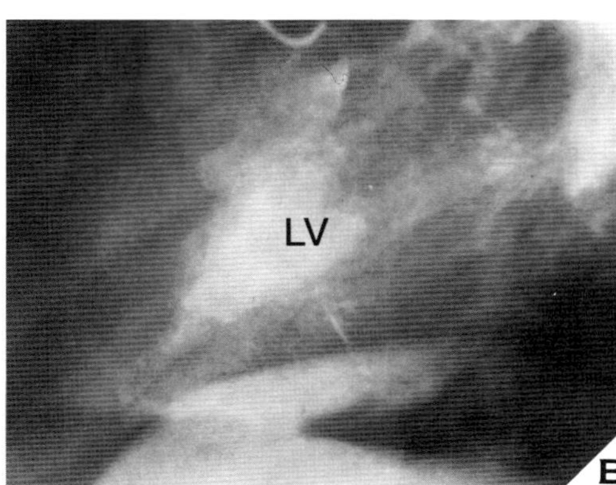

Fig. 21.61 Coronary–left ventricular fistula. (A) Early and (B) late phase of selective left coronary arteriogram (lateral projection) shows complete opacification of the left ventricle (LV) by contrast material which passed from the coronary arteries into the ventricular cavity during systole. (Ao = aorta; CX = circumflex artery; LAD = left anterior descending artery)

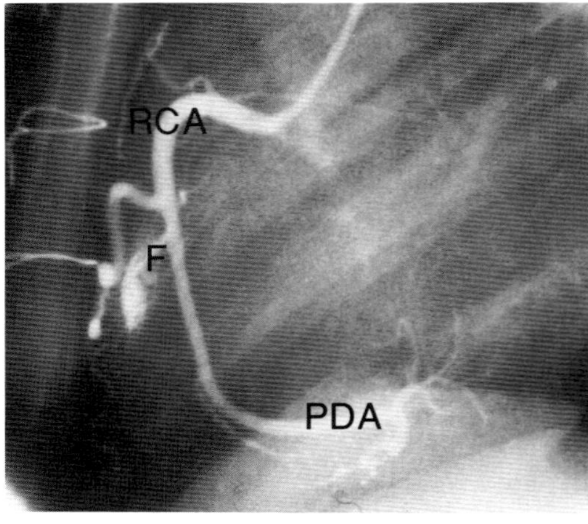

Fig. 21.62 Iatrogenic right coronary–right ventricular fistula. This patient had multiple right ventricular endocardial biopsies after cardiac transplantation. Right coronary arteriogram (RAO projection) demonstrates a large channel connecting an enlarged right marginal artery with the right ventricular cavity. (F = fistula; RCA = right coronary artery; PDA = posterior descending artery)

CHAPTER 22

Pericardial Disease

ANATOMY

The pericardium consists of two layers: a thin serous membrane which covers the epicardium (serous or visceral pericardium) and a relatively thick outer fibrous layer (fibrous or parietal pericardium) which encloses the heart and the proximal portions of the great vessels. The two layers of the pericardium enclose a potential space that normally contains about 20 to 25 mL of pericardial fluid. The latter is an ultrafiltrate of serum which has the function of lubricating the pericardial surfaces.

The relations of the fibrous pericardium are shown schematically in Fig. 22.1. The fibrous pericardium extends cephalad to the middle segment of the ascending aorta; it covers the entire pulmonary trunk, the proximal segments of the right and left pulmonary arteries, and a portion of the superior vena cava, but does not extend over the aortic arch. Inferiorly, it extends to the proximal segment of the inferior vena cava and merges with the superior surface of the diaphragm. Posteriorly, the fibrous pericardium is related to the trachea, the right and left main bronchi, and the esophagus, and is attached to the caval veins, the pulmonary veins (at their entrance into the left atrium), and the hilar portions of the pulmonary arteries. Inferiorly, the fibrous pericardium is supported by the central tendon of the diaphragm; anteriorly, by ligamentous attachments to the body and xiphoid process of the sternum; and posteriorly, by the pulmonary veins and the superior and inferior venae cavae.

The posterior and superior aspects of the pericardial sac contain several recesses and sinuses that are formed by the reflections of the fibrous pericardium over the great vessels (Fig. 22.1).

The *superior (anterior) pericardial recess* extends superiorly along the anterior aspect of the aorta, pulmonary trunk, and superior vena cava (Fig. 22.1). It extends cephalad to reach the upper part of the ascending aorta (it is separated from the thymic lymph nodes by a thin layer of parietal pericardium and

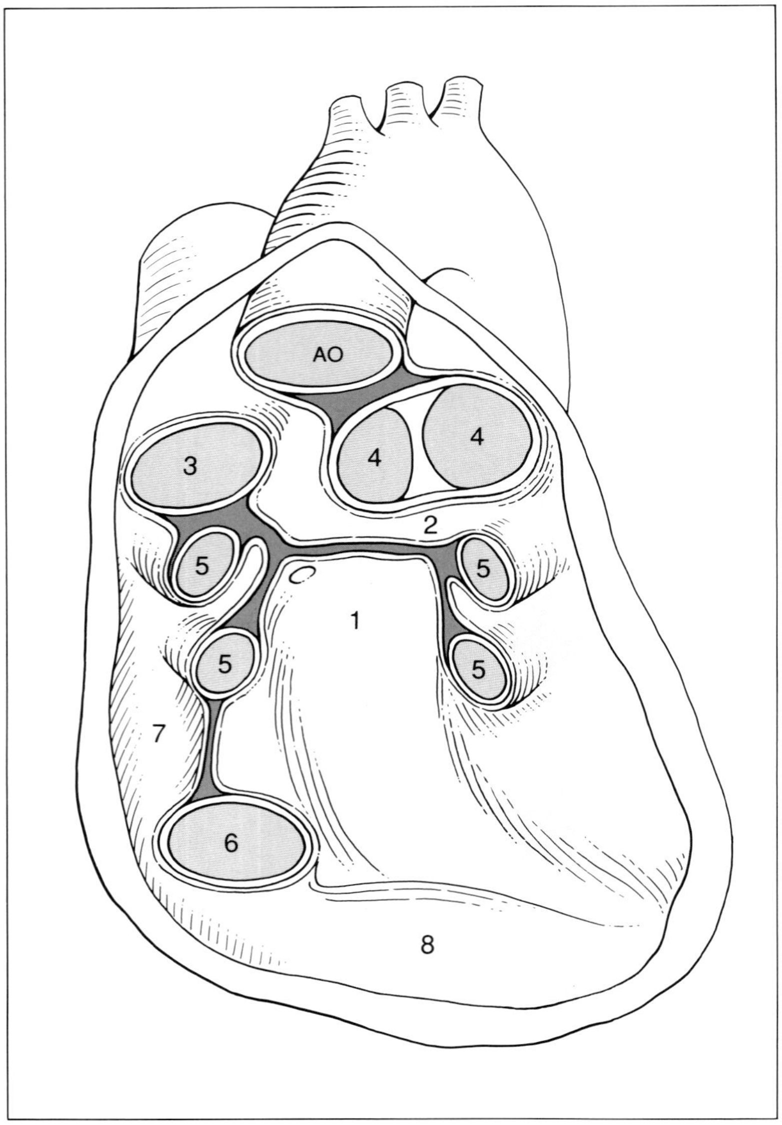

Fig. 22.1 Anatomy of the pericardium. Schematic representation of the posterior aspect of the fibrous pericardium (pericardial sac), showing the pericardial recesses. The heart is attached to the mediastinum by the pulmonary veins, superior and inferior venae cavae, pulmonary arteries, and the ascending aorta. The pericardial recesses occur where these structures enter or leave the heart. A transverse reflection of the pericardium between the right and left superior pulmonary veins divides the posterior aspect of the pericardium into two segments: the superior (transverse) sinus and the inferior (oblique) sinus. A vertical reflection of the pericardium encompassing the superior vena cava, right superior pulmonary vein, right inferior pulmonary vein, and the inferior vena cava separates the oblique sinus from the right paracardial recess. On the left, the superior and inferior pulmonary veins and the left border of the pericardium form the left pericardial recess. The transverse sinus is limited inferiorly by the junction between the right and left superior pulmonary arteries; superiorly by the right and left pulmonary veins; and anteriorly by the aorta and pulmonary trunk. On the right, the transverse sinus communicates with the superior pericardial recess; on the left, it communicates with the left paracardial recess. (The superior pericardial recess, not shown in this illustration, lies anterior and superior to the pulmonary trunk and the ascending aorta.) The inferior paracardial recess lies between the inferior wall of the heart and the diaphragmatic surface of the fibrous pericardium.

1 inferior (oblique) recess
2 superior recess
3 superior vena cava
4 pulmonary arteries
5 pulmonary veins
6 inferior vena cava
7 right pericardial recess
8 inferior pericardial recess
AO aorta

mediastinal fat). It extends to the right to connect with the transverse sinus. On the left, it surrounds the pulmonary trunk, extending posteriorly to reach the anterior aspect of the left pulmonary artery.

The *transverse sinus* lies posterior to the aorta and pulmonary trunk. Its posterior–inferior boundary is formed by pericardial reflection which extends transversely between the right and left superior pulmonary veins at their junction with the left atrium (Fig. 22.1). Its posterior boundary is formed by the superior portion of the left atrium (just above the entrance of the superior pulmonary veins and behind the ascending aorta); above this point it is contiguous with the carinal lymph nodes. As the transverse sinus extends laterally to reach the right hilum, the right pulmonary artery protrudes into it from behind. (Because the right pulmonary artery is almost completely covered by pericardium, for practical purposes it can be considered to lie within the transverse sinus.) Just posterior to the right pulmonary artery, and posterior to the transverse sinus, is the bronchus intermedius.

The transverse sinus is divided into two regions: the *pericardial transverse sinus (recess)* and the *cardiac (anatomical) transverse sinus (recess)*. The pericardial transverse sinus lies behind the aorta and is bounded posteriorly by the pericardium overlying the carina, it is formed by the reflection of the pericardium between the right and left pulmonary veins (ie, at the point where the pericardium is attached to the mediastinum and the superior aspect of the left atrium). The cardiac (anatomic) transverse sinus is situated between the posterior wall of the aorta and the anterior walls of the artria. Its floor is formed by the junction of the ventricles and the great arteries. It extends to the right to join the retrocaval recess, and to the left and superiorly to join the left pulmonary recess (Figs. 22.2 and 22.3).

The *oblique sinus* extends behind the atria (mainly the left atrium), coursing medial to the inferior vena cava to reach the pericardial reflection over the right and left superior pulmonary veins. The most superior and medial aspects of the oblique sinus are immediately adjacent to the carinal and subcarinal lymph nodes (Fig. 22.1).

The *paracardiac recesses* are the portions of the pericardial space adjacent to the ventricular chambers. Therefore, when describing the portion of the pericardial space adjacent to the right or left ventricle, one refers to the corresponding anterior, posteroinferior, or lateral paracardiac recess.

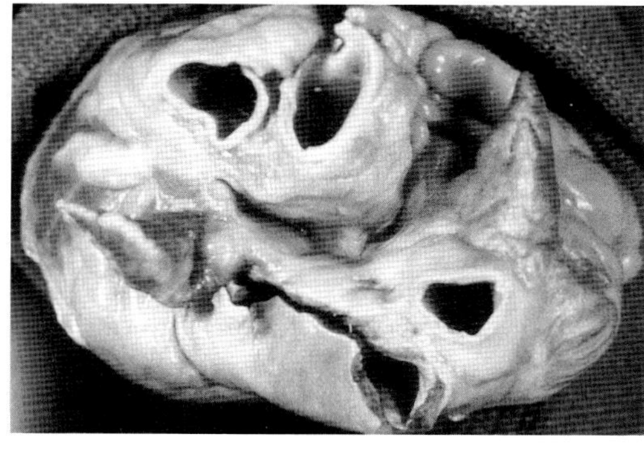

Fig. 22.2 Relations of transverse sinus. In this anatomic specimen (viewed from above), the aorta and pulmonary trunk have been displaced anteriorly to demonstrate the transverse sinus, which lies between the aorta and the anterior wall of the left atrium. Laterally, the groove-like transverse sinus communicates with the superior pericardial recess (on the right) and the left paracardial recess (on the left).

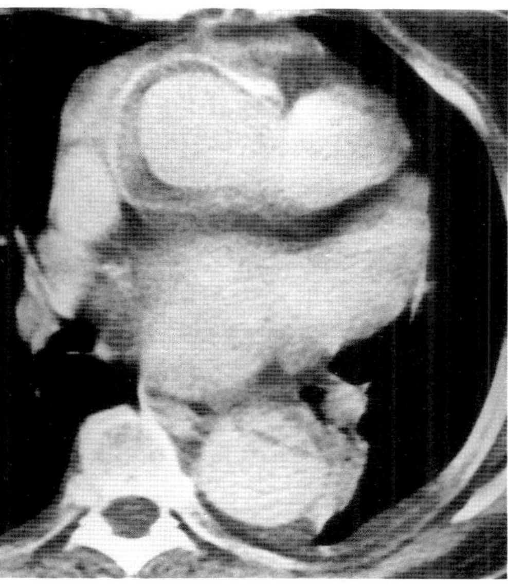

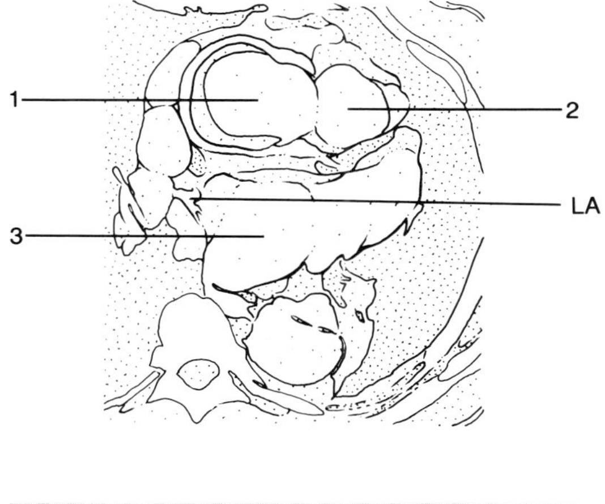

1 ascending aorta
2 pulmonary trunk
3 transverse sinus
LA left atrium

Fig. 22.3 Relations of transverse sinus. Contrast-enhanced axial CT scan in a patient with a pericardial effusion secondary to aortic dissection shows the transverse sinus, which is distended with fluid. The transverse sinus lies posterior to the aorta and the pulmonary trunk and anterior to the left atrium.

IMAGING OF THE NORMAL PERICARDIUM

PLAIN FILMS

It is usually possible to identify the anterior aspect of the pericardium on frontal and lateral chest films. This is because of the normal contrast between the pericardium (soft tissue density) and the epicardial and extrapericardial fat, which lie on either side of it (Fig. 22.4). On the lateral film, the pericardium appears as a thin layer just beneath the sternum; it is most conspicuous in individuals with large accumulations of epicardial and extrapericardial fat (Fig. 22.5).

CT AND MRI

On gated high-contrast CT scans the fibrous pericardium appears as a thin white line interposed between the epicardial and extrapericardial fat (Figs. 22.6 and 22.7). The normal pericardium is almost always demonstrated on CT owing to the excellent contrast between the normal pericardium and the surrounding fat. (When the extrapericardial fat is lacking, the external surface is demarcated by the adjacent air-filled lung.)

On MRI the fibrous pericardium appears as a curvilinear structure of low signal intensity between the high-intensity extrapericardial fat and the medium-intensity myocardium or high-intensity epicardial fat (Fig. 22.8). The fibrous pericardium

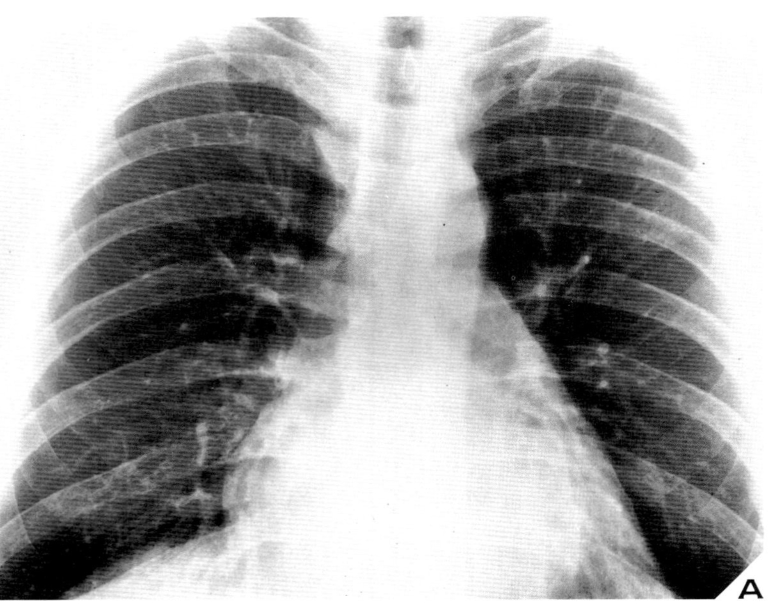

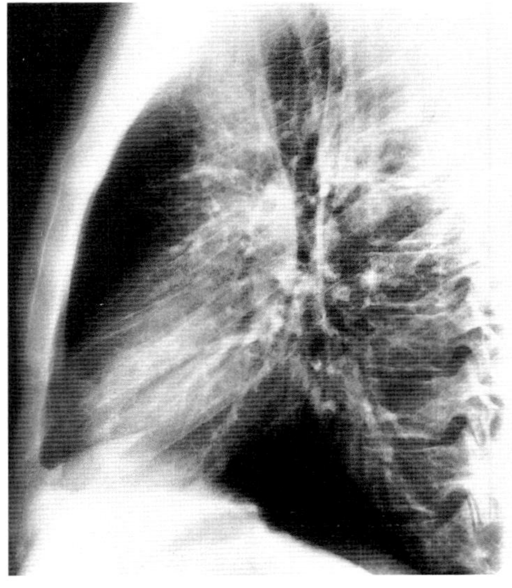

Fig. 22.4 Pericardium outlined by epicardial fat. (A) Posteroanterior and (B) lateral chest films of a patient with an excessive accumulation of epicardial fat along the left heart border. The epicardial fat is interposed between the myocardium and the visceral layer of the pericardium. The outer surface of the parietal pericardium is silhouetted against the adjacent lung.

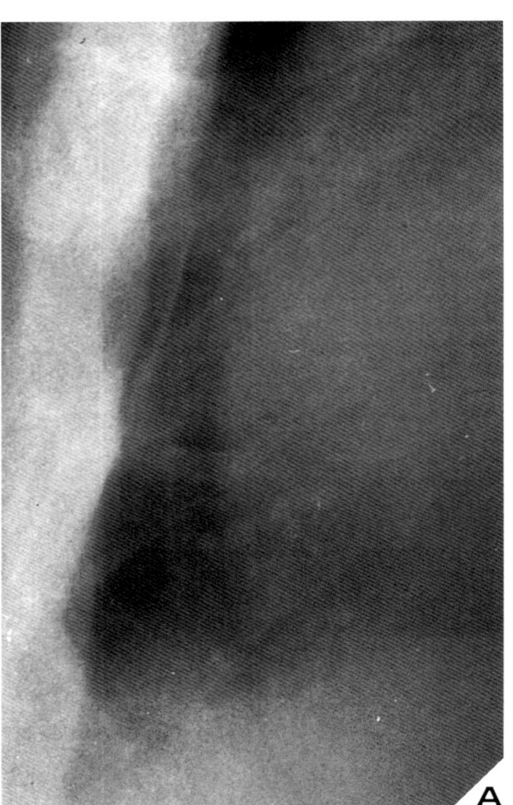

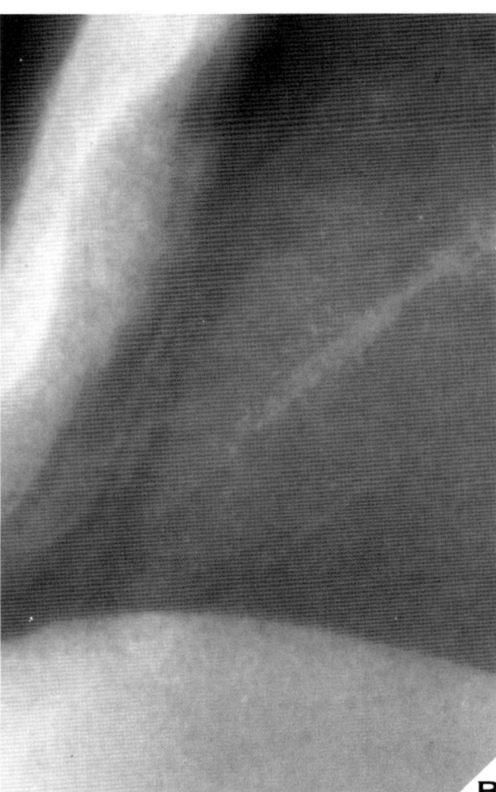

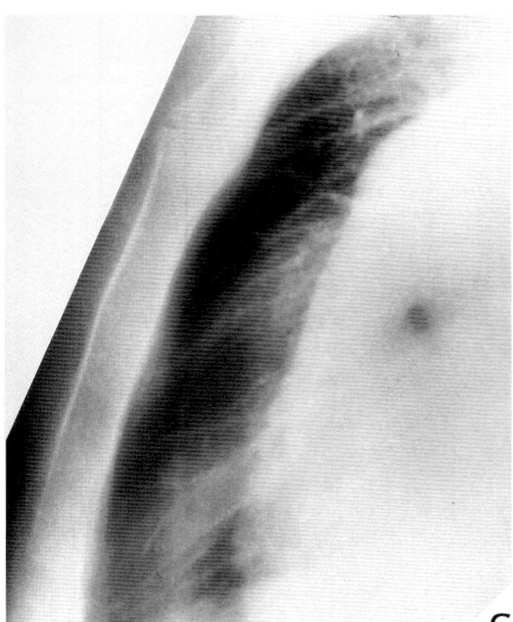

Fig. 22.5 Normal anterior pericardium. Detail of lateral chest films in three different patients show the normal variation in the appearance of the anterior pericardium. (A) The pericardium appears as a thin line between the epicardial and extrapericardial fat. (B) The pericardium is thicker but still within normal limits. (C) The thin pericardium is outlined by a large amount of epicardial and extrapericardial fat.

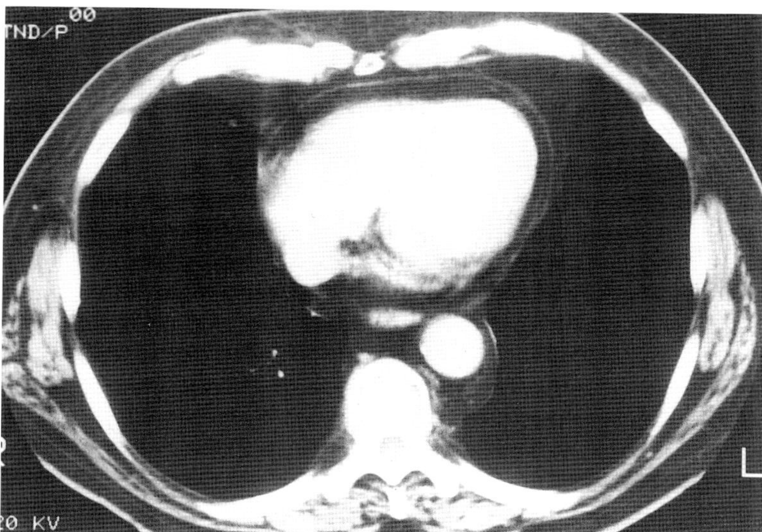

Fig. 22.6 Normal pericardium demonstrated by CT. Transverse section of the heart at the level of the cardiac chambers demonstrates the normal pericardium (which measures 1 mm in thickness) outlined by epicardial and extrapericardial fat.

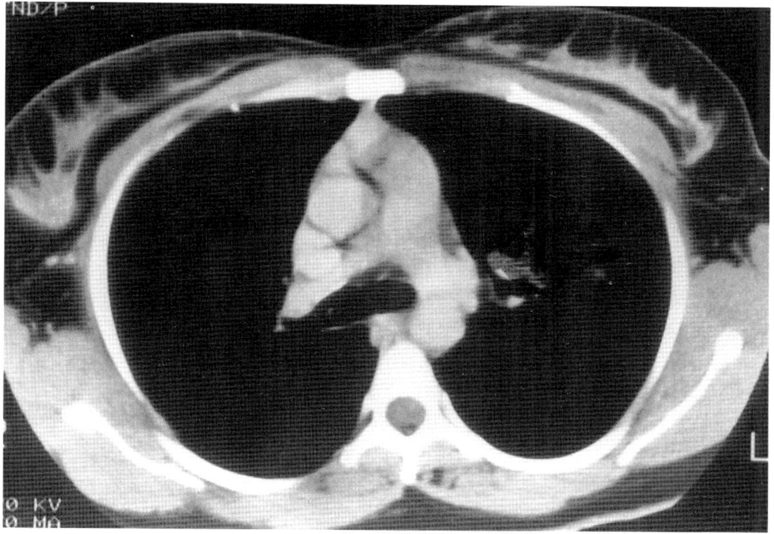

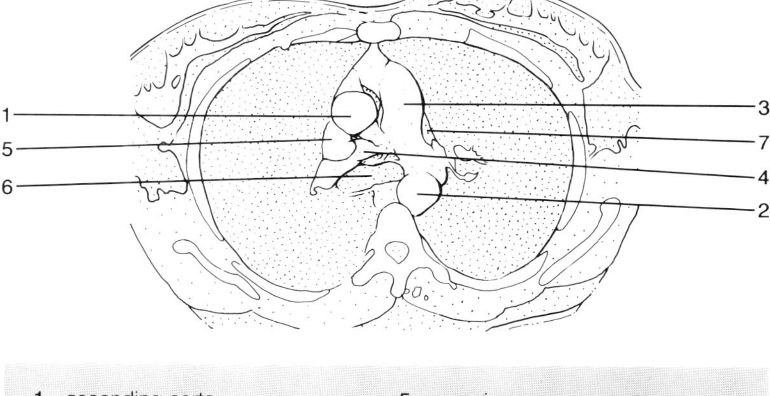

1	ascending aorta	5	superior vena cava
2	descending thoracic aorta	6	tracheal bifurcation
3	pulmonary trunk	7	pericardium over left pericardial recess
4	right pulmonary artery		

Fig. 22.7 Normal pericardium demonstrated by CT. Section through the aortic root and pulmonary trunk. At this level the fibrous pericardium is adherent to the vessels except at the periphery of the left pericardial recess, where it appears as a thin line separated from the pulmonary trunk by fat.

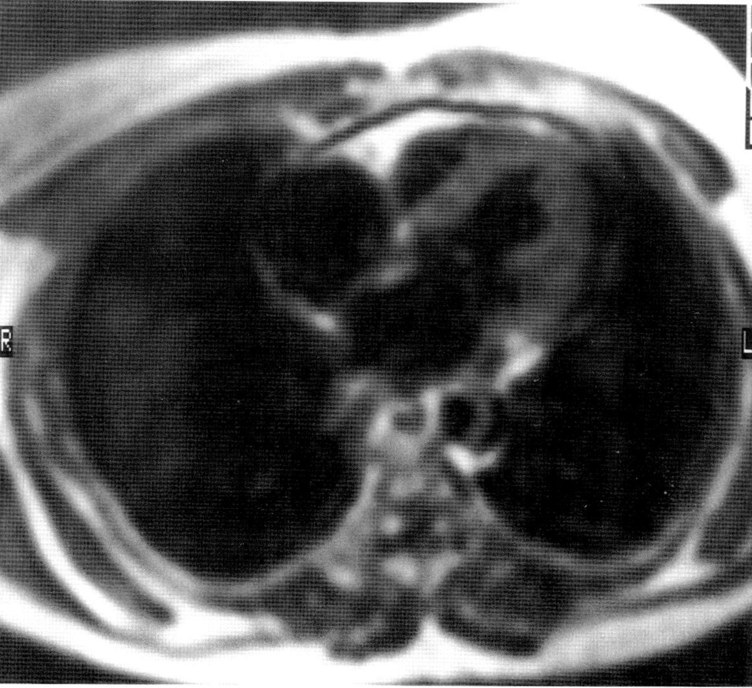

Fig. 22.8 Normal pericardium demonstrated by MRI. T1-weighted spin–echo image of the heart at the level of the ventricular chambers. The anterior pericardium appears as a linear 1–2-mm low-signal band between two regions of high signal, which represent the epicardial and extrapericardial fat.

has a long T1, short T2, and low spin density, and thus appears dark on both T1- and T2-weighted images. Measurements of pericardial thickness should be interpreted with caution, as they tend to be falsely high; in one study the mean pericardial thickness observed on MR images in normal subjects was 1.9 mm compared with a mean value of 1.0 mm in anatomic specimens.

ECHOCARDIOGRAPHY

On transesophageal echocardiograms the normal pericardium measures 1 to 3 mm in thickness; however, there is considerable variation owing to technical factors. In general, an echocardiographic measurement of 5 mm or greater is considered abnormal.

NORMAL DISTRIBUTION OF PERICARDIAL FAT

The distribution of pericardial and epicardial fat is important for identifying the normal pericardium and detecting pathologic conditions. The normal accumulation of epicardial fat in the anterior interventricular sulcus and the atrioventricular groove appears as a long, thin strip between the myocardium and pericardium on both CT and MRI (Figs. 22.6 and 22.8). Extrapericardial fat tends to accumulate at the cardiac apex and along the anteroinferior aspect of the heart. On plain films, apical fat collections typically have a triangular configuration (see Fig. 22.4A), whereas fat deposits along the anteroinferior aspect of the heart usually appear as a thick layer.

NORMAL PERICARDIAL FLUID

The small amount of fluid normally present in the pericardial space cannot be detected on plain films or by echocardiography. MRI and high-resolution CT can sometimes detect small amounts of normal pericardial fluid in the recesses adjacent to the less mobile structures (eg, vessels). Pericardial fluid cannot normally be detected in the paracardiac recesses by CT or MRI in normal subjects.

CONGENITAL MALFORMATIONS

CONGENITAL PERICARDIAL DEFECT

Congenital pericardial defect is defined as a discontinuity in the fibrous pericardium which allows the pericardial and pleural spaces to communicate. Such defects may be small and localized or may involve the entire pericardium.

Although congenital defects may occur anywhere in the fibrous pericardium, the great majority are on the left. In a review of 47 cases of partial pericardial defect collected from the literature, 40 occurred on the left, 5 on the right, and 2 at the base (diaphragmatic aspect) (Glover et al, 1969). Total absence of the pericardium—which can affect the right, left, or inferior portion—is a rare anomaly. Because they are usually asymptomatic and seldom verified anatomically, the true incidence of congenital pericardial defects is unknown.

Associated abnormalities of the heart and/or lungs (eg, patent ductus arteriosus, bronchogenic cyst) have been present in approximately half the reported cases of total or partial absence of the pericardium and have sometimes led to the discovery of the pericardial defect. Although congenital pericardial defects are usually asymptomatic, chest pain has been documented in a small percentage of cases. Fatal cardiac torsion has been reported as a rare complication in individuals with complete absence of the pericardium.

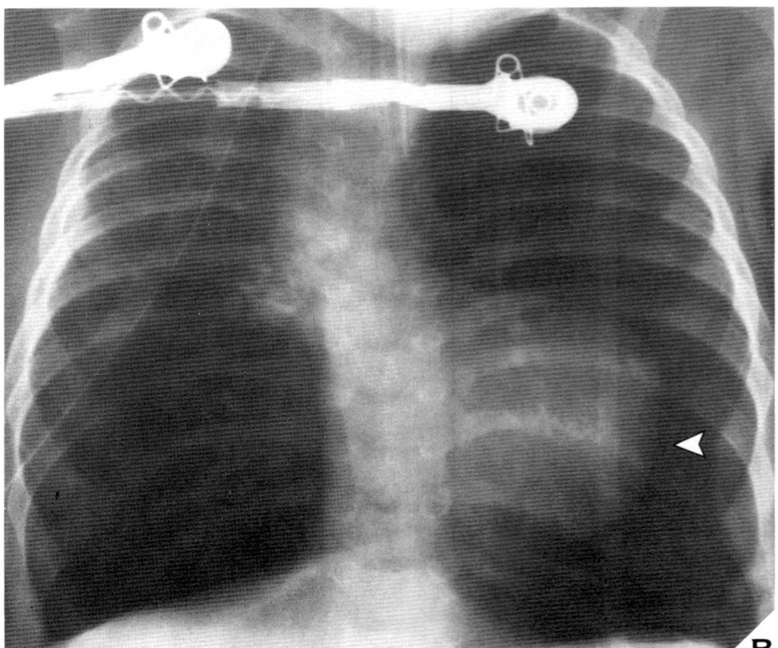

Fig. 22.9 Complete absence of the left pericardium. Erect chest films in two different patients. (A) The normal-sized heart is displaced to the left; the mediastinum is in normal position. (B) In a patient with pulmonary atresia (note absence of pulmonary trunk) and VSD and a right Blalock anastomosis, the heart is markedly displaced to the left; however, the mediastinum is in normal position. The right heart border is obscured by the spine. The indentation of the left heart border (*arrow*) represents the interventricular groove, an anatomic detail that is not visible when the pericardium is intact.

IMAGING AND INVASIVE DIAGNOSIS

Plain Films

Partial or complete absence of the pericardium is usually an incidental finding on chest radiographs obtained for an unrelated reason. In patients with complete absence of the left pericardium, the normal-sized heart is displaced into the left hemithorax, while the mediastinal structures remain in normal position (Fig. 22.9). The right border of the heart is projected over, or even to the left of, the spine. The pulmonary trunk, left atrial appendage, and left ventricular border appear unusually prominent. When the patient is turned into the left decubitus position, the heart is displaced even further into the left hemothorax (Fig. 22.10). Chest films of patients with partial absence of the left pericardium reveal prominence of the subjacent cardiovascular segment, which protrudes through the defect. The most common location of partial pericardial defects is the area overlying the left atrial appendage and pulmonary trunk (Fig. 22.11). In such cases the differential diagnosis includes enlargement of the left atrial appendage secondary to left atrial enlargement, and left juxtaposition of the atrial appendages. (The latter is usually associated with complex cyanotic congenital malformations.)

In patients with partial absence of the right pericardium, the

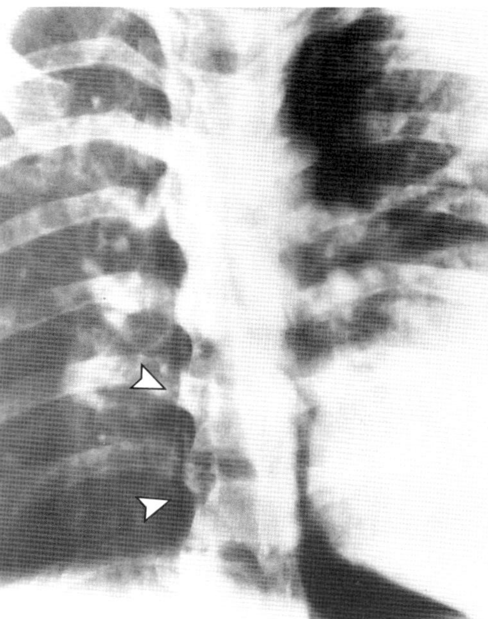

Fig. 22.10 Complete absence of the left pericardium. Left lateral decubitus projection following injection of a small amount of air into the left pleural space (diagnostic pneumothorax) shows the heart markedly displaced to the left. The normal right pericardium appears as a thin line (*arrows*) demarcated by air in the pericardial sac and the right lung. Note that although the heart lies entirely in the left hemithorax, the mediastinum is not displaced.

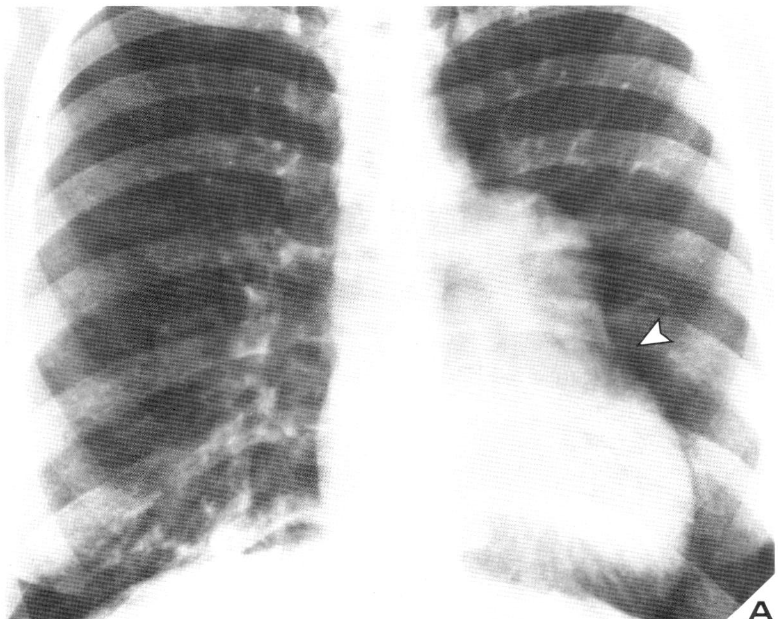

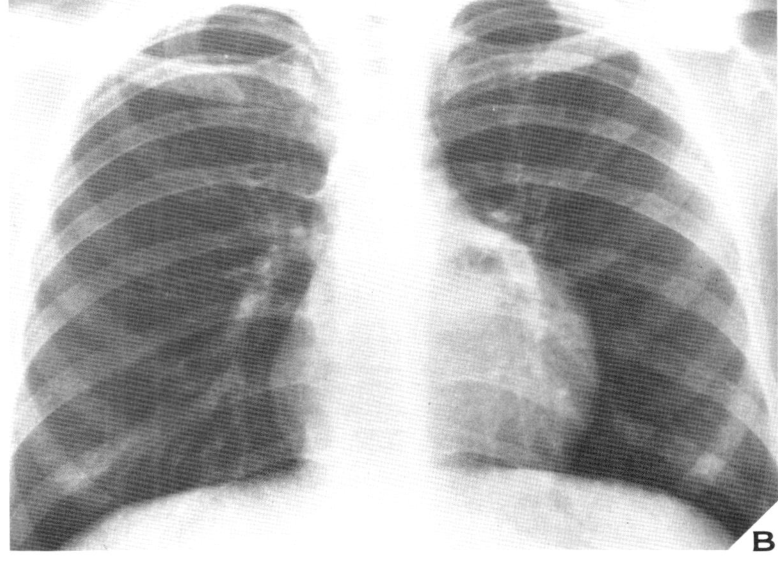

Fig. 22.11 Partial absence of the left pericardium. Plain film findings in two different patients. (A) The pericardial defect is located between the left superior attachment of the pericardium (above the pulmonary trunk) and the left atrial appendage. The prominent bulge along the left upper heart border represents the pulmonary trunk, which protrudes through the pericardial defect. (The margins of the defects are indicated by *arrows*.) (B) The pericardial defect is located inferiorly, between the level of the left atrial appendage and the cardiac apex.

frontal film reveals an abnormal bulge along the right heart border resulting from protrusion of a portion of the right atrium through the defect (Fig. 22.12). The differential diagnosis of this radiographic pattern includes right atrial dilatation secondary to right heart failure, a cardiac tumor involving the right atrium or pericardium, and bronchogenic carcinoma. Complete absence of the right pericardium is extremely rare.

Echocardiography

Echocardiography demonstrates the lack of normal pericardial continuity. However, owing to the low resolution of transthoracic echocardiography, the echocardiographic findings may suggest a small partial pericardial defect even when the pericardium is intact. (Transesophageal imaging improves diagnostic accuracy, although false positives are not uncommon.) Complete absence of the left or right pericardium is easily diagnosed by the characteristic displacement of the heart seen when the patient lies on his side with the pericardial defect in a dependent position.

CT and MRI

There have been few reports on CT and MRI findings associated with partial or complete absence of the pericardium. Characteristic alterations in the axis of the pulmonary trunk have been observed in patients with the common type of partial left pericardial defect. Direct contact of various cardiac structures with the lung has been described in other kinds of congenital pericardial defects.

Invasive Diagnosis

In the past, a diagnostic (ie, induced) pneumothorax was commonly used to confirm the presence of a pericardial defect; modern diagnostic methods have obviated the need for this technique (Fig. 22.10). Although cardiac catheterization and angiocardiography are diagnostic (Fig. 22.13), these invasive procedures are now seldom indicated.

PERICARDIAL CYSTS AND DIVERTICULA

Pericardial cysts are fluid-filled sacs that are related to the pericardium. (When the lumen is continuous with the pericardial space, the sac is called a *pericardial diverticulum.*) Although their etiology remains in doubt, most authors believe that pericardial cysts and diverticula represent congenital defects resulting from abnormal persistence of the parietal pericardial recesses normally present in the fetus.

Most pericardial cysts and diverticula occur in the right

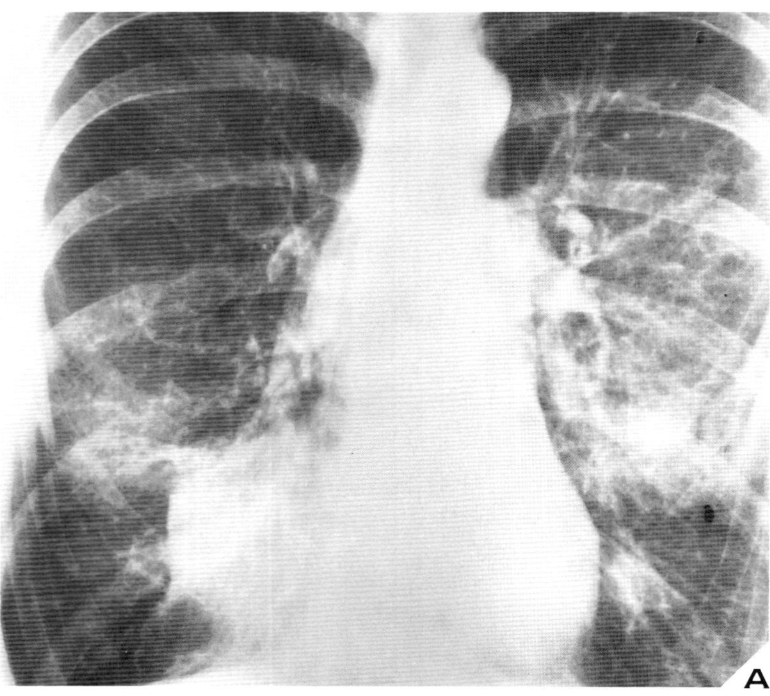

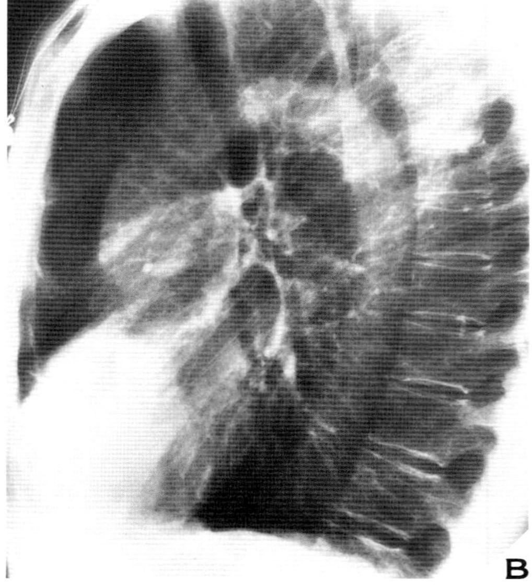

Fig. 22.12 Partial absence of the right pericardium. (A) Posteroanterior chest film of an asymptomatic patient demonstrates deformity of the right heart border at the level of the right atrium, which protrudes through a partial pericardial defect into the right pleural space. On the lateral projection (B), the protruding right atrium appears as an area of increased density just below the aortic valve.

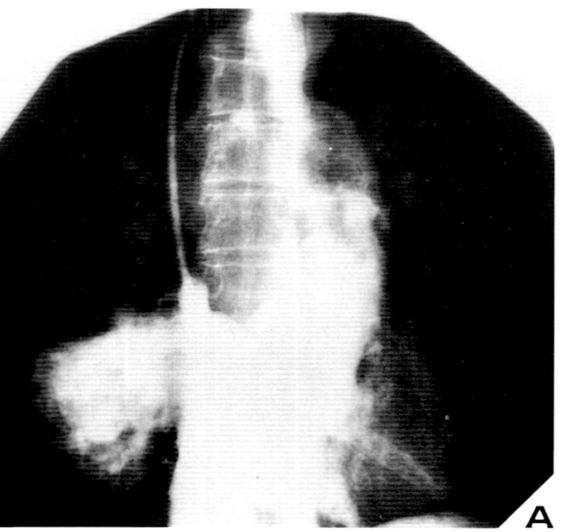

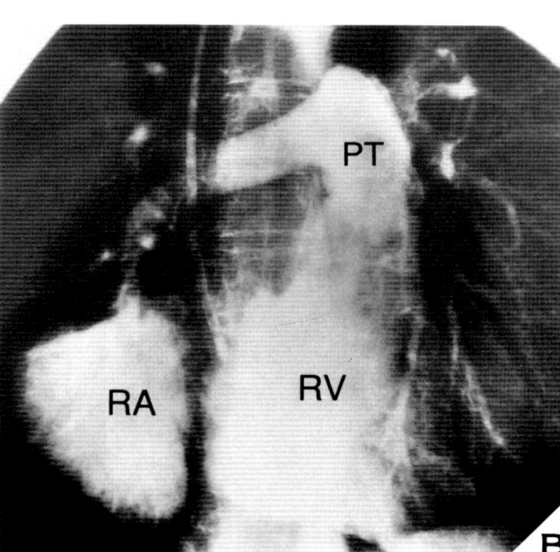

Fig. 22.13 Partial absence of the right pericardium. Same patient as shown in Fig. 22.12. (A) Early and (B) late phases of right atriogram (frontal projection) show the right atrium protruding through the pericardial defect. There is a wide communication between the non-herniated and herniated portions of the right atrium. There was no evidence of obstruction on angiography or cardiac catheterization. (PT = pulmonary trunk)

cardiophrenic angle (70 percent). Less often they occur in the left cardiophrenic angle (22 percent). Rarely, they are bilateral or occur at a site remote from the cardiophrenic angle. Pericardial cysts and diverticula vary in size from 2 cm to more than 16 cm in diameter. The lesion has a smooth outer border; internally, it may be unilocular or multilocular. The cyst wall is composed of connective tissue, with abundant collagen and scattered elastic fibers. The lining typically consists of a single flattened layer of mesothelial cells.

CLINICAL FEATURES

Most often, pericardial cysts and diverticula are discovered incidentally. In one series, more than one third of the patients had nonspecific symptoms (chest pain, dizziness); however, these complaints were probably due to the condition that led them to seek medical attention rather than to the pericardial abnormality (Feigin et al, 1977).

IMAGING AND INVASIVE DIAGNOSIS

Chest Films

Although large pericardial cysts and diverticula are easily detected on plain films, small lesions may not be noted on standard projections. On the frontal chest film the lesion typically appears as a smooth, round, homogeneous density in the right or left cardiophrenic angle; on the lateral projection it is contiguous with both the anterior chest wall and the diaphragm (Fig. 22.14). Cysts and diverticula overlying the cardiac apex typically have a round or triangular appearance (Fig. 22.15). A pericar-

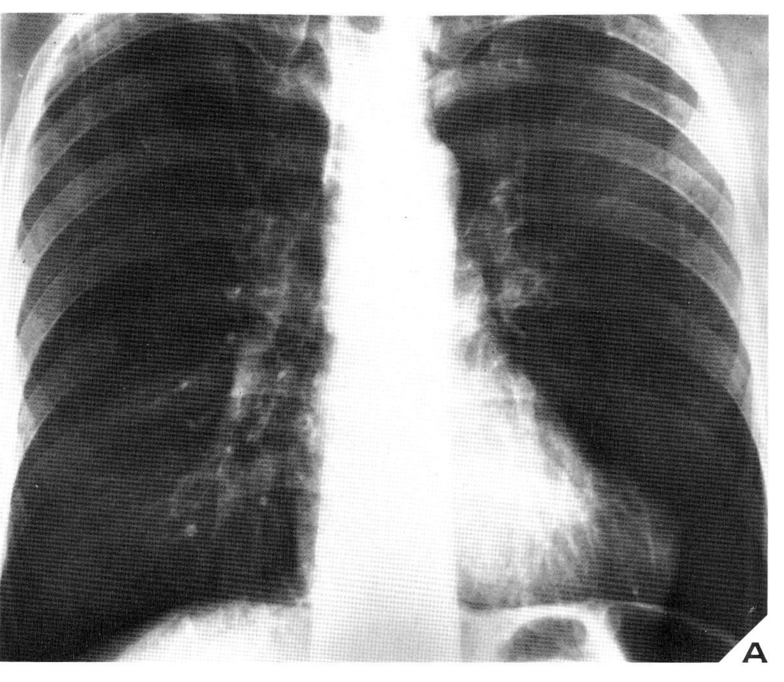

Fig. 22.14 Pericardial cyst. (A) Posteroanterior chest film shows a deformity of the cardiac silhouette at the level of the left cardiophrenic angle. Heart size is normal. On the lateral projection (B), a mass density is seen in the anterior cardiophrenic angle. This appearance is typical of pericardial cysts, which are usually located in the left cardiophrenic angle.

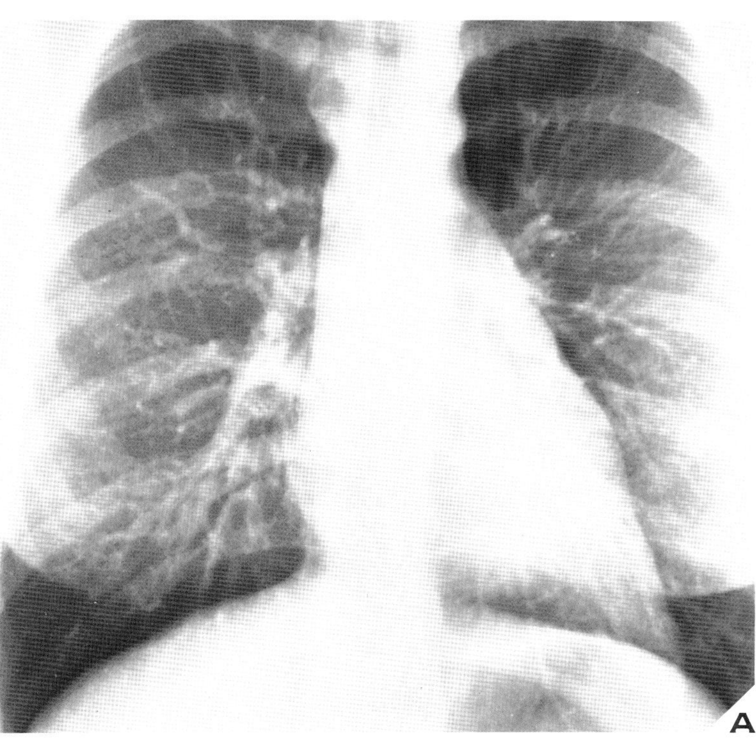

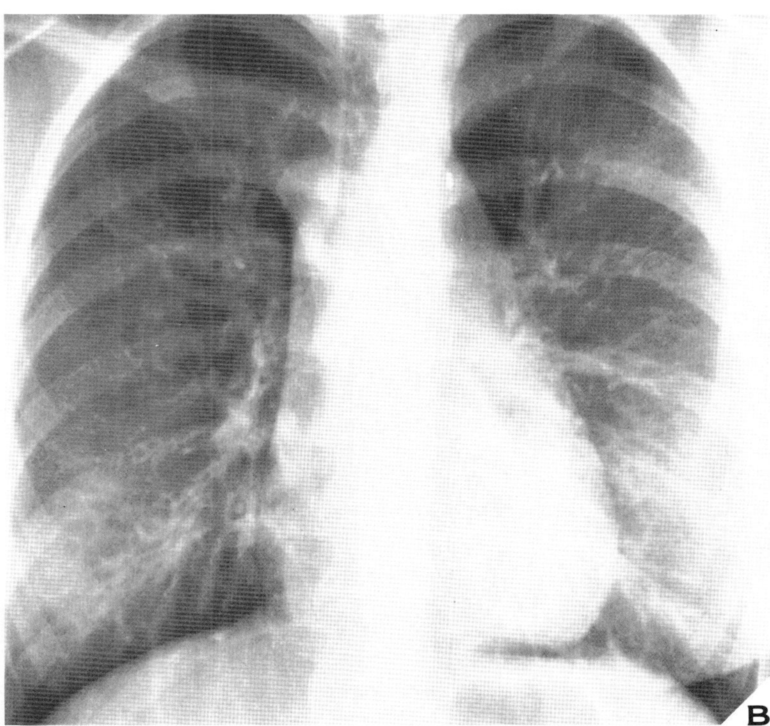

Fig. 22.15 Small pericardial cyst. (A) Posteroanterior chest film shows a triangular density at the level of the apex, which extends downward towards the diaphragm. This patient subsequently underwent repair of an aortic coarctation, at which time a small pericardial cyst was resected. (B) Postoperative chest film.

dial cyst or diverticulum in an unusual location can be mistaken for hilar lymphadenopathy or a mediastinal mass.

Echocardiography

Two-dimensional echocardiography is highly sensitive and specific for diagnosis of pericardial cysts and diverticula. Both the cystic nature of the lesion and its relation to the heart are clearly depicted by this modality. Cysts and diverticula in the costophrenic angle or at the apex are best seen on apical and subxiphoid views; the transesophageal approach is more suitable for lesions arising from the posterior aspect of the pericardium. In general, there is no associated pericardial effusion.

CT and MRI

CT and MRI are more sensitive and specific than chest radiography in the diagnosis of pericardial cysts and diverticula. On CT, pericardial cysts and diverticula appear as nonenhancing water-density masses (Fig. 22.16 and 22.17). On MRI, the lesion has a low-intensity signal on T1-weighted (short TR, short TE) and a high-intensity signal on T2-weighted (long TR, long TE) spin–echo images.

Angiocardiography

Because pericardial cysts and diverticula are accurately diagnosed by noninvasive techniques, angiocardiography can be omitted.

DISEASES OF THE PERICARDIUM

PERICARDIAL EFFUSION

NATURE AND DISTRIBUTION OF THE FLUID

The term *pericardial effusion* denotes any fluid collection (exudate, transudate, chyle, blood) within the pericardial space. It may result from lesions of the pericardium itself or may be a manifestation of a systemic disorder.

The various types of pericardial effusion and their usual etiology are shown in Fig. 22.18. The most frequent cause of a serofibrinous exudate is an inflammatory process (pericarditis). Hemopericardium is usually due to penetrating trauma, aortic dissection, myocardial infarction, or cardiac surgery.

Owing to the small capacity of the posterior pericardial space, pericardial fluid tends to collect anteriorly and laterally rather than posteriorly. With the patient in the supine position, pericardial fluid initially accumulates in the anterior paracardiac recess; as the volume of pericardial fluid increases, fluid accumulates in the lateral or paracardiac recesses, as well as in the posteroinferior paracardiac recess. When the patient is prone, the fluid tends to collect in the lateral paracardiac recesses.

CLINICAL FEATURES

Patients with pericardial effusion typically present with exertional dyspnea and a sensation of heaviness or fullness in the chest (which may be aggravated by exercise). A massive pericardial effusion may be associated with cough or hoarseness when the distended pericardium impinges on the phrenic nerve, or with dysphagia when it compresses the esophagus. Physical examination typically reveals a diffuse or absent apical impulse. Owing to the redistribution of the fluid with changes in position, the apical impulse may be palpable when the patient is supine but not when the patient is sitting. Auscultation typically reveals muffled heart sounds. Other auscultatory findings include an early diastolic sound and a pericardial friction rub.

ECG changes occur in 80 percent of patients with acute pericarditis. The most common finding in such cases is low-voltage QRS-complexes. Low voltage is not specific for acute pericarditis, however, as it may also be seen in patients with pleural effusion. The second most common ECG abnormality is ST-segment elevation (usually in leads I, II, V5, and V6), which typically appears within a few hours after the onset of chest pain and fever. (ST-segment depression also occurs, but is less

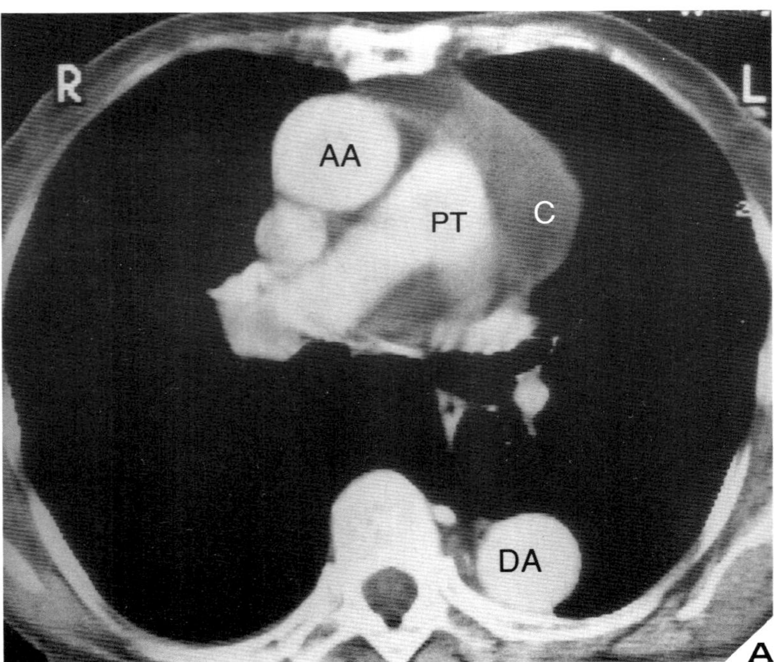

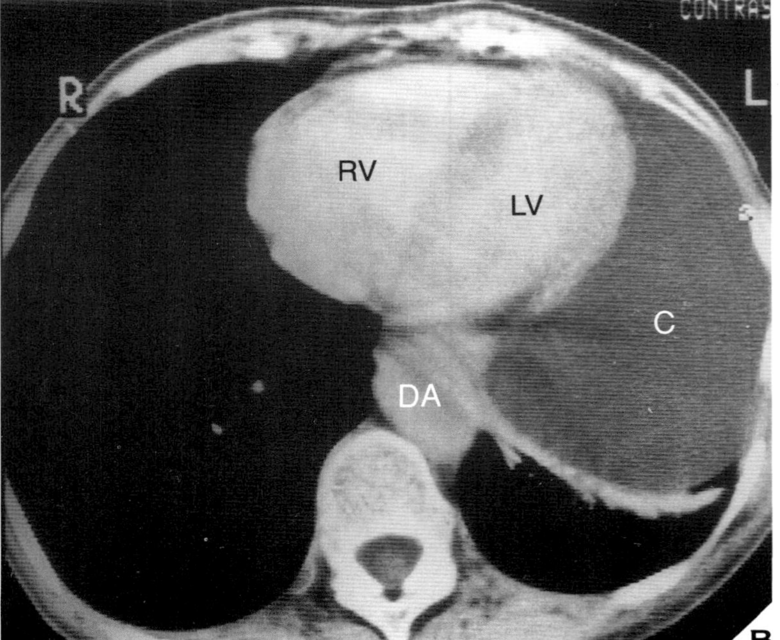

Fig. 22.16 Large pericardial cyst. In this patient the plain film showed a typical large pericardial cyst extending upward from the left cardiophrenic angle to the level of the pulmonary trunk. Contrast-enhanced CT scans (A) at the level of the bifurcation of the pulmonary arteries and (B) through the inferior portion of the ventricles demonstrate the unopacified cyst (C), which appears as a large low-density structure. The most cephalic portion of the cyst, which is separated from the lung by pericardium, lies anterior to the pulmonary trunk (PT) and ascending aorta (AA). (DA = descending thoracic aorta; RV = right ventricle; LV = left ventricle)

common.) ST-segment elevation typically persists for a few hours up to several days, during which time the T-waves become flat and then inverted.

Two syndromes in which pericardial effusion is a prominent feature deserve mention.

Dressler's syndrome (postmyocardial infarction syndrome) is an inflammatory disorder of the pericardium which typically occurs 4 to 6 weeks after myocardial infarction. It is characterized by fever, chest pain, leukocytosis, pleural effusions (60 percent), and pericardial effusions (70 percent). Pneumonitis is

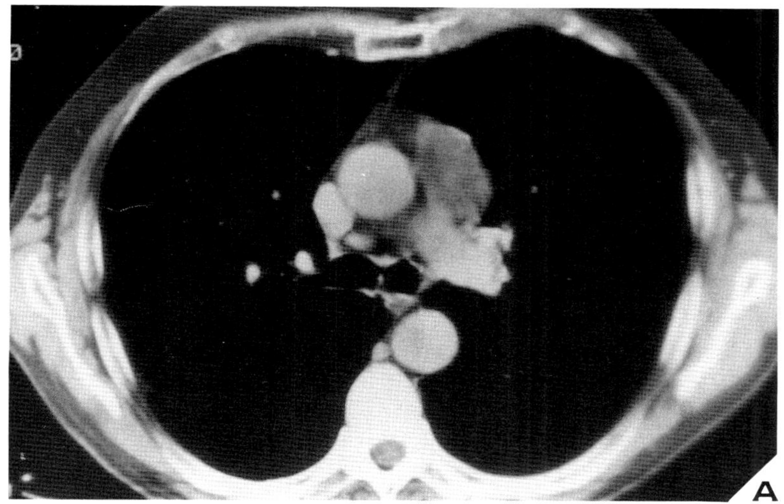

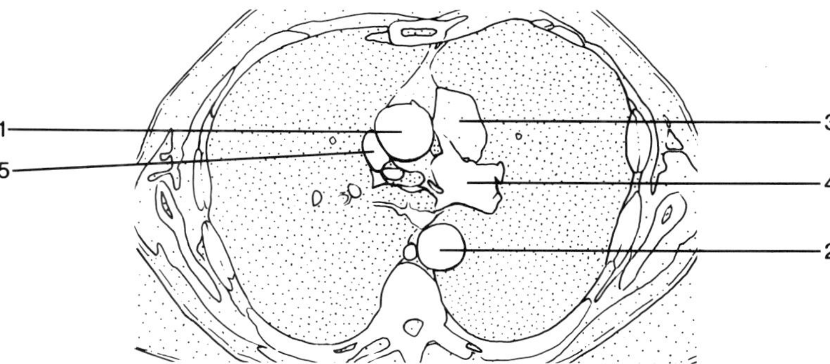

1	ascending aorta	4	left pulmonary artery
2	descending thoracic aorta	5	superior vena cava
3	pulmonary trunk	6	pericardial cyst

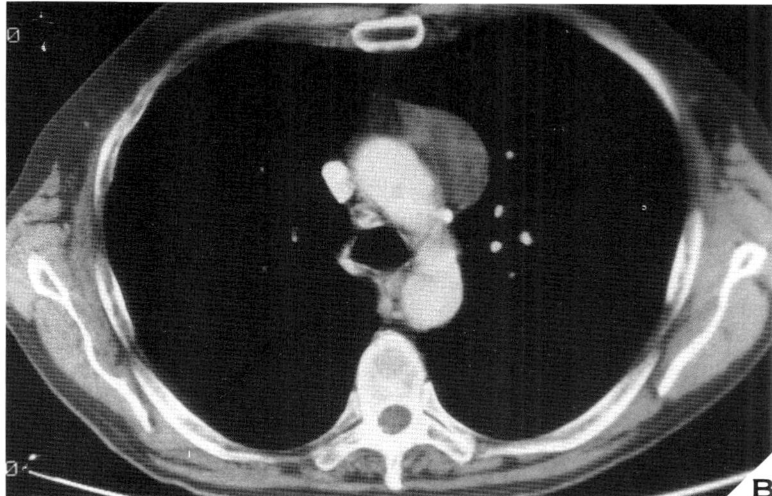

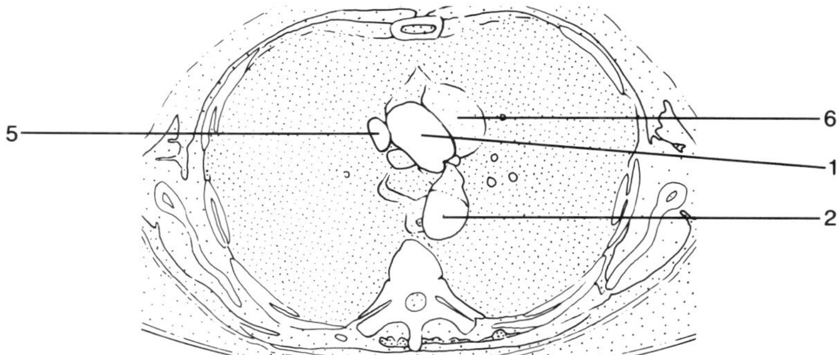

Fig. 22.17 Pericardial cyst in an atypical location. Contrast-enhanced CT scans at the level of the left pulmonary artery (A) and at the level of the inferior aspect of the aortic arch (B) demonstrate a nonenhancing fluid-filled structure along the left side of the ascending aorta and the inferior aspect of aortic arch. Although the location is unusual, this appearance is typical of a pericardial cyst.

FIG. 22.18 CAUSES OF PERICARDIAL EFFUSION

Serous

Congestive heart failure
Hypoalbuminemia
Previous thoracic irradiation
Recurrent viral pericarditis
Myocardial infarction (Dressler's syndrome)
Cardiac surgery, penetrating trauma (postpericardiotomy syndrome)

Serosanguinous

Uremia
Neoplastic infiltration
Blunt chest trauma
Cholesterol (idiopathic)

Serofibrinous

Bacterial pericarditis
Tuberculous pericarditis
Systemic lupus erythematosus
Myxedema

Hemorrhagic

Cardiac surgery
Myocardial infarction plus anticoagulant therapy
Penetrating trauma
Vascular pericardial neoplasms

Chylous

Idiopathic
Cardiac surgery (damage to major lymphatic channels)
Malignant neoplasms (lymphatic obstruction)
Benign intrathoracic masses (compression of lymphatic channels)

Fig. 22.18 Causes of pericardial effusion.

also common, occurring in about one third of the cases. The possibility of Dressler's syndrome should be considered in any patient who presents with pleural and pericardial effusions several weeks after a myocardial infarction (see Fig. 22.20). The etiology of Dressler's syndrome is unknown, although it is believed to have an autoimmune basis.

Postpericardiotomy syndrome is an inflammatory disorder of the pericardium which manifests after an interval ranging from days to months after surgical procedures in which the pericardium is incised. (It has been reported to occur in approximately 25 percent of children and 15 percent of adults who undergo open cardiac surgery.) It can also occur after penetrating or blunt trauma or perforation of the ventricular wall by a diagnostic catheter. Although the etiology is uncertain, it is believed to represent an autoimmune response to a viral infection. Patients with the postpericardiotomy syndrome typically present with fever, chest pain that becomes more intense with deep inspiration, and radiographic evidence of a pericardial effusion. As in the case of Dressler's syndrome, the diagnosis is based on exclusion of other conditions with similar clinical features (eg, postoperative infective endocarditis, surgically induced hemopericardium, pulmonary embolism) and the benign course of the disorder. Infective pericarditis secondary to a wound infection or sternal osteomyelitis can also cause a pericardial effusion. Pericardial involvement after median sternotomy is best studied by CT (see Fig. 22.27; see also Chapter 16.)

IMAGING AND INVASIVE DIAGNOSIS

Plain Films

Characteristic plain film findings can usually be appreciated when the volume of pericardial fluid exceeds 200 mL. Classically, frontal and lateral projections reveal a globular cardiovascular silhouette ("water-bottle heart") (Figs. 22.19 and 22.20). On the frontal projection, the borders of the cardiovascular silhouette are smooth and continuous, and the contours of normal border-forming structures [eg, the left atrial

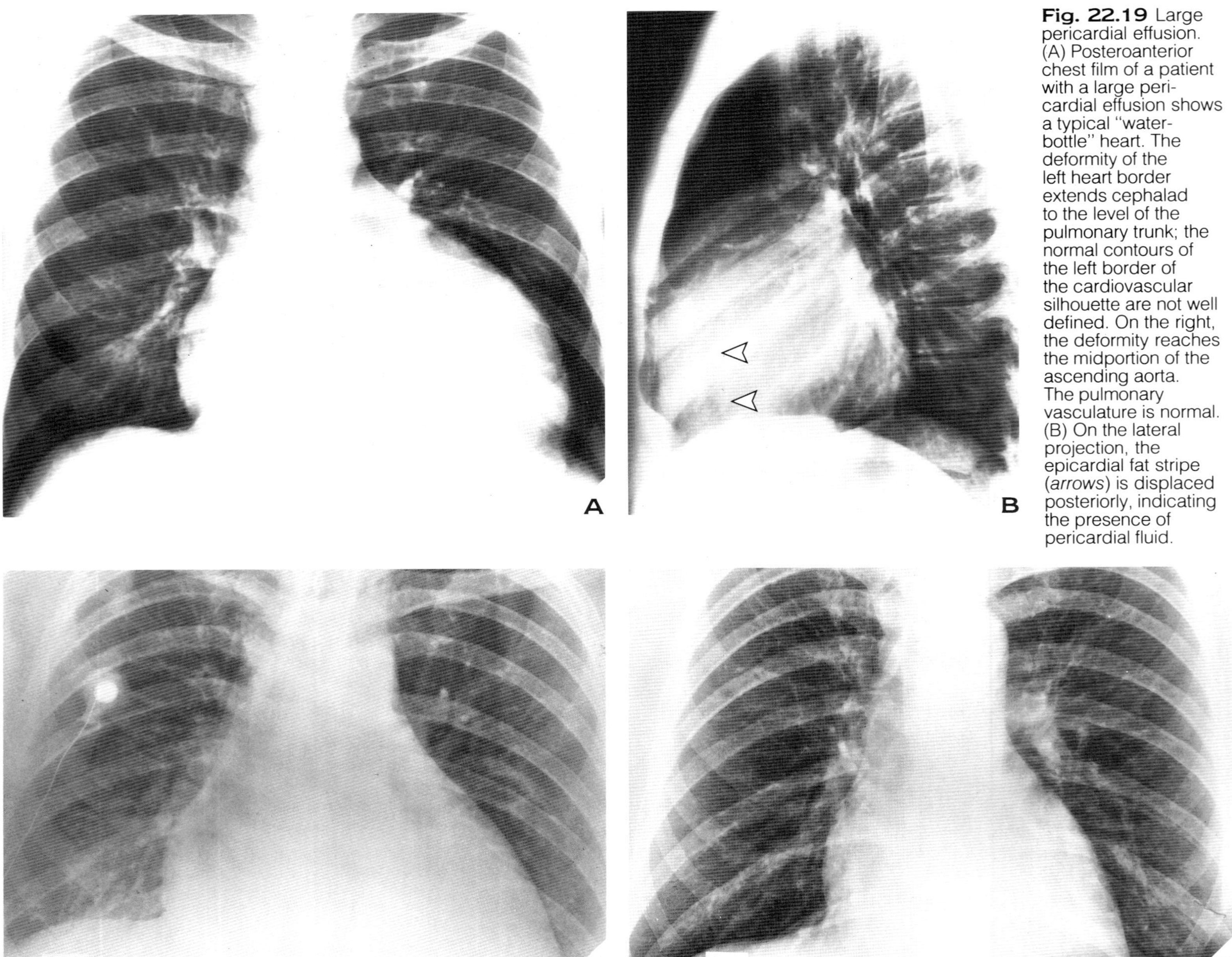

Fig. 22.19 Large pericardial effusion. (A) Posteroanterior chest film of a patient with a large pericardial effusion shows a typical "water-bottle" heart. The deformity of the left heart border extends cephalad to the level of the pulmonary trunk; the normal contours of the left border of the cardiovascular silhouette are not well defined. On the right, the deformity reaches the midportion of the ascending aorta. The pulmonary vasculature is normal. (B) On the lateral projection, the epicardial fat stripe (*arrows*) is displaced posteriorly, indicating the presence of pericardial fluid.

Fig. 22.20 Dressler's syndrome. (A) Frontal chest film in a patient with fever, chest pain, and leukocytosis shows deformity of cardiovascular silhouette with loss of normal contours, indicating the presence of a pericardial effusion, and pulmonary venous hypertension. The patient had had a myocardial infarction three weeks before. (B) Four months later the chest film is normal.

appendage and pulmonary trunk (on the left) and the junction between the right atrium and the superior vena cava or ascending aorta (on the right)] are effaced. The deformity extends upward to include the middle segment of the ascending aorta on the right and the pulmonary trunk, but not the aortic arch, on the left. On the lateral projection, there is widening of the zone of contact between the cardiovascular silhouette and the anterior chest wall, with partial obliteration of the retrosternal space.

Plain film findings indicating that the heart is displaced by an extracardiac density are very helpful in the radiographic diagnosis of pericardial effusion. Displacement of the epicardial fat from the borders of the cardiovascular silhouette ("positive epicardial fat pad sign") is particularly important in this context. Posterior displacement is appreciated on the lateral projection; the epicardial fat in the anterior inverventricular sulcus, which is normally in contact with the anterior chest wall, is projected over the middle portion of the cardiac silhouette (Figs. 22.19B and 22.21). Significant displacement of the epicardial fat from the anterior chest wall (10 mm or more) indicates the presence of either pericardial fluid or abnormal tissue (eg, tumor) or other material (eg, exudate) in the pericardial sac. On the frontal projection, separation of the epicardial fat from the left or right border of the cardiovascular silhouette has the same significance.

The deformity of the cardiovascular silhouette produced by a pericardial effusion is not always uniform. For example, a patient with pericarditis secondary to radiation therapy may have unusual cardiac configuration resulting from a localized accumulation of pericardial fluid.

The pulmonary vascularity is usually normal in patients with pericardial effusion, However, radiographic evidence of pulmonary venous hypertension may be seen in patients in whom the fluid has accumulated rapidly (Fig. 22.20), or when there is an excessive amount of pericardial fluid. Dilatation of the superior vena cava and/or azygos vein, indicating systemic venous hypertension, also may be seen in such cases. The pulmonary vasculature may be diminished in patients with cardiac tamponade (see below).

It should be emphasized that conditions other than pericardial effusion (eg, dilated cardiomyopathy, Ebstein's malformation with severe tricuspid insufficiency, polyvalvular disease with severe ventricular dysfunction) are associated with globular enlargement of the cardiovascular silhouette. A careful analysis of the pulmonary vasculature may suggest the correct diagnosis in such cases. Whereas the pulmonary vasculature is usually normal in patients with pericardial effusion, it is usually decreased in patients with Ebstein's malformation owing to the presence of a right to left shunt at the atrial level. In patients with congestive failure secondary to dilated cardiomyopathy, as well as in those with polyvalvular disease, pulmonary venous hypertension is the rule.

Fluoroscopy with cine or videotape recording can confirm the presence of a large pericardial effusion (eg, 200 mL or more). A positive epicardial fat pad sign, which may be difficult to see on plain films, is easily appreciated on fluoroscopy in the frontal, lateral, or oblique projection. Another classical finding is the disparity between the motion of the heart and the motionless borders of the cardiovascular silhouette. The heart, which floats in the pericardial fluid, is animated by exaggerated displacement during the cardiac cycle (the "swimming sign").

Echocardiography

Echocardiography can detect all but the smallest pericardial effusions. With a sensitivity of 100 percent and a specificity of 98 percent, echocardiography is indicated whenever the clinical and/or plain film findings suggest the presence of pericardial

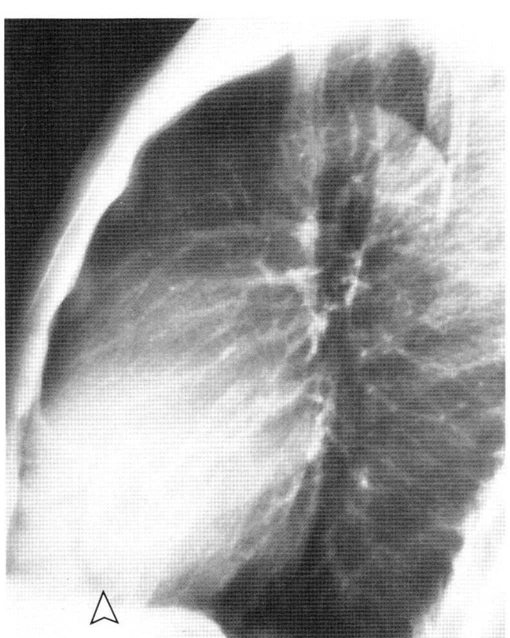

Fig. 22.21 Large pericardial effusion. Lateral chest film demonstrates marked increase in the distance between the epicardial fat pad (*arrow*) and the anterior chest wall, which measures more than 10 mm (normal, less than 5 mm).

fluid. As fluid collects in the pericardial sac it separates the fibrous pericardium from the serous pericardium, creating an echo-free space in between (Figs. 22.22 and 22.23). Small amounts of pericardial fluid in the posteroinferior and anterior pericardial recesses are readily identified by echocardiography. The posterior wall of the left ventricle is seen to move normally, whereas the posterior wall of the pericardial sac remains fixed and immobile. With larger effusions, fluid collects behind the left atrium. Fluid in the transverse and retrocaval pericardial recesses can also be detected. Reflection of the incident beam by the sternum prevents visualization of the superior pericardial recess, where pericardial fluid tends to collect first; therefore, some small pericardial effusions may not be detected by echocardiography.

CT and MRI

On CT, pericardial fluid can be identified as a fluid-filled space separating the heart (outlined by epicardial fat) from the fibrous pericardium. Pericardial fluid in the anterior, posterior, inferior, paracardial, and retrocaval recesses, as well as in the transverse and oblique pericardial recesses is readily detected by CT (Fig. 22.24). Most observers agree that pericardial fluid accumulates first in the anterior paracardial recess, anterior to the right ventricle. It then collects in the posteroinferior and lateral recesses before spilling into the other pericardial recesses.

When the patient with a small- or moderate-sized pericardial effusion is studied in the supine position, most of the pericardial fluid can be seen to collect in the superior and anterior paracardiac recesses. In patients with larger effusions, fluid can be seen in the right or left paracardiac recess. When the patient is turned prone, most of the fluid that was in the anterior pericardial recess shifts into the right pericardial or retrocaval recess.

Unlike echocardiography, CT clearly depicts the retrosternal space and can detect small effusions limited to the anterior paracardiac recess (Fig. 22.25). CT can also identify localized accumulations of pericardial fluid which may be difficult to evaluate on echocardiography (Fig. 22.26). CT is the modality

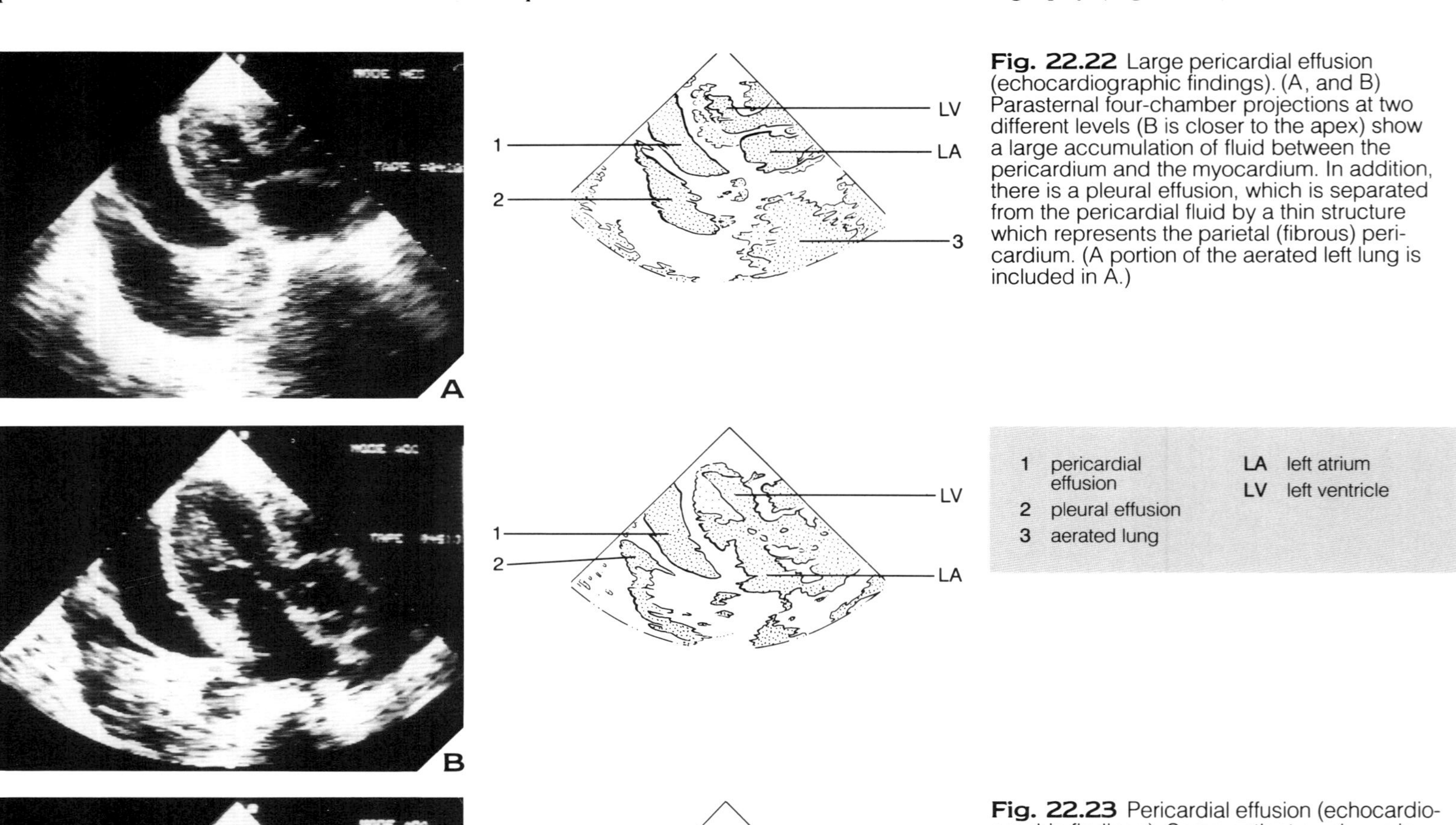

Fig. 22.22 Large pericardial effusion (echocardiographic findings). (A, and B) Parasternal four-chamber projections at two different levels (B is closer to the apex) show a large accumulation of fluid between the pericardium and the myocardium. In addition, there is a pleural effusion, which is separated from the pericardial fluid by a thin structure which represents the parietal (fibrous) pericardium. (A portion of the aerated left lung is included in A.)

1	pericardial effusion	LA	left atrium
2	pleural effusion	LV	left ventricle
3	aerated lung		

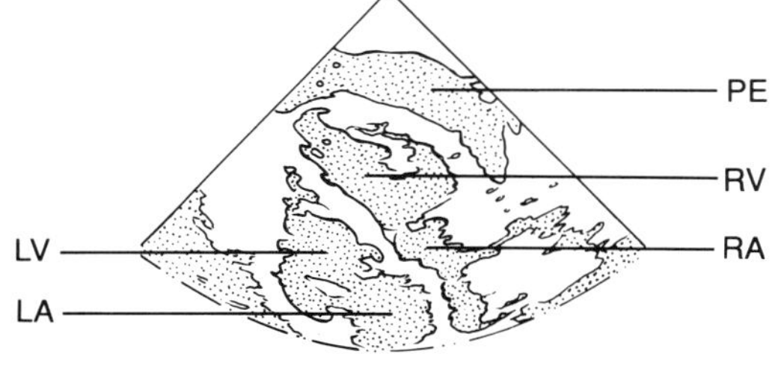

Fig. 22.23 Pericardial effusion (echocardiographic findings). Same patient as shown in Fig. 22.17. Apical four-chamber projection demonstrates an accumulation of fluid anterior to the right ventricle, which represents a pericardial effusion (PE). The fluid collection extends upward towards the right atrium.

RA	right atrium	LV	left ventricle
RV	right ventricle	PE	pericardial effusion
LA	left atrium		

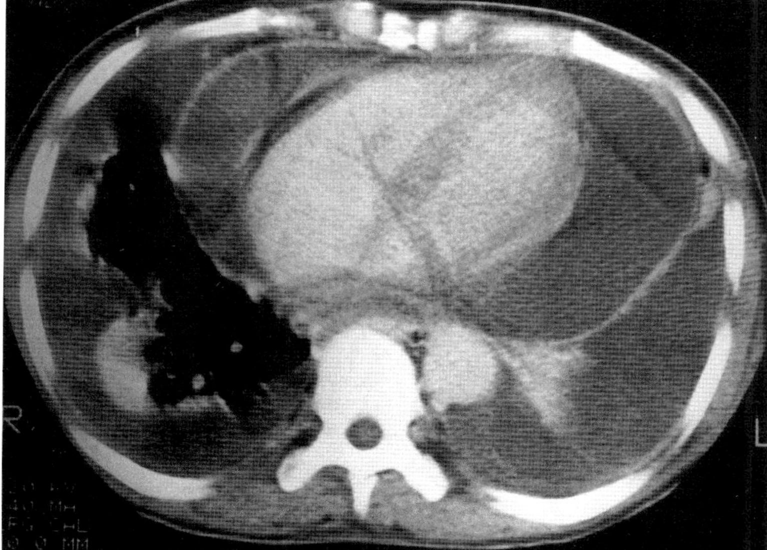

Fig. 22.24 Large pericardial effusion (CT findings). Contrast-enhanced scan through the midportion of the ventricles shows fluid (low density) in the right and left paracardiac recesses, as well as anterior to the heart. There is a large left pleural effusion. The visceral pericardium can be identified as a thin layer between the epicardial fat and the fluid in the right paracardiac recess. On the left, the fibrous pericardium is seen as a thin layer between the fluid in the left paracardiac recess and the fluid in the left pleural space.

1 fluid in left pericardial recess
2 fluid in right pericardial recess
3 epicardial fat
4 fibrous pericardium
5 visceral pericardium
6 left pleural effusion
7 descending thoracic aorta

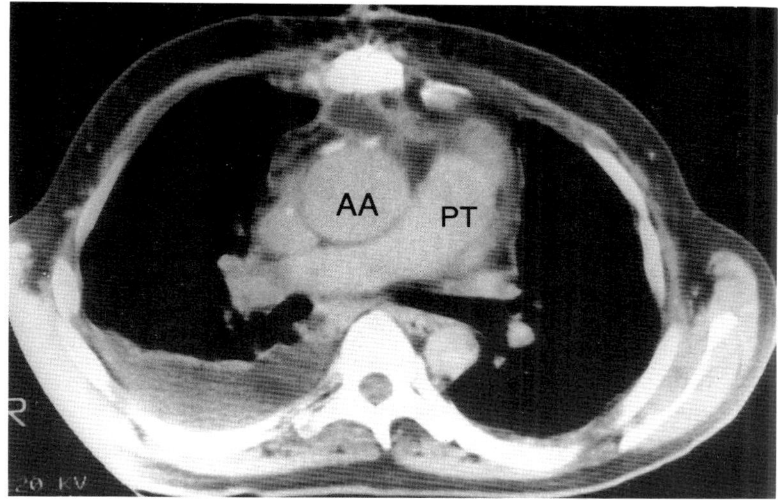

Fig. 22.25 Localized pericardial effusion in anterior recess (CT findings). Contrast-enhanced scan at level of pulmonary trunk demonstrates pericardial fluid anterior to the ascending aorta (AA) and pulmonary trunk (PT). A right pleural effusion is also present.

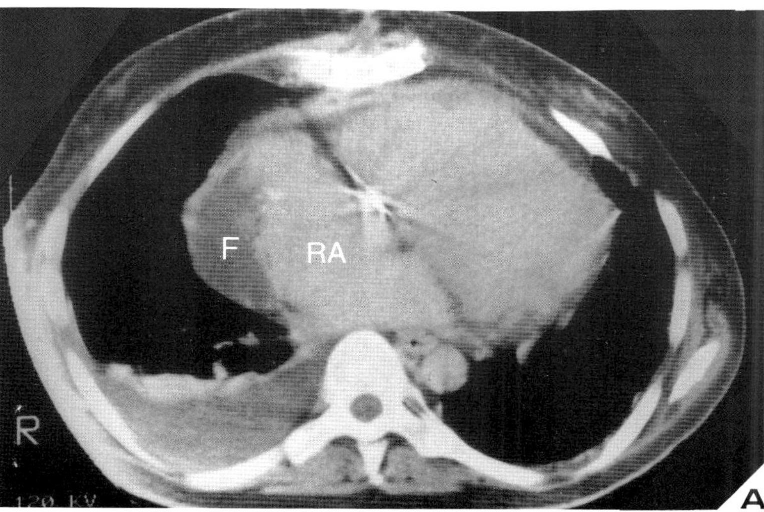

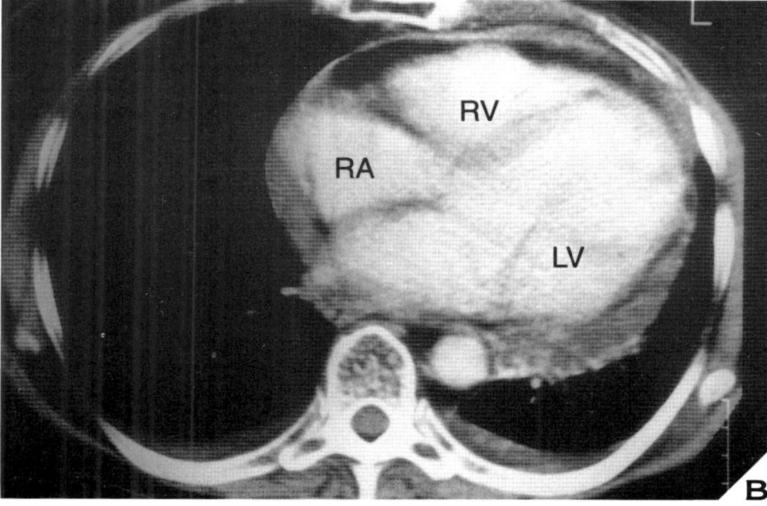

Fig. 22.26 Localized pericardial effusion (CT findings). (A,B) Contrast-enhanced CT scans of two different patients. (A) The pericardial fluid (F) is collected around the right atrium. (B) The fluid (F) is collected in the anterior recess, in front of the right atrium and right ventricle, and posterior to the left ventricle. Pleural effusions are present in both patients.

of choice for diagnosing infective pericarditis following median sternotomy (Fig. 22.27). In such cases the pericardium is thickened and typically enhances with intravenous contrast material; unlike simple effusions (transudates), which shift with changes in patient position, pericardial exudate is often loculated.

Pericardial fluid has a low-intensity signal on T1-weighted (short TR, short TE) spin–echo images; the signal becomes brighter as TR and TE (ie, T2 weighting) increase. The thickness of the pericardium is usually normal; however, it may be increased in patients with pericarditis or neoplastic involvement. The distribution of fluid is similar to that seen on CT (Fig. 22.28). MRI appears to be more sensitive than CT for detecting small amounts of fluid in the anterior pericardial recess.

MRI offers no advantage over echocardiography and is therefore not indicated as the initial imaging study in patients in whom pericardial effusion is suspected. MRI may be useful in the differential diagnosis of simple and inflammatory pericardial effusions. The latter may exhibit increased signal intensity on short TR/short TE images, presumably reflecting the high fibrin content of inflammatory exudates.

Cardiac Catheterization

The atrial, ventricular, aortic, and pulmonary arterial pressure curves are normal in the absence of pericardial tamponade (see below) or underlying cardiac disease.

Angiocardiography

Because the diagnosis of isolated pericardial effusion is easily confirmed by noninvasive means (echocardiography), angiocardiography is no longer used for this purpose. However, pericardial fluid may be detected on an angiographic study performed for another reason.

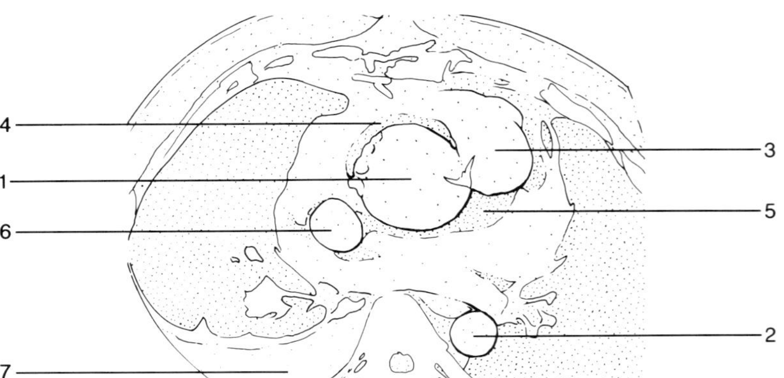

1 ascending aorta
2 descending thoracic aorta
3 pulmonary trunk
4 pericardial fluid in superior recess
5 pericardial fluid in transverse sinus
6 superior vena cava
7 right pleural effusion

Fig. 22.27 Pericarditis following median sternotomy. Contrast-enhanced CT scan at the level of the great arteries shows marked thickening of the pericardium, with fluid in the superior pericardial recess and transverse sinus. There is a right pleural effusion.

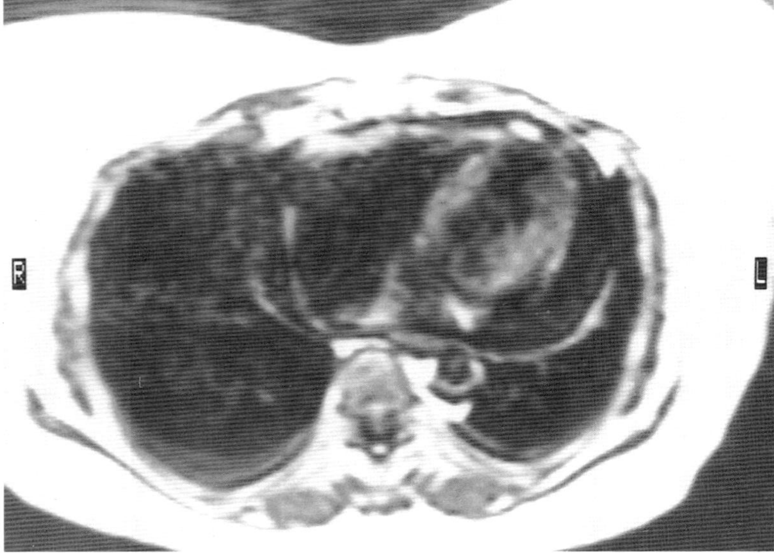

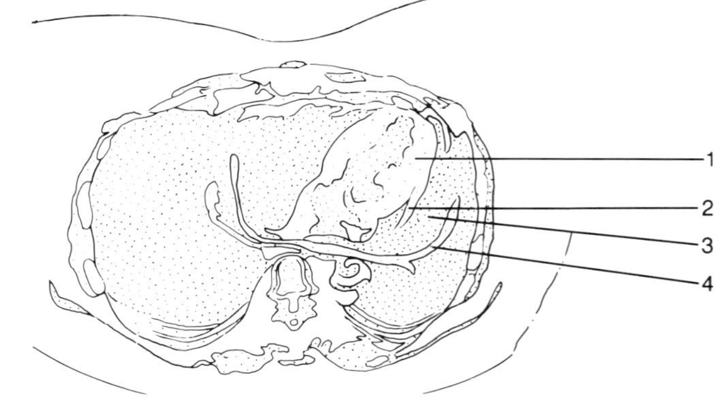

1 left ventricular wall
2 epicardial fat over left ventricle
3 pericardial effusion
4 parietal layer of pericardium

Fig. 22.28 Pericardial effusion (MRI findings). Axial T1-weighed spin–echo image shows a large pericardial effusion, which appears as a signal void between the epicardial fat overlying the wall of the left ventricle and the extrapericardial fat.

The angiographic diagnosis of pericardial effusion is based on the demonstration of a gap between the opacified cardiac chambers and the pericardium. On the frontal projection, a gap of 5 mm or more between the opacified right atrium and the border of the cardiac silhouette is reliable evidence of pericardial fluid or pericardial thickening due to another cause (Figs. 22.29 and 22.30). (Owing to the morphology of the right atrium and the normal laxity of the pericardial reflections, measurements of pericardial thickness are unreliable unless the right atrium is completely opacified.) Pericardial thickening can also be demonstrated by right or left ventriculography (Figs. 22.30 and 22.31). Two landmarks that indicate the position of the anterior heart border on the lateral projection are the left anterior descending coronary artery and fat in the anterior interventricular sulcus; a gap of 8 mm or more between either of these landmarks and the anterior chest wall can be taken as evidence of pericardial effusion or abnormal pericardial thickening. Excessive mobility of the heart within a relatively fixed cardiovascular silhouette is indicative of a large pericardial effusion. A small amount of pericardial fluid in the transverse or oblique sinus or the retrocaval pericardial recess cannot be detected by angiocardiography.

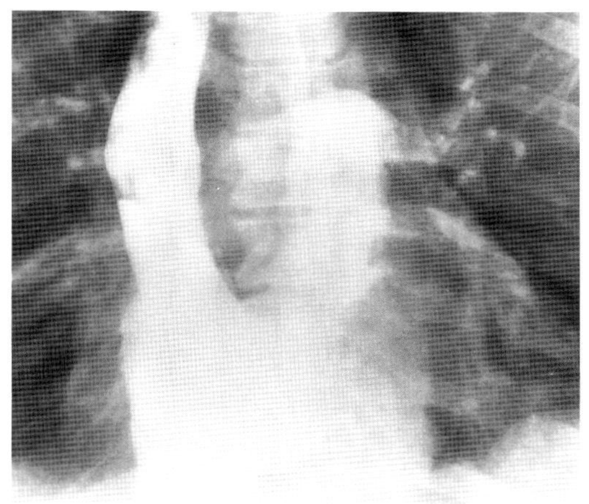

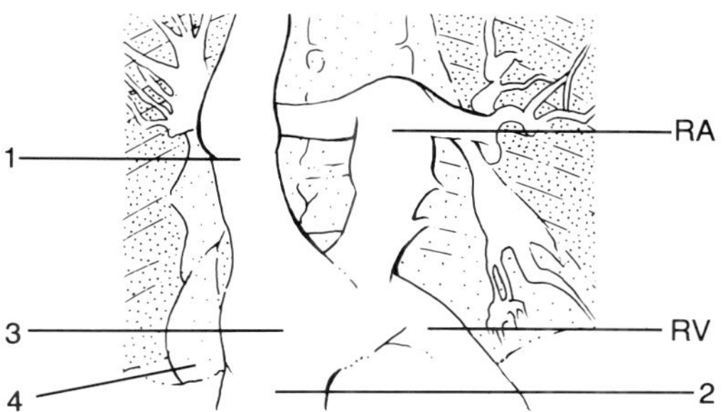

Fig. 22.29 Large pericardial effusion (angiocardiographic findings). Frontal projection of right atriogram demonstrates a wide separation between the lateral margin of the opacificed right atrium and the right border of the cardiac silhouette indicating the presence of fluid in the right lateral paracardiac recess. The lateral margin of the right atrium is flattened.

1	superior vena cava	**4**	pulmonary trunk
2	inferior vena cava	**RA**	right atrium
3	pericardial effusion	**RV**	right ventricle

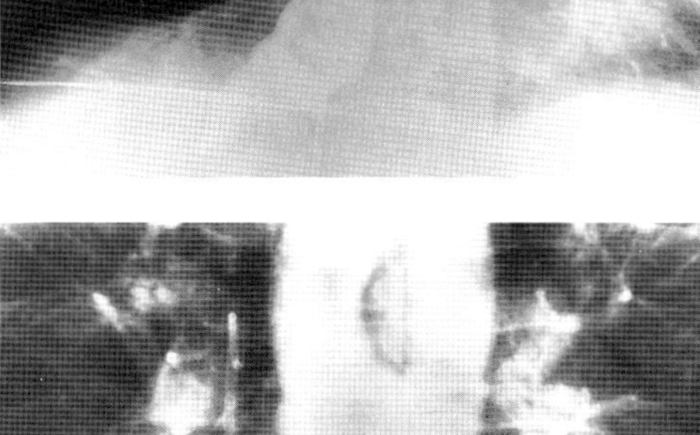

Fig. 22.30 Large pericardial effusion (angiocardiographic findings). Right atriogram shows medial displacement of the right atrium and upward displacement of the right ventricle by the pericardial fluid (PE) (note the wide space between the diaphragm and the inferior border of the right ventricle). The pulmonary arteries are normal.

1	inferior vena cava	**PE**	pericardial effusion
2	pulmonary trunk		
RA	right atrium	**RV**	right ventricle

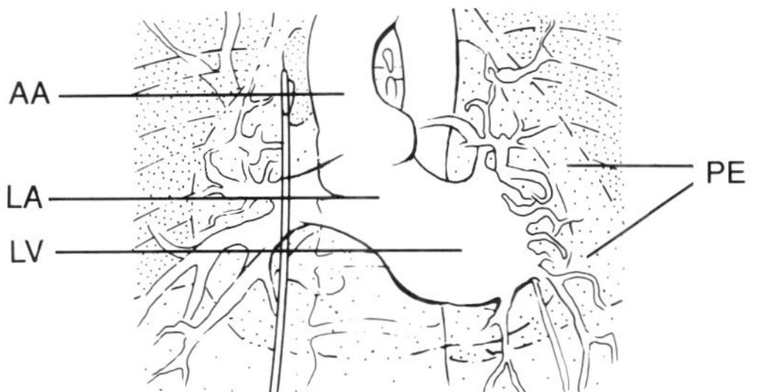

Fig. 22.31 Large pericardial effusion (angiocardiographic findings). Left ventricular phase of right atriogram. Note the wide separation, measuring 3 cm, between the left border of the opacified left ventricle and the border of the cardiac silhouette, indicating the presence of a large pericardial effusion (PE). (AA, ascending aorta)

LV	left ventricle	**AA**	ascending aorta
LA	left atrium	**PE**	pericardial effusion

CARDIAC TAMPONADE
PATHOPHYSIOLOGY AND CLINICAL FEATURES

Cardiac tamponade is defined as a hemodynamic state in which increased intrapericardial pressure causes an elevation of right atrial and systemic venous pressures and threatens to decrease, or actually decreases, cardiac output (Fig. 22.32). A rapid increase in the pericardial contents leads to a marked increase in intrapericardial pressure, which may reach 20 to 30 mm Hg, resulting in a severe, and sometimes fatal, decrease in cardiac output. Compensatory mechanisms include reflex vasoconstriction, catecholamine release, and the immediate retention of water and sodium by the kidneys. These compensatory mechanisms, which increase systemic venous and right atrial pressure, maintain cardiac output at a level compatible with life. If,

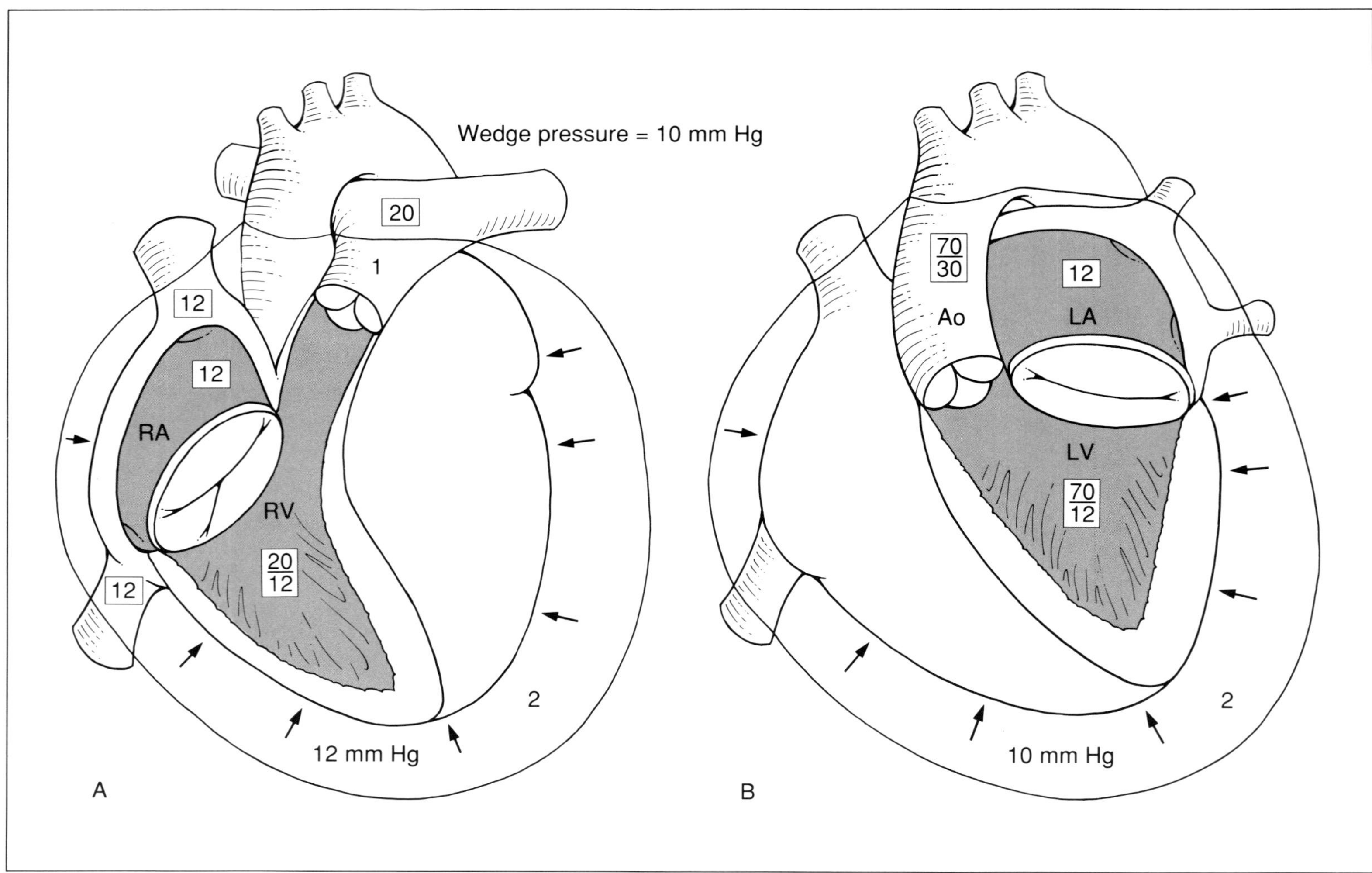

Fig. 22.32 Hemodynamic changes in cardiac tamponade. (**A**) Right heart chambers. (**B**) Left heart chambers. In this example, the hypostatic pressure in the pericardial space is 10 mm Hg. The right atrial and right ventricular end diastolic pressures are increased. The left atrial and left ventricular end diastolic pressures are also increased. Systemic blood pressure is decreased. The pulmonary wedge pressure is elevated.

1 pulmonary trunk
2 pericardial space
RA right atrium
RV right ventricle
LV left ventricle
LA left atrium
AO aorta

despite treatment, intrapericardial pressure continues to exceed right atrial pressure, cardiac output will drop to levels incompatible with life and the patient will die.

Clinically, patients with cardiac tamponade present with increased systemic venous pressure, a small heart, and low systemic arterial pressure (Beck's triad). Because atrial filling is largely confined to ventricular systole, when total cardiac blood volume is the smallest, paradoxical waves are seen in the jugular veins. The jugular venous pressure tracing reveals attenuation of the "Y" descent and preservation, or even exaggeration, of the "X" descent (Fig. 22.33).

"Pulsus paradoxicus" is a classic sign of cardiac tamponade. It denotes a decrease in blood pressure of 10 mm Hg or more during quiet inspiration. Pulsus paradoxicus is believed to result from displacement of the ventricular septum towards the left ventricle during inspiration, which results in decreased left

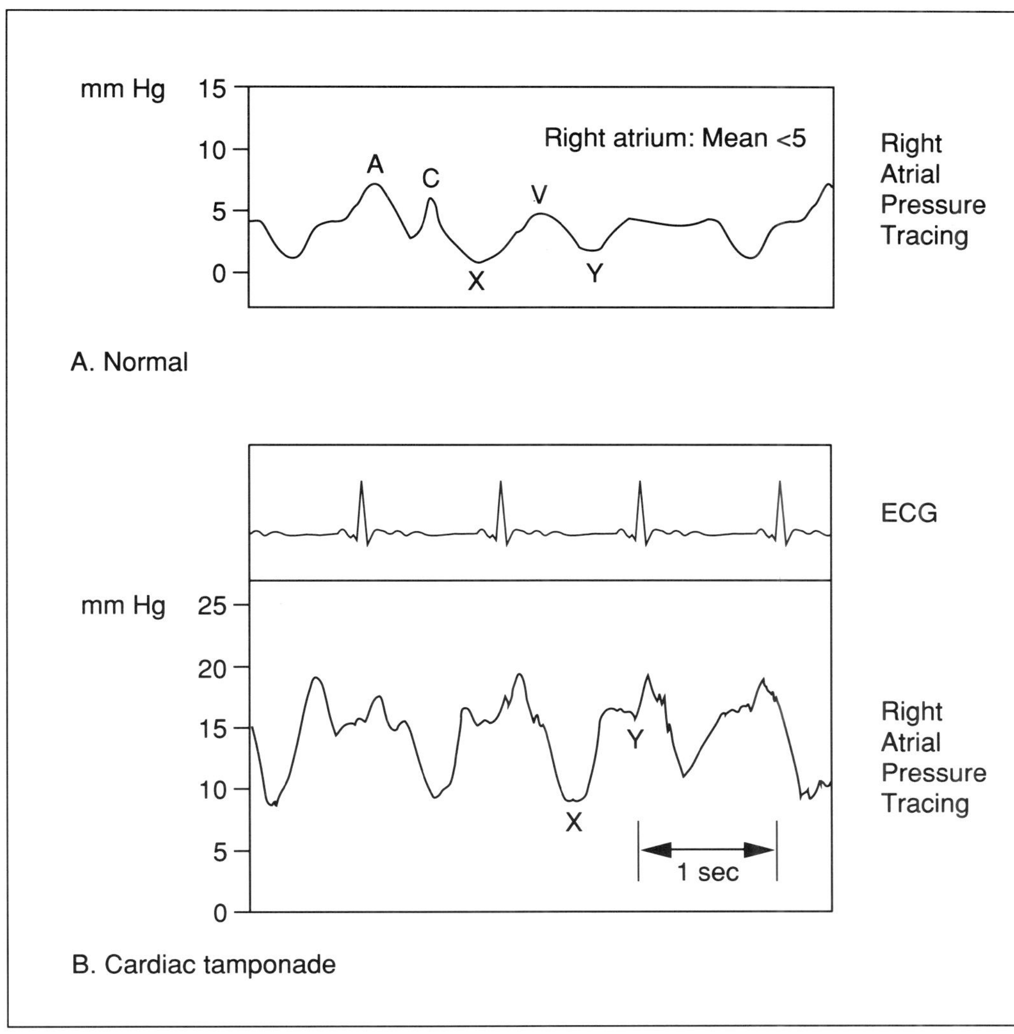

Fig. 22.33 Right atrial pressure tracing in cardiac tamponade. (**A**) Normal tracing (mean pressure 5 mm Hg or less). (**B**) Cardiac tamponade. The right atrial tracing is characterized by a prominent systolic dip (X) and a very small diastolic dip (Y). Because right ventricular filling is restricted, right atrial pressure remains elevated; in this patient the right atrial pressure is 15 mm Hg.

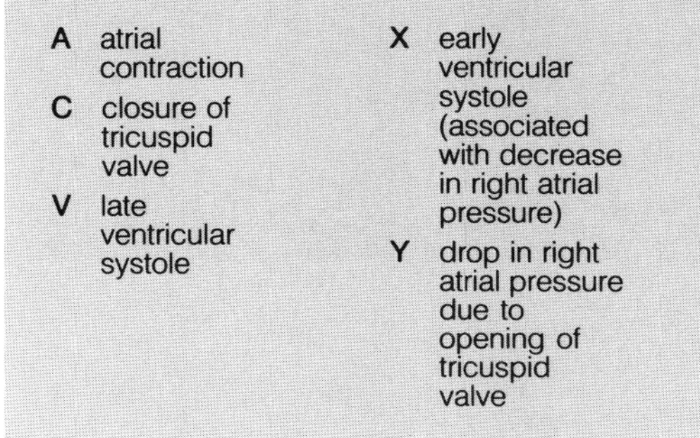

A	atrial contraction	**X**	early ventricular systole (associated with decrease in right atrial pressure)
C	closure of tricuspid valve	**Y**	drop in right atrial pressure due to opening of tricuspid valve
V	late ventricular systole		

ventricular filling and reduced stroke volume (Fig. 22.34). Although right ventricular volume increases during inspiration, total cardiac volume is decreased.

IMAGING AND INVASIVE DIAGNOSIS

Plain Films

The plain film findings in cardiac tamponade are nonspecific; they depend on the rate at which pericardial fluid has been accumulating and the compliance ("stretchability") of the pericardium. When pericardial fluid has been accumulating at a slow rate and pericardial compliance is normal, a large volume of pericardial fluid may accumulate before cardiac tamponade occurs. In these patients, chest films may show a typical pericardial effusion. On the other hand, when the pericardial fluid has accumulated rapidly and the pericardium has not had time to stretch (eg, rupture of the aorta into the pericardium), the cardiac silhouette is usually normal or only slightly enlarged. Calcification or fibrosis of the pericardium may prevent the pericardial cavity from enlarging, in which case cardiac tamponade may occur with a normal or nearly normal cardiovascular silhouette. To sum up, the most common radiographic pattern in patients with cardiac tamponade is a normal cardiovascular silhouette and decreased pulmonary vascularity (Fig. 22.35). A minority of patients have typical plain film findings of pericardial effusion, asymmetrical enlargement of the cardiac silhouette, or generalized cardiomegaly.

Echocardiography

The echocardiographic diagnosis of cardiac tamponade is based on the anatomic and hemodynamic changes associated with this disorder. Diastolic collapse of the free wall of the right ventricle is the most sensitive indicator of cardiac tamponade (Fig. 22.36). However, this finding may not be present in patients with right ventricular hypertrophy or constrictive pericarditis. Other echocardiographic signs of cardiac tamponade include decreased cross-sectional area of the mitral valve orifice, decreased diameter of the left ventricle in diastole, increased diameter of the right ventricle during inspiration, and displacement of the ventricular septum to the left during inspiration.

Cardiac Catheterization and Angiocardiography

Invasive diagnostic procedures are indicated in patients with suspected cardiac tamponade only when noninvasive studies have failed to establish the diagnosis. Cardiac catheterization

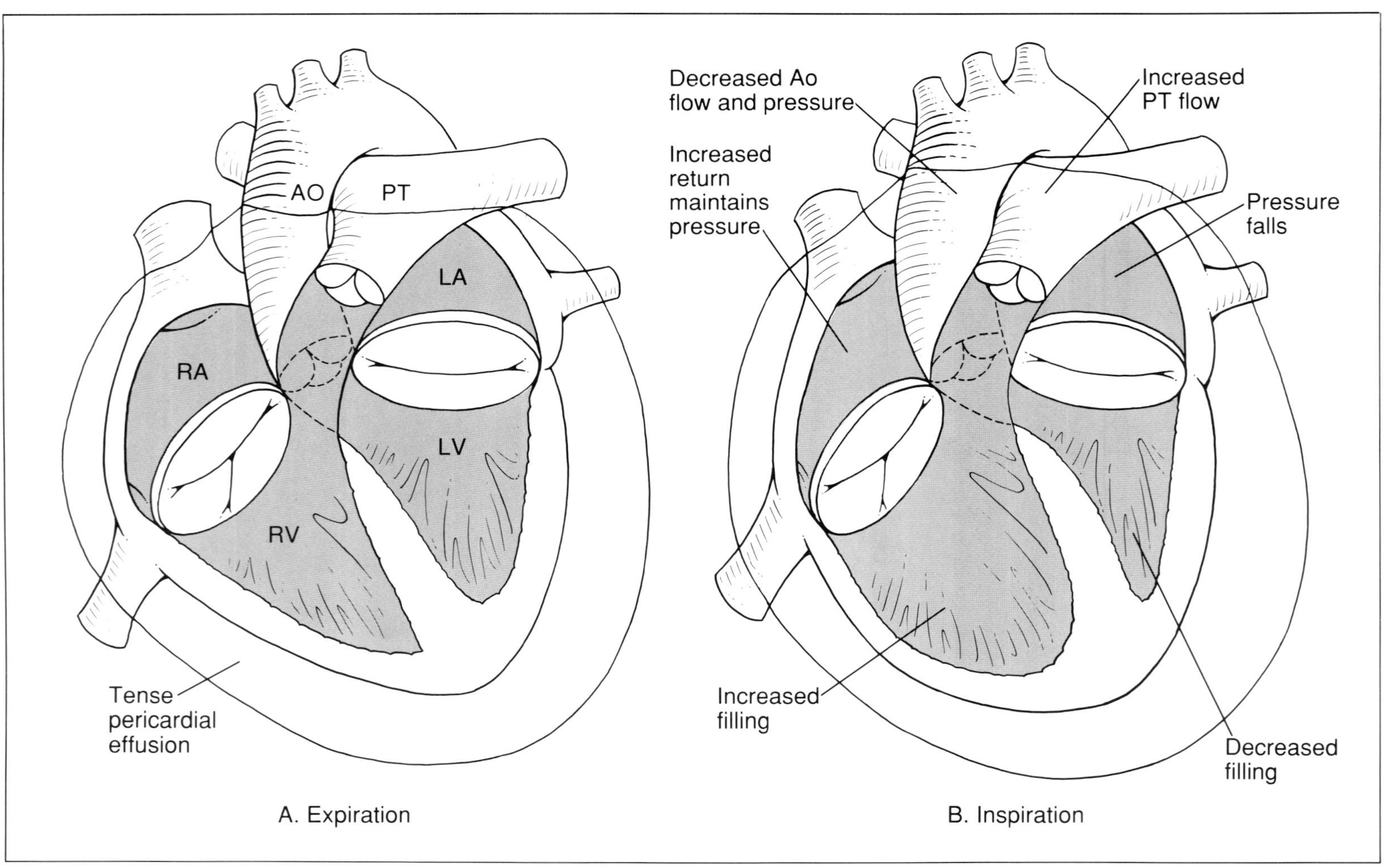

Fig. 22.34 Proposed mechanism for pulsus paradoxicus in cardiac tamponade. Schematic representative of postulated changes in ventricular size and hemodynamics resulting from competitive filling of the ventricles caused by a tense pericardial effusion. During inspiration the increased pressure in the right ventricle causes the ventricular septum to be displaced to the left, decreasing the end diastolic left ventricular volume. This leads to a decrease in aortic flow and a decrease in systemic blood pressure. (Adapted with permission from Cosio FG et al, Chest 71:787, 1977)

AO aorta
LA left atrium
LV left ventricle
PT pulmonary trunk
RA right atrium

reveals a decrease in systemic arterial pressure during expiration. The right atrial and right ventricular end diastolic pressures are both elevated, exceeding the elevated intrapericardial pressure. Throughout most of the cardiac cycle the pulmonary arterial wedge pressure is approximately equal to the intrapericardial pressure (it is lower in early inspiration and higher during expiration). The venous pressure required to maintain a given ventricular diastolic volume and pressure is determined primarily by pericardial rather than ventricular compliance, while the rate at which the right and left ventricles fill is determined by the pulmonary and systemic venous pressures, respectively. As these pressures vary during respiration, they alternately favor right and left ventricular failure, thereby contributing to the development of pulsus paradoxicus.

PNEUMOPERICARDIUM

Pneumopericardium (gas in the pericardial sac) may result from a gas-forming intrapericardial infection; most often, however, it is the result of a spontaneous communication with an adjacent air-containing viscus (esophagus or stomach) or penetrating trauma. Pneumopericardium is a common finding after open

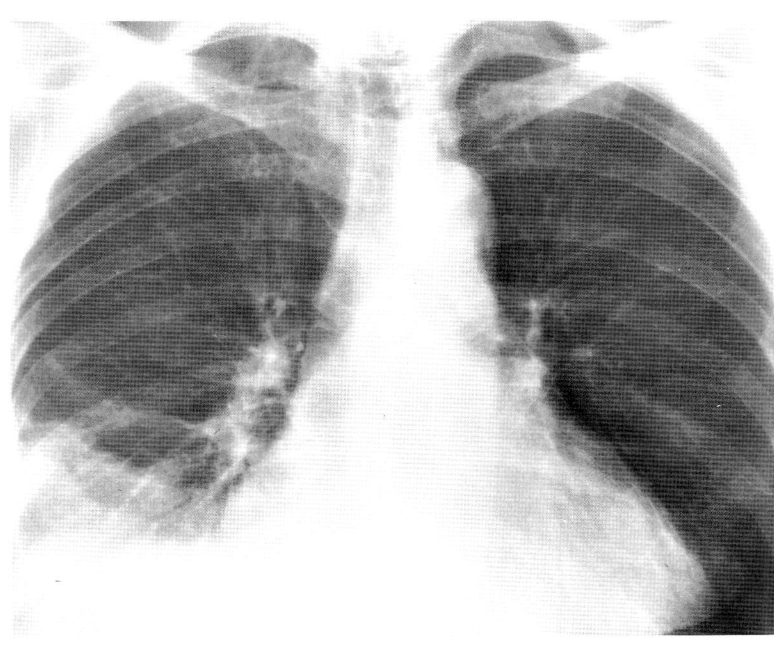

Fig. 22.35 Cardiac tamponade. Frontal chest film shows a normal-sized heart and normal pulmonary vascularity. There is a right pleural effusion. The heart and pulmonary vasculature usually appear normal in patients with cardiac tamponade.

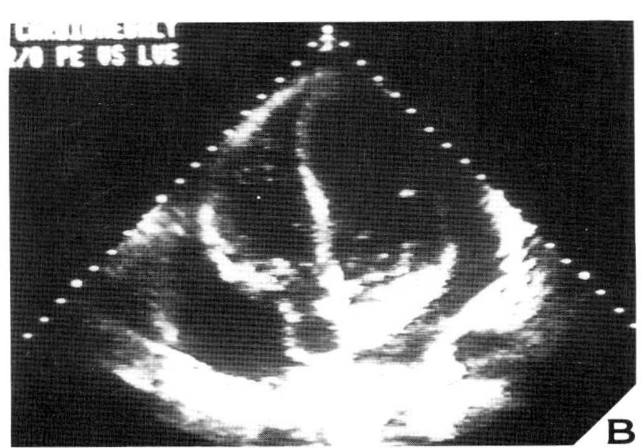

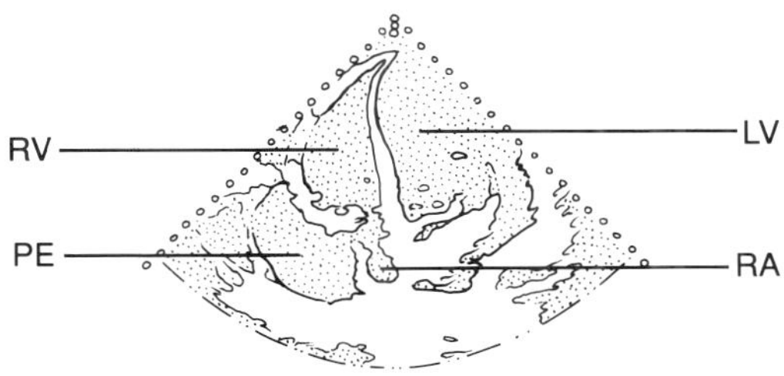

Fig. 22.36 Cardiac tamponade (echocardiographic findings). Apical four-chamber view in (A) systole and (B) diastole. During diastole, the right atrial border and right ventricles are displaced medially and both chambers are partially collapsed. The ventricular septum is displaced to the right.

RV	right ventricle	LA	left atrium
LV	left ventricle	PE	pericardial effusion
RA	right atrium		

cardiac surgery. It may also occur in neonates undergoing mechanical ventilation for respiratory distress syndrome (hyaline membrane disease).

HEMODYNAMICS AND CLINICAL FEATURES

A small pneumopericardium does not produce signs or symptoms, whereas a large one may cause increased intrapericardial pressure with cardiac tamponade (tension pneumopericardium). Such patients present clinically with chest pain and dyspnea. Ausculation typically reveals a loud metallic, splashing sound synchronous with systole (which results from the displacement of gas within the pericardial space as the heart contracts). Other manifestations of tension pneumopericardium include systemic hypotension and jugular venous distension, which reflect the increased right atrial pressure and increased right ventricular end diastolic pressure.

IMAGING

A small amount of air (less than 10 ml) in the pericardial sac of an adult cannot be detected on chest films or CT; however, larger amounts are easily detected with either modality.

Intrapericardial air tends to accumulate in the left subpulmonic recess, an extension of the transverse sinus. Air in this recess appears on the frontal projection as a lucency along the left heart border; the left atrial appendage and pulmonary trunk (structures that are not sharply outlined in the absence of intrapericardial air) are displayed in exquisite detail (Fig. 22.37). Intrapericardial air also accumulates in the superior and anterior paracardiac recesses, which are bounded posteriorly by the anterior wall of the aorta and inferiorly by the anteroinferior aspect of the right ventricle. Air in the superior and anterior paracardiac recesses is easily identified on the lateral projection (Fig. 22.38). Air tends to collect beneath the anterior chest wall in a supine patient; therefore, a small pneumopericardium may not be appreciated unless a cross-table lateral or lateral decubitus projection is obtained.

The possibility of a tension pneumopericardium should be strongly considered when there is a large amount of intrapericardial air and the heart appears unusually small (Fig. 22.39). The volume of gas needed to produce cardiac tamponade varies from patient to patient, depending on the rate at which it is accumulating and the distensibility of the pericardium.

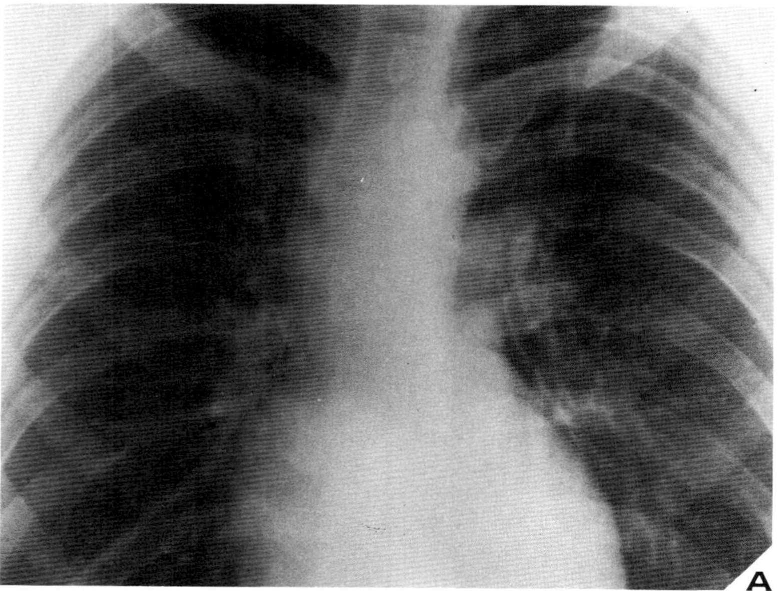

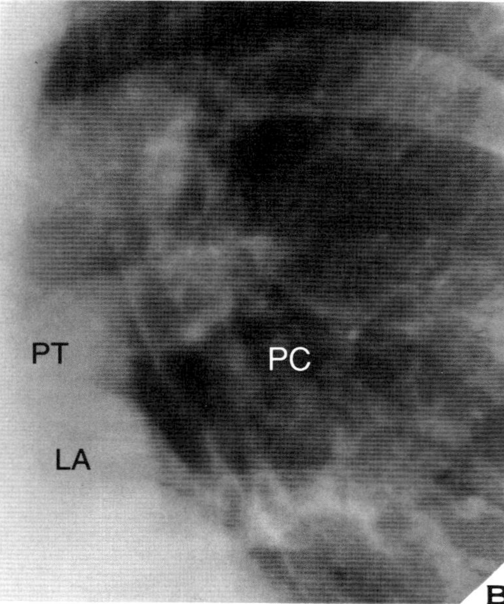

Fig. 22.37 Traumatic pneumopericardium. (A) Frontal chest film (obtained shortly after a penetrating chest injury) shows a small air collection along the left upper heart border. (B) Close-up view shows unusually sharp definition of the pulmonary trunk (PT), left atrial appendage (LA), and the parietal pericardium (PC), indicating that air is present in the left paracardiac recess.

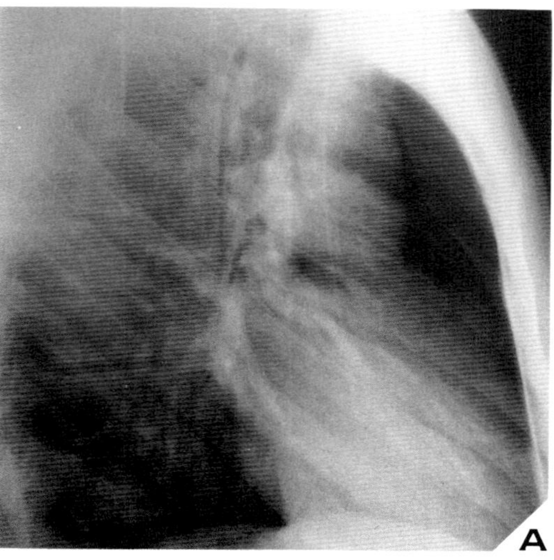

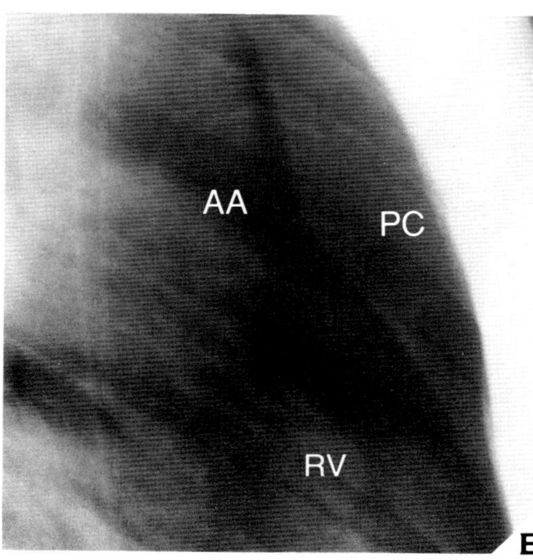

Fig. 22.38 Localized pneumopericardium. (A) Lateral chest film shows the anterior border of the ascending aorta (AA) and the superior and inferior aspects of the right ventricle (RV), indicating that the air is in the superior pericardial and right paracardiac recesses. Note that the intrapericardial air does not extend beyond the midascending aorta. (B) Close-up of A. (PC = parietal layer of pericardium).

CONSTRICTIVE PERICARDITIS

In this disorder, scarring of the parietal and visceral pericardium secondary to pericardial inflammation is severe enough to compress the heart and interfere with cardiac filling.

PATHOLOGY

The pericardial layers are fused together, producing a fibrotic, thickened pericardium measuring more than 5 mm in thickness; the pathologic process typically extends into the epicardium. Although the entire pericardium is involved, the areas over the left atrium and left ventricle tend to be most severely affected. Approximately 50 percent of patients with constrictive pericarditis have pericardial calcification; however, it should be emphasized that the *absence* of pericardial calcification does not exclude this disorder, and that some patients with a thick, heavily calcified pericardium do not have clinical manifestations of constrictive pericarditis. When pericardial calcification occurs over the left ventricle it is usually extensive.

PATHOPHYSIOLOGY AND HEMODYNAMIC FEATURES

The thick, nondistensible pericardium restricts ventricular filling; because the ventricles cannot fully expand during diastole, stroke volume is decreased. The mode of ventricular filling is also abnormal. In early diastole, ventricular filling is rapid; ventricular capacity is quickly reached and late diastolic filling is decreased or absent. The ventricular pressure curve displays an early deep decline followed by a high end diastolic plateau ("square root sign"), reflecting the restricted distensibility of the ventricular chamber (see Chapter 19).

CLINICAL FEATURES

The severity of the clinical manifestations depends on the degree of hemodynamic impairment. The usual symptoms are weakness, peripheral edema, and abdominal swelling. Physical examination typically reveals neck vein distension, hepatomegaly, ascites, and peripheral edema. Pulsus paradoxicus is occasionally observed, although less commonly than in cardiac tamponade.

Constrictive pericarditis may be associated with pericardial effusion and pericardial thickening, a complex that has been termed "effusive constrictive pericarditis." This disorder is particularly common in patients with nephrogenic ("uremic") pericarditis. The hemodynamic pattern is the same as that of noneffusive constrictive pericarditis: however, unlike the latter condition, diastolic ventricular restriction persists even after the fluid is removed. There is thus no change in the jugular venous pulse wave, which reflects the variation of right atrial pressure with respiration, after the fluid is removed.

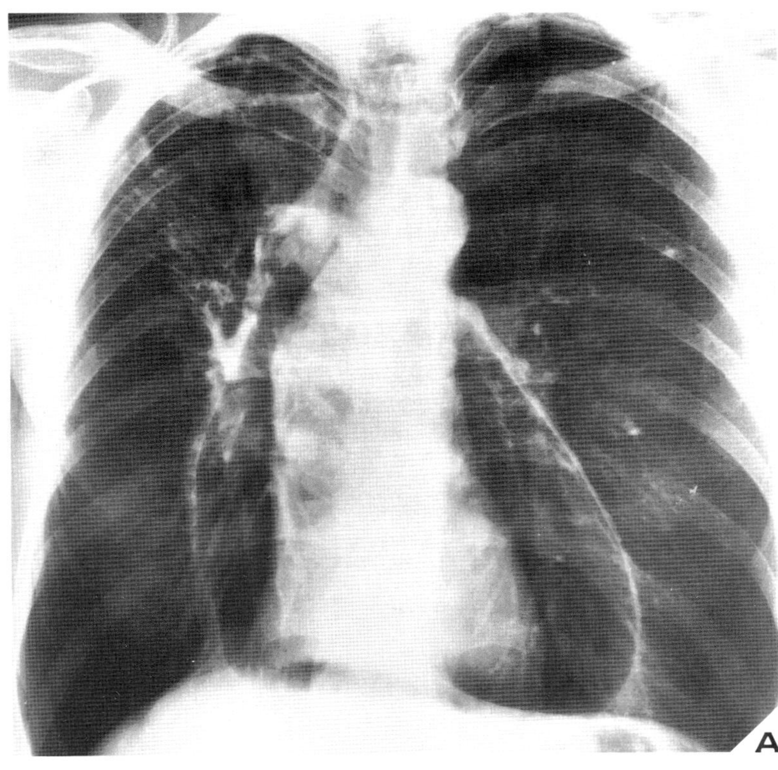

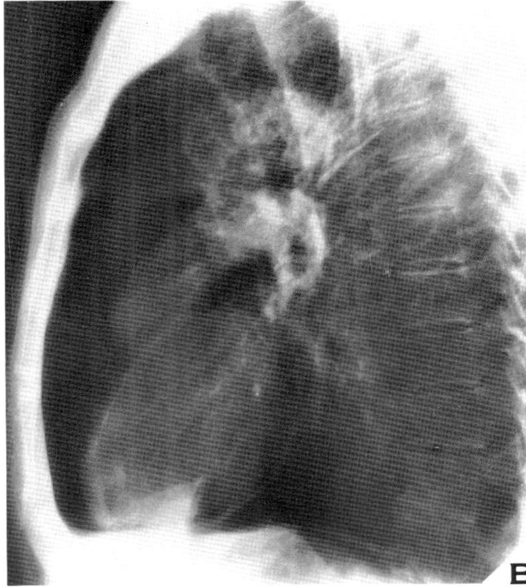

Fig. 22.39 Cardiac tamponade secondary to tension pneumopericardium. Erect (A) posteroanterior and (B) lateral chest film show a massive pneumopericardium with air surrounding the heart; the ascending aorta and pulmonary trunk are sharply outlined by the intrapericardial air most of which is in the superior right paracardiac and the lateral pericardial recesses. (Only a small amount of air has collected behind the left ventricle, in the posterior portion of the pericardial sac.) The heart is very small and the pulmonary vasculature is decreased, indicating the presence of cardiac tamponade.

IMAGING AND INVASIVE DIAGNOSIS

Plain Films

Thickening of the pericardium can often be appreciated on plain films (the radiographic findings are the same as those described for pericardial effusion). Pericardial calcification can be detected radiographically in approximately 50 percent of patients with constrictive pericarditis, typically appearing as a curvilinear opacity that conforms to the contours of the pericardial sac on frontal and lateral projections (Fig. 22.40). It may be difficult to differentiate pericardial from myocardial calcifica-

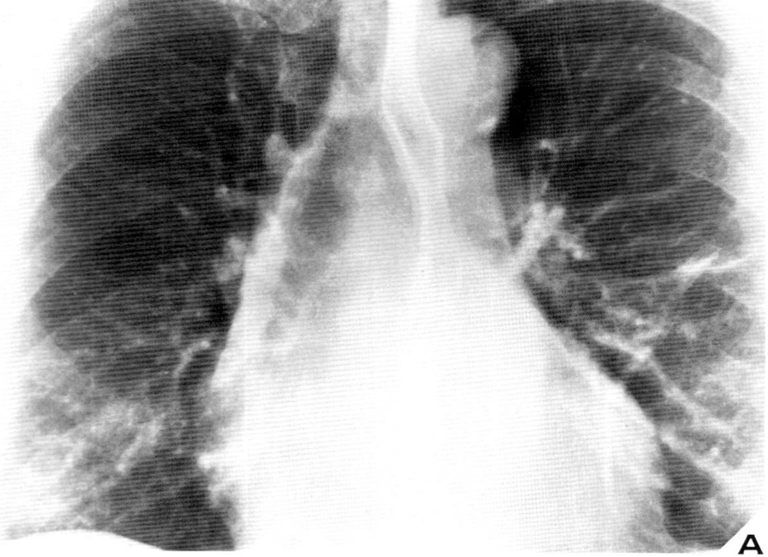

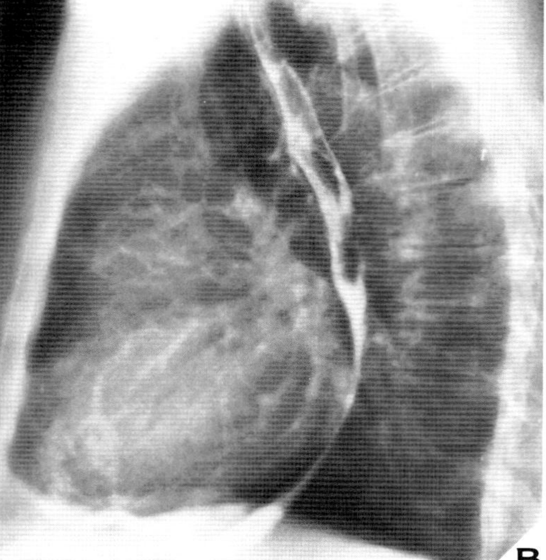

Fig. 22.40 Constrictive pericarditis. (A) Frontal- and (B) lateral chest films show mild cardiomegaly with left atrial enlargement (note posterior displacement of the exophagus) and evidence of pulmonary venous hypertension (note cephalization pattern). There is extensive calcification of left, inferior, anterior and posterior portions of the pericardium in this patient, who had clinical evidence of constrictive pericarditis.

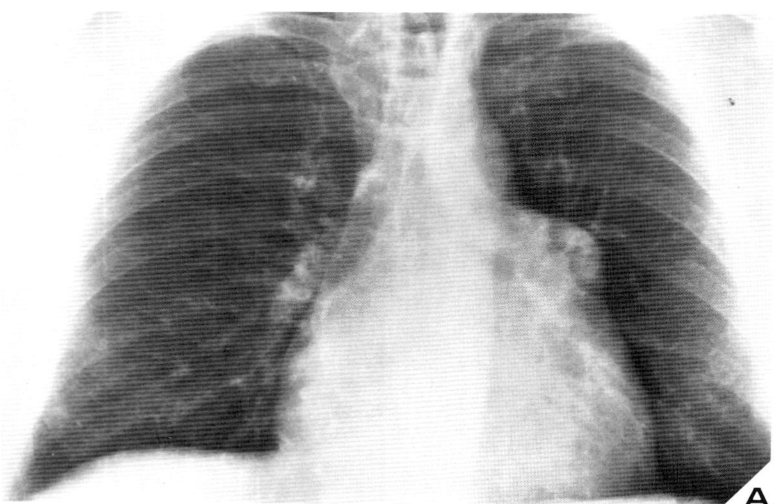

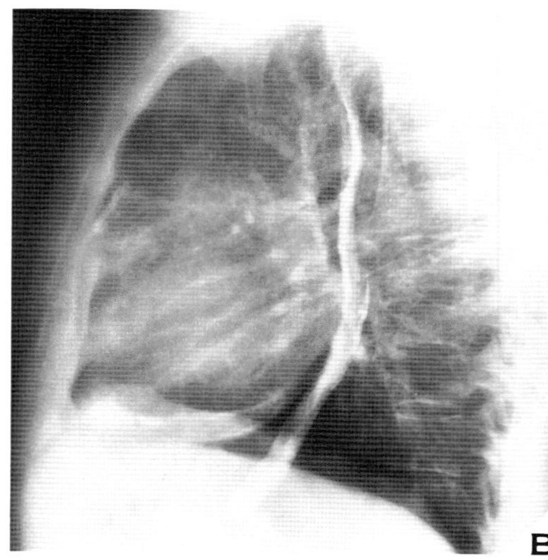

Fig. 22.41 Pericardial calcification without constrictive pericarditis. (A) Frontal and (B) lateral chest films show calcifications in the anterior, inferior, and posterior aspects of the pericardium. The pulmonary vasculature is normal and the left atrium is only minimally enlarged. There were no clinical manifestations of constrictive pericarditis.

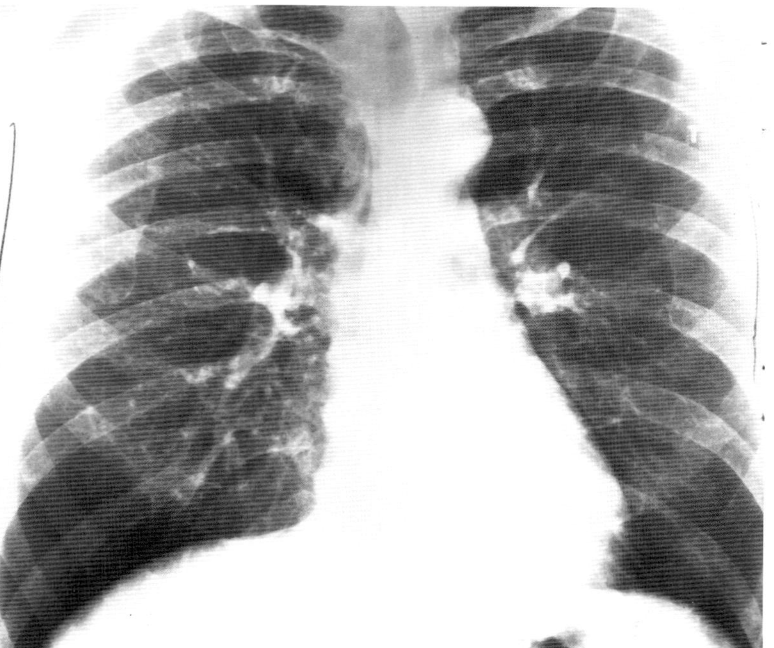

Fig. 22.42 Constrictive pericarditis. Frontal chest film shows a small heart with diminished pulmonary vascularity. No calcifications are identified.

tion in certain locations (eg, over the left ventricle). The pericardium over the anterior and inferior surfaces of the heart is the most frequent site of calcification. Calcification over the left ventricle is less common, and is typically associated with severe ventricular restriction. Pericardial calcification over the left atrium is rare.

The heart is usually of normal size, although it may be slightly enlarged. The left atrium is often enlarged. There is usually evidence of pulmonary venous hypertension (cephalization pattern), and interstitial pulmonary edema is sometimes apparent (Fig. 22.40). The differential diagnosis of this radiographic pattern includes constrictive pericarditis, mitral valvular stenosis, and restricted cardiomyopathy. Although the presence of pericardial calcification favors the diagnosis of constrictive pericarditis, these conditions usually cannot be differentiated on the plain film findings alone. As noted above, pericardial calcification may be seen in patients without clinical evidence of constrictive pericarditis (Fig. 22.41) and is absent in approximately 50 percent of patients with this disorder (Fig. 22.42). Although distension of the superior vena cava and/or azygos vein favors the diagnosis of constrictive pericarditis, this radiographic sign is often absent even in patients with obvious jugular venous distension on physical examination.

Echocardiography

On echocardiography, pericardial thickening appears as two parallel moving echoes of equal intensity, 1 to 3 mm apart. Poor resolution can sometimes lead to an incorrect diagnosis of pericardial thickening. Pericardial calcification appears as an echogenic line over the surface of the heart. Acoustic shadowing may be present. Other echocardiographic findings include flattening of the posterior wall of the right ventricle during diastole (Fig. 22.43), abnormal septal motion, early opening of the pulmonic valve, and dilatation of the superior and inferior venae cavae. However, these signs are not specific for constrictive pericarditis (they may also be seen in restricted cardiomyopathy). Restriction of ventricular wall motion, particularly that of the free walls of both ventricles, increases the apparent displacement of the septum, a phenomenon analogous to the increased motion of the septal arteries observed on coronary arteriography (Figs. 22.47 and 22.48). An abnormal pericardial echo may indicate the presence of abnormal tissue (eg, tumor) or other accumulated material in the pericardial sac, another cause of systolic ventricular restriction.

CT and MRI

CT has become an important tool in the diagnosis of constrictive pericarditis. The normal fibrous pericardium appears as a 1- to 2-mm band of soft tissue density overlying the surface of the heart (delineated by the epicardial fat). In most cases of early constrictive pericarditis, the thickened pericardium can be identified as a curvilinear band 5 to 20 mm thick. A similar appearance can be seen in patients with neoplastic infiltration of the pericardium, which produces a similar hemodynamic distur-

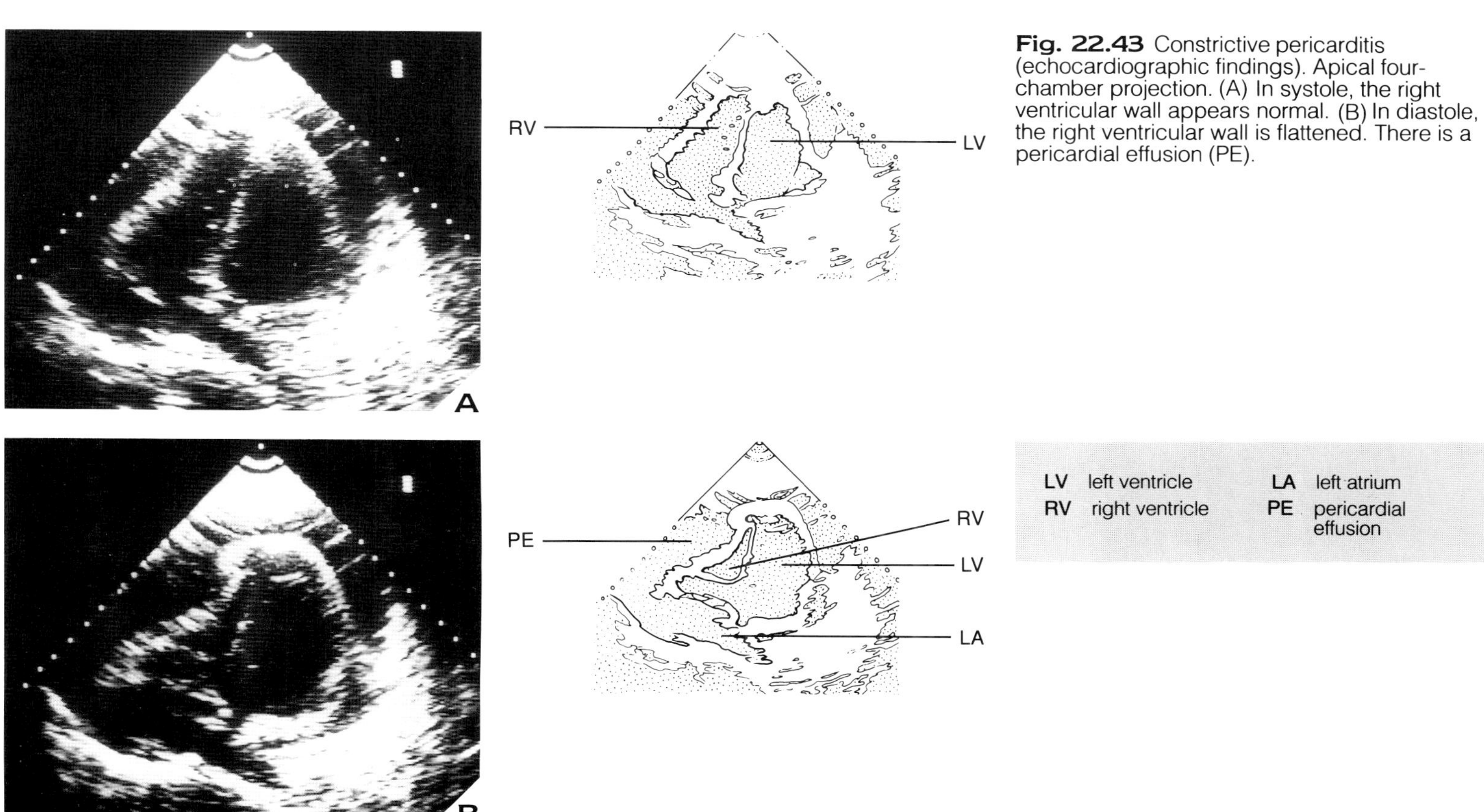

Fig. 22.43 Constrictive pericarditis (echocardiographic findings). Apical four-chamber projection. (A) In systole, the right ventricular wall appears normal. (B) In diastole, the right ventricular wall is flattened. There is a pericardial effusion (PE).

bance (Fig. 22.44). Pericardial calcification, particularly in the vicinity of the atrioventricular groove, is clearly shown by CT (Fig. 22.45). As noted earlier, a thickened or calcified pericardium does not necessarily indicate the presence of a dynamic functional disturbance.

Other CT findings associated with constrictive pericarditis include dilatation of the inferior and/or superior venae cavae, deformity of the right ventricular contour, and abnormal angulation of the ventricular septum. These findings, all of which can also be seen in restricted cardiomyopathy, are more clearly depicted by echocardiography.

Pericardial thickening of 2 mm or greater is clearly shown by MRI. On T1-weighted spin–echo images, the thickened pericardium has a signal of low, intermediate, or high intensity. Thickening of the visceral and parietal pericardium is easily distinguished from pericardial fluid, which has a decreased or very low signal intensity. (Both pericardial fluid and thickened pericardium are seen in patients with effusive constrictive pericarditis.) Another feature useful in differentiating pericardial fluid from the thickened pericardium associated with constrictive pericarditis is the distribution of the signal: whereas pericardial fluid tends to accumulate in the anterosuperior recess, thickened pericardium is mainly related to the ventricles.

Cardiac Catheterization

The presence of characteristic intracardiac hemodynamic changes is important in establishing the diagnosis of constrictive pericarditis. Classically, the end diastolic pressure is elevated to an equal degree in the right atrium, right ventricle, left atrium, and pulmonary trunk. The atrial pressure curve demonstrates an exaggerated "X" descent, attenuation or absence of the "Y" descent, and elevated "a" and "v" waves. The right ventricular pressure tracing reveals a short early diastolic filling phase with a low peak pressure, followed by a sustained elevation of the diastolic filling pressure; late in diastole there is equalization of right and left ventricular pressures. This pattern, which is also seen in other disorders associated with restricted ventricular filling (eg, restricted cardiomyopathy), has been called the "square root sign" (see Chapter 19).

Combined echocardiographic–manometric techniques have been used to assess constrictive pericarditis and other disorders associated with ventricular restriction; although these new techniques show promise, they have not yet been validated in clinical practice.

Angiocardiography

The degree of pericardial thickening is assessed by examining the contour, thickness, and motion of the right atrial wall after a

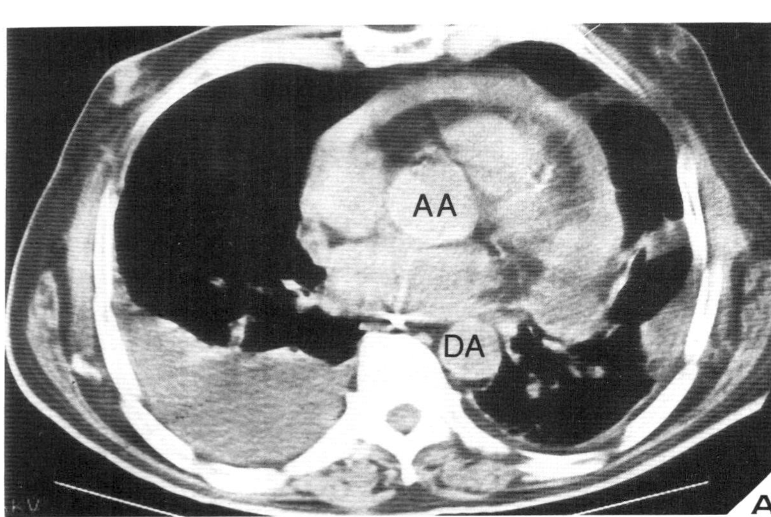

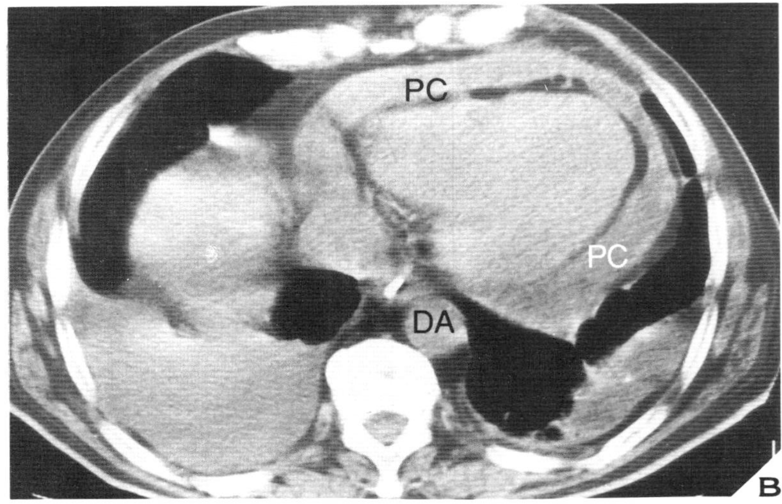

Fig. 22.44 Constrictive pericarditis (CT findings). Contrast-enhanced CT (A) at the level of the mediastinum and (B) at the level of the ventricles in a patient with lymphomatous infiltration of the pericardium demonstrate marked thickening of the pericardium (PC), particularly over the ventricles. Fluid is present in the anterior paracardial recess. Cardiac catheterization revealed diastolic ventricular restriction. (AA = ascending aorta; DA = descending thoracic aorta)

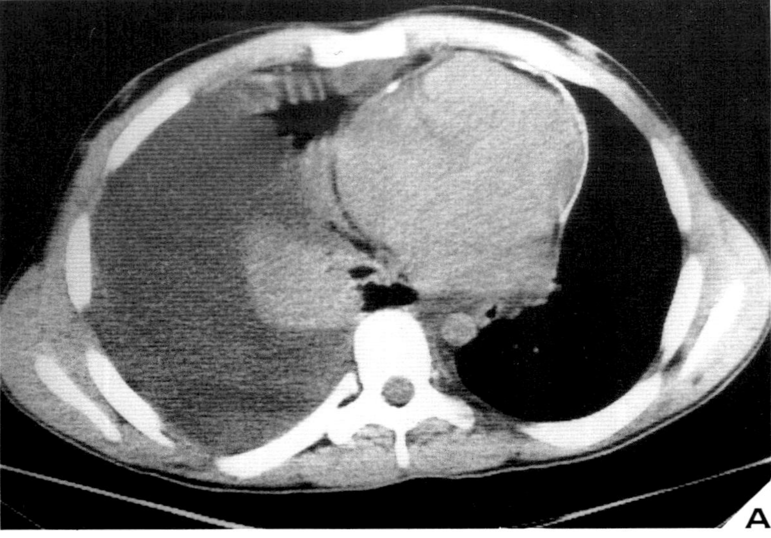

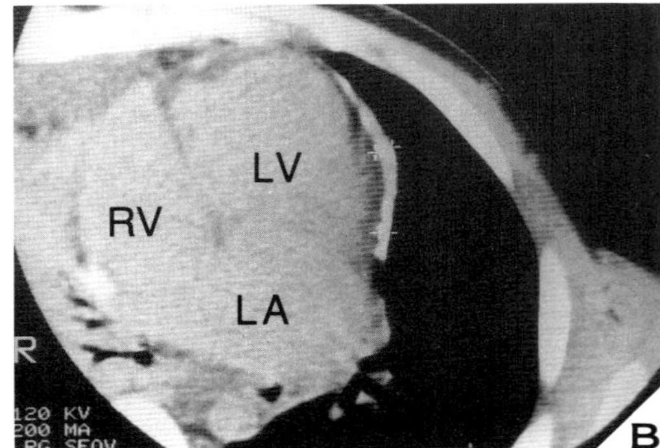

Fig. 22.45 Constrictive pericarditis with calcification of the pericardium (CT findings). (A) Conventional and (B) magnified images of contrast-enhanced CT at the level of the ventricles demonstrate calcification of the anterior and lateral pericardium. The calcification is densest over the free wall of the left ventricle (LV). The calcified pericardium measures 5 mm in thickness. There is a large right pleural effusion. (LA = left atrium; RV = right ventricle)

right atrial injection. Separation of the right atrial lumen from the cardiac contour by 5 mm or more can be taken as evidence of pericardial thickening (Fig. 22.46). Medial displacement of the right atrial wall during diastole is another important angiographic sign of constrictive pericarditis; in severe cases, the right atrial border becomes concave during diastole. This finding is not specific for constrictive pericarditis, however, and may occasionally be seen in the absence of cardiac or pericardial disease. Abnormal filling of the ventricles, which is clearly shown by cardiac catheterization, is not well demonstrated by angiocardiography.

Coronary arteriography may be helpful in differentiating constrictive pericarditis from restricted cardiomyopathy. Exaggerated displacement of the septal arteries is characteristic of constrictive pericarditis, which spares the ventricular septum (Figs. 22.47 and 22.48). Conversely, diminished excursion of the septal arteries is a common finding in restricted cardiomyopathy, which almost always involves the ventricular septum.

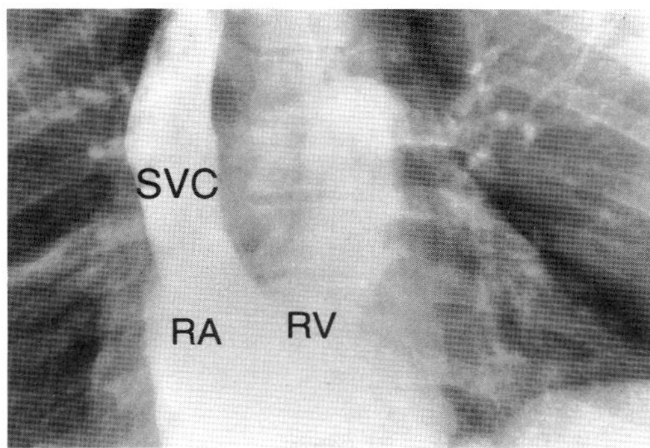

Fig. 22.46 Constrictive pericarditis (angiocardiographic findings). Right atriogram demonstrates abnormal separation (more than 5 mm) between the border of the opacified right atrial chamber (RA) and the border of the cardiac silhouette. The right atrial border is unusually straight. (Its normally convex contour is usually preserved in patients with unconstrictive pericardial effusions.) When the constriction is more severe, the right atrial deformity is more pronounced; in the most severe cases, the right atrial border may be concave. (SVC = superior vena cava)

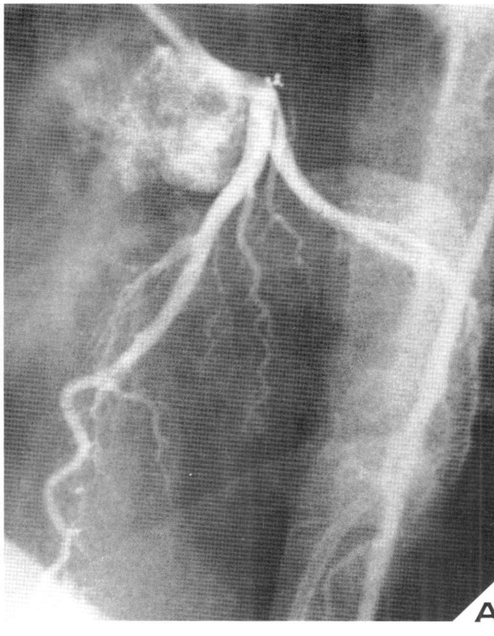

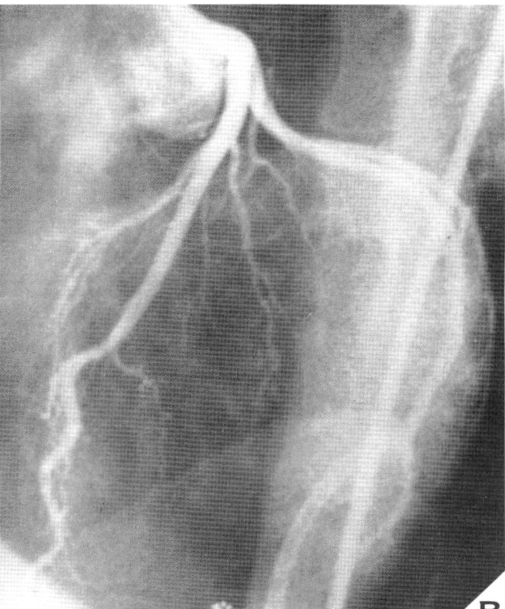

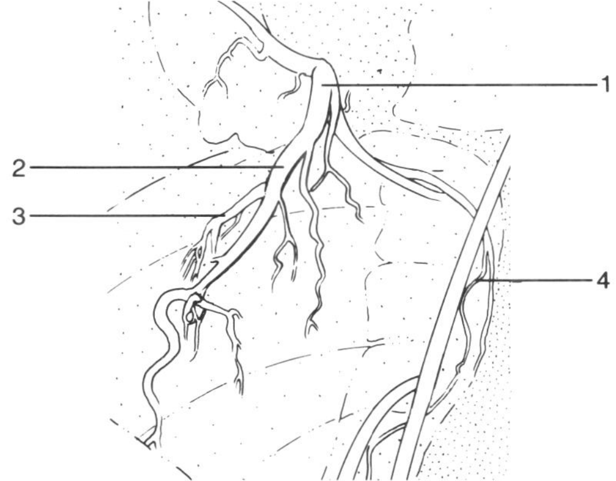

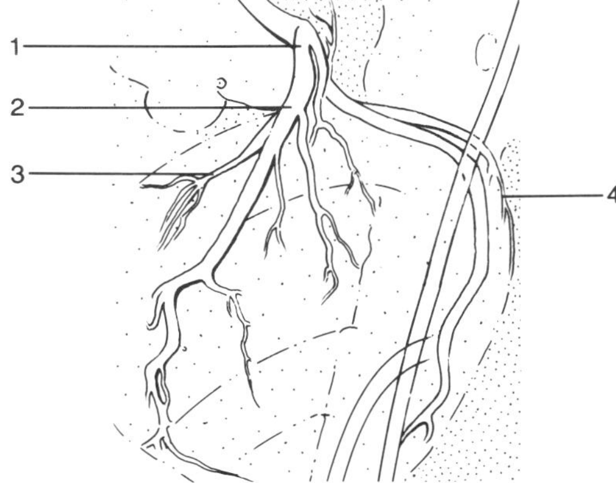

Fig. 22.47 Normal displacement of the septal arteries. Left coronary arteriograms (left anterior oblique projection with craniocaudal angulation) in (A) systole and (B) diastole show moderate displacement of the septal branches of the left anterior descending coronary artery with respect to the main trunk and the marginal branches of the circumflex coronary artery.

1 left main coronary artery
2 left anterior descending coronary artery
3 septal arteries
4 marginal arteries

DIAGNOSIS OF CONSTRICTIVE PERICARDITIS

The diagnosis of constrictive pericarditis is suggested by the clinical history, laboratory data, and the physical signs observed at the bedside. Typical plain film findings—pericardial calcification and pulmonary venous hypertension associated with a normal cardiac silhouette or left atrial enlargement—lend further support. (In the absence of pericardial calcification, these findings would favor mitral valvular stenosis or restrictive cardiomyopathy.) Echocardiography, which can exclude mitral valvular disease, dilated cardiomyopathy, pericardial effusion, and other processes causing similar symptoms, can therefore narrow the differential diagnosis. If angiocardiography demonstrates normal systolic ventricular function, the only remaining possibilities are restrictive cardiomyopathy and constrictive pericarditis. The demonstration of thickened pericardium by CT or MRI is strong evidence in favor of constrictive pericarditis; if the pericardium is of normal thickness, a transcutaneous endocardial biopsy may be necessary to identify an infiltrative process causing restricted cardiomyopathy. On occasion, it may not be possible, even after exhaustive diagnostic evaluation, to differentiate constrictive pericarditis and restrictive cardiomyopathy. In such cases thoracotomy may be needed to establish the diagnosis.

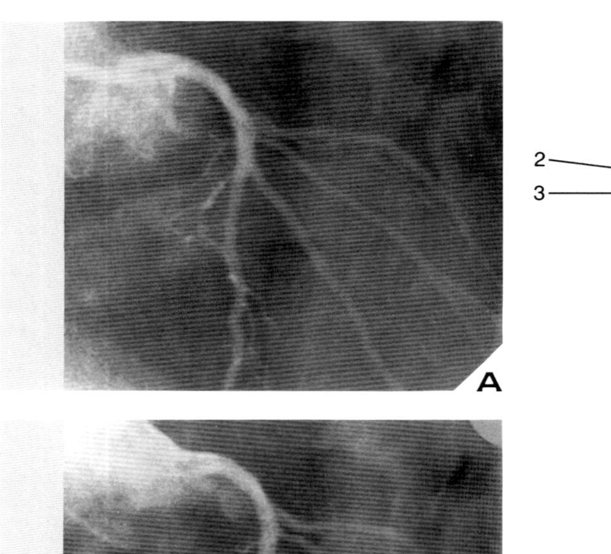

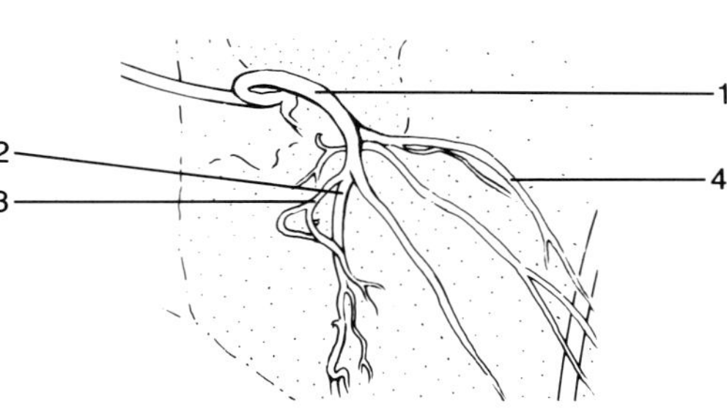

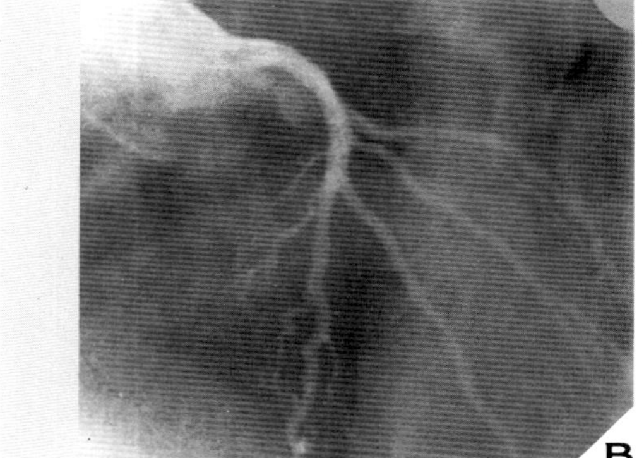

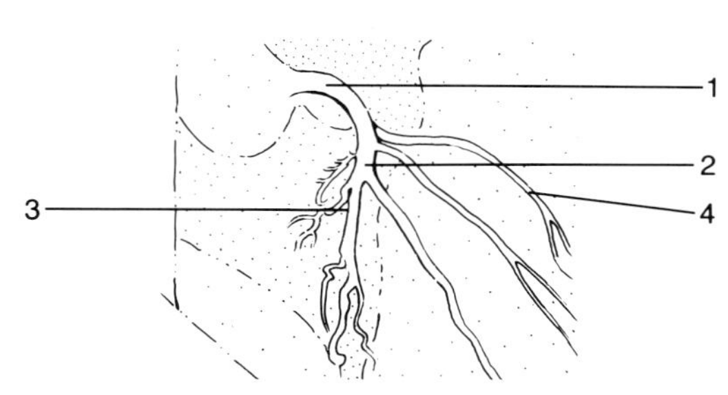

Fig. 22.48 Exaggerated displacement of septal arteries in constrictive pericarditis . Left coronary arteriograms (left anterior oblique projection with craniocaudal angulation) in (A) systole and (B) diastole show exaggerated displacement of the septal branches, some of which overlap the left anterior descending artery during diastole.

1 left main coronary artery
2 left anterior descending coronary artery
3 septal arteries
4 marginal arteries

CHAPTER 23

Infective Endocarditis

BACTERIAL ENDOCARDITIS

Bacterial endocarditis is an infectious process of the endocardium which almost always involves the cardiac valves. Caused by bacteria of varying pathogenicity, it commonly results in malfunction of the affected valve and the adjacent myocardium and is associated with a variety of systemic sequelae.

PATHOLOGY

Bacterial endocarditis occurs in two varieties: acute bacterial endocarditis (ABE) and subacute bacterial endocarditis (SBE).

ACUTE BACTERIAL ENDOCARDITIS

The acute form is characterized by vegetations which nearly always cluster on the surface of a valve; more than one valve may be affected (Fig. 23.1). The vegetations may be small and granular or large and polypoid. The lesions are typically located along the line of closure of the leaflets, but other portions of the structure may be affected. When the aortic valve is involved, the vegetations are usually found on the ventricular aspect of the affected leaflets; when the mitral valve is involved, they typically occur on the atrial surface. Vegetations may extend from the margin of the valve to the adjacent endocardium (mitral or tricuspid valve) or intima (aortic or pulmonic valve), or from one valve surface to another. Vegetations on the aortic cusps

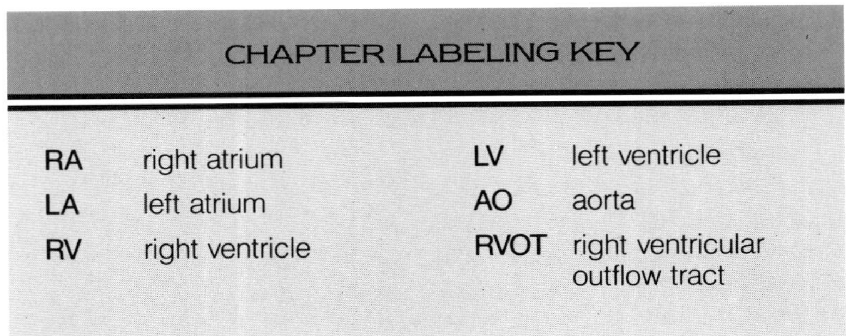

CHAPTER LABELING KEY

RA	right atrium	LV	left ventricle
LA	left atrium	AO	aorta
RV	right ventricle	RVOT	right ventricular outflow tract

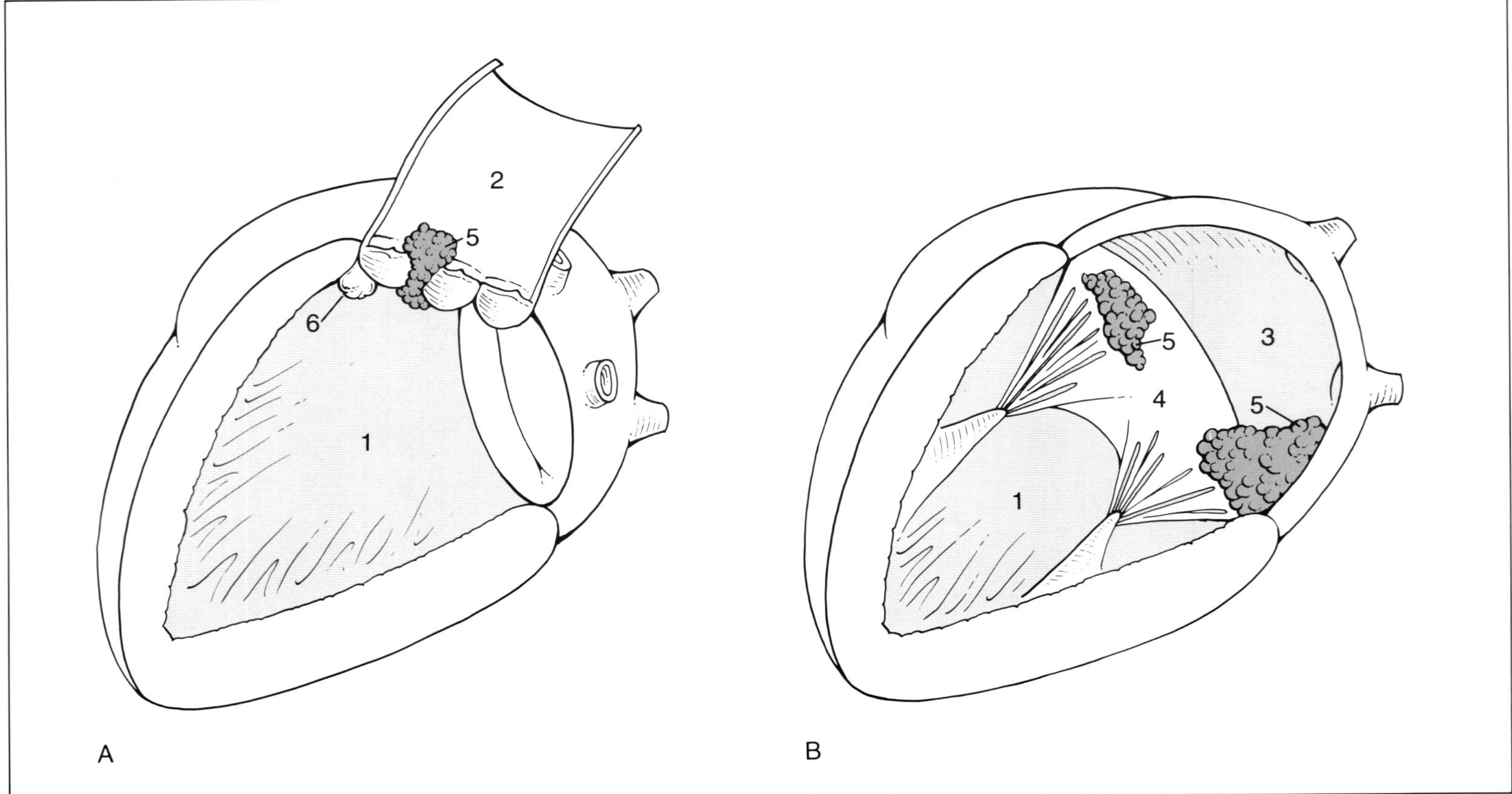

1	left ventricle	4	anterior leaflet of mitral valve
2	aorta	5	vegetations
3	left atrium	6	abscess

Fig. 23.1 Acute bacterial endocarditis. Typical lesions are shown diagramatically. (A) Aortic valve. Note vegetations at the commissures between right and left coronary cusps. In addition, there is an abscess beneath the left coronary cusp. (B) Mitral valve. Note vegetations in the anterolateral and posteromedial commissures, one of which extends into the left atrium.

may extend to the ventricular endocardium and the anterior leaflet of the mitral valve. Vegetations may also occur on the endocardium near the affected structure, or on the ventricular septum, chordae tendineae, or papillary muscles; rarely, the vegetations are confined to the mural endocardium, sparing the valves.

Typically, acute vegetations are broadly implanted and their surface is soft and friable. Pieces of necrotic valve tissue and vegetations may break off, leaving behind an irregular surface to which fresh thrombus will occasionally adhere. The free margin of the affected leaflet or leaflets may become frayed and irregular. The chordae tendineae may become ulcerated and eventually rupture, and perforation of the leaflets or even of the ventricular septum may occur. The valve tissue itself may become grossly inflamed and edematous. The necrotic process often results in thinning of the valve leaflets and/or endocardium, which can lead to rupture or aneurysm formation (Fig. 23.2). Some aneurysms actually represent abscesses, which become cavities within the endocardium in the process of healing. (Most abscesses secondary to ABE of the mitral and tricuspid valves develop at the insertion of the leaflets.) Aneurysms of the aortic cusps are more properly termed "pseudoaneurysms," because they result from destruction of the wall of the sinus of Valsalva; progression of the destructive process may lead to perforation into the pericardial space or a cardiac chamber (usually the right atrium or right ventricle) (see Chapters 9 and 27).

SUBACUTE BACTERIAL ENDOCARDITIS

The lesions of SBE are similar to those of ABE; however, the vegetations are smaller. Not infrequently, the vegetations extend beyond the borders of the leaflet onto the adjacent mural endocardium. In time, the vegetations become less friable and are more firmly incorporated into the underlying valve. During the healing process the valve leaflets become fibrotic, often with focal calcium deposits. The deformed leaflets do not effectively seal the valvular orifice, resulting in valvular incompetence.

CLINICAL FEATURES

ACUTE BACTERIAL ENDOCARDITIS

Seventy-five percent of cases of ABE involve normally formed valves. Risk factors in such cases include alcohol abuse, drug abuse and underlying malignancy. ABE involving a normal valve has a worse prognosis than ABE involving a malformed valve, even in immunocompromised patients.

Many microorganisms have been implicated as causative

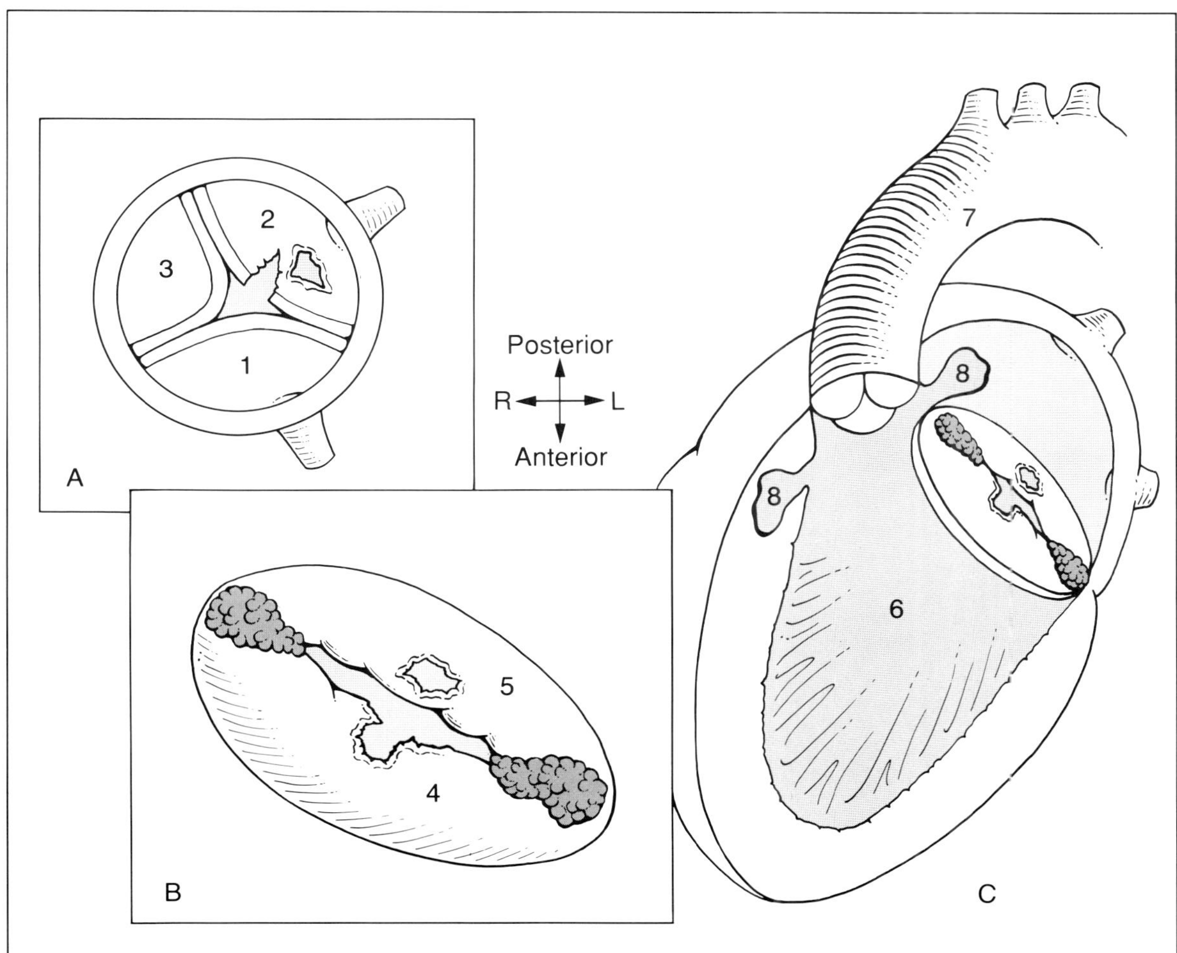

Fig. 23.2 Late sequelae of acute bacterial endocarditis. Typical late lesions are illustrated diagrammatically. (A) Aortic valve. Note perforation of the left coronary cusp, with perforation also of its free borders. (B) Mitral valve. Note perforation of the posterior and anterior leaflets. Granulations are present in the commissures. (C) Left ventricle and aorta (viewed from lateral aspect). Two pseudoaneurysms are shown: one is excavating the septum and the other is extending from beneath the aortic valve towards the posterosuperior portion of the mitral valve. These lesions most likely represent healed abscesses.

1 right coronary cusp of aortic valve
2 left coronary cusp of aortic valve
3 non coronary cusp of aortic valve
4 anterior mitral leaflet
5 posterior mitral leaflet
6 left ventricle
7 aorta
8 pseudoaneurysm

agents in ABE (Fig. 23.3). The most common is *Staphylococcus aureus*. ABE should be considered whenever this organism is recovered from a blood specimen; the diagnosis of ABE is virtually certain when positive blood cultures are repeatedly obtained over a period of several days. (Blood cultures obtained before the institution of antibiotic therapy are positive in more than 95 percent of cases.) *S. aureus* is usually the causative agent in right-sided ABE, which occurs almost exclusively in intravenous drug abusers.

Patients with ABE typically present with signs of sepsis; however, owing to the abrupt onset of the disease, splenomegaly is uncommon. There is usually evidence of congestive heart failure (rales), and auscultation reveals a new or intensified heart murmur. Many patients present with intractable heart failure secondary to valvular insufficiency, particularly when the aortic valve is involved (Fig. 23.4). Congestive heart failure may develop acutely when a previously normal aortic valve is infected with *S. aureus* or another highly virulent organism.

Patients with ABE of the mitral or aortic valve frequently have signs and symptoms of peripheral vascular occlusion secondary to systemic embolization. Any part of the body, including the eyes, central nervous system, and kidneys, may be affected. Splinter hemorrhages of the nailbeds and Osler's nodes—classical features of both ABE and SBE—result from the vasculitis caused by infected emboli. An occasional patient may present with a pulsatile mass representing a mycotic aneurysm. Laboratory tests commonly reveal evidence of hemolytic anemia (eg, reticulocytosis), an elevated erythrocyte sedimentation rate, and urinary abnormalities compatible with a focal nephritis. Other clinical manifestations of ABE include arrhythmias and heart block due to involvement of the conduction system, as well as signs of pericardial inflammation (effusion or friction rub).

Patients with ABE of the tricuspid and/or pulmonic valves typically present with signs of right ventricular failure (ie, an enlarged, pulsatile liver with dilated pulsatile neck veins). A systolic murmur along the right sternal border, indicating tricuspid

CAUSATIVE ORGANISM IN 70 PATIENTS WITH ACUTE BACTERIAL ENDOCARDITIS

Positive Blood Culture (n = 63)	
Staphylococcus aureus	34%
Streptococcus viridans	18%
Streptococcus fecalis	9%
Gram negative	9%
Staphylococcus epidermidis	3%
Others	10%
Negative Blood Culture (n = 7)	
Staphylococcus [cultured from valve]	1%
Gram-positive cocci on valve	1%
Valve histology consistent with infection	4%

(From Jaffe et al; Infective endocarditis 1983–1988. J Am Coll Cardiol 1990; 15:1227, with permission)

Fig. 23.3 Causative organism in 70 patients with acute bacterial endocarditis.

VALVULAR REGURGITATION IN ACUTE BACTERIAL ENDOCARDITIS

Severity	Aortic	Mitral	Tricuspid	Pulmonary
Absent	1	0	0	0
1+	3	2	1	1
2+	7	7	6	0
3+	5	4	5	0
4+	14	6	4	0
Total	30	19	16	1

(From Jaffe et al; Infective endocarditis 1983–1988. J Am Coll Cardiol 1990; 15:1227, with permission)

Fig. 23.4 Valvular regurgitation in patients with acute bacterial endocarditis.

insufficiency, is usually audible in such cases. Not infrequently the major manifestations are related to repeated septic pulmonary emboli. Although the clinical manifestations of right-sided ABE may be subtle, this diagnosis should be strongly considered in a high-risk patient (eg, an intravenous drug abuser) who presents with fever, hemoptysis, and pulmonary infiltrates.

SUBACUTE BACTERIAL ENDOCARDITIS

SBE (endocarditis lenta) is manifested clinically by a persistent low-grade fever and a heart murmur that is often of low intensity. Splenomegaly and evidence of peripheral septic embolization (eg, splinter hemorrhages, Osler's nodes) are usually but not always present. Most patients have systemic symptoms, including anorexia, weight loss, and anemia. (If the murmur is unimpressive, it may be erroneously ascribed to the anemia that is commonly present.)

A history of dental extractions, urinary tract instrumentation, or other invasive procedure in the weeks preceding the onset of symptoms should suggest the diagnosis of SBE. Blood cultures may be negative in patients who received inadequate antibiotic therapy before diagnosis; however, blood cultures usually became positive several weeks after antibiotics are discontinued.

To sum up, the diagnosis of ABE or SBE should be strongly considered in a patient with any of the following:

1. Valvular vegetations demonstrated by imaging techniques (see below).
2. Two or more positive blood cultures in the presence of a heart murmur.
3. Fever in the presence of a heart murmur and peripheral emboli.
4. Fever, hemoptysis, and lung infiltrates in an intravenous drug abuser.

IMAGING AND INVASIVE DIAGNOSIS

PLAIN FILMS

The utility of the plain film in the diagnosis of bacterial endocarditis depends on the valve affected, the presence of myocardial or pericardial involvement, the presence of pulmonary involvement, and evidence of systemic embolization (mycotic aneurysms). Chest films of patients with aortic insufficiency, the most common functional derangement in both ABE and SBE, typically reveal left ventricular and left atrial enlargement and pulmonary venous hypertension. However, the cardiomegaly may be less impressive in patients with aortic insufficiency of acute onset; dilatation of the aorta is notably absent in such cases (Fig. 23.5). A similar radiographic pattern is seen in patients with combined aortic and mitral insufficiency and those with isolated mitral insufficiency.

In patients with pericardial involvement, chest films may show evidence of pericardial effusion or, less often, constrictive pericarditis (see Chapter 22). Deformity of the ascending aorta arch or descending thoracic aorta suggests the presence of a mycotic aneurysm (see Chapter 27).

Patients with right-sided involvement typically have radiographic evidence of congestive heart failure, often with unilateral or bilateral pleural effusions. The heart is usually large, with prominence of the right atrium and right ventricle. The

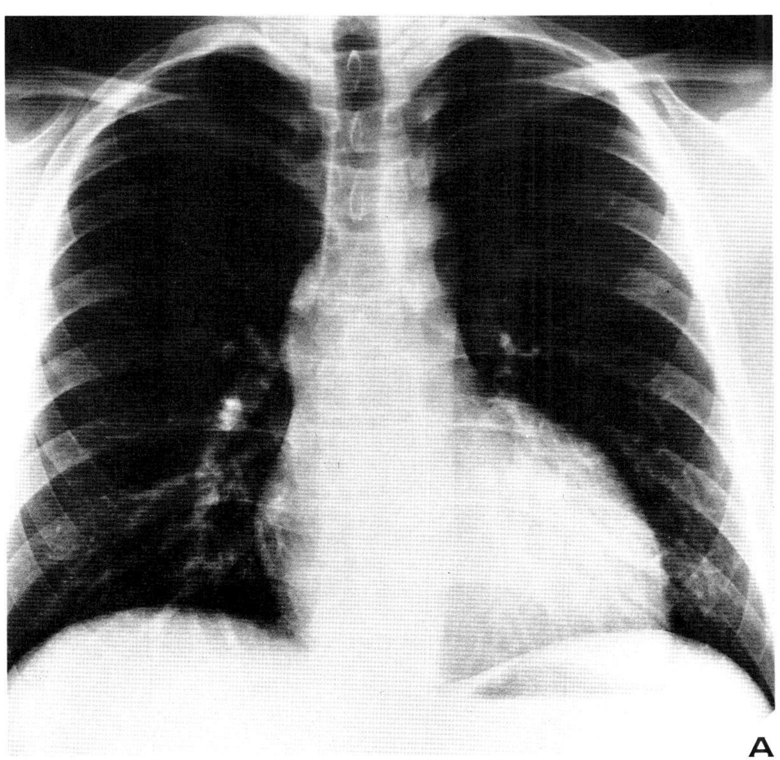

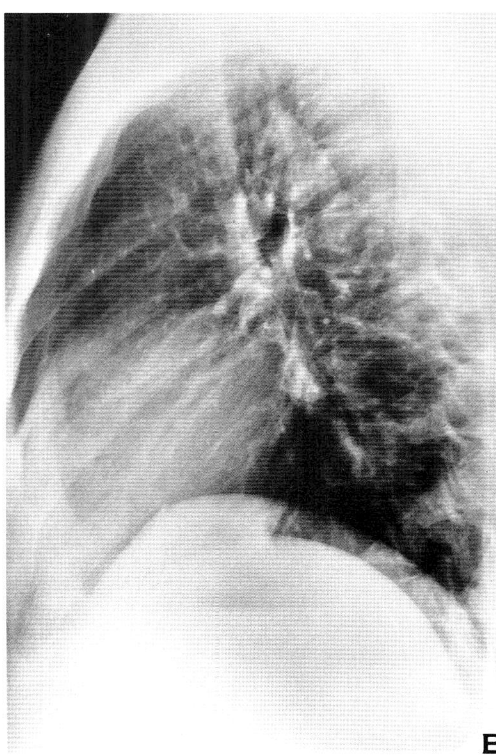

Fig. 23.5 Acute bacterial endocarditis in a patient with acute aortic insufficiency. (A) Posteroanterior and (B) lateral chest films show moderate cardiac enlargement with prominence of the left ventricle. The ascending aorta, aortic arch, and descending thoracic aorta are unremarkable.

azygos vein may be distended, reflecting tricuspid insufficiency and/or right ventricular failure. Many patients with right-sided involvement have patchy opacities or lung nodules. The latter may evolve into thin-walled cysts, the finding of which is virtually pathognomonic of septic pulmonary emboli in this context (Fig. 23.6). Chest films of patients with pulmonic insufficiency show dilatation of the pulmonary trunk and main pulmonary arteries, which is most dramatic during systole.

ECHOCARDIOGRAPHY

When it is correlated with the clinical findings, echocardiography is highly accurate in the diagnosis of both ABE and SBE; the presence of vegetations on the valves or endocardial surfaces and various sequelae (eg, rupture of the leaflets, chordae tendineae, or papillary muscles) are nicely demonstrated with this modality. Vegetations typically appear as one or more echo-dense masses contiguous with the leaflets or at the commissures (Figs. 23.7 to 23.9). Criteria for the echocardiographic

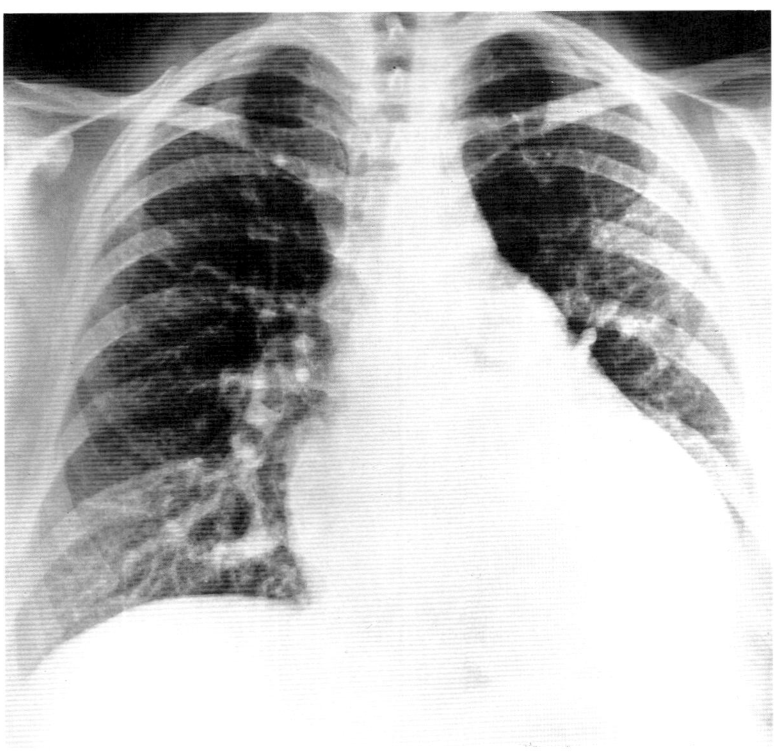

Fig. 23.6 Acute bacterial endocarditis involving mitral and tricuspid valves. Posteroanterior chest film of an intravenous drug abuser shows cardiomegaly with biventricular enlargement and prominence of the pulmonary trunk. Note the cavitating nodule in the right lower zone, which represents a septic embolus.

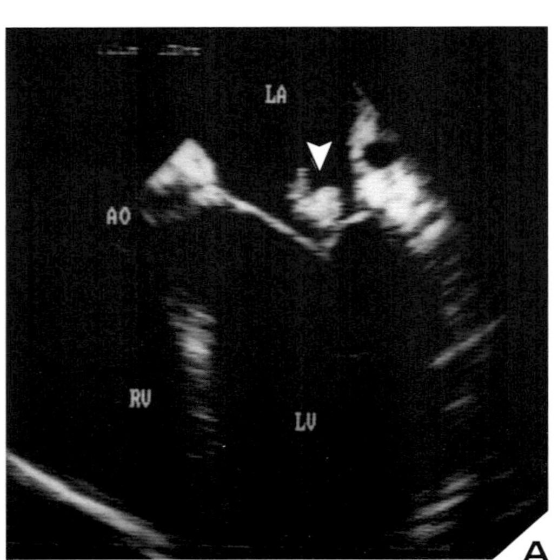

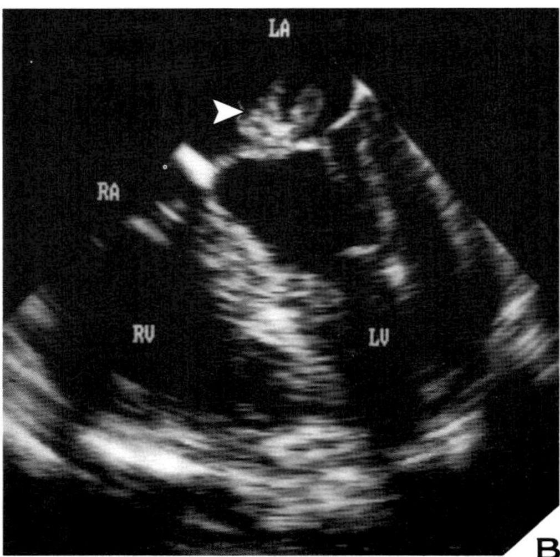

Fig. 23.7 Acute bacterial endocarditis involving mitral valve. Echocardiographic findings in two different patients. (A) Long-axial view demonstrates an echogenic mass (*arrow*) on the posterior mitral leaflet. (B) Four-chamber view demonstrates an echogenic mass (*arrow*) on the septal leaflet. The echogenic masses, which represent vegetations, were seen to move with the corresponding mitral valve leaflet.

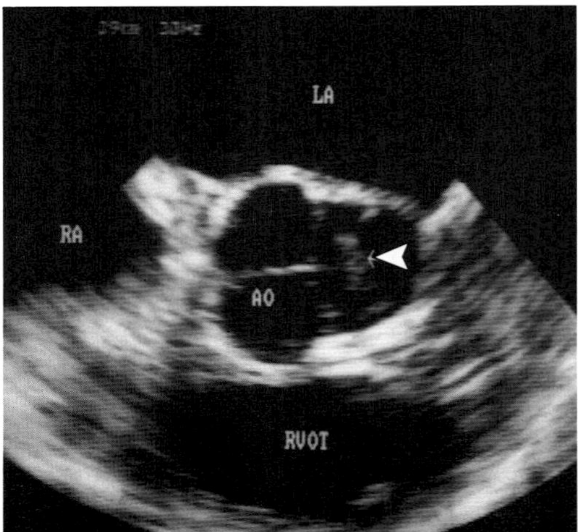

Fig. 23.8 Vegetation on the aortic valve. Short-axis view of echocardiogram at level of aortic valve shows an echogenic mass (*arrow*) attached to the left coronary cusp.

diagnosis of vegetations include attachment to the endocardial surface, consistent visualization throughout the cardiac cycle, demonstration in multiple views, and motion independent of other cardiac structures. Doppler imaging is helpful in assessing valvular function (Figs. 23.10 and 23.11; see Appendix). Color Doppler is especially useful for evaluating the tricuspid valve; vegetations on the leaflets, as well as such complications as perforation and fistulae, are clearly seen on the four-chamber projection (Fig. 23.10; see Appendix). Lesions of the pulmonic valve are best appreciated on the short-axis view.

An endocardial pseudoaneurysm, which often represents an abscess that has healed after treatment, appears as an echo-free space within the endocardium in the vicinity of the valve; an intramural fistula or sinus tract has a similar appearance (Figs. 23.12 and 23.13). These lesions typically occur in the ventricle in patients with lesions of the aortic valve and in the atrium in patients with mitral lesions. Other complications that can be demonstrated by echocardiography include mycotic aneurysms of the aorta and branches of the aortic arch, and pseudoaneurysms of the sinuses of Valsalva and their sequelae.

The echocardiographic findings in patients with suspected bacterial endocarditis must be interpreted in light of the clinical picture, as somewhat similar images can be seen in patients with rheumatic valvular disease. Echocardiographic findings suggestive of bacterial endocarditis can also be seen in patients with myxoma, myxomatous valvular degeneration secondary to mitral valve prolapse, and spontaneous rupture of the chordae tendineae.

Echocardiography will fail to demonstrate vegetations or destructive changes in the leaflets in some patients with typical clinical findings of bacterial endocarditis. This is likely to be the case in a patient who has recently received intensive antibiotic therapy. In one large study (Stewart et al, 1980), vegetations were rarely detected after two weeks of appropriate antibiotic treatment.

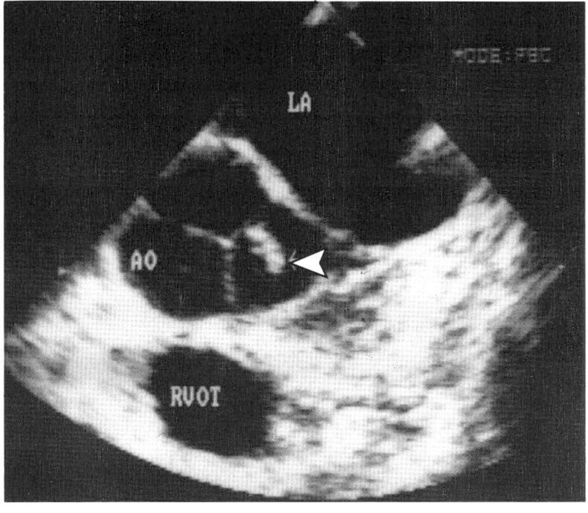

Fig. 23.9 Vegetation of the aortic valve. Short-axial view of echocardiogram shows an echogenic mass (*arrow*) adherent to the noncoronary cusp, which lies anterior and to the left of the left coronary cusp.

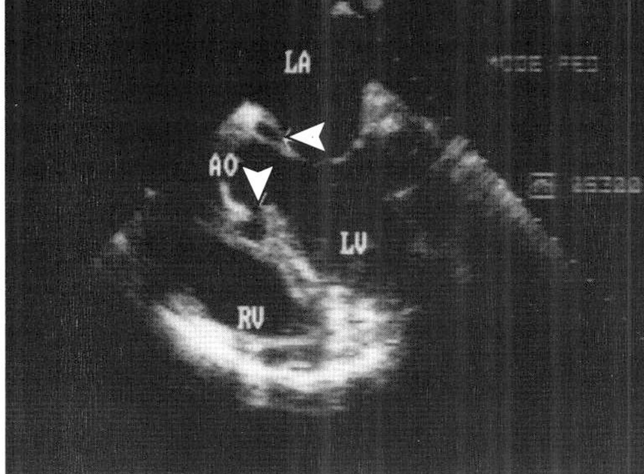

Fig. 23.12 Healed abscess or fistula tract secondary to fungal endocarditis. Four-chamber section of echocardiogram demonstrates an echo-free space (*horizontal arrow*) in the ventricular septum. A second echo-free space (*vertical arrow*) is seen at the junction of the anterior mitral leaflet and the aortic valve. These spaces could represent a fistula tract resulting from the destruction of infected tissue or a healing abscess.

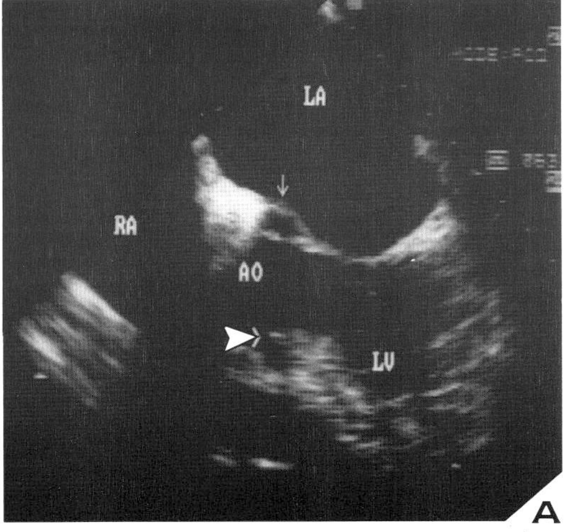

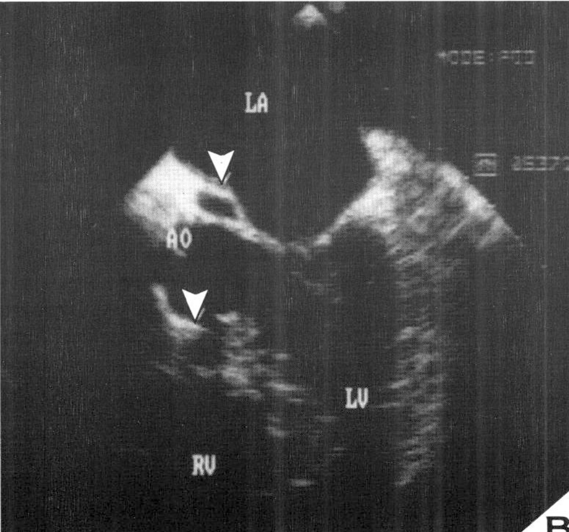

Fig. 23.13 Healed abscess or fistula tract secondary to fungal endocarditis. (A, B) Long axial projection of patient shown in Fig. 24.12. The two echo-free areas are again seen. The one at the junction of the aortic and mitral valves (*upper vertical arrows* in A and B) has the configuration of a healed abscess. The other is now clearly identified as a fistula tract. Its communication (*horizontal arrowhead*) with the left ventricular cavity is best appreciated in A, while its extension into the ventricular septum (*lower vertical arrow*) is clearly seen in B. The echocardiographic findings in fungal endocarditis and bacterial endocarditis are indistinguishable.

CT AND MRI

Although CT has low sensitivity in detecting ABE or SBE, it may be useful in evaluating such complications as mycotic aneurysm of the aorta and its branches (Fig. 23.14), left ventricular aneurysm, and large intracavitary vegetations. MRI is capable of demonstrating abscesses in the vicinity of the cardiac valves; however, experience with this modality is limited. At the present time, neither CT nor MRI offers any advantage over echocardiography in the diagnosis of bacterial endocarditis.

ANGIOGRAPHY

The angiocardiographic diagnosis of bacterial endocarditis depends on demonstration of secondary anatomic changes (eg, abscess, pseudoaneurysm, fistula or sinus tract, valve destruction). Therefore, the study is likely to be normal in many patients diagnosed clinically as having bacterial endocarditis. Angiography is particularly useful in patients who develop bacterial endocarditis following valve replacement (Fig. 23.15). Coronary arteriography is indicated when there is evidence of ischemic heart disease (which may result from extension of a mycotic aneurysm or embolization of the coronary arterial tree).

Lesions of the mitral valve are best evaluated by cine left ventriculography in the long axial and elongated right anterior oblique projections. Lesions of the aortic valve are best demonstrated by cine left ventriculography in the lateral and left anterior oblique projections. Vegetations appear as filling defects contiguous with the aortic or mitral leaflets (small vegeta-

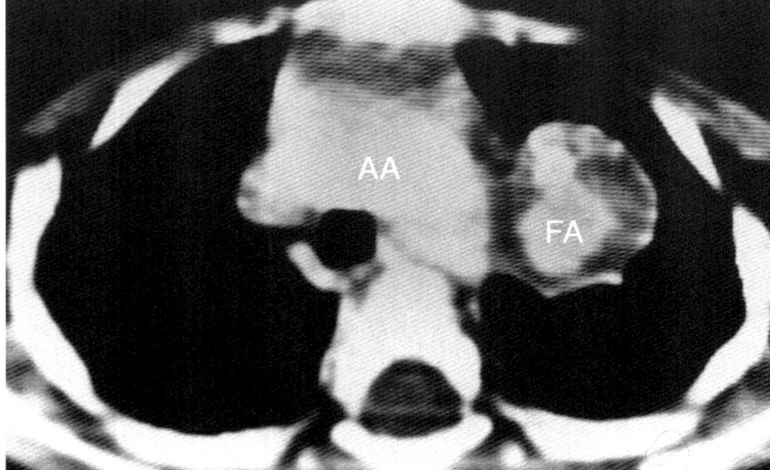

Fig. 23.14 Mycotic aneurysm of the aortic arch secondary to bacterial endocarditis. Contrast-enhanced CT scan at the level of the aortic arch demonstrates a false aneurysm (FA) arising from the left side of the distal aortic arch (AA). The relatively narrow neck is a typical feature of false aneurysms. The filling defects within the false aneurysm represent thrombus.

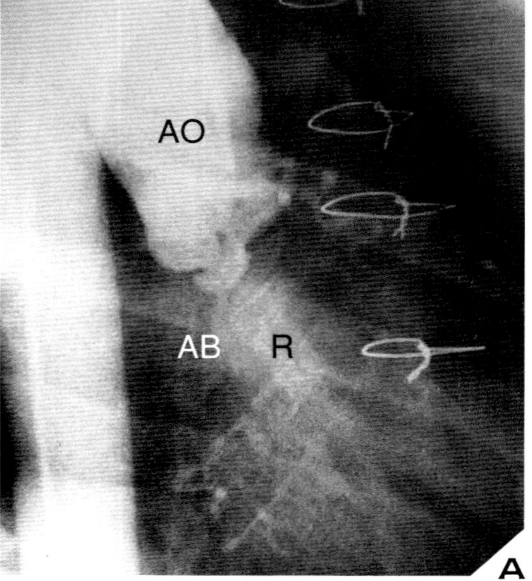

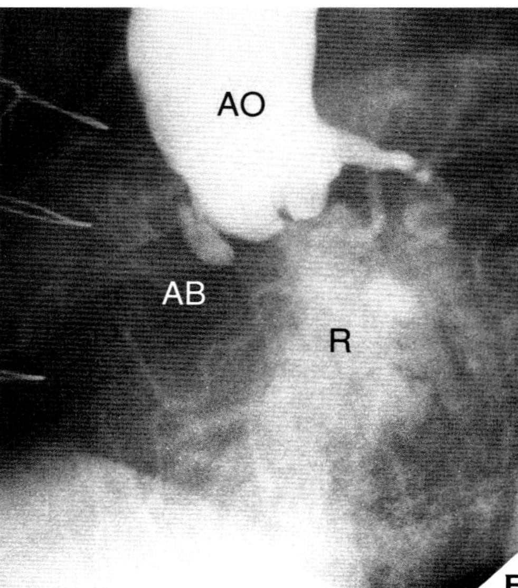

Fig. 23.15 Subacute bacterial endocarditis associated with a prosthetic aortic valve. (A) Right and (B) left anterior oblique projections of thoracic aortogram (in diastole) show an abscess (AB)arising from the right coronary cusp and extending anteriorly and inferiorly to it. A small amount of contrast material refluxes (R) into the left ventricle indicating moderate aortic insufficiency.

tions are unlikely to be detected unless one has a high index of suspicion). The anterior (septal) leaflet of the mitral valve is seen in profile in the long axial projection; vegetations, as well as rupture of the anterior leaflet, can often be identified in this projection. Severe mitral insufficiency, although uncommon, may indicate perforation of the anterior or posterior mitral leaflet (Fig. 23.16). Perforation of the ventricular septum is best demonstrated on left ventriculography in the long axial projection (Fig. 23.17).

Thoracic aortography is usually performed in conjunction with left ventriculography in patients with aortic valve involvement. The combined study is necessary to assess the degree of aortic insufficiency and to detect complications such as aortic root abscess and pseudoaneurysm of the sinuses of Valsalva

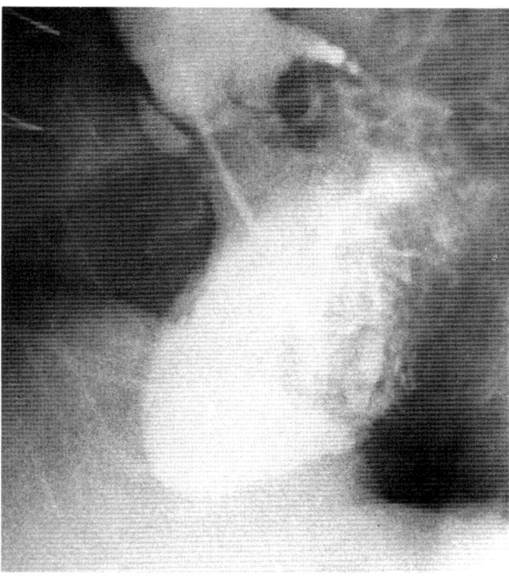

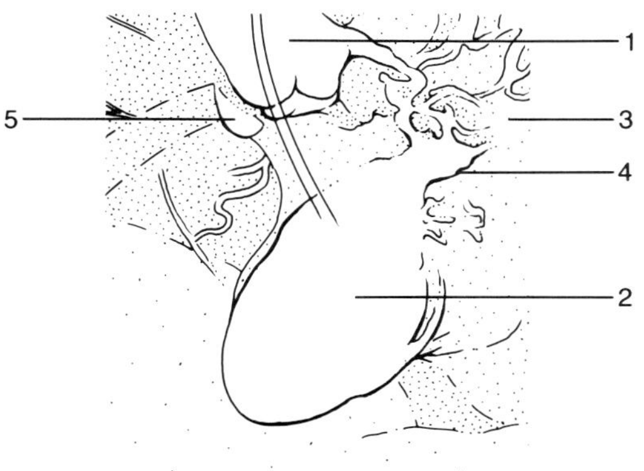

Fig. 23.16 Subacute bacterial endocarditis involving aortic and mitral valves. Long-axial projection of left ventriculogram (in systole) demonstrates reflux of contrast material into the left atrium through a narrow channel at the level of the posteromedial commissure of the mitral valve (probably related to a ruptured posterior leaflet). In addition, there is an abscess related to the right coronary cusp of the aortic valve.

1 aorta
2 left ventricle
3 left atrium
4 regurgitant jet through ruptured posterior leaflet of mitral valve
5 abscess of right coronary cusp

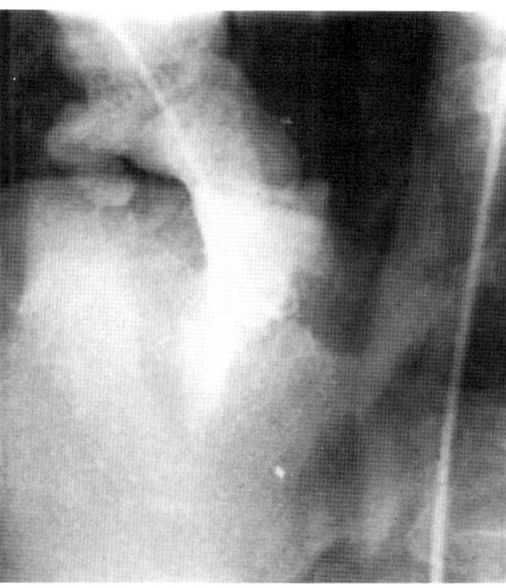

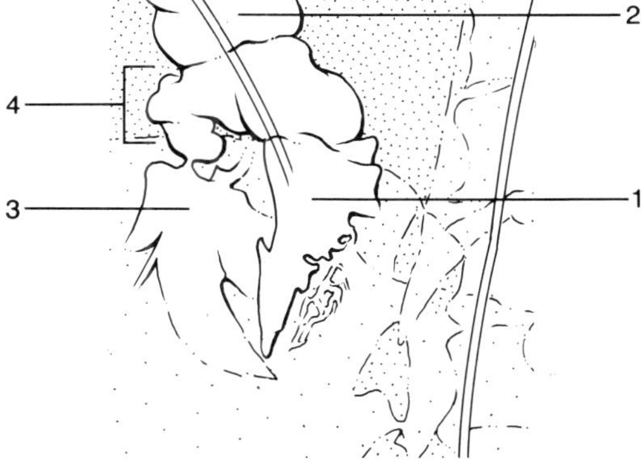

Fig. 23.17 Intramural fistula secondary to bacterial endocarditis. Long-axial projection of left ventriculogram demonstrates a fistula tract between the left and right ventricles. The tract arises below the aortic valve very close to the right coronary cusp. It enters the ventricular septum, runs for a short distance in an apical direction, and communicates with the right ventricle through a narrow opening.

1 left ventricle
2 aorta
3 right ventricle
4 fistula

(Figs. 23.15, 23.18, and 23.19). Thoracic aortography may also reveal a deformed or bicuspid aortic valve, both of which are associated with a significantly increased incidence of bacterial endocarditis. Aortic abscess and postinfective pseudoaneurysm produce a saccular deformity of the aortic root, sinuses of Valsalva, or surrounding structures. Such deformities may be present even when the aorta appears intact. Postinfective pseudoaneurysms of the sinuses of Valsalva have a typical "windsock" appearance (Fig. 23.19); like congenital sinus of Valsalva aneurysms, they may rupture into surrounding cavities. Angiographically, an aortic root abscess appears as a round, extraluminal collection of contrast material within the periaortic soft tissues (Figs. 23.15 and 23.16). Although this appearance can suggest a congenital aneurysm of the sinuses of Valsalva, the latter condition is usually associated with a single large sinus which prolapses below the plane of the aortic valve (see Chapter 9). Another disorder that can simulate an aortic root abscess angiographically is a congenital fistula between the aorta and the left ventricle (see Chapter 13). However, this condition should present no problem in differential diagnosis, since it presents very early in life with signs and symptoms of aortic insufficiency.

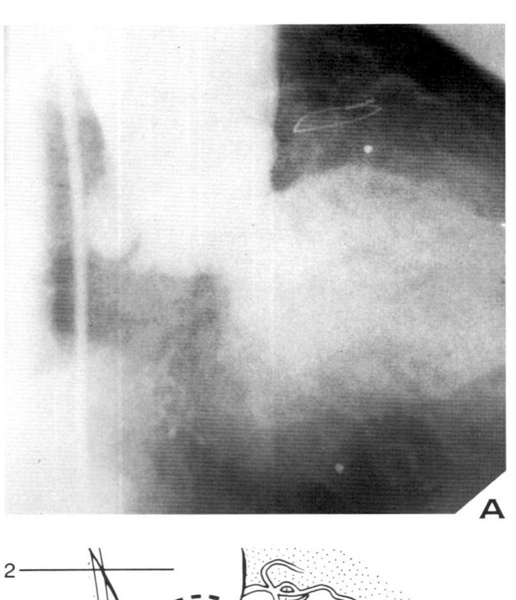

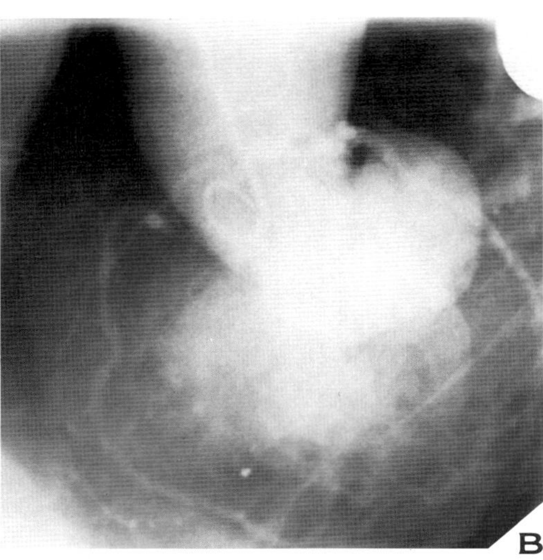

Fig. 23.18 Severe aortic insufficiency and saccular aortic aneurysm secondary to bacterial endocarditis. (A) Right anterior oblique and (B) lateral projections of thoracic aortogram (in diastole) show marked reflux of contrast material, with opacification of the entire left ventricle. The saccular structure at the junction between the aortic and mitral valves represents an aneurysm. The aneurysm overlies the aorta on the right anterior oblique projection and is best seen on the lateral. The site of origin of the aneurysm is not demonstrated on the angiogram; at operation, it was found to arise from the posterior aspect of the left ventricular outflow tract.

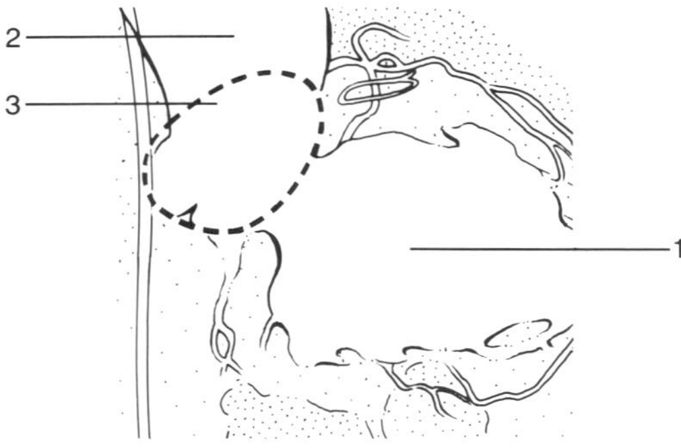

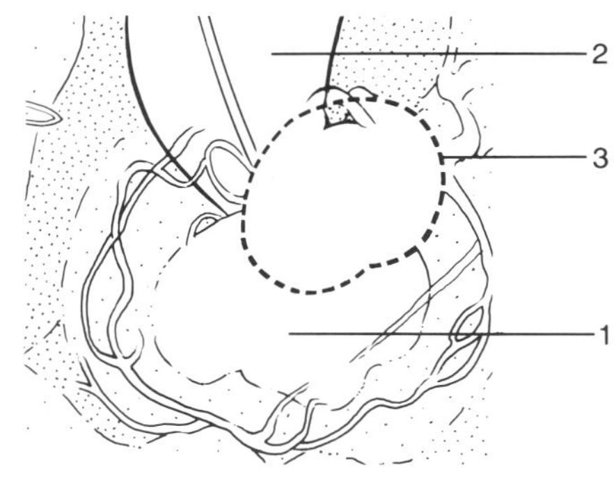

1 left ventricle	3 aneurysm
2 aorta	

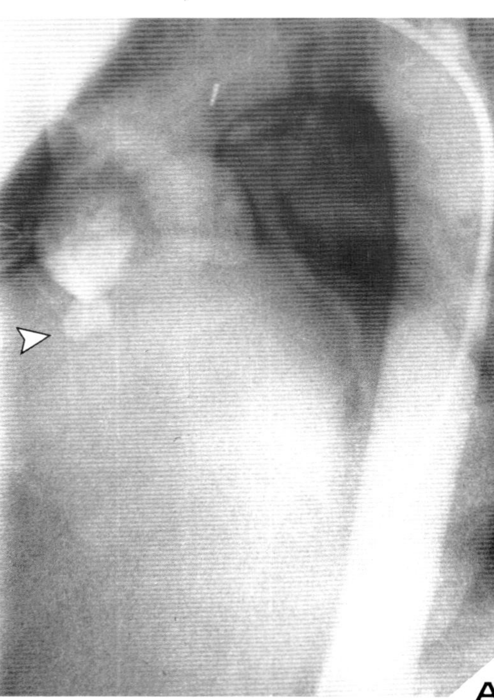

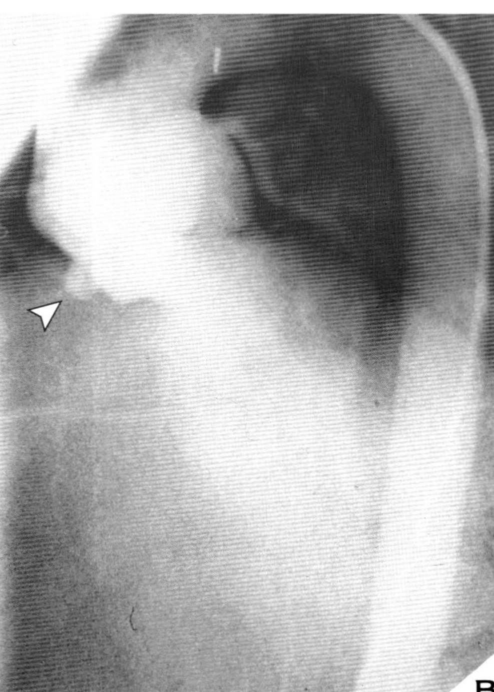

Fig. 23.19 Aneurysm of the right coronary sinus of Valsalva secondary to bacterial endocarditis. Right anterior oblique projection of thoracic aortogram in (A) systole and (B) diastole demonstrates a pseudoaneurysm (*arrow*) arising from the wall of the right sinus of Valsalva, which probably represents a healing abscess. Note complete opacification of left ventricle indicating grade IV/V aortic insufficiency.

Angiocardiography is of little value in evaluating the tricuspid valve in patients with right-sided bacterial endocarditis. Right ventriculography demonstrates right ventricular enlargement and tricuspid insufficiency. However, the degree of tricuspid insufficiency cannot be accurately assessed because the catheter traverses the tricuspid valve. For the same reason, the degree of pulmonic insufficiency cannot be reliably assessed by injecting contrast material into the pulmonary trunk. Echocardiography remains the modality of choice for evaluating the complications of right-sided bacterial endocarditis.

FUNGAL ENDOCARDITIS

Fungal endocarditis, usually caused by saprophytic organisms such as *Candida,* most often occurs as a nosocomial infection ("line sepsis"). The pathological and imaging features are similar to those of bacterial endocarditis.

CARDIAC INFECTIONS IN THE IMMUNOCOMPROMISED PATIENT

Although immunocompromised patients are at increased risk for myocardial and pericardial infections, they do not appear to be at increased risk for infective endocarditis. In one series of 70 patients with HIV infections, the most common cardiac abnormalities were dilated cardiomyopathy and pericarditis; none had evidence of infective endocarditis (Himelman et al, 1989).

CHAPTER 24

Cardiac Manifestations of Lung Disease

The common denominator of cardiac disorders associated with lung disease is increased pulmonary arterial pressure and the effect it produces on the right ventricle. Lung disorders associated with increased pulmonary arterial pressure include various types of lung disease, primary pulmonary hypertension, and pulmonary embolism.

CHRONIC COR PULMONALE

This condition, which is usually a consequence of pulmonary emphysema, chronic bronchitis, or chronic parenchymal disease, accounts for 20 to 30 percent of all hospital admissions for "heart failure." Chronic cor pulmonale secondary to chronic obstructive pulmonary disease (COPD) (ie, pulmonary emphysema or chronic bronchitis), is most common in men between 50 and 60 years of age, particularly in those with a significant smoking history.

PATHOLOGY

The underlying pathologic change in pulmonary emphysema is loss of lung elasticity, which is accompanied by destruction of the walls of the bronchioles and terminal airways (respiratory ducts and alveoli). The net effect is a decrease in total alveolar capacity resulting in alveolar hypoxia and pulmonary arteriolar vasoconstriction. The resultant increase in pulmonary vascular resistance leads to pulmonary hypertension.

Medial hypertrophy of muscular pulmonary arteries is a constant finding in all forms of pulmonary hypertension, including that resulting from lung disease. Microscopically, there is increased thickness of the muscular layers in the acinar and preacinar arteries, resulting in various degrees of luminal obstruction. These changes, which represent the structural response to the vasoconstriction caused by chronic hypoxemia, tend to be more severe in patients with primary pulmonary hypertension than in those with pulmonary thromboembolism or COPD. Di-

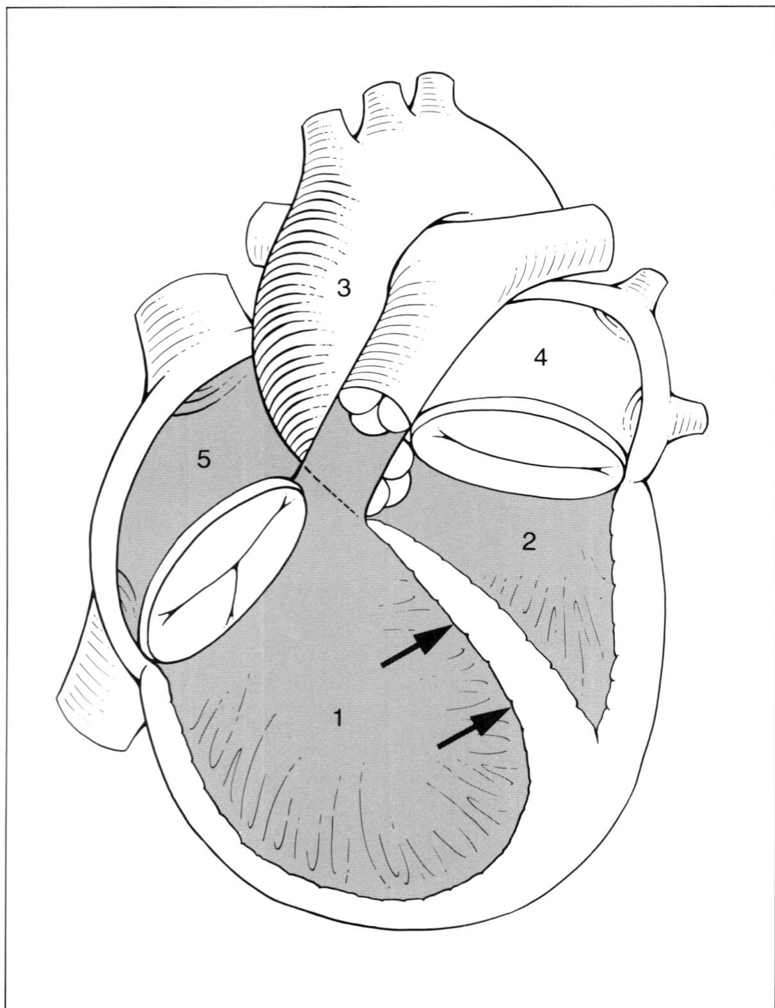

Fig. 24.1 Left ventricular dysfunction secondary to chronic cor pulmonale. Right ventricular overload during diastole causes displacement of the ventricular septum, restricting the size of the left ventricular chamber. In severe cases, the left ventricle may be compressed against the posterior aspect of the pericardium.

1 right ventricle
2 left ventricle
3 aorta
4 left atrium
5 right atrium

latation of the central pulmonary arteries can cause compression of the left main bronchus and bronchus intermedius, leading to recurrent pneumonias.

HEMODYNAMIC EFFECTS

The increase in pulmonary artery pressure causes increased afterloading of the right ventricle, which undergoes hypertrophy, becomes dilated, and ultimately fails. The tricuspid valve frequently becomes incompetent. The right atrium is usually dilated secondary to right ventricular pressure overload and tricuspid insufficiency (if present).

Left ventricular dysfunction, manifested by increased end diastolic pressure during exercise testing, is not uncommon in patients with moderate to severe COPD. Alterations in the structure and function of the right ventricle and ventricular septum are believed to be the main reason for left ventricular dysfunction. Dilatation and hypertrophy of the right ventricle cause the septum to shift, altering the configuration and compliance of the left ventricle, decreasing its efficiency, and making it abnormally stiff (Fig. 24.1). Other factors contributing to left ventricular dysfunction include coronary artery hypoxemia and increased cardiac output. (The latter reflects the increased respiratory effort needed to overcome the peripheral hypoxemia.) Progressive left ventricular failure results in pulmonary vascular congestion and pulmonary edema, which compound the ventilatory disturbance produced by the underlying lung disease.

CLINICAL FEATURES

The clinical manifestations of chronic cor pulmonale are often obscured by the underlying lung disease. Peripheral edema is often the first sign of chronic cor pulmonale. Physical examination usually reveals an anterior sternal lift during systole, indicating right ventricular hypertrophy. Patients with tricuspid insufficiency typically exhibit neck vein distension with a prominent "V" wave.

End-stage cor pulmonale is characterized by hepatic congestion and ascites secondary to right ventricular failure and tricuspid insufficiency. Pulmonary vascular congestion and pulmonary edema—the classic signs of left ventricular failure—are not uncommon at this stage. (Pulmonary vascular congestion and pulmonary edema are not seen in patients with "pure" right-sided heart failure.)

The electrocardiogram typically shows evidence of right ventricular hypertrophy (low QRS voltage, right axis deviation of the mean QRS vector) and right atrial dysfunction ("P pulmonale"). Mild degrees of left ventricular dysfunction cannot be appreciated on the ECG; however, patients with severe left ventricular ischemia exhibit ST-segment changes in leads V5 and V6.

IMAGING AND INVASIVE DIAGNOSIS

Frontal and lateral chest films show the typical features of the underlying lung disease (Fig. 24.2). The enlarged right ventricle projects anteriorly and to the right. (Mild degrees of right ven-

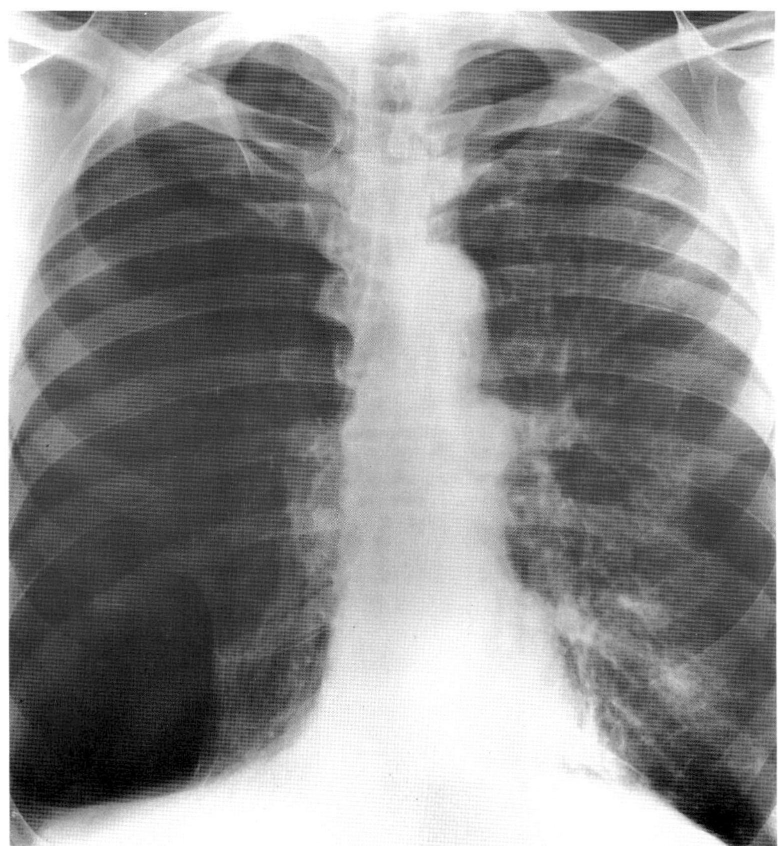

Fig. 24.2 Chronic cor pulmonale secondary to COPD. Frontal chest film shows severe emphysema. The pulmonary vasculature is sparse in both lungs, particularly the posterior segment of the right lower lobe. Note the small size of the heart and the relative enlargement of the right and left pulmonary arteries. The patient had clinical manifestations of chronic cor pulmonale. The right ventricular systolic pressure was 50 mm Hg.

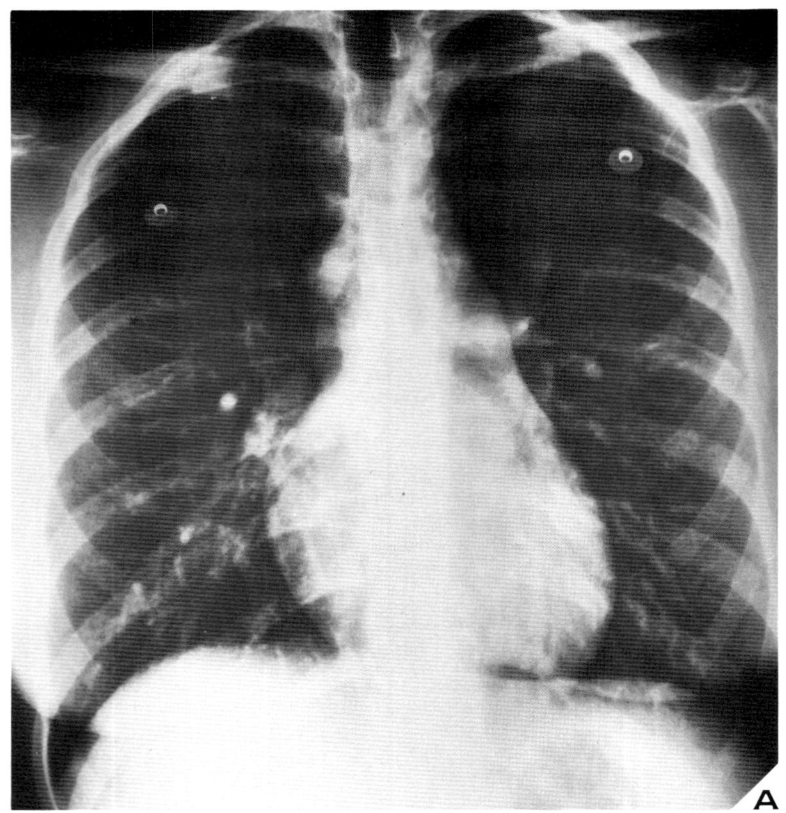

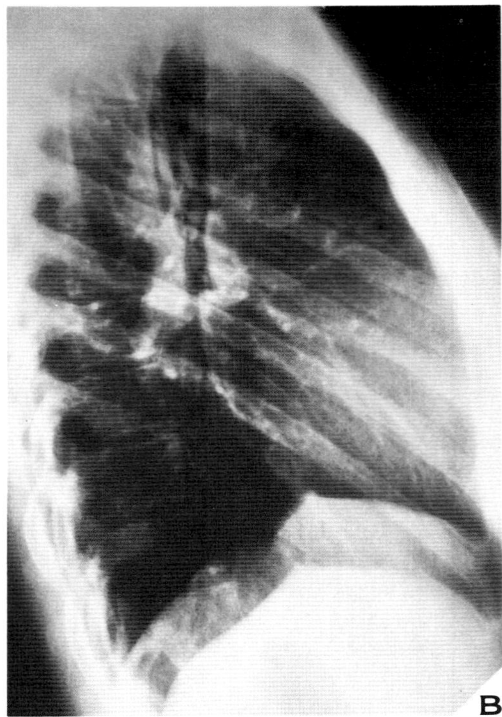

Fig. 24.3 Chronic cor pulmonale secondary to COPD. (A) Posteroanterior and (B) lateral chest films shown moderately severe lung disease. Although the heart is of normal size, there is increased contact with the anterior chest wall (B), indicating right ventricular enlargement. The right atrium is enlarged and the pulmonary trunk is dilated. The azygos vein is also dilated, reflecting increased pressure in the systemic veins.

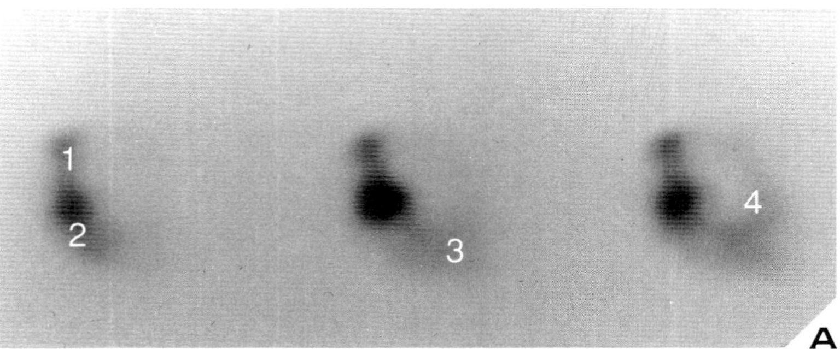

1	superior vena cava	5	right pulmonary artery
2	right atrium	6	left atrium
3	right ventricle	7	left ventricle
4	pulmonary trunk	8	aorta

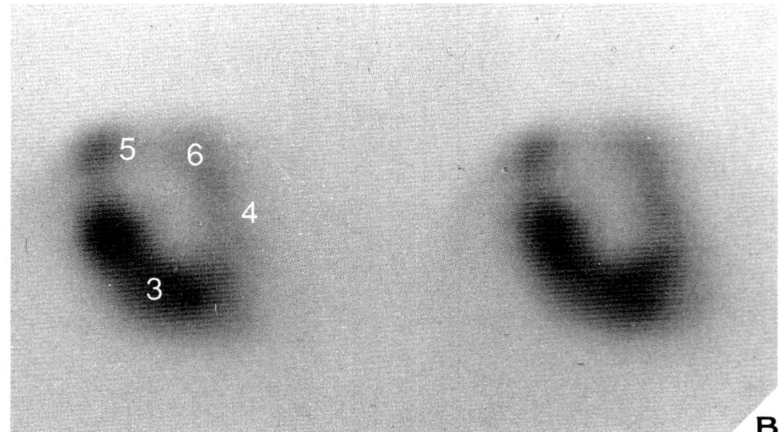

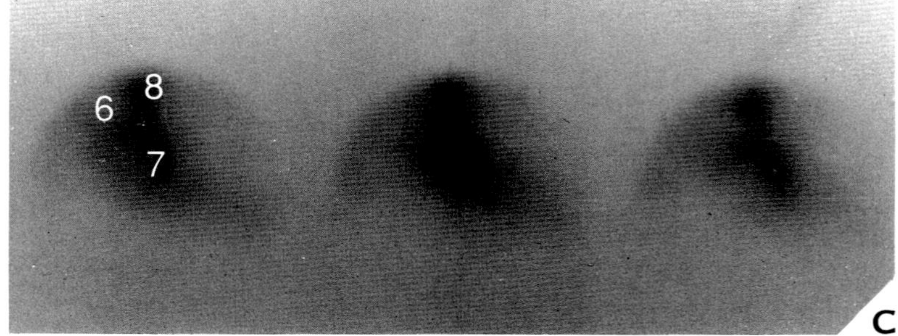

Fig. 24.4 Radionuclide angiography in chronic cor pulmonale. First-pass study using ^{99m}Tc-tagged albumin macroaggregates. (A) In the first set of three images, the right atrium, right ventricle, and a portion of the pulmonary trunk are visualized. The right ventricular cavity is enlarged. (B) In the second set of images the enlarged right ventricle is again demonstrated. The pulmonary trunk and main pulmonary arteries are now seen to be enlarged. (C) In the third set of images, the left atrium, left ventricle, and aorta are visualized and appear normal. The disparity between the size of the right and left ventricles indicates right ventricular overload.

tricular enlargement may be difficult to appreciate if the lungs are markedly hyperinflated.) When the right ventricle is greatly enlarged it forms the left heart border, including the apex. The pulmonary trunk and main pulmonary arteries are markedly dilated. There is often a gross disparity in the size of the central and peripheral pulmonary branches. Prominence of the right atrium and superior vena cava (due to right ventricular failure and tricuspid insufficiency) are the rule in patients with advanced disease (Fig. 24.3).

NUCLEAR MEDICINE

The cardiovascular abnormalities associated with COPD are clearly shown by radionuclide angiography. The first-pass technique demonstrates the configuration of right ventricle. The gated equilibrium technique, which entails labeling of the entire circulating blood volume with [^{99m}Tc]-albumin or tagged autologous erythrocytes, demonstrates right ventricular size and contractility. The information thus gained can be combined with echocardiography to provide a dynamic display of the contracting heart. When images are obtained in the appropriate oblique projection, it is possible to differentiate the right and left ventricles and to assess right ventricular contractility (Fig. 24.4). Radionuclide angiography has largely been superseded by echocardiography and MRI in the assessment of right ventricular function.

By labeling the myocardium with ^{201}Tl (thallium), it is possible to estimate the severity of right ventricular hypertrophy and dysfunction in patients with pulmonary hypertension secondary to chronic lung disease or other disorders. The myocardium of the normal right ventricle is thin and does not take up thallium, either at rest or with exercise, whereas the myocardium of the hypertrophied right ventricle exhibits moderate to marked uptake (Fig. 24.5). A sustained decrease in pulmonary artery pressure after medical treatment or other therapy often leads to a decrease in thallium uptake by the right ventricular myocardium.

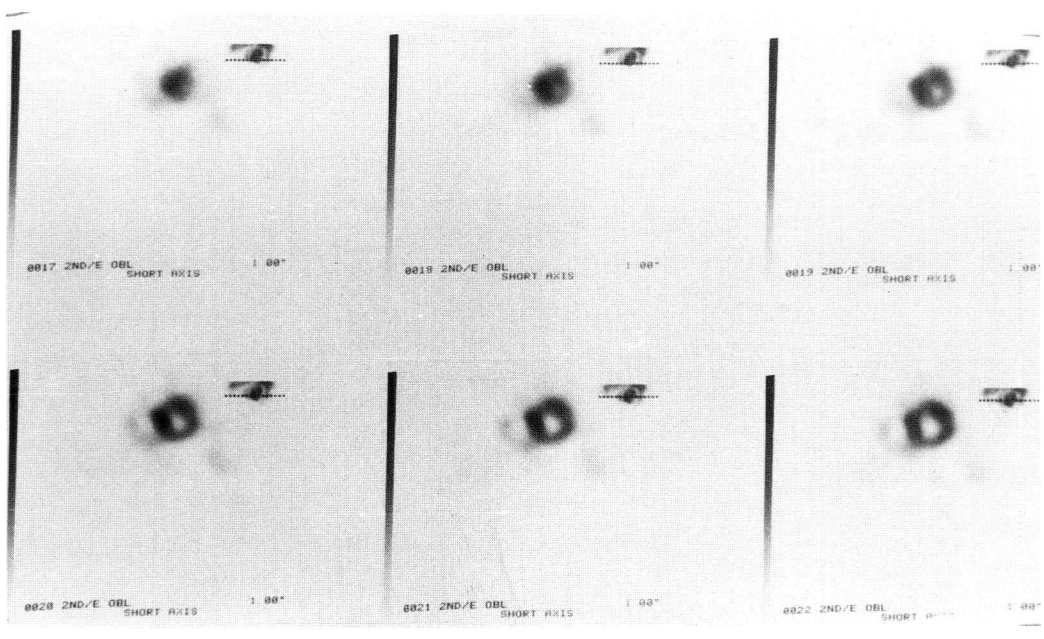

Fig. 24.5 Abnormal thallium uptake due to pulmonary hypertension (chronic cor pulmonale secondary to COPD). Tomographic (SPECT) images in short axis projection demonstrate a significant increase in the uptake of the radionuclide (^{201}Tl) by the right ventricular myocardium, indicating right ventricular hypertrophy. There is abnormal distribution of activity in the left ventricular myocardium, with increased uptake in the ventricular septum.

Perfusion and ventilation scans are commonly used to assess pulmonary function and morphology in patients with COPD (Fig. 24.6). They are particularly helpful in differentiating COPD from pulmonary thromboembolism (see below).

ECHOCARDIOGRAPHY

Transthoracic and transesophageal echocardiography provide important information regarding right ventricular function and the size of the pulmonary arteries; the cross-sectional display enables one to evaluate the entire right ventricle in several planes. Conventional and color Doppler imaging document the severity of associated pulmonic and tricuspid valvular insufficiency (Fig. 24.7, Appendix). The most commonly employed projection is the four-chamber view, obtained via a subcostal or parasternal window. The apical two-dimensional approach, recently developed for the study of right ventricular volume and ejection fraction, yields data that correlate well with those obtained by other techniques and is gaining wide acceptance as a clinical tool.

CT AND MAGNETIC RESONANCE IMAGING

Spin–echo and cine MRI can detect secondary morphologic changes in the right ventricle and right atrium; these features can also be detected by cine CT. However, these changes are nonspecific, and can be seen in patients with pulmonary hypertension of any etiology (see below). Conventional and thin-section CT demonstrate characteristic parenchymal abnormalities in patients with COPD.

CARDIAC CATHETERIZATION

In patients with relatively mild COPD without hypoxemia, cardiac catheterization demonstrates normal right atrial and right ventricular end diastolic pressure, low to normal cardiac output, normal or slightly increased pulmonary arterial pressure, normal capillary wedge pressure, and normal to slightly elevated pulmonary vascular resistance at rest. With exercise, there is an increase in pulmonary arterial pressure, right ventricular end diastolic pressure, and stroke volume; however, the capillary wedge pressure remains normal. (The normal capillary wedge pressure, which is often significantly lower than the diastolic pulmonary arterial pressure, excludes left heart failure as the cause of the pulmonary hypertension.) Resting end diastolic pressure remains normal for a long time in many patients with pulmonary hypertension secondary to chronic lung disease. Patients with pulmonary infection or other superimposed lung disease may exhibit right ventricular failure at rest.

Progression of the pulmonary disease leads to severe chronic hypoxemia and is usually associated with chronic hypercapnia and moderate pulmonary hypertension. At this stage the sys-

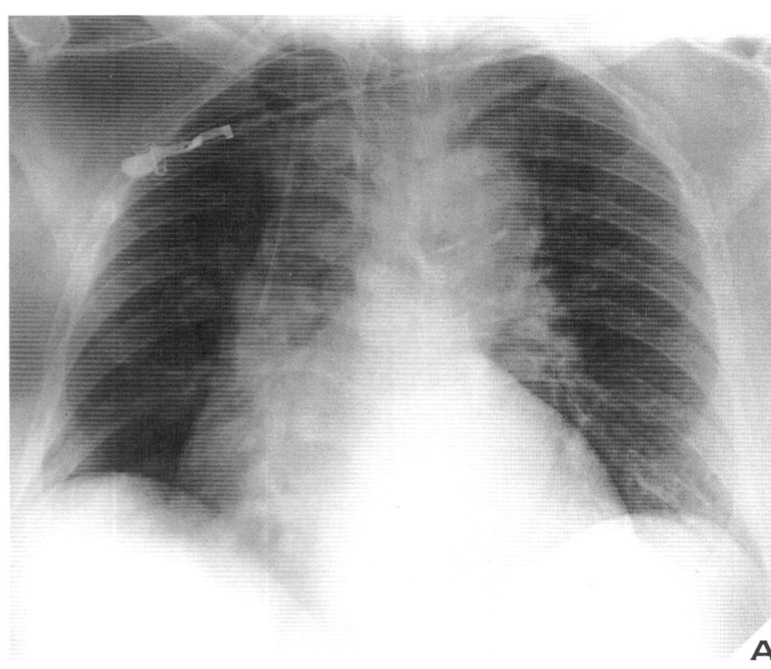

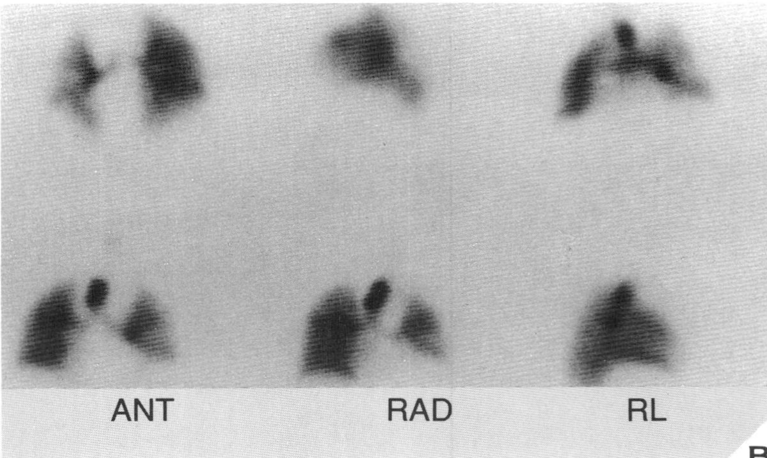

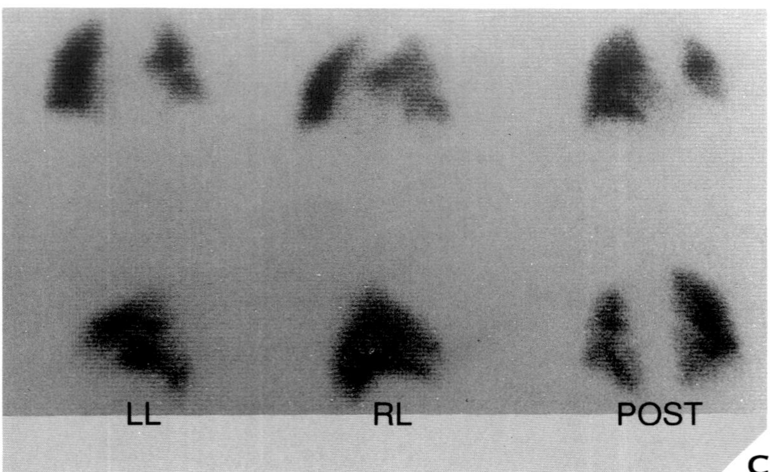

Fig. 24.6 Abnormal perfusion–ventilation scan in COPD (A) Chest film shows overinflation of right lower lobe. The heart is slightly enlarged with right ventricular hypertrophy. The main pulmonary arteries are dilated. (B) Ventilation scan (aerosol technique) demonstrates poor ventilation of the mid and posterior portions of the left lung and deposition of the aerosol in the large airways. (C) Perfusion scan (^{99}Tc-macroaggregated albumin; MAA) demonstrates areas of decreased uptake in the left lung corresponding to those seen on the aerosol scan. Matching defects on ventilation and perfusion scans are commonly seen in patients with COPD.

tolic pulmonary arterial pressure is elevated at rest (to 60 to 80 mm Hg) and rises further during exercise, accompanied by a rise in the right ventricular filling pressure. Cardiac output is usually normal at rest but does not exhibit a normal increase with exercise. Left ventricular dysfunction, commonly present in patients with moderate to severe COPD, is manifested by an increase in left ventricular end diastolic pressure during exercise.

ANGIOCARDIOGRAPHY

Although right ventriculography may be performed in conjunction with cardiac catheterization, it can usually be omitted in patients with chronic cor pulmonale. The right ventricle appears uniformly enlarged, with an increased zone of contact between its anterior margin and the chest wall on the lateral projection. The pulmonary trunk and main pulmonary arteries are usually markedly enlarged. The peripheral pulmonary arterial branches are small and sparsely distributed, and the small parenchymal vessels are decreased in size and number (Fig. 24.8). The abnormal vascular pattern, which is most conspicuous in areas of extensive parenchymal destruction, is believed to result from thrombosis and/or compression of small arteries by the hyperinflated lung (Fig. 24.9). Pulmonary venous return is poor owing to the lack of perfusion of the lung parenchyma.

Aortography with selective bronchial arteriography usually demonstrates dilated bronchial arteries, often associated with

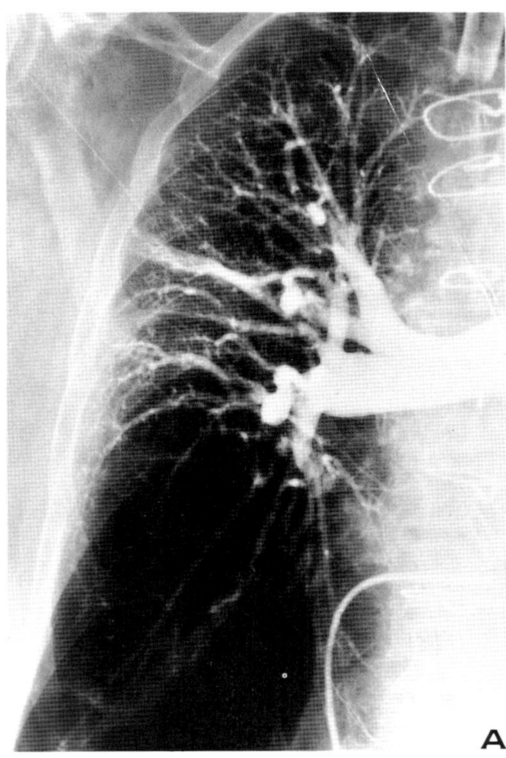

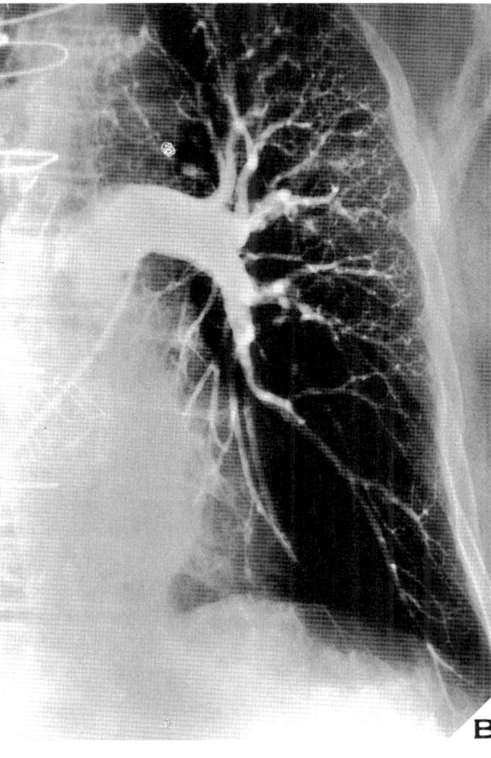

Fig. 24.8 Pulmonary arteriography in chronic cor pulmonale secondary to COPD. (A) Right and (B) left selective pulmonary arteriograms. The right main pulmonary artery is of normal size, but the lobar, segmental, and subsemental branches to the right lower lobe are very small. Similar changes are present on the left.

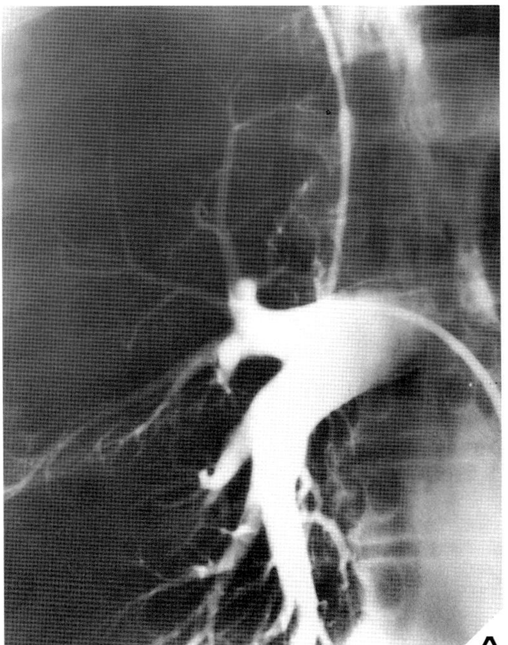

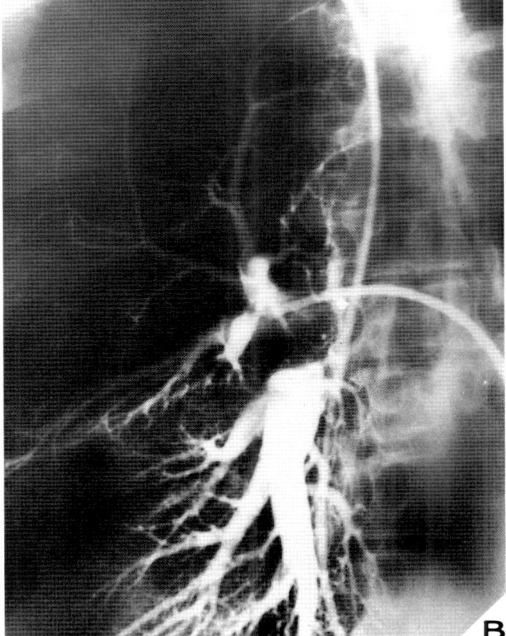

Fig. 24.9 Pulmonary arteriography in chronic cor pulmonale secondary to pulmonary emphysema. (A, B) Selective right pulmonary arteriogram. On the early arterial phase (A) the arteries supplying the right upper lobe are smaller than those supplying the lower lobe. The segmental and subsegmental branches of the right upper lobe are widely spaced and the middle lobe arteries are displaced inferiorly. The peripheral branches of the lower lobe artery are abnormally small. The late arterial phase (B) shows lack of perfusion of the right upper lobe, which is almost entirely replaced by bullae. Portions of the right lower lobe are normally perfused.

aneurysm formation. Rupture of these abnormal channels can lead to hemoptysis or massive pulmonary hemorrhage (Fig. 24.10). Percutaneous transvascular embolization techniques can be lifesaving in such cases (see Chapters 16 and 31).

DIAGNOSTIC APPROACH TO CHRONIC COR PULMONALE

The diagnosis of chronic cor pulmonale is suggested by the clinical history and typical findings on physical examination, ECG, and chest films. Echocardiography provides significant information concerning right ventricular function and demonstrates tricuspid and pulmonic insufficiency (if present). The main role of nuclear imaging is to detect pulmonary thromboemboli, which may be a cause of pulmonary hypertension (see below). Thallium scintigraphy can demonstrate right ventricular hypertrophy and dysfunction; however, this technique is rarely used at the present time. Although echocardiography or MRI may suggest the presence of pulmonary hypertension, the definitive diagnosis is made by cardiac catheterization, which allows measurement of right ventricular and pulmonary artery pressures; physiologic measurements during exercise are crucial in

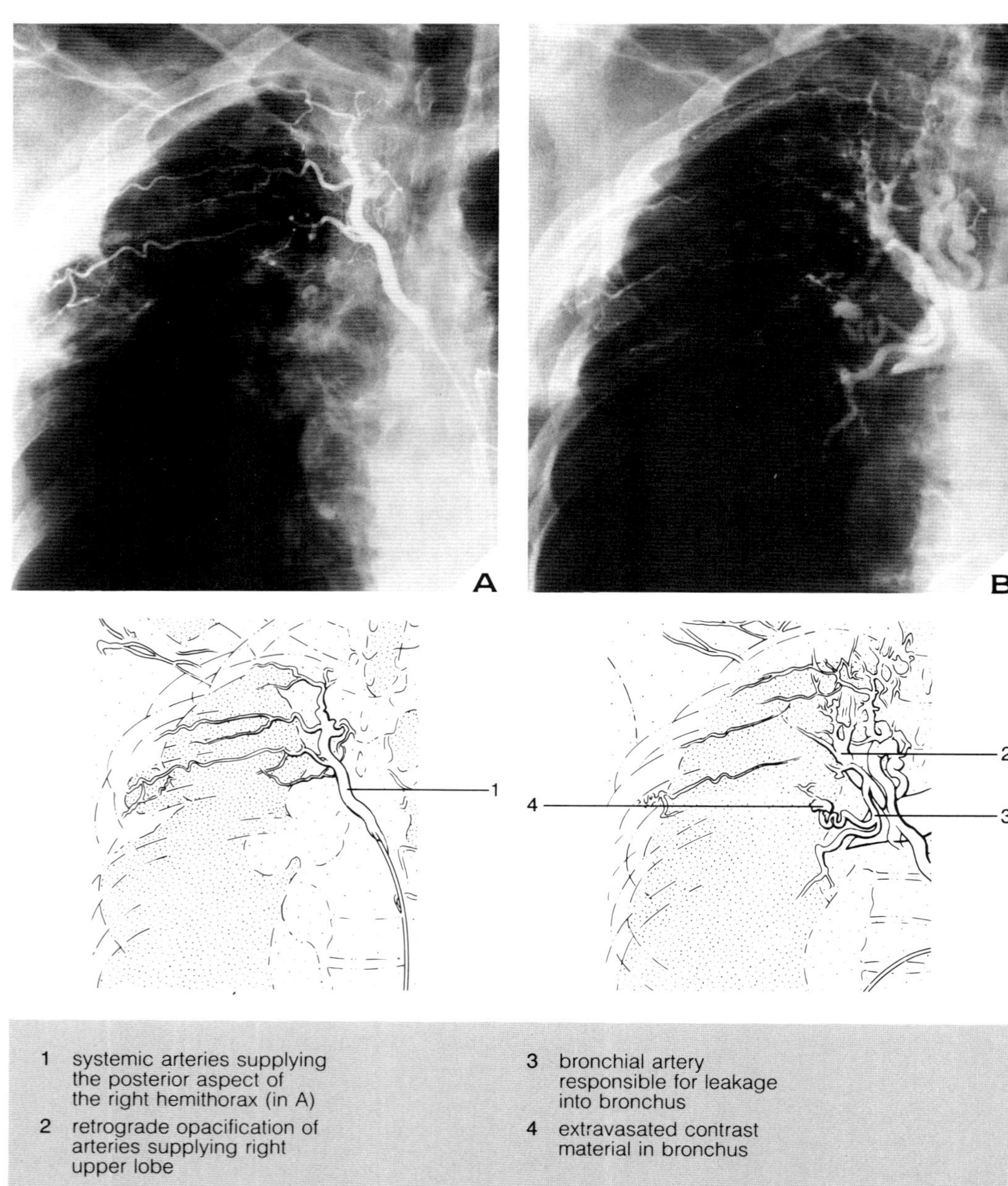

Fig. 24.10 Systemic perfusion of lungs in chronic cor pulmonale resulting in hemoptysis. Selective arteriogram of a parietal artery arising from the thoracic aorta in a patient with COPD who presented with hemoptysis. (A) Early arterial phase; branches of the markedly dilated parietal artery are distributed to the posterior aspect of the thoracic wall and to the mediastinum. (B) Late arterial phase; the contrast material has passed through the capillaries and opacifies distal branches of the pulmonary arteries to the right upper lobe. Dilated branches of the parietal artery remain opacified. A bronchial artery has ruptured into a bronchus, which is outlined by extravasated contrast material.

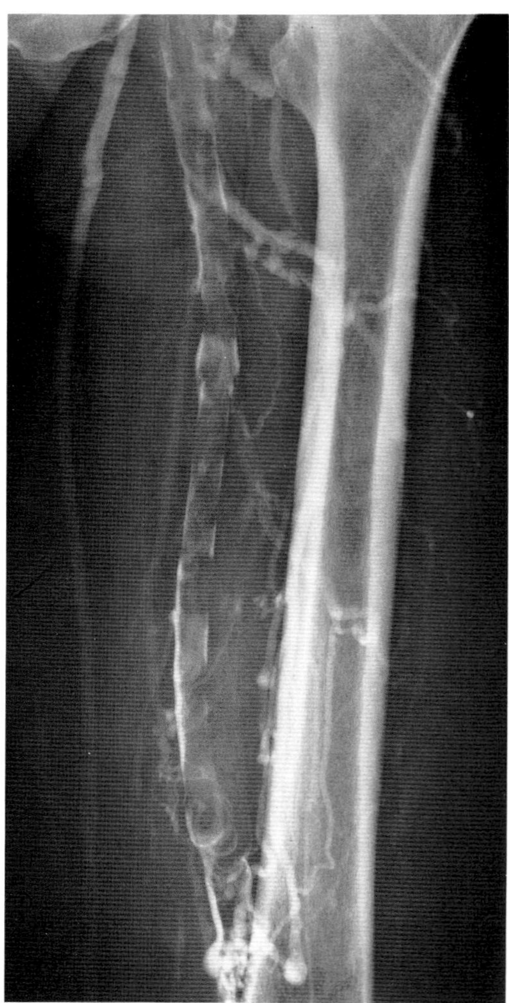

Fig. 24.11 Deep venous thrombosis. Venogram of left lower extremity in a patient with pulmonary embolism reveals a large filling defect involving the entire femoral vein. In some patients with DVT, venography demonstrates complete obstruction of the deep veins.

detecting elevated pulmonary resistance. Pulmonary arteriography demonstrates typical changes in the peripheral vessels. Although no longer routinely employed, pulmonary arteriography is sometimes performed to exclude pulmonary thromboembolism when the diagnosis of chronic cor pulmonale is in doubt or when a coexisting pulmonary embolus is suspected; to exclude infiltration of the pulmonary arteries by neoplasm or inflammatory disease; or to detect focal stenoses that may be amenable to correction either by angioplasty or surgery.

PULMONARY EMBOLISM

Pulmonary embolism is an acute process in which a clot (thromboembolus) or other material becomes lodged in the pulmonary arterial tree, resulting in localized hypoperfusion. When the hypoperfused region is large enough, a significant portion of the lung is deprived of respiratory and nutritional support, which may lead to pulmonary infarction. Although the great majority of pulmonary emboli originate in peripheral veins, they may occasionally arise in the vena cavae, right atrium, right ventricle, or main pulmonary arteries.

Pulmonary embolism is a common cause of death, accounting for about 600,000 deaths per year in the United States. It often goes undetected, reflecting the nonspecificity of the clinical and laboratory findings; in one large retrospective study, the correct diagnosis was not established prior to autopsy in more than two thirds of the cases (Rosenow, 1981). Almost 90 percent of patients with pulmonary thromboembolism survive the acute event.

CLINICAL FEATURES

Individuals with a predisposition to develop deep venous thrombosis are at greatest risk for pulmonary thromboembolism. Major risk factors include recent surgery, major trauma, prolonged bed rest, malignant disease, paralysis of the lower extremities, congestive heart failure, and advanced age.

Patients with acute pulmonary emboli typically present with dyspnea, tachypnea, and pleuritic pain. These symptoms are nonspecific, however, as they also occur in a wide spectrum of cardiopulmonary disorders. In one large series, the classic triad of acute pleuritic pain, dyspnea, and hemoptysis was observed in only 28 percent of cases (Bettman et al, 1984). Findings on physical examination include rales, pleural friction rub, fever, tachycardia, and signs of deep venous thrombosis in the lower extremities; although these findings are suggestive of acute pulmonary embolism they are nonspecific.

The ECG changes associated with acute pulmonary embolism are notoriously transient and nonspecific. The most frequently observed abnormalities are ST-segment and T-wave changes and QRS changes, each occurring in about two thirds of cases. Other abnormalities include T-wave inversion (40 percent), right bundle branch block (12 percent), and left axis deviation (12 percent). Although the clinical picture and ECG findings are nonspecific, they nevertheless play an important role in diagnosis because they indicate the need for further evaluation.

The results of routine laboratory tests (eg, WBC, sedimentation rate) are inconsistent and of little value in differential diagnosis. Although serum creatine phosphokinase and lactic acid dehydrogenase levels are frequently elevated, neither test is sufficiently sensitive or specific to serve as a screening test for acute pulmonary embolism.

Pulmonary function tests typically demonstrate decreased arterial oxygen saturation. Values of 60 percent or less are the rule in patients with extensive pulmonary thromboembolism. It must be emphasized, however, that a normal arterial oxygen saturation does not exclude a small pulmonary embolus.

As noted below, chest films frequently demonstrate a pleural effusion. In such cases thoracentesis may be helpful in differential diagnosis. The presence of a bloody pleural effusion strongly suggests the diagnosis of pulmonary thromboembolism. Bloody pleural fluid usually indicates the presence of a large embolus. Small emboli are typically associated with a simple transudate, a finding of relatively little value in differential diagnosis.

The demonstration of deep venous thrombosis (DVT) in the pelvis or lower extremity in a patient with suggestive clinical and plain film findings greatly increases diagnostic certainty. The diagnosis of DVT may be straightforward; sometimes, however, it is extremely difficult. The diagnostic evaluation begins with careful physical examination of the lower extremities. Tenderness, induration, and/or thickening along the course of the femoral vein allow a confident diagnosis of DVT in the thigh; however, physical examination is much less reliable in detecting DVT of the calf veins. [Homan's sign (calf tenderness on foot dorsiflexion) is nonspecific.]

Various imaging modalities can be used in the diagnosis of DVT. These include:

1. *Venous Doppler sonography with compression.* Although the Doppler technique accurately detects thrombi at the level of the femoral and popliteal veins, it is less reliable in detecting DVT below the knee. Sonography also allows assessment of the integrity of the venous valves.
2. *Fibrinogen scintiscan.* This test is based on the observation that intravenously administered fibrinogen which has been tagged with a suitable radioisotope (usually ^{125}I) is incorporated into a fresh thrombus and can be detected by scintigraphic techniques. Although this test is highly sensitive and specific in high-risk patients, it is of limited value in patients who are acutely ill because 6 to 24 hours are required to obtain definitive results. Fibrinogen scintigraphy is more accurate in DVT below the knee than for DVT of the ileofemoral veins. In general, however, a negative study excludes the possibility of acute DVT.
3. *Radionuclide venography.* In this technique, [^{99m}Tc]-albumen-labeled microspheres are injected into the dorsal veins of the feet and serial scintigrams of the thighs and pelvis are obtained. Radionuclide venography accurately detects thrombi in the femoral and iliac veins and the inferior vena cava. It is much less reliable in detecting thrombi below the knee.
4. *Venography (phlebography).* Venography remains the "gold standard" in the diagnosis of DVT; it is both more sensitive and more specific than sonographic and scintigraphic techniques (Fig. 24.11). The disadvantages of venography are its invasive nature, the risk of exacerbating an existing phlebitis, and tissue damage secondary to extravasation of contrast material.

IMAGING AND INVASIVE DIAGNOSIS

CHEST FILMS

Chest films occasionally show a triangular, pleural-based infiltrate (''Hampton's hump'') in one or both lower lobes, in association with a pleural effusion (Fig. 24.12). Although such infiltrates are nonspecific (they are also seen in pneumonia and congestive heart failure, among other conditions), their presence in both lungs suggests pulmonary thromboembolism, which is bilateral in 85 percent of cases. Pleural-based infiltrates nearly always indicate occlusion or peripheral arteries. (The lungs are usually clear in patients with thromboemboli of the central pulmonary arteries.) Anatomic studies have shown that such infiltrates, which may take weeks to resolve radiographically, represent localized hemorrhage and edema rather than pulmonary infarction.

Chest films demonstrate pleural fluid in about one third of patients with large pulmonary emboli; the effusion is bilateral in about 10 percent of cases. Pleural effusions associated with pulmonary emboli are usually transient; they are almost never massive (Fig. 24.13). Although pleural fluid (when present) is usually evident on the initial chest film, it may not appear until further episodes of pulmonary embolization have occurred.

Other plain film findings associated with pulmonary embolism include elevation of the ipsilateral hemidiaphragm, enlargement of the right descending pulmonary artery (Fleishner's sign), oligemia of the affected segment or segments, atelectasis, and line shadows (Fig. 24.14); none of these signs is very sensitive, however. Chest films are normal in 20 to 30 percent of patients with acute pulmonary thromboembolism.

NUCLEAR MEDICINE

The ventilation–perfusion scan (''lung scan'') is a useful noninvasive screening procedure in patients with suspected pulmonary embolism. Although a normal perfusion scan excludes an acute embolus, an abnormal study does not necessarily confirm it, as areas of decreased or absent perfusion (''perfusion defects'') can be caused by other conditions (e.g, COPD). In such cases one must determine whether there is a corresponding defect on the ventilation scan or a parenchymal abnormality (eg, bulla) in the same region on the chest film.

The diagnosis of pulmonary embolism can be made with a high degree of certainty when the ventilation–perfusion scan demonstrates an area of decreased or absent perfusion that is normally ventilated *(ventilation–perfusion mismatch)*. The diagnosis is less certain when the the ventilation–perfusion scan demonstrates areas of abnormal ventilation as well as areas of abnormal perfusion *(ventilation–perfusion match)*. In such cases the scintigraphic pattern is classified as having a low, intermediate (indeterminate), or high probability for the diagnosis of pulmonary embolism. The probability is *low* when the area of ventilation-perfusion matching is small and limited to

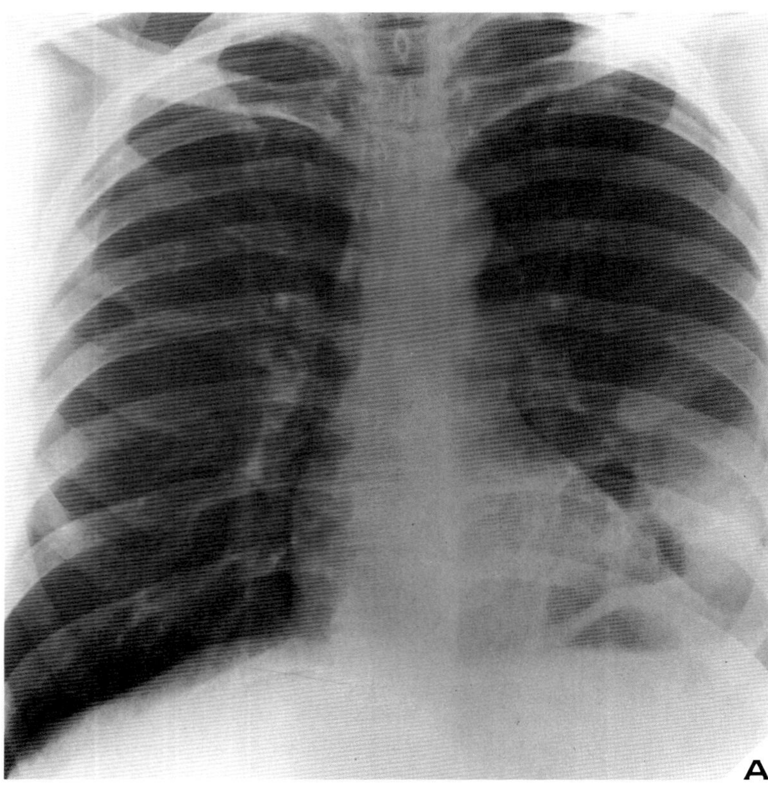

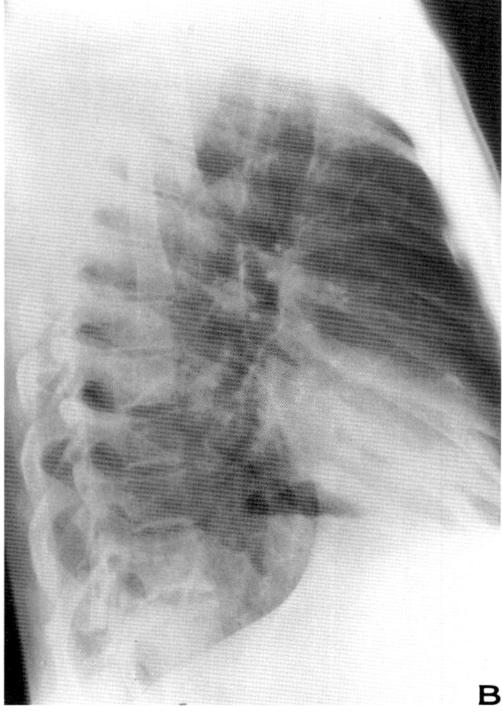

Fig. 24.12 Acute pulmonary embolism. (A) Frontal and (B) lateral chest films show a triangular-shaped infiltrate in the posterior portion of the left lower lobe (''Hampton's hump''), which presumably represents an area of hemorrhage. Pulmonary arteriography demonstrated thromboembolus in the lower lobe arteries.

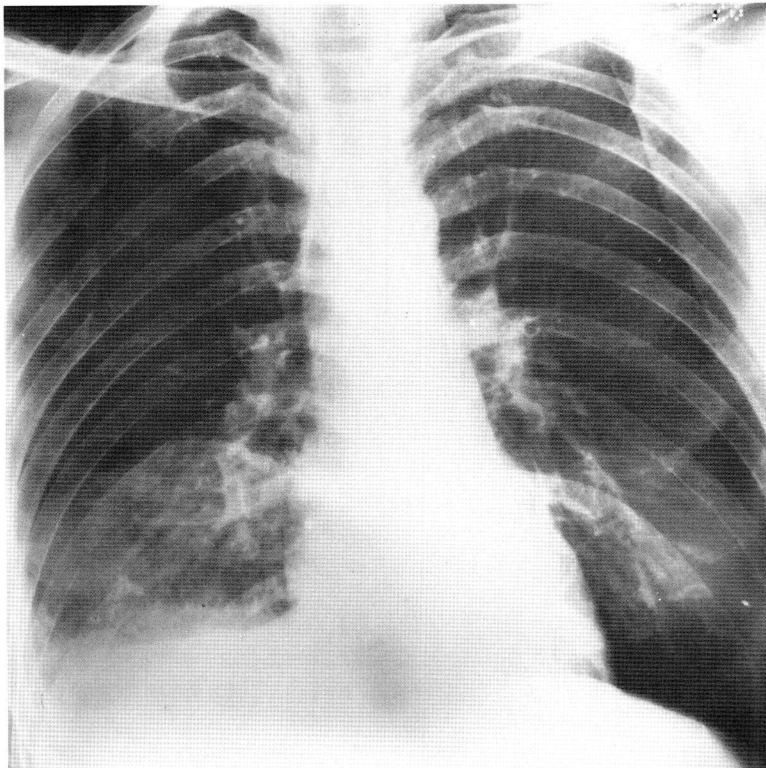

Fig. 24.13 Acute pulmonary embolism. Frontal chest film demonstrates a triangular density in the right lower lobe which abuts the diaphragm. Parenchymal densities of this type presumably represent focal hemorrhage. There is a small right pleural effusion.

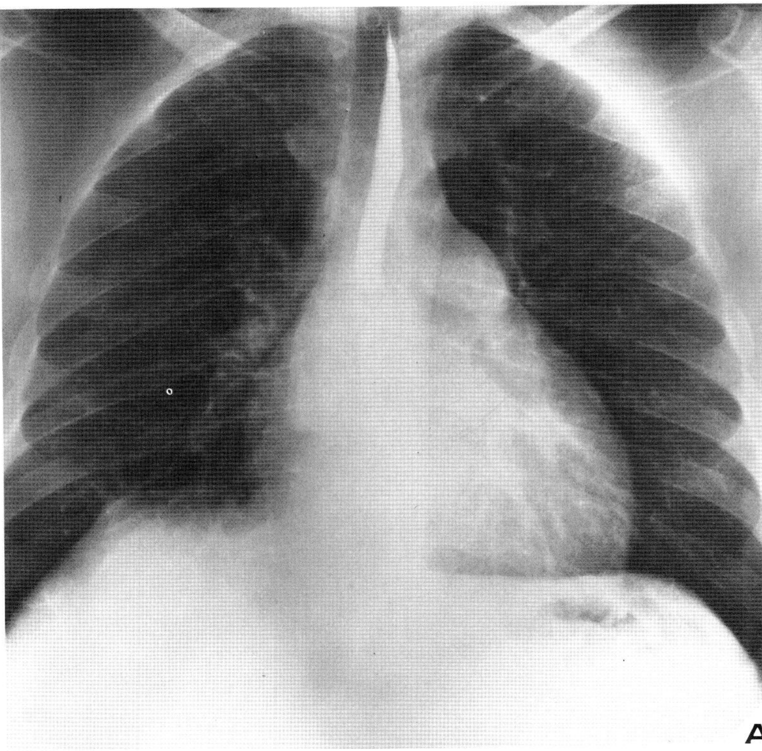

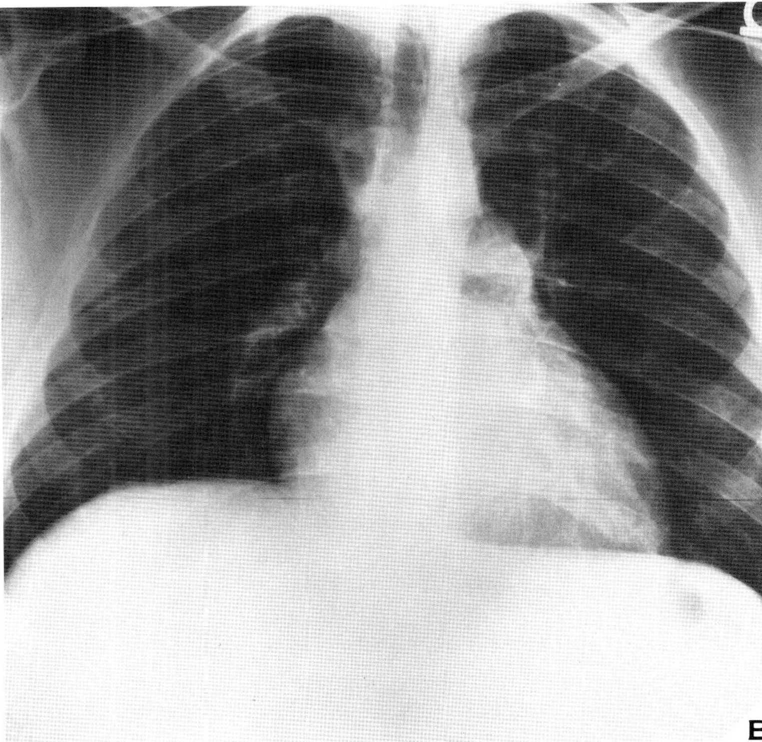

Fig. 24.14 Acute pulmonary embolism. (A) Initial chest film is normal. (B) Repeat chest film (obtained after the onset of symptoms) shows diminished vascular markings in the right lower zone. The right descending pulmonary artery is slightly larger than in A. Pulmonary arteriography demonstrated an embolus in the branches supplying the right lower lobe. Although these findings are suggestive of pulmonary embolism, plain films are not very sensitive in the diagnosis of this condition.

the area of mismatch (Fig. 24.15). (In most instances the perfusion defect is smaller than the abnormality seen on the chest film.) The probability is *intermediate* or *indeterminate* when there is a single segmental perfusion defect with a mismatch, or a multisegmental or lobar perfusion defect with either a match or mismatch. The probability is *high* when there are multiple segmental or lobar perfusion defects with a mismatch (Fig. 24.16). Generally speaking, the likelihood of a pulmonary embolus is 10 percent in the "low" group, 25 to 50 percent in the "intermediate" group, and 90 percent in the "high" group.

Many disease processes (eg, neoplasms, pneumonia, atelectasis) can simulate pulmonary infarction on the plain film. On lung scans the affected areas will be neither perfused nor ventilated (ie, there is a ventilation–perfusion match); in such cases there is a low probability that the abnormalities are due to a pulmonary embolus. This is also true when the perfusion defect is substantially smaller than the area of abnormality seen on the chest film. Conversely, the probability of a pulmonary embolus is high when the perfusion defect is much larger than the radiographic abnormality.

Once the possibility of pulmonary embolism is considered, lung scans should be obtained as soon as possible, preferably within 48 hours. This is because the size of the perfusion defect decreases over time, decreasing the predictive power of the examination (ie, a high-probability scan will become an intermediate- or low-probability one). If pulmonary angiography is subsequently performed, the scintigraphic findings will direct the angiographer to the specific area to be studied, thereby increasing diagnostic accuracy.

ECHOCARDIOGRAPHY

Echocardiography can detect hemodynamic changes that indirectly suggest the diagnosis of pulmonary embolism (eg, increased pulmonary artery pressure, right ventricular hypertension, pulmonic and tricuspid valvular insufficiency). Only rarely does echocardiography allow a specific diagnosis of pulmonary embolism, ie, when the embolus is lodged in the pulmonary trunk or in the most proximal segment of the right or left pulmonary artery (Fig. 24.17, Appendix).

COMPUTED TOMOGRAPHY

CT provides a noninvasive means of detecting pulmonary emboli that are located centrally, ie, in the pulmonary trunk or the proximal segment of the right or left pulmonary artery.

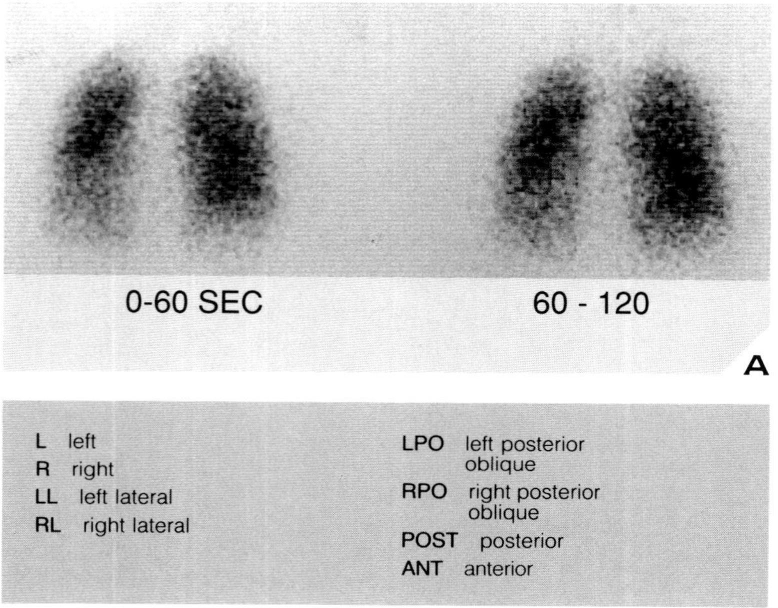

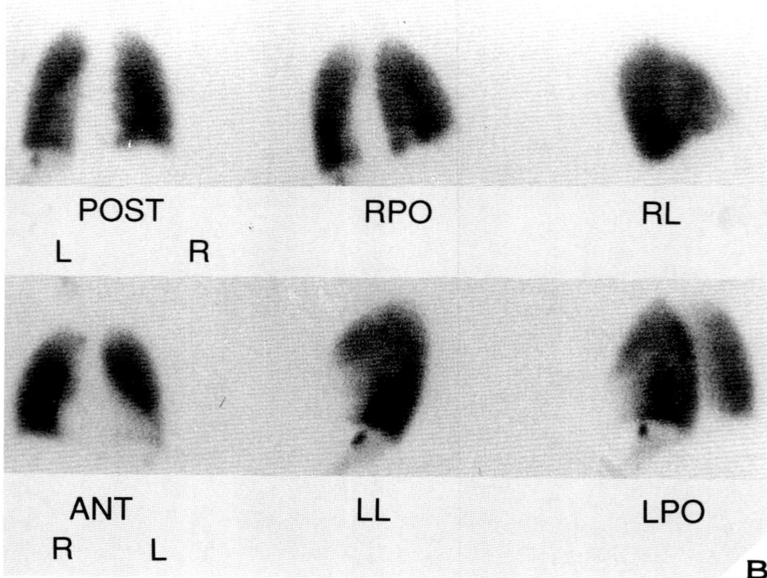

Fig. 24.15 Low probability ventilation–perfusion scan. (A) ^{133}Xe ventilation scan at 1 and 2 minutes (equilibrium phase) demonstrates even distribution of the radionuclide throughout both lungs, reaching the terminal airways and alveoli. (B) Perfusion scan (^{99m}Tc-MAA) demonstrates areas of decreased perfusion in the left lower lobe and right middle lobe. Chest films (not illustrated) were normal.

MAGNETIC RESONANCE IMAGING

Spin–echo ECG-gated MR images demonstrate the filling defect in the pulmonary trunk or large pulmonary arteries which is associated with a central pulmonary embolus. With the gradient-rephasing technique, it is possible to visualize more distal branches; in animal experiments, pulmonary emboli have been identified in vessels as small as 3 mm in diameter. In theory, MRI should be able to differentiate the hemorrhagic infiltrate associated with a pulmonary embolus from parenchymal consolidation caused by infection or atelectasis; however, preliminary studies have yielded inconsistent results. Although MRI may ultimately play a role in the diagnosis of pulmonary thromboembolism, it is not as sensitive as angiography and is not suitable for clinical application at this time.

ANGIOGRAPHY

Selective pulmonary arteriography is the definitive study in patients with suspected pulmonary embolus. It is indicated in the following situations:

1. When the ventilation–perfusion scan is of intermediate or low probability and the clinical picture is suggestive of pulmonary embolism.
2. When pulmonary embolus is suspected in the presence of parenchymal lung disease or congestive failure, both of which render the lung scan inaccurate.
3. In patients in whom anticoagulant therapy is associated with a significant risk.
4. In patients with a past history of unconfirmed "recurrent pulmonary embolism."
5. In patients with massive pulmonary embolism in whom embolectomy is contemplated.

Pulmonary arteriography should be performed within 24 to 72 hours of the onset of symptoms; otherwise, spontaneous resolution of the clot makes interpretation of the angiograms difficult. Both the left and right pulmonary arteries should be selectively opacified and images obtained in the right and left anterior oblique projections. In our experience, 35-mm cineangiography and large films are equally sensitive in detecting emboli in medium and small branches. The mortality rate of the procedure is less than 0.25 percent and the morbidity is approximately 4 percent.

The typical angiographic appearance of a pulmonary embolus is an intraluminal filling defect or cut-off of a pulmonary ar-

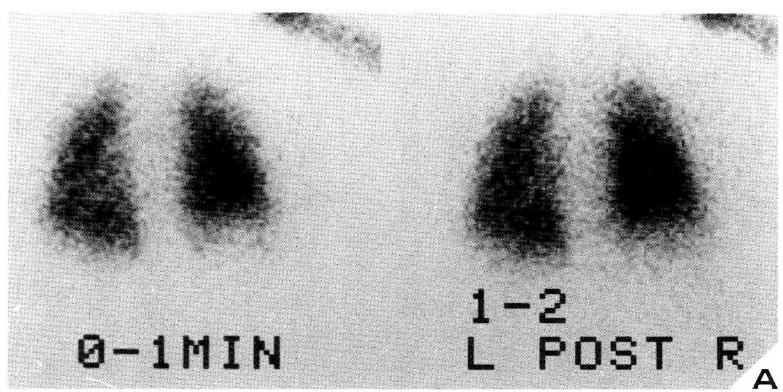

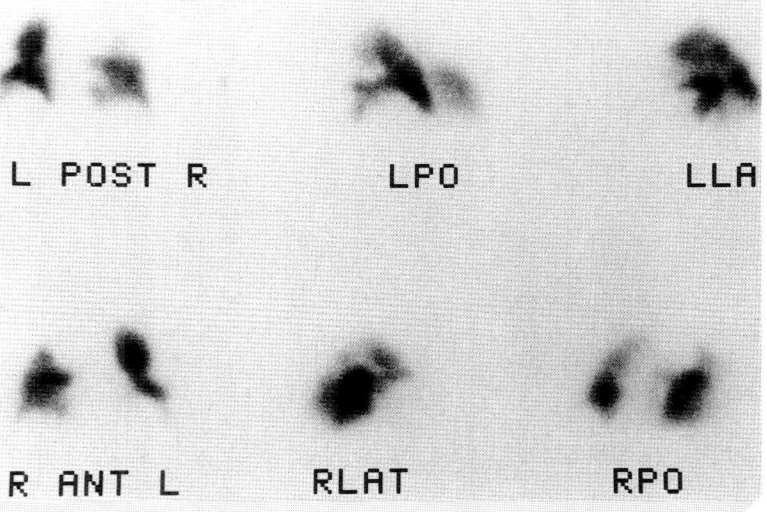

Fig. 24.16 High probability ventilation–perfusion scan. (A) ^{133}Xe ventilation scan at 1 and 2 minutes (equilibrium phase) shows uniform distribution of the radionuclide throughout both lungs. There are no findings to suggest obstruction of abnormal airway ventilation. (B) Perfusion scan (^{99m}Tc-MAA) demonstrates perfusion defects in both lungs. There is no perfusion of the right upper lobe and there are several subsegmental peripheral defects in the left lung. The chest film was normal.

tery; both may be present (Figs. 24.18 to 24.20). Localized slowing or asymmetry of blood flow is suspicious but not diagnostic; when either of these phenomena is identified, a more selective arteriogram is needed to confirm the presence of an embolus.

When pulmonary arteriography is properly performed and interpreted, false negatives are rare. In one study, none of 167 patients with suspected pulmonary thromboembolism died of the disorder or subsequently exhibited evidence of recurrent pulmonary embolism or deep venous thrombosis.

PULMONARY HYPERTENSION

Pulmonary arterial hypertension ("pulmonary hypertension") is defined as a condition in which the pressure in the pulmonary artery is higher than normal in the presence of normal left atrial pressure, ie, the mean pressure is greater than 20 mm Hg at rest or 30 mm Hg with exercise. Pulmonary hypertension results from a decrease in the effective size of the pulmonary arterial bed, which is accompanied by an increase in pulmonary resistance. There are two major types

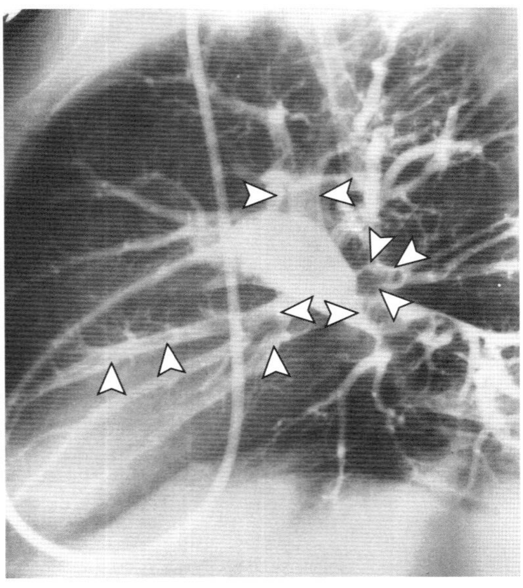

Fig. 24.18 Angiographic demonstration of multiple pulmonary emboli. Lateral projection of selective right pulmonary arteriogram reveals filling defects (*arrows*) in arteries supplying the right upper, middle, and lower lobes.

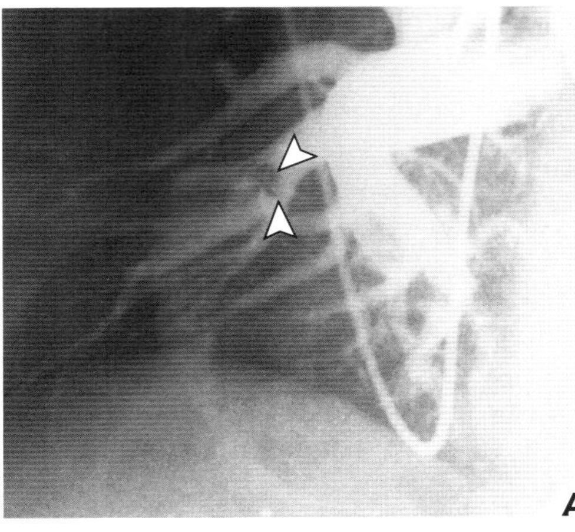

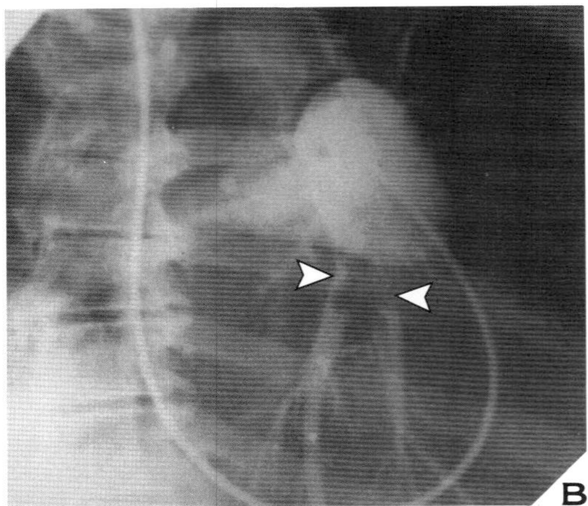

Fig. 24.19 Angiographic demonstration of multiple pulmonary emboli. (A) Selective right pulmonary arteriogram shows a filling defect (*arrows*) in the artery supplying the right middle lobe. (B) Selective left pulmonary arteriogram demonstrates filling defects (*arrows*) in arteries supplying the left lower lobe.

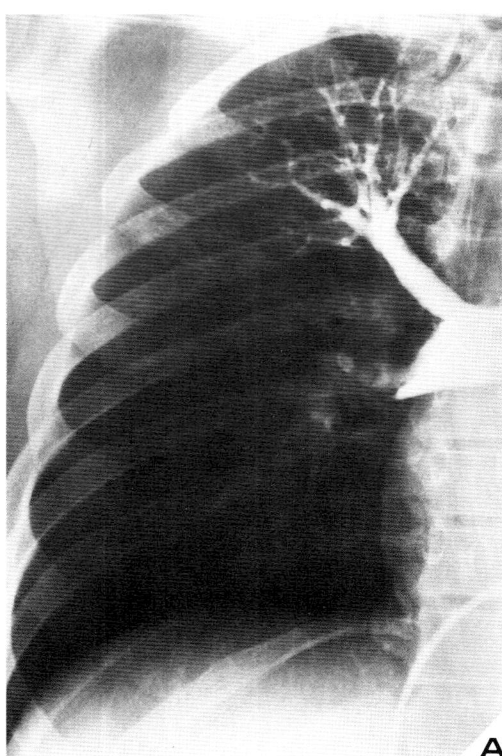

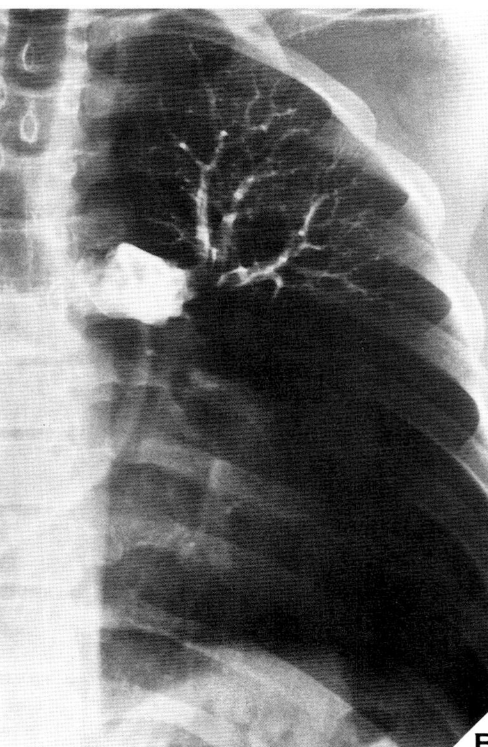

Fig. 24.20 Angiographic demonstration of massive bilateral pulmonary embolism. (A) Selective right pulmonary arteriogram shows complete occlusion of the right pulmonary artery just beyond the origin of the right upper lobe artery. Filling defects are also seen in the branches to the right upper lobe. (B) Selective left pulmonary arteriogram shows patency of the proximal segment. However, the lower lobe artery is completely occluded and there are multiple filling defects in the upper lobe branches.

of pulmonary hypertension: primary and secondary. In the former, the cause of increased pulmonary resistance is unknown; in the latter, causative factors can be identified either in the pulmonary vascular tree or in the surrounding structures.

MORPHOLOGY OF THE PULMONARY ARTERIAL SYSTEM

The pulmonary arterial tree consists of the pulmonary trunk, main pulmonary arteries, and the intraparenchymal branches (ie, lobar, segmental, subsegmental, and peripheral pulmonary arteries). The distribution of the pulmonary arteries corresponds closely with that of the cartilaginous and noncartilaginous airways.

At the peripheral level, the arteries are called *preacinar* or *intra-acinar,* according to which type of airway they accompany. The former are located at the level of the terminal bronchi (the smallest noncartilaginous division of the bronchial tree); the latter are located at the level of the respiratory bronchioles.

The walls of the pulmonary arteries can be elastic or muscular, or a combination of the two. Arteries with elastic walls (pulmonary trunk, main pulmonary arteries, lobar and segmental branches) have a diameter greater than 2000 μm. The preacinar arteries, which have a diameter of 150 to 2000 μm, are predominantly muscular. The smallest branches of the pulmonary arterial tree are the intra-acinar arteries, which measure less than 150 μm in diameter. The walls of the larger intra-acinar branches (at the level of the respiratory bronchi and alveolar ducts) contain both muscular and elastic tissue. The smaller intra-acinar branches (at the level of the alveoli arteries) lack both muscle and elastic tissue, their walls consisting of a basement membrane, endothelial cells, pericytes, and intermediate cells (Fig. 24.21).

Pulmonary resistance is predominantly produced by the preacinar and intra-acinar (acinar) muscular arteries, the so-called *pulmonary resistance arteries*. The pathologic changes associated with primary pulmonary hypertension are at the level of

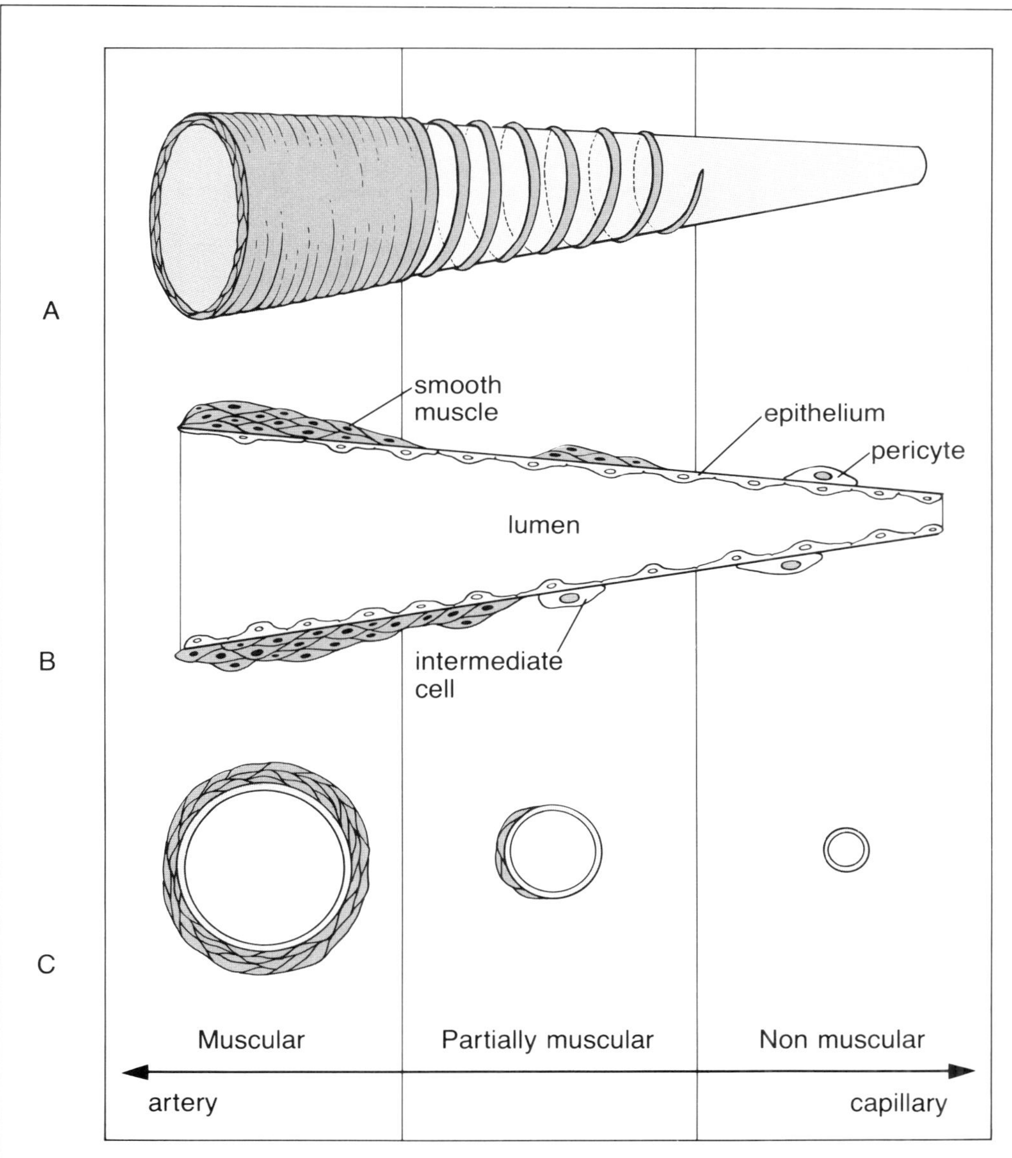

Fig. 24.21 Morphology of the preacinar and acinar arteries. (A) Light microscopy; at the distal end of the arterial tree the complete muscular coat is replaced by a spiral (partial) muscle coat. Arteries still larger than capillaries are entirely devoid of muscle. The muscular proacinar and acinar arteries represent the pulmonary resistance arteries, the usual site of the lesions in pulmonary arterial hypertension. (B) Electron microscopy domonstrates pericytes and intermediate cells in the nonmuscular part of the partially muscular artery and muscle-free region of the nonmuscular artery. These are precursors of smooth muscle cells. (C) Cross-section of the walls of muscular, partially muscular, and nonmuscular arteries indicating their relative diameter and wall thickness. (Adapted with permission from Meyrick B. Reid L: Pulmonary hypertension, Anatomic and physiologic correlates. *Clin Chest Med* 1983; 4:99)

these arteries, which normally have significant amounts of muscle in their walls (Fig. 25.22).

Pulmonary hypertension also can result from occlusion of small or large pulmonary veins. Obstructive lesions at this level produce secondary muscular hypertrophy of the peripheral muscular arteries.

PATHOGENESIS AND PATHOLOGIC ANATOMY

PRIMARY PULMONARY HYPERTENSION

The cause of the increased pulmonary resistance in this condition is unknown. The pathologic lesions are in the preacinar and intra-acinar arteries; in some instances lesions of the pulmonary venules are present as well. The lesions are of three main types: plexiform, thromboembolic, and veno-occlusive. Although any of the three lesions may predominate, they are usually present in various combinations. *Plexogenic pulmonary arteriopathy* is characterized by intimal cell proliferation and secondary fibrosis of the peripheral muscular arteries, which become dilated and take on the appearance of a vascular plexus; the muscular component of the arterial walls is usually increased. *Thromboembolic arteriopathy* is characterized by thrombi in different stages of organization within the preacinar and intra-acinar arteries. *Veno-occlusive disease* is characterized by organized or, rarely, fresh thrombi within small pulmonary veins or venules. Neomuscularization of small arteries, which produces lesions resembling plexogenic arteriopathy, is a constant finding. Medial hypertrophy of larger muscular and elastic pulmonary arteries is frequently present. Veno-occlusive disease may lead to neomuscularization of the vein walls and chronic interstitial edema, which may culminate in fibrosis of the subpleural lymphatics and/or interlobular septa. Medial hypertrophy of muscular pulmonary arteries is common in such cases.

A special variety of increased pulmonary resistance seen in the newborn is "persistent fetal circulation" ("pulmonary hypertension of the newborn"), which results from abnormal in-

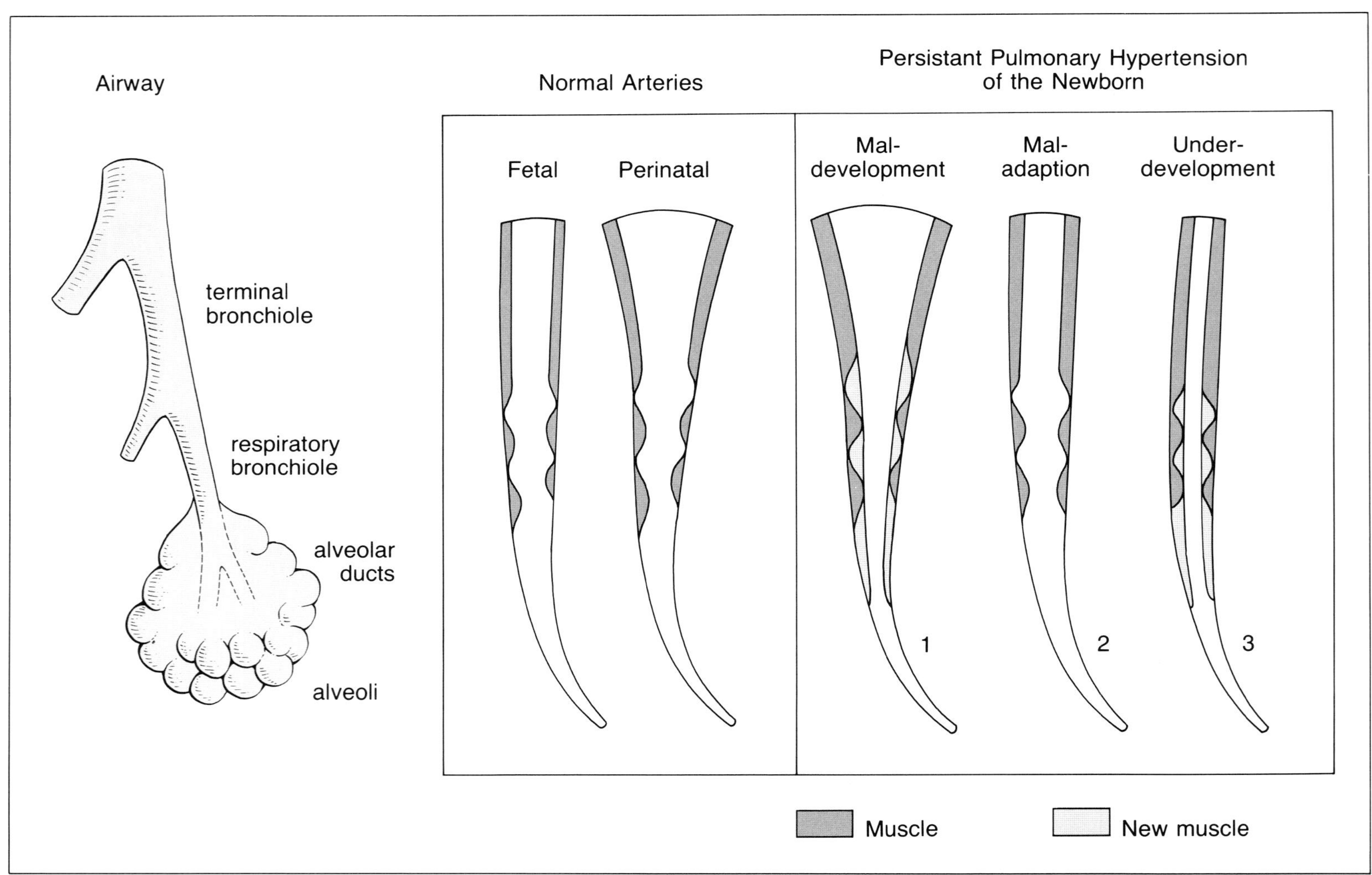

Fig. 24.22 Pulmonary hypertension of the newborn. In the normal fetus and neonate the arteries accompanying the terminal bronchioles have a complete muscle coat, whereas the arteries accompanying the respiratory bronchioles and proximal alveolar ducts have an incomplete muscle coat. The arteries at the level of the distal alveolar ducts and the alveoli are normally devoid of muscle. Pulmonary hypertension of the newborn ("persistent fetal circulation") is characterized by the precocious appearance of smooth muscle in arteries at the level of the distal alveolar ducts and alveoli, resulting in maldevelopment, maladaption, or underdevelopment of these arteries. (Adapted with permission from Meyrick B. Reid L: Pulmonary hypertension. Anatomic and physiologic correlates. *Clin Chest Med* 1983; 4:199)

trauterine development of the precapillary arterial unit (Fig. 24.22). Anatomically, there is precocious muscularization of the alveolar arteries, which may begin several weeks before birth. (Normally, arteries at the preacinar and acinar level are not as well muscularized in the newborn as they are in the child or adult.) Although this disorder is usually idiopathic, it may be associated with congenital diaphragmatic hernia, meconium aspiration syndrome, and certain types of lung dysplasia.

SECONDARY PULMONARY HYPERTENSION

Pulmonary arterial hypertension can also develop as a sequela of various disorders of the mediastinum or lung. For example, neoplasms (eg, carcinoma, Hodgkin's disease) or granulomatous disease (eg, tuberculosis, histoplasmosis, sarcoidosis) can compress or obstruct the pulmonary trunk or a main pulmonary artery. Rarely, a sarcoma may arise in a pulmonary artery. Several forms of arteritis, including giant cell arteritis, rheumatoid arthritis, lupus erythematosus, and Takayasu's disease have been associated with acquired pulmonary artery stenosis (see Chapter 27). Stenosis or occlusion of lobar and segmental arteries may also occur, leaving large portions of the lung underperfused. Although the etiology of acquired branch stenoses is obscure, it is believed that these lesions are usually caused by inflammation or pulmonary thromboembolism.

As noted in the chapters on congenital heart disease, pulmonary hypertension is a common sequela of congenital left to right shunts (Fig. 24.23). The pathologic changes in such cases are similar to those seen in primary pulmonary hypertension.

CLINICAL MANIFESTATIONS

Patients with primary pulmonary hypertension typically present with dyspnea, fatigue, chest pain, syncope, peripheral edema, and palpations. Physical examination usually reveals an increase in the pulmonic component of the second heart sound (P2), an increase in the right-sided third heart sound, and an increase in the right-sided fourth heart sound. Signs of tricuspid and pulmonic insufficiency are frequently present. ECG findings include right axis deviation, right ventricular hypertrophy, and a right ventricular strain pattern.

Pulmonary parenchymal malfunction, characterized by a reduction in both total lung capacity and forced vital capacity, is common in primary pulmonary hypertension. Hypoxemia and hypocapnia are frequently present in such cases.

IMAGING AND INVASIVE DIAGNOSIS

PLAIN FILMS

Chest films of patients with severe primary pulmonary hypertension typically reveal a prominent pulmonary trunk, enlargement of the main pulmonary arteries and lobar branches, and

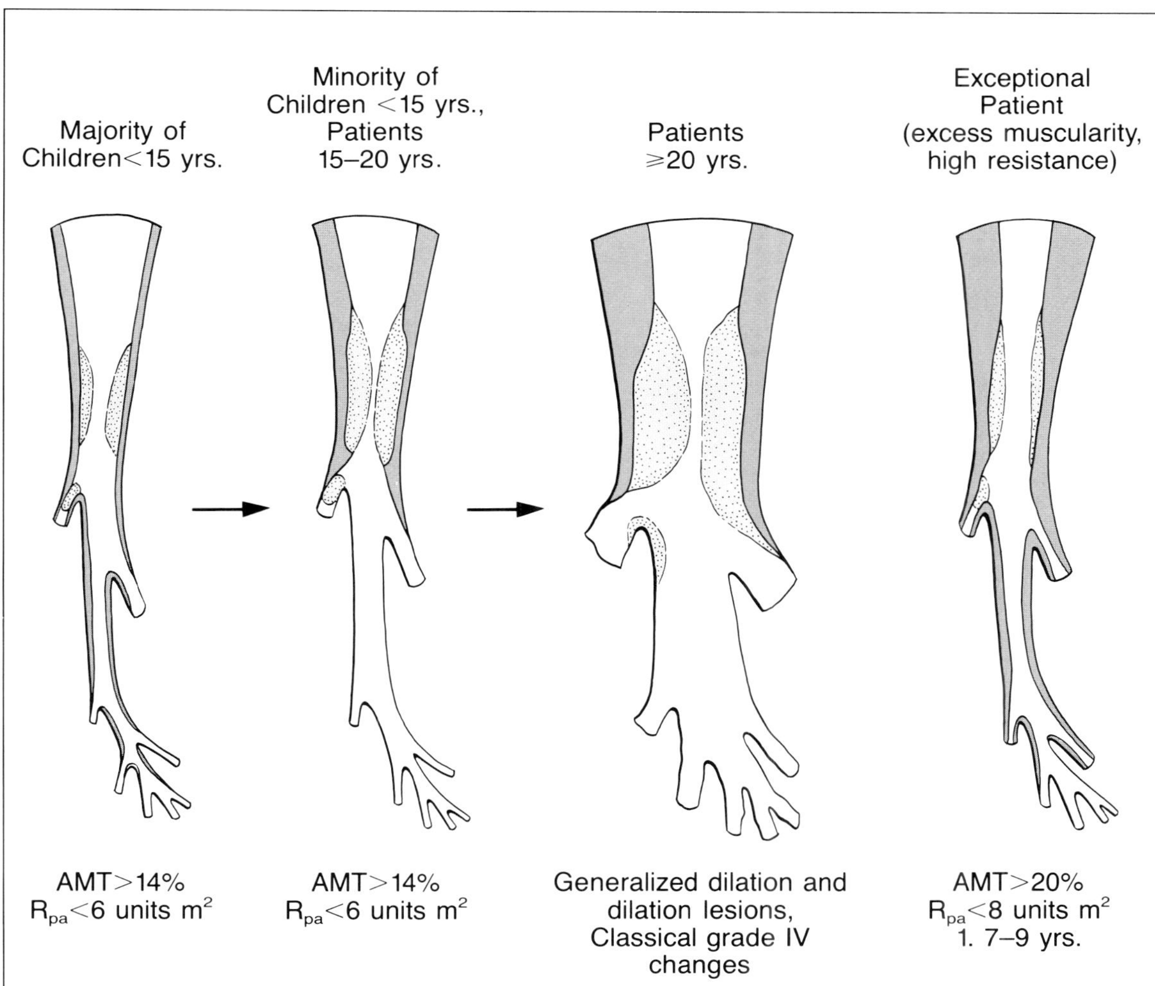

Fig. 24.23 Pathological changes related to age and pulmonary arterial resistance in patients with ventricular septal defects. The principal pathologic changes in pulmonary arteries 50–100 μm in diameter are shown schematically. An increase in the number of muscular cells in the arterial wall reduces the size of the lumen. Intimal proliferation further contributes to the obstructive pulmonary vascular disease. AMT = arterial medial thickness; R_{pa} = pulmonary arteriolar resistance. Stippling indicates intimal proliferation and fibrosis. (Adapted with permission from Haworth SG. Understanding pulmonary arterial disease in young children. *Int J Cardiol* 1987; 15:101)

decreased size of the peripheral arterial branches (Figs. 24.24 to 24.26). A similar pattern is seen in patients with secondary pulmonary hypertension resulting from congenital heart disease (Fig. 24.27). The chest film is normal in approximately 6 to 10 percent of patients with primary pulmonary hypertension.

Calcification of the wall of the pulmonary artery is an occasional finding (Fig. 24.25). Although it usually indicates longstanding severe pulmonary hypertension, pulmonary artery calcification occurs in a small number of patients with reversible pulmonary hypertension. Redistribution of pulmonary blood flow ("cephalization"), similar to that seen in pulmonary venous hypertension, is occasionally seen. This phenomenon is apparently related to the uneven distribution of the pulmonary arterial disease. Whereas pulmonary venous hypertension commonly leads to interstitial and alveolar pulmonary edema, primary pulmonary arterial hypertension does not result in increased permeability of the alveolar–capillary membrane.

ECHOCARDIOGRAPHY

Two-dimensional echocardiography demonstrates an enlarged right ventricle, a normal or small left ventricle, and paradoxical

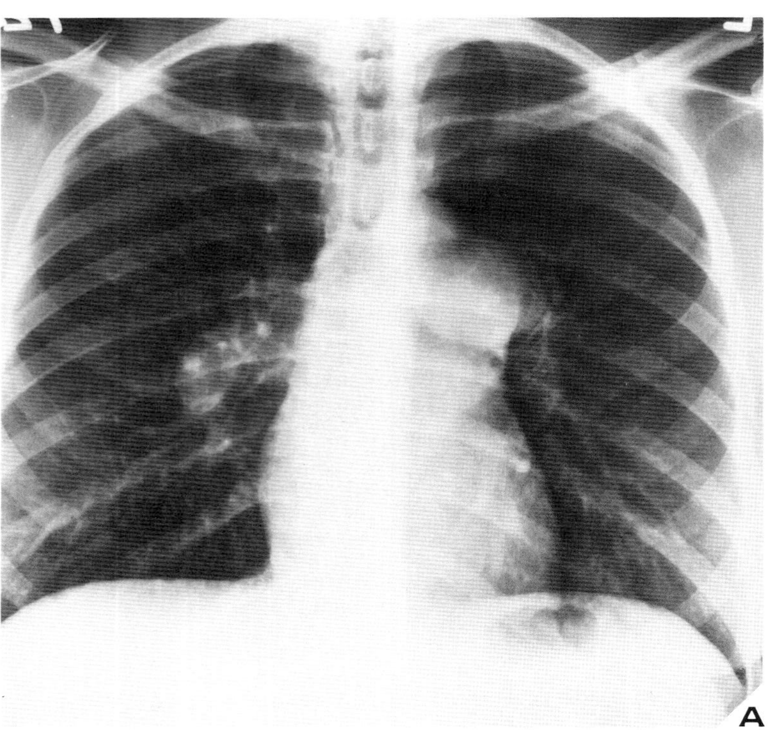

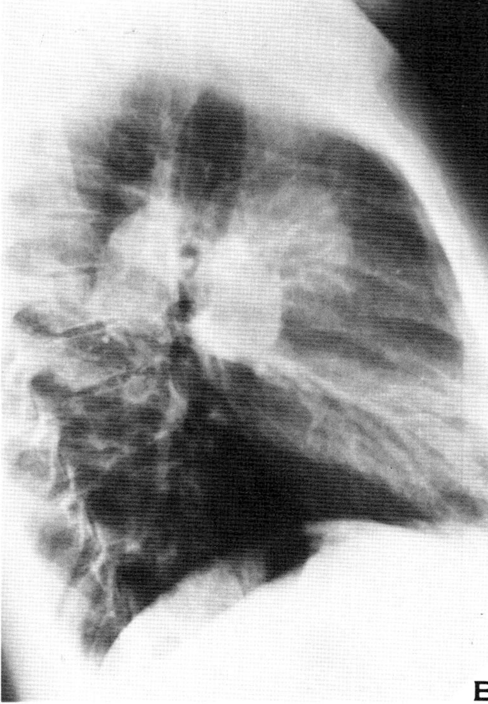

Fig. 24.24 Primary pulmonary hypertension. (A) Posteroanterior and (B) lateral chest films show massive dilatation of the pulmonary trunk and the right and left pulmonary arteries. The peripheral vasculature is diminished, whereas the central (lobar and segmental) arteries are dilated. The aortic arch is normal in size. Although the heart is of normal size, the zone of contact with the anterior chest wall is increased (B), indicating right ventricular hypertrophy. The pulmonary arterial pressure was 100/20 mm Hg.

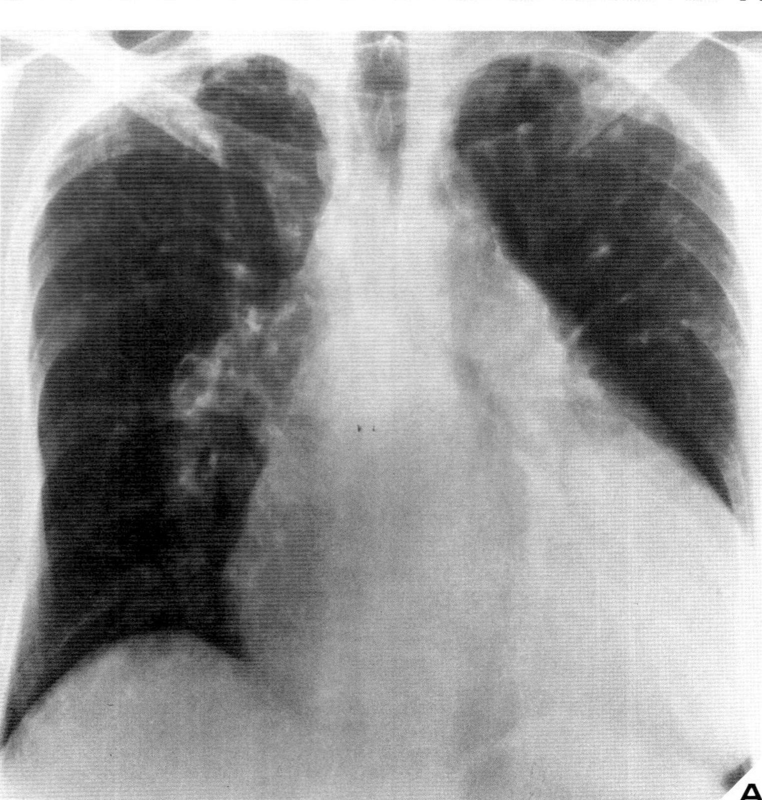

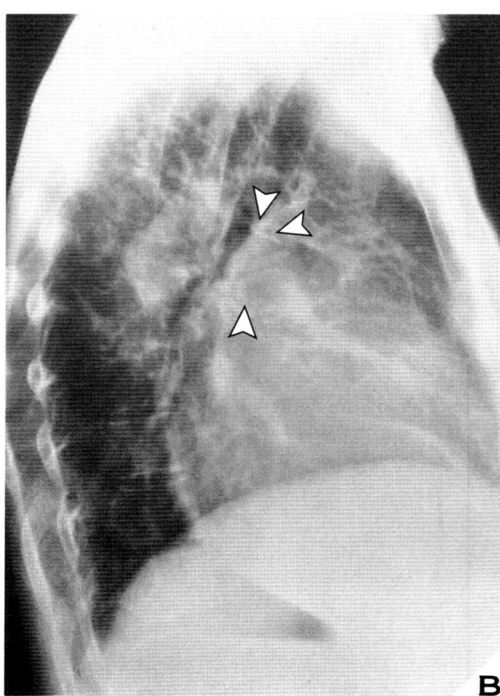

Fig. 24.25 Longstanding severe primary pulmonary hypertension (A) Posteroanterior and (B) lateral chest films show marked cardiomegaly with right ventricular and right atrial enlargement. The pulmonary trunk, as well as the right and left pulmonary arteries, are dilated. The presence of calcification (*arrows*) in the wall of the pulmonary trunk and right pulmonary artery reflects longstanding pulmonary hypertension. The azygos vein is enlarged, indicating increased pressure in the systemic veins.

motion of the ventricular septum (Fig. 24.28, Appendix). The pulmonary vascular resistance (pressure drop across the pulmonary vascular bed divided by flow), which is 1.5 to 2.0 in normal individuals, is increased 10- to 15-fold in patients with primary pulmonary hypertension. With Doppler imaging, it is possible to estimate the severity of any pulmonic and/or tricuspid valvular insufficiency that may be present. This assessment is facilitated by the use of color Doppler.

NUCLEAR MEDICINE

Ventilation–perfusion scans are sometimes used to exclude pulmonary embolism, which can mimic primary pulmonary hypertension. Most patients with primary pulmonary hypertension have normal ventilation–perfusion scans. However, some may exhibit a diffuse patchy pattern or single or multiple discrete defects. The great majority of patients with primary pulmonary hypertension fall into the low-probability group. A small number fall into the high-probability group, in which case

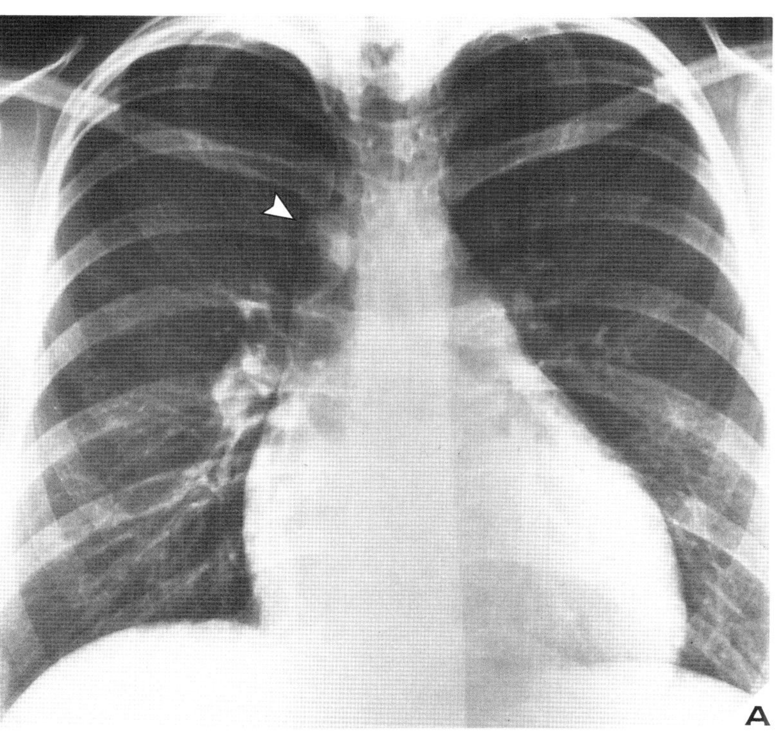

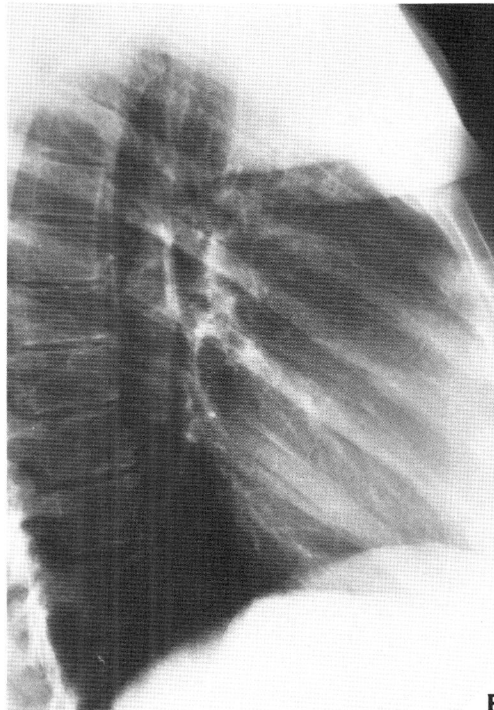

Fig. 24.26 Primary pulmonary hypertension with right ventricular failure. (A) Posteroanterior and (B) lateral chest films show cardiomegaly with right ventricular enlargement. The right and left pulmonary arteries are moderately enlarged as well. Note dilatation of azygos vein (*arrow* in A) reflecting increased pressure in the systemic veins.

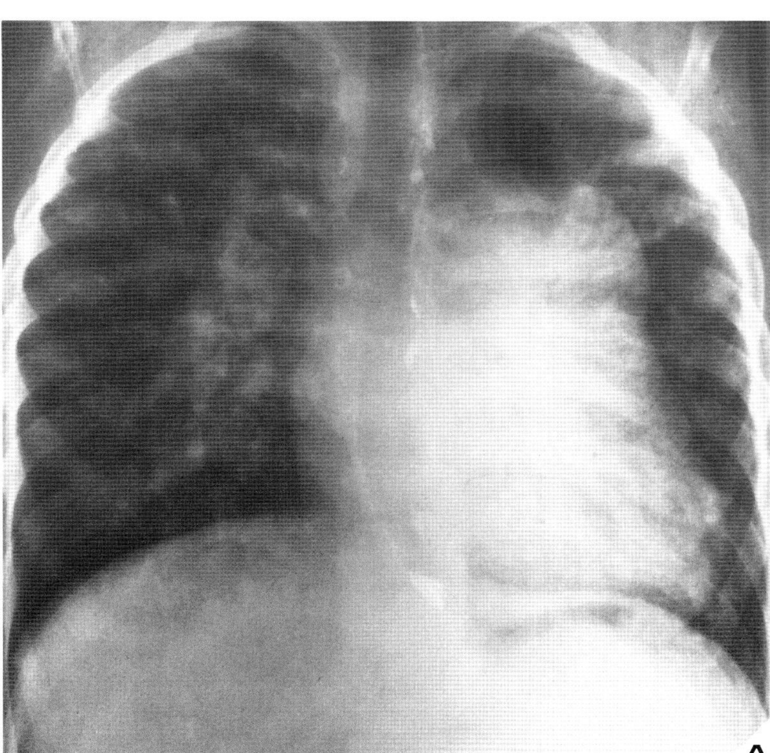

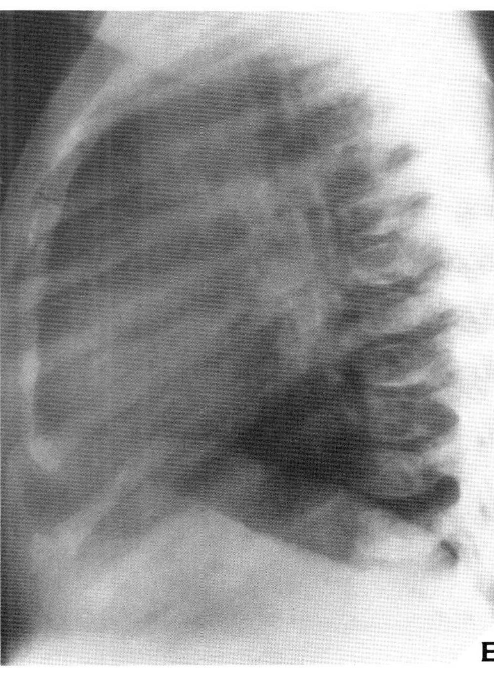

Fig. 24.27 Secondary pulmonary hypertension secondary to congenital heart disease. (A) Posteroanterior and (B) lateral chest films in a patient with severe pulmonary hypertension with increased pulmonary vascular resistance secondary to a VSD reveal cardiomegaly with right ventricular enlargement. The pulmonary trunk is markedly dilated. The right and left pulmonary arteries, as well as the lobar and segmental branches, are also enlarged; however, there is a paucity of peripheral branches. Note the hypoplastic aortic arch resulting from the left to right shunt.

pulmonary arteriography may be needed to exclude pulmonary embolus, particularly when anticoagulant therapy is contemplated.

COMPUTED TOMOGRAPHY

Although CT does not provide the definitive diagnosis, the marked disparity in the size of the central arteries and peripheral arteries typically seen in patients with primary pulmonary hypertension is dramatically shown by this technique (Figs. 24.29 and 24.30).

MRI

Preliminary studies suggest that MRI may be helpful in the differential diagnosis of primary pulmonary hypertension and pulmonary embolism. In normal subjects, ECG-gated spin–echo images show intraluminal signal in the pulmonary trunk and main pulmonary arteries only during diastole. The presence of intraluminal signal during systole indicates slow flow or thrombus. Thus, intraluminal signal is present during both systole and diastole in patients with pulmonary embolus, whereas it is present only during diastole in patients with primary pulmonary hypertension. Although these observations are provocative, the clinical efficacy of MRI in this setting remains to be confirmed.

CARDIAC CATHETERIZATION

Mean pulmonary artery pressure is significantly elevated (>20 mm Hg at rest and >30 mm Hg with exercise). The magnitude of the pressure elevation varies over a considerable range. In one series, the average mean pulmonary artery pressure was 60 mm Hg, although some patients had systolic pressures as high as 100 mm Hg. Right ventricular end diastolic pressure is often elevated, indicating right ventricular failure. (It may be normal in patients who are compensated hemodynamically.) The right atrial pressure, which reflects the right ventricular end diastolic pressure, is mildly to moderately elevated (9 mm Hg or greater). The pulmonary capillary wedge pressure is normal. Cardiac output is usually reduced (cardiac index less than 2.2 $L/min/m^2$). In general, the degree of hemodynamic disturbance demonstrated by catheterization correlates with the severity of the symptoms.

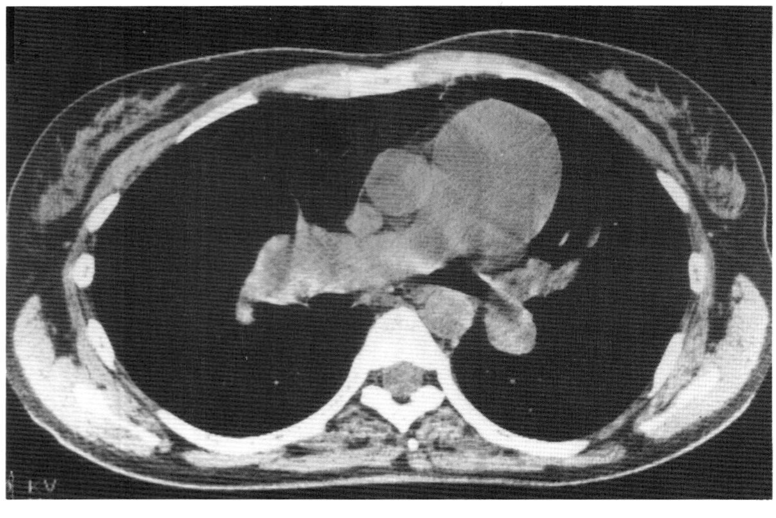

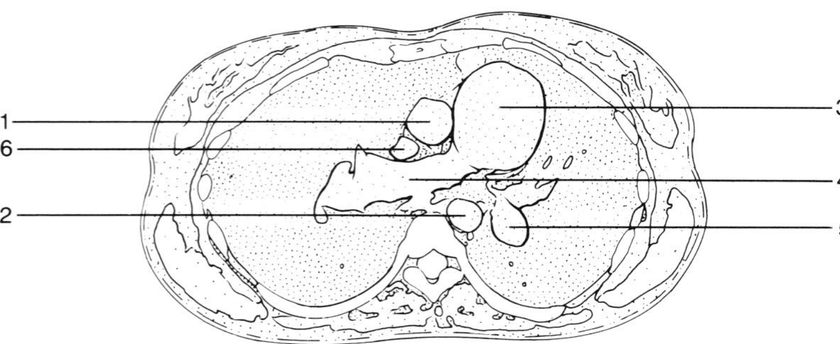

1 ascending aorta
2 descending thoracic aorta
3 pulmonary trunk
4 right pulmonary artery
5 left pulmonary artery
6 superior vena cava

Fig. 24.29 CT findings in pulmonary hypertension. Contrast-enhanced axial section at the level of the pulmonary artery bifurcation shows marked enlargement of the pulmonary trunk, which is almost three times larger than the aorta. The right and left pulmonary arteries are also enlarged. The ascending aorta is normal in size but the superior vena cava is dilated.

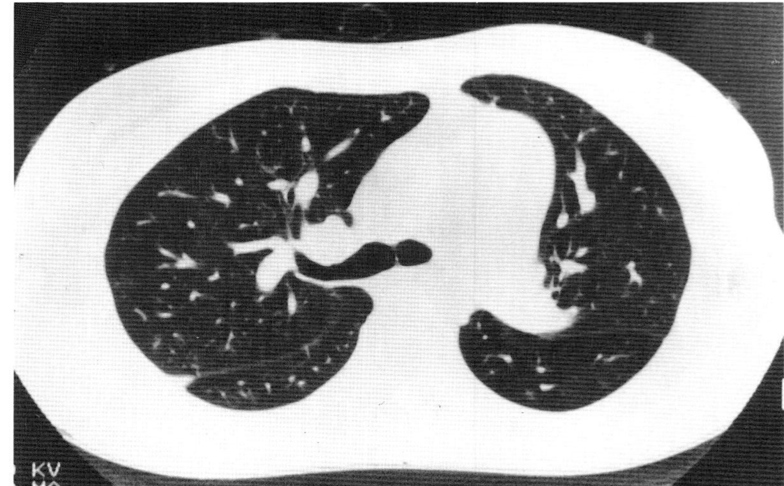

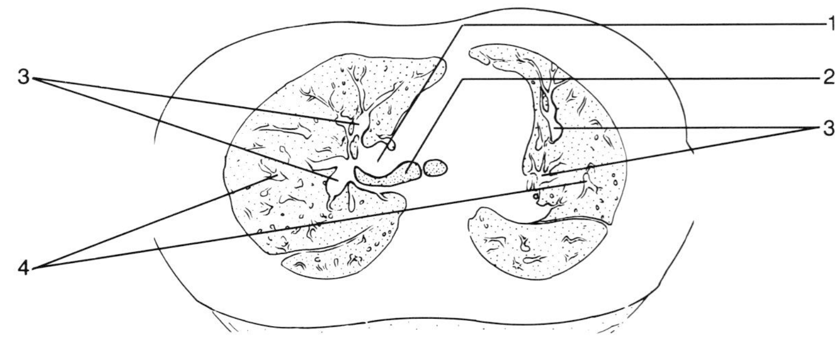

1 right pulmonary artery
2 right main bronchus
3 lobar arteries
4 segmental arteries

Fig. 24.30 Pulmonary vasculature in primary pulmonary hypertension demonstrated by high-resolution thin-section CT. Transverse section at the level of the right main bronchus shows moderate enlargement of the right pulmonary artery and dilatation of lobar and segmental arteries. The peripheral arterial branches are smaller and fewer in number than normal.

ANGIOGRAPHY

Pulmonary arteriography is indicated in patients with primary pulmonary hypertension only to rule out pulmonary embolus or other treatable conditions that might produce increased pulmonary vascular resistance (eg, stenosis of the main pulmonary arteries, peripheral pulmonary stenosis). Pulmonary arteriography is associated with significant morbidity and mortality in patients with pulmonary hypertension; a 2 percent death rate was recorded in one recent series (Rich, 1987). The risk is greatest in patients with right ventricular failure, most complications occurring in those in whom the right ventricular end diastolic pressure is 15 mm Hg or greater.

Selective arteriography of each pulmonary artery is recommended, using low-osmolality contrast material to reduce the risk of complications. A bolus of 20 mL will usually define the morphology of the pulmonary circulation in patients with pulmonary arterial hypertension and exclude pulmonary thromboembolus or other lesions that may cause increased vascular resistance.

Some authors advocate the use of selective capillary wedge injections to evaluate the rate of tapering of the small pulmonary arteries; extreme tapering indicates markedly increased pulmonary vascular resistance, whereas lesser degrees of tapering indicate normal or only moderately increased vascular resistance. Owing to limitations imposed by technical factors, this technique is not widely employed.

In patients with primary pulmonary hypertension, selective pulmonary arteriography reveals dilatation of the pulmonary trunk, main pulmonary arteries, and lobar and segmental arteries. Dilated arteries can be followed to the middle third of the lung field; beyond this point they become markedly narrowed and cannot be traced to the periphery. In some areas, arterial branches may be lacking altogether. The parenchymal branches are usually more prominent in the lower zones than in the upper zones; however, the converse may sometimes be true owing to the uneven distribution of occlusive vascular disease. Medium-sized and small pulmonary arteries often have fewer branches than those of normal lungs, an observation which indicates that some branches have been occluded by the pathologic process. Typical angiographic findings in patients with primary pulmonary hypertension are illustrated in Figs. 24.31 and 24.32.

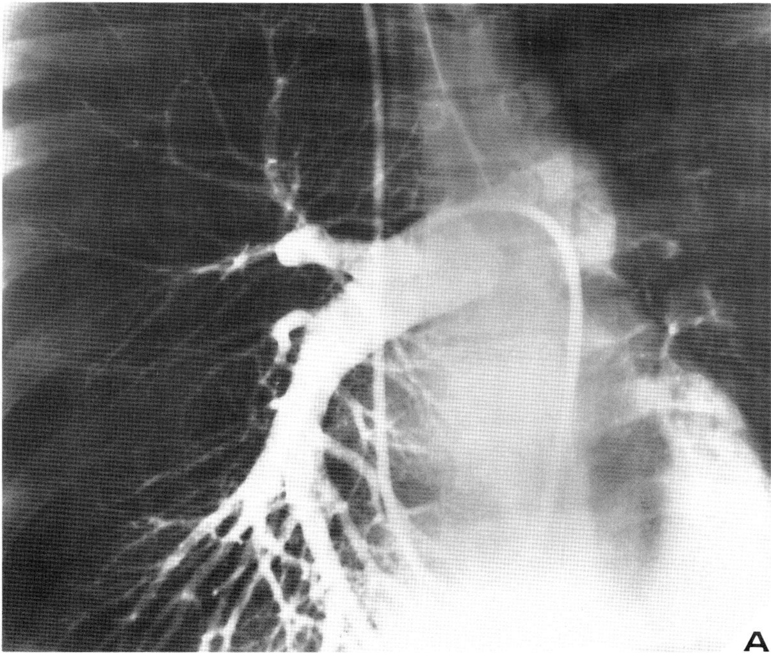

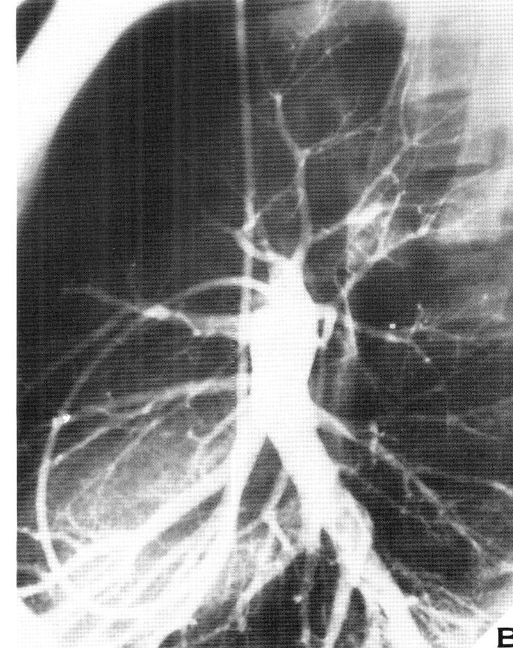

Fig. 24.31 Angiographic features of primary pulmonary hypertension. (A) Frontal and (B) lateral projectiona of selective right pulmonary pulmonary arteriogram. The right pulmonary artery is only slightly enlarged; however, the branches supplying the right upper and middle lobes are sparse and have fewer branches than normal. In contrast, the arteries supplying the right lower lobe have a normal appearance. Inhomogeneous involvement is not uncommon in patients with primary pulmonary hypertension.

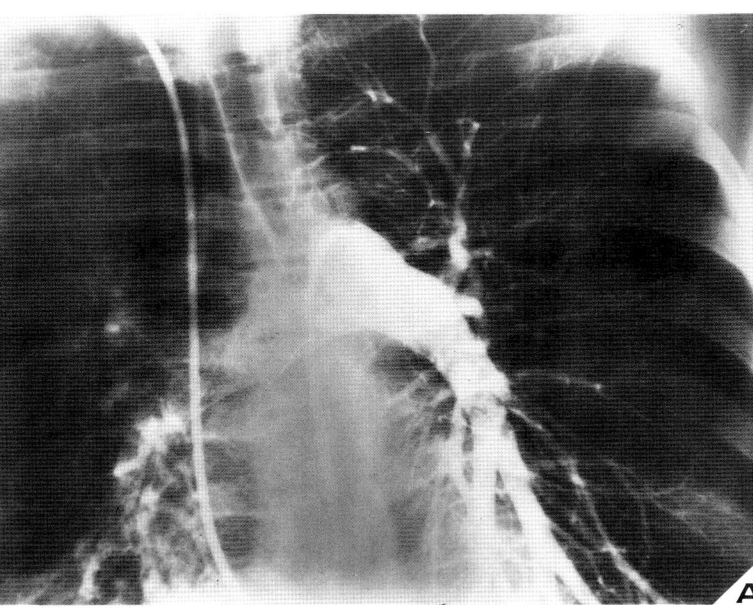

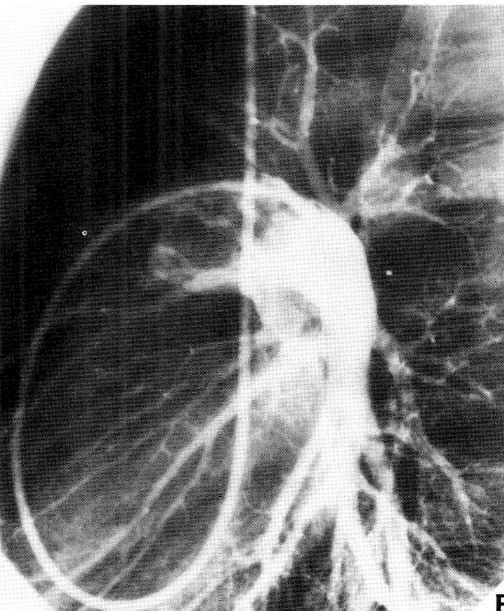

Fig. 24.32 Angiographic appearance of primary pulmonary hypertension (A) Frontal and (B) lateral projections of selective right pulmonary arteriogram demonstrate a paucity of branches to the left upper lobe, particularly to the lingula. Some of the arteries supplying the basilar segments of the lower lobes appear normal, indicating that the vascular obliterative process is unevenly distributed in the lower lobes.

During the late (venous) phase, the pulmonary veins are poorly opacified; in extreme instances, where flow through the lungs is markedly retarded, the pulmonary venous return may not be visualized. However, there is no apparent correlation between the severity of the pulmonary hypertension and the rapidity with which the pulmonary veins become opacified on selective pulmonary arteriograms.

A similar pattern may be seen in patients with secondary pulmonary hypertension accompanying a left to right shunt. In such cases, left ventriculography may fail to demonstrate a left to right shunt or may show reversal of the shunt (Eisenmenger syndrome) (Fig. 24.33). Pulmonary hypertension may also be seen in patients with peripheral pulmonary stenosis (congenital or acquired), Takayasu's disease (see Chapter 27), and neoplastic disease. Pulmonary arteriography accurately depicts the extent and severity of involvement in such cases (Fig. 24.34).

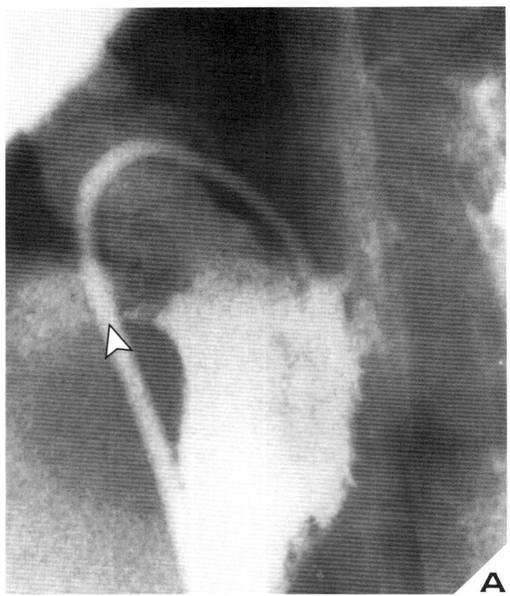

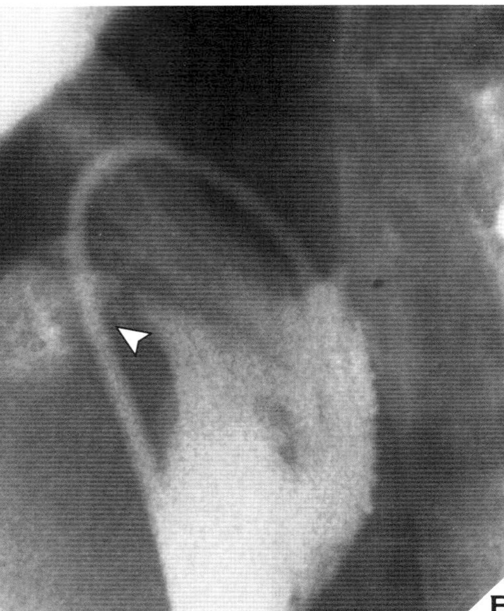

Fig. 24.33 Angiocardiographic findings in secondary pulmonary hypertension. Long axial projections of left ventriculogram in (A) systole and (B) diastole demonstrate a perimembranous VSD (*arrows*), which is bordered superiorly by the right coronary cusp. Contrast material does not flow freely into the right ventricle in either systole or diastole, indicating that right ventricular pressure is higher than left ventricular pressure throughout the cardiac cycle. Pulmonary artery pressure was higher than systemic pressure.

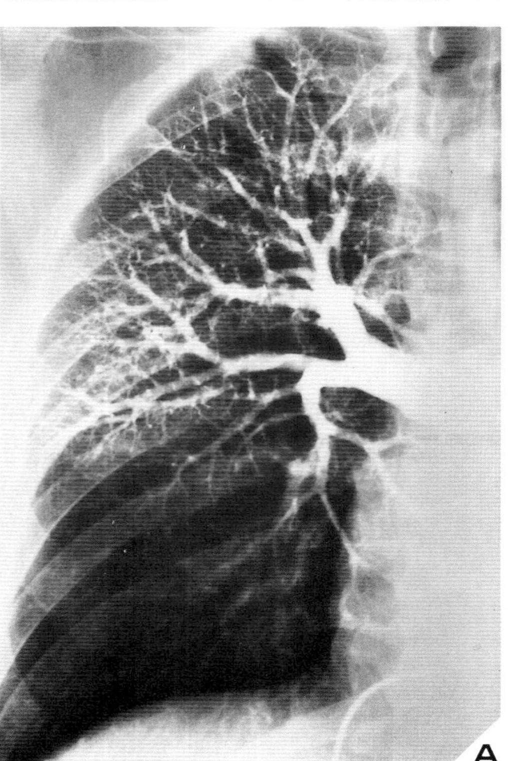

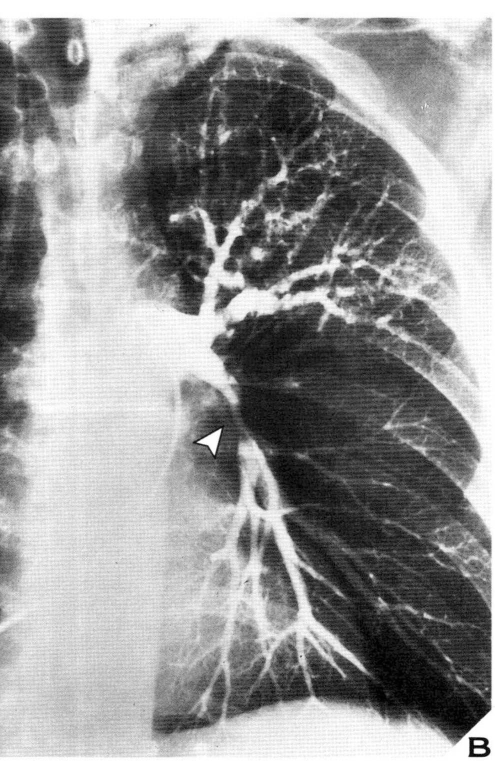

Fig. 24.34 Pulmonary hypertension secondary to obstructive vascular disease of the large pulmonary arteries. This patient had clinical manifestations of right ventricular overload. On cardiac catheterization both the right ventricular and the pulmonary artery pressure were elevated (70 mm Hg); the right ventricular pressure was also elevated (70 mm Hg). (A) Selective left pulmonary arteriogram demonstrates absence of the branch supplying part of the lingula and severe stenosis (*arrow*) of the left lower lobe artery. (B) Selective right pulmonary arteriogram shows absence of the branches to the right lower lobe. The arterial pattern of the middle and upper lobes is normal. Although this patient did not have a history of recurrent pulmonary embolism, this would be the most likely explanation for these angiographic findings.

CHAPTER 25

Cardiovascular Manifestations of Systemic Disorders

RHEUMATIC DISEASES

Cardiovascular involvement is an integral feature of this group of systemic disorders that affect connective tissues throughout the body. Although the precise etiology is unknown, they are believed to share an autoimmune pathogenesis. The cardiovascular lesions, characterized pathologically by exudation and fibrosis, affect such structures as the pericardium, myocardial interstitium, valve rings, septa, and the arterial wall, in various combinations and with variable severity.

RHEUMATIC FEVER

Cardiac involvement is the rule in rheumatic fever, which results from an abnormal immune response of connective tissues after an infection with group A streptococci. [Acute rheumatic fever, which almost always affects children and teenagers, is discussed in Chapter 29. The late sequelae of rheumatic fever (rheumatic heart disease) are discussed in Chapter 18.]

RHEUMATOID ARTHRITIS

PATHOLOGIC AND CLINICAL FEATURES

Cardiovascular manifestations occur in approximately 50 percent of patients with rheumatoid arthritis (RA). Pathologically, nodular granulomas characteristic of RA can be found in the pericardium, myocardium, endocardium (particularly the cardiac valves), and coronary arteries.

The most frequent cardiac manifestation of RA is pericarditis. The clinical manifestations are similar to those of acute pericarditis due to other causes, although cardiac tamponade is rare. The pericardial fluid typically has a high cholesterol content.

The endocardial lesions, which can occur in both the acute and the chronic phase of the disease, typically involve the leaflets and the annulus of the cardiac valves. Granuloma formation is most prominent in the leaflets, particularly at the level of the commissures. Small granulomas usually do not interfere with valvular function; however, a large granuloma can destroy the base or free border of a leaflet, leading to valvular regurgitation. Occasionally the valvular insufficiency may be of sufficient magnitude and rapidity of onset to cause severe cardiac decompensation and death. Clinically significant endocardial involvement is relatively uncommon, occurring in about 6 percent of patients with RA. The mitral valve is most frequently affected, followed (in order of frequency) by the aortic, tricuspid, and pulmonic valves.

Interstitial myocardial involvement is relatively common in patients with RA. Occasionally it is severe enough to cause cardiomegaly and congestive heart failure.

RA is occasionally associated with generalized vasculitis which can affect the coronary arteries, causing ischemic heart disease. Although the coronary arteries are involved in 20 percent of cases, the incidence of myocardial infarction in patients with RA is comparable to that in the general population.

The physical findings and ECG changes reflect the distribution of lesions (eg, pericarditis, valvular insufficiency, myocardial infiltration, ischemic heart disease). The most common ECG abnormalities are first degree atrioventricular block, complete heart block (manifested clinically by the Adams–Stokes syndrome), and left bundle branch block.

IMAGING AND INVASIVE DIAGNOSIS

In the acute phase of RA the plain film findings are nonspecific, the radiographic pattern reflecting the distribution of the lesions (eg, pericardial effusion secondary to pericardial infiltration, CHF secondary to myocardial involvement, chamber enlargement and/or pulmonary venous hypertension secondary to valvular insufficiency). Echocardiography may demonstrate pericardial fluid and/or evidence of valvular incompetence. Angiocardiography demonstrates evidence of valvular insufficiency. Patients with mitral insufficiency exhibit left ventricular and left atrial enlargement. Patients with aortic insufficiency demonstrate left ventricular enlargement and aortic dilatation.

SERONEGATIVE SPONDYLOARTHROPATHIES

This heterogeneous group of disorders has many clinical and pathologic manifestations in common with RA. Cardiovascular involvement is not uncommon in patients with two of these conditions: Reiter's disease and ankylosing spondylitis.

REITER'S DISEASE

Pathology and Clinical Features

Cardiac involvement is not uncommon in Reiter's disease, a systemic disorder characterized by arthritis, nonsuppurative migratory polyarthritis, conjunctivitis, and keratoderma blenorrhagica. The initial attack usually subsides spontaneously. Recurrent episodes occur in about 15 percent of cases.

In the acute phase the cardiac manifestations are related to involvement of the pericardium and myocardium. The latter may be severe enough to cause CHF. The ECG typically shows prolongation of the P-R interval and flattening of the P-waves, indicating myocardial involvement.

The cardiac manifestations of the late stage are primarily due to mitral and/or aortic insufficiency and atrioventricular block secondary to involvement of the conducting system. The leaflets of the affected valves are thickened, with rolled borders. The aortic valve is typically deformed, with thickened cusps and rolled edges.

Imaging and Invasive Diagnosis

As with RA, the findings on imaging studies are nonspecific and reflect the distribution of the lesions.

ANKYLOSING SPONDYLITIS

Pathologic Features

Cardiovascular involvement occurs in about 3 percent of patients with ankylosing spondylitis. The pathologic process has a predilection for the region adjacent to the aortic valve ring, including the sinuses of Valsalva, aortic leaflets, anterior mitral leaflet, and left ventricular outflow tract; the myocardium and pericardium may also be affected (Fig. 25.1).

The aortic lesions consist of focal degeneration of the elastica and muscularis (medial necrosis) and patchy inflammation of all layers of the aortic wall. The weakened aortic cusps sag into the left ventricular cavity and the sinuses of Valsalva undergo dilatation, resulting in widening of the aortic annulus and various degrees of aortic insufficiency. The aortic cusps are short and thick but are not fused. The pathologic process typically extends caudally to involve the left ventricular outflow tract, causing some degree of stenosis, and the anterior mitral leaflet, leading to mitral insufficiency. Infiltration of the membranous septum and atrioventricular bundle by fibrous tissue leads to conduction defects of variable severity.

An occasional patient exhibits dilated cardiomyopathy secondary to generalized myocardial involvement. Usually, however, myocardial dysfunction in patients with ankylosing spondylitis is secondary to aortic valve involvement. The myocardial lesions are nonspecific, consisting of perivascular lymphocyte infiltration, an increased amount of mucinous ground substance, and fibrosis. Grossly, the heart is enlarged without evidence of hypertrophy, a constellation of findings similar to that of idiopathic dilated cardiomyopathy.

Extensive pericardial involvement, with fibrous obliteration of the pericardial space, is a rare manifestation.

Clinical Features

There is no correlation between the clinical and radiologic severity of spondyloarthropathy and the degree of cardiovascular involvement. An occasional patient with clinical evidence of spondyloarthropathy exhibits signs and symptoms of cardiovascular involvement before the appearance of classical radiographic findings of ankylosing spondylitis. Marked eleva-

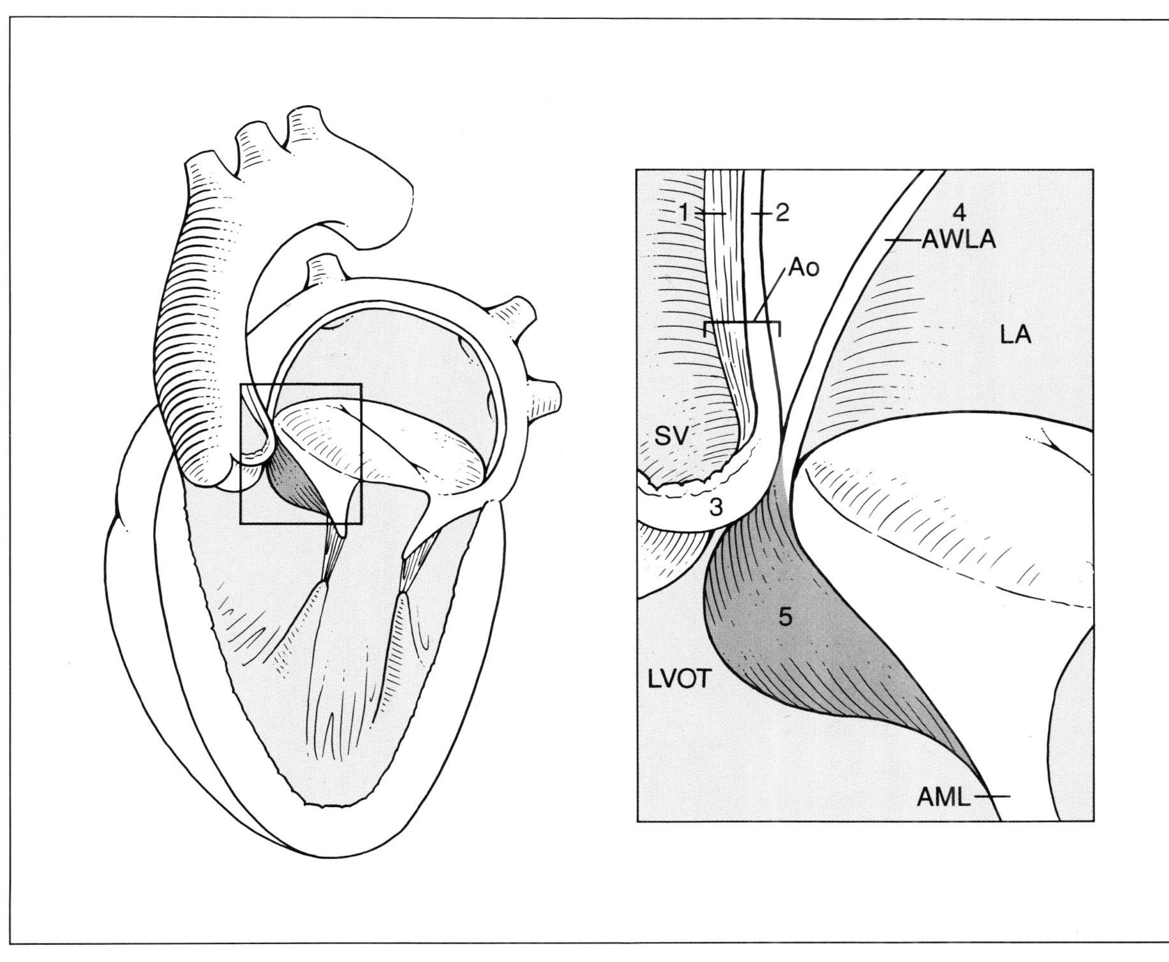

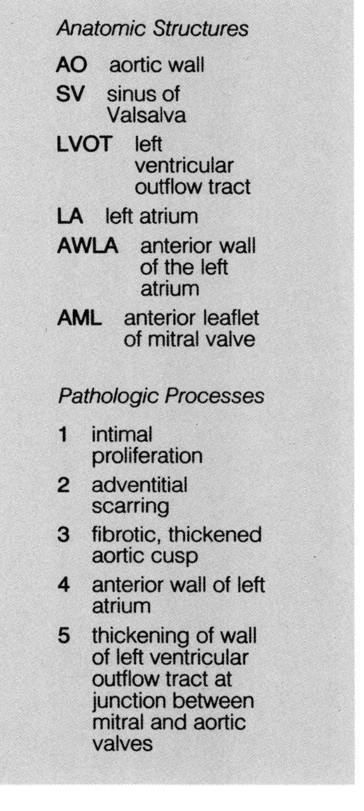

Fig. 25.1 Cardiovascular pathology in ankylosing spondylitis. Diagrammatic cross-section of the heart at the level of the junction between the aorta, mitral valve, and left atrium. There is thickening of the aortic wall due to intimal proliferation and adventitial scarring. The latter extends into the groove between the aortic valve cusp and the anterior mitral leaflet, creating a ridge beneath the aortic valve and the attachment of the anterior mitral leaflet. Adventitial scarring can also extend for a variable distance into the muscular portion of the ventricular septum. The commissures of the fibrotic, thickened aortic valve are typically displaced downward into the left ventricular outflow tract.

tion of the ESR or seropositivity for the HLA-27 antigen on tissue typing studies may suggest the correct diagnosis in such a case. The ESR is elevated in most patients with ankylosing spondylitis, although the level correlates poorly with the activity of the disease (it is normal in about 20 percent of patients with mild disease). The HLA-27 titer tends to be positive in patients with long-standing spondylitis and/or peripheral joint involvement. It is positive in 10 percent of patients with a history of spondylitis for 30 years or longer and in 18 percent of those with peripheral joint involvement.

Physical examination typically reveals cardiomegaly and signs of aortic insufficiency (less often, there is evidence of mitral insufficiency). A pericardial friction rub may be present. However, pericardial involvement is often clinically silent. The most common ECG abnormality is atrioventricular block secondary to involvement of the conducting system, which is present in about 15 percent of cases.

Imaging and Invasive Diagnosis

Plain film findings are nonspecific, reflecting the various combinations of pericardial involvement, cardiomyopathy, and valvular insufficiency that can occur in this disorder. Radiographic changes of ankylosing spondylitis can often be appreciated on the chest film (Fig. 25.2). Echocardiography demonstrates dilatation of the aortic annulus and deformity of the aortic leaflets. There may also be thickening of the septal leaflet of the mitral valve with mitral insufficiency, and narrowing of the left ventricular outflow tract (Fig. 25.3).

Angiographic findings are distinctive. Aortography in the lateral or left anterior oblique projection typically shows dilatation of the aortic annulus with moderate or severe aortic insufficiency, and a normal-sized or only slightly dilated ascending aorta (Fig. 25.4). When there is significant stenosis of the left ventricular outflow tract, the angiographic appearance may suggest the presence of an accessory cusp or valve leaflet.

CONNECTIVE TISSUE DISEASES

In this group of conditions, which includes systemic lupus erythematosus, periarteritis nodosa, scleroderma, polymyositis, and dermatomyositis, the cardiovascular system may be affected primarily or secondarily. Although the serological and immunological features of these disorders overlap, it is appropriate to discuss each separately.

SYSTEMIC LUPUS ERYTHEMATOSUS

PATHOLOGIC FEATURES

The cardiac manifestations of systemic lupus erythematosus (SLE) are caused by the diffuse microvasculitis which is the hallmark of this multisystemic disease. Although the heart is almost always affected in advanced SLE, the clinical picture is usually dominated by involvement of other organ systems.

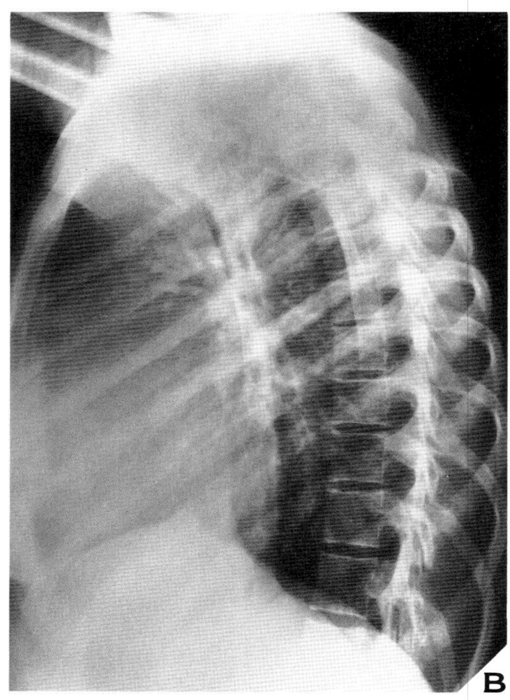

Fig. 25.2 Aortic insufficiency in a patient with ankylosing spondylitis. (A) Posteroanterior and (B) lateral chest films of a 40-year-old woman show moderate cardiomegaly with left ventricular enlargement. The ascending aorta is dilated, appearing as a prominent bulge along the right upper mediastinal border and displacing the pulmonary trunk to the left. Note squaring of the vertebral bodies in B. This appearance, which is characteristic of the early stages of ankylosing spondylitis, typically progresses to a classical "bamboo spine" over a period of many years.

Grossly, the ventricular cavities are usually enlarged owing to myocardial involvement or valvular disease. The valves are typically studded with wart-like excrescences consisting of degenerated valve tissue (Libman–Sachs lesions). These lesions, which range from pinhead size to 3 to 4 cm in diameter, may be discrete or may occur in clumps; typically, Libman–Sachs lesions extend deep beneath the endocardial surface, producing fibrosis of the valve (Fig. 25.5).

Pericardial involvement is very common in SLE. At some time in their course more than 75 percent of patients with severe SLE exhibit clinical evidence of acute pericardial inflammation with fluid accumulation. The pericardial effusion may be large enough to cause cardiac tamponade. Analysis of the pericardial fluid reveals a fibrinous exudate with a high protein content.

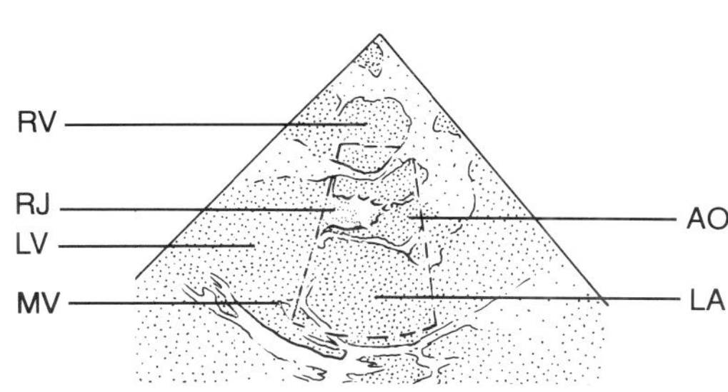

Fig. 25.3 Aortic insufficiency in a patient with ankylosing spondylitis. Parasternal long axial section of echocardiogram (in systole) demonstrates dilatation of the aortic valve with severe aortic insufficiency (note regurgitant jet in left ventricular outflow tract).

AO	aorta	**RV**	right ventricle
LA	left atrium	**MV**	mitral valve
LV	left ventricle	**RJ**	regurgitant jet

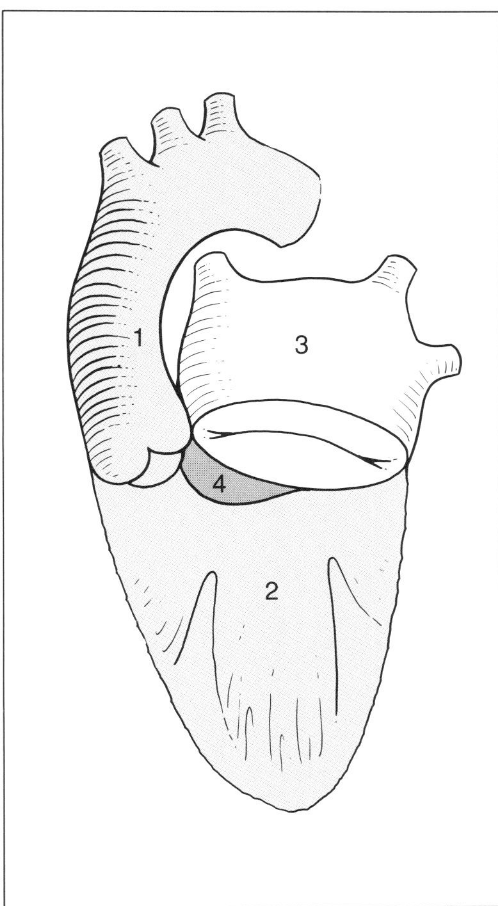

1 aorta
2 left ventricle
3 left atrium
4 fibrous proliferation

Fig. 25.4 Ankylosing spondylitis. Schematic representation of typical aortographic findings in the left anterior oblique projection. There is marked insufficiency of the aortic valve with opacification of the entire left ventricular cavity. Fibrous proliferation at the junction of the aortic valve and anterior mitral leaflet produces a filling defect along the posterior aspect of the left ventricular outflow tract. The aorta is only minimally enlarged.

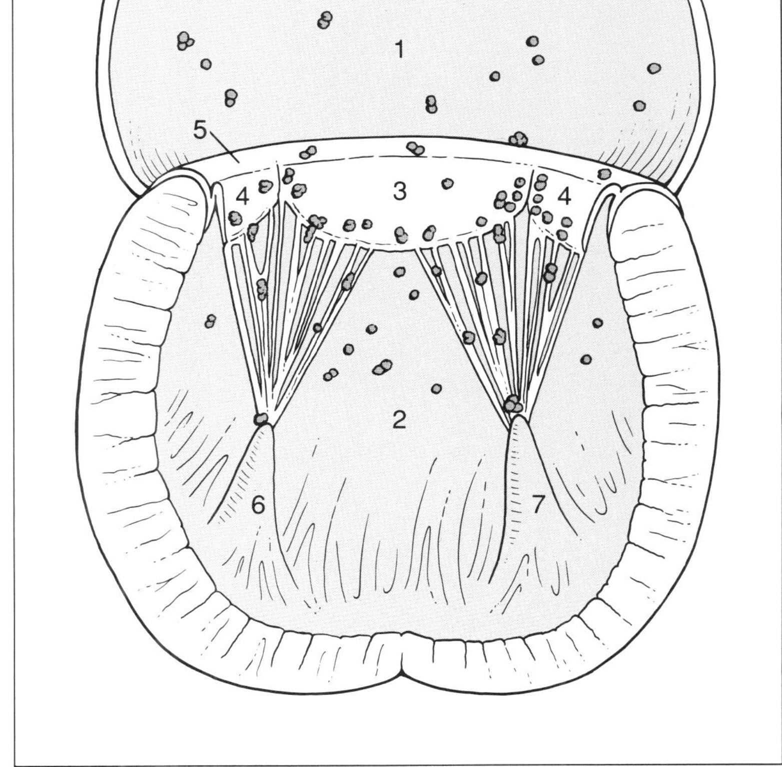

1 left atrium
2 left ventricle
3 anterior leaflet of mitral valve
4 posterior leaflet of mitral valve
5 mitral annulus
6 anterior papillary muscle
7 posterior papillary muscle

Fig. 25.5 Libman–Sachs lesions of SLE. Schematic representation of opened left ventricle and left atrium. Libman–Sachs lesions are small sterile, dry, pink, granular vegetations which may be solitary or multiple. The lesions typically occur in the endocardium of the left atrium and left ventricle, chordae tendinae, mitral annulus, and mitral leaflets. The mitral commissures are usually spared. Tiny vegetations may be obscured by the overlying chordae tendinae or trabeculations.

CLINICAL FEATURES

The usual presenting symptom in patients with cardiac involvement is chest pain secondary to pericardial inflammation. Many patients have systolic or diastolic murmurs related to valve dysfunction. Although the myocardial involvement is seldom severe enough to produce clinical signs, some degree of left ventricular dysfunction can usually be documented by echocardiography or cardiac catheterization.

IMAGING AND INVASIVE DIAGNOSIS

Plain Films

Chest films frequently show pulmonary infiltrates, usually due to pneumonitis but occasionally representing focal hemorrhage. Unilateral or bilateral pleural effusions are very common and are sometimes the initial radiographic abnormality. The amount of pleural fluid is usually small but on occasion may be massive. The heart is usually of normal size. The pulmonary vasculature is usually normal, reflecting the low incidence of significant myocardial involvement; however, pulmonary venous hypertension may be present in patients with myocardial or valvular involvement (Fig. 25.6). Typical plain film findings of pericardial effusion may be evident from time to time in a patient with active SLE (Fig. 25.6).

Echocardiography

Echocardiography is frequently used to detect pericardial fluid, a common finding in patients with SLE. Conventional two-dimensional echocardiography, augmented by color Doppler imaging, clearly demonstrates the aortic stenosis or aortic insufficiency that is commonly present in patients with SLE. Echocardiography can also detect evidence of subclinical left ventricular dysfunction (eg, increased systolic volume, decreased ejection fraction, decreased diastolic compliance).

Cardiac Catheterization and Angiography

Cardiac catheterization and left ventriculography are performed in selected cases to evaluate valvular dysfunction and assess myocardial function. The cardiomyopathy associated with SLE is typically of the dilated type; initially, however, there may be impairment of diastolic function suggestive of

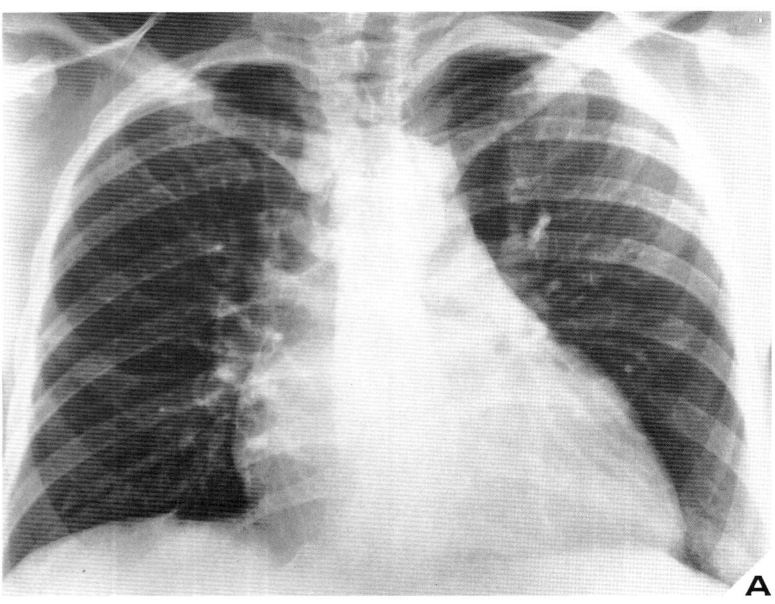

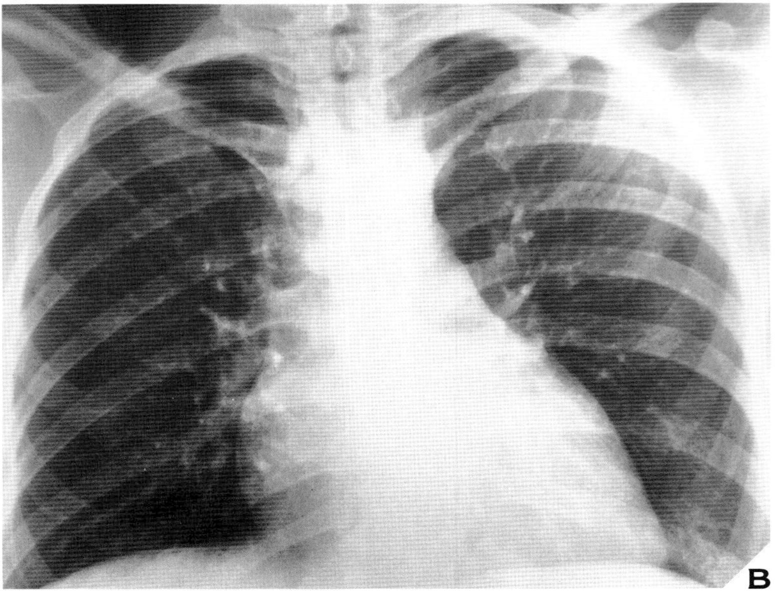

Fig. 25.6 Systemic lupus erythematosus. (A) Posteroanterior chest film in a 45-year-old woman with acute SLE shows a small pericardial effusion and mild pulmonary venous hypertension (cephalization pattern). (B) Ten weeks later, after treatment, there is no radiographic evidence of pericardial fluid and the pulmonary vasculature appears normal.

restricted cardiomyopathy. Coronary arteriography may be indicated in patients with myocardial dysfunction to exclude coronary artery involvement, which characteristically affects small epicardial branches in patients with SLE.

PERIARTERITIS NODOSA

PATHOLOGIC AND CLINICAL FEATURES

Periarteritis nodosa is a necrotizing vasculitis of the vasa vasorum of medium-sized and small arteries and veins. It can result in aneurysm formation and inflammation (leading to rupture) of the affected vessels. The clinical manifestations are mainly related to involvement of the coronary and renal arteries.

The major cardiovascular manifestations of periarteritis nodosa are related to systemic hypertension (secondary to renal artery involvement) and CHF (secondary to ischemic heart disease caused by coronary artery involvement). Pericarditis, pleuritis, and chest pain are rare. Rupture of an arterial aneurysm can occur in a relatively asymptomatic patient, leading to massive hemorrhage.

A distinctive form of periarteritis nodosa that occurs in children is associated with aneurysm formation and thrombosis of muscular arteries, with a predilection for the coronary arteries. This disorder, known as Kawasaki disease, is discussed in Chapter 29.

IMAGING AND INVASIVE DIAGNOSIS

Plain film and echocardiographic findings are nonspecific. Both may demonstrate pericardial fluid in the occasional patient with significant pericardial involvement. Coronary arteriography reveals localized dilatation and saccular aneurysms of the affected vessels (usually the proximal) portions of the three major coronary arteries (see Chapters 21 and 29). (Similar lesions can be demonstrated angiographically in the renal and other visceral arteries.) Periarteritis nodosa may also cause arterial occlusion. The coronary artery lesions may regress spontaneously, in which event follow-up angiography may show no abnormality.

DIFFUSE SCLERODERMA

Scleroderma, a chronic fibrosing condition of the skin and other soft tissues, occasionally involves the heart and pericardium. Pericardial involvement is associated with signs and symptoms of pericarditis, the most common clinical manifestation. Involvement of small branches of the coronary arteries can result in myocardial infarction or myocardial sclerosis. Signs and symptoms of myocardial involvement (eg, CHF) indicate extensive disease and connote a poor prognosis.

IMAGING

Chest films and other radiologic studies may show typical signs of scleroderma (eg, diffuse interstitial lung disease, esophageal dilatation with dysmotility, dilated bowel). The cardiovascular silhouette is usually normal. Occasionally there is evidence of a pericardial effusion. In patients with extensive myocardial involvement, echocardiography reveals evidence of left ventricular enlargement (eg, increased end systolic volume, decreased ejection fraction).

POLYMYOSITIS AND DERMATOMYOSITIS

Polymyositis and dermatomyositis are inflammatory processes of striated muscle. Both conditions can affect the heart, involving the conduction system, myocardium, and pericardium. Typically, there is swelling and degeneration of the collagen of the sinus node, which is eventually replaced by fibrous tissue. Myocardial involvement characteristically leads to fibrosis of the atria and ventricles.

The most common clinical manifestations are arrhythmias and dilated cardiomyopathy. The ECG typically reveals supraventricular tachycardia and/or complete heart block. Plain chest films, echocardiography, cardiac catheterization, and angiocardiography reveal features typical of dilated cardiomyopathy (see Chapter 19).

SYSTEMIC HYPERTENSION

Systemic hypertension is defined as elevation of the systemic blood pressure above normal limits (140/90 in adults, 110/75 in young children). The increased pressure is the result of increased systemic resistance. So-called "essential" hypertension accounts for approximately 90 percent of cases. In the remainder, systemic hypertension is caused by a wide variety of underlying disorders, including chronic renal disease, renal vascular disease, coarctation of the aorta, primary aldosteronism, Cushing's syndrome, and pheochromocytoma (Fig. 25.7).

PATHOPHYSIOLOGY

The sequence of events leading to systemic hypertension is initiated by excessively high arterial wall tension in small arteries and arterioles (resistance vessels). The resultant narrowing of the resistance vessels increases peripheral resistance, which in turn leads to fibromuscular hyperplasia of the intima and media of large and medium-sized arteries and elevation of diastolic pressure. Sustained arterial hypertension damages small arteries and arterioles throughout the body, producing functional impairment and structural changes in kidneys, CNS, coronary circulation, and peripheral circulation. The left ventricle, which must work to overcome the increased peripheral resistance, becomes hypertrophied and dilated and eventually may fail.

The hemodynamic changes produced by sustained systemic hypertension vary with the peripheral resistance and the degree of left ventricular impairment. Initially there is a high-output state, which may last for years. With progressive left ventricular failure, cardiac output decreases and pulmonary resistance increases.

Systemic hypertension accelerates the development of coronary atherosclerosis, leading to the early onset of obstructive coronary artery disease (manifested clinically by angina, myocardial infarction, or sudden death). Elevated diastolic pressure is clearly associated with an increased risk for ischemic myocardial events. In one large series, a rise in systolic pressure was more strongly correlated with ischemic heart disease than an initially high systolic pressure.

CLINICAL FEATURES

Uncomplicated systemic hypertension, which can lead to significant cardiovascular impairment over a period of 10 to 20 years, is almost always asymptomatic; however, some patients may

FIG. 25.7 CAUSES OF SECONDARY SYSTEMIC HYPERTENSION

Renal

Renal parenchymal disease
- Acute glomerulonephritis
- Chronic nephritis
- Polycystic disease
- Connective tissue diseases
- Diabetic nephropathy
- Hydronephrosis

Renovascular disease
Renin-producing tumors
Renoprival disease

Endocrine

Acromegaly
Hypothyroidism
Adrenal
- Cortical
  - Cushing's syndrome
  - Primary aldosteronism
- Medullary (pheochromocytoma)

Extraadrenal chromaffin tumors
Hypercalcemia
Exogenous
- Estrogen
- Glucocorticoids
- Mineralocorticoids (licorice, carbenoxolone)
- Sympathomimetics
- Tyramine-containing foods and MAO inhibitors

Coarctation of the aorta

Pregnancy-induced

Neurogenic

Psychogenic
Increased intracranial pressure
- Respiratory acidosis (lung or CNS disease)
- Encephalitis
- Brain tumor

Lead poisoning
Familial dysautonomia
Acute porphyria
Quadriplegia
Postoperative

Miscellaneous

Increased intravascular volume
- Polycythemia vera
- Postoperative

Burns
Carcinoid syndrome

Fig. 25.7 Causes of systemic hypertenson.

experience headache, nosebleeds, tinnitus, dizziness, and/or syncope. Untreated hypertension tends to become worse over time. (Rarely, an adult with established hypertension may become normotensive without treatment.) The first clinical manifestations of long-standing "silent" hypertension are usually related to cardiovascular impairment. It is estimated that untreated hypertension can decrease life expectancy by 10 to 20 years.

Clinical evaluation of patients with long-standing hypertension typically reveals physical findings and clinical evidence of left ventricular hypertrophy. The ECG typically shows increased QRS voltage and ST-segment depression greater than 0.5 mm. Patients with advanced disease may present with clinical manifestations of coronary artery disease or CHF. Other common complications of severe, long-standing systemic hypertension include stroke (hemorrhagic or arteriothrombotic), nephrosclerosis, aortic dissection, and peripheral vascular disease.

Structural and functional renal abnormalities are usually present, even in patients with mild hypertension. The main functional derangement is loss of concentrating ability, clinically manifested by nocturia, albuminuria, and, in patients with long-standing hypertension, decreased creatinine clearance.

Vascular changes are commonly observed in the ocular fundi and are useful to monitor the progress of vascular damage. The abnormalities seen on fundoscopic examination reflect the hypertensive neuroretinopathy and arteriosclerotic retinopathy caused by long-standing hypertension. The earliest change is narrowing of the lumen of small arteries and arterioles. Later, arteriovenous nicking (produced by sclerosis of the adventitia and/or thickening of the arteriolar walls) can be observed. As narrowing of the fundal vessels progresses, the veins that normally accompany the arteries and arterioles can no longer be identified (in time they may become completely obstructed). Worsening of the hypertension leads to rupture of small vessels, manifested fundoscopically by hemorrhages and exudates. Eventually papilledema may develop.

Initial diagnostic evaluation of any hypertensive patient should attempt to exclude renovascular hypertension and other potentially curable causes of hypertension. Renovascular hypertension results from decreased renal perfusion secondary to obstruction of one or both renal arteries or one of their major branches. After age 40 it is usually caused by atherosclerosis, whereas in children or young adults it is usually caused by so-called medial fibroplasia, a pathologic process that involves all layers of the arterial wall. The diagnosis is confirmed if the systolic pressure returns to normal after the stenosis is relieved.

IMAGING AND INVASIVE DIAGNOSIS

PLAIN FILMS

Most patients with uncomplicated systemic hypertension have normal chest films. Some patients with uncomplicated long-standing hypertension exhibit mild cardiomegaly and left ventricular enlargement (usually with prominence of the ascending aorta and aortic arch and tortuosity of the descending thoracic aorta) (Fig. 25.8). Calcification of the aortic arch in patients under 50 years of age should raise the question of systemic hypertension. Plain films or fluoroscopy may reveal calcification of the coronary arteries, which usually indicates secondary ischemic heart disease.

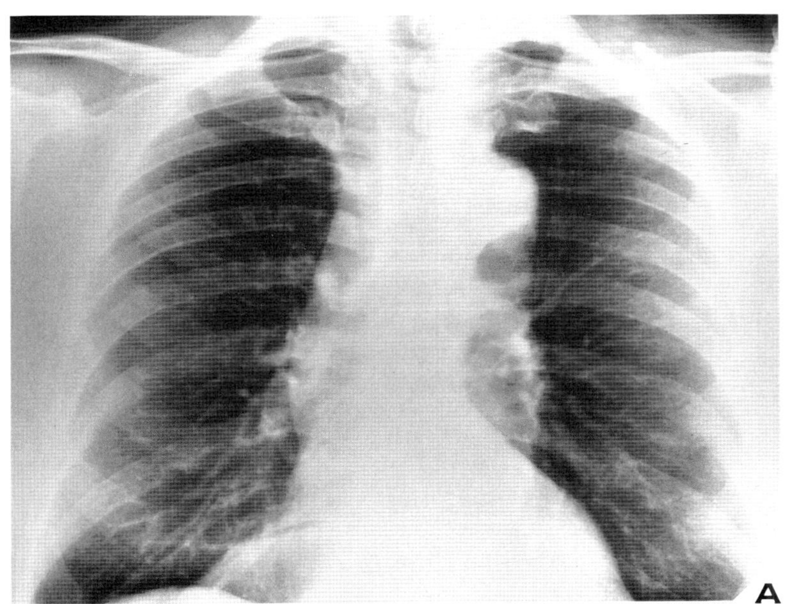

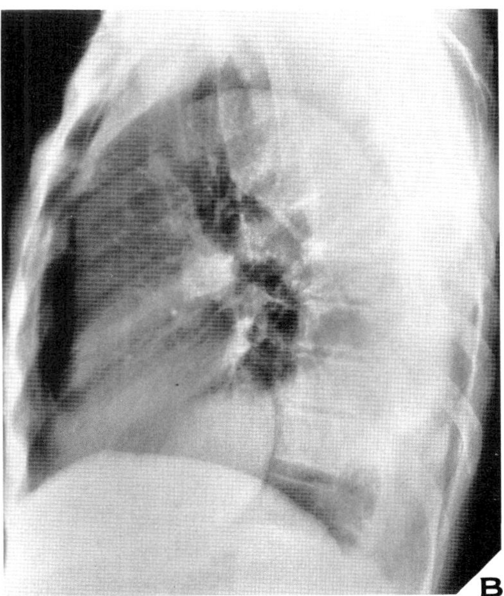

Fig. 25.8 Systemic hypertension. (A) Frontal and (B) lateral chest films of a patient with long-standing systemic hypertension. The left ventricular border projects posteriorly, inferiorly, and to the left, indicating moderate left ventricular enlargement. The dilated ascending aorta projects anteriorly and to the right. The aortic arch and descending thoracic aorta are unusually prominent.

ECHOCARDIOGRAPHY

Echocardiography reveals increased thickness of the septum and/or left ventricular wall and unusual prominence of the papillary muscles in patients with left ventricular hypertrophy secondary to long-standing hypertension (Fig. 25.9). Echocardiography also demonstrates abnormal left ventricular function. Although the aortic valve is usually competent, some patients with hypertension of relatively short duration exhibit mild aortic insufficiency, best appreciated on color Doppler images.

CT AND MRI

ECG-gated CT and spin–echo MRI demonstrate concentric hypertrophy of the left ventricle in patients with long-standing systemic hypertension. Left ventricular dysfunction and aortic insufficiency (if present) are clearly shown by cine CT or cine MRI (Fig. 25.10).

INVASIVE DIAGNOSIS

Cardiac catheterization is seldom indicated in patients with isolated systemic hypertension, since comparable data can be obtained noninvasively by echocardiography. Initially, before the onset of left ventricular failure, left ventricular systolic pressure is increased; however, the left ventricular end diastolic pressure is normal. In patients with left ventricular failure, the end diastolic pressure and end diastolic volume are both increased.

Coronary arteriography is indicated when there is clinical evidence of ischemic heart disease. Many authors believe that this should be performed in any patient over 50 years of age with severe or accelerated hypertension.

CARDIAC MANIFESTATIONS OF RENAL DISEASE

Cardiovascular disease is the principal cause of death in patients with chronic renal failure, accounting for 50 to 60 percent of deaths in this cohort compared with 15 percent in age-matched controls without renal disease. Myocardial infarction is the cause of death in 25 to 30 percent of these patients. Cerebrovascular accidents (strokes) account for an additional 10 to 15 percent.

Systemic hypertension increases the cardiovascular morbidity in patients with chronic renal failure. Not only does it increase the left ventricular workload, but it accelerates the development of obstructive coronary artery disease and ischemic heart disease. Other factors adversely affecting cardio-

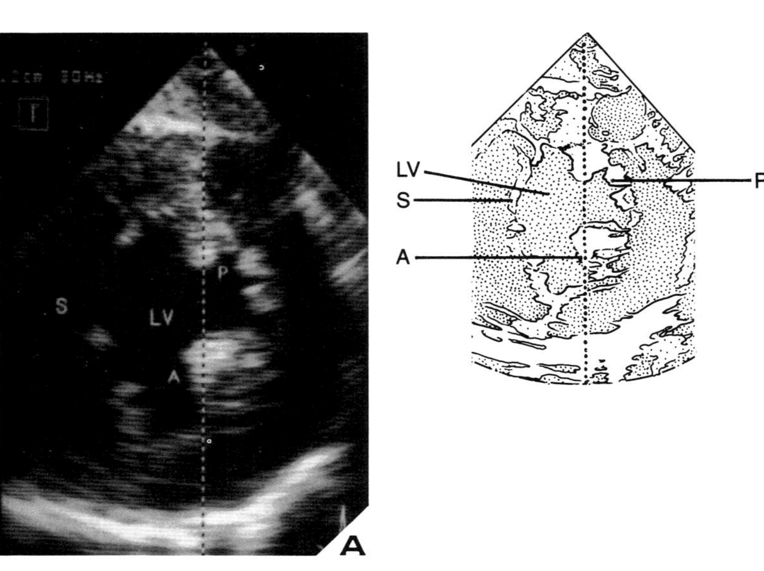

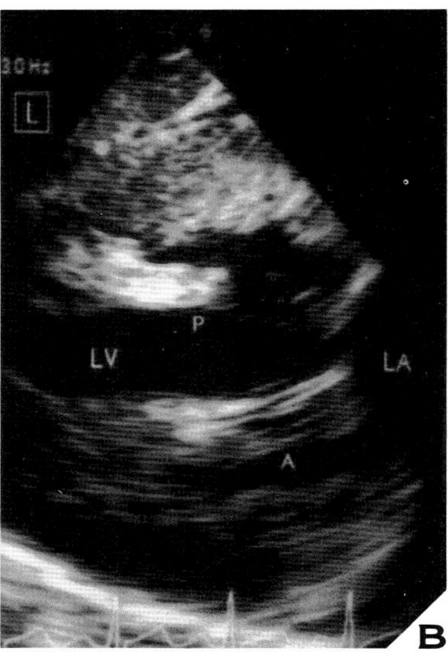

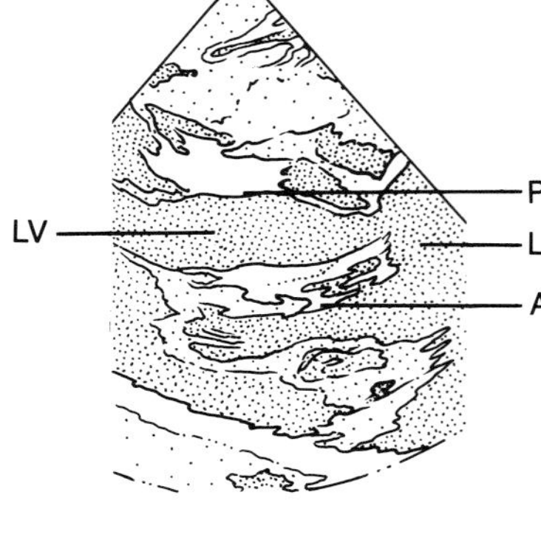

Fig. 25.9 Systemic hypertension. (A) Short-axis and (B) long-axis views of a patient with long-standing systemic hypertension demonstrate increased thickness of left ventricular wall and papillary muscles.

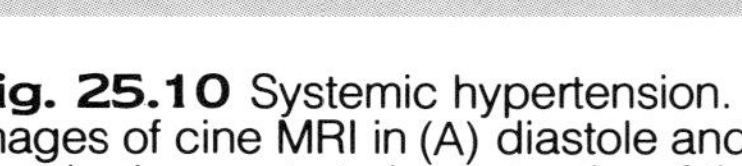

A anterior papillary muscle
P posterior papillary msucle
S ventricular septum
LA left atrium
LV left ventricle

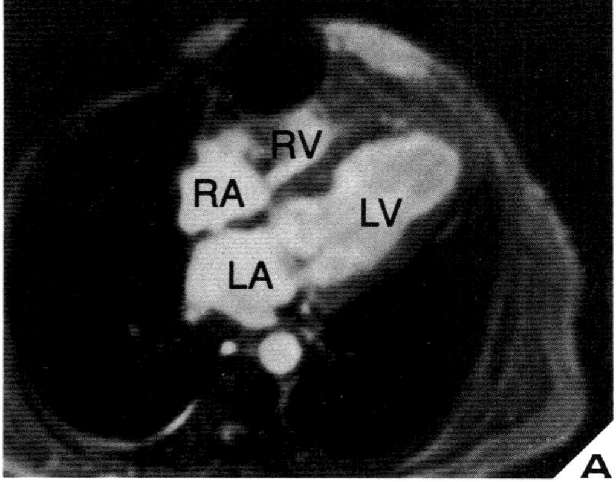

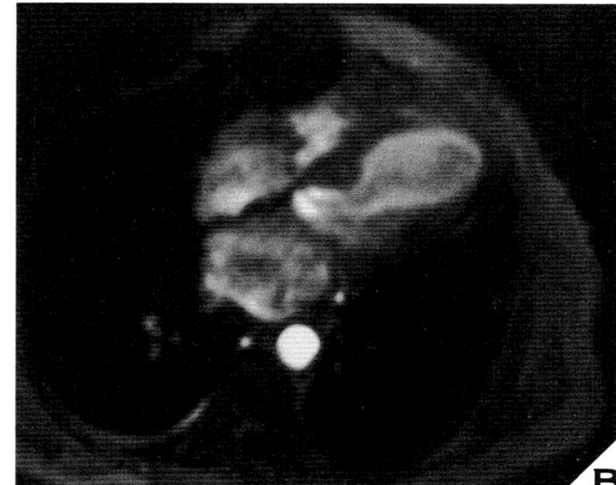

Fig. 25.10 Systemic hypertension. Axial images of cine MRI in (A) diastole and (B) systole demonstrate hypertrophy of the ventricular septum and free wall of the left ventricle (LV), which are most evident in B. (RA = right atrium; RV = right ventricle; LA = left atrium)

vascular performance in these patients are anemia, intolerance for cardiac drugs, and the increased cardiac workload imposed by the arteriovenous shunts used for dialysis. Finally, the inability of these patients to tolerate invasive diagnostic and therapeutic procedures usually makes it difficult to correct their coronary artery disease.

Chronic renal failure impairs cardiovascular performance by a number of other mechanisms, some of which are poorly understood. For example, increased pulmonary blood flow and overt pulmonary edema may occur without elevation of the pulmonary capillary wedge pressure. The mechanism is believed to be increased permeability of the pulmonary capillaries secondary to uremia. Because of the high incidence of coronary artery disease and ischemic heart disease in patients with end-stage renal failure, CHF is quite common, especially when there is coexisting valvular disease.

UREMIC PERICARDITIS

Uremic pericarditis is a common complication of chronic renal failure. Although its etiology is uncertain, it is believed to represent an inflammatory response to a circulating toxin. The serositis may be limited to the pericardium, or may also involve the pleura. Uremic pericarditis typically presents with chest pain; however, if the fluid accumulates rapidly it may cause cardiac tamponade. Chronic constrictive pericarditis develops in 4 percent of patients with uremic pericarditis.

IMAGING AND INVASIVE DIAGNOSIS

Plain films may reveal evidence of pericardial effusion or constrictive pericarditis (see Chapter 22). Chest films of patients with congestive heart failure show cardiomegaly and pulmonary venous hypertension (cephalization pattern). Because pulmonary edema in a uremic patient is not necessarily caused by CHF, it is difficult to exclude the latter on plain films alone. Echocardiography is very sensitive for detecting small amounts of pericardial fluid and can identify any associated myocardial or valvular dysfunction.

Although not always feasible, coronary arteriography may be indicated to assess the status of the coronary arteries, particularly in patients with evidence of ischemic heart disease. The potential toxic effects of the contrast material on the kidney are an important consideration when angiography is performed in patients with chronic renal failure.

CARDIAC EFFECTS OF RADIATION THERAPY

The incidence of cardiovascular complications of radiation therapy depends on how carefully they are looked for. Acute or chronic pericarditis is the most commonly reported cardiovascular complication of radiation therapy. Acute pericarditis occurs in 10 to 15 percent of patients with Hodgkin's disease who receive a dose to the mediastinum of 4000 rads or more. The incidence of this complication is dose related. Radiation-induced myocardial and endocardial damage has only rarely been documented.

Obstructive coronary artery disease, which typically develops 6 to 12 years after exposure, may cause ischemic heart disease. The coronary arterial lesions are characterized by adventitial fibrosis which merges with the fibrous tissue of the overlying epicardium, and by a notable paucity of lipid (atheroma) in the intima. This histologic pattern is distinctly different from that of coronary atherosclerosis.

Radiation-induced mediastinal fibrosis may cause obstruction of the superior vena cava (resulting in a superior vena caval syndrome) and/or stenosis of the pulmonary veins at their junction with the left atrium. Differentiation from persistent or recurrent tumor (usually Hodgkin's or non-Hodgkin's lymphoma) is often difficult.

IMAGING AND INVASIVE DIAGNOSIS

In patients with postirradiation pericarditis, various imaging studies (echocardiography, CT, MRI) demonstrate pericardial fluid or a thickened pericardium, depending on the stage of disease. In patients with radiation-induced mediastinal fibrosis, various imaging techniques (eg, venography, angiocardiography, CT, MRI) can demonstrate the venous obstruction. However, differentiation from residual or recurrent tumor is often impossible, in which case biopsy is needed for definitive diagnosis. MRI may be helpful in some instances, since lymphomatous tissue that has been entirely replaced by fibrotic tissue classically has a low signal on T1- and T2-weighted spin–echo images. The converse is not true, however: although a bright signal on T2-weighted images is generally regarded as evidence of persistent or recurrent tumor, recent studies have shown that some lesions without viable tumor cells may also have a bright signal on T2-weighted images.

ENDOCRINE AND NUTRITIONAL DISORDERS

ACROMEGALY

Excessive production of growth hormone by the anterior pituitary gland produces many adverse effects on the cardiovascular system, including cardiomegaly, systemic hypertension, coronary artery disease, conduction disturbances, and CHF. The clinical manifestations are related to the systemic hypertension, coronary artery disease, and congestive heart failure. (Although some investigators have shown that the myocardial collagen content is abnormally high in this disorder, available evidence indicates that systemic hypertension, rather than "acromegalic cardiomyopathy," is the cause of CHF in most cases.) Precocious coronary artery disease may lead to myocardial infarction in young adults with acromegaly.

IMAGING AND INVASIVE DIAGNOSIS

Chest films demonstrate cardiomegaly with left ventricular enlargement, with elongation and tortuosity of the aorta and its branches reflecting the systemic hypertension. Coronary arteriography demonstrates typical findings of obstructive coronary artery disease (see Chapter 21).

HYPERTHYROIDISM

Cardiovascular signs and symptoms are a prominent clinical feature of hyperthyroidism (Graves' disease). Patients with this disorder—which is caused by excessive production of thyroid hormones (triiodothyronine, thyroxine, or both)—commonly present with palpitations, dyspnea, tachycardia, and systemic hypertension. Physical examination typically reveals a hyperactive precordium with augmentation of the first heart sound, accentuation of the pulmonic component of the second heart sound, and a third heart sound. A metabolic flow murmur is commonly heard along the left sternal border. A distinctive systolic scratch ("Means–Lerman scratch") is occasionally heard in the left second intercostal space during expiration.

The hemodynamic manifestations reflect the increased metabolic demands of the peripheral tissues: increased stroke volume, widened pulse pressure, increased mean systolic ejection rate, increased coronary flow, shortening of the systolic ejection period, and shortening of the pre-ejection period. The high-output state can lead to CHF, which may be aggravated by underlying cardiac or cardiovascular disease.

IMAGING

Plain films typically show prominence of the left ventricle, aorta, and pulmonary arteries. Some patients exhibit generalized cardiomegaly. The pulmonary vasculature may appear plethoric owing to the increased blood content of the lungs. In the most severely affected patients, plain films may show evidence of CHF (cephalization, pulmonary edema).

HYPOTHYROIDISM

Severe hypothyroidism (myxedema) results in profound cardiomyopathy. The "myxedema heart" is typically pale, flabby, and grossly dilated. Microscopically there is myofibrillary swelling, loss of striations, and interstitial fibrosis.

The clinical findings include cardiac enlargement, marked bradycardia, weak arterial pulses, systemic hypotension, and facial and peripheral edema. Severely affected patients may have signs and symptoms of CHF. The ECG findings are characteristic: prolongation of the QT-interval, very low-amplitude P-waves, and prolongation of the QRS with decreased amplitude.

Severe hypothyroidism is associated with altered lipid metabolism, which increases the risk for coronary atherosclerosis and precocious onset of obstructive coronary artery disease. (The latter may first become apparent when total body metabolism increases after treatment of the hypothyroidism.) Chronic hypothyroidism is commonly associated with pericardial effusion, which is often quite large and may cause cardiac tamponade. The pericardial fluid typically has a high cholesterol content.

IMAGING AND INVASIVE DIAGNOSIS

Plain films typically show cardiomegaly with left ventricular enlargement. There may be evidence of pericardial effusion ("waterbottle heart"); often, however, the pericardial effusion is too small to be seen on chest films. Echocardiography can detect pericardial fluid that is not apparent on chest films and may also detect impaired left ventricular contractility.

Owing to the precocious development of coronary artery disease, chest films or cineflouroscopy may detect coronary artery calcification in relatively young individuals. Coronary arteriography confirms the presence of obstructive coronary artery disease, which tends to be most severe in patients with long-standing myxedema.

BERIBERI HEART DISEASE

Vitamin B_1 deficiency results in a dilated cardiomyopathy which may affect both ventricles. A pericardial effusion is commonly present.

DIABETES MELLITUS

The major cardiovascular sequelae of diabetes mellitus are coronary artery disease, stroke, systemic hypertension, and nephropathy. These sequelae reflect both the primary microangiopathy and the accelerated, generalized atherosclerosis and arteriosclerosis which are associated with this complex metabolic disorder. Obstructive disease of large arteries (mainly in the lower extremities, branches of the abdominal aorta, heart, and brain) is mainly seen in the elderly, whereas diabetic microangiopathy can occur at any age. "Diabetic cardiomyopathy" has been diagnosed in a small number of patients in whom no other cause of CHF could be found.

Diabetes is an additive risk factor for all types of cardiovascular disease and has a profound negative effect on the prognosis. Myocardial infarction, stroke, CHF, and hypertension are often more difficult to treat or manage in patients with diabetes.

IMAGING

Plain films typically demonstrate excessive calcifications of the coronary arteries. The heart may be normal or enlarged, depending on the associated pathology.

DISORDERS OF CONNECTIVE TISSUE, MUSCLE, AND THE CENTRAL NERVOUS SYSTEM

MUCOPOLYSACCHARIDOSES

The mucopolysaccharidoses are rare, inherited metabolic disorders caused by deficiencies of lysosomal enzymes, which result in abnormal accumulation of mucopolysaccharides throughout the body. Cardiovascular abnormalities are relatively common in Hurler syndrome [mucopolysaccharidosis (MPS) I], a recessively inherited disorder characterized by dwarfing, corneal clouding, mental retardation, skeletal malformations, and hepatosplenomegaly. They have also been documented in MPS II (Hunter syndrome), MPS I-S (Scheie syndrome, "adult" Hurler syndrome), and MPS IV (Morquio syndrome).

PATHOLOGIC FEATURES

The leaflets of the aortic, mitral, and tricuspid valves are thick, with collagenous nodules at the closure lines. Microscopically, the valvular thickening is due to the accumulation of "Hurler cells" (connective tissue cells laden with heparan sulfate and dermatan sulfate) and an increase in extracellular collagen matrix. The chordae tendinae are short and thick. Accumulations of Hurler cells are often present in the myocardial interstitium; however, the myocytes are relatively spared. The condition also affects systemic arteries, resulting in thickening of the endothelium with progressive obliteration of the lumen; involvement of the coronary arteries commonly leads to ischemic heart disease.

CLINICAL FEATURES

The cardiovascular manifestations reflect the cardiomyopathy and the valvular dysfunction. Congestive heart failure secondary to ischemic heart disease and valvular dysfunction, manifested hemodynamically by increased left ventricular end diastolic pressure, eventually occurs in approximately 10 percent of patients with Hurler's disease. The affected valves are incompetent and/or stenotic to a variable degree, the clinical manifestations reflecting the specific functional abnormality (eg, pulmonary venous hypertension secondary to mitral insufficiency and/or mitral stenosis, left ventricular failure secondary to aortic insufficiency or aortic stenosis). Aortic stenosis is common in adults with MPS I-S. Many patients have systemic hypertension, which contributes to left ventricular dysfunction; its cause is unknown. Sudden death, possibly due to arrhythmia caused by infiltration of the conducting system, occurs in a small percentage of cases.

PSEUDOXANTHOMA ELASTICUM

PATHOLOGIC FEATURES

Pseudoxanthoma elasticum (PXE), a heterogeneous group of inherited elastic tissue disorders, is characterized pathologically by fibrous proliferation of the media and intima of medium-sized arteries, which may severely narrow the lumen. The affected vessels are often extensively calcified. The coronary, renal, and other muscular arteries are commonly affected. (The lesions in the coronary arteries are indistinguishable from those in the peripheral arteries.) The endocardium and heart valves are also affected; the valve leaflets typically have rolled or thickened edges. The conducting system may also be involved.

CLINICAL FEATURES

The clinical cardiovascular manifestations of PXE usually appear in the second and third decades and are related to peripheral obliterative arterial disease (eg, intermittent claudication), systemic hypertension, coronary artery disease (angina pectoris, premature myocardial infarction), valvular dysfunction (usually aortic and/or mitral insufficiency), and restricted ventricular filling due to subendocardial fibroelastosis. Congestive heart failure, which occurs in a small percentage of cases, is probably multifactorial, reflecting the hemodynamic burdens imposed by the peripheral vascular disease, subendocardial fibroelastosis, systemic hypertension, and coronary artery disease. Sudden death, possibly due to arrhythmia, is not uncommon. Mitral valve prolapse is a common finding in one form of PXE.

IMAGING AND INVASIVE DIAGNOSIS

Chest films and echocardiography demonstrate various patterns of chamber enlargement reflecting the valvular disease and myocardial ischemia (see Chapters 18 and 20). Plain films often reveal calcification of peripheral arteries. Angiography demonstrates the lesions of the coronary arteries and visceral branches (eg, renal arteries).

EHLERS–DANLOS SYNDROME

Ehlers–Danlos syndrome comprises a heterogeneous group of connective tissue disorders characterized by hyperelasticity and fragility of the skin, hyperextensibility of the joints, ocular abnormalities, and various abnormalities of the respiratory, digestive, and cardiovascular systems. The cardiovascular manifestations are related to involvement of the mitral valve and ascending aorta. Prolapse of the anterior and/or posterior mitral leaflets, with typical findings on imaging studies, is very common (Fig. 25.11; see also Chapter 18). Dilatation of the aortic root, resulting in aortic insufficiency, is also quite common. Dissection or spontaneous rupture of the aorta and other large arteries has also been documented. Lesions resembling cystic medial necrosis have been described in the aorta. The fragility of the arteries is reported to increase the risk of arterial catheterization. Arrhythmias secondary to involvement of the conducting system are not uncommon.

OSTEOGENESIS IMPERFECTA

Osteogenesis imperfecta is a heterogeneous disorder of connective tissue involving the bones, teeth, and related structures. At least six different types, with variable patterns of genetic transmission, are currently recognized. The cardiovascular manifestations are related to involvement of the connective tissues of the aorta, valve leaflets, and mitral apparatus. The age at onset of these manifestations varies, probably reflecting the severity of the disorder.

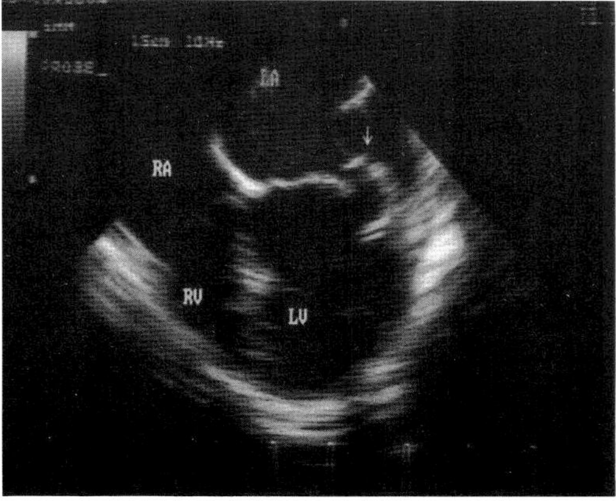

Fig. 25.11 Prolapse of posterior mitral leaflet in a patient with Ehler–Danlos syndrome. Transesophageal echocardiogram (four-chamber view, systole) demonstrates prolapse of the posterior leaflet of the mitral valve resulting from myxomatous degeneration. The posterior leaflet of the mitral valve (*arrow*) is displaced into the left atrium (LA). The entire leaflet, including the free border and the portion adjacent to the mitral annulus, is markedly thickened. The left atrium and left ventricle (LV) are markedly enlarged secondary to severe mitral insufficiency. (RA = right atrium; RV = right ventricle)

PATHOLOGIC AND CLINICAL FEATURES

The aortic annulus is commonly dilated. Cystic medial necrosis of the aorta results in aneurysms of the ascending aorta and sinuses of Valsalva and, rarely, in aortic dissection. Changes identical to those of idiopathic myxomatous degeneration are commonly observed in the aortic and mitral valves; marked thickening of the leaflets may lead to aortic and/or mitral insufficiency. The hemodynamic burden imposed by the aortic valve disease may be progressive, necessitating valve replacement. Mitral insufficiency secondary to rupture of the chordae tendinae may lead to abrupt onset of CHF.

IMAGING

The findings on imaging studies are similar to those seen in aortic aneurysms and valvular insufficiency of other etiologies (Fig. 25.12; see also Chapters 18 and 27). Chest films occasionally reveal marked aortic dilatation in patients without clinical evidence of aortic insufficiency.

MARFAN SYNDROME

Marfan syndrome is an inherited (autosomal dominant) disorder of connective tissue with highly variable phenotypic expression, which predominantly affects the skeleton, eyes, and cardiovascular system. Cardiovascular complications occur in 30 to 60 percent of patients and are the usual cause of death. Before 1970, the median age at death was 32 years; the wider use of composite grafts to replace the aortic root and aortic valve has improved long-term survival in recent years.

PATHOLOGY

The most striking changes occur in the ascending aorta and the cardiac valves. Disruption of the elastica of the proximal aorta and other large arteries leads to weakening of the arterial wall and aneurysm formation. The major histologic findings include severe loss of elastic fibers, deposition of mucopolysaccharides, and focal tears of the aortic wall; cystic medial necrosis is a prominent feature in patients who die as a result of acute aortic dissection. Another characteristic finding is myxomatous degeneration of the leaflets of the aortic, mitral, and tricuspid valves.

Involvement of the coronary arteries has been demonstrated at autopsy in a small number of patients with arrhythmias and ECG evidence of conduction abnormalities. The major pathologic findings were medial degeneration, hyperplasia, and intimal proliferation, with luminal narrowing in the arteries supplying the sinoatrial and atrioventricular nodes and small intramyocardial branches.

CLINICAL FEATURES

The first clinical manifestations of cardiovascular involvement usually appear during adolescence or early adulthood; occasionally there is clinical evidence of cardiovascular involvement during the first decade. Most patients present with aortic and/or mitral insufficiency. The initial clinical manifestations are usually related to aortic insufficiency, which is almost always secondary to dilatation of the aortic root. Initially mild, it may progress to severe aortic regurgitation, eventually culminating in left ventricular failure. As the aortic dilatation worsens, the risk of aortic dissection or rupture increases. Silent aortic dissection is not uncommon; an occasional patient may present with CHF of abrupt onset caused by dissection of the aortic root.

Although there is usually auscultatory evidence of mitral insufficiency, severe mitral regurgitation is rare. Adult patients with isolated, mild mitral dysfunction (eg, systolic click syndrome) appear to have a relatively good prognosis. Rupture of the chordae tendinae or valve can lead to abrupt onset of severe mitral insufficiency and CHF. Bacterial endocarditis involving the mitral valve is a well-documented complication, and not infrequently is the cause of death.

Once signs and symptoms of cardiovascular involvement appear, progressive functional deterioration is the rule; concurrent aortic and mitral insufficiency beginning in childhood is a particularly ominous finding.

From a clinical standpoint, the main differential diagnosis is homocystinuria, an autosomal recessive disorder that shares many phenotypic features with Marfan syndrome. However, unlike Marfan syndrome, the cardiovascular manifestations are mainly those of precocious coronary artery disease and intravascular thrombosis.

IMAGING AND INVASIVE DIAGNOSIS

Chest films typically show evidence of valve dysfunction and abnormalities of the aortic root. Dilatation of the pulmonary trunk is occasionally seen in children with Marfan syndrome. Deformity of the right cardiovascular border and filling in of the retrosternal space suggest an aortic aneurysm (Fig. 25.13), which can be confirmed by echocardiography, CT, or MRI (Fig. 25.14). MRI, which allows serial examinations of the entire aorta and avoids radiation exposure, is especially useful for long-term management of patients with Marfan syndrome, especially those who have undergone valve replacement. Aortic dissection can be detected by each of these modalities (Fig. 25.14). However, as in non-Marfan patients, MRI is more sensitive than CT or echocardiography for detection of aortic dissection.

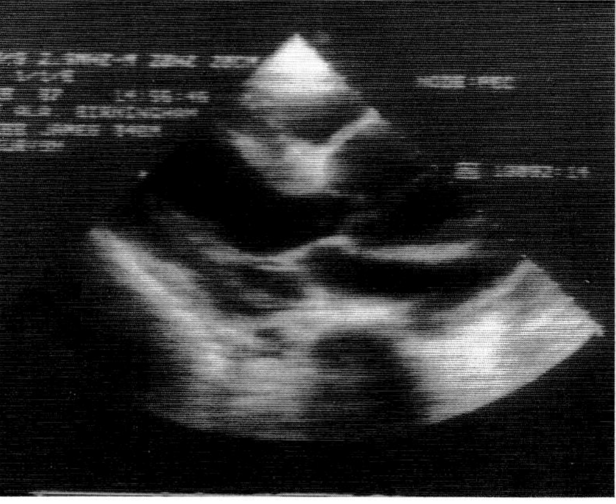

Fig. 25.12 Aortic aneurysm in a patient with osteogenesis imperfecta. Echocardiogram (subcostal long-axis projection) demonstrates marked dilatation of the aortic root and the sinuses of Valsalva. The left ventricle is slightly enlarged secondary to aortic insufficiency.

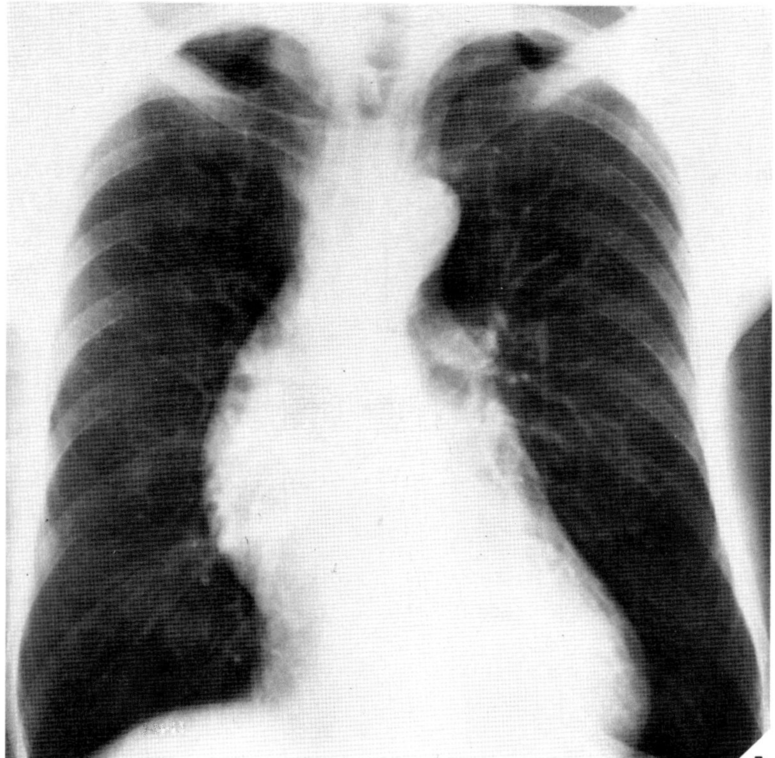

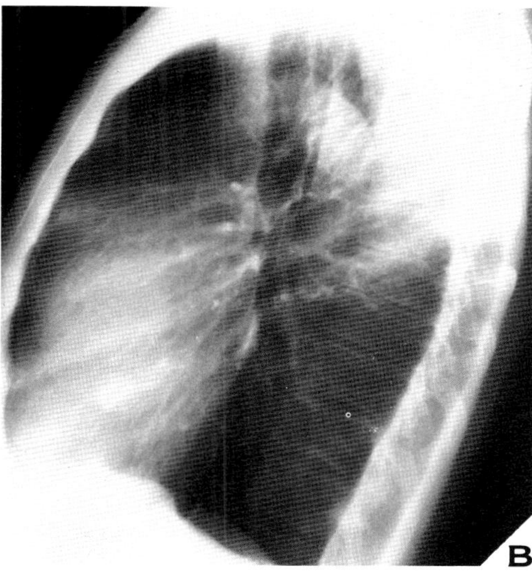

Fig. 25.13 Aortic root aneurysm in a patient with Marfan syndrome. (A) Frontal and (B) lateral projections of chest demonstrate increased height of the thorax in this very tall patient. The heart is slightly enlarged, with left ventricular prominence. The most impressive abnormality is dilatation of the aortic root, which projects anteriorly and to the right. The pulmonary outflow tract is displaced to the left by the dilated aortic root. The aortic arch and pulmonary vasculature are normal.

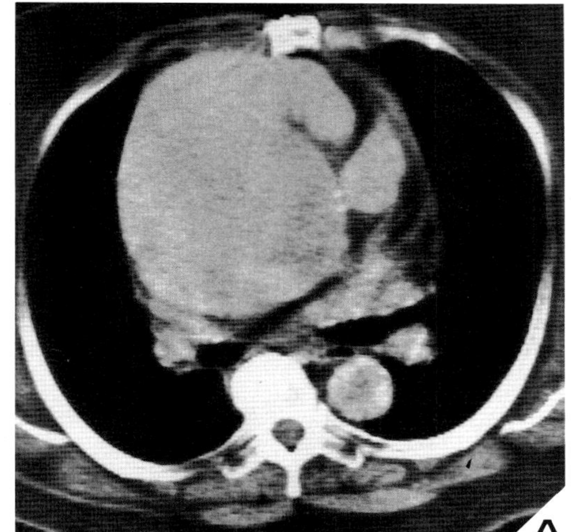

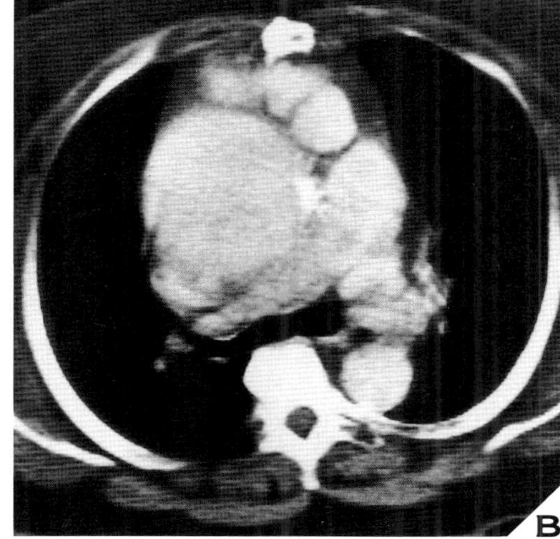

Fig. 25.14 Aortic root aneurysm and aortic dissection in a patient with Marfan syndrome. (A, B) Contrast-enhanced CT scans. (A) Section at the level of the aortic valve demonstrates marked enlargement of the aortic root, which makes contact with the anterior chest wall and displaces the surrounding structures. There is a dissection along the left anterior aspect of the aorta. (B) Section at the level of the pulmonary artery bifurcation. Although the aorta is smaller than in A, it compresses the pulmonary trunk and left pulmonary artery. At this level the dissection is seen anteriorly.

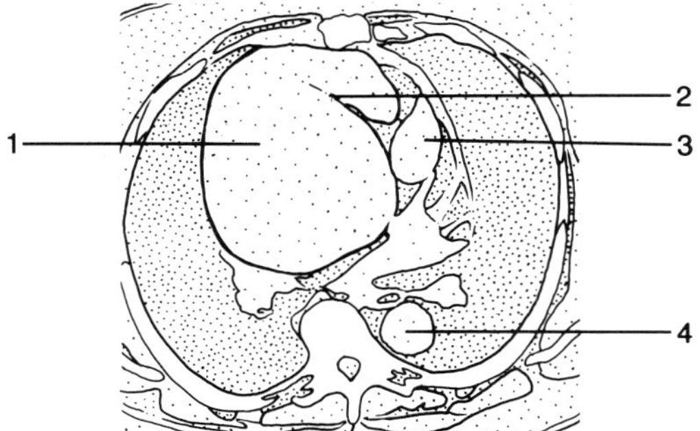

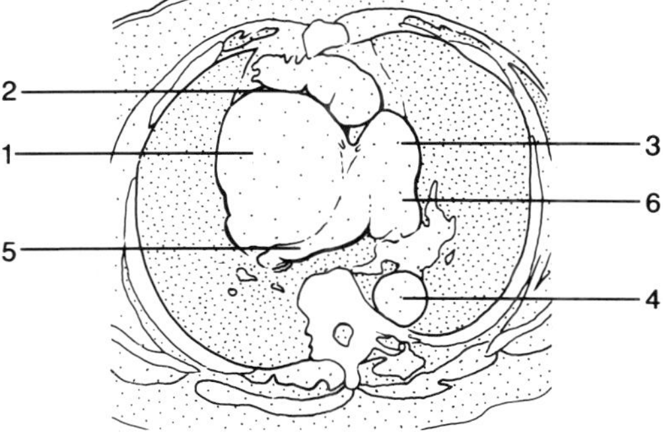

1 aneurysm of ascending aorta
2 flap separating true channel from false channel (aortic dissection)
3 pulmonary trunk
4 descending thoracic aorta
5 right pulmonary artery
6 left pulmonary artery

The angiographic findings in Marfan syndrome are characteristic. Thoracic aortography or left ventriculography demonstrates dilatation of the aortic root, including the aortic annulus. The sinuses of Valsalva are also enlarged, the aortic leaflets typically protruding into the left ventricle. The aortic aneurysm seldom extends beyond the mid-ascending aorta and only rarely extends beyond the origin of the innominate artery (Fig. 25.15). Differentiating Marfan aneurysms from luetic or arteriosclerotic aneurysms is seldom difficult, since the latter do not involve the aortic annulus. Aneurysms of the aortic arch and descending thoracic aorta can occur in Marfan syndrome but are uncommon.

The imaging findings in Marfan syndrome are discussed further in Chapters 5 and 27.

MUSCULAR DYSTROPHY

Cardiomyopathy is characteristic of certain types of progressive muscular dystrophy; not infrequently it is the cause of death. The myocardial scarring in patients with X-linked Duchenne dystrophy is almost always limited to the posterolateral wall of the left ventricle. Medial hypertrophy, with luminal narrowing of small intramural coronary arteries, is also commonly observed in patients with Duchenne dystrophy; however, the distribution of the myocardial scarring is unrelated to the arteriopathy.

Cardiac involvement should be suspected when a patient who has been clinically stable presents with dyspnea, tachycardia, and signs of CHF. In classic Duchenne dystrophy the ECG typically shows tall R-waves over the right precordium, with increased R/S amplitude ratios and deep Q-waves in the limb leads and over the left precordium. Affected siblings and asymptomatic female carriers may have similar ECG findings.

IMAGING

In the initial stages of cardiac decompensation, plain films demonstrate cardiomegaly with left ventricular enlargement; later there is generalized cardiac enlargement with evidence of congestive heart failure (Fig. 25.16). The echocardiographic findings are similar to those in other dilated cardiomyopathies.

MYOTONIC MUSCULAR DYSTROPHY

Clinical evidence of cardiac involvement is common in myotonic muscular dystrophy (myotonia atrophica, Steinert's disease), a slowly progressive, multisystemic autosomal dominant disorder which typically presents during the third or fourth decade. The major noncardiac features of this disorder include myotonia (delayed relaxation after contraction, which can be evoked by voluntary, mechanical, or electric stimulation of certain muscle groups); dystrophy or atrophy of the forearm muscles, sternocleidomastoid, and facial muscles, the latter producing an expressionless "myopathic" facies; bilateral cataracts; frontal baldness; testicular atrophy; infertility; hyperinsulinemia; and low levels of serum IgG. The earliest cardiac manifestations are related to conduction disturbances (sinus bradycardia, prolonged P-R interval, bundle branch block) which can be considered a type of "sick sinus syndrome." Some

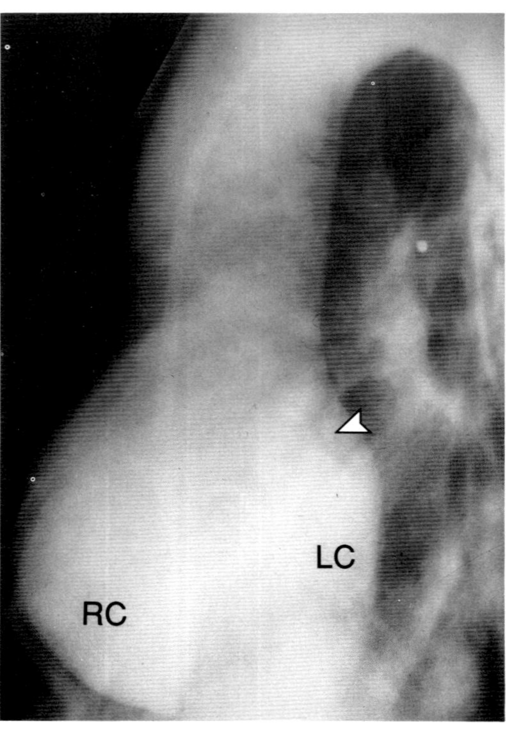

Fig. 25.15 Aortic root aneurysm and aortic dissection in a patient with Marfan syndrome. Lateral projection of thoracic aortogram demonstrates marked dilatation of the aortic root (including the sinuses of Valsalva). The dilatation extends into the ascending aorta. The aortic leaflets are enlarged. Other images showed moderate aortic insufficiency. Note the linear filling defect (*arrow*) along the posterior aspect of the ascending aorta, which represents a dissection. (RC = right coronary cusp of aortic valve; LC = left coronary cusp of aortic valve)

patients present with asymptomatic cardiomegaly, whereas others manifest overt congestive heart failure (which may be provoked or aggravated by the inappropriately slow heart rate). The cause of the cardiac manifestations is uncertain. Clinical and anatomic studies have documented myocardial abnormalities similar to those of systemic muscular dystrophy in a small percentage of cases. Although an abnormal left ventricular contraction pattern has been angiocardiographically documented in one case report, there is no convincing proof that the myotonic process affects the myocardium. [Cardiac involvement does not occur in myotonia congenita (Thomsen's disease), in which the myotonia is not associated with muscular dystrophy.] Most of the available evidence suggests a degenerative process of the specialized conduction system, the cardiac fibroskeleton. The findings on imaging studies are nonspecific.

FRIEDREICH'S ATAXIA

Significant cardiac involvement, which may begin in childhood, is common in this recessively inherited neurologic disorder; in as many as 10 percent of cases the cardiac manifestations precede the neurologic manifestations. Pathologically, the predominant cardiac lesion is a hypertrophic cardiomyopathy which can affect all four chambers; occasionally there is associated round-cell infiltration. Coronary artery involvement has also been described. Congestive heart failure secondary to progressive myocardial fibrosis is frequently the terminal event.

IMAGING

Chest films show nonspecific cardiac enlargement. The findings on cross-sectional imaging techniques and angiogcardiography

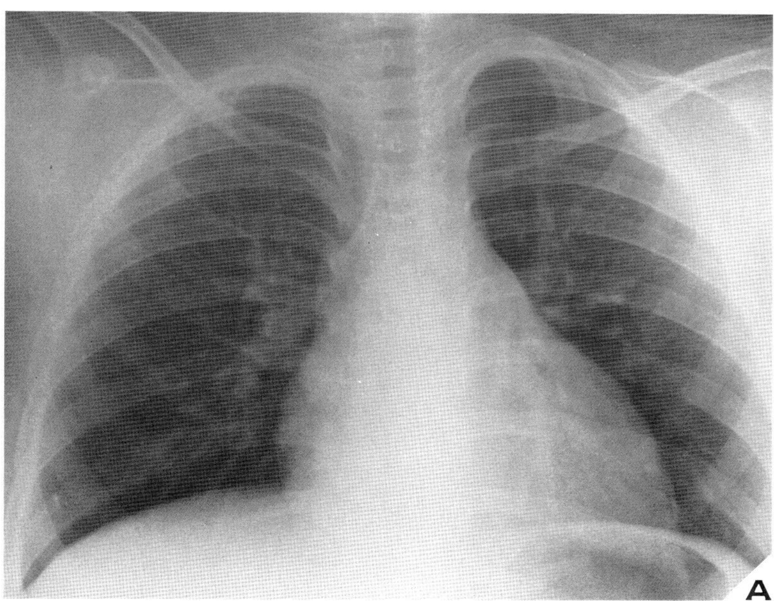

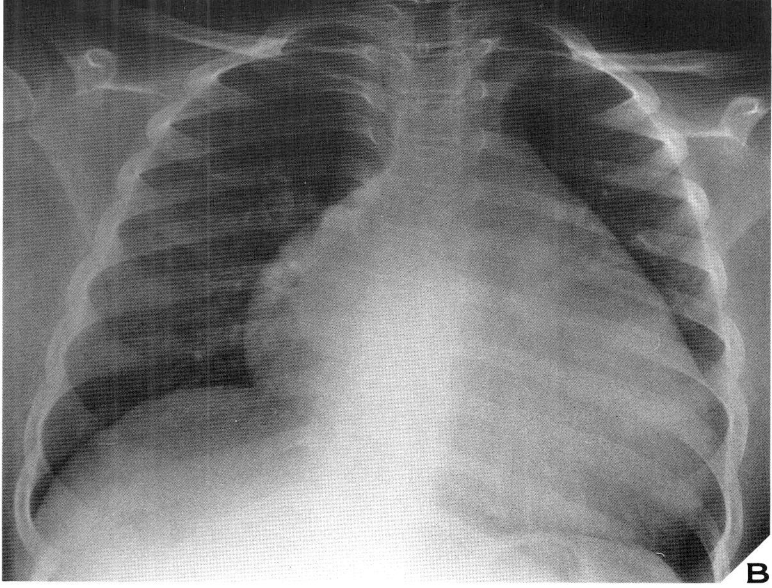

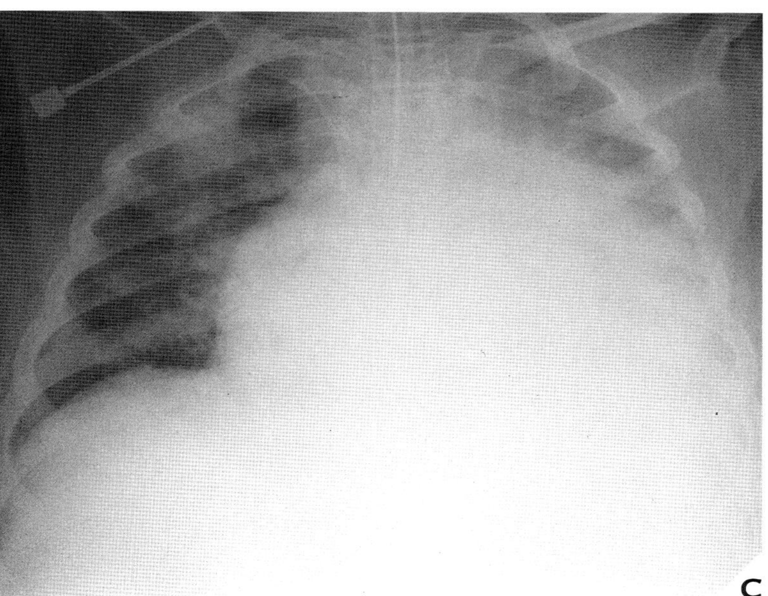

Fig. 25.16 Cardiomyopathy in a patient with Duchenne muscular dystrophy. (A) Chest film at 10 years 9 months of age demonstrates minimal cardiomegaly with left ventricular prominence. The pulmonary vasculature is normal. (B) Chest film at 12 years 6 months of age shows marked increase in cardiac enlargement. The pulmonary vasculature is normal. (C) Portable chest film obtained 2 weeks later shortly before death from CHF and respiratory failure, shows bilateral pulmonary edema.

are typical of hypertrophic cardiomyopathy (Fig. 25.17). Subaortic stenosis has been detected echocardiographically in some patients.

ACQUIRED IMMUNE DEFICIENCY SYNDROME (AIDS)

The cardiovascular manifestations of AIDS are due to opportunistic infections, nonspecific dilated (congestive) cardiomyopathy, and neoplastic involvement of the heart. Although cardiovascular pathology was not mentioned in the initial descriptions, subsequent experience has shown that it contributes to the morbidity of AIDS and is occasionally the cause of death. Often, however, cardiac involvement is masked by the other clinical manifestations of this protean multisystemic disorder and is not detected during life.

PATHOLOGIC FEATURES

Cardiomegaly is commonly found at autopsy. Various patterns (right ventricular hypertrophy with or without right ventricular dilatation, biventricular dilatation, four-chamber enlargement) have been described, reflecting the functional disturbance observed during life (see below). The cardiac enlargement is usually due to dilated cardiomyopathy. (A variable degree of left ventricular hypertrophy is usually present as well.) Right ventricular hypertrophy secondary to chronic pulmonary hypertension is a common finding in patients with severe lung disease.

INFLAMMATORY AND INFECTIOUS DISORDERS

Myocarditis, often accompanied by pericarditis, is occasionally found at autopsy in patients with AIDS (isolated pericarditis is very rare). The causative organisms include bacteria (eg, *Mycobacterium tuberculosis, Mycobacterium avium intracellulare,* fungi (cryptococcus), protozoa (eg, *Toxoplasma gondii*), and viruses (eg, cytomegalovirus). The myocarditis may be focal or diffuse. Microscopic examination reveals lymphocyte infiltration with variable degrees of myocardial necrosis. (The extent of the lymphocyte infiltration is believed to indicate active myocarditis.) Intracellular inclusions characteristic of CMV infection are commonly seen in patients with myocardial necrosis without associated inflammation. Tuberculous myocarditis is characterized by a moderately intense diffuse interstitial infiltrate of neutrophils and lymphocytes.

Although in some instances there is unequivocal evidence of an opportunistic infection, the etiology of the myocarditis is often obscure. The role of human immunodeficiency virus (HIV) is unclear. HIV is known to replicate within lymphocytes and macrophages in the myocardial interstitium; however, it is not known whether HIV replication in the myocytes themselves can cause cell injury and cell death.

The most commonly encountered endocardial lesion is nonbacterial thrombotic endocarditis ("marantic endocarditis"). The vegetations, which consist of a fibrin mesh containing a few inflammatory cells, resemble those seen in patients with protracted wasting diseases and malignant neoplasms, and probably have a similar pathogenesis. The vegetations are typically very friable and tend to embolize systemically. Infective endocarditis caused by *Aspergillus fumigatus* has been reported in a small number of patients with AIDS.

DILATED CARDIOMYOPATHY AND IDIOPATHIC MYOCARDIAL NECROSIS

Dilated (congestive) cardiomyopathy is the most common cardiac abnormality associated with AIDS. The etiology is poorly understood. Possible causative factors include drug toxicity (eg, pentamidine), cachexia, selenium deficiency secondary to malnutrition, and immunologic abnormalities. Noninflammatory myocardial necrosis, attributed by some investigators to chronic stress resulting from prolonged and excessive secretion of catecholamines, has been observed in some patients with AIDS. In some instances dilated cardiomyopathy may represent the aftermath of a burned-out viral myocarditis.

NEOPLASTIC DISORDERS

Cardiac involvement by AIDS-related neoplasms (eg, Kaposi's sarcoma, non-Hodgkins lymphoma) is not uncommon. Kaposi's sarcoma typically metastasizes to the epicardium, often spreading to the myocardium and/or pericardium. Extension of the tumor into the ventricular cavity (which interferes with ventricular filling) is a rare complication. AIDS-related lymphomas are generally of B-cell origin, often of Burkitt type. Cardiac involvement in patients with AIDS-related lymphoma may be primary or secondary. Primary cardiac lymphoma can involve the myocardium diffusely or can be multifocal, in which case it

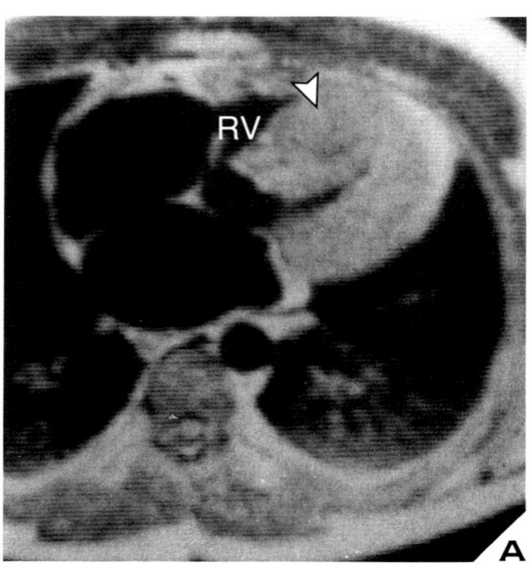

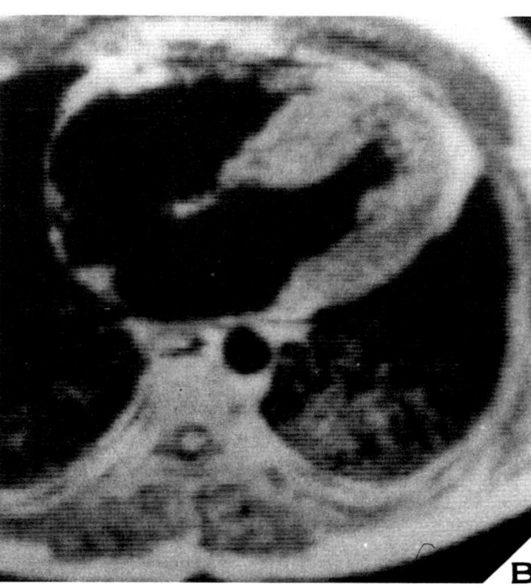

Fig. 25.17 Hypertrophic cardiomyopathy in a patient with Friedreich's ataxia. Axial spin–echo MR images through midportion of heart in (A) systole and (B) diastole demonstrate marked hypertrophy of the free wall of the left ventricle and the ventricular septum (*arrow*). During systole the left ventricular chamber is obliterated. The right ventricular wall is of normal thickness. (RV = right ventricle)

may occur as multiple discrete tumor nodules throughout the endocardium, myocardium, and epicardium, or as white "fish flesh" infiltrates in the ventricular walls and interventricular septum.

ARTERIAL LESIONS

Arteriopathy has been reported in a small number of children with AIDS. Two types of arterial lesion, inflammatory and fibrocalcific, have been described. The former can take the form of a vasculitis or perivasculitis, whereas the latter is characterized microscopically by intimal fibrosis, fragmentation of elastic tissue, and fibrosis and calcification of the media. Fibrocalcific arteriopathy affects small and medium-sized arteries in various organs, including the heart, and typically leads to a variable degree of luminal narrowing. However, aneurysms of the coronary arteries associated with intraluminal thrombosis and myocardial infarction have also been reported.

CLINICAL FEATURES

Although cardiovascular involvement is present in about two thirds of hospitalized patients with AIDS, clinical evidence of cardiovascular dysfunction can be detected in less than 10 percent of ambulatory patients. The most common clinical manifestations are related to dilated (congestive) cardiomyopathy and pericardial effusion. Arrhythmias due to inflammation or neoplastic invasion of the conducting system are not uncommon and have occasionally been associated with sudden death.

In patients with AIDS-related dilated cardiomyopathy, there is no correlation between the degree of chamber enlargement and the extent of the myocarditis observed at autopsy. (Indeed, microscopic evidence of myocarditis is commonly absent.) As with dilated cardiomyopathy of any cause, the signs and symptoms are mainly those of CHF (see Chapter 19). The ECG typically reveals evidence of left ventricular hypertrophy. Many children and adults with AIDS eventually develop pulmonary hypertension (cor pulmonale) secondary to the severe lung disease commonly present. The ECG in such cases shows typical features of right ventricular hypertrophy (see Chapter 24). Children with AIDS-related cardiovascular dysfunction typically present with shortness of breath, easy fatigability, tachypnea, sinus tachycardia with gallop rhythm, and hepatomegaly.

Pericardial effusion has been reported in 18 to 40 percent of adult patients with AIDS, occasionally resulting in cardiac tamponade (cardiac tamponade has not been documented in children). The pericardial fluid may be clear or serosanguineous. Although bacteria or fungi can sometimes be isolated from the pericardial fluid, the etiology of the effusion is often obscure.

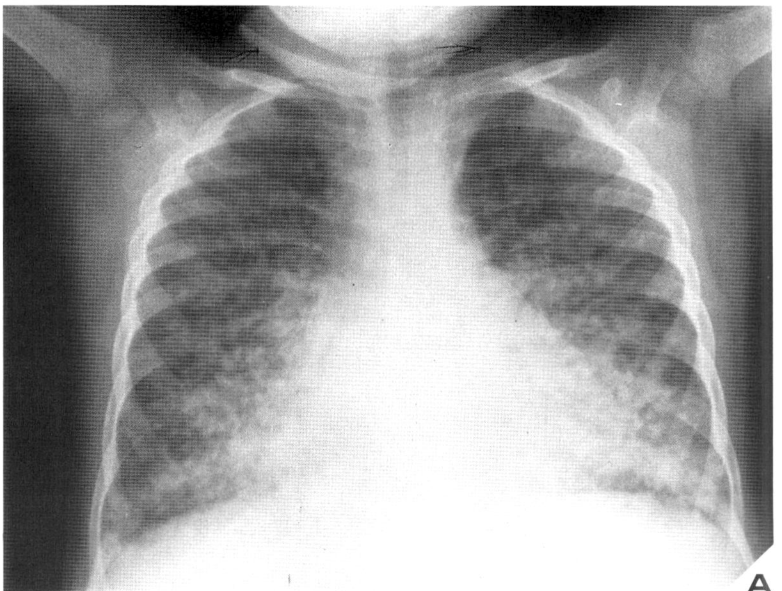

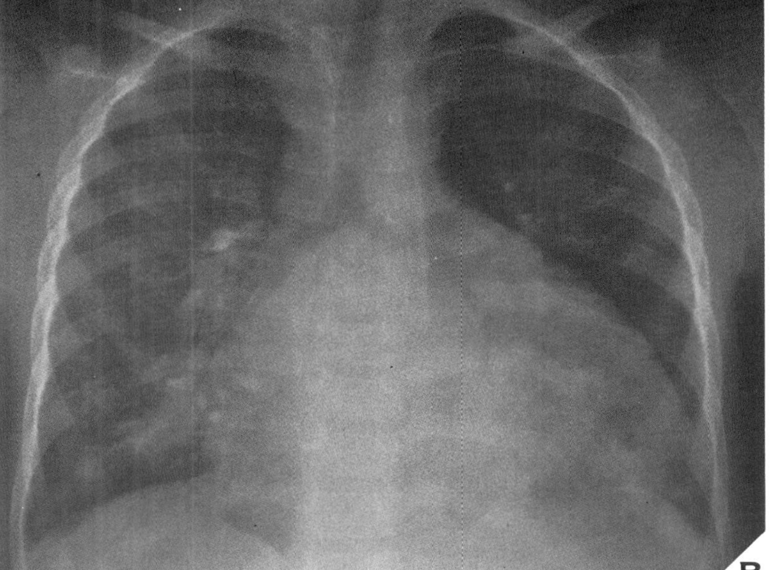

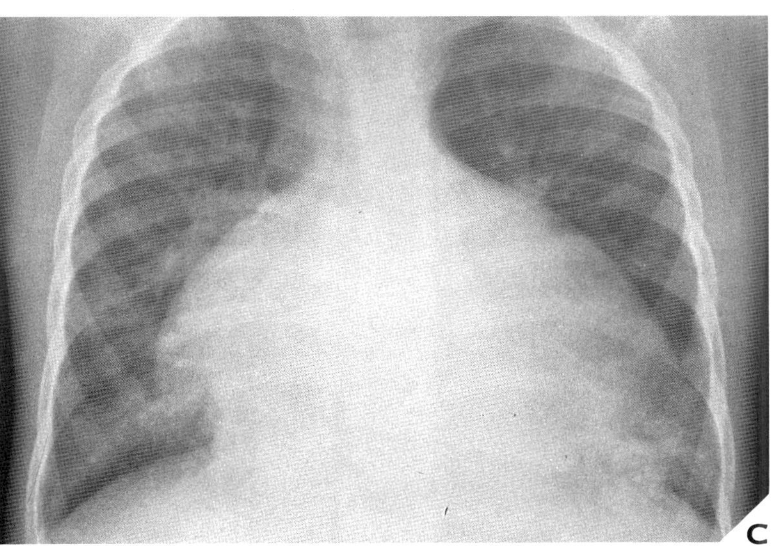

Fig. 25.18 Dilated cardiomyopathy in a child with AIDS. (A) Chest film at 17 months of age shows confluent bilateral nodular intiltrates compatable with lymphoid interstitial pneumonitis (LIP). The heart is normal. (B) Chest film at 4 years of age shows marked cardiomegaly with left ventricular and left atrial enlargement. The pulmonary vasculature is normal. There has been considerable regression of the lung lesions. (C) Chest film obtained 2 weeks later, after abrupt onset of CHF, shows further cardiac enlargement with evidence of pulmonary venous hypertension (note cephalization pattern) and alveolar and interstitial pulmonary edema. An echocardiogram showed a small pericardial effusion without tamponade and poor myocardial contractility. Despite pressor support and adequate ventilation the patient remained persistently acidotic and died the following day. At autopsy the heart weighed 140 grams (30 percent above normal). The left ventricular cavity was markedly dilated. The left ventricular wall was minimally hypertrophied. Microscopically, there was variation of myocardial fiber size and interstitial myocardial edema. There was no evidence of myocardial infarction or acute or chronic myocarditis.

CHAPTER 26

Cardiac Neoplasms

Growth of neoplastic tissue in the heart causes abnormal cardiac function by interfering with myocardial contractility or valve function, or by obstructing the great vessels. Cardiac tumors are classified, according to their origin, as primary or secondary. Most cardiac neoplasms in adults are secondary, whereas the great majority of cardiac neoplasms in children and adolescents are primary (Figure 26.1).

GENERAL CHARACTERISTICS

CLINICAL MANIFESTATIONS

The clinical manifestations of cardiac tumors are determined by the cardiac segment or segments affected and by the tumor growth pattern. The latter may be primarily (or exclusively) pericardial, intramural, or intracavitary.

PERICARDIAL INVOLVEMENT

Pericardial involvement is almost always metastatic, usually from a primary in the breast or lung. The clinical manifestations result from pericardial effusion and/or constriction.

The patient with a malignant pericardial effusion typically presents with nonspecific chest pain and shortness of breath, usually of insidious onset. However, sudden distension of the pericardium may be accompanied by hypotension, syncope, or shock; rupture of the heart or bleeding into the tumor can lead to cardiac tamponade. The physical findings are similar to those of a non-neoplastic effusion and are determined by the size and

CHAPTER LABELING KEY

RA	right atrium	RV	right ventricle
LA	left atrium	LV	left ventricle

FIG. 26.1 TUMORS OF THE HEART, PERICARDIUM, AND GREAT VESSELS

I. Embryonic Rests and Developmental Cysts
- Pericardial cyst
- Dermoid cyst
- Thyroid rest
- Parathyroid rest
- Inclusion cyst

II. Primary Neoplasms
- A. Benign
  - Myxoma (heart)
  - Rhabdomyoma (heart)*
  - Fibroma (heart, pericardium)
  - Teratoma (heart, pericardium)
  - Mesothelioma (pericardium)
  - Angioma, hemangioma (heart, pericardium)
  - Lipoma (heart, pericardium)
  - Lymphangioendothelioma (heart, pericardium)
  - Endothelioma (great vessels)
  - Tumors of the cardiac valves (neoplastic and nonneoplastic)
    - Fibroma
    - Myxoma
    - Blood cyst
- B. Malignant
  - Mesothelioma (pericardium)
  - Angiosarcoma (heart, great vessels)
  - Rhabdomyosarcoma (heart)
  - Teratoma (heart, pericardium)
  - Liposarcoma (pericardium)
  - Fibrosarcoma (pericardium, great vessels)
  - Neurosarcoma (heart, pericardium)
  - Leiomyosarcoma (heart, great vessels)
  - Malignant endothelioma (great vessels)
  - Giant cell sarcoma (great vessels)
  - Chondrosarcoma (great vessels)
  - Osteogenic sarcoma (great vessels)
  - Intimal sarcoma (great vessels)

III. Secondary (metastatic) neoplasms
- A. Contiguous spread from lung, pleura, mediastinum, or diaphragm
- B. Hematogenous and lymphogenous
  - Carcinoma (especially breast and lung)
  - Sarcoma (various)
  - Lymphosarcoma
  - Leukemia
- C. Transvenous
  - Hepatoma
  - Renal cell carcinoma
  - Bronchogenic carcinoma

**Classified as a hamartoma by some authors*

Fig. 26.1 Neoplasms of the heart and pericardium.

chronicity of the effusion. A pericardial friction rub may be detected in the initial stage. Pulsus paradoxicus and elevated jugular venous pressure indicate the presence of a large effusion. The ECG, which may demonstrate various arrhythmias and nonspecific ST-segment and T-wave changes, is not diagnostic. Definitive diagnosis is made by pericardial aspiration, which typically yields a bloody fluid containing tumor cells.

Growth of the tumor or intralesional hemorrhage may lead to pericardial constriction, manifested by dyspnea, orthopnea, chest pain, hepatomegaly, and/or dependent edema; the severity of the symptoms varies with the degree of pericardial thickening. As in the case of constrictive pericarditis, the signs and symptoms associated with neoplastic pericardial constriction result from restricted diastolic filling (see Chapter 22). If necessary, a transcutaneous or open pericardial biopsy can be obtained to confirm the diagnosis.

MYOCARDIAL INVOLVEMENT

Myocardial involvement by a primary or secondary malignancy can present with a wide spectrum of clinical manifestations, of which arrhythmias and congestive heart failure are the most common. The most frequent rhythm disturbances are premature ventricular contractions, ectopic atrial tachycardia, and minor conduction defects; these may occur alone or in various combinations. An occasional patient may develop a severe, life-threatening arrhythmia (eg, ventricular tachycardia or ventricular fibrillation). Patients with myocardial involvement may exhibit signs and symptoms of congestive heart failure, such as pulmonary congestion, hepatomegaly, and/or edema of the lower extremities.

ENDOCARDIAL INVOLVEMENT

Neoplasms that arise in the endocardium or myocardial neoplasms that extend intraluminally are associated with valvular malfunction, functional stenosis of one or more chambers, and/or tumor emboli. The clinical manifestations of left atrial myxoma resemble those of mitral stenosis. Patients with rhabdomyoma involving the left ventricle commonly present with congestive heart failure or with right or left ventricular outflow obstruction.

Peripheral embolization of an intracavitary tumor is an infrequent but serious complication. A neoplasm arising in the left atrium or left ventricle can embolize to any part of the systemic circulation, whereas right-sided lesions can embolize to the lungs. Repeated showers of pulmonary emboli can lead to pulmonary hypertension and right ventricular hypertrophy.

PRIMARY CARDIAC TUMORS

MYXOMA

Cardiac myxomas are primary intracavitary neoplasms of endocardial origin. Although the great majority arise in the left atrium, cardiac myxomas can also originate in the left or right ventricle, right atrium, or in a cardiac valve. Atrial myxomas typically arise in the atrial septum; however, they may occur anywhere in the atrial wall. Cardiac myxomas are much more common in females (sex ratio 3:1). The usual age at presentation is 30 to 60 years.

Cardiac myxomas may be pedunculated or broad-based, ranging from 1 to 15 cm in diameter (Fig. 26.2). The external surface is usually smooth, although on occasion it has a frosted appearance. Microscopically, the tumor consists of small polygonal cells in a myxoid stroma. The luminal surface may exhibit areas of necrosis, fibrosis, or hemorrhage. Although cardiac myxoma is usually considered a benign neoplasm, local recurrence and distant metastases have been reported.

LEFT ATRIAL MYXOMA

Left atrial myxomas almost always involve the left atrial chamber; 75 percent originate from the atrial septum and 25 percent arise elsewhere in the left atrium. The tumor may be multicentric or bi-atrial in origin.

Left atrial myxomas may be sporadic or familial, or they may occur as part of the "myxoma complex." Most left atrial myxomas occur sporadically. About 50 percent of patients with left atrial myxoma are 50 to 60 years of age at time of diagnosis; 12 percent are over 70 years of age. Patients with the familial form of left atrial myxoma usually become symptomatic before 40 years of age; the pattern of genetic transmission has not been established. The "myxoma complex" refers to a constellation of extracardiac abnormalities (multiple lentigines, cutaneous myxomas, mammary myxoid fibroadenomas, and pituitary tumors) associated with left atrial myxoma; no genetic pattern has been identified. As with familial left atrial myxoma, most patients with the "myxoma complex" are under 40 years of age.

Unlike sporadic left atrial myxoma, which is almost always solitary, the lesions in familial left atrial myoxma and the "myxoma complex" are usually multiple. Therefore, sporadic left atrial myxoma is the most likely diagnosis in a patient over 50 years of age with a solitary left atrial mass. Surgical excision is usually curative in patients with sporadic left atrial myxoma; however, postoperative recurrence is not uncommon in patients with familial left atrial myxoma and the "myxoma complex."

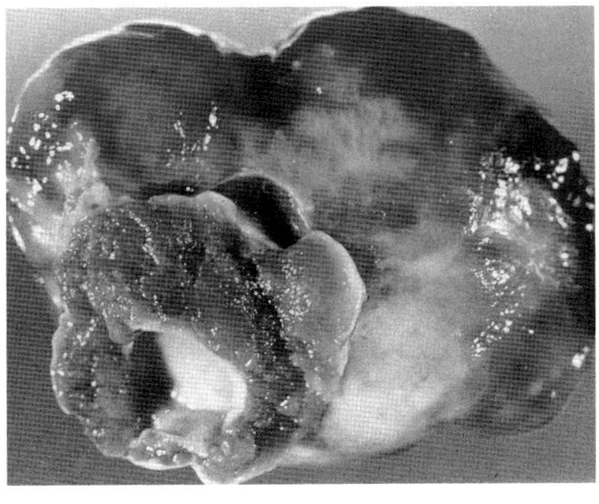

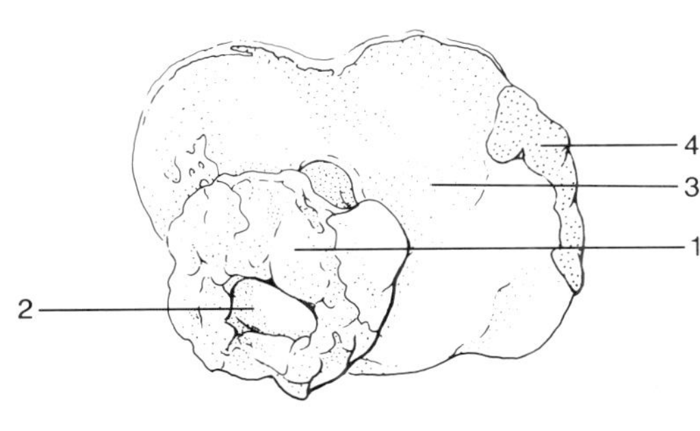

Fig. 26.2 Atrial myxoma. Surgical specimen of large left atrial myxoma showing its attachment to the atrial septum. The tumor, which occupied three fourths of the left atrial cavity, has been resected along with a portion of the atrial septum. The surface of the tumor is smooth and glistening except for scattered areas of hemorrhage.

1 atrial septum (resected)
2 fossa ovalis
3 myxoma
4 focal hemorrhage

Hemodynamic Features

Large left atrial myxomas restrict the capacity of the atrial chamber. In addition, the tumor may obstruct the mitral valve or the orifices of the pulmonary veins. A tumor that is partially detached or covered by thrombus may be the source of systemic emboli. Small lesions produce no significant hemodynamic effect.

Clinical Features

The clinical manifestations of left atrial myxoma vary according to the size of the lesion. Small tumors are asymptomatic, and are discovered incidentally on a chest radiograph, which may demonstrate cardiac calcifications, or on echocardiography. Patients with large lesions present with signs and symptoms of mitral stenosis (dyspnea, orthopnea, acute pulmonary edema, paroxysmal nocturnal orthopnea, orthopnea), some or all of which may be brought on by changes in position. Constitutional symptoms (eg, fever, pallor, anemia, fatigue, weight loss) have also been described. Physical examination commonly reveals elevated jugular venous pressure, right ventricular enlargement, and accentuation of the pulmonary component of the second heart sound. Anemia, leukocytosis, and an increase in the erythrocyte sedimentation rate have also been observed.

Imaging and Invasive Diagnosis

Plain Films Chest films are normal in patients with small lesions that do not interfere with mitral valve function. Patients with large, hemodynamically significant lesions have left atrial enlargement and evidence of pulmonary venous hypertension, a radiographic pattern indistinguishable from that seen in mitral stenosis, which is much more common (Fig. 26.3). The presence of calcification is very helpful in differential diagnosis (Fig. 26.4). The calcification associated with a left atrial myxoma is typically round or oval; most of the calcium is concentrated at the surface of the lesion, producing a curvilinear appearance. Flouroscopy reveals wide excursion of the lesion as it moves from the left atrium into the left ventricle. Differentiation from calcification of the mitral leaflets or mitral annulus usually presents no difficulty. The location of mitral valvular calcification corresponds to the anatomic location of the anterior or posterior leaflet. On fluoroscopy there is limited excursion of the calcified leaflets, particularly when mitral stenosis is present, and the calcifications remain within the left atrial cavity throughout the cardiac cycle. A calcified mitral annulus has a typical "C" shape and exhibits little motion during the cardiac cycle. The differential diagnosis between left atrial myxoma and mitral stenosis is less certain when calcification is absent. However, because the left atrium is only slightly to moderately enlarged in patients with left atrial myxoma, marked left atrial enlargement favors the diagnosis of mitral valvular disease.

Echocardiography The lesion is clearly shown by two-dimensional echocardiography, which can be performed via a transthoracic or transesophageal approach. The latter yields high-resolution images which increase diagnostic certainty. The tumor appears as an echo-dense mass within the left atrial chamber. Although the tumor usually arises from the septum, it may originate from other portions of the left atrial wall. When the tumor is pedunculated, it can be seen to move during the cardiac cycle, often protruding into the left ventricle during diastole (Fig. 26.5). Although other lesions may have a similar appearance on static images (eg, thrombus, calcified mitral leaflets, vegetations), none exhibits the mobility of a pedunculated atrial myxoma. Further diagnostic studies can usually be omitted in patients with typical echocardiographic findings.

MRI Left atrial myxoma is clearly depicted on ECG-gated spin–echo images; the lesion appears as a high-signal density against the signal-free background produced by flowing blood (Fig. 26.6). Images obtained at different phases of the cardiac

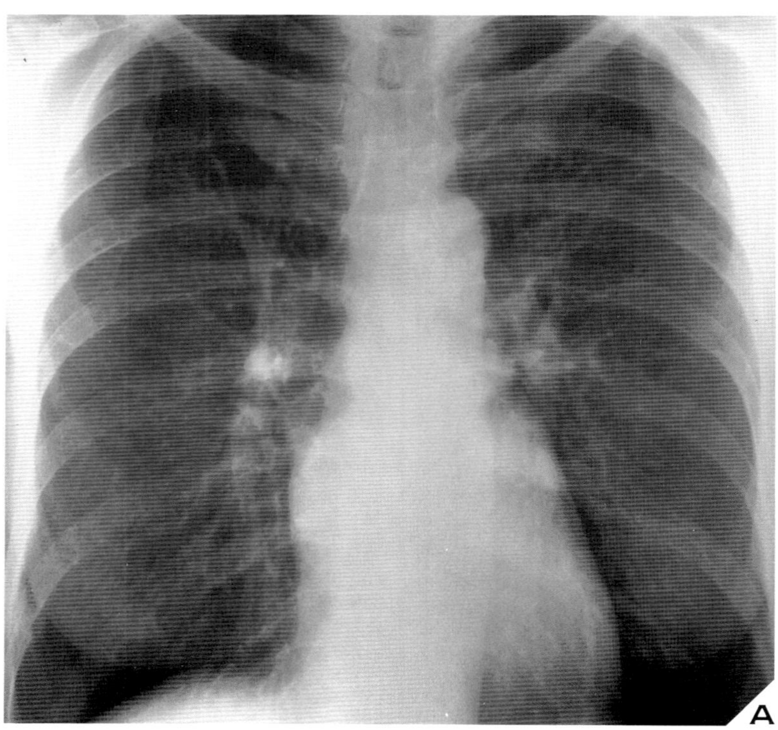

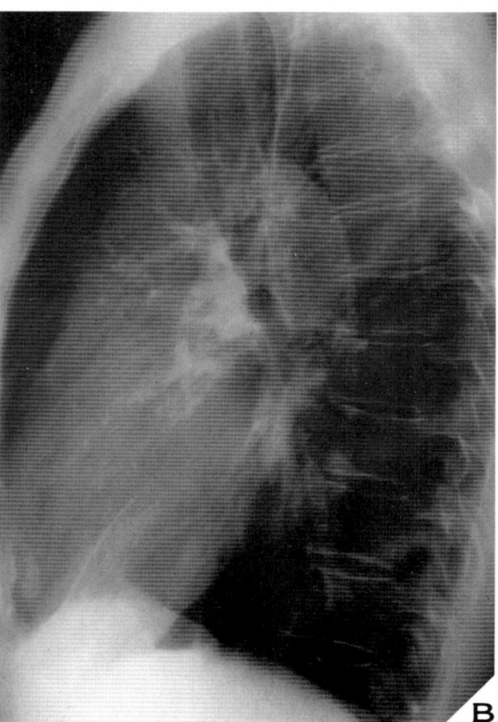

Fig. 26.3 Left atrial myxoma. (A) Posteroanterior and (B) lateral chest films of a 43-year-old woman show a normal-sized heart with marked left atrial enlargement. (note double density within right heart border, prominent left atrial appendage, and posterior displacement of left main bronchus) and evidence of pulmonary venous hypertension (cephalization pattern). No cardiac calcifications can be identified. The radiographic findings are entirely compatible with a diagnosis of mitral stenosis.

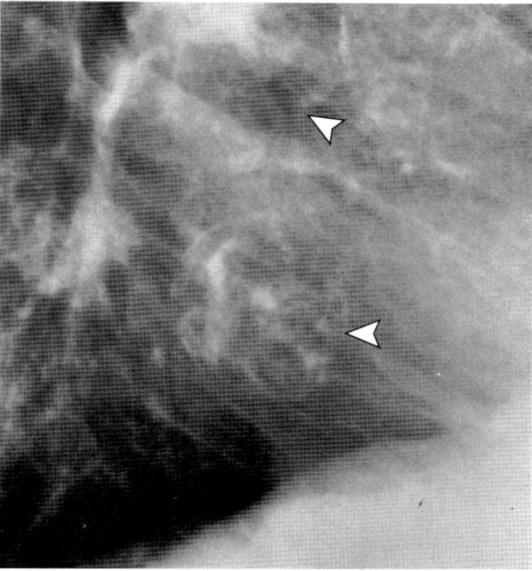

Fig. 26.4 Calcified left atrial myxoma. Close-up of lateral chest film shows a round amorphous calcification in the left atrium. The posterior margin of the calcification is well defined (*arrows*). Marked excursion of the calcification during the cardiac cycle was noted fluoroscopically. A 3 × 5 cm calcified myxoma arising from the atrial septum was surgically resected.

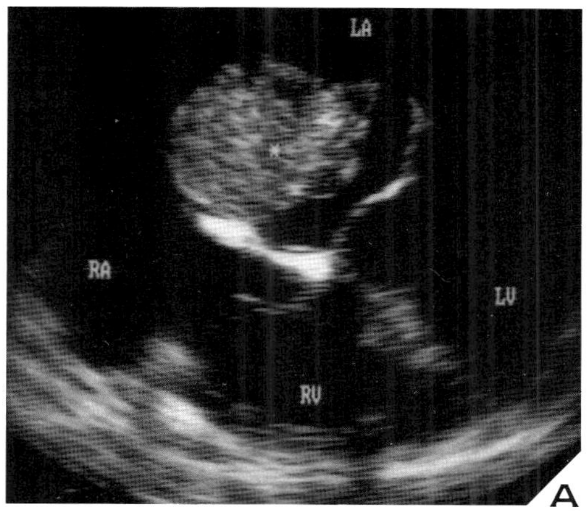

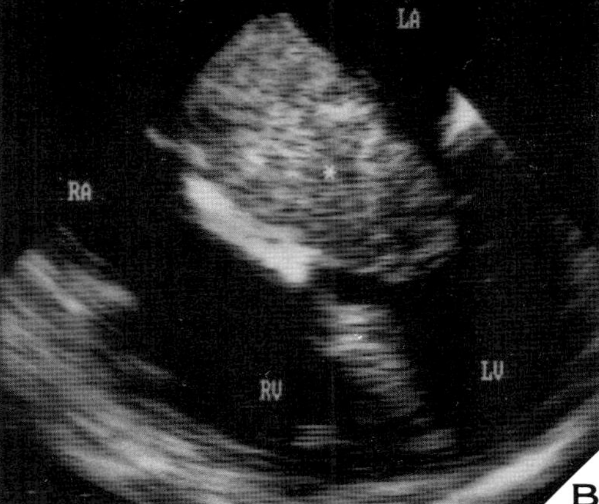

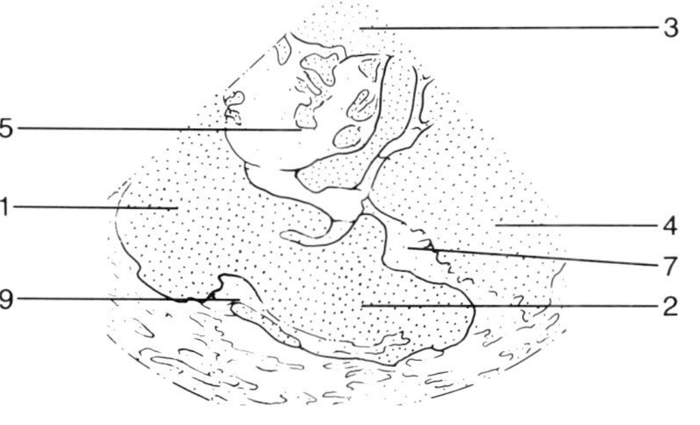

Fig. 26.5 Left atrial myxoma. Four-chamber projection of echocardiogram in (A) systole and (B) diastole demonstrates an echogenic intracavitary mass of the left atrium. A portion of the tumor, which is attached to the atrial septum, moves into the left ventricle during diastole, almost completely occluding the mitral valve orifice during this portion of the cardiac cycle.

1 right atrium
2 right ventricle
3 left atrium
4 left ventricle
5 left atrial myxoma
6 atrial septum
7 ventricular septum
8 mitral valve
9 tricuspid valve

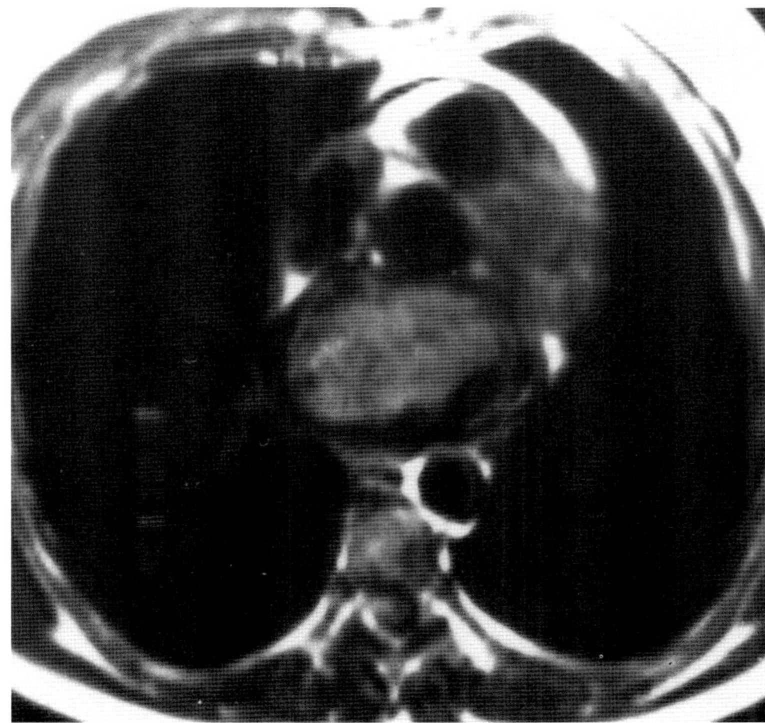

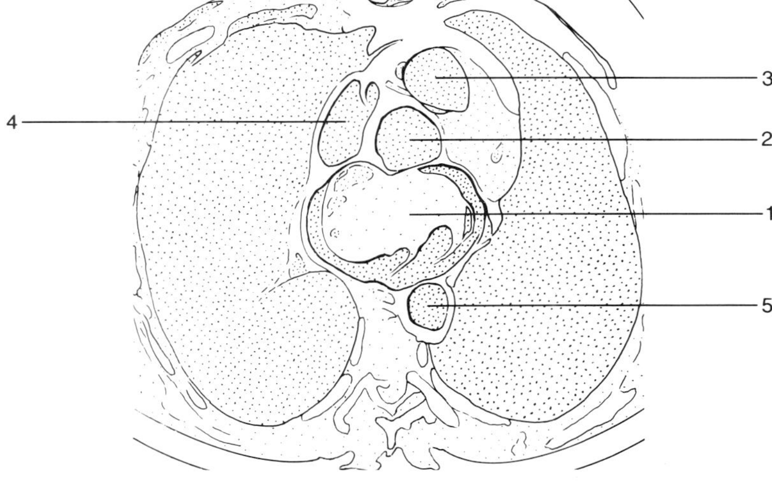

1 left atrial myxoma
2 ascending aorta
3 pulmonary trunk
4 right atrial appendage
5 descending thoracic aorta

Fig. 26.6 Left atrial myxoma (MRI findings). Axial T1-weighted spin–echo image at the level of the left atrium demonstrates a mass completely filling the left atrium. The mass, which is attached to the atrial septum, has a relatively bright signal when compared with normal myocardium and skeletal muscle. The scattered areas of brighter signal within the tumor probably represent hemorrhage. Owing to their high mucopolysaccharide content, myxomas have a relatively bright signal on T1-weighted images.

cycle demonstrate displacement of the mass and its relationship to the mitral valve and pulmonary veins. The excursion of the mass during the cardiac cycle is clearly seen on cine MRI.

CT On contrast-enhanced scans, the lesion appears as a low-density mass within the left atrial chamber (see Fig. 26.12). Conventional CT is not as accurate as echocardiography or MRI in the diagnosis of left atrial myxoma. Although cine CT has comparable sensitivity and specificity, its dependence on ionizing radiation and intravenous contrast material has relegated this modality to a secondary role in the diagnosis of left atrial myxoma.

Angiography Angiocardiography is occasionally employed in the diagnosis of left atrial myxoma. We prefer 35 mm cine at 60 frames per second for this purpose. Contrast material is injected into the pulmonary trunk and the opacified left atrium is evaluated on the levophase. The frontal and lateral projections have classically been employed for the diagnosis of left atrial myxoma; however, we prefer to use the right and left anterior oblique projections, which project the left atrium away from other cardiac structures. The tumor appears as a filling defect within the left atrial chamber (usually attached to the septum) which moves during the cardiac cycle (Figs. 26.7 and 26.8). When the bulky portion of the tumor is on a long pedicle it may protrude through the mitral orifice during diastole (Fig. 26.7). (Simultaneous pressure measurements will demonstrate a diastolic gradient in such cases.) A tumor that arises from the posterior or superior wall of the left atrium may transiently occlude the orifices of the pulmonary veins, resulting in stasis of contrast material in these vessels.

Coronary arteriography is usually performed in patients over 40 years of age to exclude coronary artery disease before surgical excision of the tumor. Occasionally, selective coronary

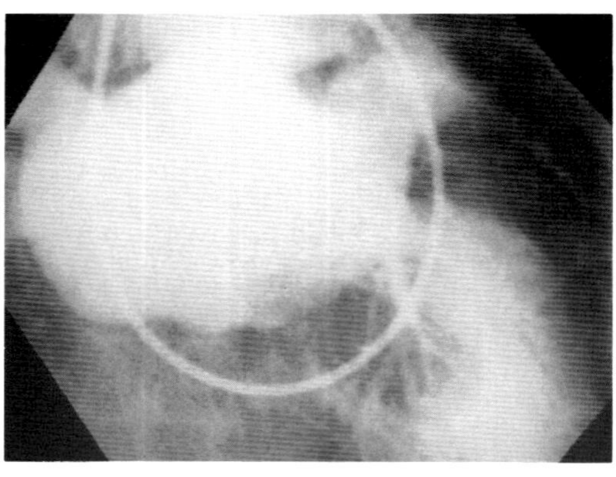

Fig. 26.7 Left atrial myxoma. Levophase of cine pulmonary arteriogram (elongated right anterior oblique projection; in diastole) demonstrates marked left atrial enlargement. The filling defect in the left ventricle represents a left atrial myxoma, which is connected by a narrow pedicle to the atrial septum. During diastole, most of the tumor protrudes through the mitral valve into the left ventricle.

1	left atrium	4	left atrial myxoma
2	left ventricle	5	attachment of pedicle of tumor to atrial septum
3	mitral valve		

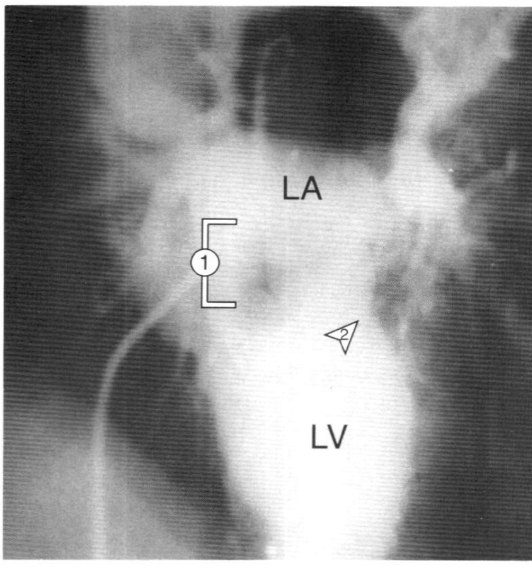

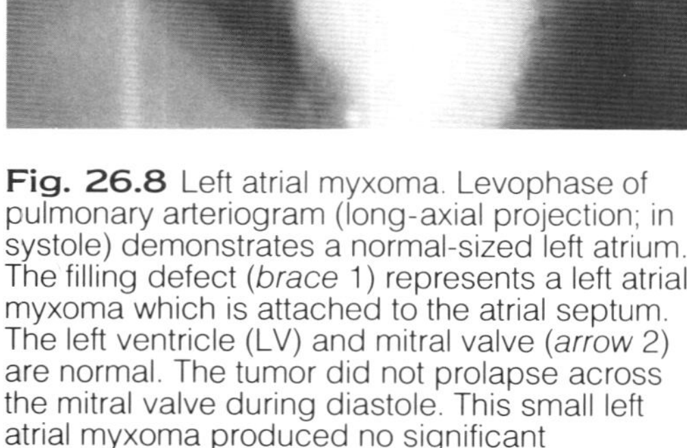

Fig. 26.8 Left atrial myxoma. Levophase of pulmonary arteriogram (long-axial projection; in systole) demonstrates a normal-sized left atrium. The filling defect (*brace* 1) represents a left atrial myxoma which is attached to the atrial septum. The left ventricle (LV) and mitral valve (*arrow* 2) are normal. The tumor did not prolapse across the mitral valve during diastole. This small left atrial myxoma produced no significant hemodynamic effect.

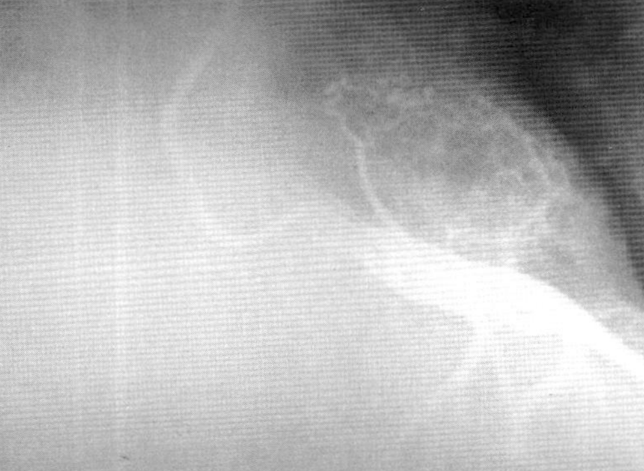

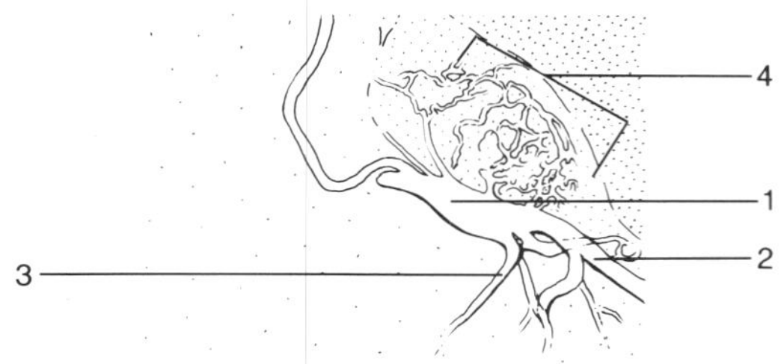

Fig. 26.9 Organized thrombus mimicking left atrial myxoma. Coronary arteriogram (left anterior oblique projection) of a 56-year-old man with rheumatic mitral valvular disease demonstrates two large branches of the circumflex artery supplying a highly vascular mass in the position of the left atrial appendage. Although the angiographic appearance is consistent with a myxoma, this is a very unusual location for this tumor; therefore, organized thrombus should be favored in this patient.

1	left main coronary artery	3	circumflex artery
2	left anterior descending coronary artery	4	organized thrombus in the left atrial appendage

arteriography may demonstrate a "tumor stain" caused by prolonged retention of contrast material in dilated capillaries within the tumor. Staining of the lesion is not pathognomonic for left atrial myxoma, however, as it may also be seen in an organized thrombus (Fig. 26.9).

RIGHT ATRIAL MYXOMA

Hemodynamic Features

Large right atrial myxomas interfere with blood flow through this chamber, producing obstruction of the caval veins or tricuspid valve. Right atrial myxomas can also give rise to pulmonary emboli.

Clinical Features

Clinically, right atrial myxoma can mimic a number of other disorders. Although most patients present with signs and symptoms of pulmonary embolism, the clinical picture may suggest tricuspid valvular disease, pulmonic stenosis, or pericarditis. An occasional patient may present with a fever of obscure origin. ECG frequently reveals rhythm disturbances (especially right bundle branch block, atrial flutter, and atrial fibrillation) and peaked P-waves. Ascites, hepatomegaly, and peripheral edema are common in patients with longstanding lesions.

Imaging and Invasive Diagnosis

Plain Films Plain films show right atrial and right ventricular enlargement, with prominence of the superior vena cava. Although these findings are also compatible with Ebstein's malformation or acquired tricuspid insufficiency, the presence of calcification or fat in the region of the right atrium—best appreciated on fluoroscopy—strongly favors the diagnosis of right atrial myxoma (Fig. 26.10).

Echocardiography Echocardiography is less sensitive and specific for right atrial myxomas than it is for left atrial myxoma. Nevertheless, most right atrial myxomas can be detected and characterized by the transthoracic approach (masses adjacent to the right border of the right atrium may not be well seen); the transesophageal approach is particularly useful for lesions close to the atrial septum. Prolapse of the tumor into the right ventricle during diastole, with partial obstruction of the tricuspid valve, is readily detected by two-dimensional echocardiography (Fig. 26.11). Owing to the relative rarity of right atrial myxoma, thrombus or metastasis is the most likely diagnosis in any adult patient in whom echocardiography reveals an uncalcified right atrial mass.

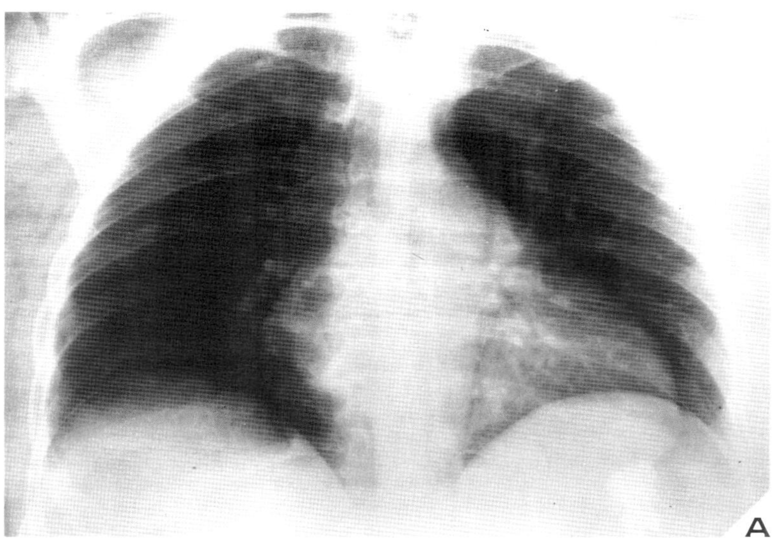

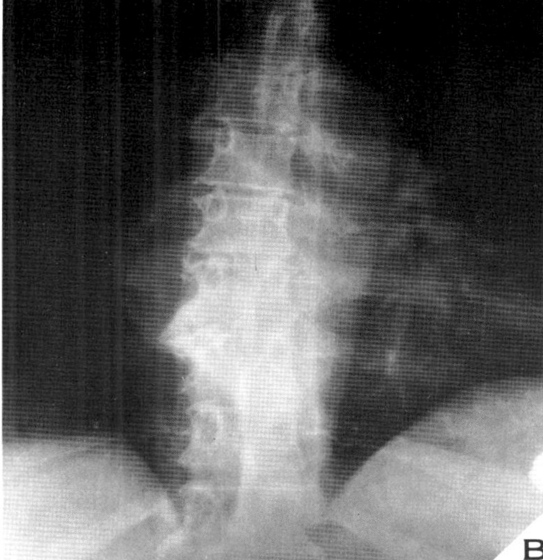

Fig. 26.10 Calcified right atrial myxoma. (A) Posteroanterior chest film demonstrates a markedly enlarged heart with deformity of the right heart border. The superior vena cava and azygos vein are dilated. Note the calcified oval density in the area of the right atrium, which is seen more closely on the overpenetrated Bucky film (B)

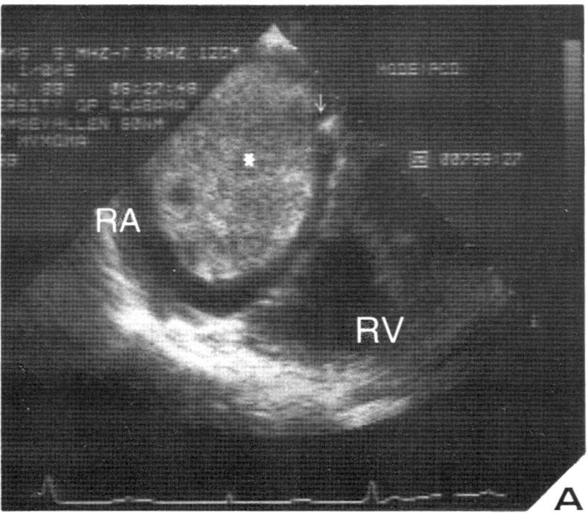

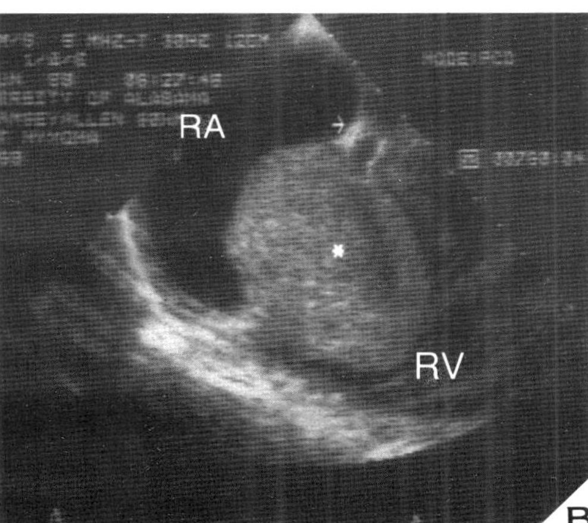

Fig. 26.11 Right atrial myxoma. Four-chamber views of echocardiogram in (A) systole and (B) diastole demonstrate a right atrial-myxoma (*), which appears as an echogenic mass attached to the atrial septum by a narrow pedicle (arrow). In systole the tricuspid leaflets are normally apposed. In diastole the mass protrudes into the right ventricular chamber (RV), resulting in marked narrowing of the tricuspid orifice. (RA = right atrium)

CT and MRI As with left atrial myxoma, the morphology and relationships of right atrial myxoma can be demonstrated by CT (Fig. 26.12). Although the dynamic relationships are clearly seen on cine CT, echocardiography is the preferred imaging modality for this tumor.

MRI provides information similar to that obtained from echocardiography. The tumor appears as a signal void on ECG-gated spin–echo MR images. Motion of the lesion during the cardiac cycle, and its relationship to the tricuspid valve and the orifices of the caval veins, are clearly depicted on cine MRI.

Angiocardiography On right atriography the tumor appears as a large filling defect attached to the septum or the right atrial wall. Frontal, lateral, and oblique projections should be obtained to completely evaluate the relationships of the lesion. The tumor typically protrudes into the tricuspid valve orifice during diastole (Fig. 26.13). The differential diagnosis of right atrial myxoma includes right atrial thrombus, intraluminal metastasis, and transcaval extension of an abdominal malignancy. A widely implanted, heavily calcified mass most likely represents thrombus. An irregularly shaped mass protruding from the orifice of the inferior vena cava is more likely to be an intraluminal metastasis or a transcaval extension of an abdominal neoplasm (eg, hepatoma, renal cell carcinoma). Pulmonary arteriography is commonly performed to rule out pulmonary embolism in patients found to have a mass in the right atrium (Fig. 26.14).

VENTRICULAR MYXOMA

The signs and symptoms of ventricular myxoma are similar to those associated with myxoma of the corresponding atrium. Left ventricular myxomas are commonly associated with peripheral emboli, and right ventricular myxomas with pulmonary emboli.

RHABDOMYOMA

Rhabdomyoma is the most common cardiac tumor in infants and children. Although cardiac rhabdomyoma may present in adulthood, the great majority of these tumors are found in children under 3 years of age.

PATHOLOGY

Cardiac rhabdomyomas, which are usually multiple, arise from the myocardium, most commonly from the ventricular septum or adjacent ventricular wall. Morphologically, the lesions are well-circumscribed, nonencapsulated, grayish-white nodules located within the myocardium; larger tumors tend to project into the ventricular lumen (Figs. 26.15 and 26.16). Microscopically, the tumor consists of round vacuolated cells with delicate protoplasmic strands which extend outward from the centrally located nucleus, an arrangement that produces a distinctive "spider-cell" appearance.

Some authors have questioned the neoplastic nature of cardiac rhabdomyoma, preferring to classify it as a form of congenital

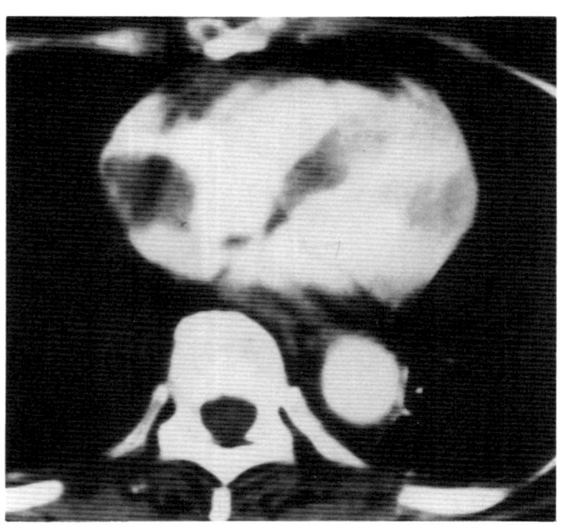

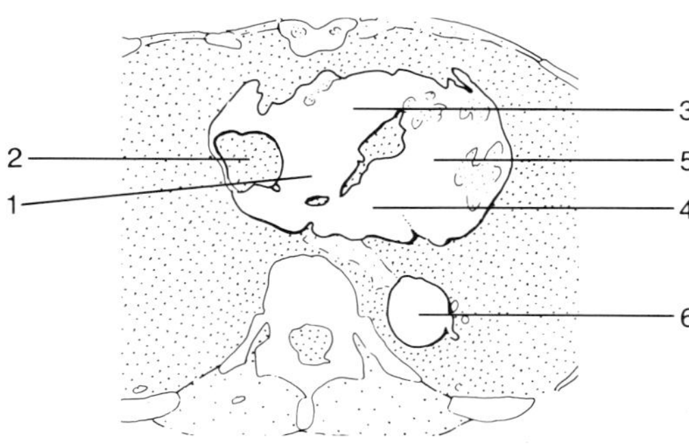

Fig. 26.12 Right atrial myxoma. Contrast-enhanced CT at the level of the right atrium demonstrates a filling defect which is unrelated to the atrial septum. The lesion, which represents a right atrial myxoma, was subsequently resected.

1 right atrium
2 right atrial myxoma
3 right ventricle
4 left atrium
5 left ventricle
6 descending thoracic aorta

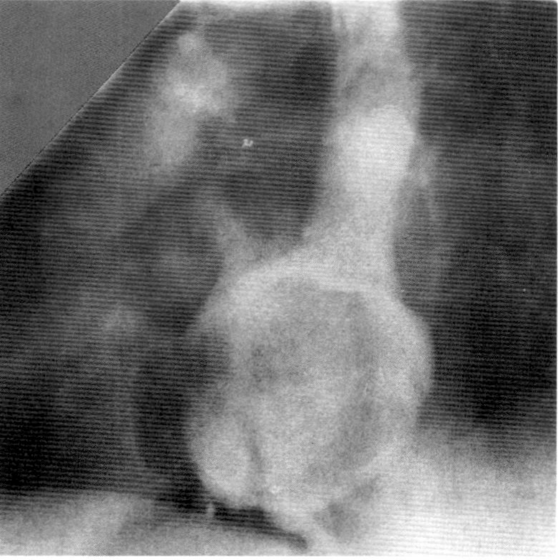

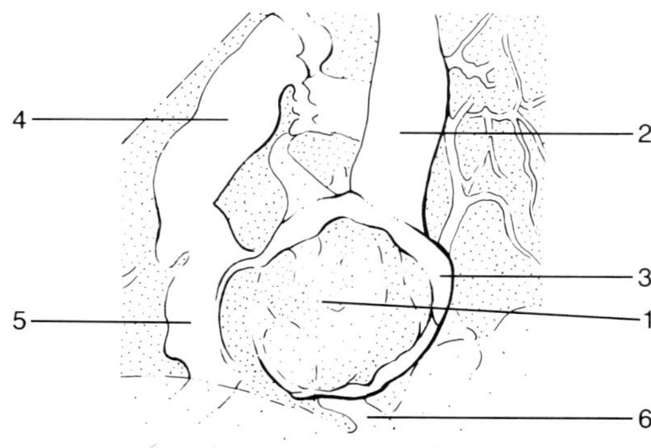

Fig. 26.13 Right atrial myxoma. Right anterior oblique projection of inferior venacavogram (in diastole) demonstrates filling defect which represents a myxoma. The tumor almost completely fills the right atrial cavity. The inferior aspect of the tumor protrudes through the tricuspid valve into the right ventricle; the site of attachment cannot be identified in this projection. The superior vena cava is completely opacified in retrograde fashion, indicating obstruction at the level of the tricuspid valve. The right ventricle and pulmonary trunk are poorly opacified.

1 right atrial myxoma
2 superior vena cava
3 right atrium
4 right ventricle
5 pulmonary trunk
6 inferior vena cava

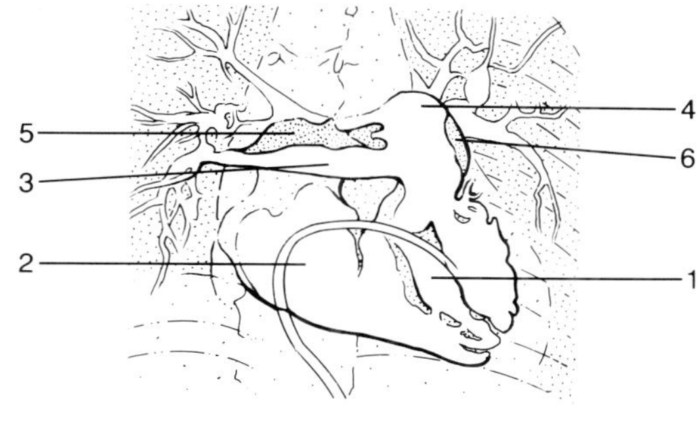

Fig. 26.14 Bilateral pulmonary emboli secondary to a right atrial myxoma. (A) Frontal and (B) lateral projections of right ventriculogram show filling defects in the proximal and distal portions of the right pulmonary artery and in the branches to the right upper lobe. In addition, there is a filling defect in the proximal segment of the left pulmonary artery. The source of the pulmonary emboli was a right atrial myxoma.

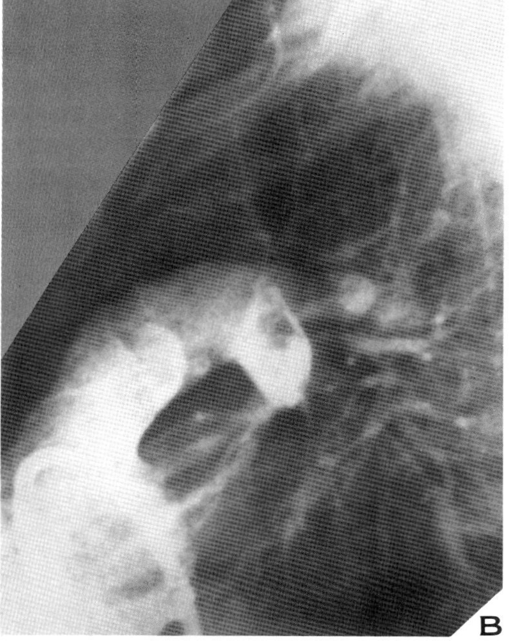

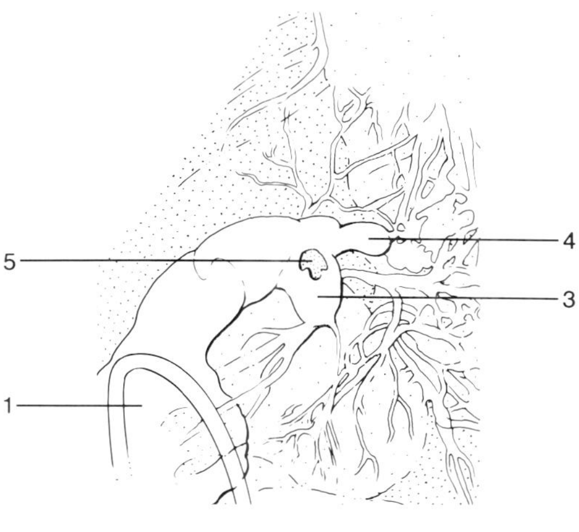

1 right ventricle
2 right atrium
3 right pulmonary artery
4 left pulmonary artery
5 embolus in right pulmonary artery
6 embolus in left pulmonary artery

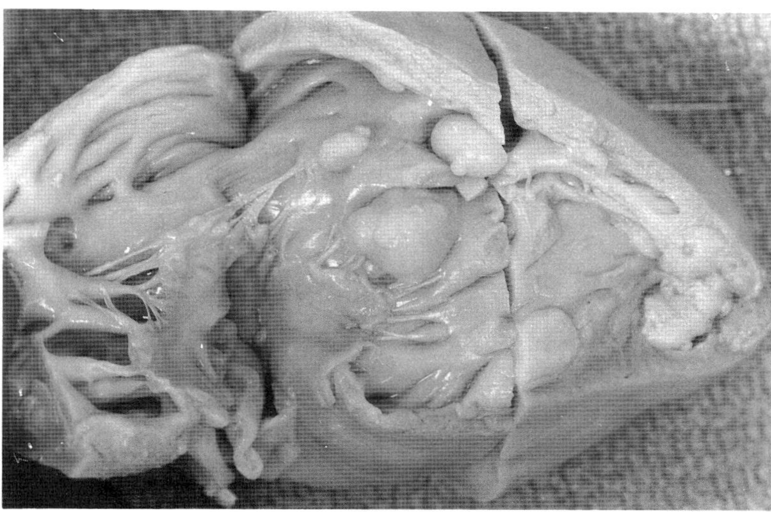

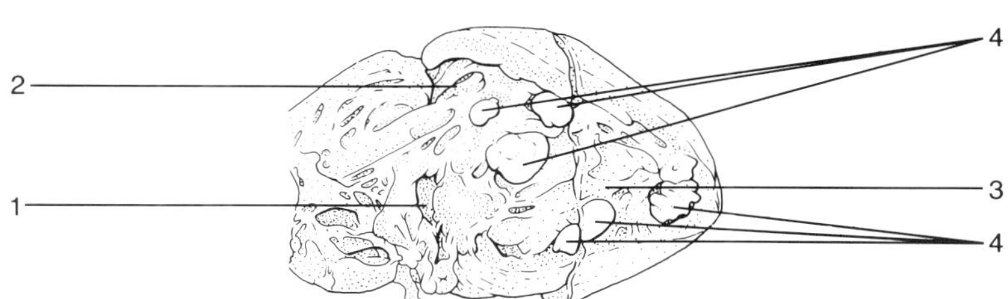

Fig. 26.15 Cardiac rhabdomyomas. Autopsy specimen of the heart (viewed through the opened right ventricle) demonstrates several tumor masses of different sizes projecting from the ventricular septum into the right ventricular cavity. The largest lesion overlies the inlet portion of the ventricular septum.

1 right atrium
2 right ventricular outflow tract
3 right ventricle
4 rhabdomyomas

hamartoma that may go into spontaneous regression. Tuberous sclerosis (epiloia, Bourneville's disease) is present in about 50 percent of patients with cardiac rhabdomyoma. Clinical manifestations of tuberous sclerosis include mental retardation, seizures, adenoma sebaceum, and (in the neonate) white spots on the skin.

CLINICAL FEATURES

The clinical presentation of cardiac rhabdomyoma depends on the size, number, and location of the tumors. Whereas small lesions are asymptomatic, large ones that project into the ventricular cavity may impair ventricular filling and/or emptying, or interfere with valve function. A patient with a large right ventricular rhabdomyoma causing tricuspid insufficiency and increased right atrial pressure may present with cyanosis secondary to right to left shunting across the foramen ovale. A strategically situated tumor may obstruct the right or left ventricular outflow tract, or it may occlude the mitral valve, producing functional mitral stenosis. Some patients present with arrhythmias secondary to involvement of the conduction pathways.

Cardiac rhabdomyomas are common in patients with tuberous sclerosis. The possibility of such a lesion should be strongly considered in a neonate with congestive heart failure who has white spots on the skin or a positive family history. The prognosis is poor for patients with intracavitary rhabdomyomas associated with tuberous sclerosis who are symptomatic during infancy.

IMAGING AND INVASIVE DIAGNOSIS

Plain films

The plain film findings are nonspecific and reflect the accompanying hemodynamic disturbance (eg, left ventricular hypertrophy secondary to left ventricular outflow tract obstruction, right atrial enlargement secondary to tricuspid insufficiency) (Fig. 26.17). In some instances the tumor may deform the cardiac contours. Calcification of the tumor is rare.

Echocardiography

Intramural tumors and their intracavitary extension are clearly depicted by two-dimensional echocardiography. The intramural component of the tumor appears as an echo-dense focus in the ventricular septum or in the ventricular or atrial wall (Fig. 26.18). The intracavitary component can be seen to move cyclically with the cardiac pulsations. Depending on their location, cardiac rhabdomyomas may interfere with the normal functioning of the mitral or tricuspid valve, producing turbulent flow on Doppler images.

CT and MRI

Both CT and spin–echo MRI accurately depict myocardial tumors and their intracavitary extension. On contrast-enhanced CT scans, the intramural component of the tumor appears as an area of decreased attenuation within the myocardium and the intracavitary portion appears as an intraluminal filling defect. The borders of the lesion, as well as its relationship to the cardiac valves, are clearly shown.

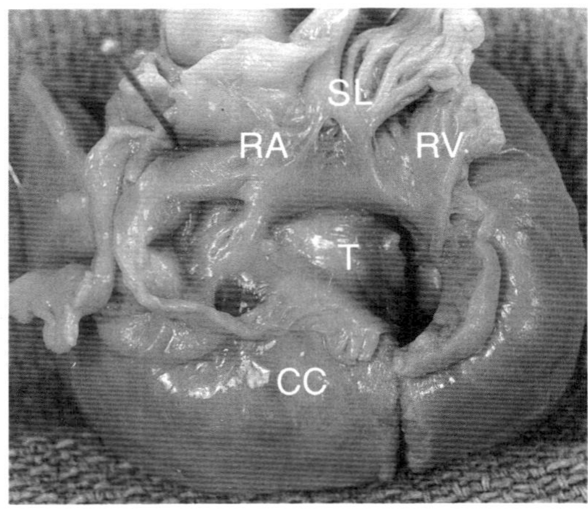

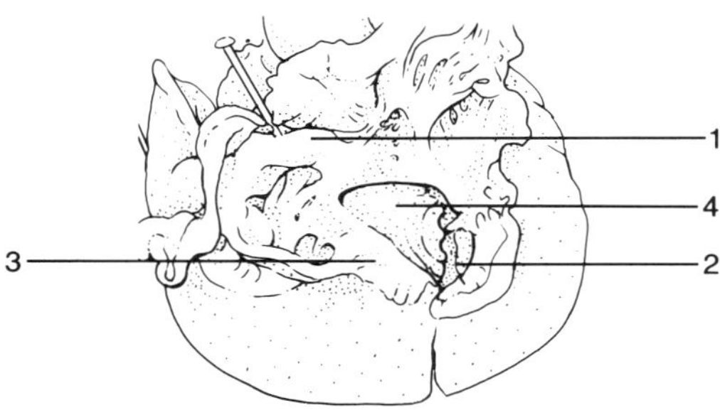

Fig. 26.16 Rhabdomyoma of the ventricular septum. In this autopsy specimen the right atrium (RA) has been opened to expose the tricuspid valve. A large rhabdomyoma (T) of the ventricular septum is seen protruding through the tricuspid valve and restricting its orifice. The septal leaflet (SL) of the tricuspid valve is displaced anteriorly. The tumor also protruded into the left ventricle, distorting the mitral valve (not seen in this view). [CC = crux cordis (junction between atrioventricular groove and interatrial septum)]

1 right atrium
2 tricuspid valve and right ventricle
3 crux cordis
4 rhabdomyoma in ventricular septum

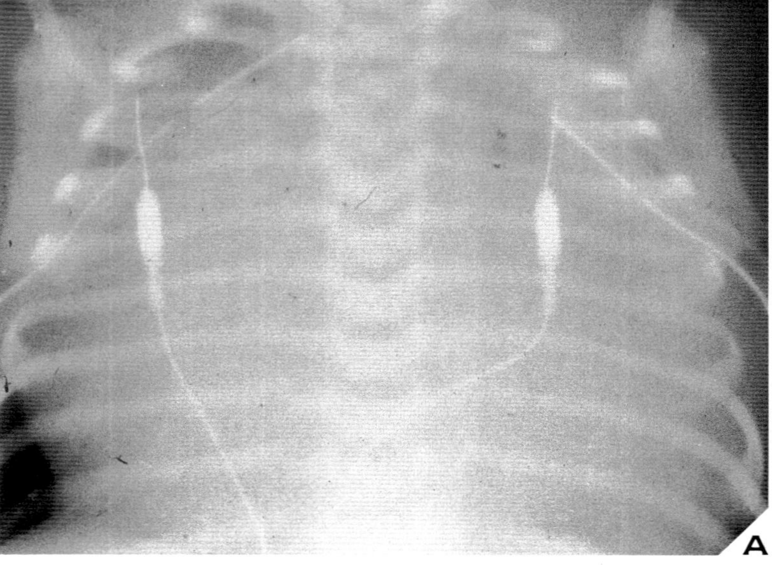

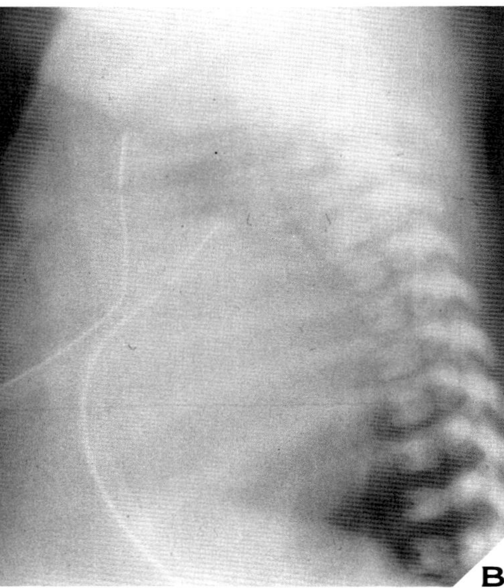

Fig. 26.17 Cardiac rhabdomyoma. (A) Frontal and (B) lateral chest films of a neonate in congestive heart failure demonstrate massive cardiomegaly. The huge heart nearly fills both hemithoraces. At autopsy, the tumor extensively involved both ventricles, accounting for the massive cardiac enlargement seen on the chest films.

Although the signal characteristics of cardiac rhabdomyomas are quite variable, the intramural component of the tumor is usually isointense with the surrounding normal myocardium on spin–echo MR images. Bulky lesions can be identified as a localized deformity of the septum or ventricular wall. The intracavitary component of the tumor appears as a discrete area of signal surrounded by the signal void produced by flowing blood. Gated spin–echo images or cine MRI depict the position of the tumor at various moments in the cardiac cycle. Cine MRI also demonstrates valvular insufficiency or stenosis caused by the tumor. The multiplanar display provided by MRI is very helpful in planning surgical resection.

Cardiac Catheterization and Angiocardiography

Cardiac catheterization is routinely performed to quantitate the hemodynamic changes produced by the tumor. Angiocardiography demonstrates the size of the mass (or masses) and its relationship to the cardiac valves (Figs. 26.19 and 26.20), and may detect associated malformations which cannot be detected

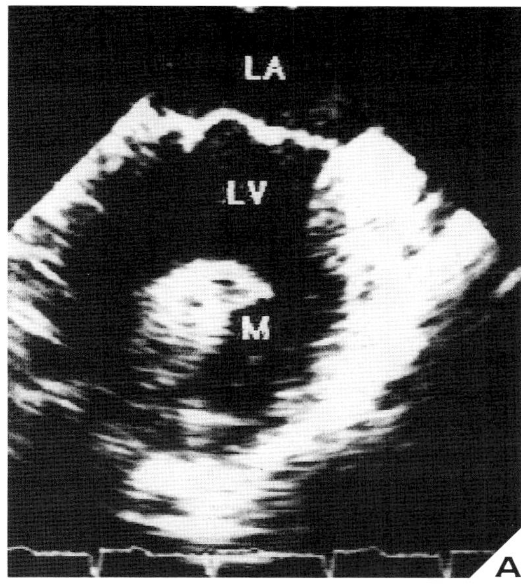

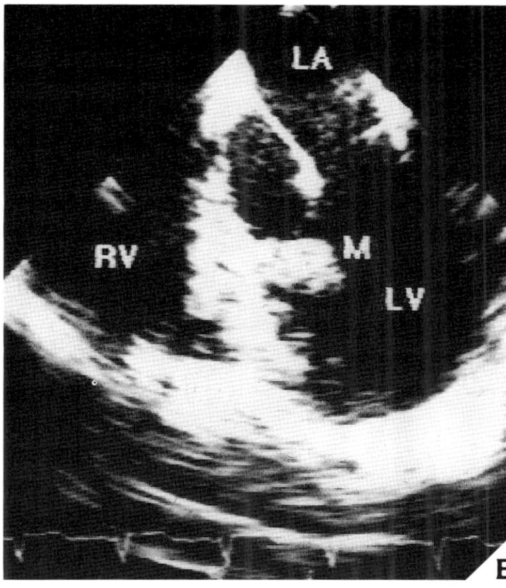

Fig. 26.18 Cardiac rhabdomyoma. (A) Two-chamber and (B) four-chamber projections of echocardiogram show an echogenic mass (M) arising from the septum and protruding into the left ventricular cavity (LV). The mass does not affect the mitral valve. The aortic valve was also spared. (LA = left atrium; RV = right ventricle).

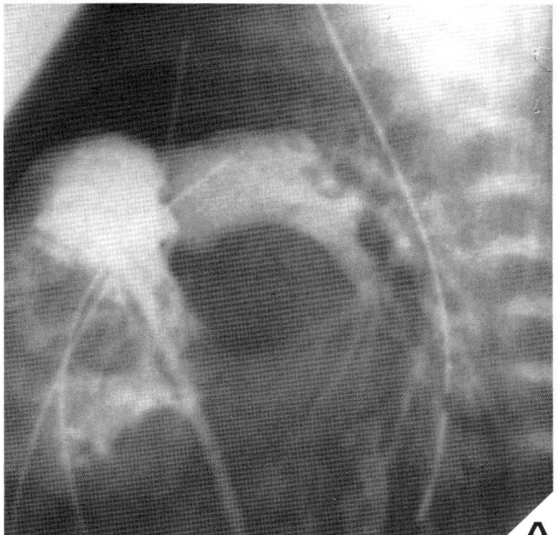

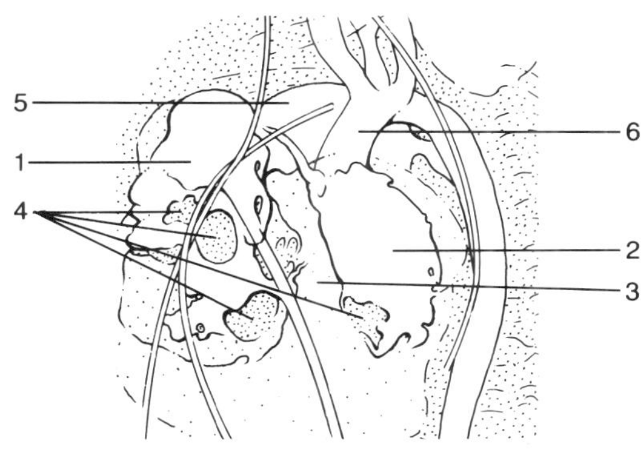

Fig. 26.19 Multiple cardiac rhabdomyomas. Lateral projections of (A) right and (B) left ventriculograms. The right ventricle is enlarged; its contours are distorted by several filling defects, which represent rhabdomyomas extending into the lumen. Although the left ventricle is of normal size, it is displaced posteriorly and superiorly (the filling defect at the apex represents a rhabdomyoma). Note the wide separation between the ventricles, indicating significant septal involvement by the tumor.

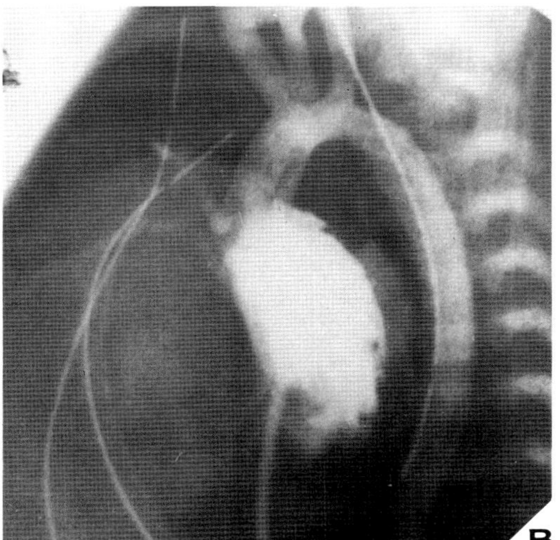

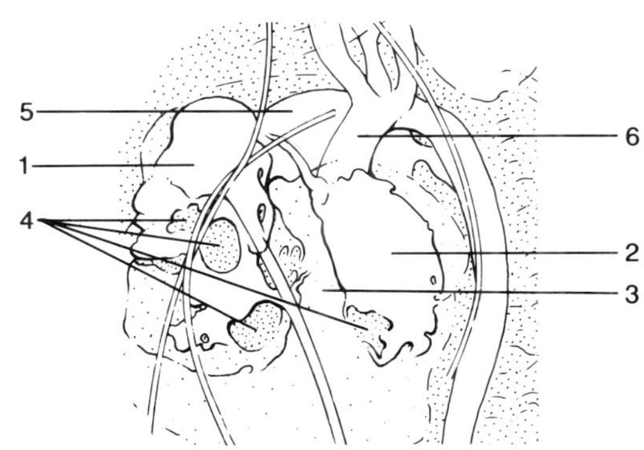

1	right ventricle	4	rhabdomyomas
2	left ventricle	5	pulmonary trunk
3	widened ventricular septum	6	aorta

by other modalities. Coronary arteriography is routinely performed in patients over 40 years of age to rule out obstructive coronary artery disease.

FIBROMA

Fibroma is the second most common cardiac neoplasm in infants and children. This benign cardiac tumor presents in children under 1 year of age, the great majority being discovered by 10 years of age.

PATHOLOGY

Cardiac fibromas are usually solitary, arising in the left ventricular wall or the ventricular septum; less often the tumor arises in the right ventricle or right atrium. Some cardiac fibromas grow primarily outside the heart, producing an extrinsic mass. On gross examination the typical lesion is a rounded, firm white intramural mass which is well circumscribed (but not encapsulated). Microscopically, the tumor consists of mature fibroblasts intermingled with cardiac muscle fibers and strands of collagen. Calcification is not uncommon, especially in older patients.

HEMODYNAMIC AND CLINICAL FEATURES

The hemodynamic and clinical manifestations depend on the extent of mural involvement and the size of the intracavitary component. Patients with marked intracavitary extension typically present with congestive heart failure.

IMAGING AND INVASIVE DIAGNOSIS

Plain Films

As with cardiac rhabdomyoma, the radiographic findings are usually nonspecific. The left ventricular contour may be deformed when the tumor involves the free wall of the left ventricle (Fig. 26.21).

Echocardiography, CT, MRI

The findings are similar to those described for rhabdomyoma.

Angiocardiography

As in the case of cardiac rhabdomyoma, angiocardiography remains useful, although not essential, for diagnostic evaluation of cardiac fibroma. Angiocardiography enables one to study the

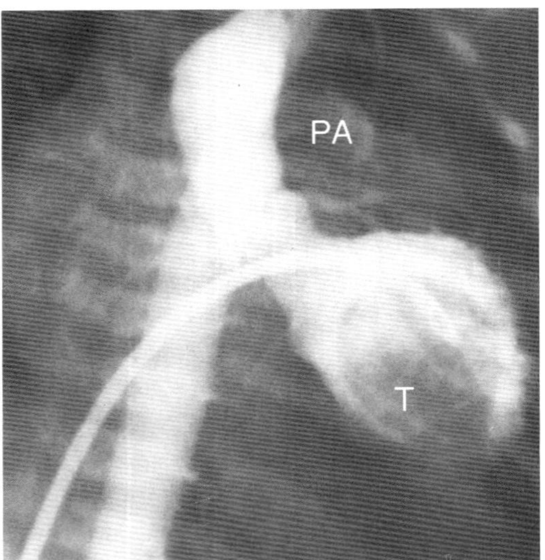

Fig. 26.20 Cardiac rhabdomyoma. Long axial view of left ventriculogram demonstrates a large filling defect (T), which represents a rhabdomyoma. The tumor occupies almost 40 percent of the left ventricular cavity. The outflow tract and aorta are normal. Note opacification of the left pulmonary artery (PA) via a patent ductus arteriosus, an incidental finding in this patient.

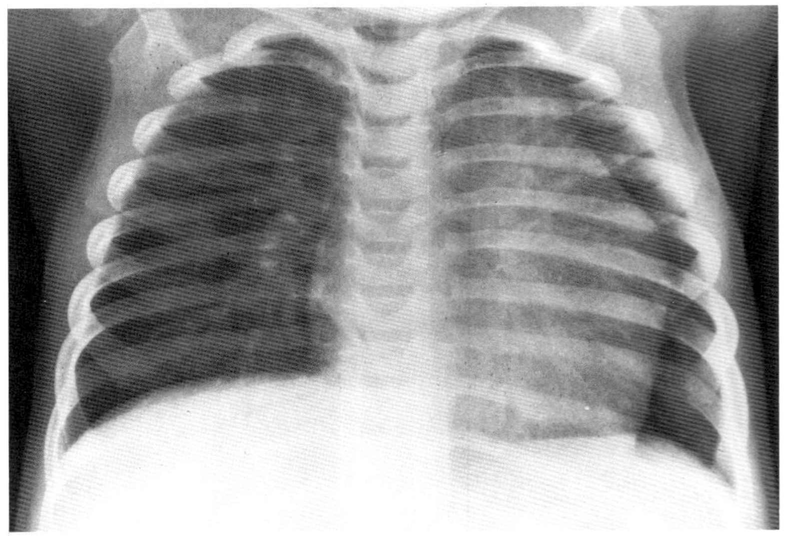

Fig. 26.21 Cardiac fibroma. Chest film of an asymptomatic 4-year-old boy shows marked deformity of the left upper heart border. The upper part of the cardiovascular silhouette is formed by the displaced pulmonary trunk. Echocardiography (not illustrated) and angiocardiography (see Fig. 27.22) confirmed the presence of a large mass in the free wall of the left ventricle, which was found at operation to be a benign fibroma.

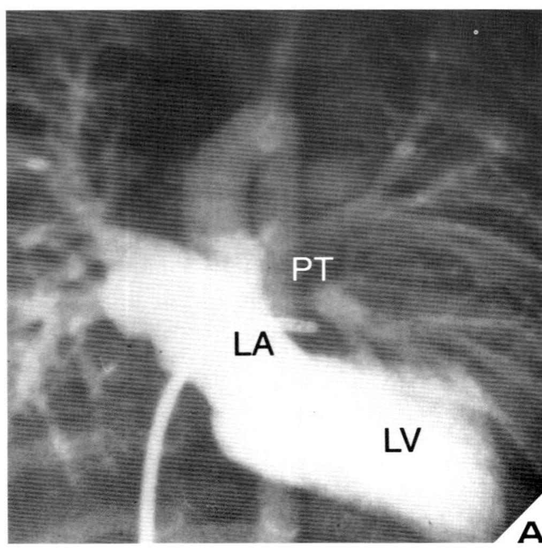

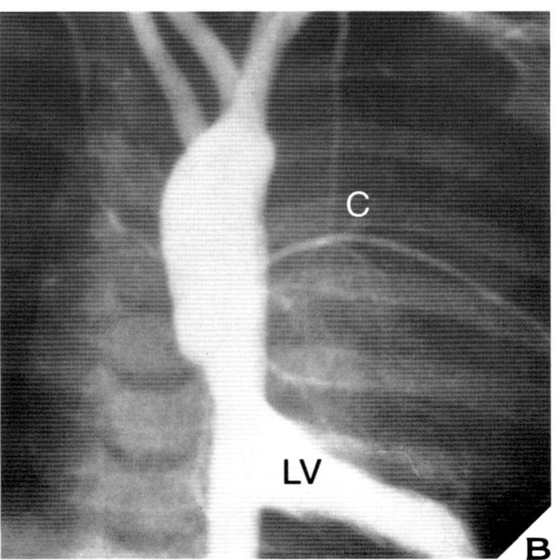

Fig. 26.22 Cardiac fibroma. Same patient as shown in Fig. 26.21. (A) Levophase of pulmonary arteriogram (frontal projection) shows a normal-sized left ventricle (LV). The left superior contour of the ventricle is deformed. The left atrium (LA) is compressed and displaced to the right, and the pulmonary trunk (PT) and left pulmonary artery are elevated. (B) Selective left ventriculogram (frontal projection) shows a wide separation between the left ventricular cavity and the left anterior descending coronary artery (C), which represents the space occupied by this benign fibroma. Despite the enormous size of the tumor, left ventricular and left atrial function were normal.

morphology of the mass, as well as its relationship to the cardiac valves and cardiac chambers. Depending on the hemodynamic effects of the lesion, the affected chambers may be either of normal size or enlarged. Tumors that involve the septum may displace the affected chamber or separate the chambers from each other (Fig. 26.22; see also Fig. 26.19). An intracavitary tumor appears angiographically as a filling defect with a broad or narrow zone of attachment (see Fig. 26.20). Left ventricular lesions can be demonstrated on the levophase of a pulmonary arteriogram or by selective left ventriculography (Fig. 26.22). Intracavitary masses are best evaluated on the long axial and elongated right anterior oblique projections.

MALIGNANT PRIMARY TUMORS

Primary malignant neoplasms of the heart and pericardium are rare. The most common primary cardiac malignancies are angiosarcoma of the right atrium and rhabdomyosarcoma, which can arise from any chamber. Mesothelioma is the most common primary malignant tumor of the pericardium.

CLINICAL FEATURES

The clinical manifestations of malignant cardiac and pericardial neoplasms vary according to the degree of myocardial involvement and whether the tumor extends into the cavities or pericardial space. Significant compromise of the left ventricle results in congestive heart failure; this can also occur when the tumor obstructs the mitral valve or fills the left atrial cavity. Signs of right-sided congestive heart failure (peripheral edema, dilatation of systemic veins) appear when the right ventricle and/or right atrium are extensively involved.

Patients with malignant pericardial tumors typically present with dyspnea, cough, and signs and symptoms of pericardial effusion. In some patients the clinical findings suggest acute pericarditis; in such cases the ECG usually reveals nonspecific ST-segment and T-wave changes. In others, the clinical picture resembles that of constrictive pericarditis with right-sided congestive heart failure. An occasional patient may present with nonspecific constitutional symptoms (eg, fever, malaise, weight loss).

Because malignant cardiac and pericardial neoplasms are quite rare, the diagnosis is usually made by exclusion and is confirmed by microscopic examination of the aspirated fluid. The prognosis for these tumors is very poor, most patients dying within 6 months irrespective of the specific histologic diagnosis.

IMAGING AND INVASIVE DIAGNOSIS

Plain films

Chest films often demonstrate massive enlargement of the heart; occasionally there is a localized deformity of the cardiovascular silhouette. A deformity differing from that produced by enlargement of the cardiac chambers suggests the possibility of a cardiac or pericardial neoplasm (Figs. 26.23 and 26.24). Patients with extensive left ventricular involvement exhibit the

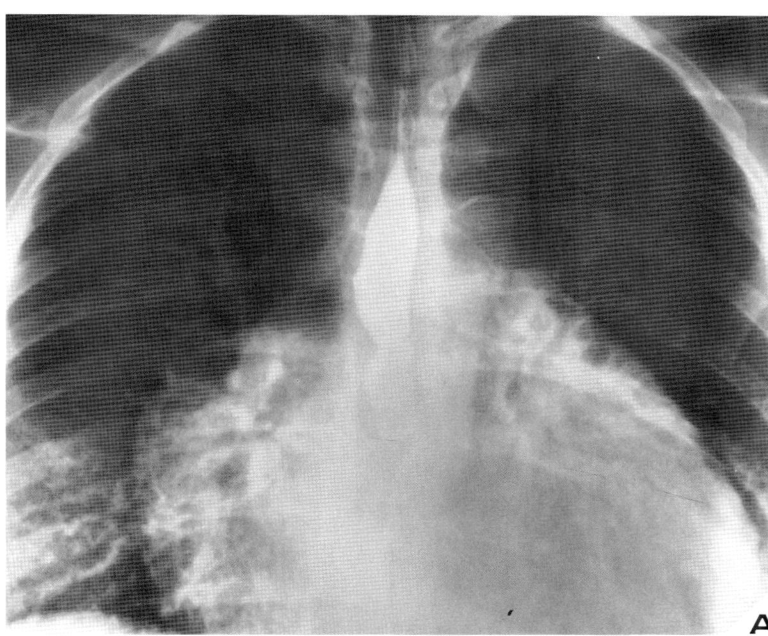

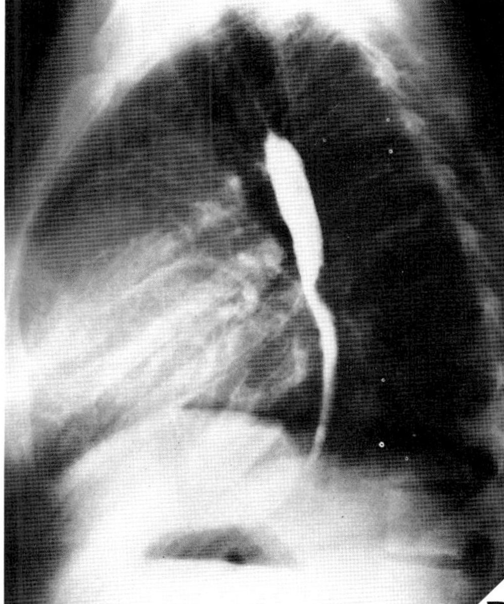

Fig. 26.23 Mesothelioma of the pericardium. (A) Frontal and (B) lateral chest films show a markedly enlarged cardiac silhouette, with deformity of both the right and left borders. The heart also bulges posteriorly (note deformity of esophagus just above the diaphragm). In addition, there is evidence of pulmonary venous hypertension (note cephalization pattern). A malignant mesothelioma was found at thoracotomy.

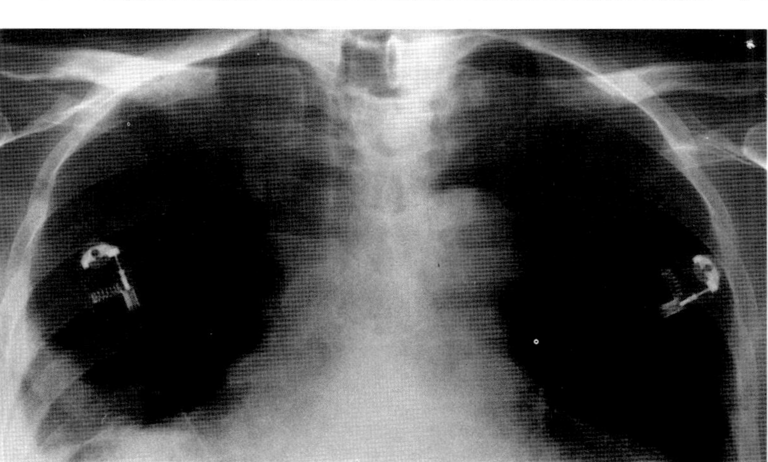

Fig. 26.24 Angiosarcoma of the right atrium. Frontal chest film shows massive cardiac enlargement and a right pleural effusion. The marked deformity of the right heart border and the normal appearance of the left heart border suggest the presence of a mass in the right atrium or a localized pericardial effusion in the right paracardiac recess. Surgical exploration revealed an angiosarcoma arising in the right atrium.

typical radiographic findings of congestive heart failure. The SVC and/or azygos vein may be dilated in patients with right-sided congestive failure secondary to right ventricular or right atrial involvement.

Echocardiography

As previously noted, echocardiography can detect and characterize both intracardiac and pericardial tumors. To completely delineate the lesion, it may be necessary to obtain multiple sections in the long axial and four-chamber projections and in various cross-sectional planes. Masses close to the lungs (eg, those in the right atrium or posterosuperior border of the left atrium) cannot be adequately evaluated by the transthoracic approach; however, such lesions are clearly seen on transesophageal images.

CT

Malignant neoplasms of the heart and pericardium are clearly depicted on contrast-enhanced CT scans. The intracavitary portion of the tumor appears as a filling defect within the cardiac chamber, while the intramural component typically appears as a bulky, low-attenuation mass that deforms the wall of the affected chamber. Primary pericardial neoplasms are associated with focal or extensive pericardial thickening, or appear as masses surrounded by pericardial fluid; this is also true of primary cardiac neoplasms that extend into the pericardial space (Figs. 26.25 and 26.26). Intracavitary masses often arise from a long pedicle. The position of the mass and its relationship to the cardiac valves can be demonstrated on ECG-gated images obtained in systole and diastole.

MRI

As noted earlier, MRI is highly accurate in detecting intracavitary, intramural, and pericardial masses. On T1-weighted spin–echo images, an intracavitary mass appears as a signal-containing area surrounded by a signal void (flowing blood). Intramural tumors deform the wall of the affected chamber. Primary cardiac tumors typically have a variable signal on T1-weighted spin–echo images and a bright signal on T2-weighted images (Fig. 26.27).

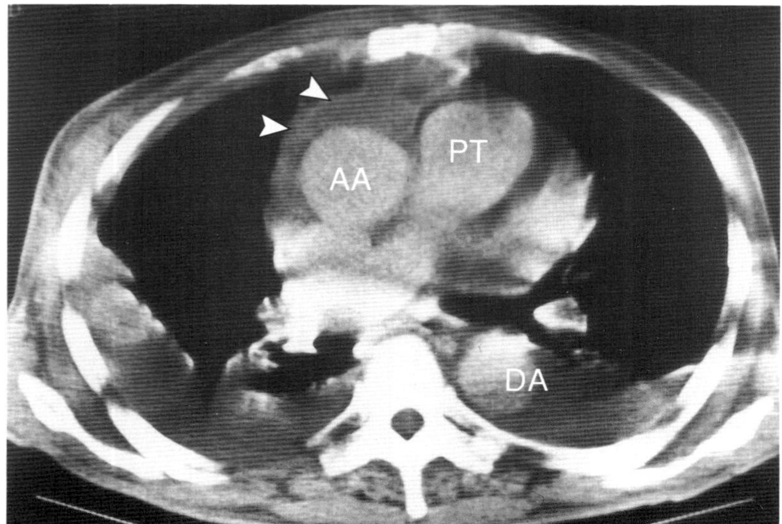

Fig. 26.25 Angiosarcoma of the right atrium. Contrast-enhanced CT at the level of the great arteries demonstrates a pericardial effusion. The soft tissue densities (*arrows*) within the pericardial space represent tumor. There are bilateral pleural effusions. (AA = ascending aorta; PT = pulmonary trunk; DA = descending thoracic aorta)

SECONDARY (METASTATIC) TUMORS

Metastatic tumors of the heart and pericardium ("cardiac metastases") are 20 to 40 times as common as primary tumors. Cardiac metastases have been observed in 1 to 5 percent of all autopsies and in 10 to 25 percent of patients dying of malignant disease. The most common primaries are carcinoma of the lung and breast, lymphoma, leukemia, and malignant melanoma; however, any malignant tumor can metastasize to the heart or pericardium. Up to 60 percent of malignant melanomas and 25 to 50 percent of bronchogenic carcinomas metastasize to the heart or pericardium. Most cardiac metastases in adults involve the pericardium. Cardiac metastases are uncommon in children, and usually represent extensions from the lung or mediastinal lymph nodes; in such cases the neoplastic involvement is usually limited to the pericardium.

Malignant tumors can also involve the heart by direct venous extension. For example, renal cell carcinoma and hepatoma can extend through the inferior vena cava into the right atrium. Squamous cell carcinoma of the lung and pleural mesothelioma can invade the left atrium via the pulmonary veins.

IMAGING

PLAIN FILMS

Plain films of patients with pericardial metastases often show deformities of the cardiac silhouette which do not resemble the configurations associated with chamber enlargement or pericardial fluid. This appearance should suggest the possibility of a cardiac metastasis in a patient with a malignant melanoma or a carcinoma of the breast or lung. Pericardial metastases are almost always associated with a pleural effusion.

ECHOCARDIOGRAPHY

Echocardiography is highly sensitive for detecting intracardiac and pericardial involvement and malignant pericardial effusions (Fig. 26.28); it is much less sensitive for detecting tumor extension beyond the heart. Intraluminal metastases that extend into the atria via the great veins appear as echo-dense intracavitary

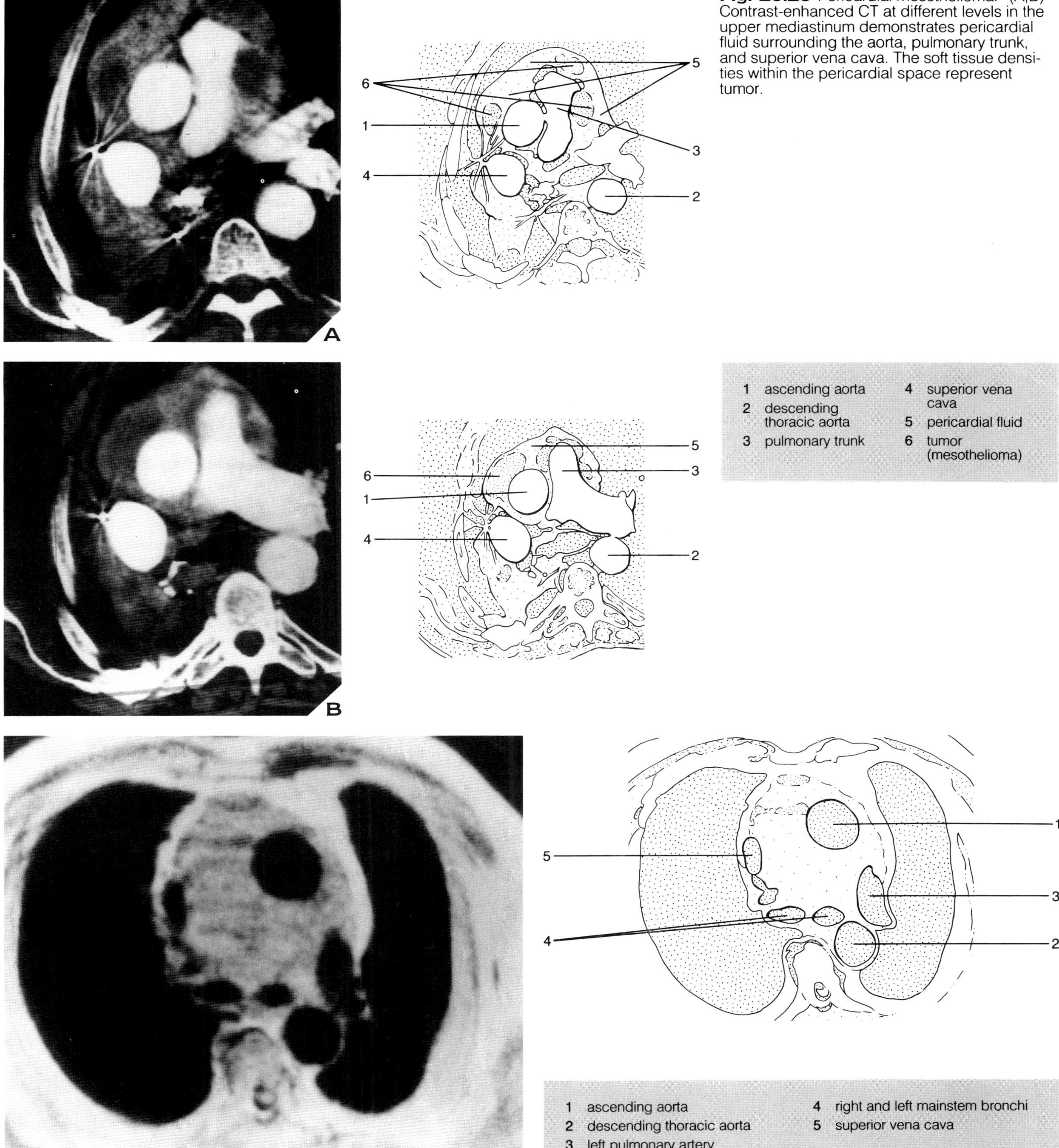

Fig. 26.26 Pericardial mesothelioma. (A,B) Contrast-enhanced CT at different levels in the upper mediastinum demonstrates pericardial fluid surrounding the aorta, pulmonary trunk, and superior vena cava. The soft tissue densities within the pericardial space represent tumor.

Fig. 26.27 Fibrosarcoma of the pericardium (MRI findings). Ungated transverse spin–echo image of the upper mediastinum demonstrates a mass within the superior recess of the pericardium. The tumor encases the mediastinal structures and displaces the bronchi posteriorly.

masses which exhibit motion during the cardiac cycle. Because echocardiography is highly accurate in detecting cardiac metastases, other diagnostic studies can usually be omitted.

CT

CT is a highly sensitive for delineation of metastatic deposits in the heart, pericardial space, and surrounding structures (Fig. 26.29). CT is particularly useful for demonstrating cardiac involvement by neoplasms originating in the lung and for extracardiac extension of cardiac metastases.

MRI

Intramural, intracavitary, and pericardial metastases are accurately depicted on spin–echo images (Fig. 26.30). Pericardial involvement by neoplasms arising in the pleura, mediastinum, or lung can usually be differentiated from pericardial metastases with this technique. On cine MRI, intracavitary metastases extending from the great veins appear as mobile masses within the affected atrial chamber, often interfering with the function of the atrioventricular valve.

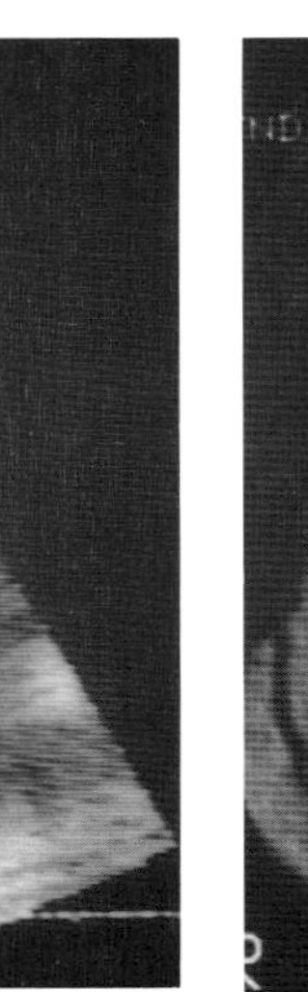

Fig. 26.28 Direct pericardial metastasis (echocardiographic findings). Long axial projection shows an echogenic mass in the pericardial space which represents direct extension from a bronchogenic carcinoma. The tumor has invaded the left atrium.

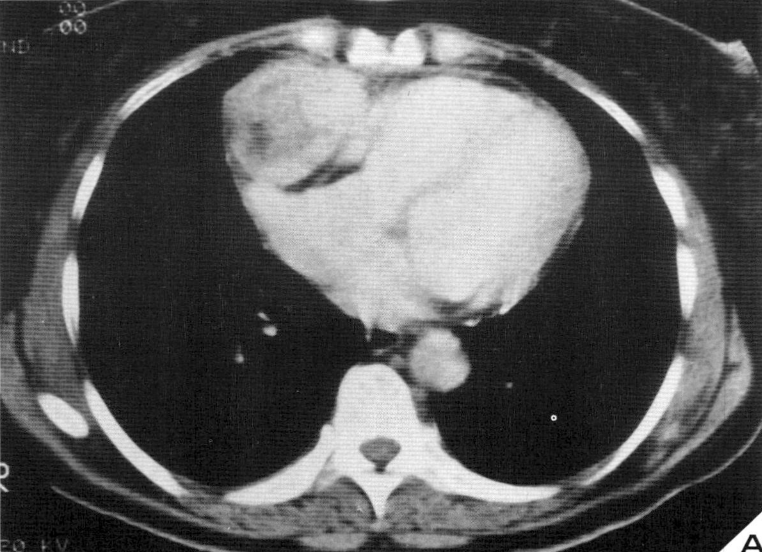

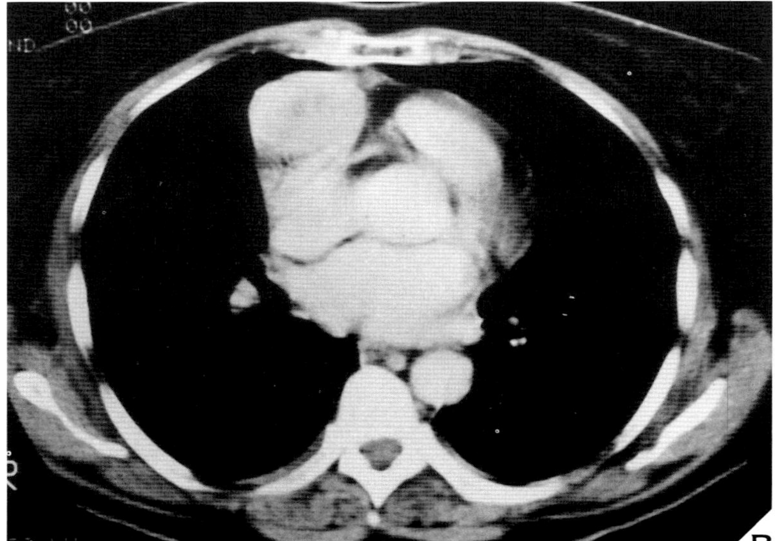

Fig. 26.29 Metastasis to the pericardium. Contrast-enhanced CT scans at the level of the ventricular mass (A) and the atria (B) demonstrate a mass in the right paracardial recess of the pericardium, compressing the right ventricle and right atrium. The right atrium is displaced posteriorly and to the left, deforming the left atrium. The patient presented with signs of restricted filling of the right cardiac chambers (see Chapter 23).

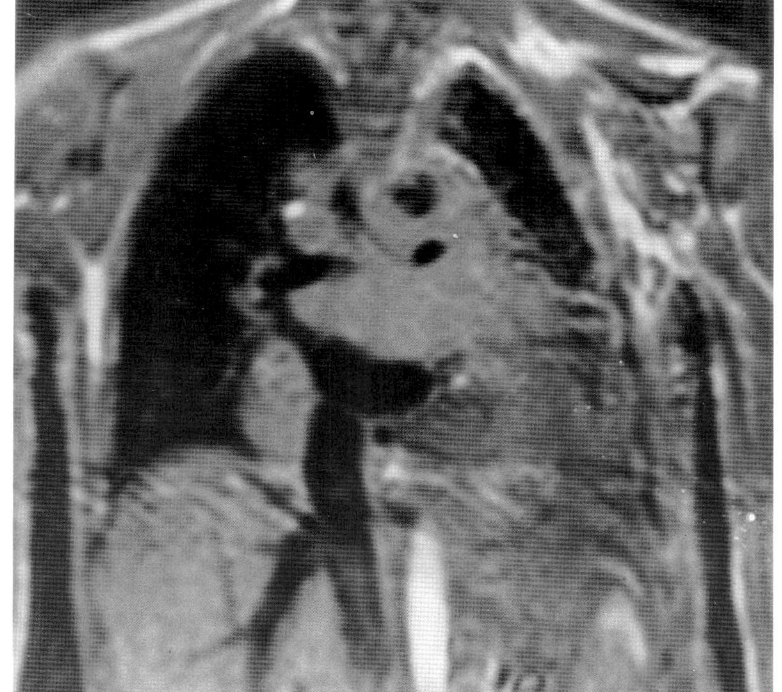

Fig. 26.30 Pericardial metastasis demonstrated by MRI. Coronal spin–echo MR image in a patient with widespread metastatic carcinoma demonstrates tumor filling the pericardial space and compressing the right atrium. The neoplastic tissue extends beyond the pericardial space (note encasement of aortic arch).

1 inferior vena cava
2 right atrium
3 right pulmonary artery
4 aortic arch
5 metastatic carcinoma within pericardial cavity
6 extrapericardial extension of metastatic carcinoma

CHAPTER 27

Diseases of the Thoracic Aorta

Among the abnormal conditions that affect the thoracic aorta, the most common are aneurysms, dissection, obstructive processes, and trauma. These conditions may also involve the arteries originating from the aorta; therefore, complete evaluation of aortic disease must include assessment of the circulatory status in the affected arterial territory.

The aorta is divided into four segments. The ascending aorta comprises the segment between the aortic valve and the origin of the first aortic branch. The aortic arch, or transverse segment, extends from the distal portion of the ascending aorta to the ductus arteriosus (which in the normal individual becomes the ligamentum arteriosus after birth). The descending thoracic aorta extends from the ductus arteriosus to the level of the diaphragm. The abdominal aorta extends from the level of the diaphragm to the point at which this artery bifurcates into the common iliac branches. The aortic arch courses in an anteroposterior direction in the upper mediastinum, extending from the right of the trachea to the posterior and superior portion of the mediastinum on the left. The segment of the aortic arch between the origin of the left subclavian artery and the ligamentum arteriosus is called the isthmus (Fig. 27.1).

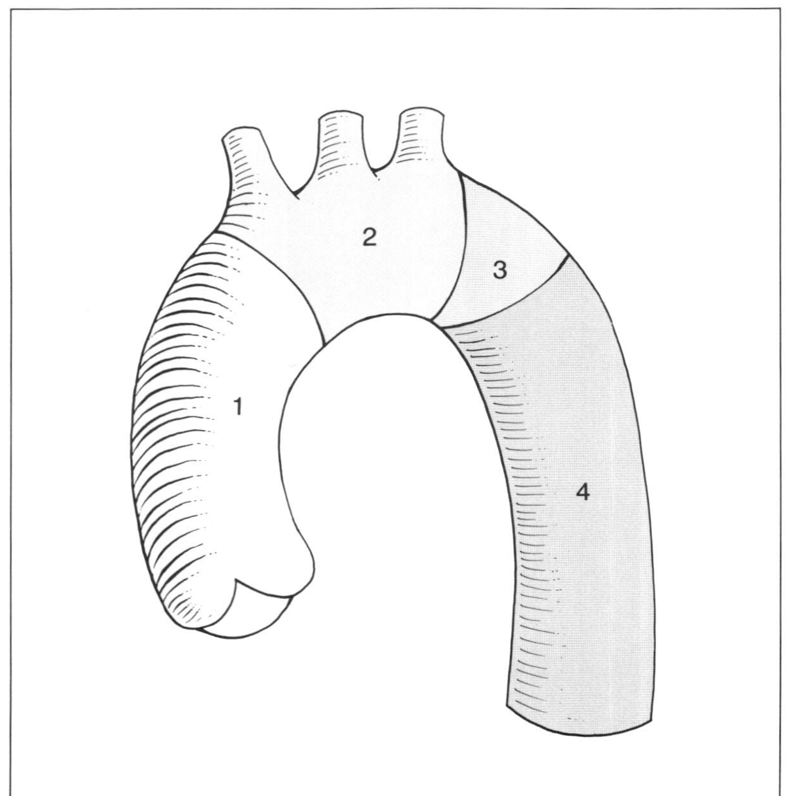

Fig. 27.1 Normal aorta.

1 ascending aorta
2 aortic arch (transverse segment)
3 descending thoracic aorta
4 aortic isthmus

DISSECTION OF THE AORTA

Aortic dissection, a spontaneous and often sudden event, occurs when the blood leaves the aortic lumen, exiting at a discrete point, and dissects the inner layer of the media from the outer layer. There may be a re-entry point downstream or upstream. When the proximal and distal connections of the dissection are patent and sufficiently large, a false channel is formed through which blood flows continuously in a manner similar to blood flow in the true aortic lumen.

PATHOGENESIS

The underlying lesion in dissection is an injury to the intima provoked by abnormal hemodynamic shear forces. The latter can be caused by several mechanisms that share a common pathway: stretching of the aorta. As the luminal diameter increases, there is a concomitant increase in stress within the aortic wall. Hypertension and/or degenerative disease of the media are common precursors of this initial stress, which triggers a chain of events leading to weakness of the aorta, dilatation, and increased tension in the vessel wall. The intima and then the media may rupture, allowing blood to dissect the aortic wall.

In patients with Marfan syndrome and certain other connective tissue disorders, severe injury to the aorta may occur at an early age because of the underlying congenital defect, which affects all the components of the media, including the ground substance, collagen, elastin, and smooth muscle cells. It is noteworthy that similar morphologic changes occur in the aorta during the course of normal aging, and also in certain types of aortic aneurysms not accompanied by dissection. Histological changes that may be observed in the aortic media include cystic medial necrosis, defined as pooling of myxoid material; elastin fragmentation, characterized by disruption of elastic lamellae; fibrosis, defined as an increase in collagen at the expense of smooth muscle cells; and medial necrosis, defined as areas containing cells that have lost their nuclei.

A rent in the intima appears to be the precipitating event in aortic dissection. Gross anatomic examination almost invariably reveals the presence of such a tear, although occasional cases have been reported in which none was found. Intimal disruption tends to occur at sites exposed to the greatest degree of hydraulic stress. Exposure of the media to pulsatile hemodynamic flow leads to cleavage of the lamellar elastic plates of the aorta, creating a false lumen. The false lumen surrounds the true lumen, usually comprising one third to two thirds of its radius. The longitudinal extension of the false lumen varies considerably (Fig. 27.2). For example, the dissection may involve the ascending segment of the aorta or the aortic arch, or may be restricted to the descending thoracic aorta.

Certain congenital malformations of the aorta predispose to aortic dissection. The incidence of dissection is 10 to 20 times greater in individuals with a bicuspid or unicuspid aortic valve than in those with a normal tricuspid valve. Coarctation of the aorta and giant cell arteritis are also risk factors. Dissection is particularly frequent in patients with Marfan syndrome, and in those with Marfan-like degenerative changes in the aorta who exhibit no overt clinical manifestations of the disorder.

CLINICAL PRESENTATION

Patients with aortic dissection typically experience the sudden onset of intense tearing or ripping pain, which is severe enough to cause them to seek medical care. The pain is typically migratory, spreading into the neck, back, and extremities as the dissection extends along the aorta. Patients with pain restricted to the anterior portion of the chest usually have proximal dissection. Pain in the back (typically in the interscapular area) is

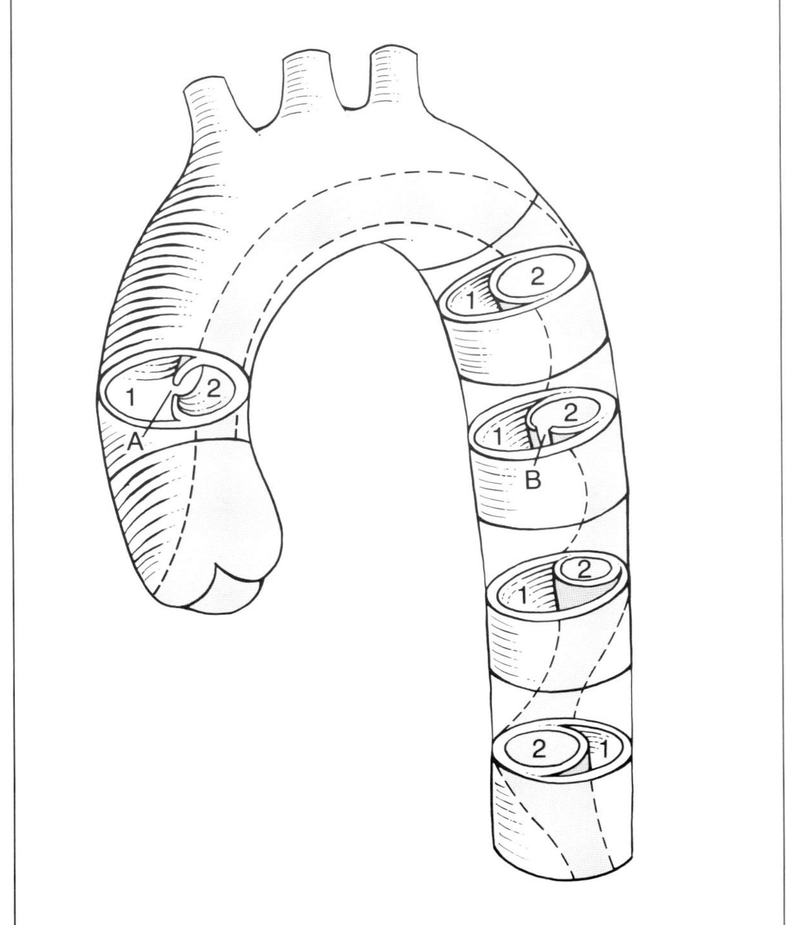

Fig. 27.2 Dissection involving the entire aorta. The internal flap separates the false and true lumens, which are usually connected at different levels.

1 false lumen
2 true lumen
A proximal entry
B distal entry

characteristic of dissection of the distal aorta. Occasionally dissection may be painless, in which case the clinical manifestations are represented by aortic valvular insufficiency or abnormal peripheral pulses. Painless dissection is most commonly seen in patients with Marfan syndrome.

On physical examination, the patient with acute aortic dissection is diaphoretic, restless, and hypertensive. Systemic hypotension may occur in patients who have complications of dissection, such as rupture into the pleural space or the pericardium. Unequal pulses are usually present in the carotid and brachial arteries, or in the arteries of the lower extremities. Clinical evidence of aortic valvular insufficiency is present in about half of patients with proximal dissections but is rarely seen in patients with distal dissection. Therefore, the recent onset of a typical aortic diastolic murmur is a strong indication of dissection. Fifteen percent of patients with dissection involving the ascending aorta have neurological disturbances secondary to compromise of the cephalic vessels.

From the clinical viewpoint, dissection of the thoracic aorta can be classified into two types (Fig. 27.3). In the first (type A), the dissection involves the ascending aorta, either localized or as a component of a more extensive dissection which involves the aortic arch and/or the descending thoracic aorta. Type B dissection affects the descending thoracic aorta beyond the origin of the left subclavian artery. Although type B dissection may be restricted to the thoracic aorta, it usually extends into the abdominal aorta.

IMAGING AND INVASIVE DIAGNOSIS

The role of diagnostic imaging is to demonstrate the dissection, its extention, and its localization, and to identify complications such as involvement of aortic arterial branches and rupture into body cavities. Complete evaluation includes assessment of aortic valvular insufficiency and the coronary arteries.

PLAIN CHEST FILMS

Chest films are abnormal in 80 to 85 percent of patients with dissection of the thoracic aorta. Although dissection is manifested by many signs, the most common are widening of the mediastinum, deformities of the aorta, and blurring of its contours (Fig. 27.4), deviation of the trachea to the right, and displacement of disruption of intimal calcification. The deformities of the aorta vary according to the area involved and the size of the false lumen. Abnormalities of the descending thoracic aorta are the rule when the dissection is restricted to this area; the lateral view usually reveals deformity of the left contour and its posterosuperior border. The diameter of the descending tho-

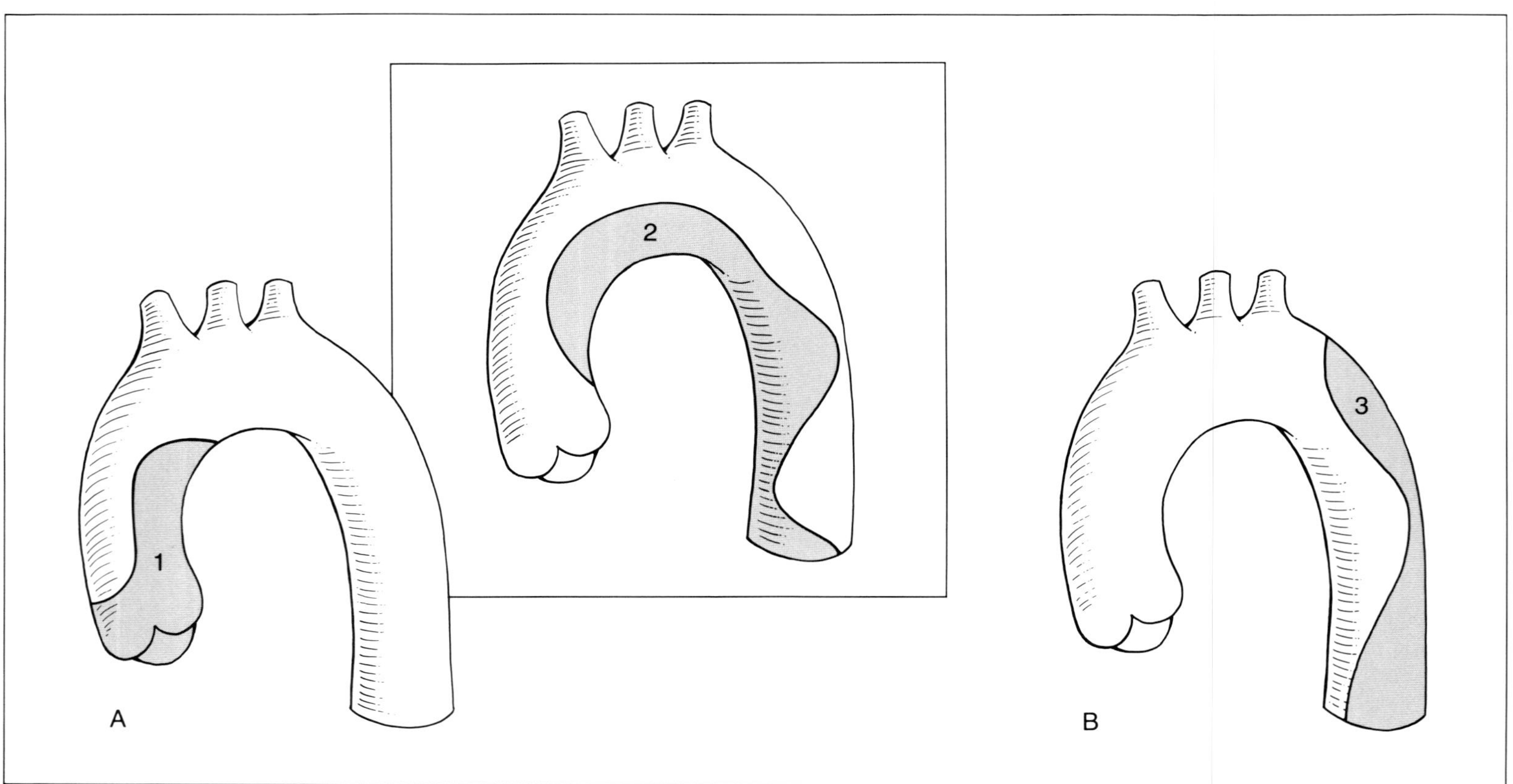

1 dissection limited to the ascending aorta
2 dissection extending to involve the entire thoracic aorta
3 dissection limited to the descending thoracic aorta

Fig. 27.3 Types of aortic dissection. (A) In Type A the proximal dissection may be limited to the ascending aorta *(1)* or it may extend into the aortic arch and descending thoracic aorta *(2)*. (B) In Type B the distal dissection affects the descending thoracic aorta exclusively *(3)*.

racic aorta is often greater than that of the ascending segment, owing to the presence of a hematoma in the dissected aortic wall or an aneurysmal dilatation of the aorta. The borders of the aorta are not clearly defined in patients with acute dissection. Left pleural effusion is a common finding.

Displacement of intimal calcification towards the lumen (ie, away from the outer border of the aorta) is a highly sensitive sign (Fig. 27.5); however, it may be difficult to evaluate in severely arteriosclerotic aortas in which the calcified intima is displaced by atheromatous plaque.

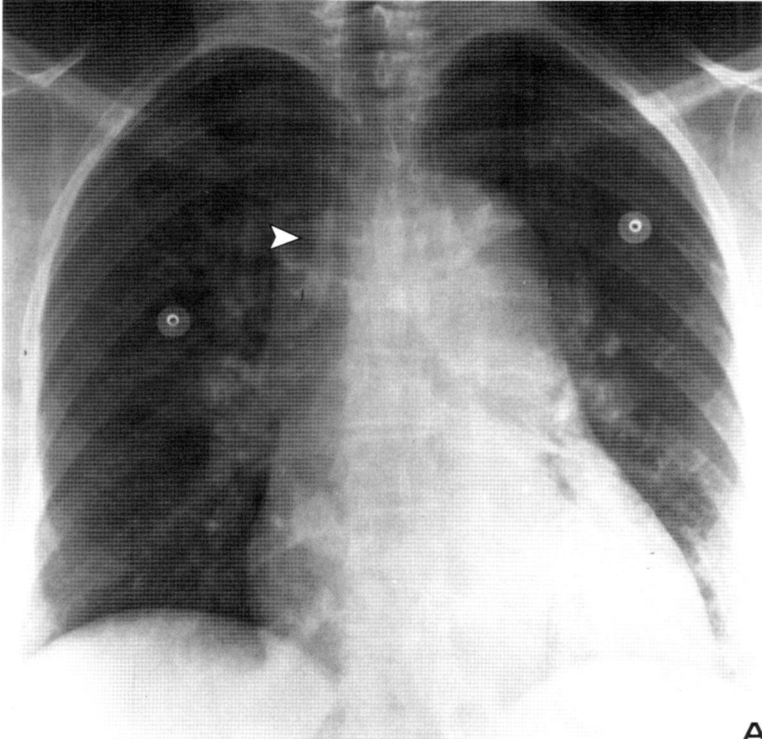

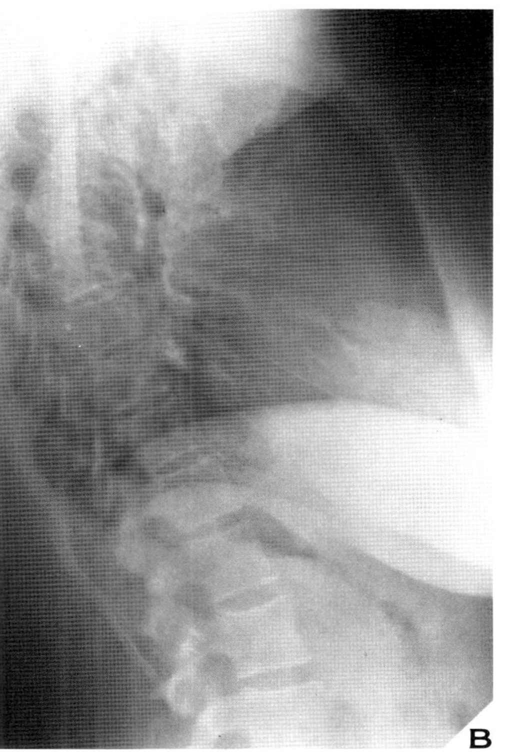

Fig. 27.4 Dissection of the entire thoracic aorta. (A) Frontal and (B) lateral chest films show a wide mediastinum (measurement made from the right border of the superior vena cava to the left border of the descending thoracic aorta). The aortic arch and descending thoracic aorta are both deformed. Other findings suggestive of dissection include downward displacement of the left main bronchus, indistinctness of the lateral margin of the descending aorta, effacement of the aortopulmonary window, and widening of the paratracheal stripe, which measures more than 5 mm *(arrow)*. In addition, there is mild pulmonary edema indicating left ventricular failure (secondary to acute aortic insufficiency caused by dissection of the aortic root).

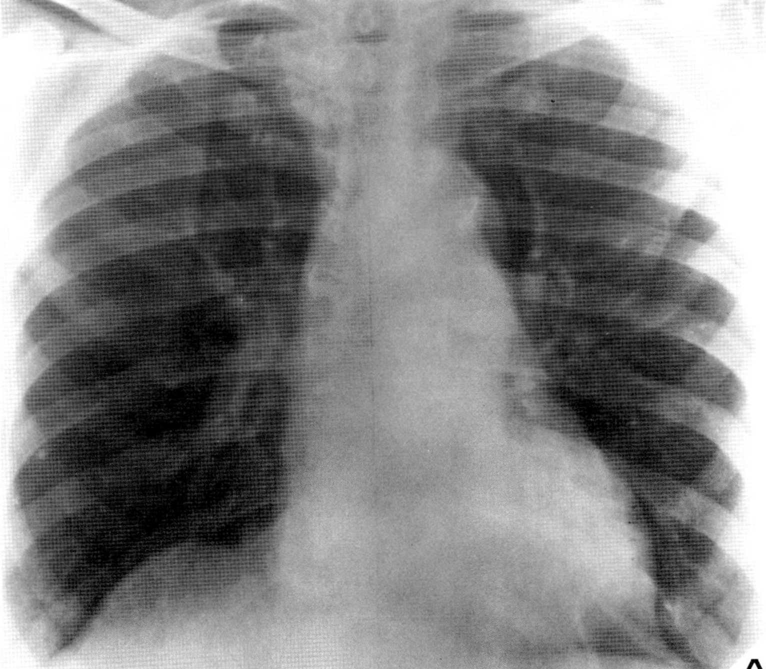

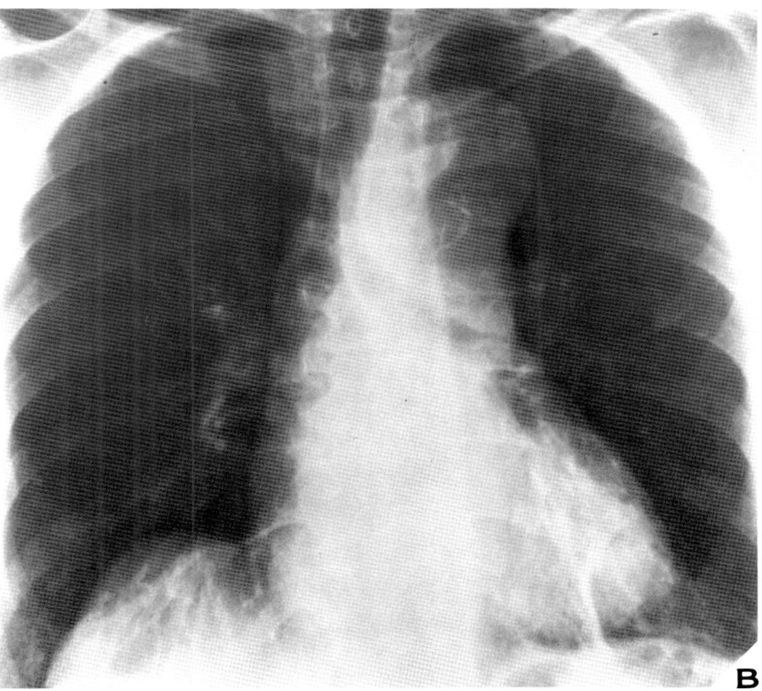

Fig. 27.5 Dissection of the aortic arch. (A) A posteroanterior chest film, obtained 2 years earlier, is normal. There is physiologic intimal calcification in the aortic arch. (B) Chest film obtained at the time of the acute episode shows medial displacement of the calcified intima and deformity of the aortic arch.

In patients with acute dissection producing aortic insufficiency, the plain chest film reveals various degrees of acute pulmonary edema; heart size is usually normal or nearly normal (Fig. 27.6). The plain chest film is normal in 15 to 20 percent of patients with aortic dissection. In patients with chronic dissection of the aorta, the chest film shows deformity of the affected segments (Figs. 27.6 to 27.10).

COMPUTED TOMOGRAPHY

Contrast-enhanced computed tomography is highly accurate for detection and assessment of aortic dissection. CT clearly demonstrates the intimal flap as well as calcification of the displaced intima. The hallmark of aortic dissection is a double lumen, with the inner (true) lumen separated from the outer (false) lumen by an intimal flap (Fig. 27.11), and aortic widen-

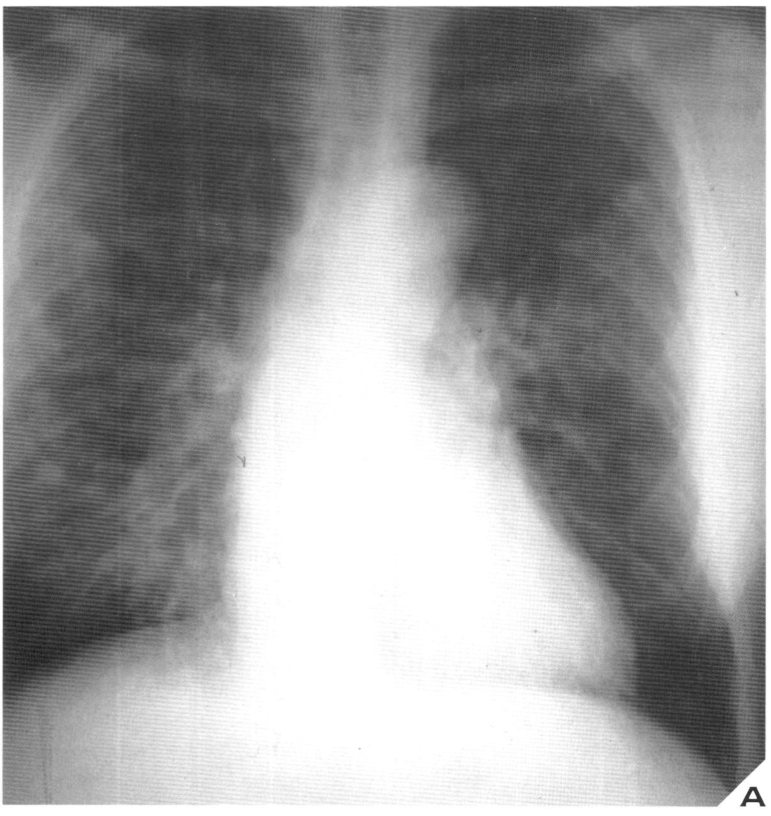

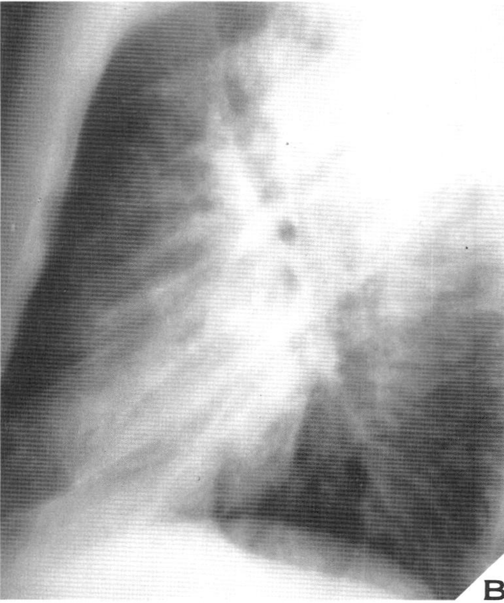

Fig. 27.6 Acute dissection of the ascending aorta with severe aortic valvular insufficiency. (A) Frontal and (B) lateral chest films reveal pulmonary edema (secondary to left ventricular failure) and minimal deformity of the ascending aorta. The heart is only minimally enlarged.

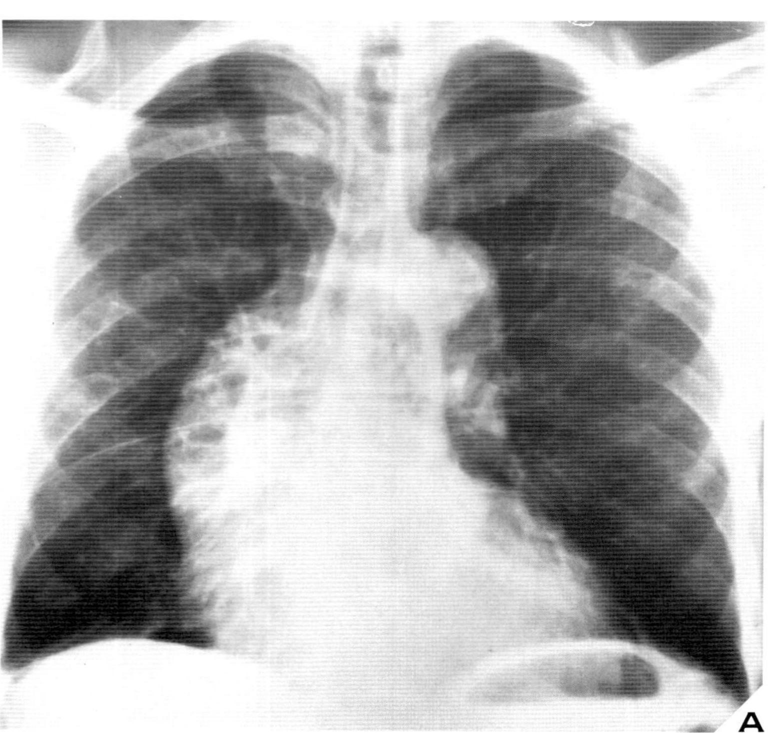

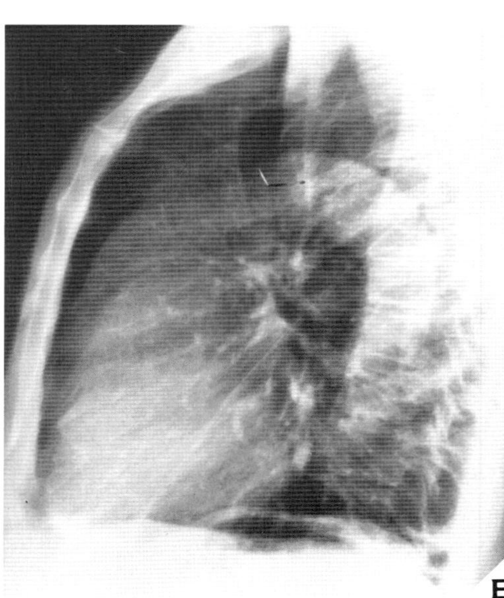

Fig. 27.7 Chronic dissection of the ascending aorta. (A) Frontal and (B) lateral chest films show marked deformity of the ascending aorta, which projects far to the right and anteriorly, obscuring the retrosternal space on the lateral projection. Both the aortic arch and the descending thoracic aorta are of normal size. The left ventricle is moderately enlarged as a result of aortic insufficiency.

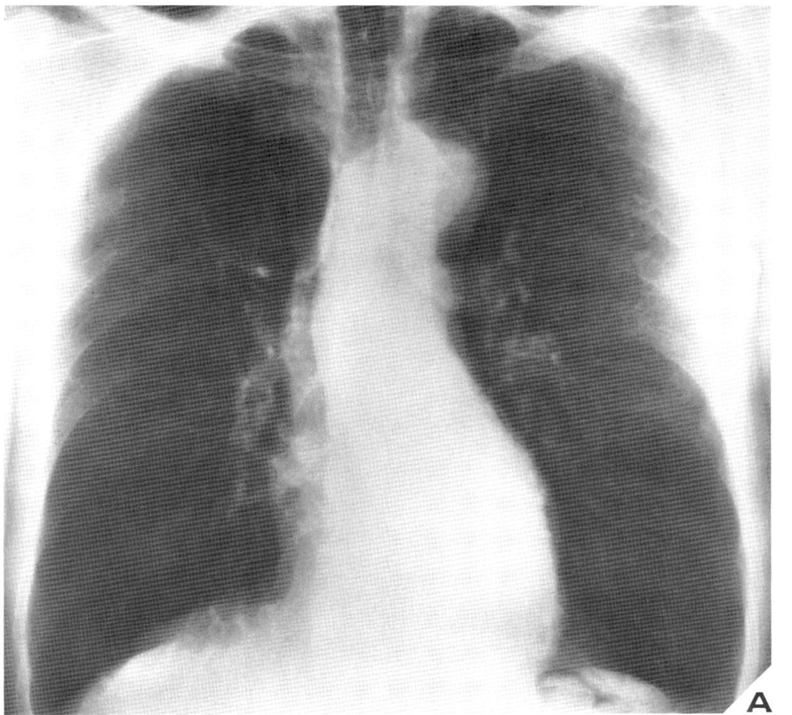

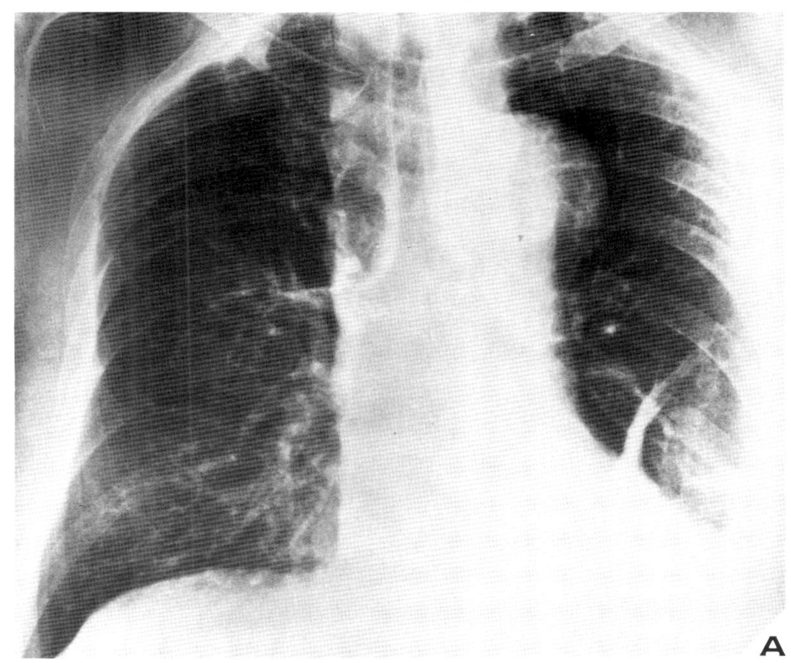

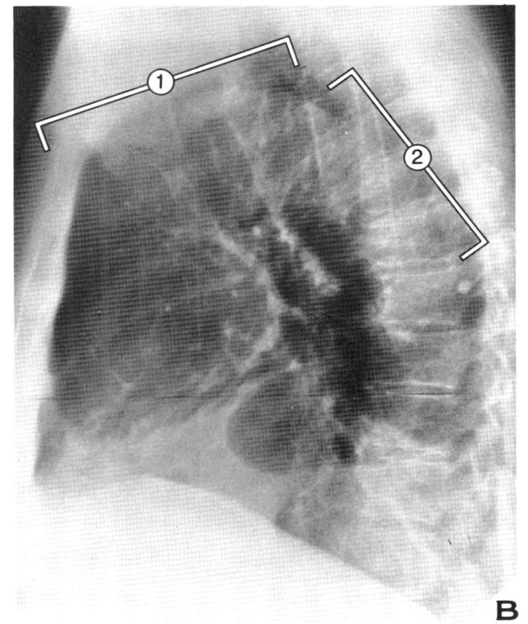

Fig. 27.8 Chronic dissection of the descending thoracic aorta. Frontal chest film demonstrates a double contour of the aortic arch. The supradiaphragmatic portion of the descending thoracic aorta is also dilated and deformed. The heart is of normal size. The pulmonary vascularity is normal.

Fig. 27.9 Dissection of the aortic arch. (A) Frontal chest film reveals a left pleural effusion and prominence of the aortic arch. (B) Lateral chest film shows unusual prominence of the anterior aspect of the aortic arch (*brace* 1). Although the descending thoracic aorta (*brace* 2) does not appear enlarged, aortography showed that dissection extended into its proximal segment.

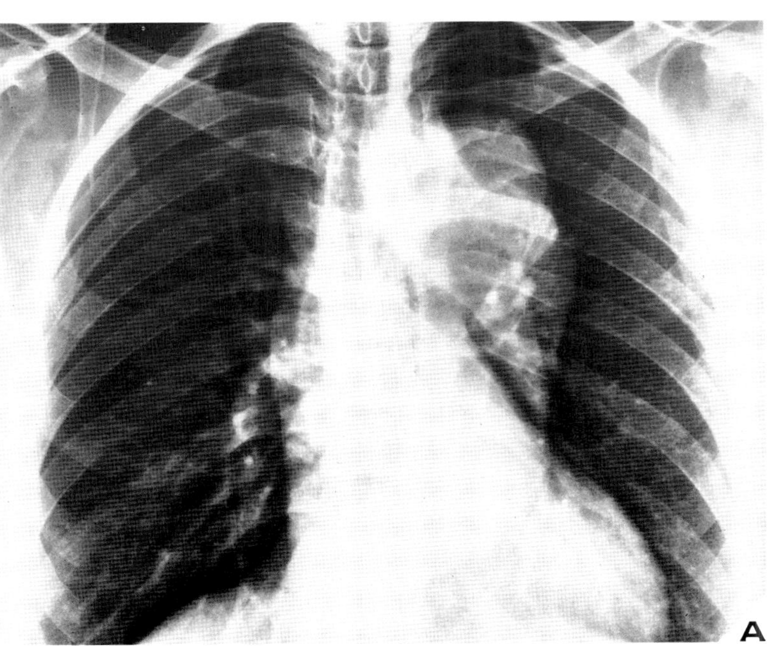

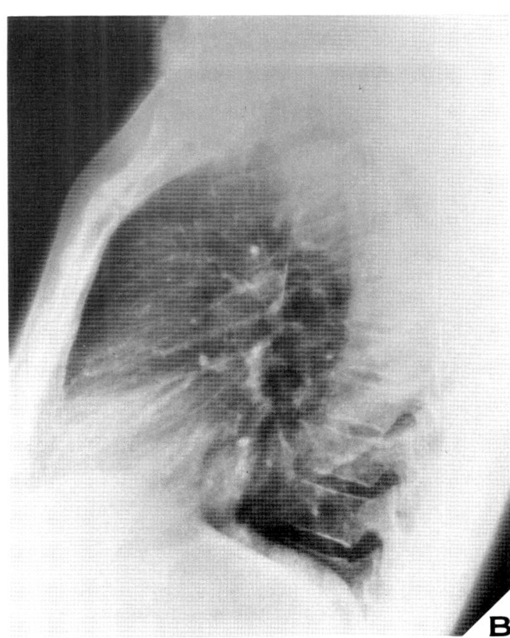

Fig. 27.10 Chronic dissection of the aortic arch and descending thoracic aorta. (A) Frontal and (B) lateral chest films show marked deformity and dilatation of the aortic arch and descending thoracic aorta. The distal segment of the descending thoracic aorta is tortuous. The left ventricle and pulmonary vascularity are normal.

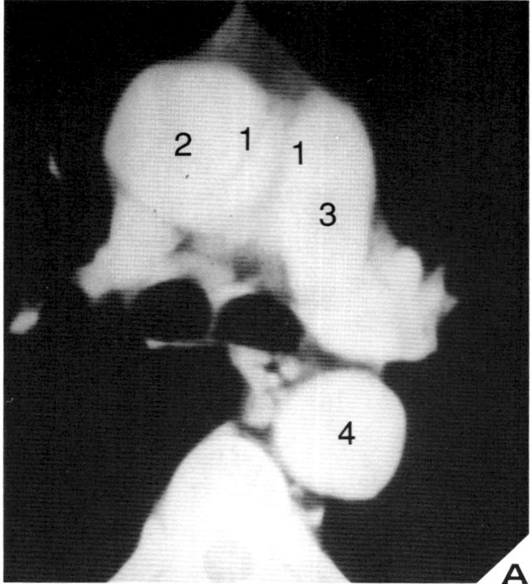

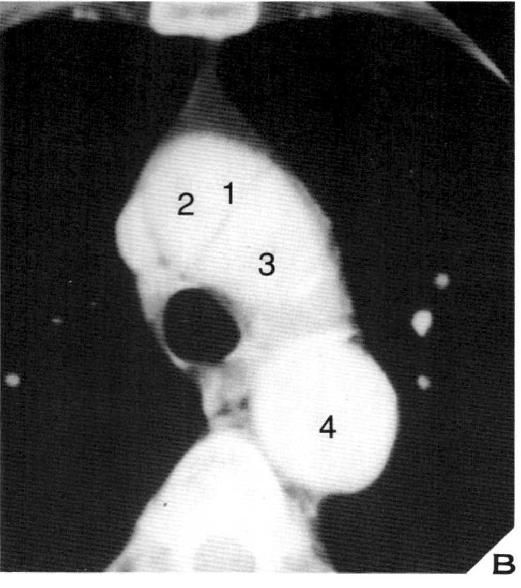

Fig. 27.11 Dissection of the ascending aorta (CT findings). Contrast-enhanced axial sections through lower (A) and upper (B) portions of the ascending aorta. The radiolucent line separating the false and true lumens is located posteriorly and on the left in A and medially in B. Note the enlargement of the ascending aorta (compare with the descending segment).

1 intimal flap	3 false lumen (ascending aorta)
2 true lumen (ascending aorta)	4 descending thoracic aorta

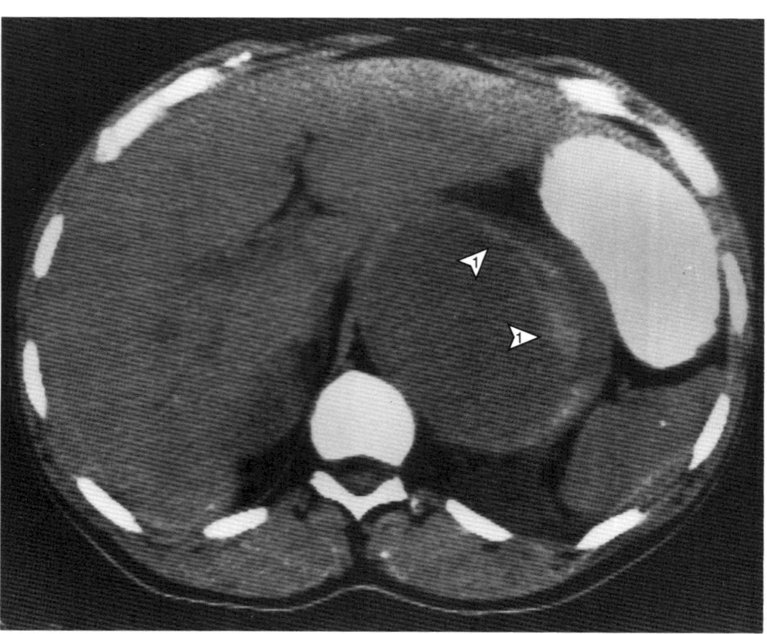

Fig. 27.12 Dissection of the upper abdominal aorta (CT findings). Unenhanced CT shows marked enlargement of the abdominal aorta. A calcified intimal flap (*arrows* 1) is displaced medially, indicating a dissection.

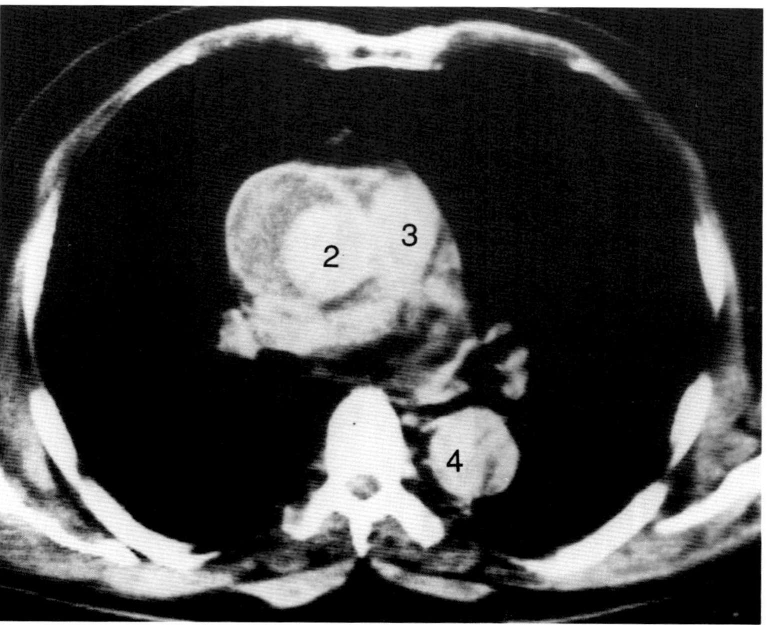

Fig. 27.13 Dissection of the ascending and descending thoracic aorta (CT findings). Contrast-enhanced CT scan at the level of the pulmonary trunk shows a dissection of the ascending aorta. The true lumen is opacified and is deformed by the false lumen, which is filled with thrombus and does not opacify. The dissection extends into the descending aorta. At this level both the false and the true lumen are opacified.

1 true lumen of ascending aorta	3 descending thoracic aorta
2 false lumen of ascending aorta	4 pulmonary trunk

ing, with medial displacement of peripheral intimal calcification and spiraling of a false lumen around the true lumen (Figs. 27.12 and 27.13). Applying the same criteria, it is possible to demonstrate extension of the dissection into the arteries arising from the aorta. Complications such as bleeding into the pericardium, the pleural space, or the mediastinum can also be demonstrated by CT (Figs. 27.14 and 27.15). Computed tomography has limited value for detecting small flaps and demonstration of aortic valvular insufficiency. Because it requires injection of contrast material, which may preclude angiography on the same day, CT may not be indicated as the initial study in patients with suspected dissection.

ECHOCARDIOGRAPHY

Echocardiography is now the modality of choice for the diagnosis of aortic dissection. Echocardiographic diagnosis depends on the demonstration of an abnormal linear echo ("intimal flap") in the lumen of the aorta in more than one scanning

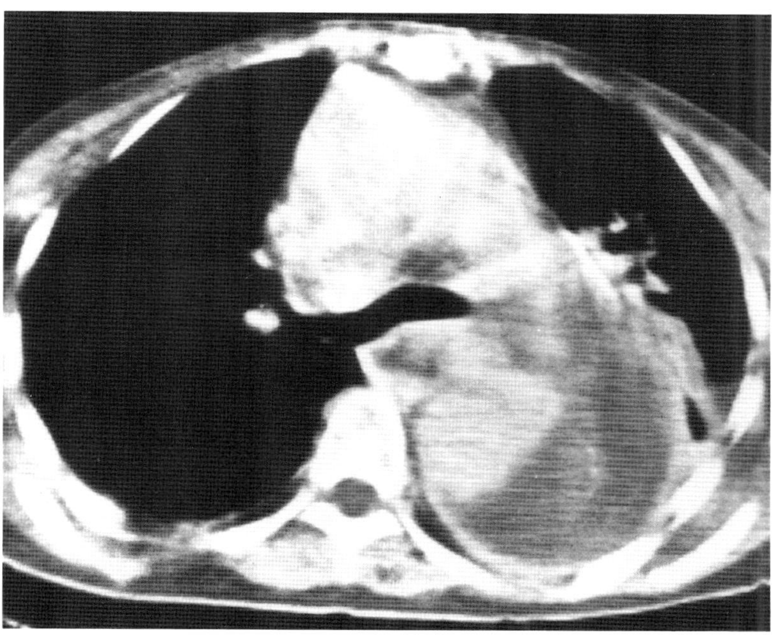

1 calcified intimal flap
2 true lumen
3 thrombus in true lumen
4 thrombus in false lumen
5 compression atelectasis

Fig. 27.14 Dissection of descending thoracic aorta (CT findings). The contrast-filled true lumen is markedly deformed by the false lumen. The calcified intimal flap is displaced medially. The filling defect in the true lumen represents thrombus. Note compression atelectasis in the left lower lobe caused by the dilated descending thoracic aorta.

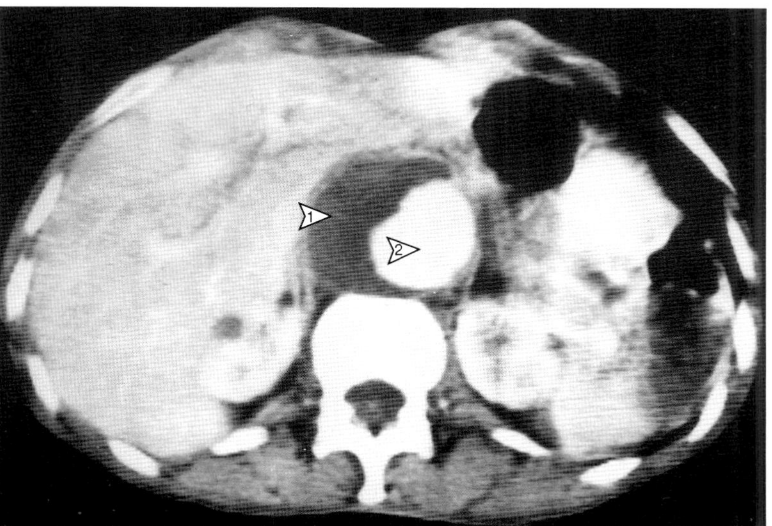

Fig. 27.15 Dissection of abdominal aorta (CT findings). Contrast-enhanced CT shows a large, thrombosed false lumen (*arrow* 1) surrounding more than 60 percent of the circumference of the true lumen (*arrow* 2), the contour of which is markedly deformed.

plane. This linear echo may be stationary or it may have an undulating motion (Fig. 27.16). Two-dimensional echocardiography demonstrates the intimal flap along a variable length of the thoracic and abdominal aorta, thus permitting accurate morphologic assessment in a large percentage of cases. Other echocardiographic signs of dissection are central displacement of the calcified intima and deformity of the aortic lumen caused by thrombus in the false channel. In the latter instance, it is important to distinguish aortic dissection from an aortic aneurysm with mural thrombus. A well defined "crescent sign" (see Fig. 27.17) strongly suggests the diagnosis of aortic dissection, whereas thrombus typically produces an irregular deformity of the lumen.

An intimal tear appears on echocardiography as a disruption in the continuity of the flap, with fluttering of the ruptured intimal borders. Color Doppler studies can identify the point at which the false and the true lumen communicate (Fig. 27.18, Appendix) and can detect blood flow within the false lumen (Fig. 27.19, Appendix). Additional echocardiographic and Doppler findings include aortic regurgitation, aortic dilatation, intracavitary rupture of the aorta, and pericardial and pleural effusion.

Transesophageal echocardiography is more sensitive than conventional 2-D echocardiography, allowing rapid, accurate visualization of the ascending aortic arch and the descending thoracic arch. False positive and false negative results are rare. A limitation of transesophageal echocardiography is its inability to visualize the upper portion of the ascending aorta owing to acoustic shadowing by the overlying air-filled trachea. Standard high left or right parasternal, suprasternal, and supraclavicular transthoracic windows are necessary to visualize this portion of the aorta.

MAGNETIC RESONANCE IMAGING

Magnetic resonance imaging is very accurate in the diagnosis of aortic dissection. Spin-echo technique with multisection acquisition of images yields a single imaging sequence of 20 axial sections covering the entire aorta, sufficient to verify the pres-

Fig. 27.16 Dissection of ascending aorta (echocardiographic findings). Transesophageal echocardiogram (frontal long-axis view at the level of the left ventricular outflow tract) shows an intimal flap in the ascending aorta, just above the sinuses of Valsalva.

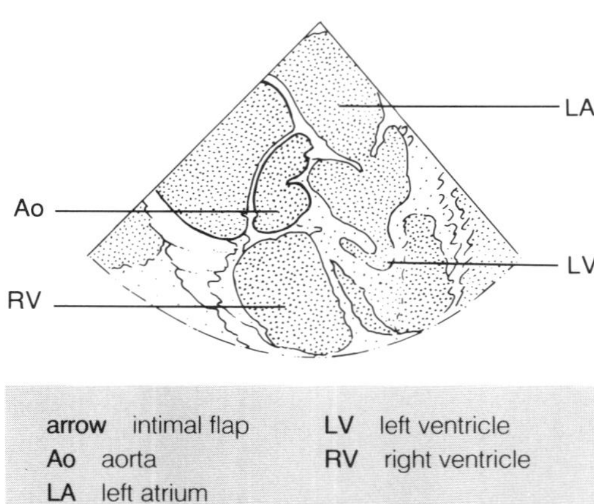

arrow	intimal flap	LV	left ventricle
Ao	aorta	RV	right ventricle
LA	left atrium		

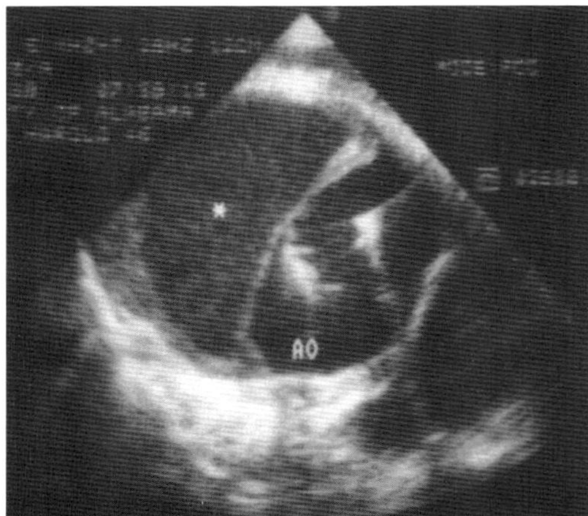

Fig. 27.17 Dissection of ascending aorta ("crescent sign"); echocardiographic findings. Transesophageal scan (short-axis projection at the level of the ascending aorta) shows true and false lumens separated by an intimal plaque. The false lumen contains mural thrombus. The true lumen contains a prosthetic aortic valve.

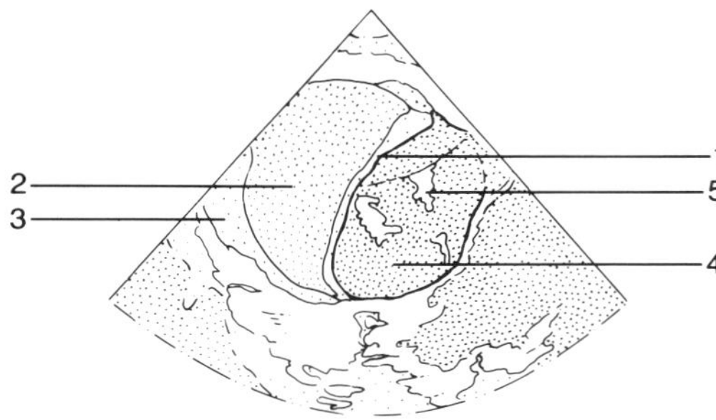

1	intimal flap	4	true lumen
2	false lumen	5	prosthetic aortic valve
3	thrombus in false lumen		

ence or absence of dissection and of an intimal flap, and to determine the type of dissection. Coronal and oblique views are used in exceptional situations (eg, when the thorax is malformed or when the aorta is extremely tortuous).

The MRI diagnosis of aortic dissection is based on demonstration of an intimal flap separating the true and the false lumens. This finding is most likely when the rates of flow through the false and true lumens are similar (Fig. 27.20). MRI may also demonstrate thrombus or a slow rate of flow in the false lumen. Extension of the dissection into the celiac artery, superior mesenteric artery, or renal arteries can also be identified; in such cases the branch artery is seen to rise from the false lumen.

When the false lumen is occluded by thrombus, MRI may show a high signal image along borders and a crescent sign, the latter resulting when dissection occurs without an intimal tear, or when the intimal tear is obliterated during the healing process (Fig. 27.21). This capability provides a significant advantage of MRI over CT and echocardiography. The crescent line associated with aortic dissection differs from that observed in aortic thrombosis.

Cine MRI has added a new dimension to the diagnosis of aortic dissection. Aortic insufficiency can be diagnosed with the cine MRI. Its only serious drawback is its inability to delineate coronary artery anatomy, information that is frequently needed to plan the surgical repair.

AORTOGRAPHY

Aortography has long been considered the "gold standard" for detection of aortic dissection. Although largely supplanted by newer modalities it remains an indispensable tool for planning the surgical repair. Aortography is performed via a femoral artery puncture using the Seldinger technique. A large volume of contrast material, usually 60 mL, is delivered into the aortic root at a rate of 30 mL per second. Biplanar imaging in the right and left anterior oblique projections will detect most thoracic aortic dissections. It is important to visualize the entire thoracic aorta. Some centers prefer the 14″ × 14″ cut-film format, which covers a larger field than the 9-inch image intensifier generally used for cineangiography. Others prefer 35 mm cine, which demonstrates small flaps as well as flaps that are obscured by unusually oriented channels on static images.

Angiographic diagnosis of aortic dissection is based on demonstration of the intimal flap separating the true and false lumens. Viewed in profile, the intimal flap appears as a linear neg-

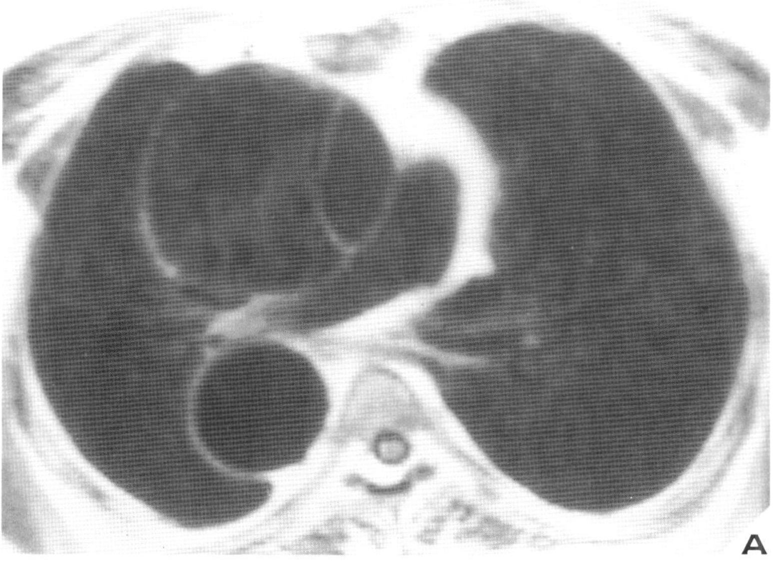

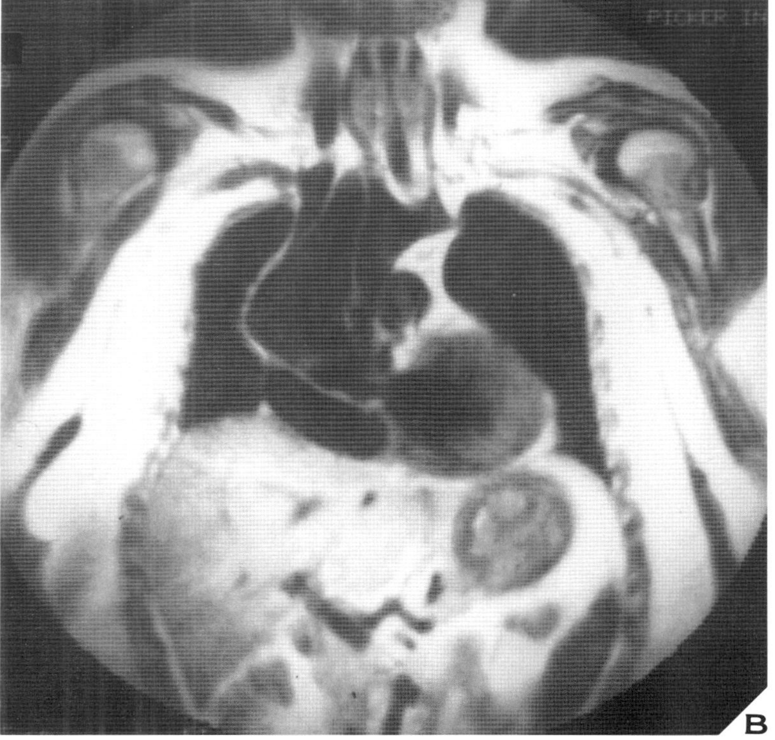

Fig. 27.20 Dissection of aortic arch (MRI findings). (A) Transverse and (B) coronal spin–echo images in a patient with a right aortic arch. (A) The intimal flap appears as a linear, high-signal image separating the true and false lumens. The false lumen is posterior and to the left of the true lumen. (B) The intimal flap is oriented vertically and extends into the innominate artery.

ative shadow located between two opacified channels (Fig. 27.21). Although the orientation of the flap is highly variable, it usually takes the form of a spiral running upward from the left posterior border of the ascending aorta towards the aortic arch, then turning posteriorly and to the left as it descends along the border of the upper descending thoracic aorta (Fig. 27.22). When a large proximal intimal tear is present, opacification of the true and false lumens occurs rapidly and almost simultaneously. The intimal tear may be located in the aortic arch; in such cases the dissection extends retrogradely into the aortic root, reaching the level of the aortic valve. This is clearly seen on cineangiography, which demonstrates contrast material passing from the true lumen into the false lumen at the level of the arch opacifying the true lumen in retrograde fashion (Fig. 27.22;

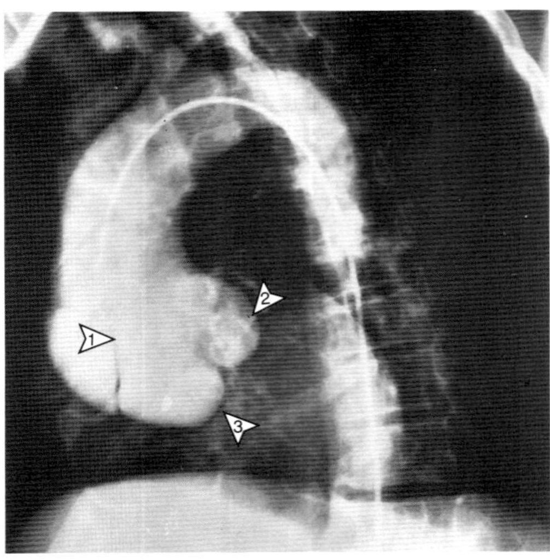

Fig. 27.21 Localized dissection of the aortic root (angiographic findings). Left anterior oblique projection of thoracic aortogram demonstrates a well-defined radiolucent line (*arrow* 1), which represents the intimal flap. There is no significant deformity of the true lumen. The aortic valve is normal (*arrow* 2 = left coronary cusp; *arrow* 3 = noncoronary cusp).

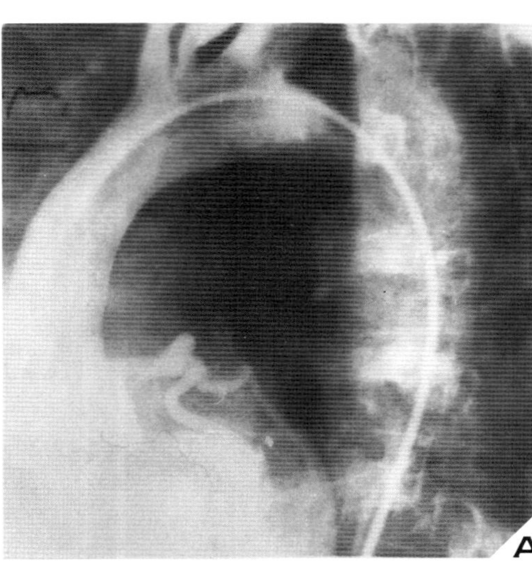

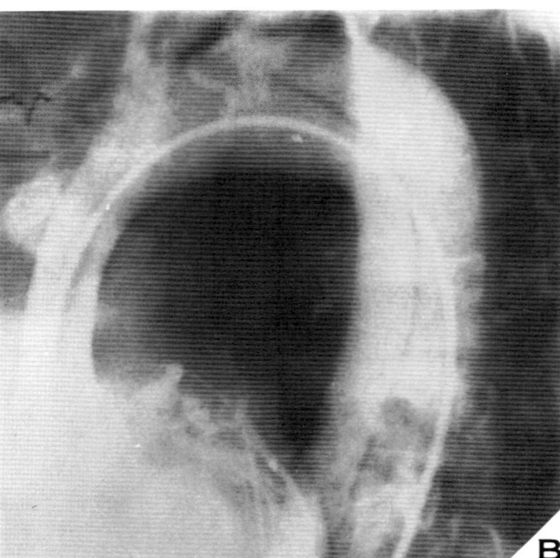

Fig. 27.22 Dissection of the entire thoracic aorta (angiographic findings); left anterior oblique projection of thoracic aortogram. (A) In the early phase, the ascending aorta is deformed but no opacification of the false lumen is seen. (B) In the late phase, the connection between the false and the true lumen is clearly seen. Contrast material opacifies the true lumen in retrograde fashion towards the ascending aorta. The upper and lower descending thoracic aorta are both well opacified, with contrast in the true and false lumens, which are separated by a large flap.

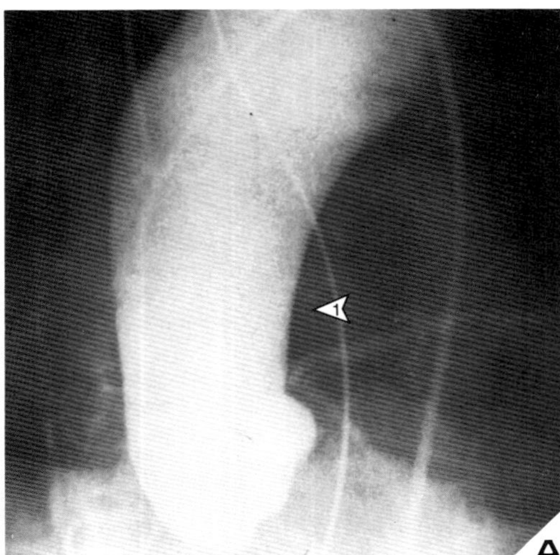

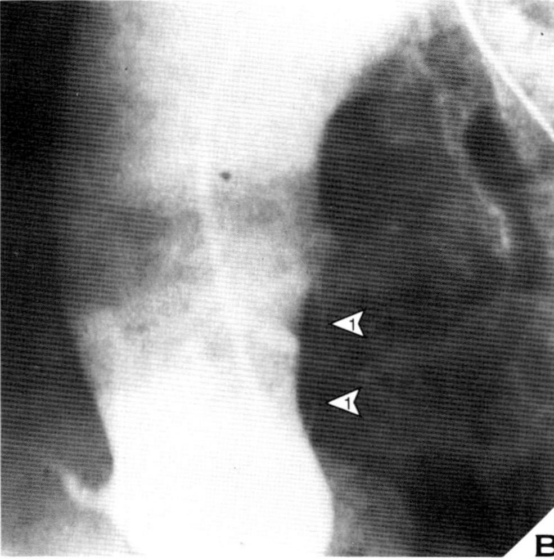

Fig. 27.23 Localized dissection of aortic root (angiographic findings). (A) Frontal and (B) lateral projections of thoracic aortogram show deformity of the left and posterior borders of the ascending aorta just above the left coronary cusp (*arrows* 1). The aortic cusps appear normal, although there is mild aortic insufficiency [note reflux into left ventricle (*arrow* 2). The upper portion of the ascending aorta appears normal.

see also Fig. 27.28). When the false lumen is not patent, deformity of the borders of the aorta indicates the presence of a dissection. A slight deformity of the aortic wall (Fig. 27.23) may be the only evidence of a minimal dissection, whereas in some large dissections the deformity is so severe that the aorta becomes a narrow channel (Figs. 27.24 and 27.25). Intimal flaps have an unusual appearance in patients with Marfan syndrome, in whom the aorta is markedly dilated. In these cases the flaps appear as linear densities that arise at different levels; in some instances they can only be visualized by cineangiography as they move during the cardiac cycle.

In some patients only the false lumen is opacified, in which case the true lumen cannot be visualized (Fig. 27.26). The morphology of the false channel is variable; although it may simulate a normal aorta, the absence of an aortic cusp (in dissections of the ascending aorta) or failure to opacify branches (in dissections of the descending segment) indicates its real nature.

Involvement of the aortic arch branches is best demonstrated by cineangiography in the left anterior oblique projection, which reveals filling defects at the origin of the innominate, left carotid, or left subclavian artery. In dissections at the abdominal level, involvement of the renal arteries or other ma-

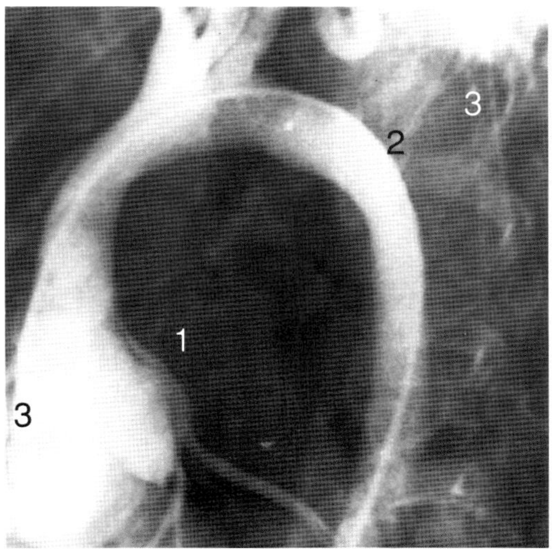

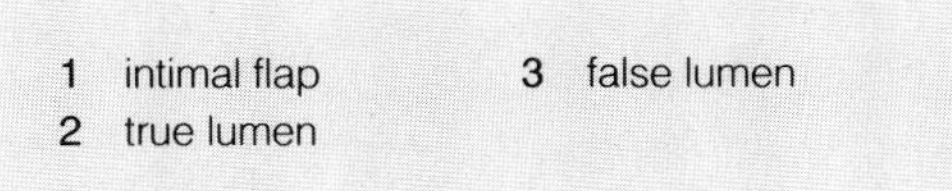

Fig. 27.24 Dissection of entire thoracic aorta (angiographic findings). Left anterior oblique projection of thoracic aortogram shows significant deformity of the aortic root, although the aortic valve appears normal. There are several connections between the true and false lumens in an area just above the sinuses of Valsalva. The aortic arch and the descending thoracic aorta are markedly deformed and appear unusually narrow.

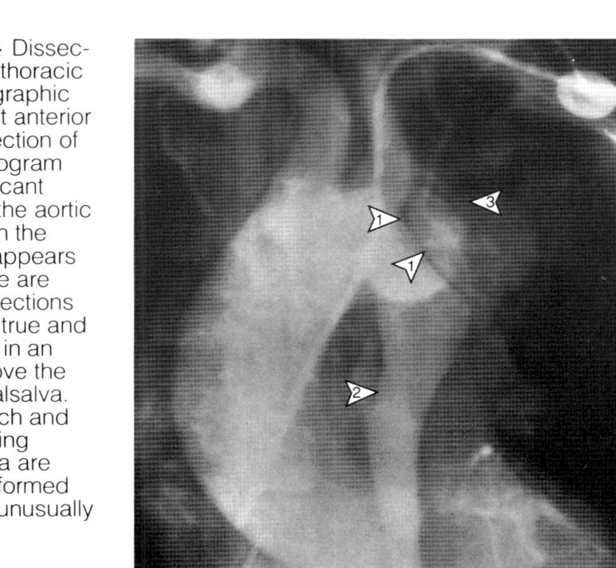

Fig. 27.25 Dissection of descending thoracic aorta (angiographic findings). Left anterior oblique projection of thoracic aortogram demonstrates marked deformity of the descending segment, beginning just beyond the origin of the left subclavian artery, with opacification of the false lumen. The intimal tear is clearly seen (*arrows* 1). (*arrow* 2 = true lumen; *arrow* 3 = false lumen)

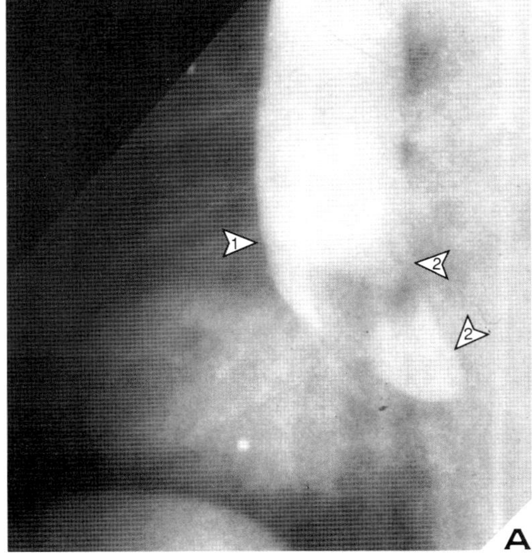

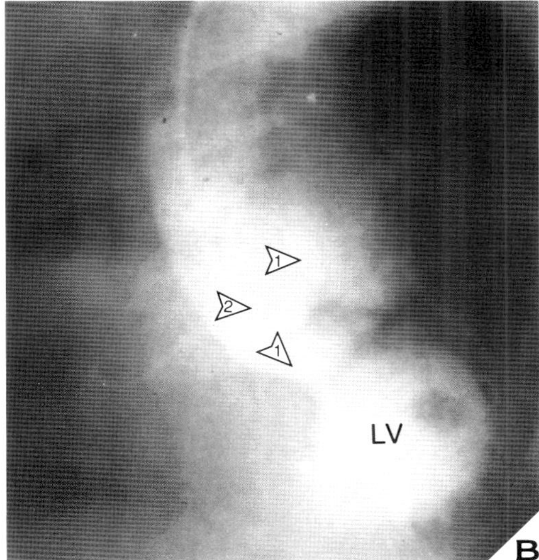

Fig. 27.26 Dissection of ascending aorta and aortic arch: inadvertent injection into false lumen. (A) Selective injection shows opacification of a tubular structure (*arrow* 1) which resembles the ascending aorta. However, the aortic cusps are not identified, indicating that the tubular structure represents the false lumen. (The expected position of the aortic cusps is indicated by *arrows* 2.) (B) The catheter was withdrawn through the intimal tear, which was at the level of the aortic arch. A repeat injection now demonstrates the aortic cusps (*arrows* 1), indicating that the catheter tip is in the true lumen (*arrow* 2). The posterior and left borders of the true lumen are slightly deformed by the adjacent false channel. Note severe aortic insufficiency, with opacification of the entire left ventricle (LV).

jor branches can be identified by selective opacification of the abdominal aorta (Fig. 27.27). Other complications of dissection, eg, rupture into the pericardium or a cardiac chamber, can also be demonstrated by aortography (Fig. 27.28).

In summary, frontal and lateral chest films should be obtained when the clinical findings suggest dissection. Although they provide important information (eg, deformity of various segments of the aorta), it must be emphasized that normal plain films do not rule out dissection. Thoracic aortography remains the most accurate method for demonstrating dissection of the aorta, its complications, and involvement of the aortic branches. Echocardiography, CT, and MRI are also highly sensitive; however, none of these modalities provides all of the information needed to plan therapy. In patients with acute dissection who are hemodynamically unstable, it may be advisable to undertake corrective surgery on the basis of the echocardiographic findings, omitting further diagnostic studies.

CHRONIC AORTIC ANEURYSM

Chronic aneurysm (true aneurysm) is defined as a localized enlargement of the aorta in which all layers of the aortic wall are present, even though one or more layers may be attenuated. A false aneurysm, on the other hand, is a localized enlargement of the aorta in which the wall consists of adventitia only. The term "chronic aneurysm" implies that the aneurysm has been present for more than 30 days.

MORPHOLOGY

Most aortic aneurysms are acquired and can be classified into two morphologic types. In the fusiform type, the aneurysm encompasses the circumference of the aorta and has a spindle shape. In the saccular type, the aneurysm protrudes from the aortic wall and resembles a pouch with a narrow neck. The basic structural change in aortic aneurysm, regardless of its cause, is weakening or destruction of the media. The aneurysm tends to enlarge, compressing the surrounding structures, and may eventually rupture.

Aneurysms of the ascending aorta are located just proximal to the origin of the innominate artery and may be associated with aortic valve insufficiency. A second type of aneurysm involves the aortic arch. Aneurysms of the descending thoracic aorta start just distal to the origin of the left subclavian artery. Thoracoabdominal aneurysms usually originate in the distal segment of the thoracic aorta, extending below the diaphragm to involve the upper and sometimes the entire abdominal aorta. The most common location of surgically treated aortic aneurysms is the ascending segment (45 percent), followed by the descending thoracic aorta (35 percent). Aortic arch aneurysms and thoracoabdominal aneurysms each account for 10 percent.

PATHOGENESIS AND ETIOLOGY

The most common cause of chronic aneurysm is arteriosclerosis or degenerative disease of the aortic wall in the setting of hypertension. The second most common cause is chronic aortic dissection. If a patent false lumen persists, it may enlarge, forming a saccular aneurysm whose wall consists of the adventitia and a layer of media. Aneurysms of this type have a tendency to weaken and enlarge.

Posttraumatic pseudo-aneurysms of the aortic arch represent 10 percent of all thoracic aneurysms. When the trauma is severe enough to rupture one wall of the aorta (usually at the level of the ligamentum arteriosus), blood may extravasate, in which case the leak is contained by the periaortic tissues. If the extravasated blood reenters the aortic lumen a false aneurysm is formed. Because the wall of the false aneurysm is weak, it tends to enlarge and display the morphology of a typical aortic arch aneurysm.

Annuloaortic ectasia, which can be isolated or associated with Marfan syndrome, leads to formation of aortic aneurysms that are usually associated with aortic valvular incompetence. The caudal portion of the aneurysm includes the aortic root and involves the annulus and the sinuses of Valsalva. The cephalic portion usually terminates at the level of the innominate artery, although cases of annuloectasia involving the aortic arch, as well as the descending aorta, have been reported.

Aortitis, which can have a specific (eg, syphilis) or a nonspecific etiology (eg, granulomatosis), is responsible for approximately 8 percent of aortic aneurysms. In syphilic aortitis, the elastic fibers of the media are destroyed and the aorta becomes enlarged. The disease process usually begins immediately above the aortic annulus, which is generally spared.

CLINICAL PRESENTATION

The clinical manifestations of thoracic aortic aneurysm are caused by compression, distortion, or erosion of surrounding structures, by intramural arterial dissection, or by rupture of the aneurysm. Some large aneurysms are entirely asymptomatic and are discovered only on routine chest films. The most common symptom is pain, usually of several months' duration; the onset of pain frequently heralds a sudden extension of the aneurysm. The location of the pain may indicate the location of the aneurysm. Pain in the anterior chest wall is usually associated with an aneurysm of the ascending aorta; transverse aortic aneurysms cause discomfort radiating to the neck; and aneurysms of the descending thoracic aorta tend to produce back pain, usually interscapular. Compression of the superior vena cava by the aneurysm, and hoarseness due to stretching the left vagus and recurrent laryngeal nerves, are typical manifestations of aneurysms of the aortic arch.

Thoracic aneurysms seldom produce direct physical signs. A large pulsatile mass eroding the anterior chest wall is a late finding. Most patients with aortic aneurysms have manifestations of arteriosclerosis, including ischemic heart disease, renal vascular disease, transient ischemic attacks or stroke, and leg claudication.

IMAGING AND INVASIVE DIAGNOSIS

PLAIN CHEST FILMS

The plain film findings in aortic aneurysm reflect the location of the disease. In patients with ascending aortic aneurysms that involve the aortic valve, chest films usually reveal localized di-

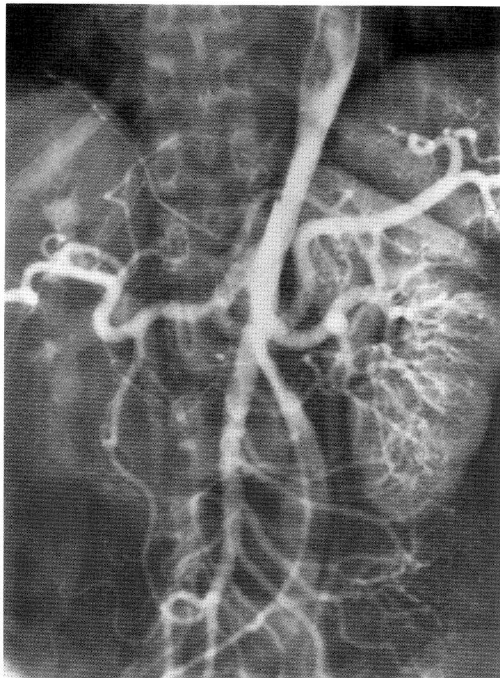

Fig. 27.27 Thoracoabdominal dissection. Transfemoral aortogram with the catheter tip at T12–L1 demonstrates marked deformity of the abdominal aorta, with opacification of the true and false lumens. Note occlusion of the right renal artery and absence of a nephrogram on the right. (The right renal collecting system is opacified from previous injections.)

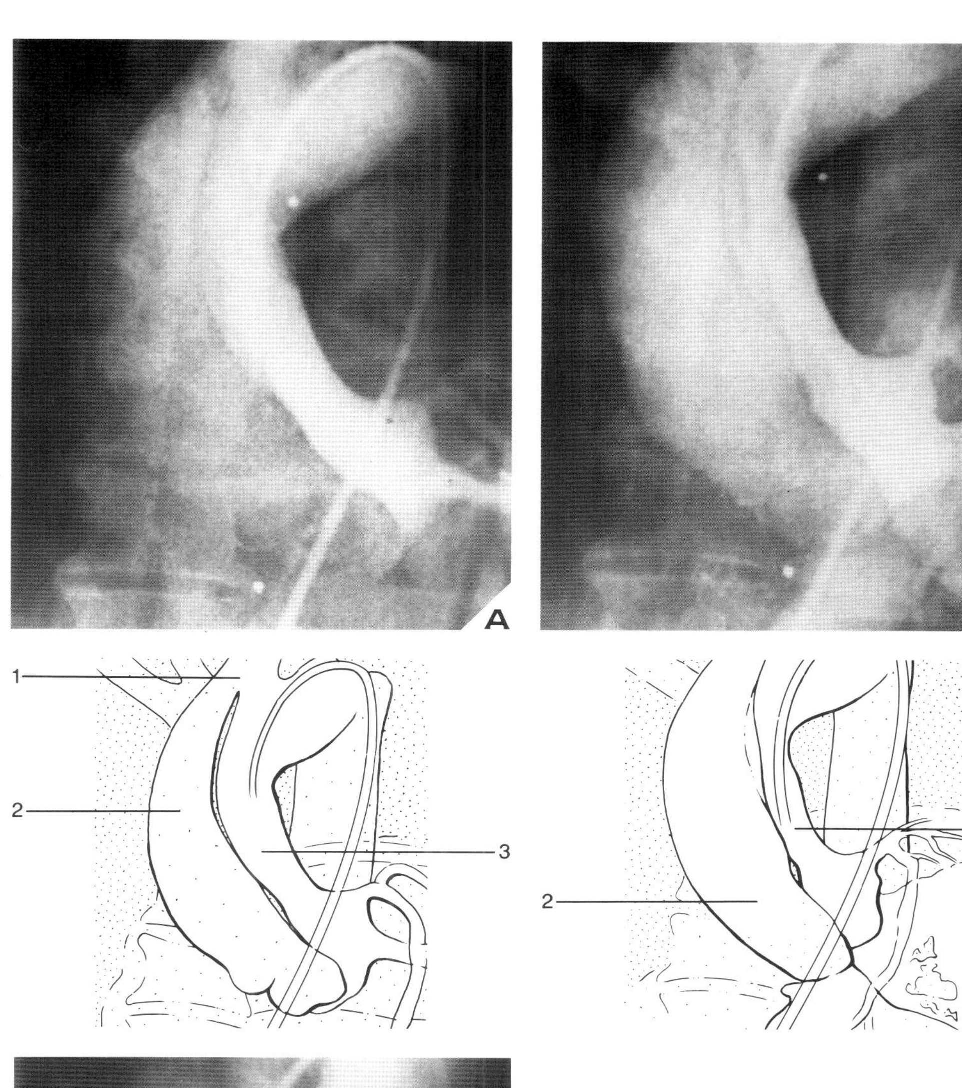

C

2
3
5
4

Fig. 27.28 Dissection of aortic root with fistula to right atrium; frontal projection of thoracic aortogram. (A) In the early phase, the ascending aorta is deformed by the false lumen, which is poorly opacified by contrast material passing through a connection at the level of the aortic arch near the origin of the innominate artery. (B) In the intermediate phase, the false lumen is opacified almost to the level of the aortic valve. (C) In the late phase, the false lumen is completely opacified. Contrast material is now present in the right atrium, indicating rupture of the false channel into the right atrium with formation of an aortoatrial fistula.

1 connection between false and true lumen
2 false lumen
3 true lumen
4 connection between aorta and right atrium
5 right atrium

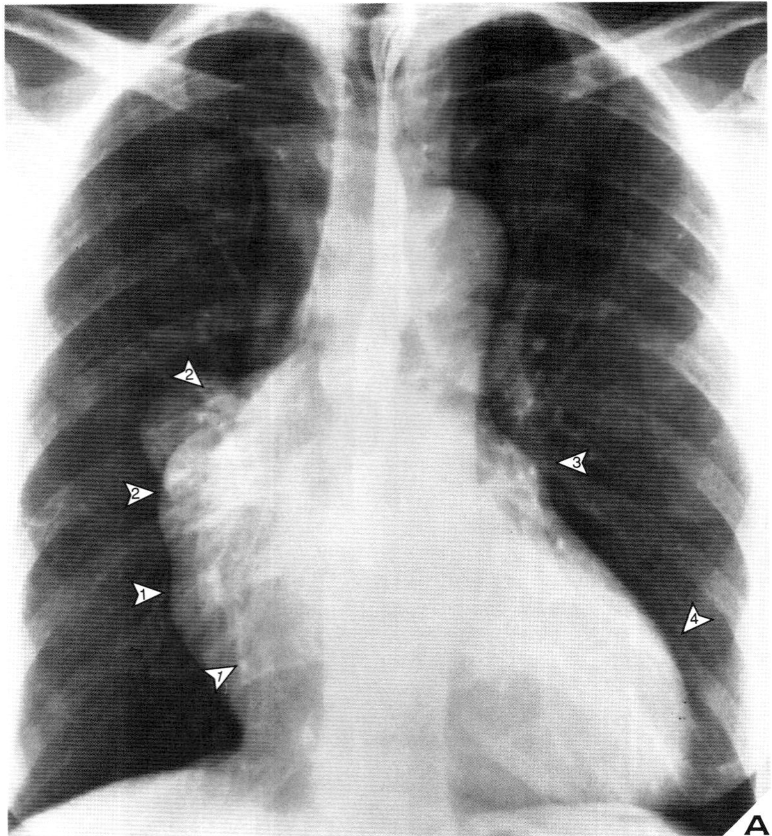

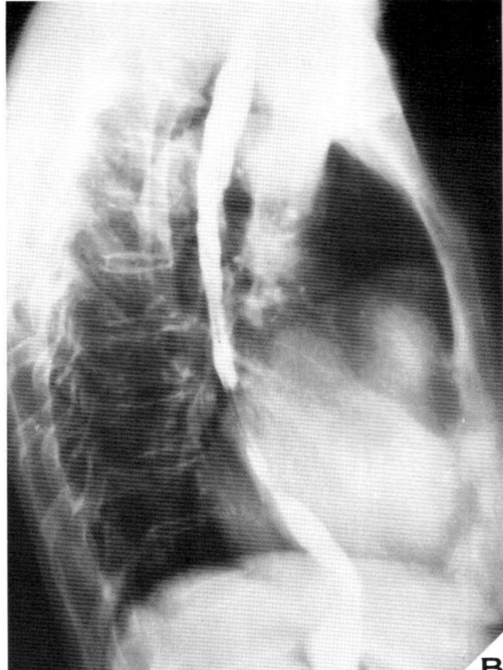

Arrows:
1 right atrial border
2 dilated aortic root and ascending aorta
3 displaced pulmonary trunk
4 left ventricular border

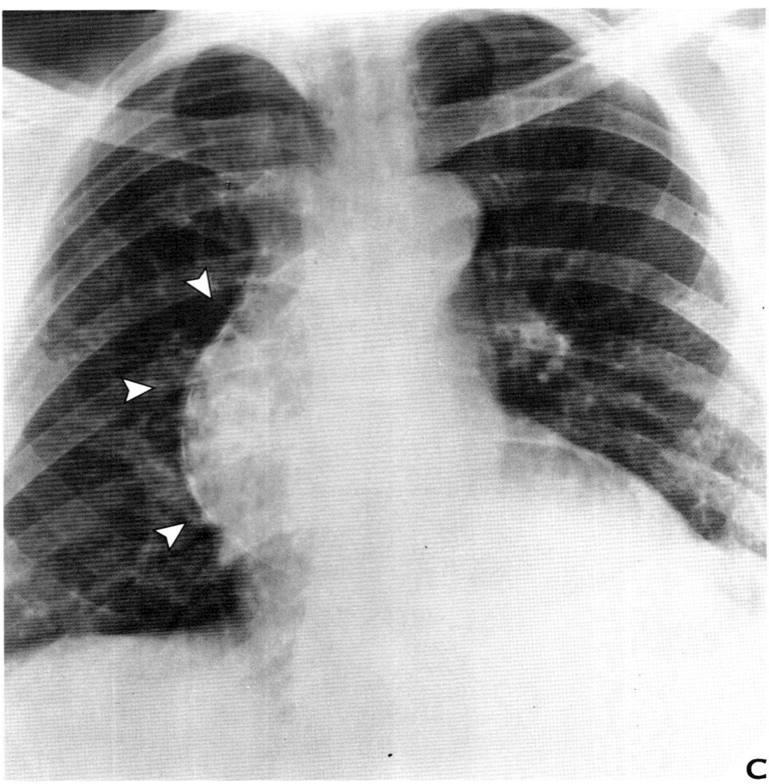

Fig. 27.29 Arteriosclerotic aneurysm of the ascending aorta (plain film findings). (A) Frontal and (B) lateral chest films demonstrate enlargement of the ascending aorta, which appears as a bulge of the cardiovascular silhouette just above the right atrial contour. The midportion of the cardiovascular silhouette is also deformed on the left, presumably due to displacement of the pulmonary trunk by the aneurysm. The left ventricle projects to the left, inferiorly, and posteriorly, indicating left ventricular enlargement (secondary to aortic insufficiency). (C) Frontal chest film of another patient demonstrates bulging of the right superior mediastinal border by a heavily calcified arteriosclerotic aortic aneurysm *(arrows)*. The aortic arch and descending thoracic aorta appear normal.

latation of the ascending aorta and left ventricle enlargement (Figs. 27.29A and 27.29B). This combination, typical of aortic-annular ectasia, is the rule in patients with Marfan syndrome. In patients with ascending aortic aneurysms the right upper border of the cardiovascular silhouette is displaced laterally. When the aneurysm is large and has grown to the left, it may displace the pulmonary trunk to the left. On the lateral view, the anterior border of the aorta is displaced anteriorly and occupies the retrosternal space. Calcifications are common in patients with arteriosclerotic aneurysms (Fig. 27.29C).

Aneurysms of the aortic arch characteristically produce enlargement and irregularity of the upper mediastinal border (Fig. 27.30). On lateral view, the deformity may extend into the ascending or descending segments. Aneurysms arising from the inferior wall of the aortic arch bulge into the aortopulmonary window. Calcification is common in aortic arch aneurysms, most of which are secondary to trauma.

Aneurysms of the descending thoracic aorta are manifested primarily by deformity and enlargement of this segment, which appears larger than the ascending aorta. The contour appears

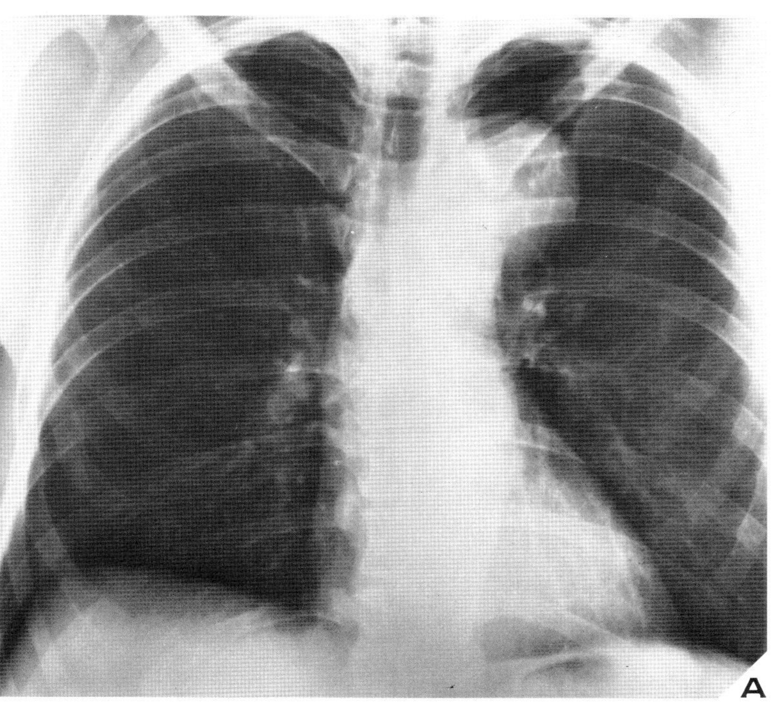

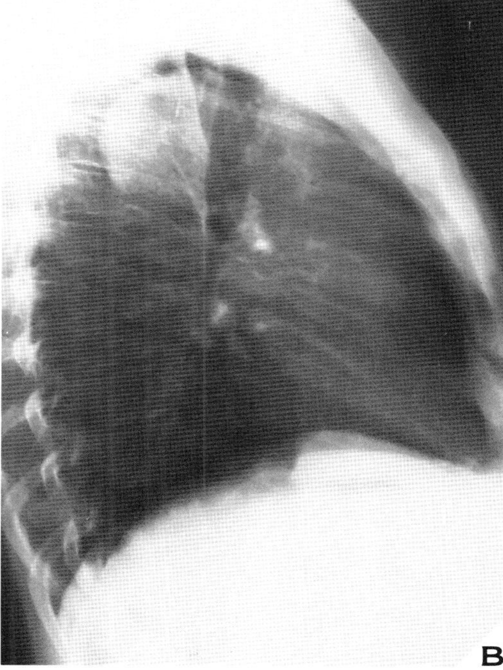

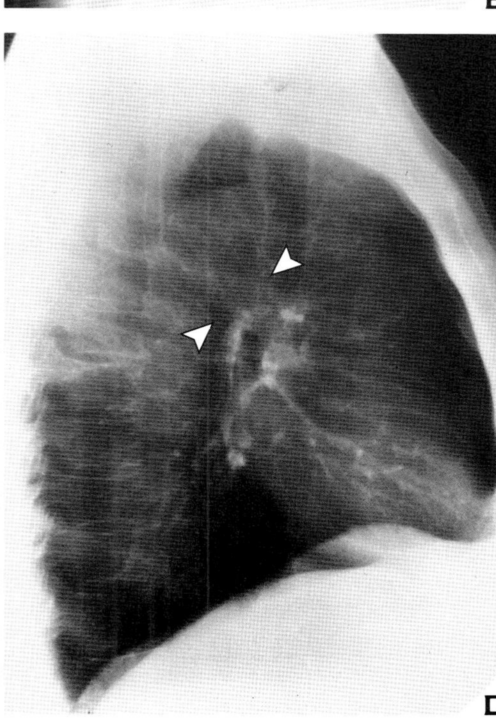

Fig. 27.30 Aneurysm of the distal aortic arch; plain film findings in two patients. (A) Frontal and (B) lateral chest films in a patient with an aneurysm of the distal aortic arch show prominence of the distal aortic arch and the adjacent portion of the descending thoracic aorta. The abnormal aortic contour is well seen on the lateral projection. (C) Frontal and (D) lateral chest films in a patient with a pseudoaneurysm of the inferior wall of the distal arch reveal abnormal prominence of the aortic arch and the adjacent portion of the descending thoracic aorta. Mass effects caused by the aneurysm are clearly seen. The trachea is displaced to the right, the left main bronchus is displaced downward, and the aortopulmonary window (*arrows* in D) is effaced.

irregular when the aneurysm is fusiform and localized when it is saccular (Fig. 27.31).

Marked tortuosity of the aorta, which is not uncommon, can be mistaken for an aneurysm (Figs. 27.32 and 27.33).

COMPUTED TOMOGRAPHY

CT is a convenient and accurate method for diagnosis of aneurysms of the thoracic aorta. It reveals the size and extent of the lesion as well as the degree of involvement of the arteries arising from the aorta. The normal ascending aorta measures 3.7 ± 0.3 cm in diameter. The aortic arch is 3.3 ± 0.6 cm, and the descending thoracic aorta is 2.4 ± 0.3 cm. An aortic diameter of more than 4.5 cm is considered to represent an aneurysm. The use of CT can create a three-dimensional display of the entire aorta, making possible an assessment of the full extent of the aneurysm. CT can detect small areas of calcification within the aneurysm, and with contrast enhancement can detect thrombus within it and differentiate between true and false aneurysms (Fig. 27.34). The thrombus within an aneurysm may occupy the entire lumen or may be localized within a dissection.

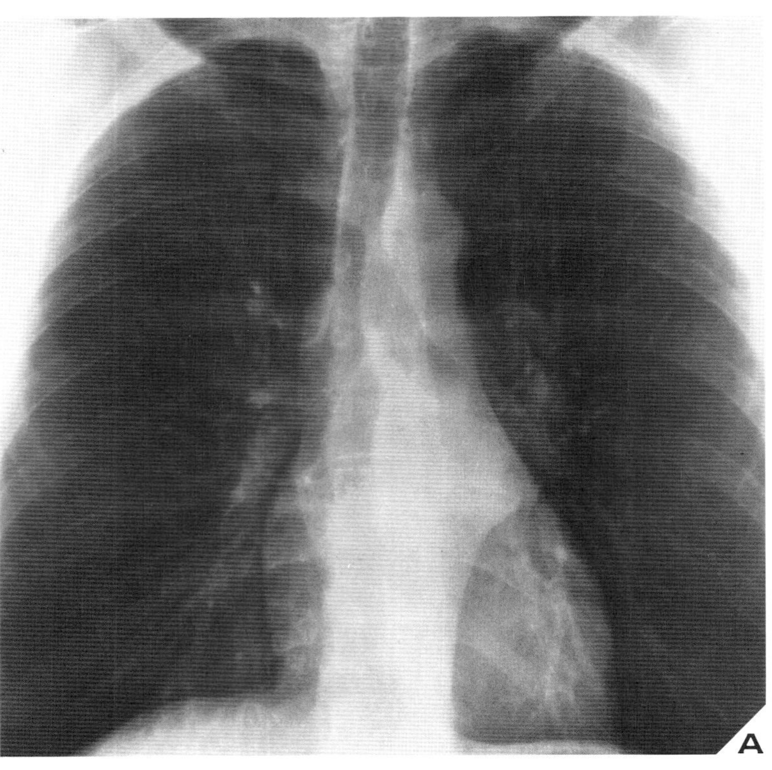

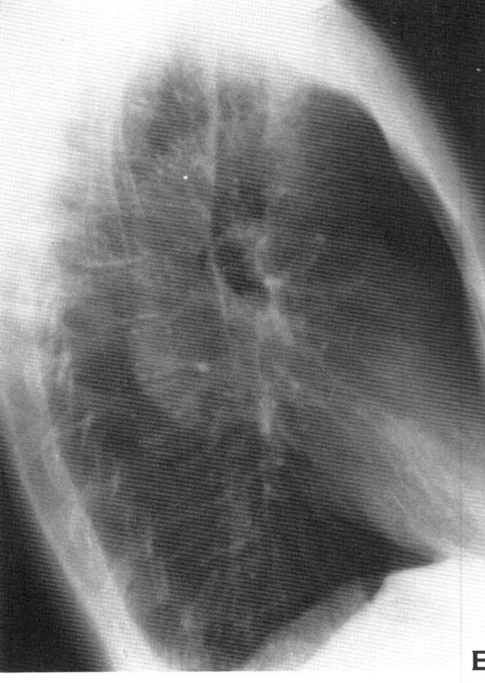

Fig. 27.31 Aneurysm of the descending thoracic aorta. (A) Frontal and (B) lateral chest films show a prominent bulge of the midportion of the descending thoracic aorta. The ascending aorta, aortic arch, and heart are normal.

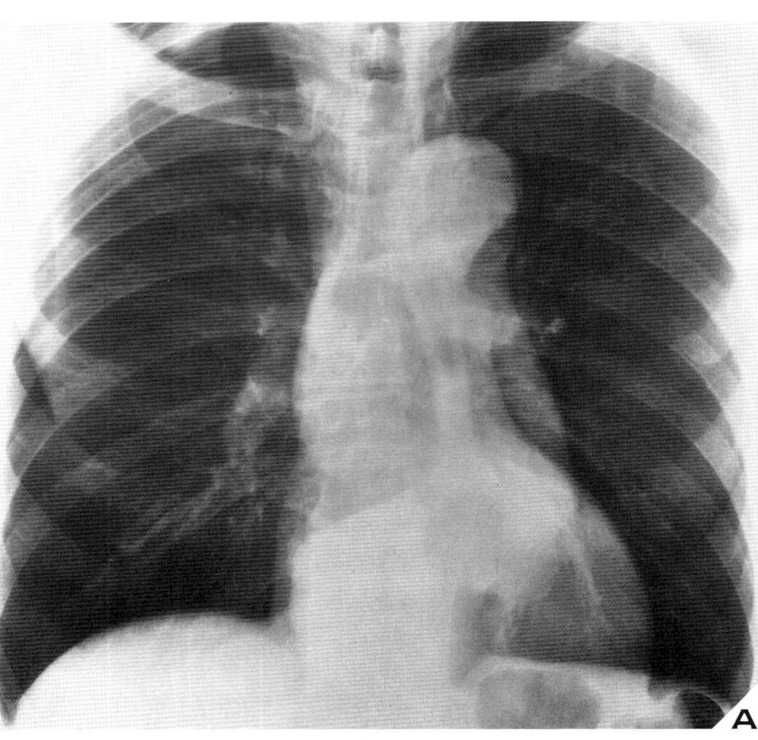

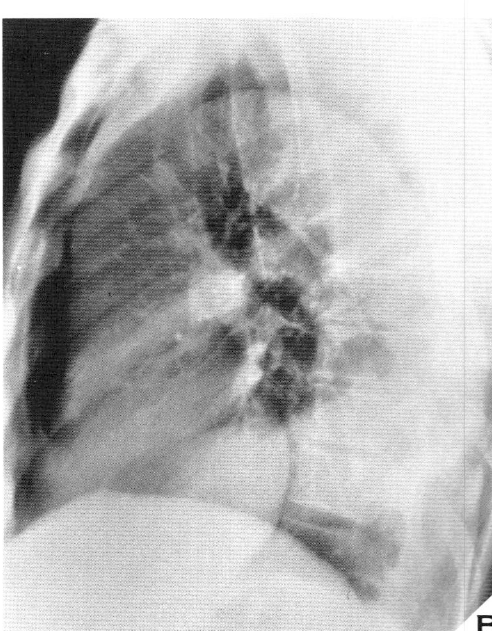

Fig. 27.32 Tortuous aorta. (A) Frontal and (B) lateral chest films show deformity of the entire descending thoracic aorta, with marked angulation at several levels. Although the aorta is very tortuous, its borders remain parallel, excluding an aneurysm. Compare with Fig. 27.33.

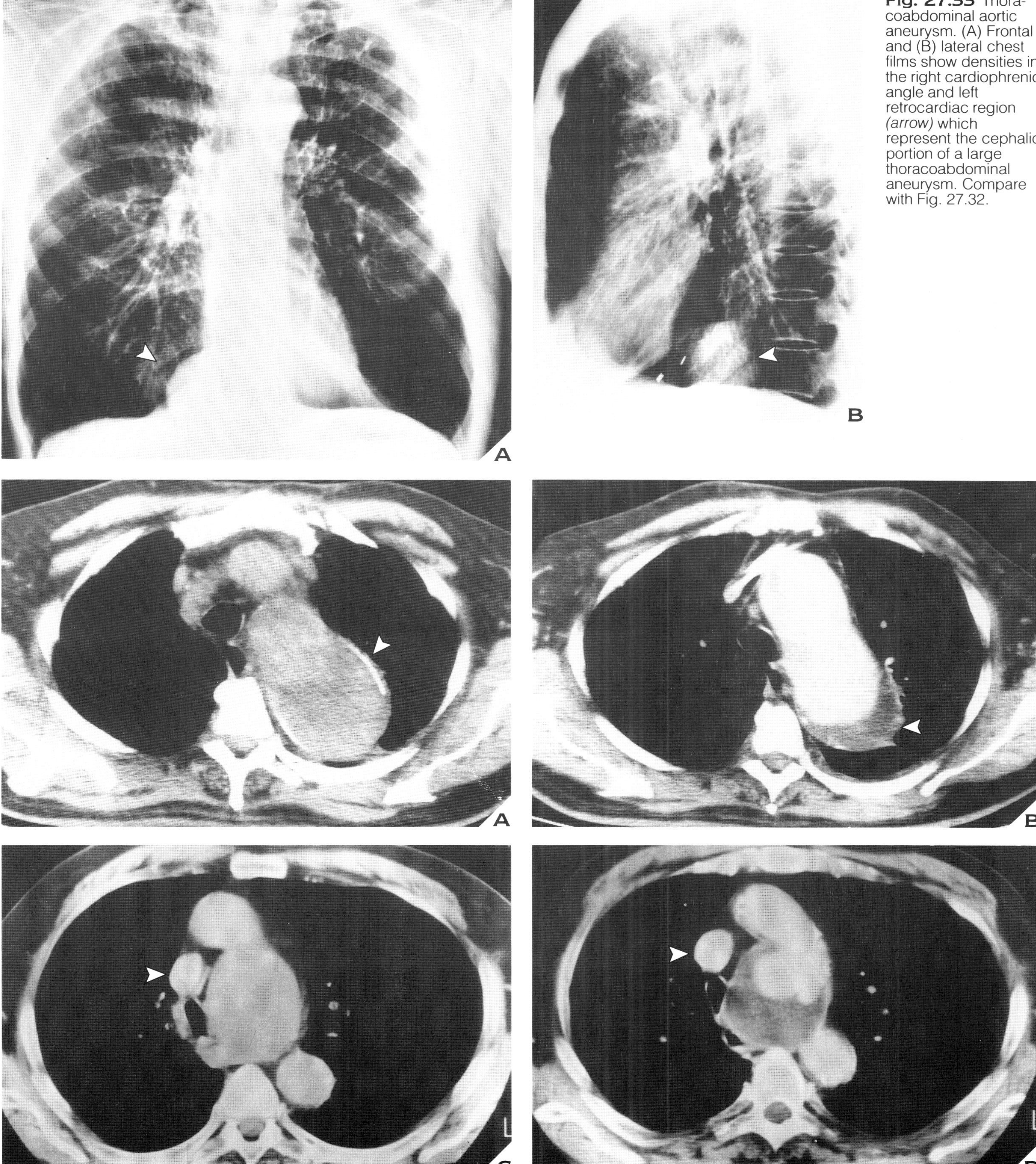

Fig. 27.33 Thoracoabdominal aortic aneurysm. (A) Frontal and (B) lateral chest films show densities in the right cardiophrenic angle and left retrocardiac region *(arrow)* which represent the cephalic portion of a large thoracoabdominal aneurysm. Compare with Fig. 27.32.

Fig. 27.34 True and false aneurysms of aortic arch (CT findings) in two patients. (A, B) True aneurysm; the unenhanced scan (A) demonstrates a calcified aneurysm measuring 7 cm in diameter *(arrows)* arising from the distal aortic arch. Contrast enhancement reveals a filling defect *(arrows)* in the left posterior portion of the aneurysm which represents mural thrombus. Note broad connection with the aortic lumen, indicating that this is a true aneurysm. (C, D) Pseudoaneurysm; in another patient, unenhanced (C) and enhanced (D) scans demonstrate a calcified aneurysm arising from the inferior aspect of the arch. The aneurysm has expanded inferiorly and to the right, compressing the right pulmonary artery (*arrow*). The narrow neck and saccular distal expansion are characteristic features of a pseudoaneurysm.

Enlargement of the descending thoracic aorta to the size of the ascending aorta indicates that an aneurysm is present (Fig. 27.35).

Rupture of an aneurysm with surrounding hematoma is also well visualized by CT. In such cases the aorta appears to be surrounded by an area of low density (Fig. 27.36). CT accurately differentiates aneurysms from pseudo-aneurysms, an important distinction in patients who have undergone aortic repair (Fig. 27.37). The major limitations of CT in the assessment of aortic aneurysms are its inability to demonstrate aortic valvular insufficiency and to identify abnormalities of the coronary arteries.

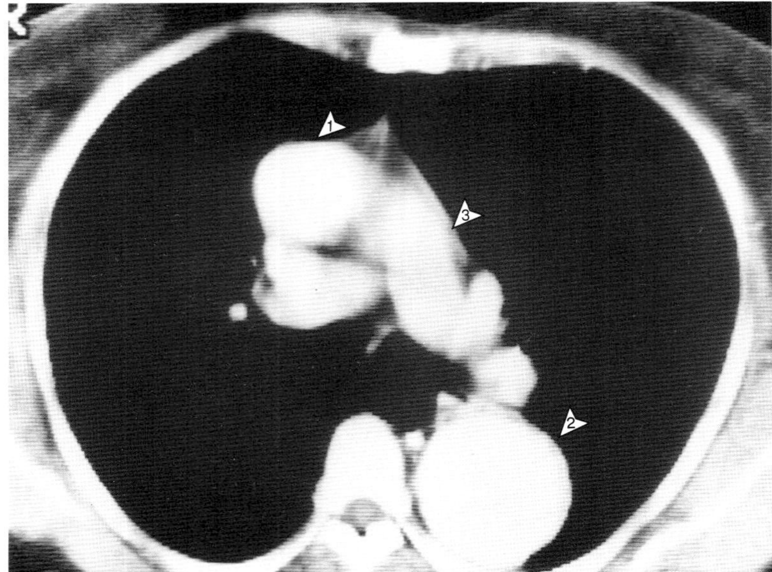

Fig. 27.35 Aneurysm of descending thoracic aorta (CT findings). A section at the level of the midportion of the ascending aorta shows a discrepancy in size between the ascending (*arrow* 1) and descending (*arrow* 2) segments of the thoracic aorta. The latter measures 6.7 cm in diameter, which is clearly normal. (*arrow* 3 = left pulmonary artery)

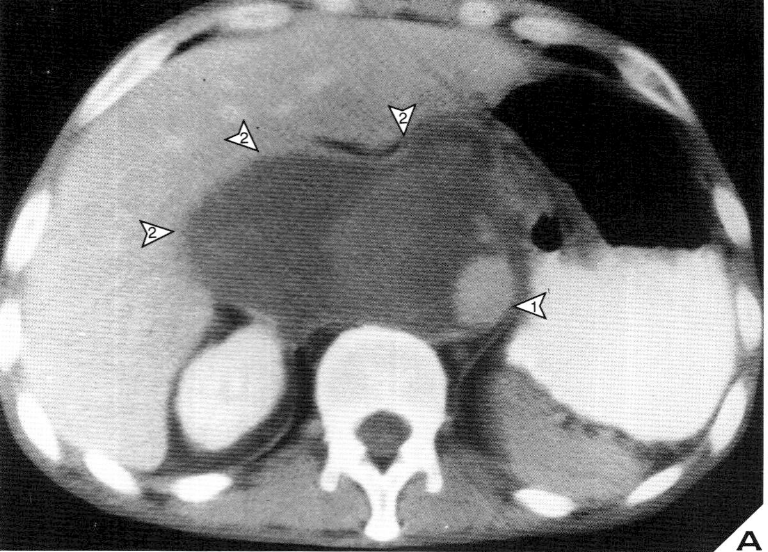

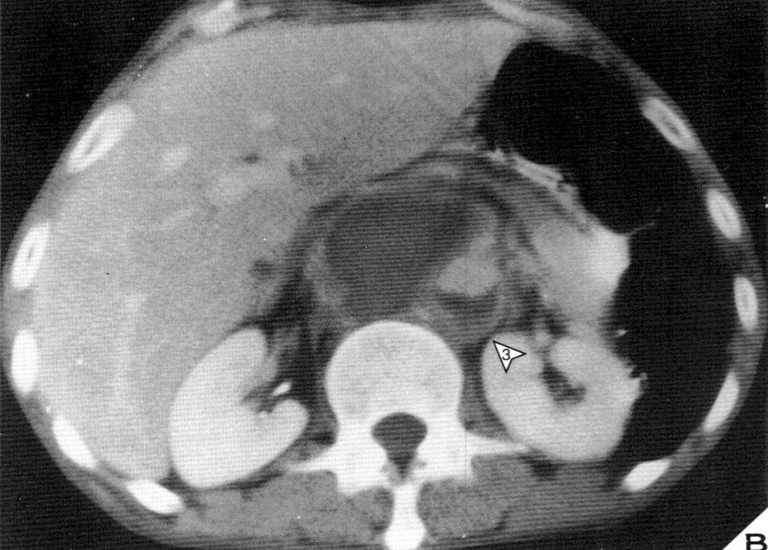

Fig. 27.36 Thoracoabdominal aortic aneurysm with rupture of the abdominal segment and periaortic hematoma (CT findings); contrast-enhanced CT scans of the upper abdomen. (A) The aorta (*arrow* 1) is displaced to the left by a large hematoma (*arrows* 2), which appears as a radiolucent space. At a more caudal level (B), the periaortic hematoma is smaller. The aneurysm appears as a bulge of the posterior portion of the aorta; the filling defect (*arrow* 3) represents mural thrombus within the aneurysm.

MAGNETIC RESONANCE IMAGING

MRI is comparable in accuracy to CT for detection and characterization of aortic aneurysms. Tranverse sections at different levels from the aortic arch to the diaphragm demonstrate the location of the aneurysm, its extent, and the involvement of arterial branches arising from it. Owing to the negative image of the circulating blood, it is possible to image the entire aorta on spin–echo images, which can be obtained in both coronal and parasagittal planes. It is thus possible to identify the origin of arteries arising at the level of the aneurysm. In asymptomatic or mildly symptomatic chronic aneurysms the pathologic alterations are accurately depicted. A limitation of MRI is its inability to demonstrate calcification. Unlike CT, however, MRI can demonstrate aortic valvular regurgitation; the use of a gradient refocused echo sequence (cine MRI) enables assessment of the severity of the aortic insufficiency and evaluation of the size and contractility of the left ventricle.

ECHOCARDIOGRAPHY

Echocardiographic diagnosis of aortic aneurysm is based on the demonstration of a dilated aorta. Using either the transthoracic or the transesophageal approach, it is possible to visualize any segment of the aorta and to determine the size and extent of the aneurysm and whether any major arterial branches are involved. The size of the aneurysm is measured and compared with the aortic diameter normally expected for the patient's

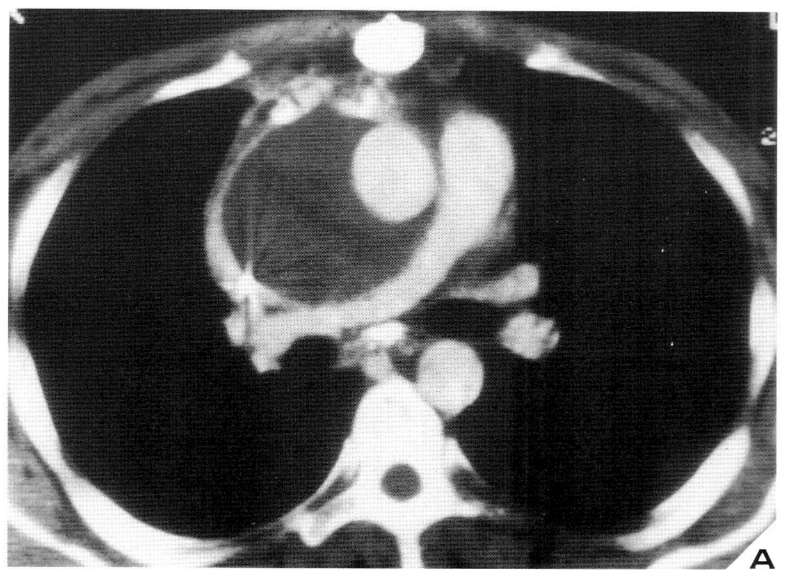

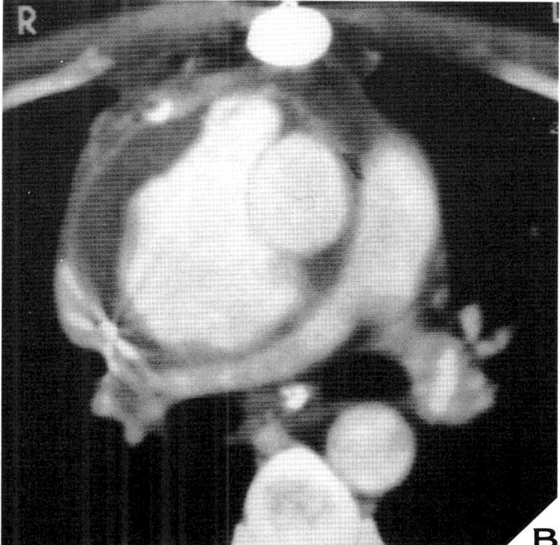

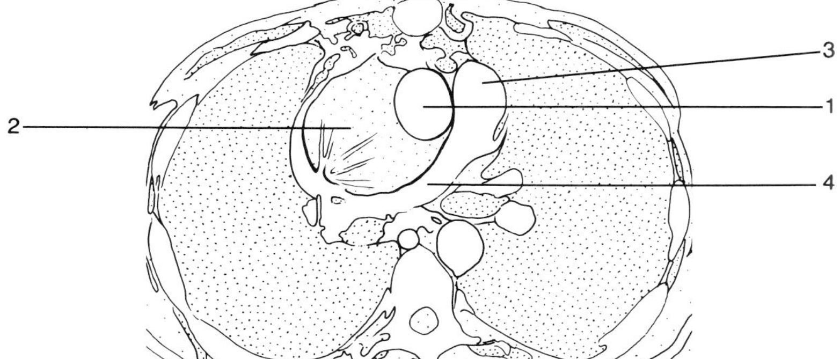

1 prosthetic tube in ascending aorta
2 false aneurysm of ascending aorta
3 pulmonary trunk
4 right pulmonary artery

Fig. 27.37 False aneurysm of the ascending aorta (CT findings). This patient developed recurrent symptoms several months after an aneurysm repair employing a conduit. (A) Contrast-enhanced CT scan obtained a few days later demonstrates the prosthetic tube surrounded by a hematoma (B) On repeat study, obtained several months after A, the area adjacent to the conduit is opacified by extravasated contrast material fills. Aortography (not illustrated) revealed a leak at the distal suture line with formation of a false aneurysm.

age. Ascending aortic aneurysms may or may not involve the aortic annulus in the same way as annular aortic ectasia (Fig. 27.38). Aneurysms of the aortic arch (Fig. 27.39; Fig. 27.40, Appendix; Fig. 27.41) and of the descending thoracic aorta (Fig. 27.42, Appendix) are accurately detected by transesophageal echocardiography.

Echocardiography also provides information about the function of the aortic valve and the performance of the left ventricle. With Doppler-image flow mapping, it is possible to evaluate the blood flow through the aneurysm as well as the patency of the arteries arising from it. (This analysis is facilitated by color Doppler imaging.) In most cases bi-directional flow can be identified; the reverse flow is usually confined to late systole or early diastole. Bi-directional flow has been attributed to the presence of eddy currents in the markedly dilatated vessel; the reversal of flow in mid-diastole indicates the presence of aortic regurgitation. Calcification and thrombosis of the aneurysm can also be identified by echocardiography.

ANGIOGRAPHY

Aortography is highly accurate in detecting aortic aneurysm. It is desirable to selectively opacify the entire segment in ques-

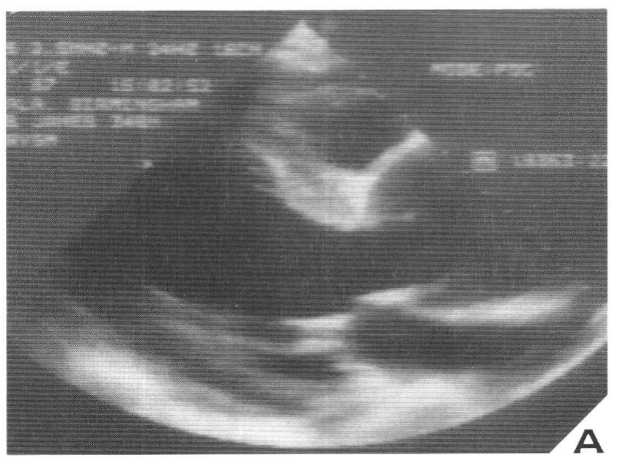

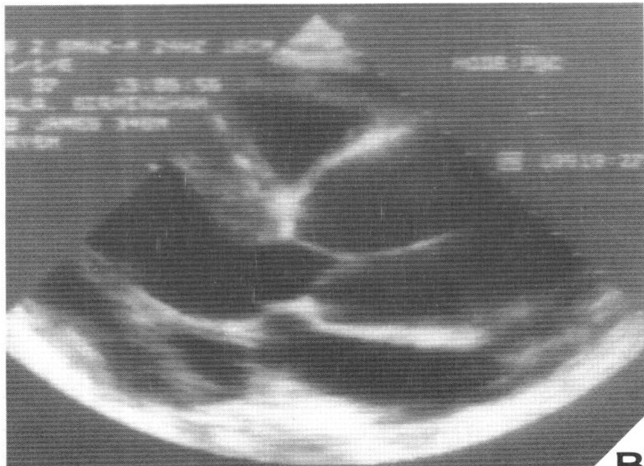

Fig. 27.38 Aortic root aneurysm (echocardiographic findings). Parasternal long axial views in (A) systole and (B) diastole demonstrate marked dilatation of the ascending aorta, including the aortic valve annulus. The sinuses of Valsalva are also enlarged. The aneurysm measures 8 cm in transverse diameter. Color Doppler images (not illustrated) demonstrated significant aortic insufficiency.

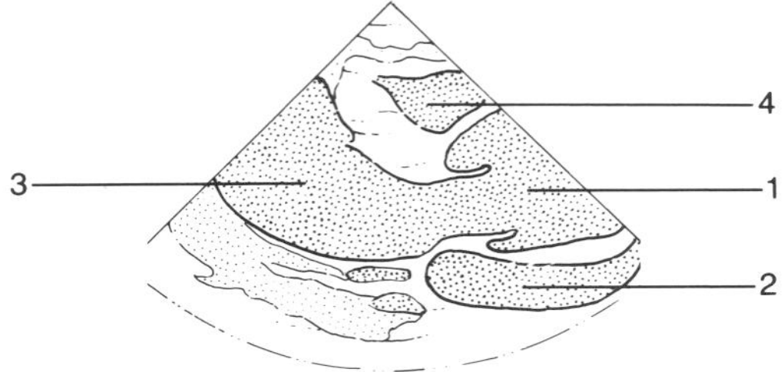

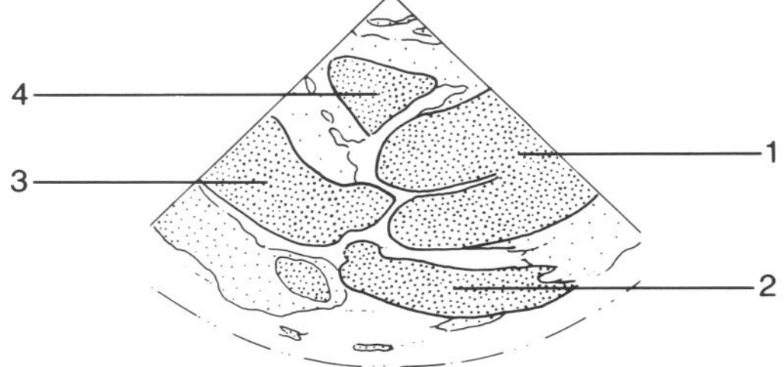

1 ascending aorta
2 left atrium
3 left ventricle
4 right ventricular outflow tract

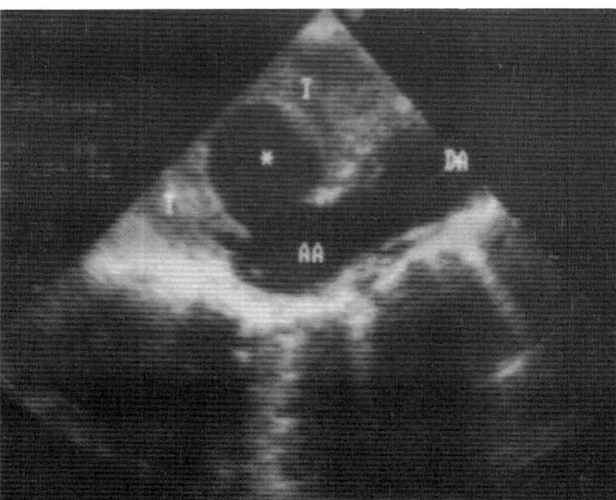

Fig. 27.39 Aortic arch aneurysm (echocardiographic findings). Transesophageal scan of aortic arch demonstrates a large aneurysm of the aortic arch that contains mural thrombus. The proximal segment of the descending thoracic aorta, included in the section, appears normal.

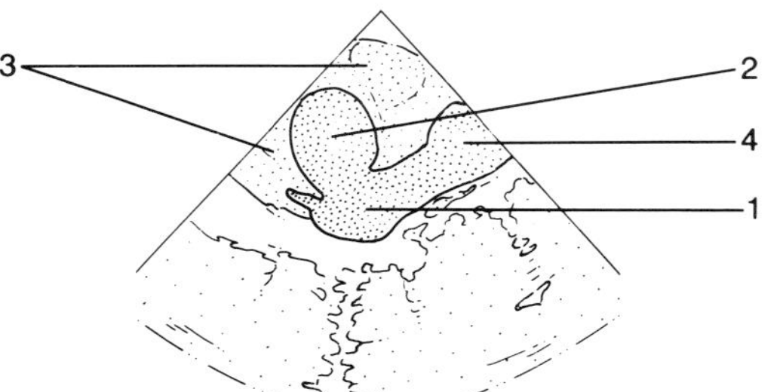

1 aortic arch
2 aneurysm
3 mural thrombus
4 normal descending thoracic aorta

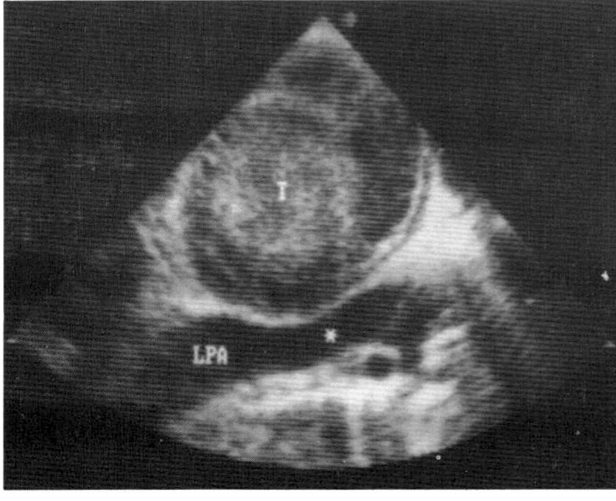

Fig. 27.41 Aortic arch aneurysm (echocardiographic findings). Transesophageal echocardiogram of aortic arch demonstrates a large aneurysm which is completely filled with thrombus (T). Note compression (*) of the left pulmonary artery (LPA) by the aneurysm.

tion. The projection and the site of injection depend on the location of the aneurysm. Either 35-mm cineangiography or the large (cut film) format can be employed.

Frontal and lateral views are optimal for demonstrating aneurysms of the ascending aorta. Left anterior oblique and right anterior oblique views can be employed when the aorta is displaced from its normal position.

Ascending aortic aneurysms are characterized by dilatation of the ascending aorta immediately above the sinuses of Valsalva (Fig. 27.43). When aortic ectasia is present, the dilatation involves the annulus of the aortic valve, and the sinuses of Valsalva appear enlarged (Fig. 27.44). The degree of aortic insufficiency is graded according to the amount of contrast material that refluxes from the aorta into the left ventricle. In patients with classical Marfan syndrome, the aortic aneurysm extends cephalad but does not reach the aortic arch. Thrombus is rarely seen in this type of aneurysm, but may appear as a filling defect in the lumen.

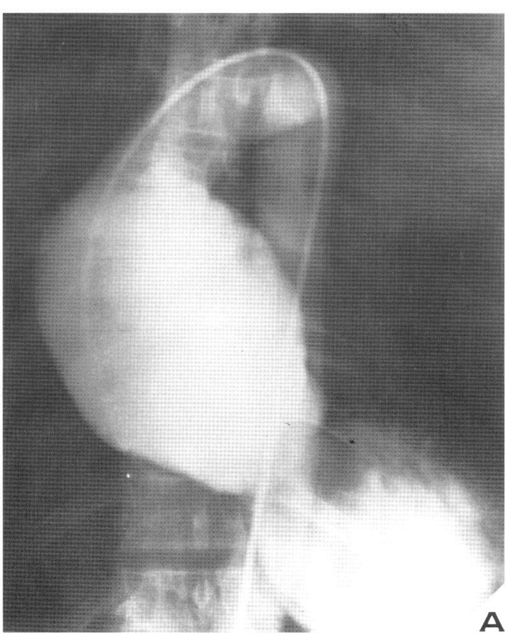

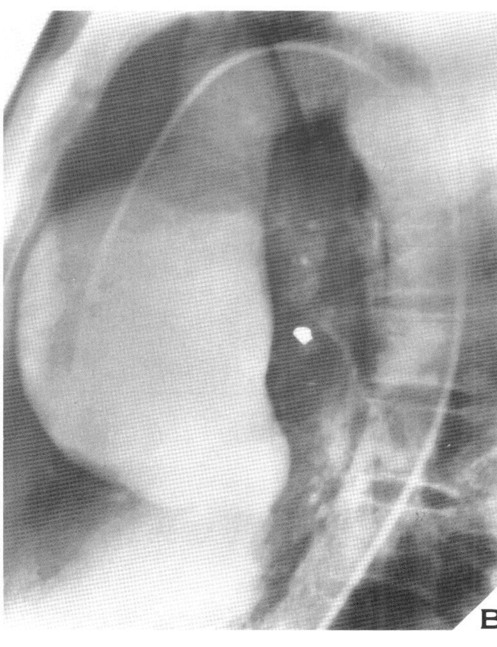

Fig. 27.43 Aortic root aneurysm (angiographic findings). (A) Frontal and (B) lateral projections of thoracic aortogram demonstrate marked dilatation of the aortic root, which extends upward but ends below the origin of the innominate artery. The direction of expansion, ie, mainly to the right and anteriorly, is characteristic of arteriosclerotic aneurysms. Although the aortic annulus is only slightly widened, there is significant aortic insufficiency.

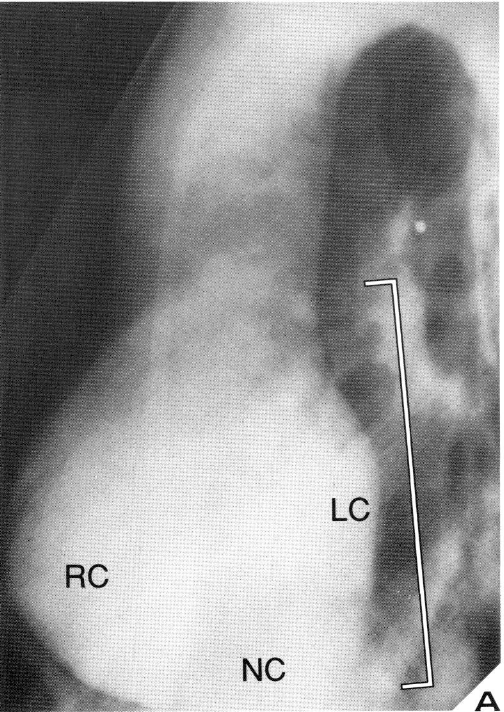

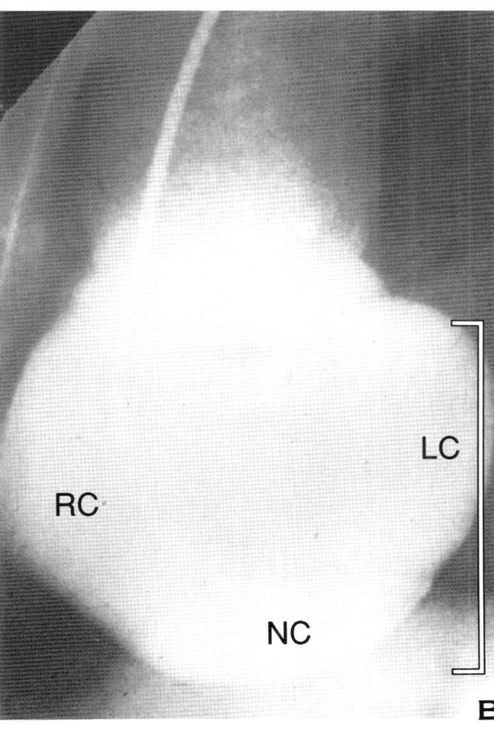

Fig. 27.44 Aortic aneurysm associated with annulo-ectasia (angiographic findings); lateral projections of thoracic aortograms in two different patients. (A) In this patient, the aortogram demonstrates a large aneurysm of the aortic root with massive enlargement of the sinuses of Valsalva. The aneurysm *(brace)* involves a short segment of the ascending aorta. (B) In this patient the aneurysm *(brace)* is almost entirely limited to the sinuses of Valsalva, almost completely sparing the ascending aorta. Although the sinuses of Valsalva are markedly dilated, there is only minimal aortic insufficiency. (RC = right coronary cusp; LC = left coronary cusp; NC = noncoronary cusp)

Aortic arch aneurysms are well visualized in the lateral and in the left anterior oblique projection, especially the latter, which tends to "open up" the aorta (Fig. 27.45). The aneurysm often arises from the concave aspect of the arch, extends downward, and may compress the pulmonary artery or other mediastinal structures. When the aneurysm arises from the convex aspect it usually involves the origin of one or more branches of the aortic arch. Most aneurysms of the aortic arch actually represent posttraumatic pseudo-aneurysms (Fig. 27.46). Calcification in the wall of the aneurysm, as well as thrombus within the aneurysmal sac, are common observations in such cases. Aneurysms of the descending thoracic aorta are well demonstrated in the left anterior oblique projection (Fig. 27.47) or in lateral projections (Fig. 27.48). These aneurysms are usually localized and saccular, but they may also be fusiform. Arteriosclerotic plaques, some of which may be ulcerated (Fig. 27.47), are commonly seen. Thrombus in the aneurysmal sac is usually easily identified. As a complementary study, coronary angiography is performed to detect associated coronary artery stenosis.

In summary, the diagnosis of aortic aneurysm can be suspected on the basis of history and physical examination. Plain chest films often demonstrate localized dilatation of the aorta. Angiography confirms the diagnosis and provides the information needed to plan treatment. Echocardiography, MRI, and CT are valuable noninvasive methods; however, each has significant limitations. All three modalities can be used to follow the progress of patients undergoing medical or surgical therapy.

INFLAMMATORY DISORDERS

TAKAYASU'S ARTERITIS

PATHOLOGY

Takayasu's arteritis is an inflammatory process of unknown etiology which mainly affects the aorta and its major branches. Large and medium-sized pulmonary arteries are also commonly affected. The initial lesion consists of intimal proliferation and degeneration of the elastic fibers of the media, accompanied by varying degrees of round-cell infiltration. The late (cicatricial) phase is characterized by marked stenosis of the affected arteries, which may progress to obliteration. Not infrequently, a dilated segment is interposed between two narrowed ones. Discrete aneurysms can occur, although they are relatively infrequent.

CLINICAL FEATURES

In its early stages, Takayasu's arteritis is characterized by systemic symptoms including fever, anorexia, malaise, weight loss, night sweats, fatigue, and pain. Late manifestations vary depending on the site (or sites) of involvement. In one large series of patients with Takayasu's arteritis, absent pulses were observed in 96 percent, systemic hypertension in 74 percent, and congestive heart failure in 24 percent (Lupi–Herrera, 1977). Retinopathy is present in only 25 percent. Takayasu's arteritis usually occurs in teenagers and young adults. There is a very strong female predilection (sex ratio 8.5:1).

There are three varieties of Takayasu's arteritis, classified according to the distribution of the arterial lesions. Type I, the most common variety, affects the ascending aorta and aortic arch and their branches (including the coronary arteries). Type II, which is less common, affects the abdominal aorta and its branches, the renal arteries in particular. Type III, the least common variety, affects the entire aorta. Stenosis or obliteration of pulmonary arteries is present in approximately 50 percent of patients with Takayasu's arteritis, often leading to pulmonary hypertension.

In patients with type I disease, physical examination typically reveals absent pulses or diminished blood pressure in the upper extremities and normal or near normal pulses and blood pressure in the lower extremities *(reverse coarctation sign)*. When the coronary arteries are affected, the initial signs are those of ischemic heart disease. Patients with Type II disease typically present with systemic hypertension secondary to renal artery involvement; longstanding hypertension may lead to congestive heart failure.

IMAGING AND INVASIVE DIAGNOSIS

Chest Films

There are no characteristic radiographic findings in the early stages of the disease. In the chronic (cicatricial) stage, calcification of the aorta and brachiocephalic arteries can often be detected on plain films; the arterial calcification may be extensive

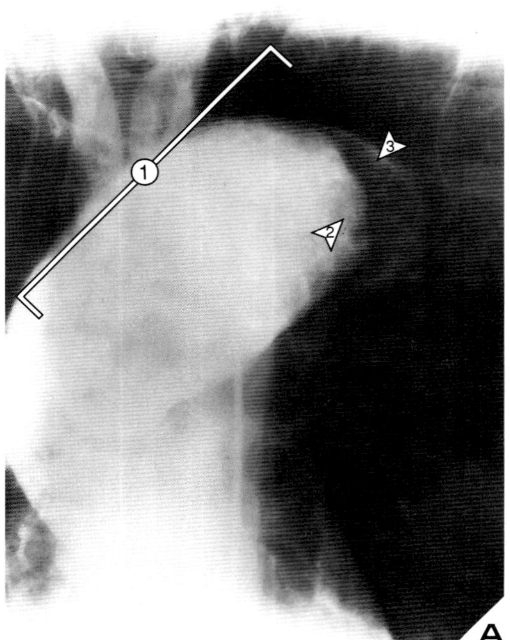

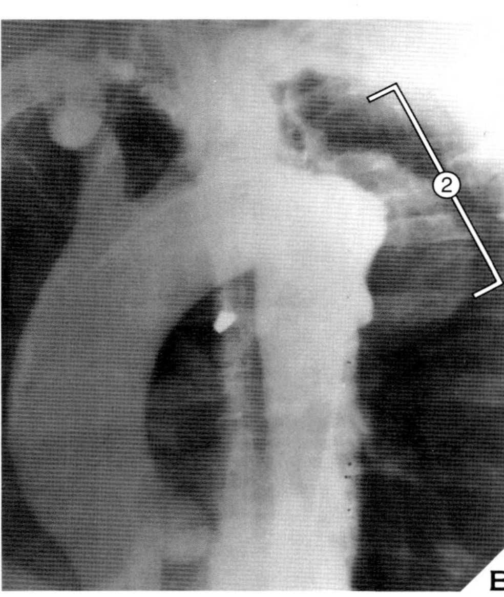

Fig. 27.45 Saccular aortic arch aneurysm (angiographic findings). Thoracic aortograms in two different patients. (A) Frontal projection of the first patient demonstrates an aneurysm (*brace* 1) involving the entire aortic arch. Note the small mural thrombus (*arrow* 2) between the opacified lumen and the calcified wall of the aneurysm (*arrow* 3). (B) In the second patient, the left anterior oblique projection demonstrates an aneurysm *(brace 2)* containing a large mural thrombus. The diameter of the aneurysm is approximately the same as that of the aorta itself. Note the irregular contour of the aorta in the area bordering the thrombus.

(Fig. 27.49) or subtle. (Even minimal arterial calcification should suggest the diagnosis in a teenager or young adult.) Patients with pulmonary arterial hypertension secondary to Takayasu's arteritis have plain film findings similar to those of primary pulmonary hypertension (see Chapter 24); the central and peripheral branches are decreased in size, sometimes asymmetrically (Fig. 27.49).

Echocardiography

Conventional two-dimensional echocardiography reliably detects narrowing of the thoracic aorta and the brachiocephalic branches. Color Doppler imaging reveals increased flow velocity in the affected arterial segments.

MRI

Spin–echo images demonstrate narrowing of the aorta and its branches. T2-weighted pulse sequences may demonstrate increased signal in the vessel walls in the acute and subacute stages of the disease. Cine MRI demonstrates turbulent flow in the stenotic segments.

Cardiac Catheterization

Right heart catheterization demonstrates typical findings of pulmonary hypertension (eg, right ventricular failure, secondary tricuspid insufficiency) in patients with severe involvement of the pulmonary trunk and its branches; the pressure gradient across the stenosis can be measured by selective catheteriza-

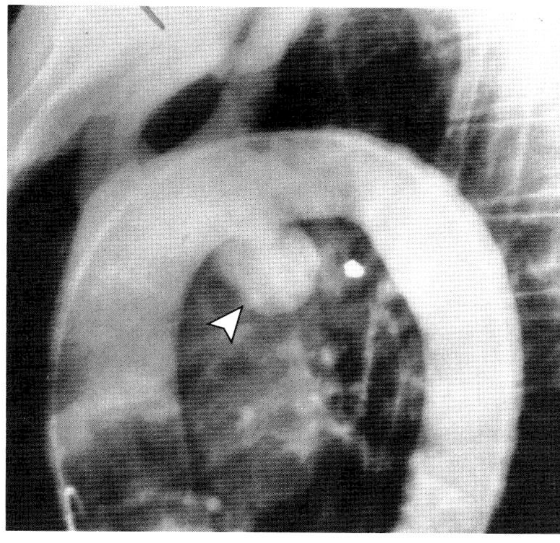

Fig. 27.46 False aneurysm of aortic arch (angiographic findings). Lateral projection of thoracic aortogram demonstrates a 3.5 cm collection of contrast material *(arrow)* extending beyond the inferior wall of the aortic arch, which has a smaller caliber than normal. The relatively narrow connection with the aortic lumen is typical of false aneurysms. The "wall" of a false aneurysm typically consists of fibrous tissue and organized thrombus.

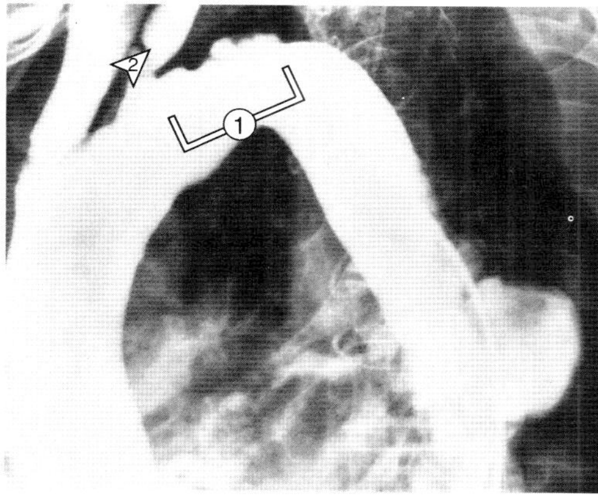

Fig. 27.47 Saccular aneurysm of the descending thoracic aorta (angiographic findings). Left anterior oblique projection of thoracic aortogram demonstrates an aneurysm of the posterior wall of mid-descending aorta. The filling defect in its cephalic portion represents mural thrombus. The marginal irregularities in the distal aortic arch (*brace* 1) most likely represent ulcerations within arteriosclerotic plaque. (*arrow* 2 = left subclavian artery)

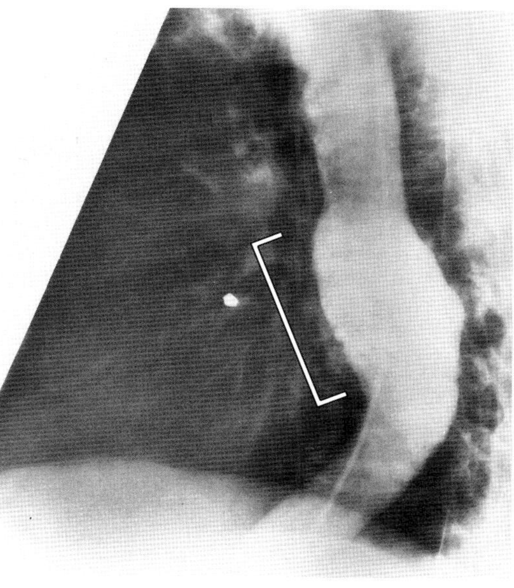

Fig. 27.48 Fusiform aneurysm of descending thoracic aorta (angiographic findings). Lateral projection of thoracic aortogram demonstrates a 4 cm aneurysm *(brace)* of the middle portion of the descending thoracic aorta. The borders of the dilated segment are uniform, indicating absence of thrombus. The configuration is typical of an arteriosclerotic aneurysm.

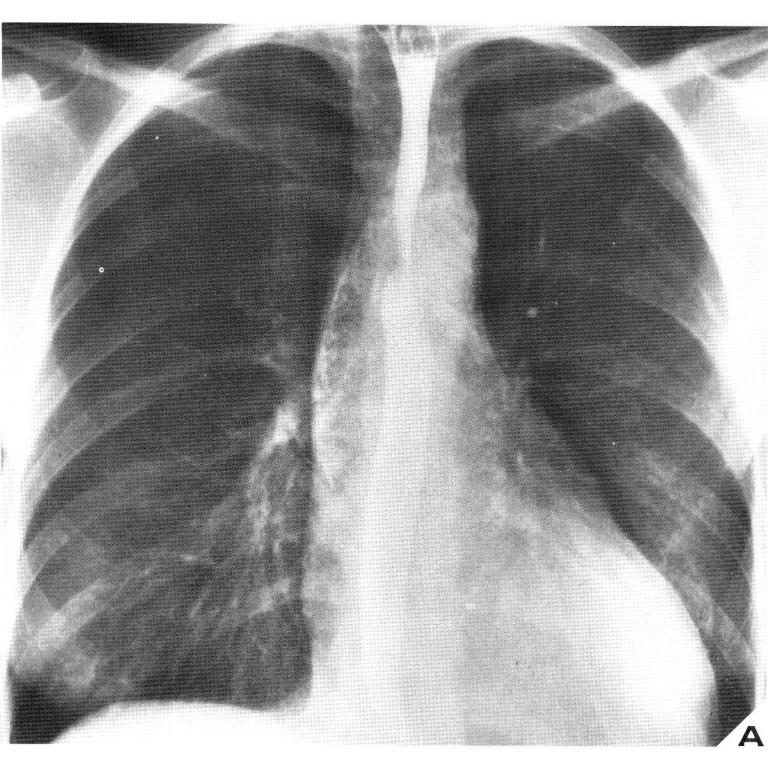

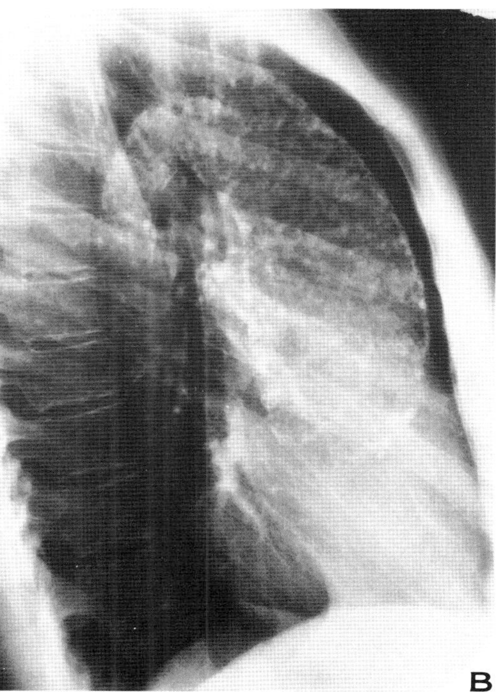

Fig. 27.49 Takayasu's arteritis. (A) Frontal and (B) lateral chest films of a 25-year-old woman demonstrate extensive calcification of the ascending aorta, aortic arch, and upper descending thoracic aorta. The innominate and right common carotid arteries are also calcified. The ascending aorta is dilated but the aortic arch and proximal descending thoracic aorts are decreased in caliber. The left pulmonary artery is smaller than the right and has fewer peripheral branches, indicating stenosis of the left pulmonary artery. There is cardiomegaly with left ventricular enlargment.

tion of the affected vessel. In similar fashion, the pressure gradients across a stenotic segment of the aorta or systemic artery can be measured at the time of aortography.

Angiography

Angiography is the method of choice for documenting the severity and extent of arterial narrowing. Involvement of the thoracic aorta and its branches, including the coronary arteries, is demonstrated by thoracic aortography in the left anterior oblique projection (Fig. 27.50). Typically, there is diffuse smooth narrowing of the affected arteries, with or without poststenotic dilatation. Narrowing of the distal aortic arch with preservation of the ascending aorta and proximal arch—the so-called *rat-tail sign*—is a common finding (see Fig. 27.49B). In some instances, it may be necessary to selectively opacify individual branches to fully document the extent of involvement (Figs. 27.51 and 27.52).

GIANT-CELL ARTERITIS

Giant-cell arteritis is an inflammatory process that involves the media of small- and medium-sized arteries, usually affecting arteries of the extremities and of the head and neck. Involvement of the ascending aorta, which is affected in about 15 percent of reported cases, may lead to aneurysm, dissection, or aortic insufficiency.

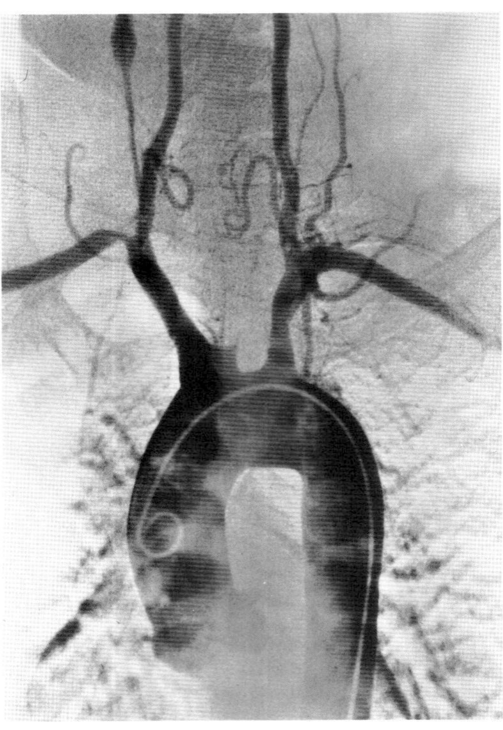

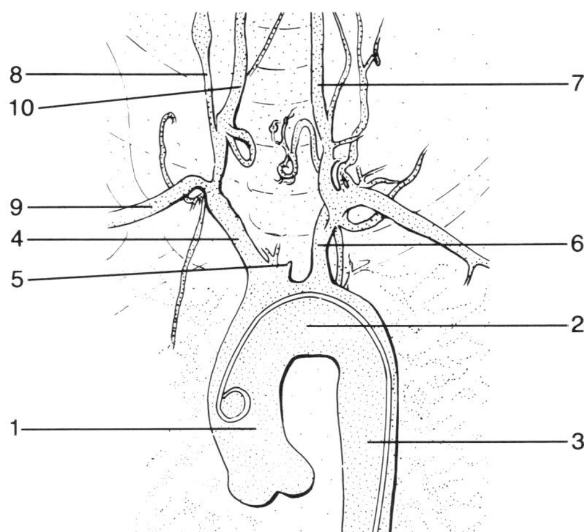

Fig. 27.50 Takayasu's arteritis involving the branches of the aortic arch (angiographic findings). Left anterior oblique projection of thoracic aortogram. The ascending aorta, aortic arch, and descending thoracic aorta are normal. There is a diffuse tubular stenosis of the proximal portion of the right common carotid artery. [Although the distal portion of this artery appears normal on the aortogram, a selective arteriogram (not illustrated) demonstrated mild stenosis.] There is localized stenosis at the takeoff of the right subclavian artery, and the left common carotid artery is occluded at its origin. The left subclavian and left vertebral arteries appear normal.

1 ascending aorta
2 aortic arch
3 descending thoracic aorta
4 right innominate artery
5 occluded left common carotid artery
6 left subclavian artery
7 left vertebral artery
8 right common carotid artery
9 right subclavian artery
10 right vertebral artery

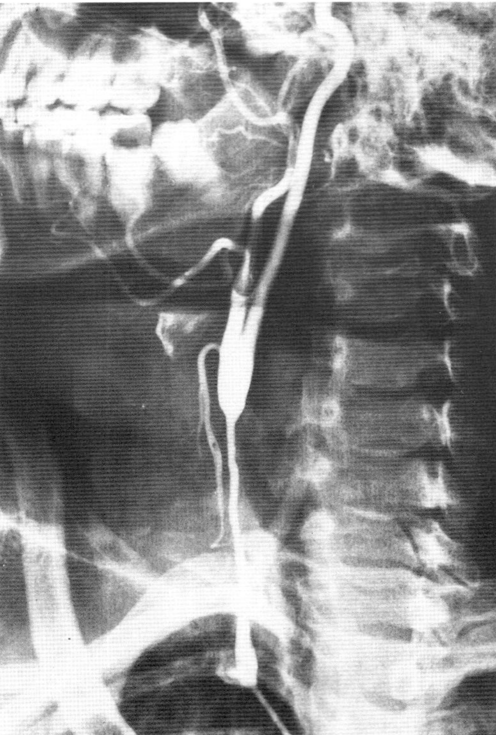

Fig. 27.51 Takayasu's arteritis involving the right common carotid artery (angiographic findings). Selective common carotid arteriogram (right anterior oblique projection) demonstrates tubular stenosis of the entire vessel. The internal and external carotid arteries are normal.

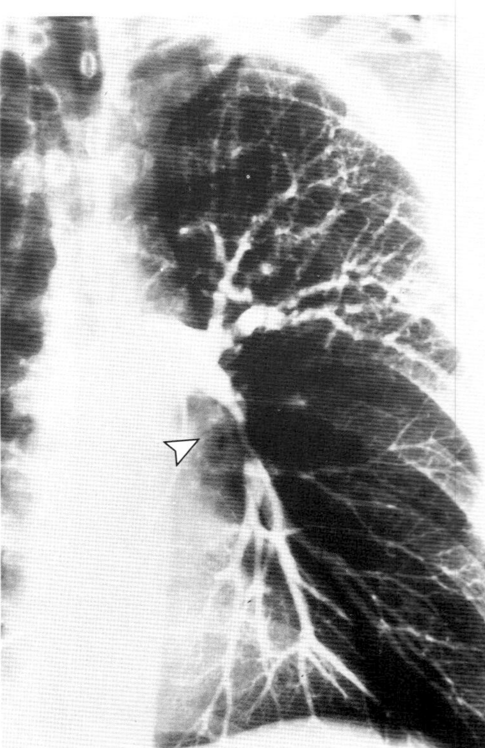

Fig. 27.52 Takayasu's arteritis involving pulmonary artery (angiographic findings). Frontal projection of selective left pulmonary arteriogram demonstrates severe segmental stenosis *(arrow)* of the branch supplying the left lower lobe. The narrowing is produced by a localized thickening of the arterial wall. Note the absence of filling defects in the lumen of the affected artery.

Giant-cell arteritis is almost exclusively a disorder of the elderly, occurring with equal frequency in both sexes. In the acute phase, the clinical picture can resemble that of Takayasu's arteritis. The patient typically presents with systemic signs (malaise, fever, headache); many patients complain of diffuse muscle aching and stiffness (''polymyalgia rheumatica''). The erythrocyte sedimentation rate is often markedly elevated. The diagnosis is usually established by biopsy of the superficial temporal artery, which is almost always involved.

Angiography demonstrates multiple segmental areas of involvement in the affected vessels. Although the disease is usually self-limited and responds dramatically to corticosteroid therapy, there may be residual narrowing of the affected vessels.

OTHER TYPES OF ARTERITIS AFFECTING THE AORTA

Arteritis, sometimes affecting the aorta and its branches, is not uncommon in patients with ankylosing spondylitis, psoriatic arthritis, ulcerative colitis, relapsing polychondritis, and Reiter's syndrome.

CHAPTER 28

Trauma to the Heart and Great Vessels

Injuries of the heart and great vessels can result from either penetrating or nonpenetrating trauma; whereas the former is usually recognized and treated promptly, the latter may be less obvious, leading to delay in diagnosis and treatment. The heart and great vessels can also be injured in the course of diagnostic and therapeutic interventions, eg, cardiac catheterization and transluminal angioplasty.

AORTIC INJURIES

NONPENETRATING INJURIES

PATHOGENESIS

Traumatic rupture of the aorta is a common sequela of deceleration injuries. Sudden deceleration in the anteroposterior plane typically causes rupture of the segment immediately distal to the origin of the ligamentum arteriosum, the aortic isthmus. The predilection for this site is explained by the difference in deceleration rates between the relatively immobile aortic arch, held in place by the great arteries and the ligamentum arteriosum, and the descending thoracic aorta, which is essentially free of attachments (Fig. 28.1) Aortic injuries resulting from other mechanisms usually do not involve the isthmus. Blunt trauma generates rotational forces that typically lead to rupture of the ascending aorta (Fig. 28.2). A fall from a great height generates powerful longitudinal deceleration forces which typically cause detachment of the aortic valve and/or laceration of the aortic root (Fig. 28.3).

Tears associated with deceleration injuries usually originate in the intima and extend outward, producing injuries that range in severity from localized intimal disruption to complete transection of the aorta. The great majority of patients with major aortic injuries die within minutes from exsanguination. In the survivors, a localized mediastinal hematoma compresses the lumen, preventing rapid exsanguination. Trauma victims with rupture of the ascending aorta or detachment of the aortic valve seldom survive long enough to receive definitive treatment.

CLINICAL FEATURES

Approximately 10 to 15 percent of trauma victims with nonpenetrating aortic injuries survive long enough to receive medical attention. Most patients with aortic injuries that are not immediately lethal have partial disruption or transection of the aortic isthmus. Approximately 2 to 5 percent of patients with such in-

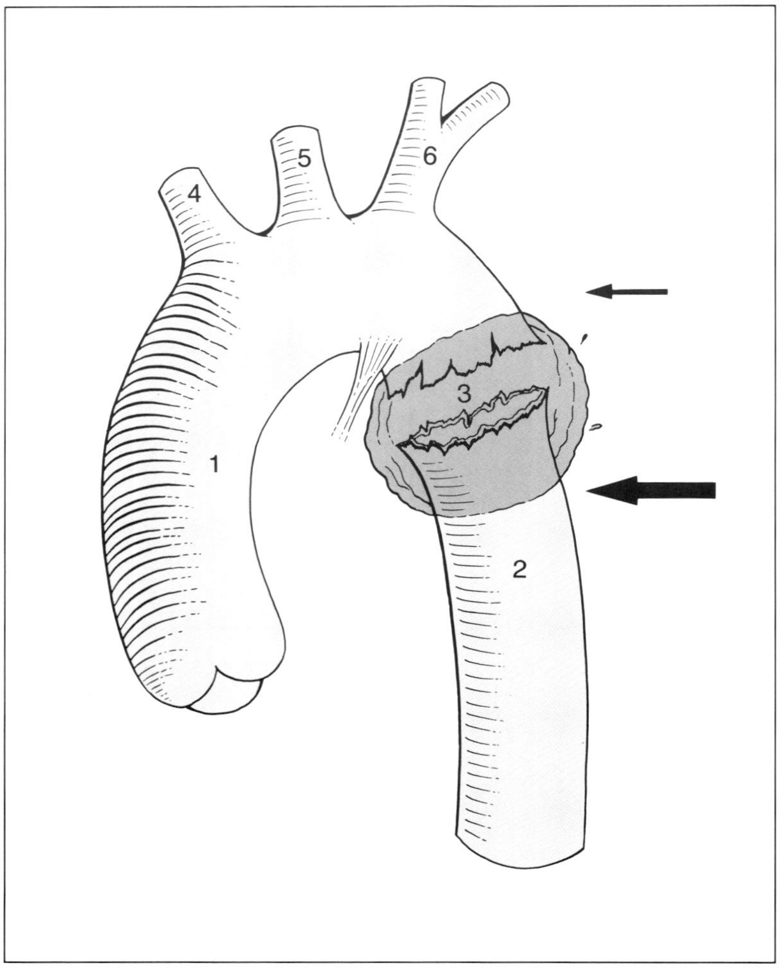

Fig. 28.1 Rupture of the aorta due to anteroposterior deceleration force. The rupture typically occurs at the aortic isthmus, ie, the short segment just distal to the ligamentum arteriosus. The difference between the deceleration rates above and below this point creates both shearing and bending stresses, resulting in partial or complete disruption of the aortic isthmus.

1 ascending aorta
2 descending aorta
3 transection with surrounding hematoma
4 innominate artery
5 left common carotid artery
6 left subclavian artery
thin arrow deceleration force above isthmus
thick arrow deceleration force below isthmus

juries survive without treatment, presenting after an interval of months or years with a chronic traumatic aortic aneurysm (see Chapter 27).

Patients with nonpenetrating aortic injuries often have other serious injuries that may divert attention from the chest. They commonly have evidence of systemic hypoperfusion (hypovolemic shock) and may appear moribund. They may complain of dyspnea, back pain, dysphagia, and/or hoarseness. Physical examination typically reveals increased pulse amplitude and blood pressure in the upper extremities and decreased pulse amplitude and blood pressure in the lower extremities. (This constellation of findings may simulate coarctation of the aorta.) A systolic or continuous murmur is sometimes audible in the infrascapular area.

IMAGING AND INVASIVE DIAGNOSIS

Plain Films

The chest film is relatively insensitive in detecting mild to moderate injuries of the aortic isthmus; it is of greater value as a screening test in patients with severe injuries. Although many radiographic signs have been described, none is pathognomonic of aortic rupture. In our experience, a combination of

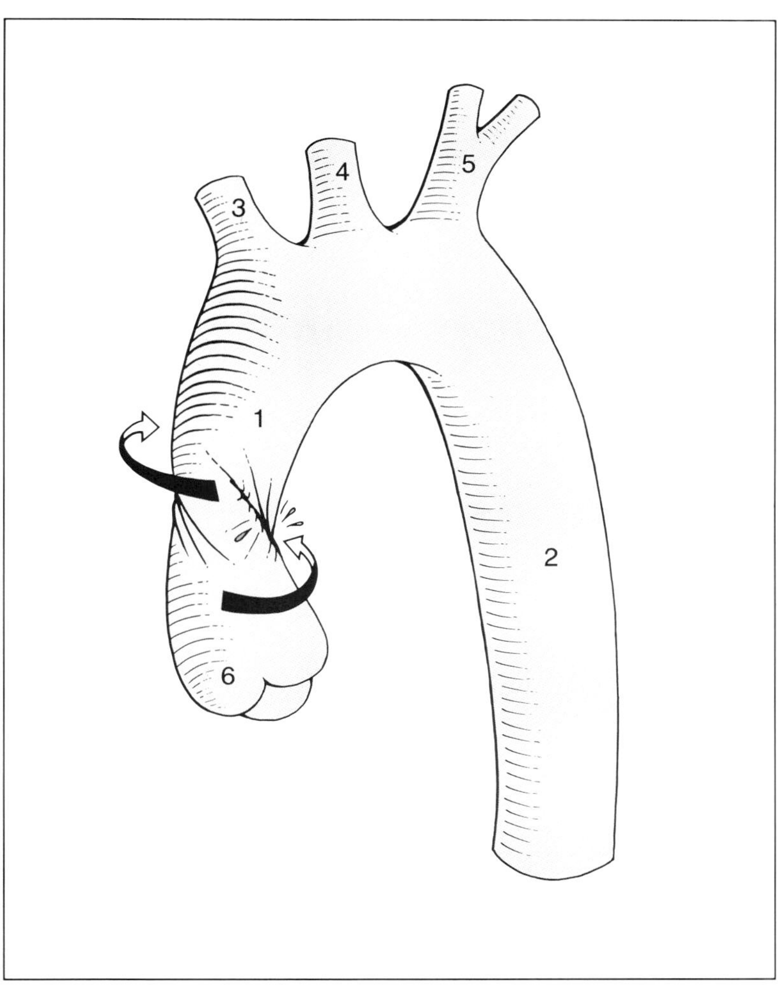

1 ascending aorta
2 descending aorta
3 innominate artery
4 left common carotid artery
5 left subclavian artery
6 aortic valve
arrow torsional force

Fig. 28.2 Rupture of the ascending aorta due to torsional force. Injuries of the ascending aorta are usually caused by blunt trauma. (Adapted with permission from Hurst J, et al: *Atlas of the Heart.* New York, London: Gower Medical Publishing, 1988:10.3)

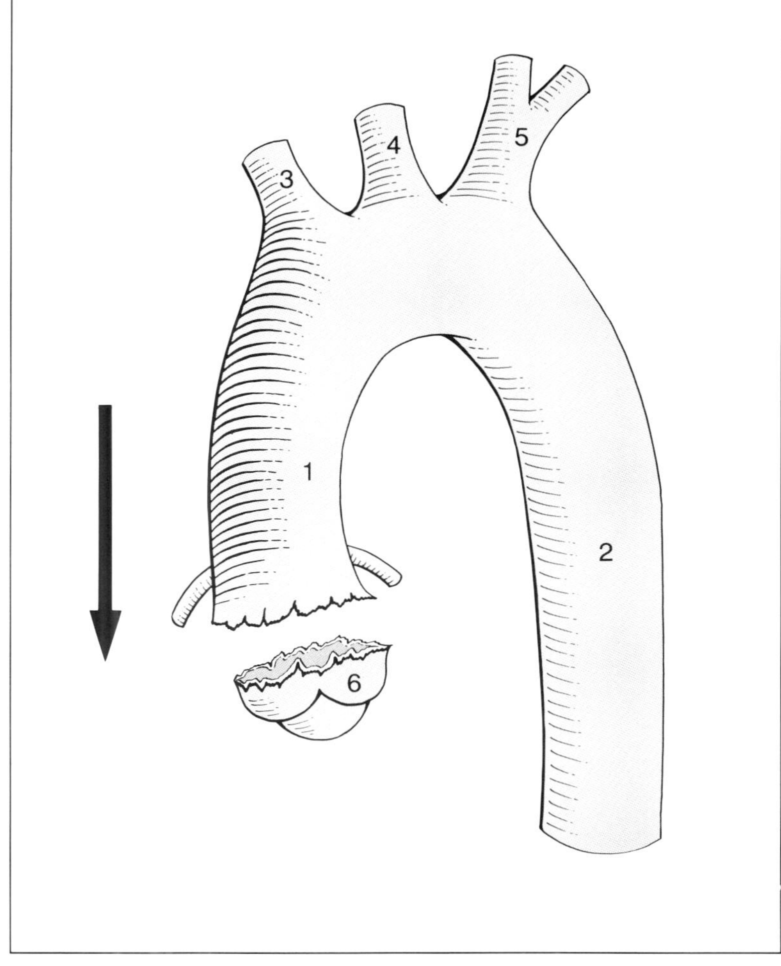

1 ascending aorta
2 descending aorta
3 innominate artery
4 left common carotid artery
5 left subclavian artery
6 aortic valve
arrow deceleration force

Fig. 28.3 Detachment of the aortic valve due to longitudinal deceleration force. Injuries of the aortic root, which result in detachment of the aortic valve, typically result from falls from a great height.

four plain film findings strongly favors this diagnosis: irregularity of the aortic contour, particularly that of the aortic arch; widening of the mediastinum; displacement of the trachea to the right with downward displacement of the left main bronchus; and widening of the left paraspinal line (Figs. 28.4 and 28.5). (Displacement of the nasogastric tube to the right, indicating displacement of the esophagus by the mediastinal hematoma, is another useful sign.) Recent studies indicate that fractures of the first and second ribs, once believed to correlate strongly with aortic trauma, are of little predictive value. Although hemothorax and pneumothorax are common in patients with major aortic injuries, they can occur with any severe thoracic injury and thus have little predictive value.

Mediastinal width cannot be accurately measured on the supine portable chest films usually obtained in patients with severe thoracic injuries; however, a mediastinal/thoracic ratio of .25 or more, as well as marked widening of the right paratracheal stripe (to 5 mm or more), indicates significant mediastinal hemorrhage and strongly favors the diagnosis of aortic rupture (Figs. 28.4 and 28.5).

Approximately 10 percent of patients with major aortic injuries have normal chest films; therefore, a normal chest film does not eliminate the need for angiography in a patient with suggestive clinical findings.

Echocardiography

Echocardiography readily demonstrates the hemopericardium associated with some aortic injuries. However, echocardiography is seldom performed in patients with acute aortic trauma, and its reliability in detecting such injuries is unknown.

Computed Tomography

Although CT accurately depicts the nonvascular injuries associated with decelerating trauma, it is far less sensitive than aortography in detecting aortic injuries. Unenhanced scans typically demonstrate a mediastinal hematoma; enhanced scans may show irregularity of the aortic wall and/or leakage of contrast material. When the CT findings suggest an aortic injury, aortography is performed before surgery to define it further.

CT performed to evaluate a mediastinal mass occasionally demonstrates findings suggestive of an old, unsuspected aortic injury, which can be confirmed by aortography.

MRI

In theory, MRI can be of value in patients with suspected aortic injuries, as spin–echo images will demonstrate mediastinal hematoma and discontinuity of the aortic wall and cine MRI will demonstrate turbulent flow at the site of the aortic injury. However, MRI is seldom an option in patients with major chest injuries, who are invariably attached to life support systems that are incompatible with strong magnetic fields and pulsed radiofrequency signals.

Angiography

Aortography in the left anterior oblique and lateral projections, with the catheter positioned in the aortic root, provides the definitive diagnosis. We prefer 35-mm cine to large-format films. Intra-arterial digital angiography is a reasonable alternative, although the false negative rate is higher than that for cine or large films. The use of digital intravenous angiography (DIVA) in patients with suspected aortic injuries has been reported; however, owing to the extreme dilution of the contrast material, some leaks may not be detected. Because of its low sensitivity, DIVA should not be used in such cases.

If the femoral pulses are good, we introduce the catheter via a femoral artery puncture, advancing it retrogradely into the aortic root. If the femoral pulses are weak or absent, we use the left or right axillary artery for access. The axillary artery approach bypasses the aortic isthmus, avoiding catheter trauma which might exacerbate the injury.

The angiographic findings reflect the degree of injury to the aortic wall. Slight irregularity of the contour of the isthmus may

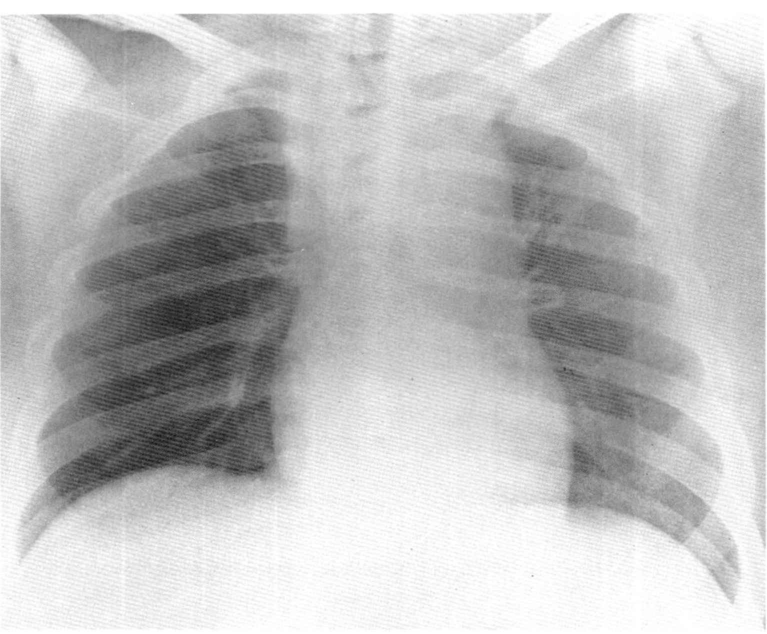

Fig. 28.4 Transection of aortic isthmus. Supine chest film of a young man involved in a motor vehicle accident demonstrates widening of the mediastinum (mediastinum/thorax ratio 0.43; normal, less than 0.25) and marked widening of the right paratracheal stripe. The left main bronchus is displaced downward. The pulmonary vasculature is normal. Aortography demonstrated a complete transection of the aortic isthmus.

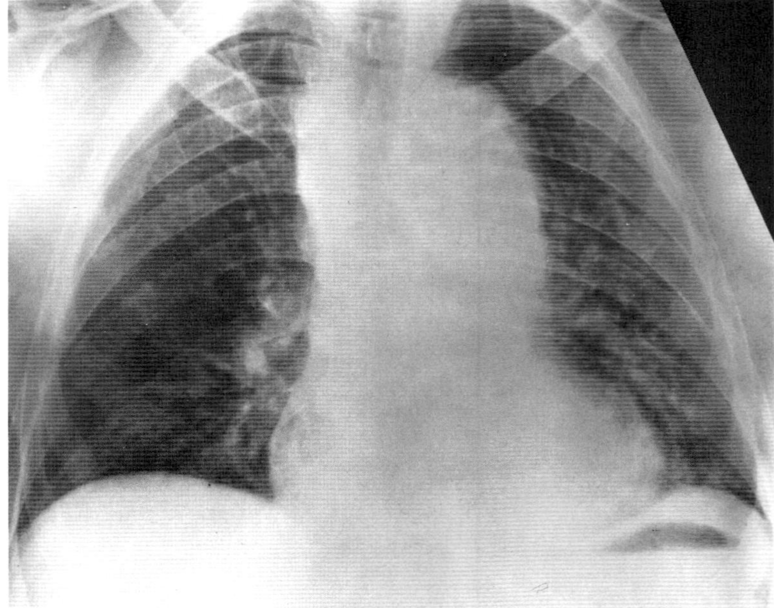

Fig. 28.5 Transection of aortic isthmus. Chest film of a patient involved in a motor vehicle accident demonstrates marked widening of the mediastinum and right paratracheal stripe and downward displacement of the left main bronchus. The borders of the aortic arch and proximal descending aorta are indistinct, reflecting mediastinal hemorrhage and/or edema. Aortography demonstrated a complete transection of the aortic isthmus.

be the only sign of a mild injury (Fig. 28.6). In patients with extensive disruption or complete transection of the aorta, aortography demonstrates periaortic leakage of the contrast material (Fig. 28.7). In patients with less severe injuries, the extravasation may be evident only on late films. The only evidence of an intimal tear may be prolonged retention of extravasated contrast material within the intima. Linear lucencies within the aortic lumen, which are best appreciated on cineangiograms, indicate disruption of the intima. In an exceptional case the hematoma may accumulate within the intima and media, in which event the angiographic appearance may simulate a localized dissection (Fig. 28.8).

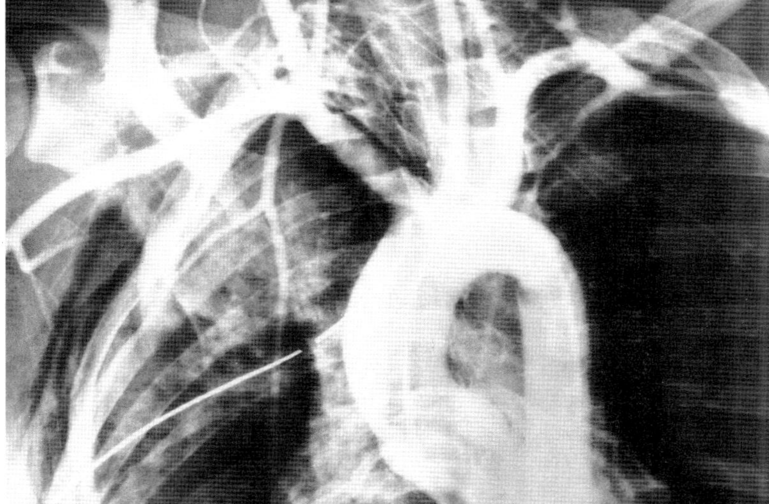

Fig. 28.6 Partial disruption of aortic isthmus. Left anterior oblique projection of thoracic aortogram shows a small irregularity of the inferior wall of the distal aortic arch indicating partial disruption of the aorta.

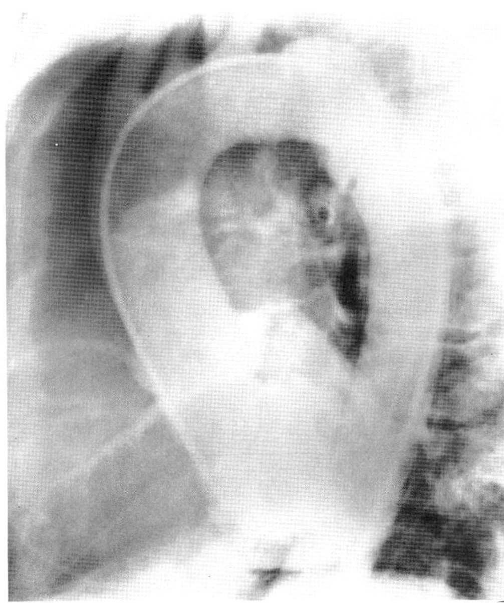

Fig. 28.7 Partial disruption of distal aortic arch. Left anterior oblique projection of left ventriculogram demonstrates marked deformity along the posterosuperior and inferior aspects of the distal aortic arch (aortic isthmus). There was no evidence of obstruction.

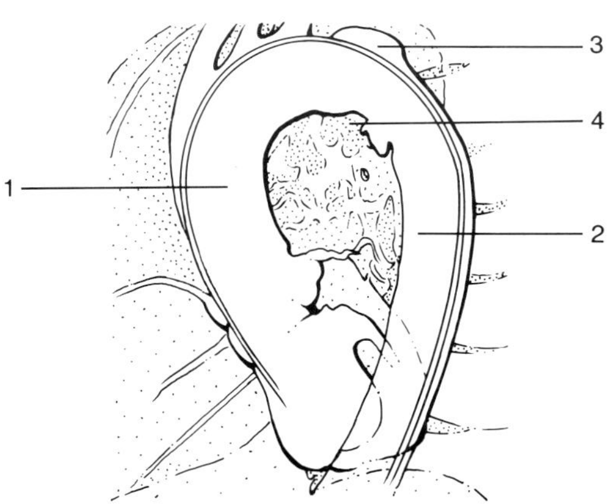

1 ascending aorta
2 descending thoracic aorta
3 deformity of posterosuperior border of aortic arch
4 deformity of inferior border of aortic arch

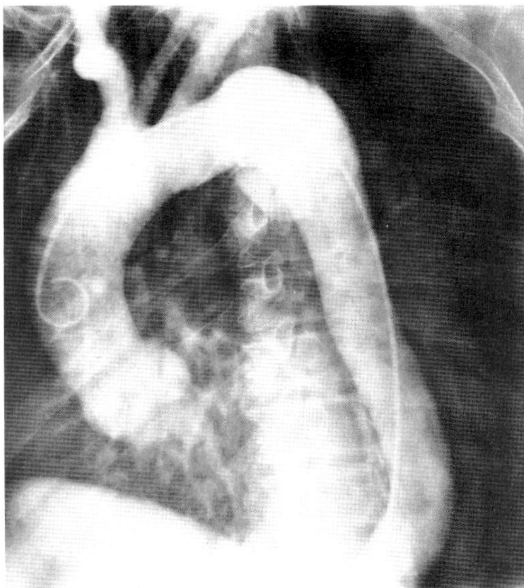

Fig. 28.8 Partial disruption of distal aortic arch simulating aortic dissection. Left anterior oblique projection of thoracic aortogram demonstrates an accumulation of contrast material along the inferior aspect of the proximal descending thoracic aorta, which simulates a localized dissection. Widening of proximal descending thoracic aorta simulates an aneurysm.

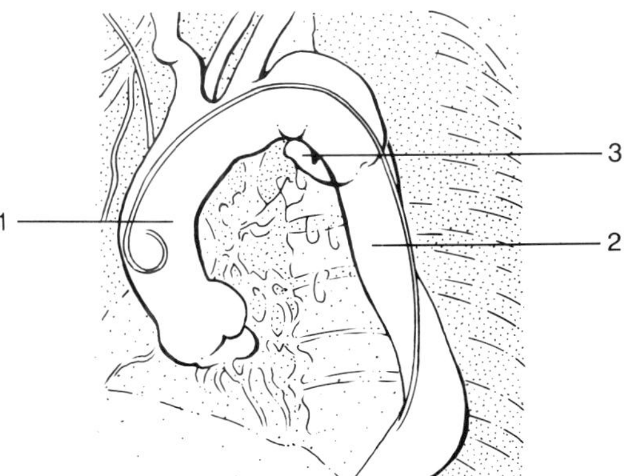

1 ascending aorta
2 descending thoracic aorta
3 extravasated contrast material (site of aortic rupture)

PENETRATING WOUNDS OF THE AORTA

PATHOGENESIS

The aorta can be injured by missile or stab wounds. Although some patients may survive long enough to receive medical attention, penetrating wounds of the aorta usually lead to rapid exsanguination; injuries of the intrapericardial segment usually cause rapidly fatal tamponade. Occasionally there is an associated penetrating injury of the heart or a great vein; in such cases an aortocardiac or aortovenous fistula may form, allowing the patient to survive for hours or days, or even longer. If the missile remains in the aortic lumen it may migrate distally (embolize) and occlude a peripheral artery.

CLINICAL FEATURES

Massive and/or continuous bleeding after a penetrating chest wound suggests the diagnosis of a penetrating aortic injury. Hypovolemic shock may be present. Patients with lacerations of the intra-aortic segment typically present with signs and

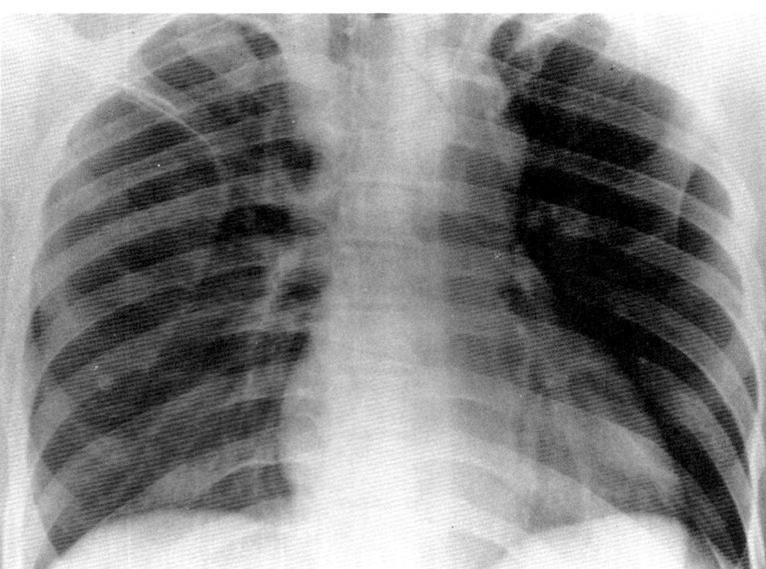

Fig. 28.9 Penetrating missile injury of the aorta with migrating bullet. Frontal chest film shows blurring of borders of the aortic arch and descending thoracic aorta. The left paraspinal stripe is displaced to the left. There is a small pneumothorax. No bullet fragment is seen. The entrance wound was in the right thoracic wall; there was no exit wound. A plain film of the abdomen (not illustrated) demonstrated the bullet in the right upper thigh; angiography showed the bullet in the right profunda femoral artery (see Fig. 28.11).

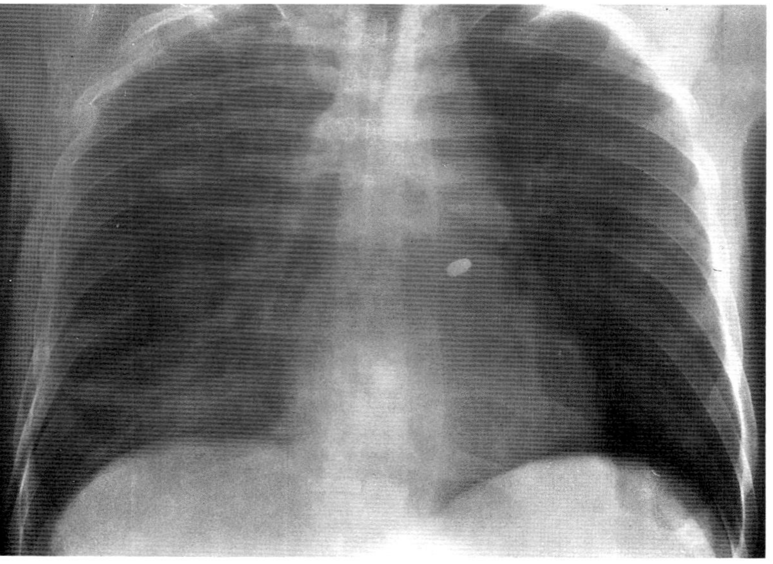

Fig. 28.10 Penetrating injury of aorta. Chest film of a patient with an entrance wound in the right hemithorax shows a bullet at the level of T8. The contour of the aortic arch and descending thoracic aorta is blurred. The left paraspinal line is displaced towards the left. The opacification of the right lower lobe is the result of a pulmonary contusion. This patient subsequently developed a fistula to the azygos vein (see Figs. 28.12 and 28.14).

symptoms of pericardial tamponade. A continuous murmur suggests the presence of an aortocardiac or aortovascular fistula or narrowing of the aortic lumen secondary to compression by extravasated blood within the adventitia. A patient with a large aortocardiac or aortovascular fistula commonly presents with signs of volume overload on the receiving chamber or vessel. A small aortovenous fistula may not be detected for weeks or months after the injury (see Fig. 28.12).

IMAGING AND INVASIVE DIAGNOSIS

Plain Films

Plain films typically show mediastinal widening secondary to hemorrhage (Figs. 28.9 and 28.10). In a patient who is bleeding into the pericardial cavity (hemopericardium), the plain film findings resemble those of an ordinary pericardial effusion. If there is no exit wound, failure to detect the missile in the chest should raise the question of intravascular migration (Fig. 28.11). A patient with a subacute or chronic aortovascular fistula usually exhibits chamber or vessel enlargement, reflecting the volume overload (Fig. 28.12).

Echocardiography

Echocardiography is rarely indicated in patients with acute penetrating injuries of the aorta. Dissections or aneurysms, which may result from untreated injuries, exhibit typical echocardiographic features (see Chapter 27).

CT

False aneurysms are readily demonstrated by CT (see Chapter 27).

MRI

Early experience indicates that MRI is of value in demonstrating traumatic aneurysms and aortovascular fistulas. In the lat-

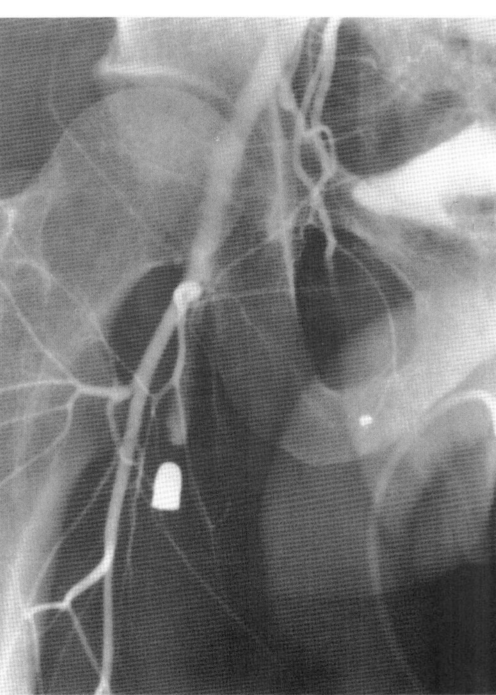

Fig. 28.11 Intravascular migration of bullet; same patient as in Fig. 28.9. Abdominal aortogram shows bullet in right profunda femoris artery, which is completely occluded. The patient was shot in the right chest, the bullet entering the distal aortic arch (see Fig. 28.13).

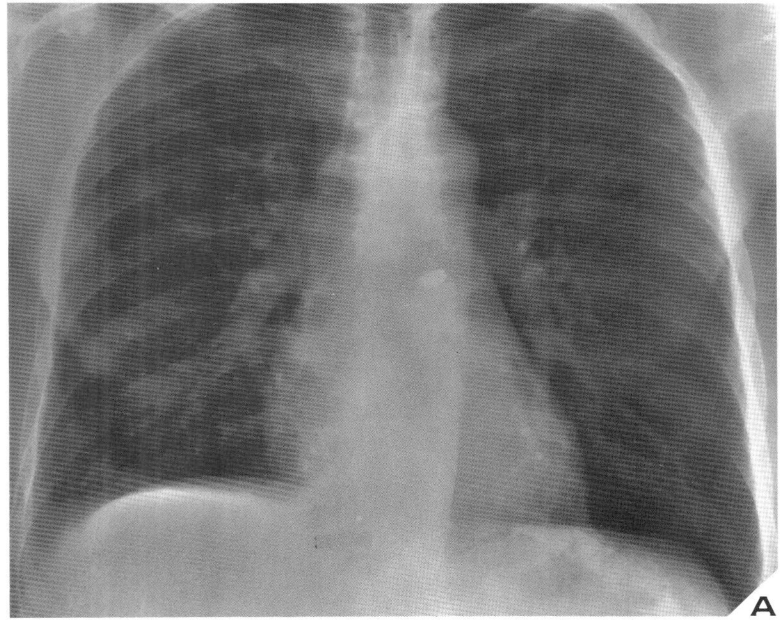

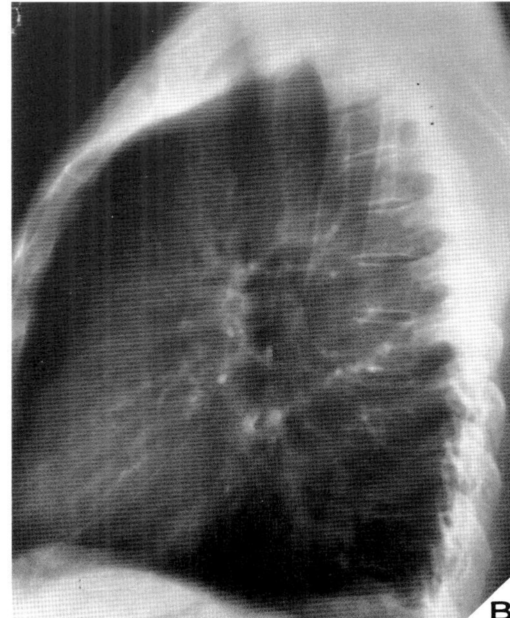

Fig. 28.12 Aortovenous fistula following penetrating injury of thoracic aorta; same patient as in Fig. 28.10. (A) Frontal and (B) lateral chest films obtained 2 months after the shooting show no change in the position of the bullet, which is anterior and to the left of T8. The contour of the descending thoracic aorta is now sharply defined. The left ventricle and azygos vein are slightly enlarged. These findings suggest the presence of a fistula between the aorta and the hemiazygos, which was confirmed by angiography (see Fig. 28.14).

ter, spin–echo images demonstrate loss of the normal contour of the affected vascular structures. In patients with aortovenous fistulas, cine MRI demonstrates abnormal flow from the aorta to the recipient vein.

Angiography

Aortography ordinarily demonstrates irregularity of the aortic wall and extravasation of contrast material (Fig. 28.13A). In some instances, deformity of the aorta caused by the adjacent hematoma may be the only finding (Fig. 28.13B). Aortography is diagnostic in patients with a suspected aortovascular fistula (Fig. 28.14).

Role of Imaging and Invasive Diagnosis in Acute Penetrating Injuries of the Aorta

In patients who are clinically unstable, the radiologic evaluation is usually limited to supine and cross-table lateral chest films. Aortography provides more specific information and is indicated if the patient's condition permits. It should be performed in a patient with a suspected penetrating aortic injury even when chest films or echocardiography are unremarkable. In patients with missile wounds, the site of the entrance wound, together with the location of the foreign body on frontal and lateral projections, suggests the site of the vascular injury and guides the angiographic examination. Angiography will also confirm (or exclude) a subacute or chronic aortovascular fistula, which may not be apparent initially. Echocardiography, CT, or MRI may be of value in detecting subacute or late complications (eg, aneurysm, aortovascular fistula).

INJURIES OF THE SYSTEMIC VEINS

Disruption of the great veins (superior or inferior vena cava) results in hemorrhage into the mediastinum. However, because of the low pressure in the systemic veins the bleeding is rarely rapid. The hematoma surrounding the disrupted vein may oc-

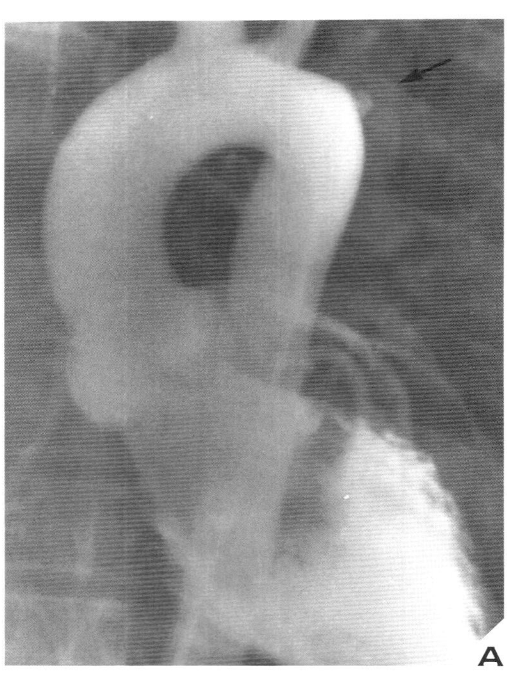

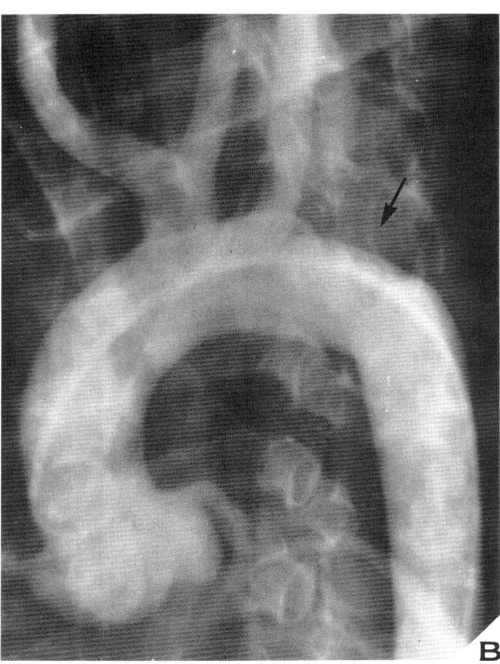

Fig. 28.13 Penetrating injury of aorta; same patient as in Figs. 28.9 and 28.11. (A) Frontal projection of left ventriculogram shows a small amount of extravasated contrast material (*arrow*) along the superior aspect of the distal aortic arch, indicating that this is the entry site. (The bullet has migrated into the right profunda femoris artery.) (B) Left anterior oblique projection of thoracic aortogram demonstrates localized flattening (*arrow*) of the superior aspect of the distal aortic arch caused by a hematoma at the entry site.

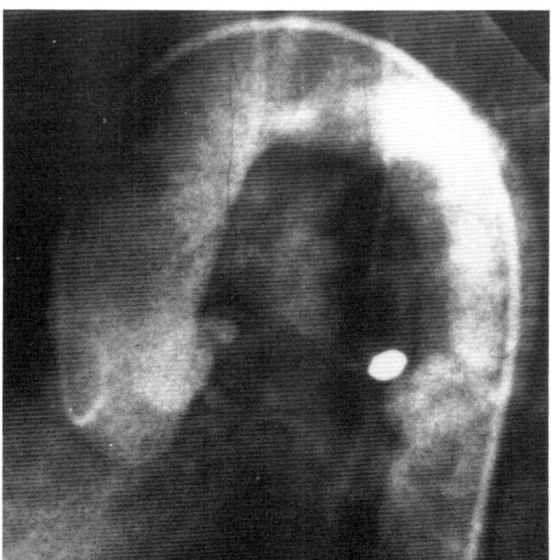

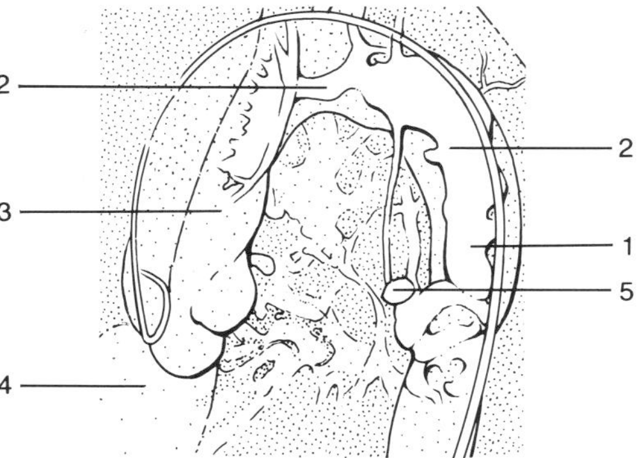

Fig. 28.14 Aortovenous fistula following penetrating wound of aorta; same patient as in Figs. 28.10 and 28.12. Lateral projection of thoracic angiogram shows opacification of the hemiazygos and azygos veins, which overlie the aorta. The fistula is to the hemiazygos vein at the level of the bullet.

1	hemiazygos vein	4	right atrium
2	azygos vein	5	bullet
3	superior vena cava		

clude it, preventing further bleeding. A large tear may lead to an exsanguinating hemorrhage, resulting in a massive mediastinal hematoma.

IMAGING

Plain films show widening of the mediastinum. CT, echocardiography, or MRI will demonstrate a large hematoma surrounding the great veins. Venography (via a brachial or femoral vein, depending on the site of injury) confirms the diagnosis.

INJURIES OF THE HEART

The heart is vulnerable to both penetrating and nonpenetrating trauma. Indirect cardiac injuries also may result from the increased intravascular pressure associated with exercise.

BLUNT INJURIES OF THE HEART

The most common cause of nonpenetrating cardiac injuries is a motor vehicle accident in which the vehicle stops suddenly and the driver's chest is hurled against the steering wheel. In deceleration injuries of this type, compression of the heart between the anterior chest wall and the spine results in a cardiac contusion (Fig. 28.15). The right ventricle is the most commonly affected cardiac structure, followed by the right atrium and the left ventricle. Trauma to the great arteries also may result from such injuries.

PATHOGENESIS

Myocardial and Pericardial Injuries

The mildest form of cardiac contusion is a small hemorrhagic focus which may be limited to the subendocardial region or a valve. Moderately severe contusions may be confined to the myocardium or may also involve the epicardium and adjacent myocardium. Severe myocardial contusions are often accompanied by lacerations of the epicardial and/or endocardial surfaces. Epicardial lacerations may lead to hemorrhage into the pericardial space, resulting in cardiac tamponade. Endocardial lacerations may be followed by thrombus formation. Severe contusions, with extensive myocardial damage, commonly cause rupture of the myocardium, which is usually acutely fatal. (Delayed cardiac rupture may occur in patients who survive the acute injury.) Pericardial involvement, manifested pathologically by hemorrhage and a fibrinous reaction and clinically by a friction rub, occurs in about 50 percent of patients with cardiac contusions of various degrees of severity. The coronary arteries, which course within the epicardium, are traumatized in a small percentage of cases.

Isolated rupture of the ventricular septum is a rare sequela of blunt cardiac injury. The rupture may result from the injury it-

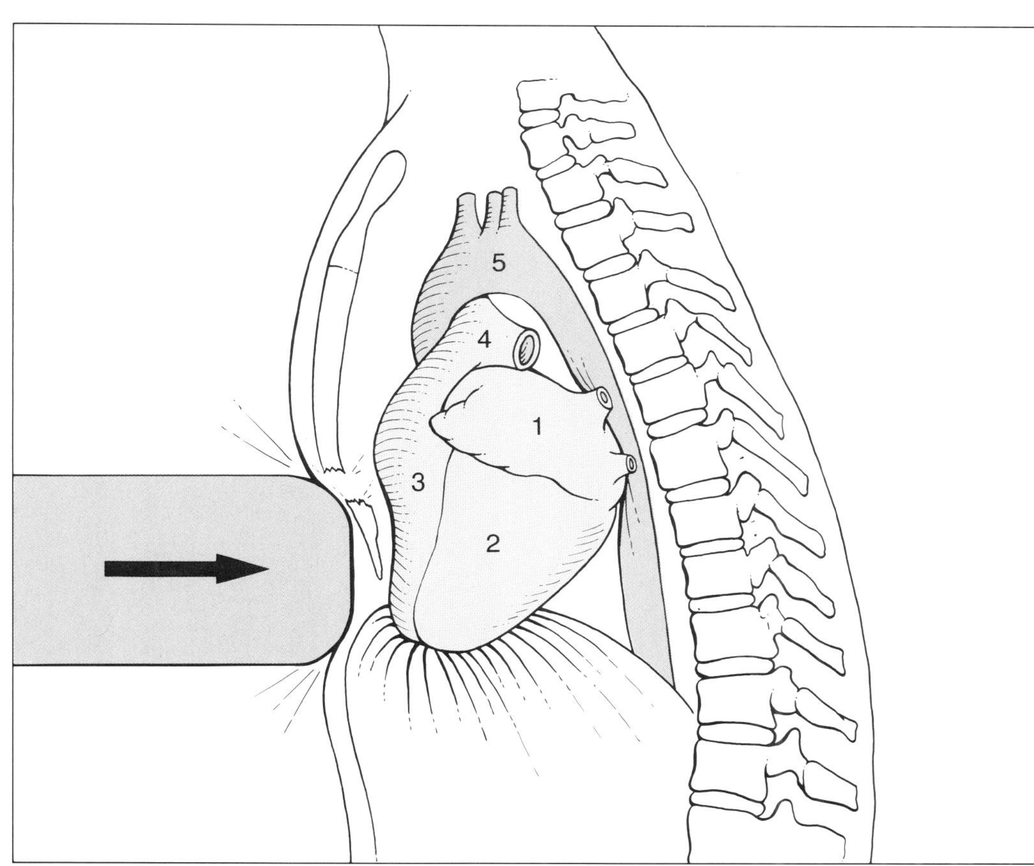

Fig. 28.15 Cardiac injury-caused external trauma. A force applied to the anterior chest wall compresses the heart between the sternum and the spine, resulting in a diffuse injury to the heart. The structures most likely to be injured by this mechanism are the right ventricle, right atrium, and the pulmonary trunk.

1 left atrium
2 left ventricle
3 right ventricle
4 pulmonary trunk
5 aorta

self or may occur weeks or months later secondary to infarction.

During the healing process, the traumatized myocardium is replaced by fibrous tissue, which may result in the formation of a ventricular aneurysm months or years after the acute injury. Other late complications include rupture of the ventricular septum and insufficiency of the mitral or tricuspid valve secondary to rupture of a papillary muscle.

Valvular Injuries

Valvular injuries can result from direct trauma; more often, however, they are due to the increased intracardiac pressure produced by the compressive force. Therefore, rupture of the aortic valve is most likely to occur when the compressive force is applied at the end of ventricular systole. Conversely, rupture of the mitral or tricuspid valves is most likely when the force is applied at the beginning of ventricular systole (Fig. 28.16). Rupture of the mitral or tricuspid valves, which is usually accompanied by rupture of the chordae tendinae, results in acute valvular insufficiency. The usual aortic valve injury involves splitting of one or more cusps, with extension of the tear into the wall of the corresponding sinus of Valsalva or the aortic annulus. In an occasional case the tear is limited to the wall of the sinus and the cusps remain intact (Fig. 28.16B).

HEMODYNAMIC FEATURES

The hemodynamic changes associated with a cardiac contusion depend on the extent of myocardial injury. Extensive myocardial damage leads to congestive heart failure, with elevation of the end diastolic ventricular pressure and decreased systolic force; the latter results in systemic hypotension. Cardiac tamponade (secondary to hemopericardium) leads to decreased end diastolic pressure in both ventricles and increased pressure in both atria. The net effect is equalization of the pressures in all four chambers. Rupture of the ventricular septum causes increased saturation of the blood in the right ventricle and pulmonary artery. The resulting right ventricular dysfunction commonly leads to tricuspid insufficiency with increased saturation in the right atrium.

CLINICAL FEATURES

The diagnosis of cardiac contusion is suggested by the history, clinical evidence of hemodynamic aberrations, electrocardiographic abnormalities, and elevation of the cardiac enzyme levels. (Patients with acute cardiac rupture seldom survive long enough to undergo diagnostic studies.) Chest pain is almost always present and is often accompanied by a pericardial friction rub. The chest pain, which may not appear until days or weeks after the injury, can closely mimic that associated with ischemic heart disease. The ECG demonstrates abnormalities of the QRS complex and ST-segment and T-wave changes similar to those seen in ischemic heart disease.

Patients with right ventricular failure secondary to an extensive right ventricular contusion exhibit jugular venous distension and a large, tender liver. Patients with a large hemopericardium have typical signs of cardiac tamponade.

In patients with rupture of the ventricular septum, physical examination reveals a holosystolic murmur and thrill along the left sternal border at the fourth or fifth interspace. The ECG findings are similar to those seen in ischemic heart disease.

Patients with valvular injuries typically present with congestive heart failure of acute onset. Physical examination reveals typical findings of aortic, mitral, or tricuspid insufficiency. Occasionally, more than one valve may be incompetent.

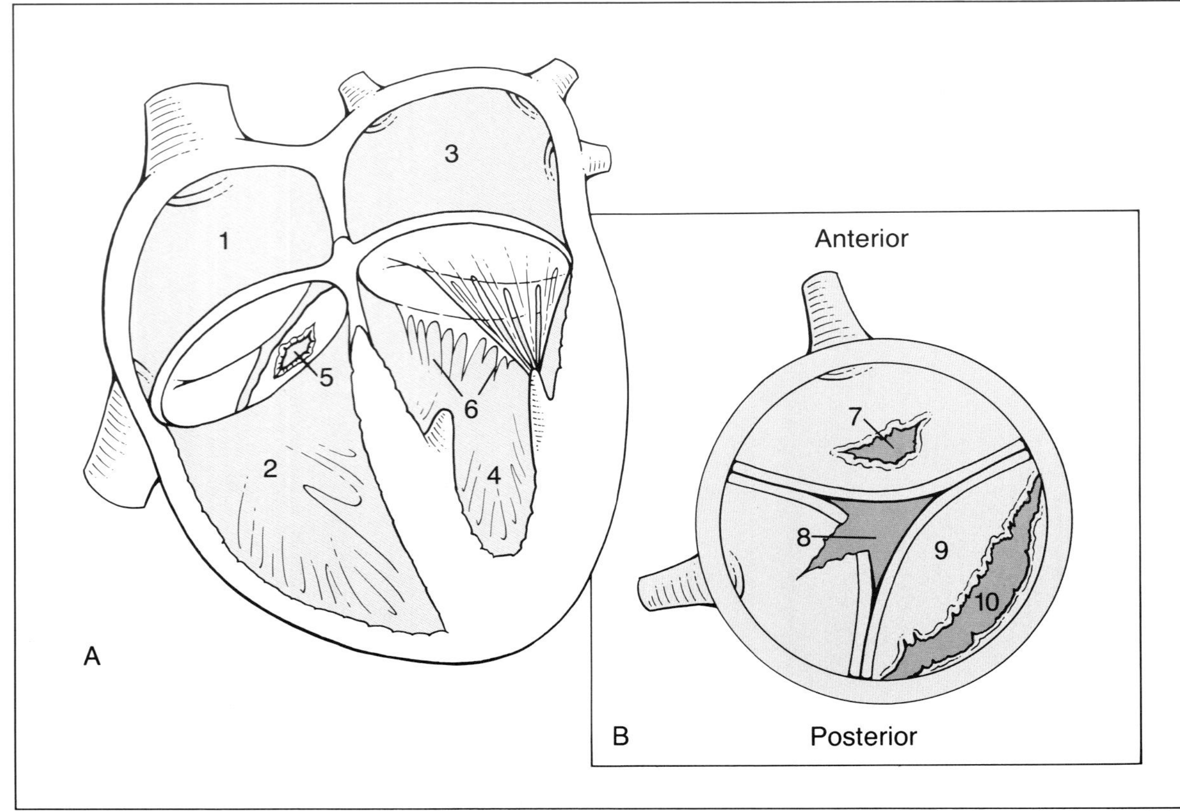

Fig. 28.16 Valvular injury associated with cardiac contusion. (A) Coronal section was taken at the level of the atrioventricular (AV) valves. Damage to the AV valves occurs during systole and results in rupture of the leaflets or chordae tendineae, or both. (B) Aortic valve is shown as viewed from above. Damage to the aortic valve occurs during diastole, and may result in rupture or perforation of the cusps or laceration of a sinus of Valsalva.

1 right atrium
2 right ventricle
3 left atrium
4 left ventricle
5 ruptured tricuspid valve leaflet
6 rupture of the chordae tendineae of the mitral valve
7 rupture of the left coronary cusp
8 marginal tear of the left coronary cusp
9 noncoronary cusp
10 rupture of the noncoronary cusp at its insertion on the aortic wall

IMAGING AND INVASIVE DIAGNOSIS

Plain Films

Plain films are seldom available in the immediate post injury period. The plain film findings in patients with hemopericardium of acute or delayed onset are similar to those of any pericardial effusion (see Chapter 22). Chest films of patients with severe right ventricular failure with tricuspid insufficiency, ie, dilatation of the right atrium, superior vena cava, and azygos vein. An occasional late complication is formation of a ventricular aneurysm, which produces a characteristic deformity of the cardiac silhouette (Fig. 28.17) (see also Chapter 20).

Echocardiography

Echocardiography is far more sensitive than chest radiography in detecting hemopericardium, and is therefore the examination of choice in the acutely injured patient. Because of its sensitivity in detecting pericardial fluid, a baseline study should be obtained as soon as possible after the injury, and repeat studies should be obtained at frequent intervals during convalescence.

In addition to demonstrating pericardial fluid, echocardiography provides important anatomic and functional information. Using either the transthoracic or transesophageal approach, one can evaluate the morphology of the atria, ventricles, and great vessels, detect abnormal contraction of the ventricular wall, and assess the integrity of the ventricular septum (Fig. 28.18). Color flow Doppler can identify damaged cardiac valves and allow their function to be assessed.

CT, MRI, and Nuclear Medicine

These modalities are rarely employed in the diagnosis of acute cardiac injuries. However, they may be of value in diagnosing late complications, such as ventricular aneurysm.

Angiocardiography

Although angiocardiography is seldom necessary in patients with acute injuries, it may be useful in diagnosing ventricular aneurysms and other chronic sequelae of blunt cardiac injury. Coronary arteriography is sometimes necessary to assess the coronary circulation in patients with severe chronic myocardial damage.

PENETRATING INJURIES OF THE HEART

Penetrating wounds of the heart may be inflicted by sharp objects, such as ice picks or knives, or by projectiles (eg, bullets or shell fragments). Gunshot victims usually die immediately from rapid and voluminous blood loss. Many victims of stab wounds die immediately from exsanguinating hemorrhage. However, a significant percentage survive long enough to

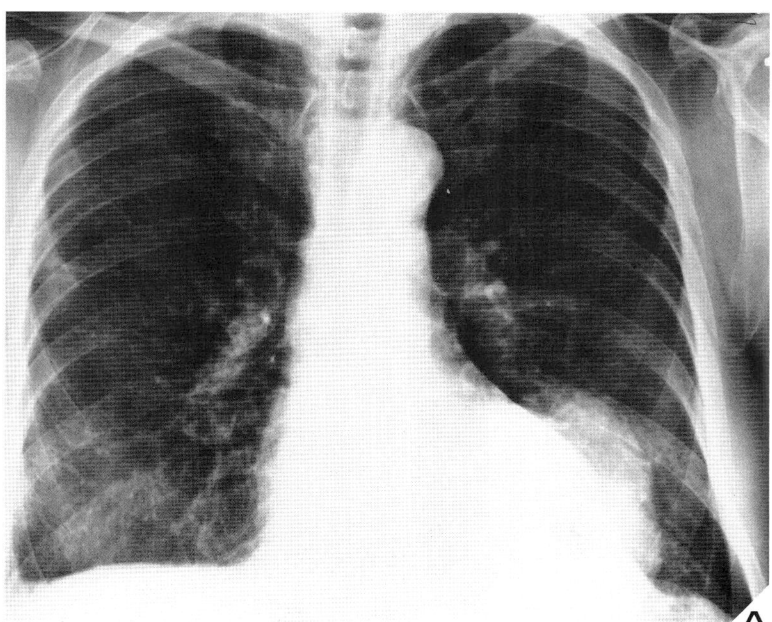

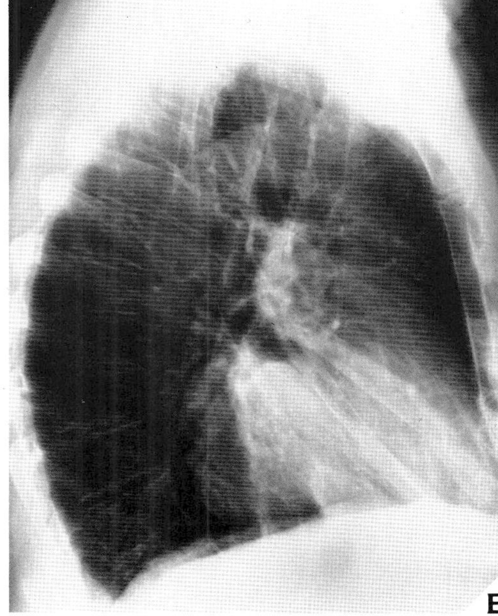

Fig. 28.17 Posttraumatic ventricular aneurysm. (A) Posteroanterior and (B) lateral chest films of a patient who had sustained severe blunt chest trauma in the past demonstrate moderate left ventricular enlargement. Note the prominent bulge extending posteriorly and to the left from the left heart border, which represents a posttraumatic aneurysm of the posteroinferior wall of the left ventricle.

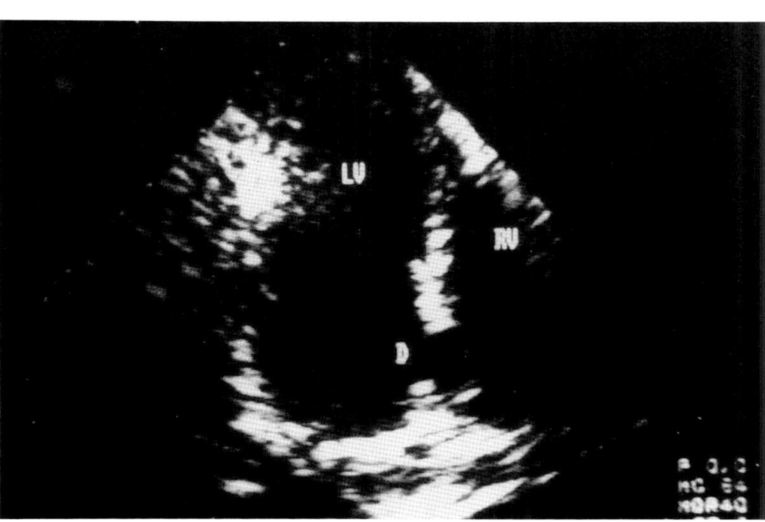

Fig. 28.18 Ruptured ventricular septum. Four-chamber view of echocardiogram demonstrates an echo-free area in the midportion of the ventricular septum. Both ventricles are enlarged. (D = defect.)

reach the hospital. Such individuals may have cardiac wounds ranging in length from a few millimeters to 2.5 centimeters or more, and present with cardiac tamponade of varying severity. A prompt, accurate clinical assessment is essential, as even patients with no detectable pulse or blood pressure can be saved if surgery is performed immediately.

The structures most likely to be injured by a penetrating injury are, in order of frequency, the right ventricle (40 percent), the left ventricle (20 percent), and the right atrium (10 percent). Injuries of the intrapericardial segments of the great vessels (ascending aorta, pulmonary trunk, and superior vena cava) account for 7 percent. Injuries of coronary arteries, as well as isolated injuries of the pericardium, are less common (Fig. 28.19). Penetrating cardiac injuries range in severity from simple lacerations that penetrate the myocardium without entering a cardiac chamber (intramural injuries) to lacerations that enter a cardiac chamber (intraluminal injuries). More than one cardiac chamber may be affected.

HEMODYNAMIC FEATURES

The fundamental hemodynamic change in acute cardiac tamponade is increased intrapericardial pressure which restricts the venous return to the right ventricle during diastole. The resulting rise in right ventricular and diastolic pressure leads to an increase in right atrial and central venous pressure. On the arterial side, the resultant cardiac compression leads to a reduction in cardiac output, followed by a fall in systemic blood pressure and decreased perfusion of the coronary arterial tree. The amount of intrapericardial blood needed to produce cardiac tamponade depends on the elasticity of the pericardium. In a previously normal individual, 150 to 200 mL of blood in the pericardial space will raise the central venous pressure high enough to decrease cardiac output. Smaller volumes usually do not cause significant compression of the cardiac chambers. In such cases, the intrapericardial blood seals the wound and contributes to spontaneous healing.

CLINICAL FEATURES

The immediate cause of death is exsanguination or cardiac tamponade. Patients who survive the immediate injury may later succumb to sepsis, infarction of the affected ventricle, cardiac failure, or constrictive pericarditis.

Some patients with penetrating cardiac injuries arrive at the hospital in remarkably stable condition. Unless the possibility of a penetrating injury is considered, a potentially salvageable patient will be lost. Careful attention to the site of the entry wound decreases the likelihood of such an error. The danger zone includes the region of the heart (precordium) and extends downward to include the left upper quadrant. It includes the midportion of the left hemithorax to the level of the clavicle, and a portion of the right parasternal region (Fig. 28.20).

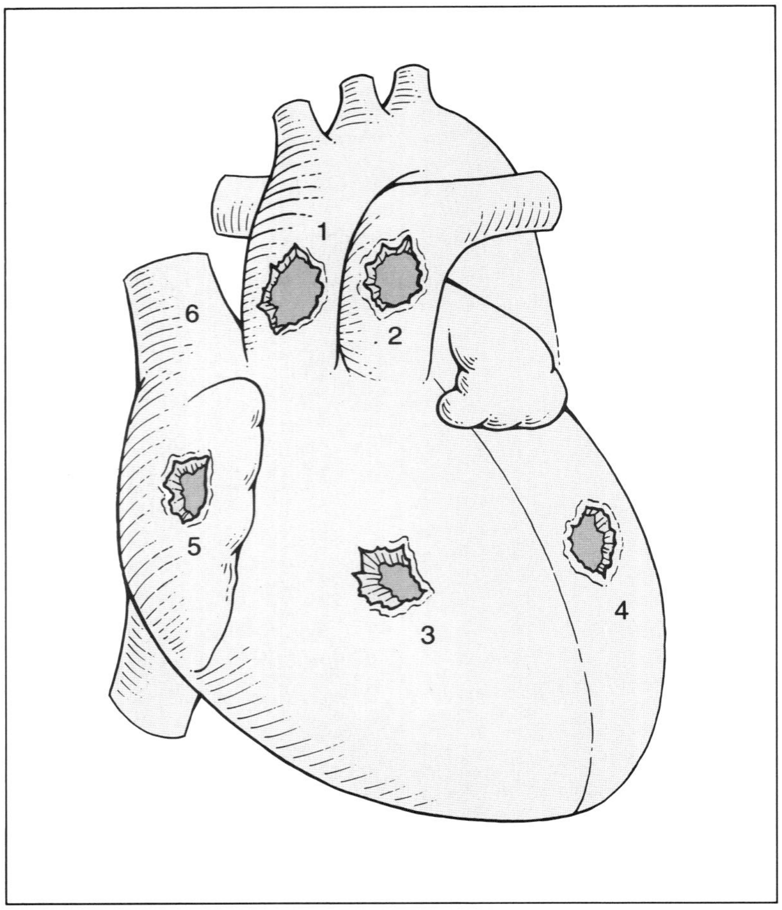

1
2
6
5
3
4

Fig. 28.19 Common sites of injury by penetrating missiles or sharp objects. The most common sites of injury (in order of frequency) are the right ventricle, left ventricle, right atrium, and intrapericardial portions of the great vessels.

1	aorta	4	left ventricle
2	pulmonary trunk	5	right atrium
3	right ventricle	6	superior vena cava

IMAGING

Plain Films

Frontal and lateral chest films will demonstrate a metallic foreign body if it is still in the thorax (Fig. 28.21). In patients with gunshot wounds, the presence of shell fragments may indicate the path of the missile and suggest the site of cardiac and/or vascular injury. Chest films may also show other evidence of thoracic injury (eg, hemothorax, pneumothorax, pulmonary contusion, fractures of the ribs or vertebrae).

The frontal chest film may show the typical appearance of a pericardial effusion (Fig. 28.21). Owing to the lack of distensibility of the normal pericardium, the cardiac silhouette may appear normal or nearly normal in some patients with a hemodynamically significant hemopericardium.

The classic radiographic signs of acute cardiac tamponade are a small heart, pulmonary underperfusion, and dilatation of the superior vena cava and azygos veins (see Chapter 22). However, owing to their precarious condition, it is often impossible to obtain a satisfactory chest film in patients with acute cardiac tamponade.

Echocardiography

Echocardiography is very sensitive in detecting both hemopericardium and acute cardiac tamponade. The latter is associated with a characteristic deformation of the right atrium and right ventricle during diastole (see Chapter 22). No further diagnostic studies are necessary, since acute cardiac tamponade demands immediate surgery.

Fig. 28.20 Penetrating injuries of the heart and great vessels: the danger zone. A missile or sharp object entering anywhere in the "danger zone" is likely to penetrate the heart or great vessels.

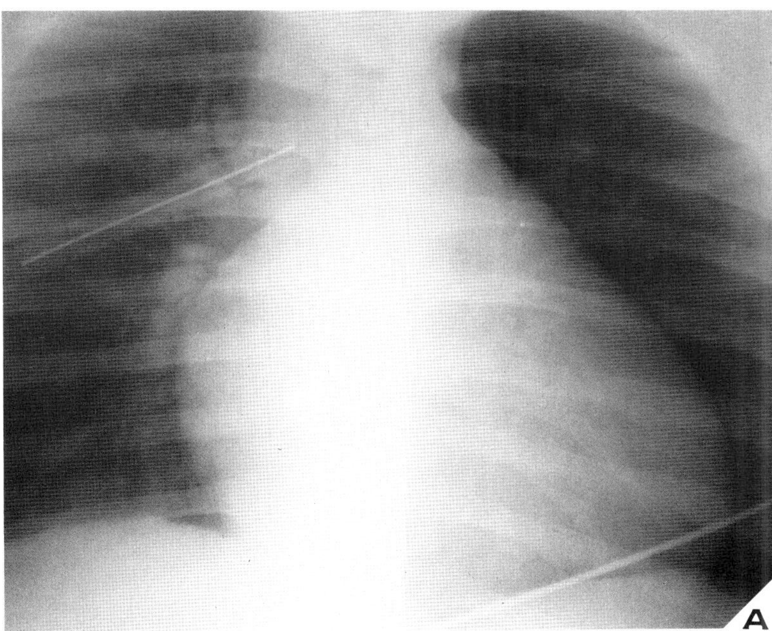

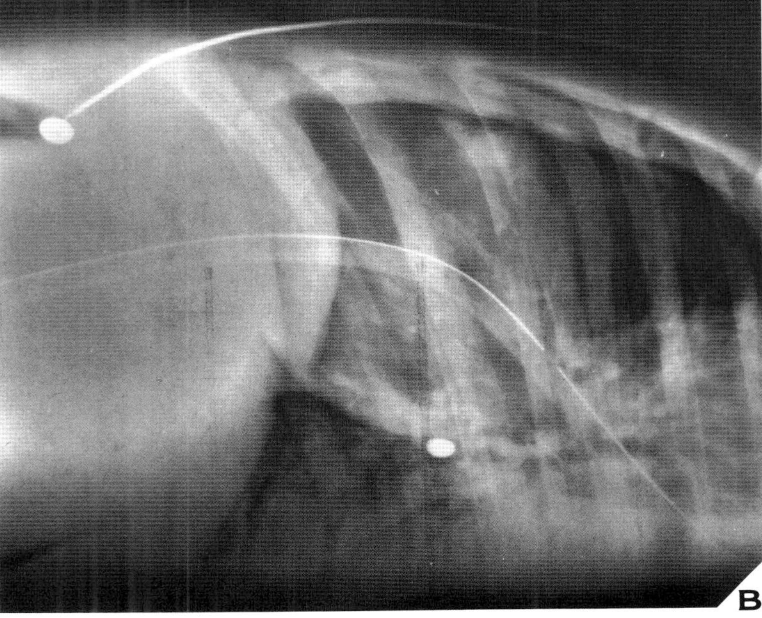

Fig. 28.21 Gunshot wound of the heart. This 10-year-old boy was shot in the chest by a playmate. (A) Supine frontal chest film shows a bullet overlying the right side of the heart. There is slight fullness of the left upper heart border, indicating the presence of a hemopericardium. There is a hemothorax on the right. (B) A cross-table lateral chest film shows the bullet projecting slightly beyond the posterior border of the heart. Thoracotomy revealed two perforating wounds of the right atrium; the bullet was in the pericardial space posterior to the right atrium. The patient made an uneventful recovery.

CHAPTER 29

Acquired Heart Disease in Children

Acquired cardiac disease is uncommon in infants and children. The cardiac disorders most frequently encountered in this age group are rheumatic fever, acute glomerulonephritis, bacterial endocarditis, pericarditis, myocarditis, and Kawasaki disease and, in the neonate, maternal diabetes-induced cardiomyopathy. Glycogenosis type II (Pompe's disease) and the primary form of endocardial fibroelastosis are rare causes of myocardial dysfunction in infants. Congenital anomalies of the coronary arteries (anomalous origin of the left coronary artery from the pulmonary trunk, coronary–cavitary fistula), a rare cause of ischemic heart disease in this age group, are discussed in Chapters 20 and 21. Systemic disorders associated with cardiac involvement in both children and adults (eg, dermatomyositis, systemic lupus erythematosus, muscular dystrophy, Ehler–Danlos syndrome, osteogenesis imperfecta, pseudoxanthoma elasticum, Marfan syndrome, mucopolysaccharidoses, acute glomerulonephritis, nephrotic syndrome) are discussed in Chapter 25.

RHEUMATIC FEVER

Rheumatic fever (RF) is caused by an abnormal immune response of connective tissue to a Group A streptococcus infection (usually of the pharynx or tonsils). The inflammatory process affects multiple organ systems, including the heart, brain, skin, and joints. Individual susceptibility appears to be an important factor in the pathogenesis of the disease.

RF is overwhelmingly a disease of children and adolescents. Nowadays, RF is uncommon, accounting for fewer than 1 percent of admissions on most pediatric services (at some centers the prevalence in hospitalized children is 0.2 percent or less). The dramatic decline in occurrence rate in the last four decades can be attributed to the prompt, effective antimicrobial treatment of Group A streptococcal infections in children and teenagers. However, recent epidemiologic data indicate that the frequency of RF and other diseases associated with Group A streptococcal infections (eg, acute glomerulonephritis) has increased in recent years.

The percentage of patients with RF who progress to chronic rheumatic heart disease (RHD) varies according to the severity of the cardiac involvement in the acute phase. In patients with minimal carditis, 96 percent had no evidence of RHD 5 years later and 94 percent had normal hearts at 10 years. Of those with moderately severe carditis in the acute phase, 80 and 70 percent had normal hearts at 5 and 10 years, respectively. The prognosis is much worse in patients who initially had severe cardiac involvement, only 30 percent of whom had normal hearts at 5 years. (Valvular dysfunction caused by RHD is discussed in Chapter 18.)

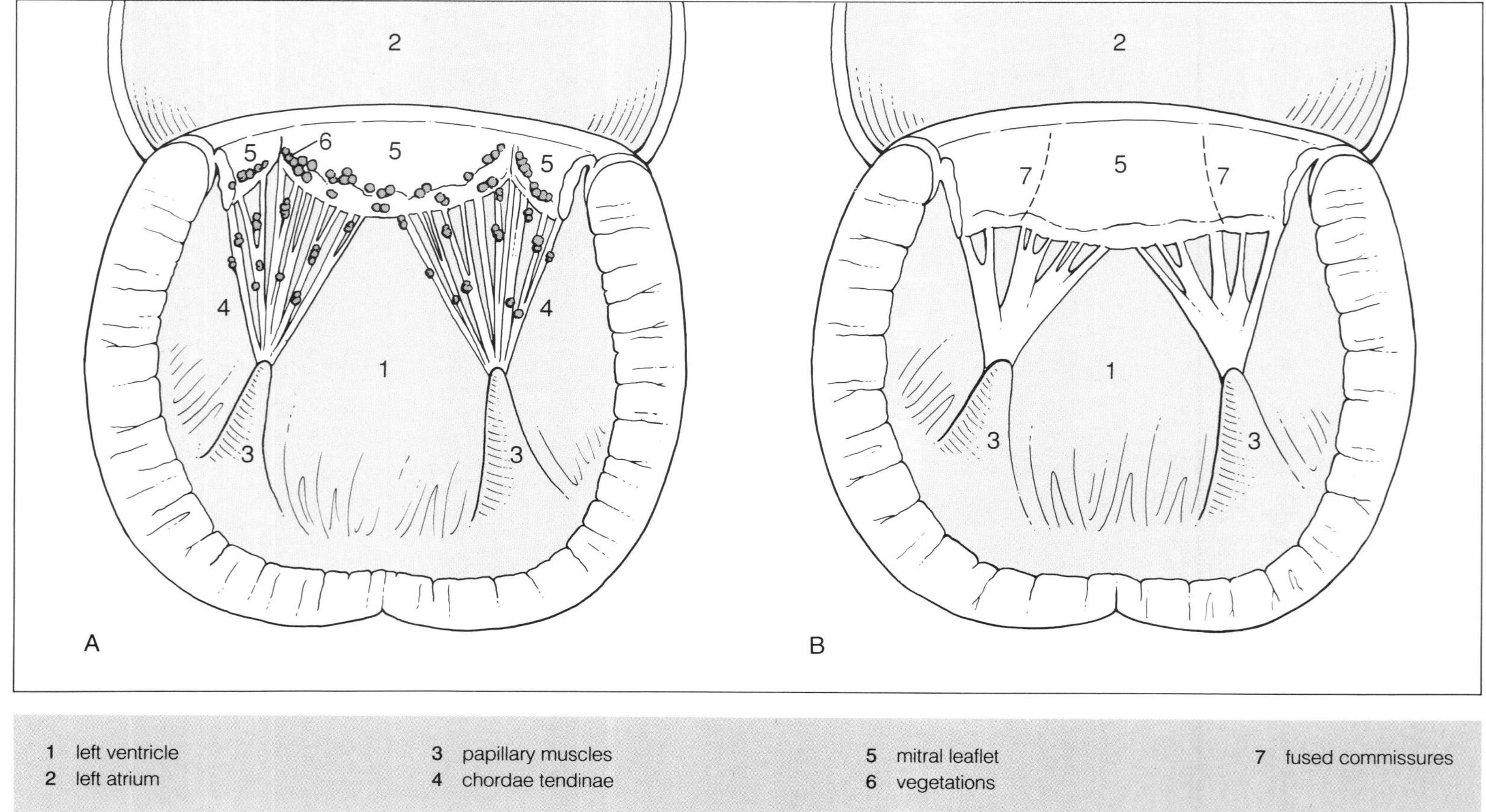

1 left ventricle
2 left atrium
3 papillary muscles
4 chordae tendinae
5 mitral leaflet
6 vegetations
7 fused commissures

Fig. 29.1 Acute rheumatic valvulitis. In this diagrammatic representation the inflammatory process involves the mitral valve. (A) Acute phase. The mitral leaflets are thickened by edema. Deposition of fibrin and platelets along the free borders of the leaflet has resulted in the formation of vegetations, producing the verrucous appearance characteristic of the acute phase. Vegetations may also occur on the adjacent portions of the chordae tendinae. (B) Chronic phase. The healing process has resulted in fusion of the commissures. The chordae tendinae are short and thick. The net effect is to narrow the mitral orifice, causing mitral stenosis.

PATHOLOGY

All three layers of the heart—endocardium, myocardium, and pericardium—are affected in the acute phase.

Myocardium. The myocardial involvement is characterized by focal interstitial myocarditis (characterized by Aschoff bodies), diffuse interstitial myocarditis, and damage to the myocardial cells of the conduction system.

Endocardium. The earliest endocardial lesions consist of minute translucent nodules (verrucae), which typically occur along the line of closure of the valve leaflets (Fig. 29.1); however, verrucae can be found in any part of the endocardium. The leaflets may become thickened and hypervascularized. Progressive fibrosis of the affected valves may lead to clinically significant valvular dysfunction, the hallmark of RHD (Fig. 29.2; see also Chapter 18). Aschoff bodies may also be seen in the endocardium.

Pericardium. Fibrinous pericarditis is a common feature of acute RF. This process mainly involves the visceral pericardium, which becomes thickened and nodular. Although a small amount of pericardial fluid is commonly present, a large pericardial effusion is very unusual.

CLINICAL FEATURES

Patients with RF typically present with signs and symptoms of multiple organ involvement (carditis, arthritis, chorea, subcutaneous nodules, erythema marginatum), arthralgia, and fever.

CARDIAC MANIFESTATIONS

Carditis is a common manifestation of RF, occurring in more than one third of the cases; it is frequently the sole major manifestation in infants and young children. The clinical manifestations reflect the valvulitis, pericarditis, and myocarditis associated with the acute phase. Acute rheumatic myocarditis commonly causes a dilated cardiomyopathy which can lead to congestive heart failure.

Most of the findings on physical examination reflect the valvulitis, which mainly involves the mitral and aortic valves (the tricuspid valve is occasionally affected). An apical systolic murmur of mitral insufficiency or a basal diastolic crescendo murmur of aortic insufficiency is frequently audible. Occasionally there is a change in an existing murmur. (A murmur of valvular stenosis nearly always indicates a preexisting congenital or acquired lesion. Such a murmur is seldom associated with the initial attack of RF.) Some patients present with (or soon develop) signs and symptoms of cardiac failure (cardiomegaly, gallop rhythm) and/or fibrinous pericarditis (friction rub). Arrhythmias secondary to involvement of the conduction system are not uncommon.

Acute rheumatic myocarditis is accompanied by characteristic ECG changes. These include: prolongation of the PR-interval to 0.18 seconds or longer (secondary to inflammation in the vicinity of the atrioventricular node); decreased amplitude of the T-waves, indicating abnormal repolarization; and (occasionally) elevation of the ST-segment.

EXTRACARDIAC MANIFESTATIONS

The most common extracardiac manifestations of RF are chorea and erythema marginatum. The former is a neurologic disorder characterized by involuntary, purposeless movements; it usually disappears early in the course of the disease. The latter is a pink macular eruption, which typically is distributed over the trunk and the inner aspect of the thighs and arms; it is commonly associated with carditis. The skin lesions may appear late in the course of the disease, after other manifestations of the acute process have abated.

Subcutaneous nodules, which are typically located over the extensor surface of the elbows, knees, knuckles, and ankles, are an infrequent manifestation of RF. The nodules are firm and nontender and are not attached to the overlying skin. There is no associated inflammation of the skin. Subcutaneous nodules typically appear several weeks after the onset of the disease and are evanescent, usually disappearing after a week or two. Occasionally, they may persist for a only a few days; only rarely do they persist for more than 1 month. There is no correlation between the presence (or absence) of subcutaneous nodules and the severity of the carditis.

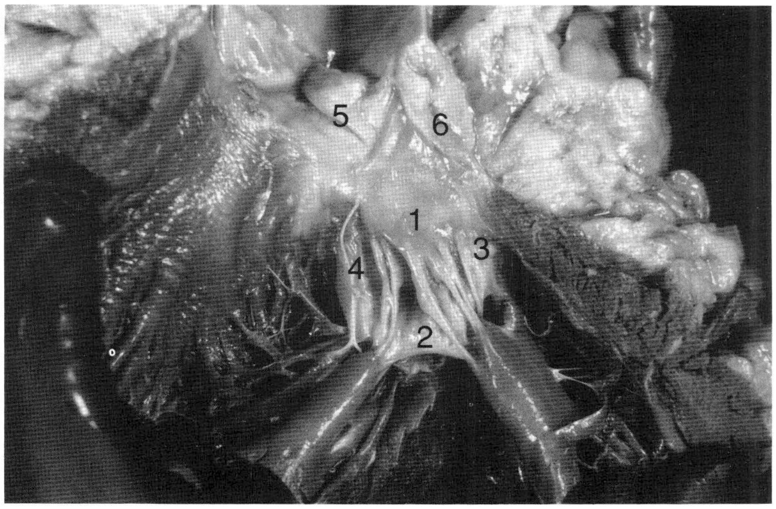

Fig. 29.2 Chronic rheumatic valvular disease. Anatomic specimen (viewed from left ventricle) shows damage to the mitral and aortic valves caused by rheumatic heart disease. The chordae tendinae are short and the mitral leaflets are thickened and fused at their commissures. The heads of the papillary muscles are closer to the mitral annulus than in normal hearts (see Chapter 18). The leaflets of the aortic valve are also abnormally thick.

1 anterior leaflet of mitral valve
2 posterior leaflet of mitral valve
3 fused posteromedial commissure
4 fused anteromedial commissure
5 noncoronary cusp of aortic valve
6 left coronary cusp of aortic valve

DIFFERENTIAL DIAGNOSIS

The clinical diagnosis of RF is based on the Jones criteria (Fig. 29.3) and on laboratory evidence indicating a recent infection with Group A streptococcus. The latter is provided by two laboratory assays for antistreptococcal antibodies.

The *antistreptolysin-O (ASO) titer* is elevated in approximately 80 percent of patients with acute RF. An ASO titer greater than 333 Dodd units in a child under 5 years of age, or greater than 250 Dodd units in an older child or teenager, favors the diagnosis of RF in a child with an indeterminate Jones score. False positives and false negatives are common. ASO titers in healthy children vary widely according to age, geographic location, and other factors that increase the likelihood of streptococcal infection; thus, titers of 200 to 300 Dodd units are common in healthy children living in crowded cities in the northern United States. (The ASO titer may also be elevated in patients with malignant tumors, acute glomerulonephritis, or rheumatoid arthritis.) False negatives occur in as many as 22 percent of patients with acute RF.

The *antideoxyribonuclease B (anti-DNAse B) titer* has proved to be an extremely useful test with highly reproducible results. A titer greater than 1:100 usually indicates RF in infants and children under 6 years of age.

The differential diagnosis of acute RF includes rheumatoid arthritis, septic arthritis, acute leukemia, bacterial endocarditis, viral myocarditis, and pericarditis, as well as lupus erythematosus and other collagen/vascular diseases. Judicious use of the Jones criteria and antistreptococcal antibody titers will decrease the number of false positive diagnoses, especially in the early stages of the disease when the Jones score may be equivocal.

FIG 29.3 JONES CRITERIA (REVISED)*

Major Manifestations	Minor Manifestations
Carditis	Fever
Polyarthritis	Arthralgia
Chorea	Previous rheumatic fever or rheumatic heart disease
Erythema marginatum	Elevated ESR or positive CRP
Subcutaneous nodules	Prolonged P-R interval

**Plus supporting evidence of preceding streptococcal infection; history of recent scarlet fever; positive throat culture for group A streptococcus; increased ASO titer or other streptococcal antibodies.*

Fig. 29.3 Jones criteria.

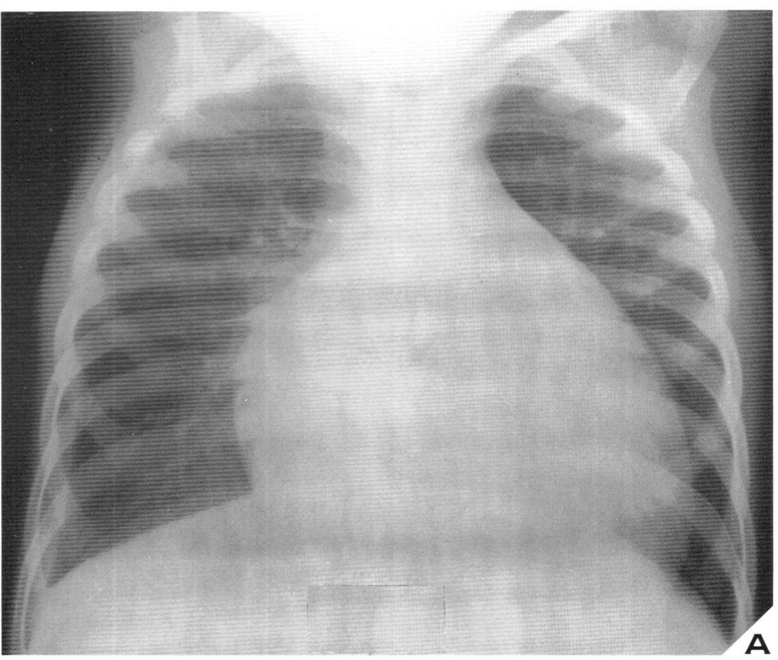

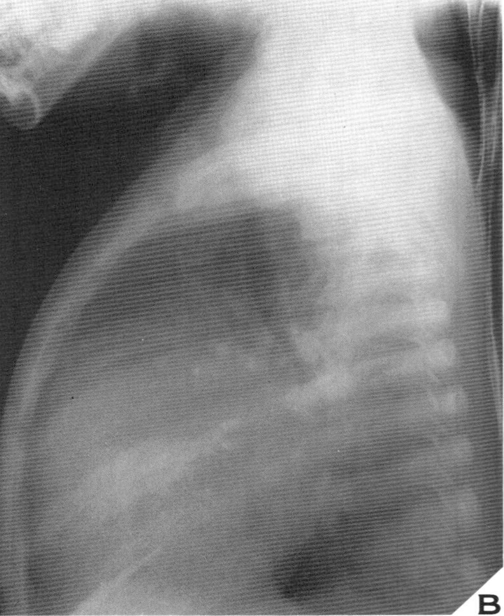

Fig. 29.4 Rheumatic pancarditis. (A) Frontal and (B) lateral chest films in a 3.5-year-old boy with acute rheumatic fever show enlargement of the cardiovascular silhouette with deformity of the right and left borders, indicating the presence of a pericardial effusion. The aortic arch and upper mediastinum are normal. There is evidence of pulmonary venous hypertension (cephalization pattern) as well as a small right pleural effusion. Further evaluation revealed dilatation of both ventricles and insufficiency of the aortic, mitral, and tricuspid valves.

IMAGING AND INVASIVE DIAGNOSIS

PLAIN FILMS

Chest films of children with minimal cardiac involvement are normal. Chest films of patients with acute, severe rheumatic pancarditis (ie, myocardial, endocardial, and pericardial involvement) typically show massive cardiomegaly accompanied by evidence of pulmonary venous hypertension (cephalization pattern) (Fig. 29.4). Chest films of patients with tricuspid insufficiency may exhibit hepatomegaly and dilations of the azygos vein and/or superior vena cava. After the acute phase the heart becomes smaller, reflecting the regression of the myocarditis and pericarditis (Fig. 29.5). (A decrease in heart size usually indicates successful medical management.)

In some patients with severe valvulitis, cardiomegaly and congestive heart failure are the predominant radiologic findings during the acute phase and afterward. On the other hand, the heart size and pulmonary vasculature eventually become normal in the great majority of patients with minimal valvular involvement in the acute phase. Progressive scarring of the affected valves, culminating in chronic RHD, is the rule in patients with severe carditis. In such cases the chest film reflects the degree of valvular dysfunction (Fig. 29.6; see also Chapter 18).

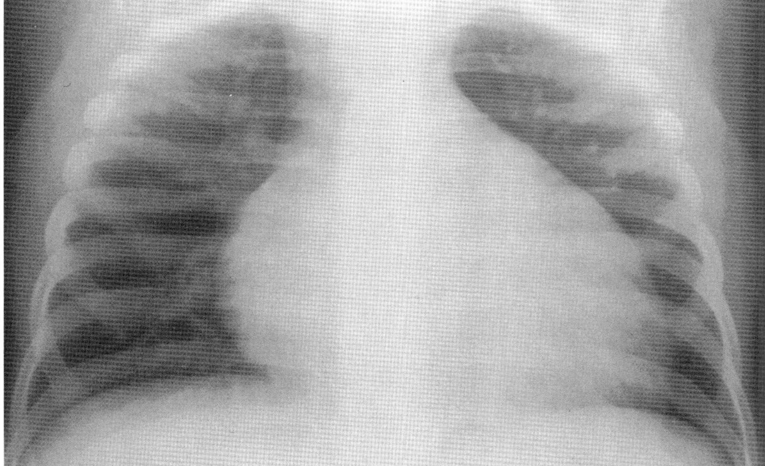

Fig. 29.5 Rheumatic pancarditis. Same patient as shown in Fig. 29.4 (5 weeks later). After treatment, the heart is smaller. However, left and right atrial enlargement and right ventricular prominence persist, suggesting mitral and tricuspid valvular dysfunction.

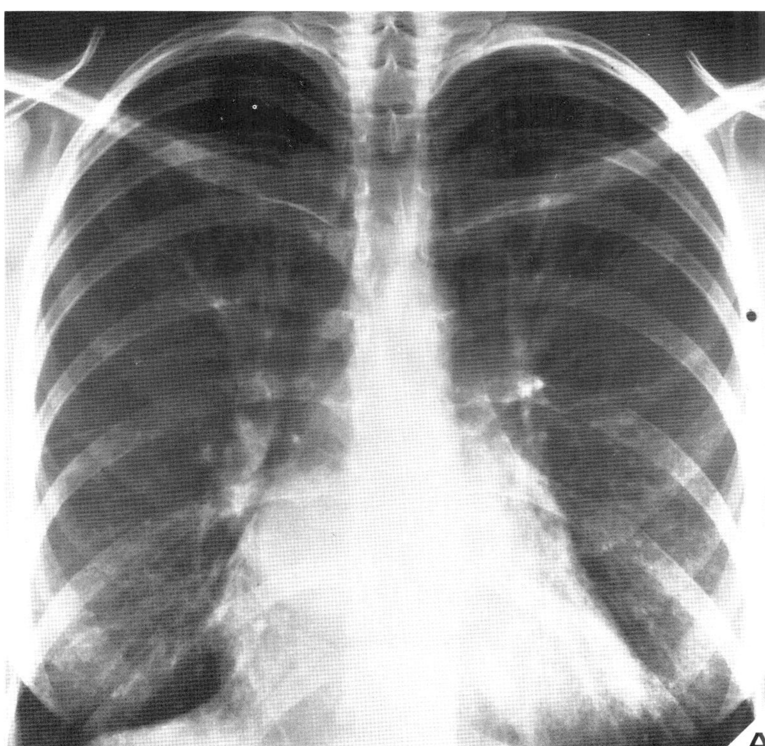

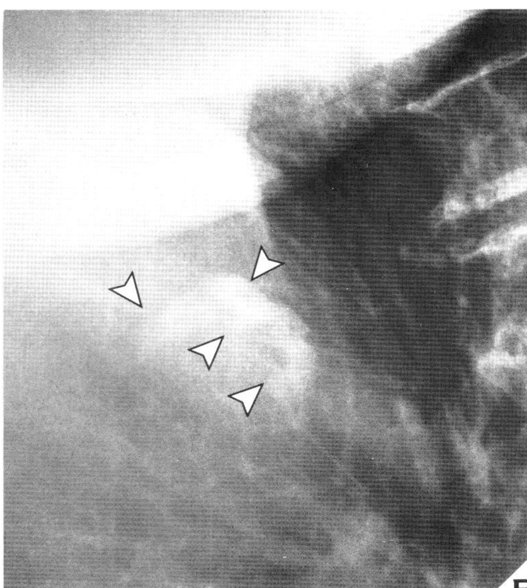

Fig. 29.6 Chronic rheumatic heart disease (mitral valvular disease). (A) Posteroanterior chest film of an adult patient shows mild cardiomegaly with left atrial enlargement (note double density), slight right ventricular enlargement, and prominence of the pulmonary trunk. Note prominence of the pulmonary veins in the upper zones (cephalization pattern) indicating pulmonary venous hypertension, ie, pulmonary venous pressure greater than 20 mm Hg. (B) Detail of lateral projection shows heavy calcification of mitral annulus and mitral leaflets (*arrows*). The plain film findings are typical of mitral stenosis (see Chapter 18).

ECHOCARDIOGRAPHY

Two-dimensional echocardiography clearly depicts the valvular and pericardial involvement associated with acute RF (Fig. 29.7; see also Chapters 22 and 23). Doppler imaging is very helpful in documenting the degree of valvular insufficiency associated with acute rheumatic endocarditis.

CARDIAC CATHETERIZATION AND ANGIOCARDIOGRAPHY

Invasive diagnosis is rarely indicated in patients with acute RF, since the diagnosis is clearly established by clinical criteria and the anatomic and functional abnormalities are accurately characterized by echocardiography.

ACUTE GLOMERULONEPHRITIS

Acute glomerulonephritis (AGN), which results from an abnormal immune response to a Group A streptococcal infection, is an important cause of transient congestive heart failure in children and adolescents. The major clinical manifestations of AGN are systemic hypertension, periorbital and peripheral edema, and various degrees of renal insufficiency. Some children present with symptoms suggesting pneumonia (cough, dyspnea) and rales may be audible in the lungs. Routine urinalysis reveals blood, protein, and casts in the urine. In the great majority of cases there is direct or indirect evidence of a preceding beta-hemolytic streptococcal infection (decreased beta 1C glomulin level, increased ASO titer). Renal biopsy, although seldom necessary, confirms the diagnosis.

The constellation of cardiac enlargement, pulmonary congestion, and peripheral edema is extremely common in children with AGN. The primary mechanism is circulatory failure secondary to fluid retention caused by a primary defect in the renal excretion of sodium. However, other factors, including increased capillary permeability, hypoproteinemia, and left ventricular failure may be contributory.

IMAGING

Chest films are abnormal in the majority of children with AGN. In a series of 104 children with AGN, 34 (33 percent) had normal chest films, 13 (12 percent) had mild cardiomegaly, 38 (37 percent) had an "incipient heart failure" pattern, and 17 (16 percent) had an "overt heart failure" pattern (Macpherson and Banerjee, 1974). The "incipient heart failure" pattern is characterized by mild cardiac enlargement, interstitial pulmonary edema ("hilar haze," septal lines), increased visibility of peripheral pulmonary vessels reflecting mild pulmonary venous hypertension, and small pleural effusions (Fig. 29.8). The "overt heart failure" pattern is characterized by gross cardiac enlargement, pulmonary vascular congestion, septal lines, and alveolar pulmonary edema (usually bilateral and symmetrical, often accentuated at the lung bases). The "incipient heart failure" pattern usually disappears within a week; in only 5/38 patients (13 percent) in this series did it progress to overt heart failure. Surprisingly, there was no significant correlation between the chest radiographic findings and any of the common clinical and laboratory features of AGN (eg, systemic hypertension, edema, uremia, proteinuria, ECG changes). In two patients there were localized parenchymal consolidations without other radiologic manifestations of cardiac failure, which were attributed to coexistent inflammation.

Other causes of the radiographic "cardiac failure pattern" include primary cardiac disease (acute rheumatic fever, acute myocarditis, other cardiomyopathies), systemic hypertension, fluid and electrolyte imbalance, and severe anemia) and certain lung diseases (eg, interstitial pneumonitis, leukemic infiltration,

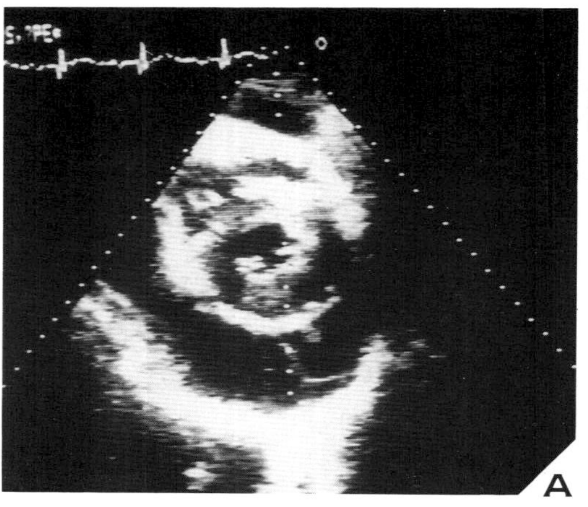

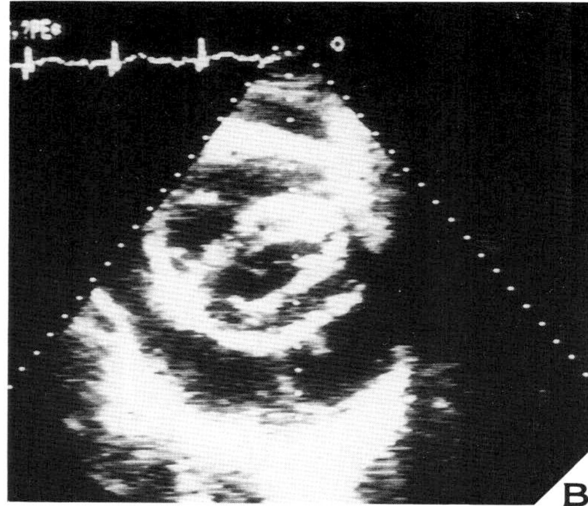

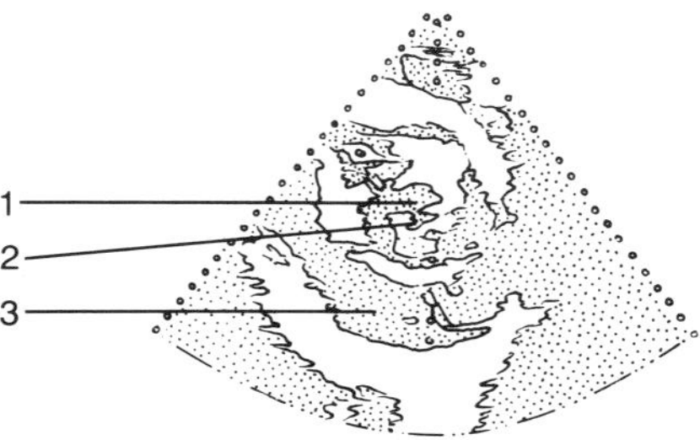

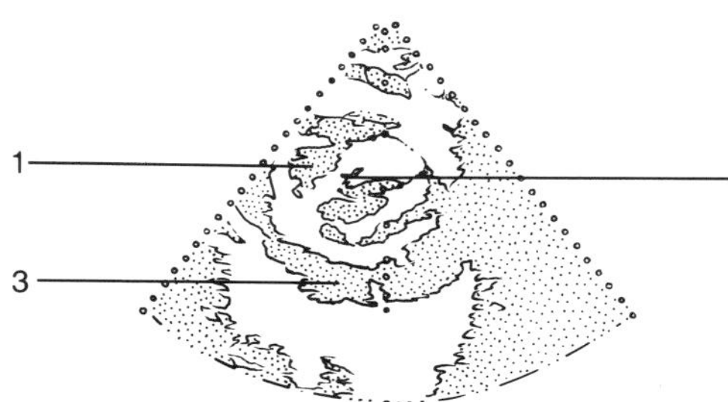

Fig. 29.7 Large pericardial effusion secondary to acute rheumatic carditis (echocardiographic findings). Transverse parasternal views at level of the base of the left ventricle in (A) diastole and (B) systole demonstrate a large pericardial effusion.

1 left ventricle
2 mitral valve
3 pericardial effusion

autoimmune diseases). Differentiation from these conditions is not possible on radiographic grounds alone. (Edema of the soft tissues of the chest wall favors the diagnosis of AGN.) However, AGN was the final diagnosis in three quarters of the children who presented with the "cardiac failure pattern" in the 1974 series. Despite the recent increase in cases of acute rheumatic fever, AGN remains the most likely cause of the radiographic "cardiac failure pattern" in a previously well child over 2 years of age.

SYSTEMIC HYPERTENSION IN CHILDREN AND ADOLESCENTS

"Essential" hypertension is uncommon in children and adolescents. The younger the child, the greater the chance that the hypertension is secondary to an underlying disorder. The etiology is renal disease in about 80 percent of prepubertal patients with systemic hypertension.

The major causes of acute hypertension in children and adolescents are acute glomerulonephritis, pyelonephritis, hydronephrosis, trauma, and collagen vascular disease (particularly systemic lupus erythematosus). The hemolytic–uremic syndrome, which usually follows an upper respiratory infection or gastroenteritis, may be associated with acute, severe hypertension in infants and children. Severe hypertension may also occur as a sequela of umbilical artery catheterization (usually due to renal artery thrombosis). Infrequent causes of systemic hypertension in children and adolescents include congenital adrenal hyperplasia and pheochromocytoma. Chronic hypertension in children and adolescents is usually due to a congenital malformation (eg, ureteropelvic junction obstruction), reflux nephropathy, unilateral renal parenchymal disease, renal artery disease, or chronic glomerulonephritis.

IMAGING

As in adults, the chest films of children with severe acute or chronic systemic hypertension may show various degrees of cardiomegaly and congestive heart failure (see Chapter 25). Although hypertension is commonly present in children with acute glomerulonephritis, the radiographic findings reflect the acute volume expansion secondary to renal failure rather than the hypertension per se.

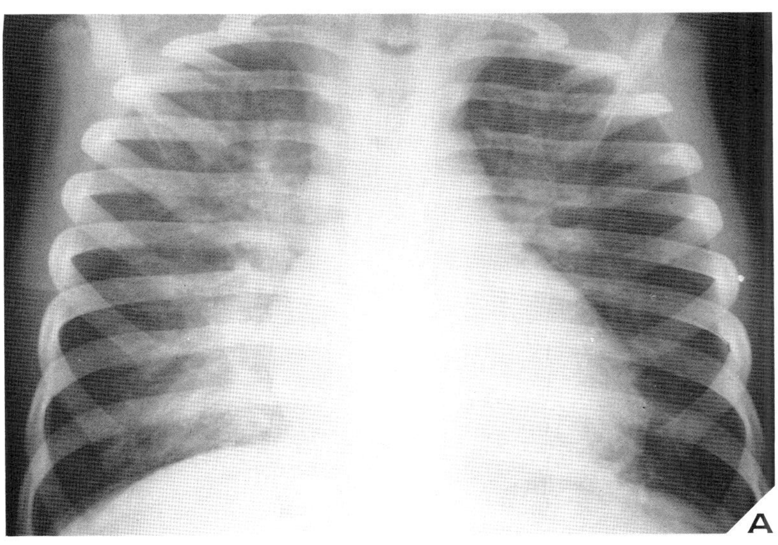

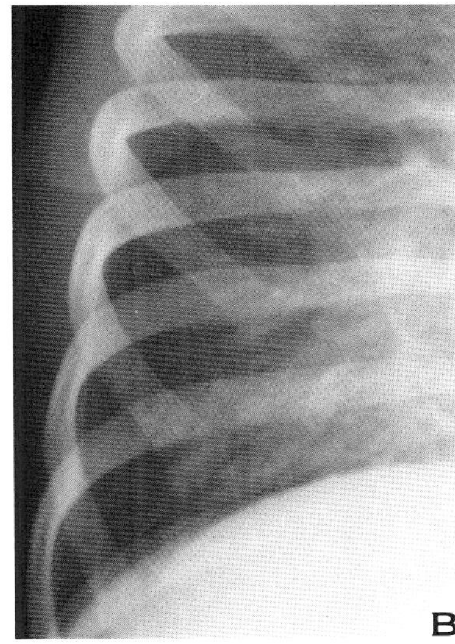

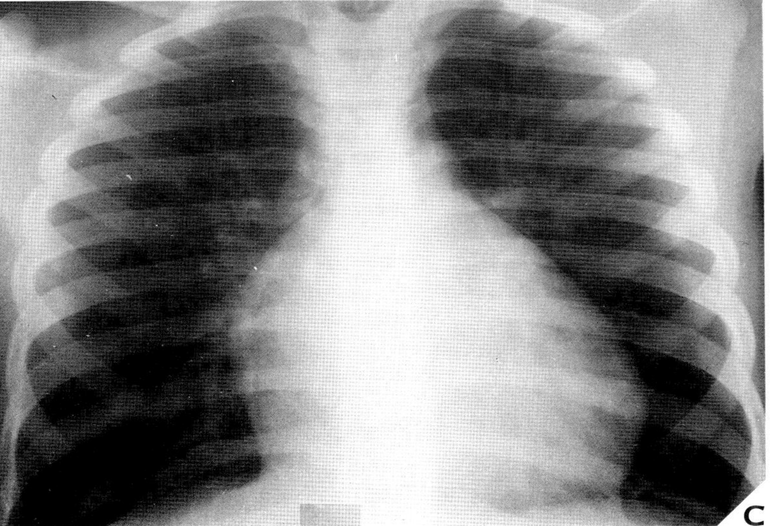

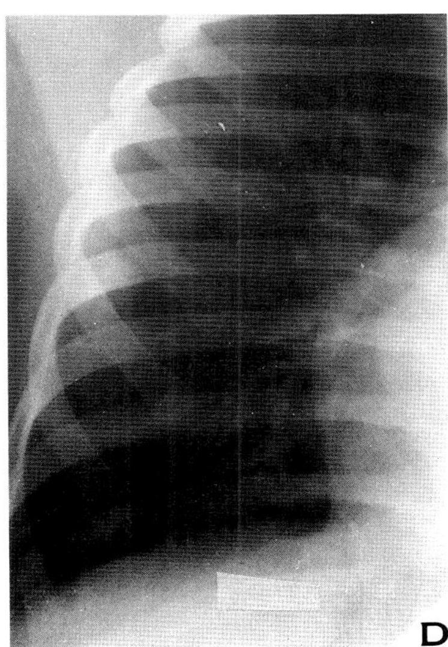

Fig. 29.8 Acute glomerulonephritis. (A, B) Initial chest film demonstrates mild cardiomegaly, pulmonary vascular congestion, and interstitial and alveolar edema. Note Kerley B lines in B, a close-up of right lung base. (C, D) Five days later, after treatment, the pulmonary vascular congestion and pulmonary edema have cleared. The heart remains enlarged.

INFECTIVE ENDOCARDITIS

Infective endocarditis is relatively infrequent in infants and children, accounting for about 0.05 percent of admissions in hospitals with active pediatric cardiology programs. *Streptococcus viridans* is the most common causative organism, accounting for approximately half the pediatric cases in one series (Fig. 29.9). Less common causative organisms include *Staphylococcus aureus (pyogenes), Streptococcus pneumoniae* (diplococcus), and saprophytic fungi such as candida and aspergillus.

The distinction between acute and subacute bacterial endocarditis—which was useful several decades ago—is no longer germane. [The diagnosis of "acute bacterial endocarditis (ABE)" was applied to untreated patients with an infection less than 6 weeks in duration; the term "subacute bacterial endocarditis (SBE)" was reserved for infections of longer duration.] Nor does the nature of causative agent warrant a distinction between "acute" and "subacute" forms of bacterial endocarditis. Formerly, certain bacterial species [eg, *Staphylococcus aureus*, *Streptococcus pneumoniae* ("pneumococcus"), *Neisseria gonorrhoeae* ("gonococcus"), *Streptococcus pyogenes*, and *Hemophilus influenzae*] were typically associated with ABE, whereas others [eg, alpha (nonhemolytic) streptococci, *Staphlyococcus epidermitis*] were typically associated with SBE. Because the course of the disease has been modified by many factors related to therapy (including host response), this distinction no longer applies. The various organisms listed in Fig. 29.9 can cause either an acute or a subacute infection. However, *S. aureus (pyogenes)* remains an important risk factor in hospital deaths. Various factors related to antibiotic therapy have altered the spectrum of causative organisms, especially for hospital-acquired endocardial infections; for example, fungal infections are now relatively common in many institutions.

To sum up: because the natural history of the endocardial infection is usually modified by antibiotic therapy, we prefer to avoid the terms "acute" and "subacute" and simply refer to "infective endocarditis." In any given clinical setting, certain organisms may be more prevalent in children than in adults, and some may be more virulent than others.

PATHOGENESIS AND PATHOLOGY

The underlying cause of infective endocarditis is believed to be turbulent flow caused by a malfunctioning valve, stenotic vessel, or septal defect. The resulting jet of blood causes superficial endothelial damage, leading to the deposition of platelets and fibrin on the endothelial surface and the formation of a sterile platelet–fibrin thrombus. Clumps of microorganisms that transiently invade the bloodstream (eg, during dental extractions or surgical procedures) lodge on the bland thrombus and multiply, forming a mass of necrotic tissue, fibrin, and microorganisms known as a vegetation. The pathology and complications of infective endocarditis are discussed further in Chapter 23.

The underlying cause of infective endocarditis differs in children and adults. In adults, the infection is usually engrafted on valves damaged by rheumatic heart disease (usually the mitral and aortic valves), whereas in children it is almost always associated with congenital heart disease (Fig. 29.10). In infective endocarditis associated with PDA, the vegetations typically

FIG. 29.9 CAUSATIVE ORGANISMS IN 196 PATIENTS WITH INFECTIVE ENDOCARDITIS

	Children[1] N = 24	Adults and Older Children N = 172
Streptococcus viridans	13	91
Nonhemolytic streptococcus, including enterococcus	1	28
Staphylococcus aureus	2	24
Staphylococcus albus	0	4
Hemolytic streptococcus	1	1
Streptococcus [Diplococcus] pneumoniae	1	0
Escherichia coli	0	3
Pseudomonas	1	5
Hemophilus influenzae	1	0
Klebsiella pneumoniae	0	0
Others	0	2
Unknown	4	14

[1] *Under 2 yr. of age*

Fig. 29.9 Causative organisms in 196 patients with infective endocarditis. (Reproduced with permission from Keith J, Rowe R, Vlad P: *Heart Disease in Infancy and Childhood*. London: McMillan Publishing Company, 1978:233)

FIG. 29.10 CONGENITAL MALFORMATIONS MOST COMMONLY ASSOCIATED WITH INFECTIVE ENDOCARDITIS IN CHILDREN

Ventricular septal defect	Patent ductus arteriosus (PDA)
Aortic stenosis	Coarctation of the aorta
Pulmonic stenosis	Tetralogy of Fallot

Fig. 29.10 Congenital malformations most commonly associated with infective endocarditis in children.

occur in the left pulmonary artery, adjacent to the ductal orifice. When infective endocarditis occurs in patients with coarctation of the aorta, the vegetations are located just distal to the stenotic segment or on leaflets of the bicuspid aortic valve that is commonly associated with this anomaly.

CLINICAL FEATURES

The clinical manifestations of infective endocarditis depend on the virulence of the organism, the host reaction, the nature and severity of the underlying heart disease, and the age of the patient. Infective endocarditis has not been documented in infants under 3 months of age, and is very rare during the first year of life. *Staphylococcus aureus (pyogenes)*, perhaps the most virulent causative organism, usually causes extensive valve destruction even with appropriate treatment.

The child with infective endocarditis typically presents with unexplained fever, malaise, and a murmur of organic heart disease, and usually appears very ill. The specific clinical manifestations reflect the location of the vegetations and the severity of the underlying heart disease. Typically, the signs and symptoms of the underlying congenital heart disease become worse (eg, decreased exercise tolerance, deepening of the cyanosis). Some patients may experience paroxysmal dyspnea or syncopal episodes. Patients with underlying aortic stenosis commonly present with evidence of aortic insufficiency. Because aortic insufficiency commonly leads to congestive heart failure, aortic valve lesions have a more ominous prognosis than right-sided valvular legions, which are more commonly associated with infective endocarditis.

The major complications of infective endocarditis are embolization and mycotic aneurysms. Embolization is much more common in adults than in children. When it does occur in children, it is usually associated with right-sided lesions and typically causes small pulmonary infarcts. Systemic embolization (to the kidneys, spleen and brain) is very unusual in children. However, "paradoxical" peripheral embolization from vegetations on the right side of the heart can occur in patients with atrial or ventricular septal defects. Embolization to large systemic arteries is very rare; when it occurs, it is usually secondary to fungal infections, which are characterized by large, friable vegetations.

Peripheral microembolization (manifested by Osler's nodules and splinter hemorrhages) is uncommon in children and teenagers with infective endocarditis. (Osler's nodules—common in the pre-antibiotic era—are ephemeral, tender, erythematous, pea-sized intradermal masses which typically occur on the pads of the fingertips and toes, the thenar and hypothenar eminences, and the soles of the feet.)

Pericarditis or cardiac tamponade resulting from rupture of a mycotic aneurysm of the aorta is an extremely rare complication of infective endocarditis in children.

IMAGING AND INVASIVE DIAGNOSIS

PLAIN FILMS

The plain film findings in children with infective endocarditis are nonspecific. In patients with aortic or mitral insufficiency, chest films show left ventricular and left atrial enlargement (Fig. 29.11). Patients with congestive heart failure exhibit pulmonary venous hypertension (cephalization pattern), sometimes associated with interstitial or alveolar edema.

ECHOCARDIOGRAPHY

Two-dimensional echocardiography, augmented by color Doppler imaging, is highly sensitive in the detection of vegetations and valvular dysfunction (see Chapter 23).

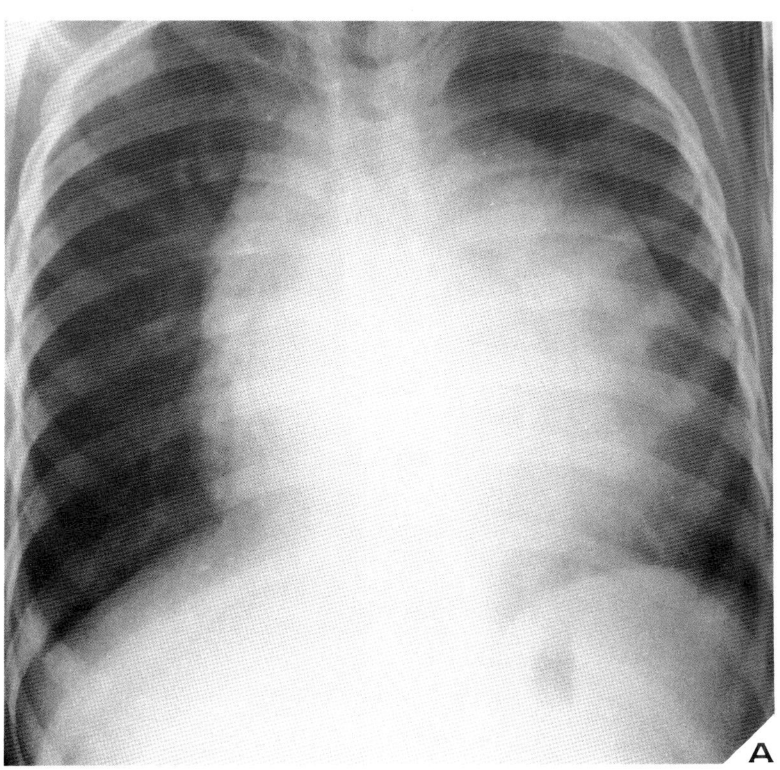

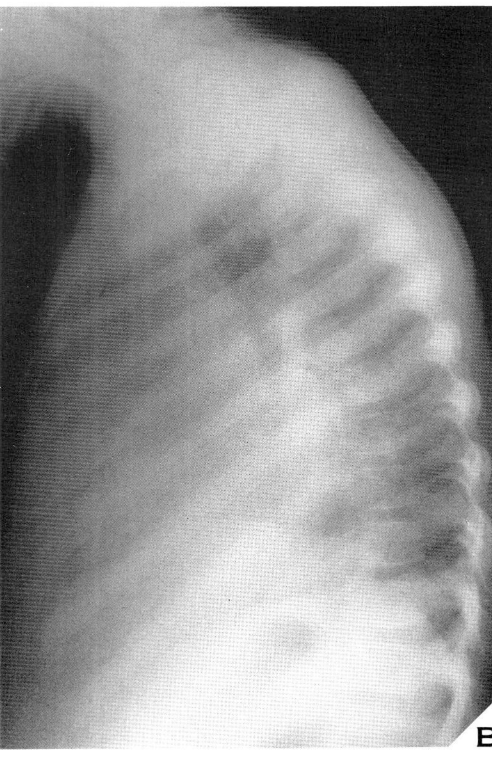

Fig. 29.11 Acute bacterial endocarditis. (A) Posteroanterior and (B) lateral chest films show cardiomegaly involving all four chambers and a small left pleural effusion. Clinical evaluation confirmed the presence of mitral, tricuspid, and aortic insufficiency. *Streptococcus viridans* was isolated from the blood.

MAGNETIC RESONANCE IMAGING

Cine MRI clearly depicts the valvular insufficiency and may demonstrate perforation of the leaflets (Fig. 29.12).

CARDIAC CATHETERIZATION AND ANGIOCARDIOGRAPHY

Invasive diagnostic procedures are not needed to confirm the diagnosis of infective endocarditis, since the anatomic changes produced by the infection, as well as the underlying cardiac malformation, are clearly shown by echocardiography. Occasionally, cardiac catheterization and angiocardiography may be necessary to completely assess the cardiac malformation.

INFECTIVE PERICARDITIS

PYOGENIC (PURULENT) PERICARDITIS

Although purulent pericarditis (a frequent cause of death in the pre-antibiotic era) is now uncommon, about one third of cases occur in children under 6 years of age. In one large series, the most common pathogens, in order of frequency, were *Staphylococcus aureus (pyogenes)* (37 percent), *Streptococcus pneumoniae* ("pneumococcus") (22 percent), and hemolytic streptococci (17 percent).

CLINICAL FEATURES

The clinical manifestations of pyogenic pericarditis are related to the organism, the age of the patient, the size of the pericardial effusion, and the presence (or absence) of associated myocarditis. Fever, tachypnea, chest pain, and dyspnea are almost always present. Substernal chest pain, typically more severe during inspiration, is a common complaint. The heart sounds are usually muffled, and there may be a pericardial friction rub. In some cases, physical examination may reveal the classical findings of cardiac tamponade (neck vein distension, hepatomegaly, pulsus paradoxicus, hypotension with a narrow pulse pressure) (see Chapter 22). The ECG is usually abnormal, exhibiting decreased QRS amplitude and ST-segment and T-wave abnormalities. Elevation or depression of the ST-segment, when present, indicate that there is an associated myocarditis.

Microscopic examination of the pericardial fluid reveals marked leukocytosis (often greater than 50,000 WBC/mm^3). Protein levels vary; however, the glucose level is usually low. The diagnosis is confirmed by isolating the pathogen from the pericardial fluid.

IMAGING

The imaging of pericardial disease is discussed in Chapter 22 and will be only briefly considered here. Plain films in patients with purulent pericarditis usually show an abnormal cardiac

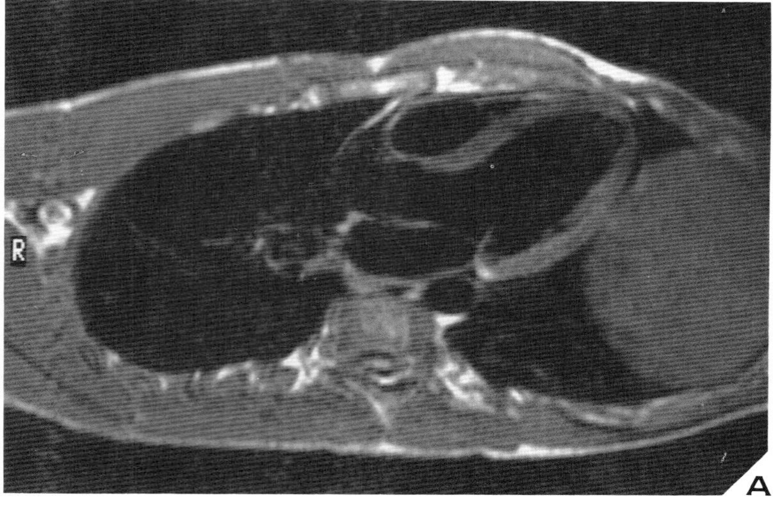

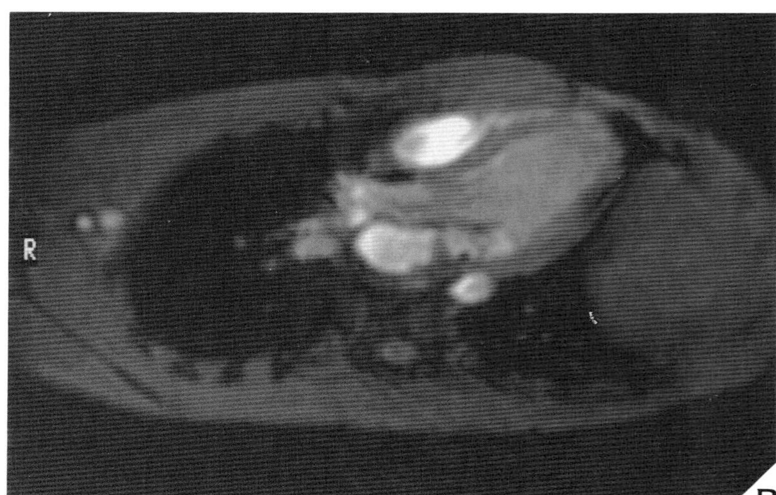

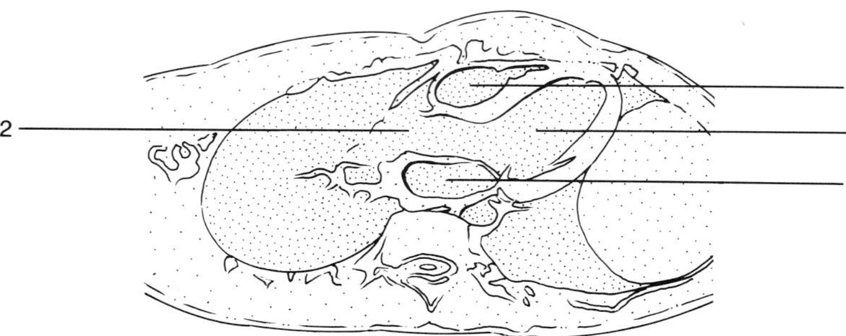

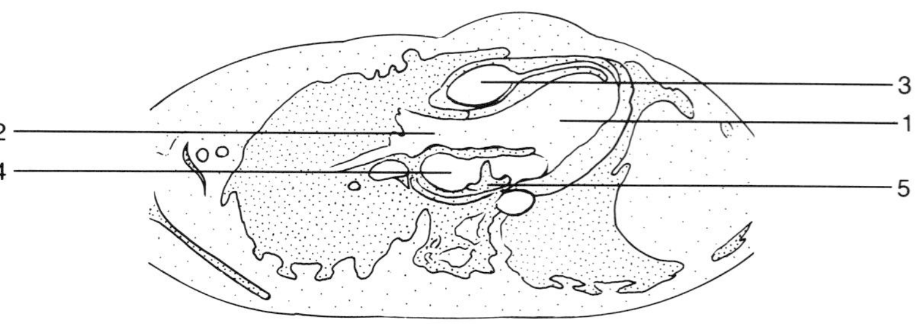

Fig. 29.12 Infective endocarditis with perforation of the mitral valve (MRI findings). Axial (A) spin–echo and (B) gradient echo (cine) images in a young adult show an enlarged left ventricle emptying into the aorta. Note the signal void in the left atrium close to the anterior mitral leaflet. A perforation of the anterior mitral leaflet was found at operation.

1 left ventricle
2 aorta
3 right ventricle
4 left atrium
5 signal void in left atrium

silhouette; often, there is a "water bottle" configuration characteristic of a large pericardial effusion. An occasional patient may have a loculated exudate, in which case chest films may demonstrate a localized deformity of the cardiac contour. Echocardiography, performed by either a transthoracic or a transesophageal approach, is highly accurate in detecting pericardial fluid, which appears as a signal void interposed between the epicardium and the fibrous pericardium.

VIRAL PERICARDITIS

Most cases of "pericarditis of unknown etiology" are probably viral pericarditis. The most frequent causative viruses are Coxsackie B, influenza, mumps, varicella, and Asian influenza.

CLINICAL FEATURES

The patient with viral pericarditis is usually between 3 and 11 years of age. Typically, the patient complains of pain in the chest, neck, shoulders, and abdomen. The onset of the pain is usually insidious; however, it may be of abrupt onset, sometimes awakening the patient at night. Fever, which usually subsides in 7 to 10 days, is a common presenting symptom.

Physical examination usually reveals evidence of a moderate-sized to large pericardial effusion. A pericardial friction rub may be present in patients with lesser amounts of pericardial fluid. The leukocyte count ranges from 7,000 to 25,000. The pericardial fluid is typically serosanguineous. The diagnosis is confirmed by positive titers and/or viral cultures, or inferred by excluding other types of pericarditis and causes of pericardial effusion.

Most patients are not acutely ill and recover uneventfully in about 2 weeks; an occasional patient may remain symptomatic for up to 3 months. Rarely, infections with Coxsackie B virus may progress to constrictive pericarditis.

IMAGING

Plain films show the typical findings of a pericardial effusion (Fig. 29.13). Pericardial fluid may accumulate rapidly; in an occasional patient serial films obtained over a period of a few hours may show a dramatic change. Echocardiography shows a normal-sized heart surrounded by pericardial fluid.

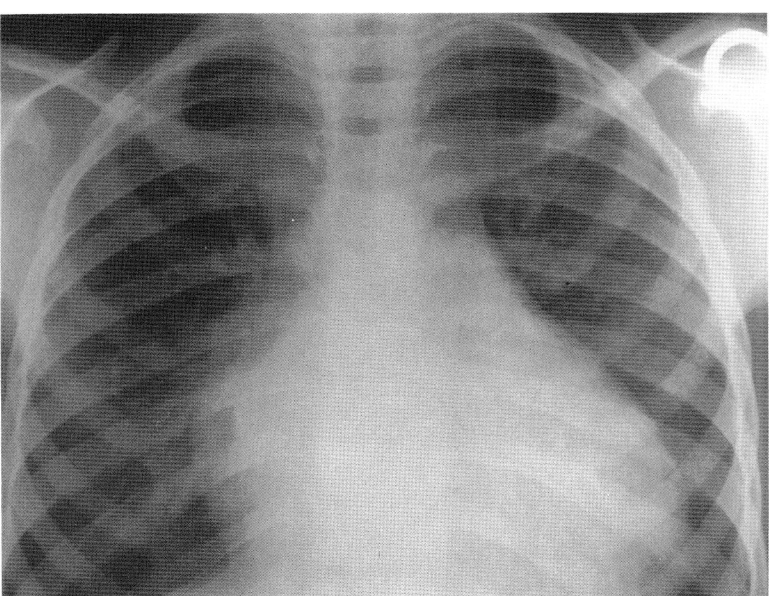

Fig. 29.13 Viral pericarditis. Posteroanterior chest film in a child with viral (Coxsackie B) pericarditis demonstrates a typical "water bottle" cardiovascular silhouette. Note dilatation of the superior vena cava, indicating restricted filling of the right ventricle caused by the pericardial effusion.

INFECTIVE MYOCARDITIS

The myocardium can be infected by bacteria, spirochetes, rickettsia, viruses, fungi, protozoa, or helminths. Primary myocardial infections are rare; in the great majority of cases infective myocarditis is associated with a systemic infection. Although the prevalence of infective myocarditis in a given population is unknown, 5.2 percent of the approximately 6,500 reported cases have occurred in children under 16 years of age.

Infective myocarditis is frequently associated with pericarditis ("myocardiopericarditis"), particularly in patients with Coxsackie B infections. The pericardial fluid in patients with viral myocardiopericarditis is typically serosanguineous. The pericardial fluid in patients with bacterial myocardiopericarditis is typically purulent.

PATHOLOGY

Viral myocarditis is usually caused by Coxsackie B virus. It is characterized pathologically by ventricular dilatation with little or no hypertrophy; dilatation of the supporting structures commonly results in incompetence of the atrioventricular valves. The myocardium is flabby to the touch and the cut surface may have a slightly pale appearance. Some hearts exhibit left ventricular hypertrophy and endocardial thickening. In such cases the mitral valve is usually involved; the leaflets typically have rolled edges and the chordae tendinae are short and thickened. Microscopic examination reveals a cellular infiltrate (usually mononuclear), usually perivascular in distribution. Occasionally the microscopic lesions are predominantly subendocardial or subepicardial in distribution. Viral myocarditis is characterized by muscle fragmentation and necrosis; characteristic inclusions are sometimes seen in the myocytes.

Bacterial infections, particularly those caused by gram-positive cocci, are associated with myocardial abscess formation. Fungal myocarditis is characterized by fibrocaseous abscesses and focal granulomas; endocardial involvement, with vegetations of the endocardial surfaces and valve leaflets, is commonly present as well. The causative organism can often be identified in the abscess or granuloma or within macrophages, or it may be free in the myocardium. In general, the pathologic findings of rickettsial infections are those of a primary vasculitis with secondary myocytic involvement.

CLINICAL FEATURES

Infants and children with viral myocarditis typically present with dyspnea, tachypnea, and CHF of relatively abrupt onset. The illness is often preceded by an acute respiratory infection. Bacterial or fungal myocarditis is nearly always associated with systemic infection; it frequently goes unrecognized until the process is far advanced. Often, involvement of other organ systems dominates the clinical picture, or there may be a long "silent" interval before clinical manifestations of cardiac involvement appear. The possibility of bacterial or fungal myocarditis should be considered whenever a patient with a systemic infection has persistent tachycardia out of proportion to the fever, develops an arrhythmia (usually premature ventricular beats or an atrial arrhythmia), or exhibits tachypnea, dyspnea, or signs and symptoms of congestive heart failure. Cardiomegaly, which reflects severe cardiomyopathy, may be present in patients with advanced disease. The ECG findings are nonspecific and include ST-segment abnormalities and arrhythmias (eg, ectopic beats secondary to atrioventricular or intraventricular conduction defects).

The diagnosis of infective myocarditis is usually one of exclusion. In patients with pericardial involvement ("myocardiopericarditis"), the causative agent can sometimes be isolated from the pericardial fluid. Transcatheter endocardial biopsy may be rewarding in some instances. More often, however, an open myocardial biopsy is required to verify the diagnosis and identify the pathogen.

IMAGING AND INVASIVE DIAGNOSIS

PLAIN FILMS

The plain film findings are nonspecific. Children with severe congestive heart failure exhibit cardiomegaly, pulmonary venous hypertension, and interstitial or alveolar pulmonary edema (Fig. 29.14). However, patients in whom the cardiac involvement is less severe may have a normal chest film.

ECHOCARDIOGRAPHY

Echocardiography typically reveals nonspecific findings of ventricular dilatation and poor contractility. Pericardial fluid may be seen in patients with pericardial involvement.

NUCLEAR MEDICINE

SPECT imaging with monoclonal ^{111}I-labeled anti-myosin F(ab) (see Chapter 20) has been reported to have a sensitivity of 83 percent and a specificity of 53 percent in the diagnosis of infective endocarditis. Further data are needed to assess the reliability of this technique.

CARDIAC CATHETERIZATION

Cardiac catheterization findings in patients with infective myocarditis are usually nonspecific. A constellation of functional aberrations suggestive of abnormal ventricular distensibility (elevated right atrial pressure associated with moderate elevation of systolic pressure in both ventricles and little or no elevation of right ventricular end diastolic pressure) has been described, but the sensitivity and specificity of this pattern remain to be confirmed.

KAWASAKI DISEASE (MUCOCUTANEOUS LYMPH NODE SYNDROME)

Kawasaki disease (mucocutaneous lymph node syndrome), first described in 1967, is an acute systemic inflammatory disorder of unknown etiology which occurs predominantly in children under 5 years of age. Initially observed in Japanese children, Kawasaki disease is now known to have a worldwide distribution. Coronary arterial involvement is relatively common and is the major cause of morbidity and late mortality in this disorder.

CLINICAL FEATURES

The clinical course of Kawasaki disease can be divided into three phases. The first phase, which lasts for about 1 to 2 weeks, is characterized by cervical and axillary (sometimes generalized) lymphadenopathy, mucocutaneous lesions, fever, and

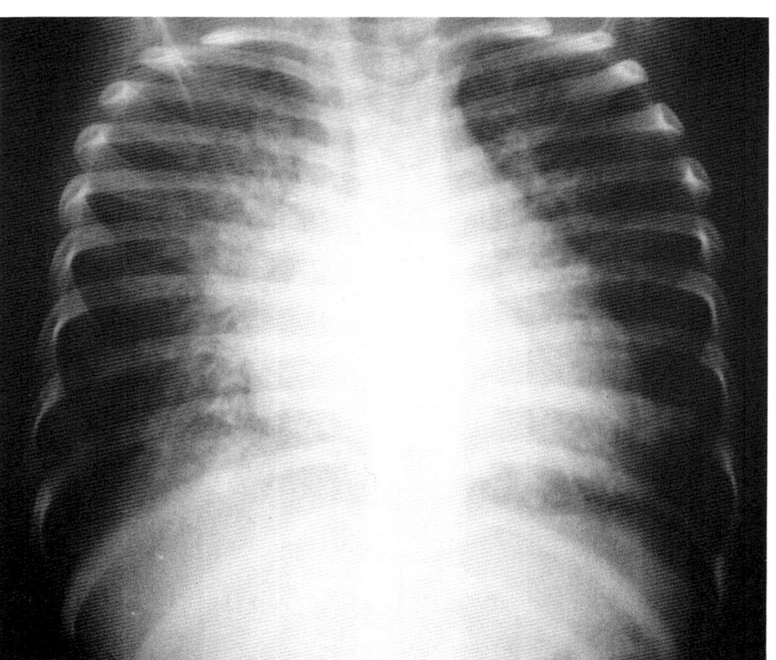

Fig. 29.14 Viral myocarditis. This previously well 14-month-old girl presented with abrupt onset of tachypnea, breathing difficulty, and vomiting. Blood gases revealed moderate desaturation in room air with improvement in 50 percent oxygen. Frontal chest film shows moderate cardiac enlargement with severe interstitial pulmonary edema. Echocardiography demonstrated decreased contractility of the left ventricle. Serological studies were compatible with a Coxsackie B viral infection.

intense leukocytosis with a predominance of neutrophils. The mucocutaneous lesions consist of erythema of the palms and feet; a polymorphous exanthem of the trunk without crusts or vesiculation; peripheral edema with induration; dryness, fissuring, and erythema of the lips; and erythema of the tongue ("strawberry tongue") and oropharyngeal mucous membranes. Other nonspecific symptoms (eg, diarrhea) may be present. The second phase, which typically lasts about 2 to 5 weeks, is characterized by desquamation of the rash, beginning at the fingertips, and joint involvement (arthritis or arthralgia). The third (convalescent) phase lasts until the sedimentation rate has returned to normal and all clinical signs have disappeared.

Cardiovascular complications, including coronary arterial lesions, myocarditis, pericarditis, valvulitis, and atrioventricular conduction abnormalities, are relatively common. Coronary arterial involvement is the most serious sequela of Kawasaki disease. Coronary artery aneurysms, which can result in left ventricular dysfunction secondary to myocardial ischemia or acute (possibly fatal) myocardial infarction, develop in 10 to 20 percent of cases. Pericardial effusion, which typically occurs during the second or third week of the illness, has been demonstrated echocardiographically in 25 percent of patients with Kawasaki disease, but is usually of little clinical importance.

PATHOLOGY

A subacute myocarditis with round cell infiltration is characteristic of the early stages of Kawasaki disease. The most severe lesions are seen in myocardial biopsies performed within 5 months of the onset of the illness. Endocardial involvement (valvulitis) can also occur.

The coronary arterial lesions, which appear within a few days after the clinical onset, consist of an arteritis with histopathologic features resembling those of infantile polyarteritis nodosa. Aneurysm formation has been detected as early as the second week after the onset of symptoms (Fig. 29.15). The large epicardial coronary arteries are the most commonly affected; small peripheral and intramyocardial branches are spared. (The most common sites of involvement, in order of frequency, are the proximal segment of the left anterior descending artery, the proximal segment of the right coronary artery, and the left main coronary artery. When the circumflex artery and distal right coronary artery are involved, more proximal segments of the arteries are invariably involved as well.) Grossly, the aneurysm may be saccular, fusiform, or diffuse; in some instances, the abnormality may consist of a localized dilatation. The wall of a mature aneurysm exhibits hyaline degeneration and intimal thickening similar to that seen in arteriosclerotic (atherosclerotic) aneurysms. Protein-like material and thrombus are commonly present within its lumen. Stenosis or occlusion of the affected artery is not uncommon. The narrowing, which results from intimal proliferation and thrombus formation, tends to occur at or adjacent to the site of the aneurysm.

The arteritis associated with Kawasaki disease also may affect extracardiac vessels, including the axillary, brachial, iliac, and renal arteries; extracardiac arterial lesions have been reported to occur in 2.4 percent of cases.

CLINICOPATHOLOGIC CORRELATION

Criteria for the diagnosis of Kawasaki disease—initially promulgated by the Research Committee on Mucocutaneous Lymph Node Syndrome in Japan and later adopted by the Centers for Disease Control in Atlanta—have allowed accurate assessment of outcome. Most of the available data come from Japan. In one large series, coronary arterial lesions were detected angiographically in 35/162 (21.6 percent) unselected Japanese children who met the diagnostic criteria for Kawasaki disease (Kuribayashi et al, 1989). Aneurysm formation is more common in infants (1 year of age) than in older patients. Two thirds of patients with coronary artery aneurysms undergo spontaneous resolution within 30 months, the caliber of the affected artery reverting to normal. Aneurysms in infant girls are more likely to resolve spontaneously than aneurysms in older boys. Small and medium-sized fusiform aneurysms, the most common type, tend to resolve spontaneously, whereas large aneurysms seldom do so. Distal aneurysms tend to be smaller than more centrally located aneurysms and tend to resolve sooner. Stenosis or occlusion, which can lead to myocardial infarction, tends to be associated with large aneurysms of long duration. In one series, coronary arterial stenosis was detected in 13 percent

FIG. 29.15 PATHOGENISIS OF CORONARY ARTERY LESIONS IN KAWASAKI DISEASE (MUCOCUTANEOUS LYMPH NODE SYNDROME)*

Stage	Interval from clinical onset	Pathologic Features
Stage 1	0–9 days	Acute perivasculitis and endarteritis.
Stage 2	12–25 days	Acute inflammation of all layers of the arterial wall (panvasculitis) with formation of thrombus-filled aneurysm, which may rupture.
Stage 3	28–31 days	Organization of thrombus and intimal proliferation lead to stenosis of the affected arteries. Acute inflammation gradually subsides and is replaced with granulation tissue.
Stage 4	After 40 days (chronic phase)	Scar formation, calcification, enlargement of aneurysm, varying degrees of stenosis.

**Adapted from data in Fujiwara and Hamishima (1978)*

Fig. 29.15 Pathogenesis of coronary artery lesions in Kawasaki disease (mucocutaneous lymph node syndrome).

of children with coronary artery aneurysms and complete occlusion in 8 percent.

A recent nationwide survey in Japan indicated that the death rate due to Kawasaki disease and its sequelae was 0.3 percent. About two thirds of the deaths were due to acute myocardial infarction, manifested clinically by vomiting, restlessness, abdominal pain, chest pain, and cardiogenic shock. In the rest, a clinically silent myocardial infarction was found at autopsy. The most common patterns of involvement in fatal cases were obstruction of the left main coronary artery and obstruction of both the left anterior descending and right coronary arteries. (Isolated right coronary arterial involvement is seldom a cause of severe morbidity or death.) Acute rupture of a coronary artery aneurysm with pericardial tamponade is an infrequent cause of death. Many children with myocardial infarction secondary to coronary arterial involvement survive with a variable degree of left ventricular dysfunction. Mitral regurgitation, presumably secondary to papillary muscle dysfunction associated with myocardial ischemia, occurs in a small percentage of cases.

To sum up: the greatest risk of a persistent aneurysm is associated with a large, centrally located aneurysm in a boy 2 years of age or older. Children with such lesions are at the greatest risk for serious cardiovascular sequelae and death.

IMAGING AND INVASIVE DIAGNOSIS

PLAIN FILMS

Chest films are usually normal in children with Kawasaki disease without cardiac involvement, as well as in the great majority of those with coronary artery aneurysms and their sequelae (Fig. 29.16). Coronary artery calcification is a rare finding. Patients with myocardial ischemia or infarction may exhibit left ventricular enlargement.

ECHOCARDIOGRAPHY

Echocardiography may demonstrate pericardial effusion in the acute and subacute phases. Some coronary artery aneurysms, mainly those arising in the proximal segments, can be detected echocardiographically. Although the transesophageal approach increases the diagnostic yield, more peripheral lesions (eg, aneurysms of the middle segment of the left anterior descending artery or the right coronary artery) are rarely detected by echocardiography.

NUCLEAR IMAGING

Scintigraphy with ^{111}I-tagged leukocytes has demonstrated diffuse myocardial uptake in a small number of children who were scanned during the initial or subacute phase of the disease (Williamson et al, 1986). This finding, which presumably reflects the acute myocarditis that commonly occurs in Kawasaki disease, may narrow the differential diagnosis in a child with a fever of unknown origin. It is not known whether the intensity of the cardiac uptake predicts the severity of the cardiovascular manifestations.

Patients with severe coronary arterial involvement demonstrate scintigraphic findings typical of chronic myocardial ischemia or myocardial infarction (see Chapter 20).

CT AND MRI

Both ultrafast (cine) CT and MRI are capable of detecting coronary artery aneurysms in infants and children with Kawasaki disease. If overlapping sections are employed, cine CT can detect aneurysms as small as 4 mm in diameter. Coronary artery aneurysms appear as areas of signal void on ECG-gated spin–echo MR images. Abnormal flow characteristics within the aneurysm can also be discerned with this technique. MRI can also detect aneurysms of the axillary, iliac, and renal arteries, which occasionally occur in patients with Kawasaki disease.

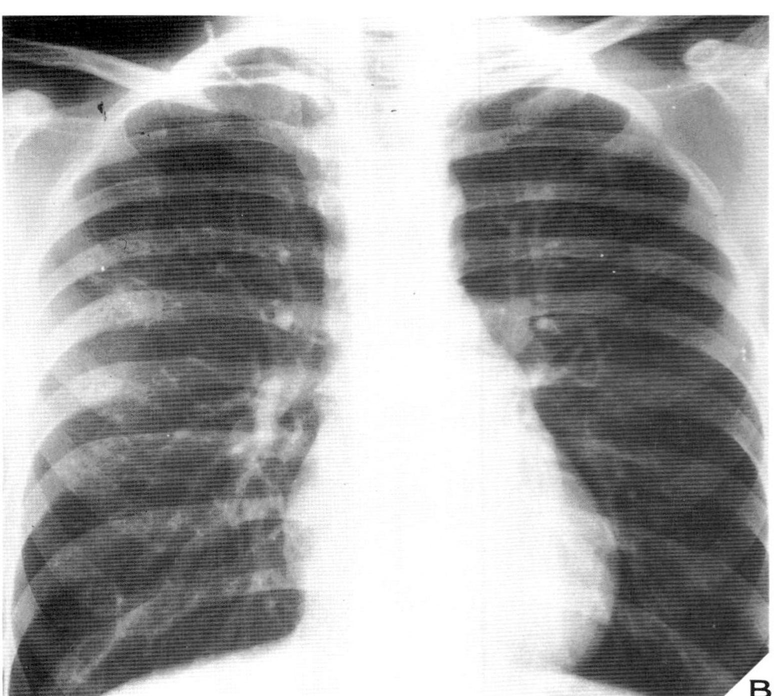

Fig. 29.16 Kawasaki disease. (A) Frontal chest film at 6 years of age (during acute phase) is normal. Subsequently, coronary arteriography demonstrated an aneurysm of the left main coronary artery extending into the left anterior descending artery and a separate, smaller aneurysm of the circumflex artery (see Fig. 29.16). (B) Chest film at 9 years of age is normal. There were no clinical signs of myocardial ischemia. Repeat coronary arteriogram demonstrated occlusion of the left anterior descending artery (see Fig. 29.17). A cine left ventriculogram showed minimal left ventricular enlargement.

ANGIOGRAPHY

Although echocardiography, cine CT, and MRI can serve as screening methods, coronary arteriography remains the method of choice for detecting coronary arterial involvement in patients with Kawasaki disease. (Arteriography will also detect aneurysms of the renal, axillary, and iliac arteries.) Selective catheterization of the right and left coronary arteries is routinely performed. The most frequent sites of involvement are the proximal segment of the left anterior descending artery (34 percent), the right coronary artery (33 percent), and the left main coronary artery (27 percent). Aneurysms of the posterior descending, posterolateral, and diagonal arteries also occur but are much less common. Aneurysms of the right coronary artery are usually limited to the proximal segment (48 percent); however, the entire artery may be involved. Saccular aneurysms typically involve one wall of an artery that is otherwise normal. The presence of an intraluminal filling defect in the aneurysm indicates thrombus. Selective arteriography will also detect stenoses or occlusions distal to the aneurysm. Typical angiographic findings in patients with Kawasaki disease are illustrated in Figs. 29.17 through 29.20 (see also Fig. 21.34).

Although left ventriculography can be used to assess left ventricular dysfunction secondary to myocardial necrosis, it has largely been supplanted by safe, noninvasive techniques such as echocardiography, scintigraphy, and MRI.

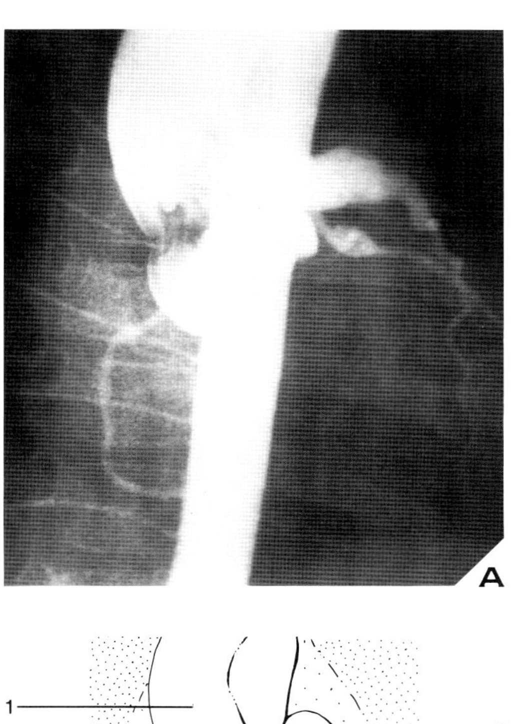

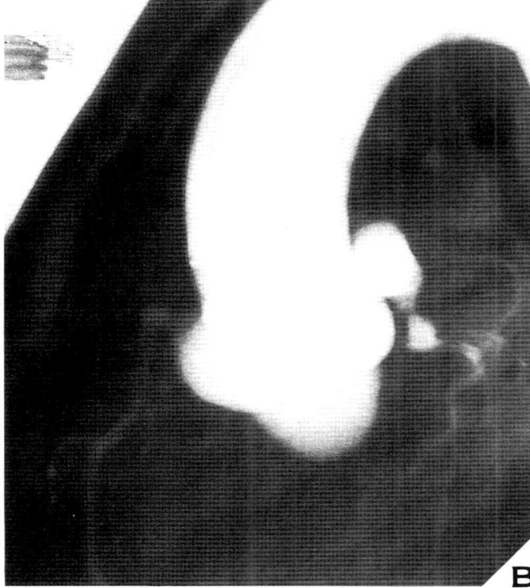

Fig. 29.17 Kawasaki disease. Same patient as Fig. 29.16. (A) Frontal and (B) lateral projections of thoracic aortogram at 6 years of age demonstrate a large saccular aneurysm of the left main coronary artery extending into the left anterior descending artery (LAD). There is also a small aneurysm of the circumflex artery (the filling defect in the aneurysm represents thrombus). Both the LAD and the circumflex artery are patent distally. The right coronary artery is normal.

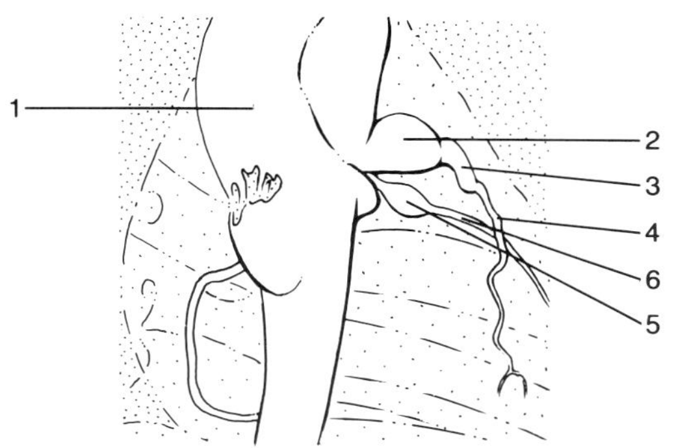

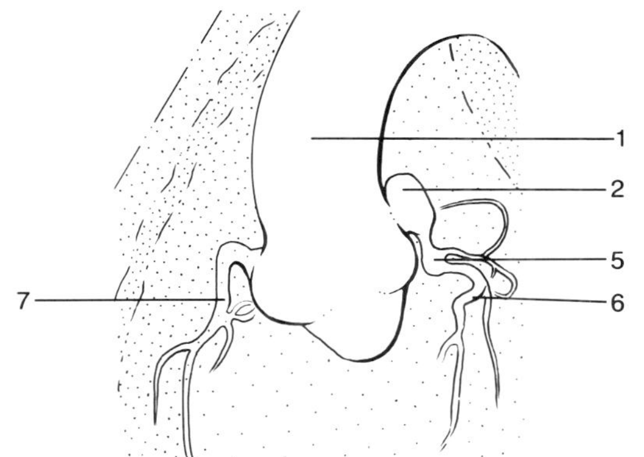

1 ascending aorta
2 aneurysm of left main coronary artery
3 aneurysm of proximal segment of left anterior descending artery
4 normal portion of left anterior descending artery
5 aneurysm of circumflex artery
6 normal portion of circumflex artery
7 normal right coronary artery

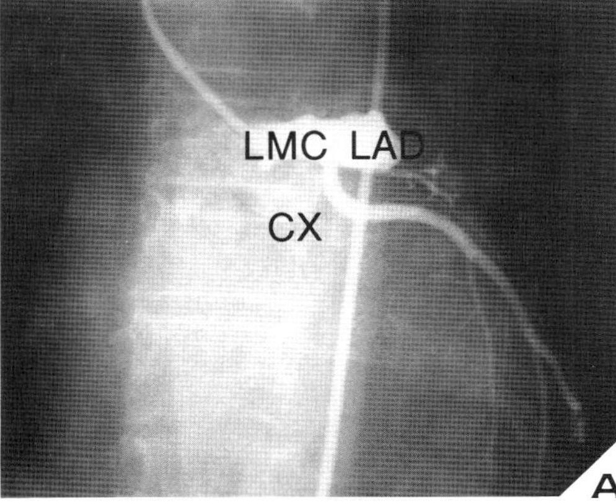

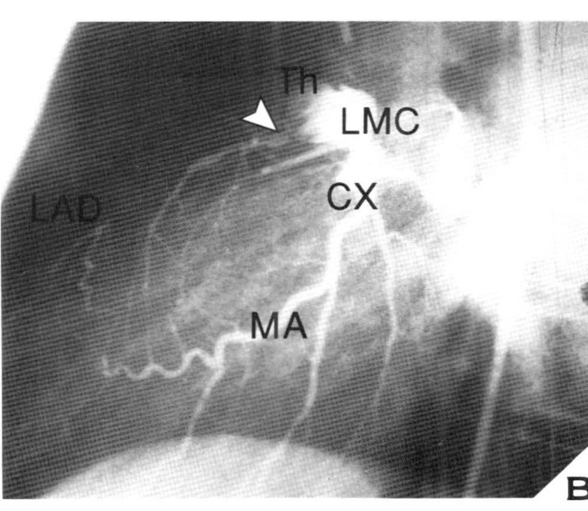

Fig. 29.18 Kawasaki disease. Same patient as Figs. 29.16 and 29.17. (A) Frontal and (B) lateral projections of left coronary arteriogram at 9 years of age show no change in the appearance of the aneurysm of the left main coronary (LMC) and left anterior descending (LAD) arteries (compare Fig. 29.16). However, the proximal segment of the LAD is occluded (*arrow*) just beyond the aneurysm. The distal LAD is supplied by collateral circulation. The filling defect (Th) in the aneurysm represents thrombus. The aneurysm of the circumflex artery (CX) has disappeared. However, the caliber of the circumflex artery is greater than normal. (MA = marginal artery).

POMPE'S DISEASE (GLYCOGENOSIS TYPE II)

Pompe's disease is an extremely rare, lethal autosomal recessive disorder caused by an inability to synthesize the enzyme alpha-1,4-glucosidase. Pathologically, it is characterized by the accumulation of glycogen in muscle (including myocardium) and other tissues throughout the body. Myocardial glycogenosis results in severe hypertrophic cardiomyopathy. The hemodynamic features are those of a hypertrophic cardiomyopathy (with or without left ventricular outflow obstruction).

CLINICAL FEATURES

Symptoms typically appear at 2 to 5 months of age and always before 18 months of age. The characteristic clinical manifestations include feeding difficulty, failure to thrive, frequent respiratory infections, cyanosis, tachycardia, and massive cardiac enlargement. The ECG typically reveals evidence of left ventricular hypertrophy, with increased QRS voltage and a shortened P-Q interval. Death typically results from intractable heart failure. Accumulations of glycogen in the ventricular septum may be responsible for arrhythmias and sudden death.

The differential diagnosis includes dilated cardiomyopathy, anomalous origin of the left coronary artery from the pulmonary trunk, and acute myocarditis. The diagnosis of Pompe's disease is confirmed by demonstrating increased muscular glycogen on a skeletal muscle biopsy and demonstrating the absence of alpha-glucosidase activity in a muscle or liver biopsy or in leukocytes.

At present, the only treatment for Pompe's disease is cardiac transplantation.

IMAGING AND INVASIVE DIAGNOSIS

Plain films typically show massive cardiac enlargement, which usually involves all four chambers (Fig. 29.21). Pulmonary vascular congestion is frequently present. Atelectasis of the left lower lobe secondary to compression by the enlarged heart is very common. Conditions with similar plain film findings include anomalous origin of the left coronary artery from the pulmonary trunk, dilated cardiomyopathy, and Ebstein's anomaly.

Echocardiography, MRI, and cine CT demonstrate increased thickness of the myocardium and small ventricular cavities. In some patients, the cavity of either ventricle may be obstructed in systole by masses projecting from the free wall of either ventricle or the ventricular septum. These masses, which at one time were mistaken for rhabdomyomas, represent nodular collections of glycogen within the myocardium.

Left or right ventriculography typically demonstrates marked hypertrophy of the ventricular wall; in extreme instances the

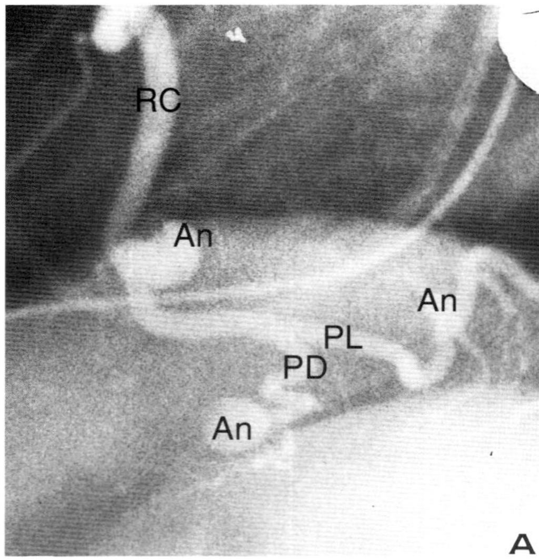

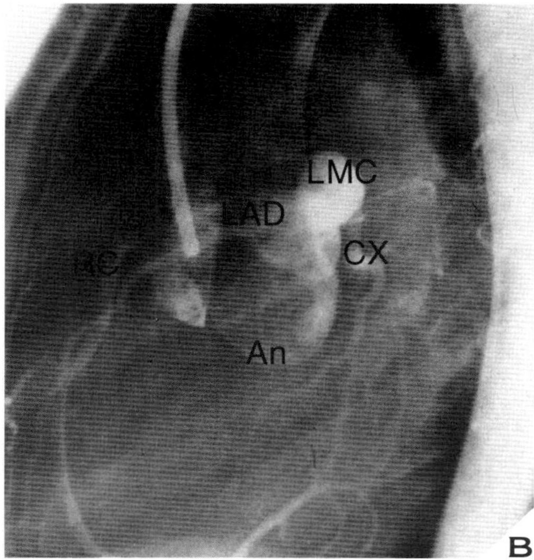

Fig. 29.19 Kawasaki disease. (A, B) Angiograhic findings in two different children. (A) Selective right coronary arteriogram shows multiple saccular aneurysms (An) involving the distal portion of the right coronary (RC), posterior descending (PD), and posterolateral (PL) arteries. (B) Lateral projection of thoracic aortogram demonstrates huge saccular aneurysms (An) of the left main coronary (LMC) and left anterior descending (LAD) arteries. The filling defect in the aneurysm represents thrombus. (CX = circumflex artery)

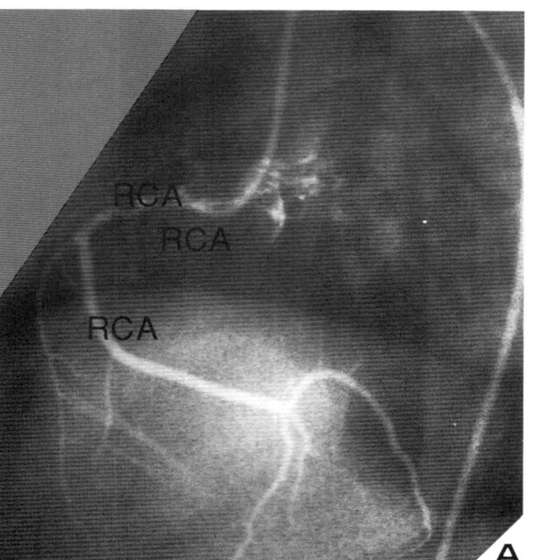

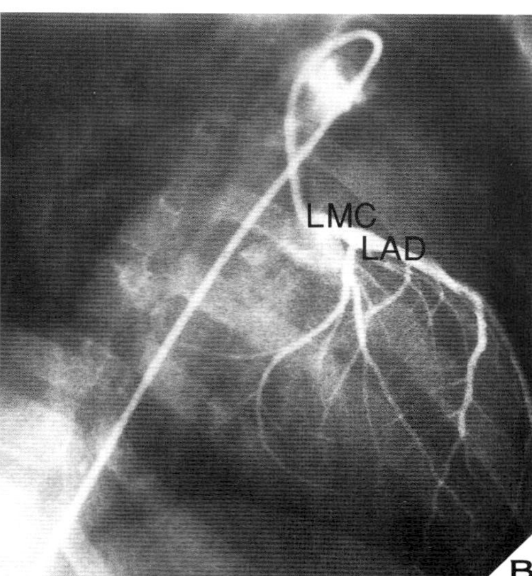

Fig. 29.20 Acute phase of Kawasaki disease. (A) Right coronary arteriogram (LAO projection) and (B) left coronary arteriogram (RAO projection) in a 1-year-old child demonstrate a long narrowed segment (60 percent stenosis) of the proximal segment of the right coronary artery (RCA). There is mild fusiform dilatation of the left main coronary (LMC) and left anterior descending (LAD) arteries.

ventricular cavity may be completely obliterated. Masses of glycogen in the free wall or ventricular septum appear angiographically as mural masses obstructing the ventricular cavity to a variable extent.

MUSCLE AND CONNECTIVE TISSUE DISORDERS

A number of muscle and connective tissue disorders may involve the cardiovascular system in both children and adults (eg, muscular dystrophy, mucopolysaccharidoses, Marfan syndrome, pseudoxanthoma elasticum, Ehler–Danlos syndrome, osteogenesis imperfecta). This group of disorders is considered in Chapter 25.

INFANTS OF DIABETIC OR PREDIABETIC MOTHERS

Infants of diabetic or prediabetic mothers (IDMs) frequently exhibit cardiomegaly, which may be due to a cardiac malformation (see Chapter 5) or cardiomyopathy. The cardiomyopathy in IDMs can be of either the hypertrophic (obstructive) type or the dilated (congestive) type. The hypertrophic (obstructive) type usually takes the form of asymmetric septal hypertrophy with left ventricular outflow tract obstruction, which is morphologically and hemodynamically indistinguishable from the adult form of idiopathic subaortic stenosis (IHSS). The muscle hypertrophy typically involves the upper two thirds of the ventricular septum and the adjacent portions of the free walls of the left and right ventricles. Occasionally there is extensive right ventricular or biventricular involvement. The muscle hypertrophy regresses spontaneously, with resolution of the left ventricular outflow tract obstruction over a period of days or weeks.

Diabetes-related dilated (congestive) cardiomyopathy is characterized pathologically by generalized hypertrophy and hyperplasia of myocardial cells; the clinical and radiographic picture can mimic that of the hypoplastic left heart syndrome. Spontaneous recovery is the rule.

IMAGING

Plain films of newborn infants with cardiomyopathy of either the congestive or hypertrophic type typically show cardiomegaly, often accompanied by vascular congestion (Figs. 29.22

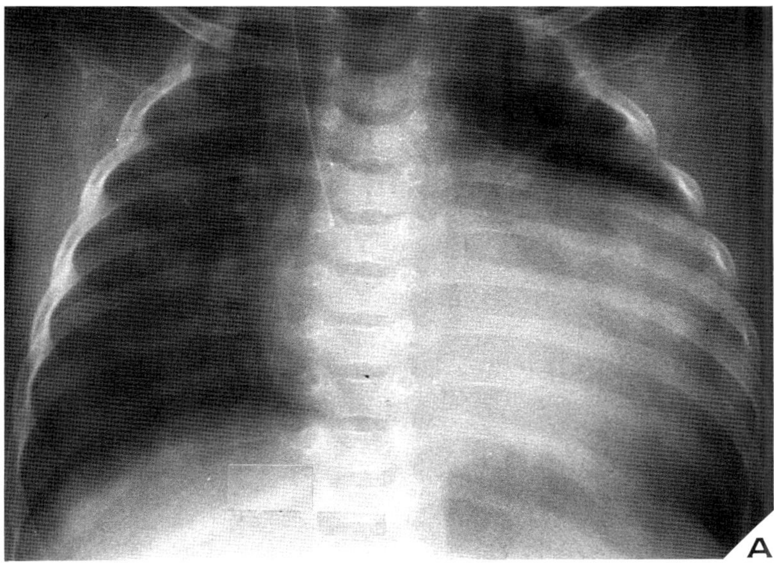

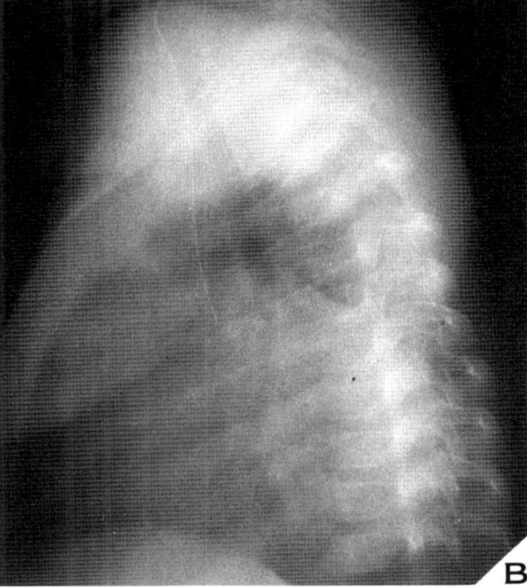

Fig. 29.21 Pompe disease. This 5-month-old infant presented with profound generalized muscle weakness, failure to thrive, hepatomegaly, and an enlarged tongue. (A) Frontal and (B) lateral chest films demonstrate massive cardiomegaly with marked left ventricular enlargement. The pulmonary vasculature is normal. There is compression atelectasis of the left lung. Muscle biopsy and subsequent autopsy (1 month later) confirmed the diagnosis of Pompe disease (glycogenosis type II).

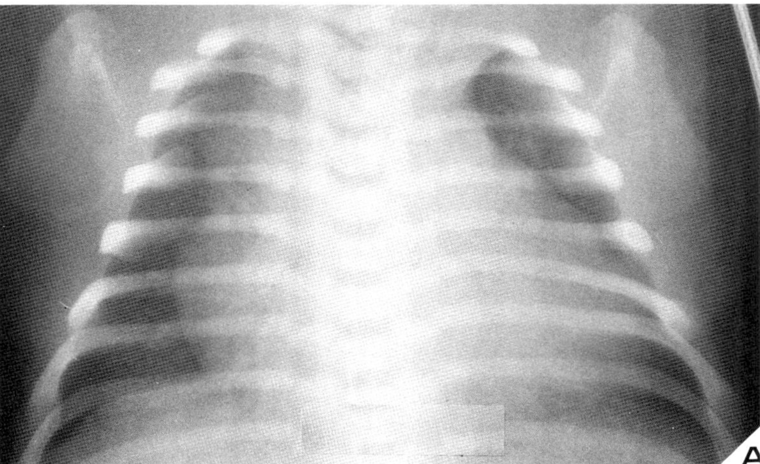

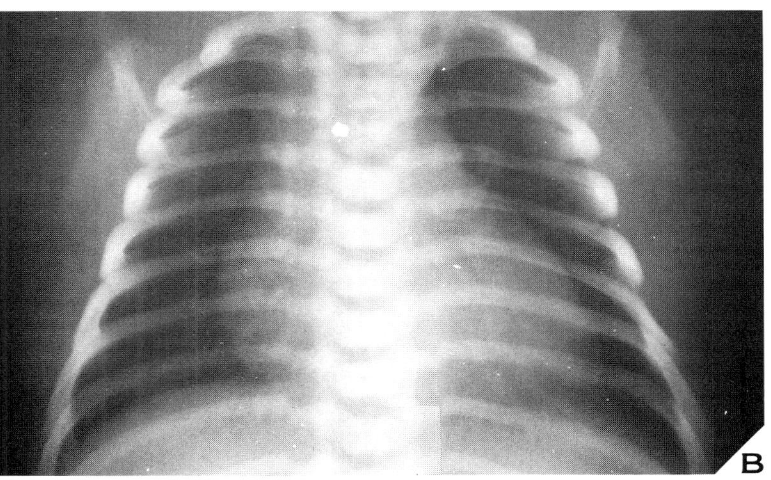

Fig. 29.22 Transient cardiomyopathy in infant of a diabetic mother. (A, B) This full-term infant had clinical signs of congestive heart failure immediately after birth, with severe hypoglycemia. (A) Initial chest film at 5 hours of age shows marked cardiac enlargement with normal pulmonary vasculature. (B) By 5 days of age there has been marked regression of the cardiomegaly. The infant had a mild tachycardia but was otherwise asymptomatic. His subsequent course was uneventful.

and 29.23). The echocardiographic findings resemble those of the adult forms of these disorders (see Chapter 19). Echocardiography is helpful in excluding congenital cardiac malformations, which occur in about 4 percent of IDMs.

ENDOCARDIAL FIBROELASTOSIS

Congenital endocardial fibroelastosis (EFE) is a rare disorder of unknown cause. Two forms of primary EFE have been described: dilated and restrictive. The dilated form, which accounts for the great majority of cases of primary EFE, can be considered a form of dilated cardiomyopathy in which the endocardial thickening is presumably secondary to inadequate subendocardial blood flow. Although the etiology is unknown, there is suggestive evidence that it may represent a "burned-out" fetal myocarditis. The restrictive ("contracted") form is characterized by a thick, fibrous endocardium, which restricts diastolic filling, and a small or normal-sized left ventricle. The restrictive form of EFE is extremely rare; indeed, its existence has been questioned by some authors.

The *dilated form of primary EFE* is characterized by marked left ventricular dilatation. The hyperplastic endocardium may be several centimeters thick. The aortic and mitral leaflets, as well as the chordae tendinae, are thickened and distorted. The patient typically presents with signs and symptoms of left ventricular dysfunction and congestive heart failure at 4 to 10 months of age (sometimes as early as the neonatal period). A murmur of mitral insufficiency is audible in about 40 percent of cases. The ECG demonstrates left ventricular hypertrophy with inverted T-waves in the left precordial leads; less common findings include myocardial infarction patterns, atrioventricular block, and arrhythmias. The clinical course is usually progressively downhill; although the prognosis is grim in infants who present with marked cardiomegaly, a number of authors have reported long-term survival with vigorous medical therapy.

In the *restrictive form of primary EFE*, the endocardial fibroelastosis is confined to the left ventricle. The atria and right ventricle are markedly enlarged and hypertrophied. The clinical picture is that of left-sided obstructive disease, particularly if the mitral valve is very small.

The *secondary form of EFE*, which is characterized by thickening of the endocardium or cardiac valves, is almost always associated with congenital left-sided obstructive lesions (eg, congenital aortic stenosis, coarctation of the aorta, hypoplastic left heart syndrome) and can be considered an integral feature of these entities. It is rarely associated with congenital obstructions on the right side of the heart. The clinical and radiologic findings in patients with secondary EFE reflect the underlying lesion (see Chapter 12).

IMAGING AND INVASIVE DIAGNOSIS

Chest films reveal marked cardiomegaly with normal pulmonary vasculature or congestive changes. Echocardiography typically demonstrates left ventricular and left atrial dilatation, decreased septal and left ventricular posterior wall motion, and mitral valve insufficiency. Cardiac catheterization reveals evidence of left ventricular dysfunction and moderate pulmonary hypertension. Left ventriculography demonstrates a markedly dilated, poorly functioning, usually thin-walled left ventricle and varying degrees of mitrial insufficiency (Fig. 29.24). The left ventricle usually has a globular configuration; however, dyskinetic or akinetic segments are occasionally seen.

DIFFERENTIAL DIAGNOSIS

The differential diagnosis of primary EFE includes anomalous (pulmonary) origin of the left coronary artery (see Chapter 20), myocarditis, idiopathic or diabetes-induced hypertrophic subaortic stenosis, malformations causing obstruction of the left ventricular outflow tract, and type II glycogen storage disease (Pompe's disease). The first four conditions usually have distinctive ECG and echocardiographic features; however, angiography may be necessary to exclude anomalous origin of the left coronary artery. Skeletal muscle biopsy is diagnostic in Pompe's disease. Although the diagnosis of primary EFE is usually established on clinical grounds, transcatheter endocardial biopsy techniques can provide the definitive diagnosis if necessary.

ENDOMYOCARDIAL FIBROSIS (EMF)

EMF is a disorder of unknown (possibly infectious) etiology, characterized by extensive endocardial fibrosis causing restrictive cardiomyopathy and atrioventricular valvular insufficiency. First described in equatorial Africa in the 1950s, it has now been recognized in tropical and subtropical regions throughout the world. EMF is a relatively frequent cause of heart failure and death in children and young adults in the affected populations, accounting for 15 to 25 percent of deaths from heart disease in equatorial Africa.

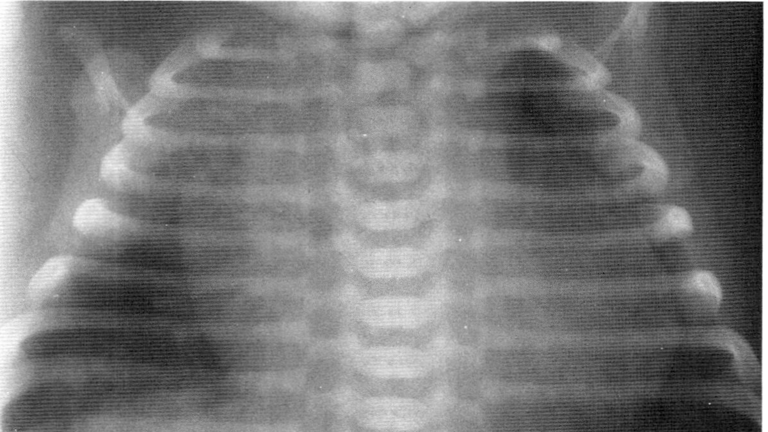

Fig. 29.23 Transient cardiomyopathy with persistent fetal circulation mimicking the hypoplastic left heart syndrome in an infant of a diabetic mother. This full-term infant was cyanotic and tachypneic since birth; the cyanosis did not improve on 100 percent oxygen. He was severely hypoglycemic. A frontal chest film shortly after birth shows generalized cardiac enlargement and pulmonary vascular congestion. Right cardiac catheterization at 2 days of age revealed a large right ventricle with marked right to left shunting across the ductus arteriosus; a hypoplastic left ventricle could not be excluded. Left heart catheterization at 4 days of age demonstrated a morphologically normal but poorly contracting left ventricle. There was no pressure gradient. The infant's condition gradually improved; his cardiac status was considered normal at 13 days of age.

PATHOLOGIC FEATURES

Grossly, the heart is normal in size or slightly enlarged; hypertrophy is typically absent and massive cardiomegaly does not occur. The fibrotic process typically affects the atrioventricular valves and the inflow portions of the ventricles (right, or left, or both). The thickened, fibrotic endocardium covers the papillary muscles and chordae tendinae and produces thickening of the atrioventricular valves. On the right, fibrosis may extend to the apex of the right ventricle, which may be obliterated by a mass of fibrous tissue and thrombus. The tricuspid valve is pulled down and distorted by the fibrotic process involving the supporting structures. Right atrial thrombi are common. In patients with left-sided involvement the fibrosis typically extends from the apex of the left ventricle to the posterior leaflet of the mitral valve; the anterior mitral leaflet is usually spared. Although mural thrombus may be present, obliteration of the left ventricular cavity does not occur.

Microscopically, the involved endocardium is represented by a thick superficial layer of hyalinized fibrous tissue and a deeper layer of collagen fibers; foci of calcification or mural thrombus may be present. Septa composed of fibrous and granulation tissue commonly extend for a variable distance into the myocardium.

CLINICAL FEATURES

Occasionally the disease is heralded by an acute febrile illness; more often, however, the clinical onset is insidious. The clinical manifestations are mainly those of progressive congestive heart failure (secondary to restricted cardiomyopathy) and mitral and/or tricuspid insufficiency (secondary to mechanical dysfunction). An occasional patient may have a large pericardial effusion. Depending on the distribution of the lesions, the physical findings are those of right ventricular, left ventricular, or biventricular failure. The ECG usually shows T-wave abnormalities and diminished QRS voltage; there may be evidence of left ventricular and right atrial enlargement. Atrial fibrillation is occasionally present. Hemodynamic studies reveal normal systolic function with diastolic impairment.

The clinical course is usually relentlessly downhill. Not infrequently, sudden, unexpected cardiovascular collapse, presumably due to an arrhythmia, is the cause of death. Patients with predominantly right-sided involvement appear to have a somewhat better prognosis than those with predominantly left-sided involvement. The results of medical therapy have been disappointing, with few patients surviving more than 10 years. Surgery appears to offer greater promise. An aggressive surgical approach, which consists of resecting the fibrotic endocardium and replacing the mitral and/or tricuspid valves, has led to significant symptomatic improvement in the small number of patients who have been operated on.

IMAGING AND INVASIVE DIAGNOSIS

Initially, heart size is normal. Later, chest films show cardiomegaly of variable degree with evidence of mitral insufficiency (left atrial enlargement, pulmonary venous hypertension). Cardiac calcification is an occasional finding. Chest films of patients with advanced left-sided disease typically reveal marked cardiomegaly with dilatation of the right ventricle and right atrium secondary to pulmonary arterial hypertension. Initially, echocardiography and cardiac catheterization demonstrate evidence of restricted cardiomyopathy and atrioventricular valvular insufficiency; later, both studies confirm the presence of left and/or right ventricular failure. Echocardiography or left ventriculography demonstrates left ventricular dyssynergy and an intracavitary filling defect representing mural thrombus.

The diagnosis of EMF is usually based on the typical clinical picture and radiographic findings. Although transcatheter endocardial biopsy can be helpful in confirming the diagnosis, it is usually omitted because of the risk of dislodging a mural thrombus, which can embolize peripherally.

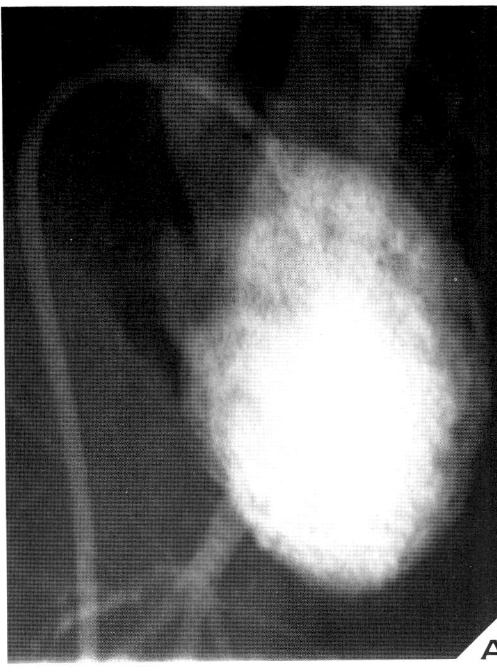

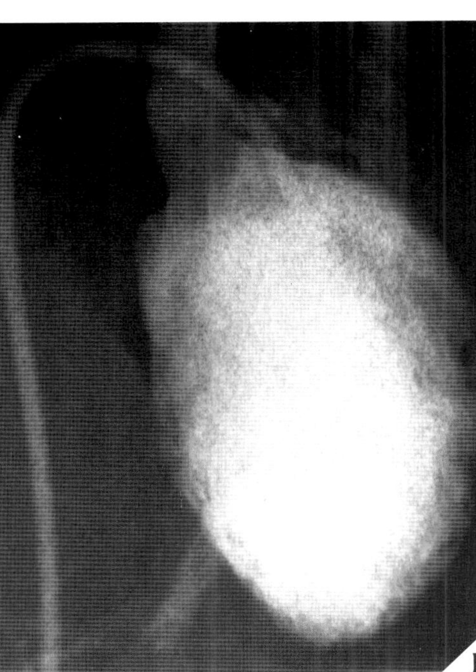

Fig. 29.24 Dilated form of primary endocardial fibroelastosis. This infant presented with congestive heart failure. Four-chamber projections of left ventriculogram in (A) systole and (B) diastole demonstrate a very large, globular left ventricle with markedly decreased contractility. The calculated ejection fraction was 20 percent. The mitral valve is competent despite the presence of the catheter.

CHAPTER 30

Treatment of Ischemic Heart Disease with Catheter Techniques and Surgery

Although surgery remains the definitive treatment for many acquired cardiovascular disorders, an increasing number of therapeutic procedures are being performed in the catheterization laboratory. For example, specially designed balloon catheters can be used to dilate stenotic portions of the cardiovascular system (eg, coronary, renal, or femoral arteries; aortic, pulmonic, or mitral valves) or to occlude an abnormal connection or vessel. Intraaortic counterpulsation balloon catheters can be used to maintain cardiac output in patients with acute left ventricular failure secondary to myocardial infarction.

Catheter techniques are also employed in thrombolytic therapy, which is gaining increasing acceptance as a treatment for acute myocardial infarction. Initially, streptokinase, the first thrombolytic agent to be used for this purpose, was introduced directly into the infarct-related artery. (With the intra-arterial catheter in place, serial coronary arteriograms were obtained to monitor the therapeutic effect.) Because it has subsequently been shown that thrombolytic agents are also effective when injected intravenously, the intra-arterial technique has largely been abandoned.

This chapter considers the treatment of ischemic heart disease with catheter techniques and surgery. The following chapter will discuss the treatment of acquired valvular disease with catheter techniques (balloon valvuloplasty) and surgery (prosthetic valve replacement) and cardiac transplantation. (Embolization techniques used in the treatment of congenital and acquired heart disease are discussed in Chapters 16 and 31. Plain film findings in the early postoperative period are discussed in Chapter 16.)

PRINCIPLES

Definitive treatment of ischemic heart disease caused by coronary artery disease is directed at revascularizing the ischemic myocardium, which can be accomplished by either surgical or nonsurgical means. (Cardiac transplantation is an option in a small number of cases; see Chapter 32.) The major nonsurgical approaches are percutaneous transluminal coronary angioplasty (PTCA) and thrombolytic therapy. PTCA is mainly used in patients with chronic ischemic heart disease, whereas thrombolytic therapy is employed in the first few hours after an acute myocardial infarction. The most widely used surgical revascularization technique is the coronary artery bypass graft (CABG).

PERCUTANEOUS TRANSLUMINAL CORONARY ANGIOPLASTY (PTCA)

Percutaneous transluminal angioplasty, introduced as a treatment for peripheral arterial atherosclerosis by Dotter and Judkins in the 1960s, was successfully applied to the treatment of coronary artery disease by Grüntzig in 1978. PTCA is now extensively employed in the treatment of coronary atherosclerosis causing myocardial ischemia.

PATHOLOGY OF CORONARY ATHEROSCLEROSIS

Before we discuss the technical aspects of the procedure, it may be helpful to review the pathogenesis and morphology of coronary arteriosclerosis (see also Chapter 20). Normal coronary

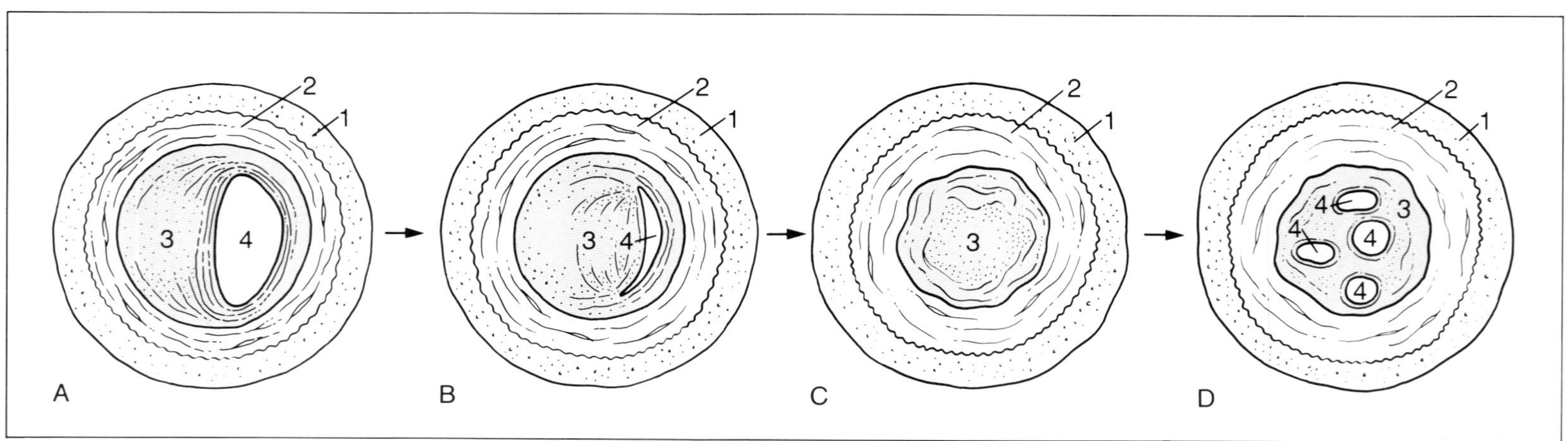

Fig. 30.1 Coronary atherosclerosis. Sequential histopathological changes are shown schematically. (A) Initially, intra- and extracellular lipid accumulates in the intimal layer, resulting in narrowing of the arterial lumen. (B) Further accumulation of lipid causes injury to the arterial wall, which leads to proliferation of smooth muscle and fibrous tissue. The resulting fibromuscular plaque causes significant narrowing of the lumen. (C) Extensive proliferation of fibromuscular tissue results in occlusion of the lumen. (D) Undermining of the fibromuscular tissue creates several channels through which blood flows (recanalization).

1 adventitia
2 media
3 intima
4 lumen

arteries have compliant walls that can be passively stretched to enlarge the lumen, which enables them to adapt to wide variations in flow and vascular tone. The arterial wall is composed of three layers: the *intima*, consisting of endothelial cells attached to a thin layer of extracellular matrix; the *media*, consisting of circumferentially oriented layers of smooth muscle surrounded by elastin and collagen fibers; and the *adventitia*, consisting of loosely arranged connective tissue, fibroblasts, and a few muscle cells.

Coronary artery obstruction is usually due to atherosclerosis, which typically involves large and medium-sized branches that course within the epicardium. Post-mortem studies have shown that atheromatous plaques are the underlying lesion in more than 90 percent of patients with signs and symptoms of ischemic heart disease, with other causes of coronary artery stenosis (eg, emboli, dissection, vasculitis, and fibromuscular dysplasia) accounting for less than 10 percent. The initial stage of atheromatous plaque formation consists of proliferation of smooth muscle in the media. This process, which is believed to be a response to local injury, is accompanied by deposition of variable amounts of intracellular and extracellular lipid in the intima (Fig. 30.1). Although the atheromatous plaque may impinge on the arterial lumen, experimental studies have shown that in a typical obstructing lesion 90 percent of the stenosis is due to splinting and muscle contraction and only 10 percent is caused by the atheromatous plaque itself. In time, the atheromatous plaque undergoes necrosis, which leads to further lipid deposition, hemorrhage, and eventually calcification. The luminal surface of a complex atheromatous plaque typically consists of a thin fibrous cap that encloses a core of necrotic debris and lipid. The process commonly extends into the media, with fraying of the internal elastic membrane and fragmentation of the media (Fig. 30.2). (Medial involvement is the usual cause of symptoms in males with ischemic heart disease.)

Mural thrombus is a common feature of coronary atherosclerosis. It is believed to result from exposure of the circulating blood to thrombogenic substances present on the surface of an ulcerated plaque. In time, the mural thrombus may undergo organization and become incorporated into the plaque, resulting in further narrowing of the arterial lumen. Hemorrhage into the plaque may cause it to rupture or ulcerate, a sequence of events that is believed to be the precipitating factor in most cases of acute thrombotic occlusion.

Coronary atherosclerosis typically leads to progressive stenosis of the affected segments. The key events are focal endothelial and intimal damage resulting in the accumulation of platelets and leukocytes at the site of endothelial injury, and infiltration of the media and adventitia by leukocytes and mast cells secondary to injury or progression of the vascular disease. It is likely that the cause of the endothelial injury varies from patient to patient. The major etiologic factors appear to be mechanical injury, hypercholesterolemia, and local changes associated with the atherosclerotic process. Immunological, inflammatory, and infectious factors may play a role in some patients. The plaque may continue to grow by accretion of platelets or fibrous material, or it may rupture. The rupture typically begins as a crack along the luminal surface of the plaque that extends into the interior of the plaque. Less often, the rupture is caused by hemorrhage within the plaque. Cor-

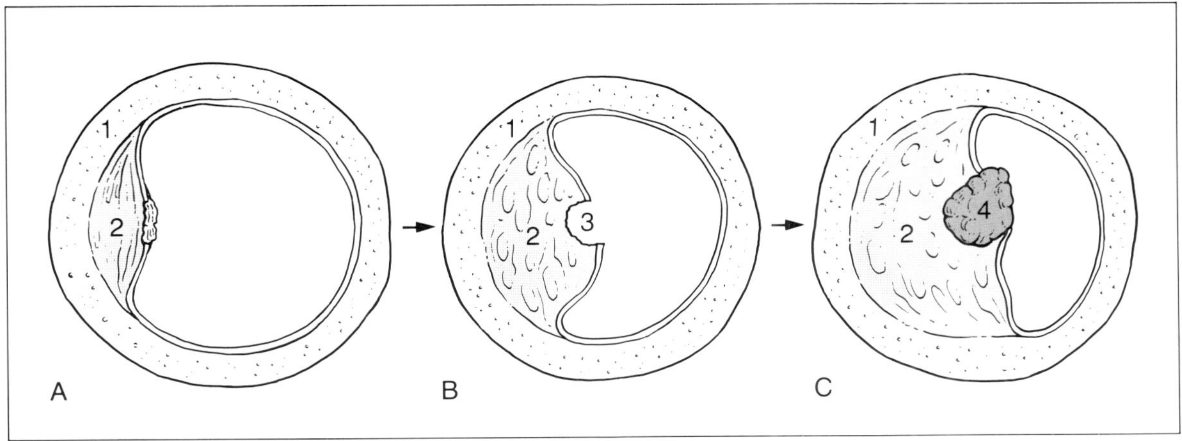

Fig. 30.2 Ulcerated atherosclerotic plaque. Sequential histopathologic changes are shown schematically. (A–C) The endothelium over the atherosclerotic plaque is disrupted, causing superficial necrosis of the plaque. The necrotic debris is removed by the action of the flowing blood, resulting in the formation of an ulcer. Proliferation of fibrous and muscle tissue leads to progressive enlargement of the atherosclerotic plaque. Fibrin and blood clot collect in the ulcer. The resulting thrombus may undergo organization or may become detached and embolize into peripheral branches of the coronary arterial tree.

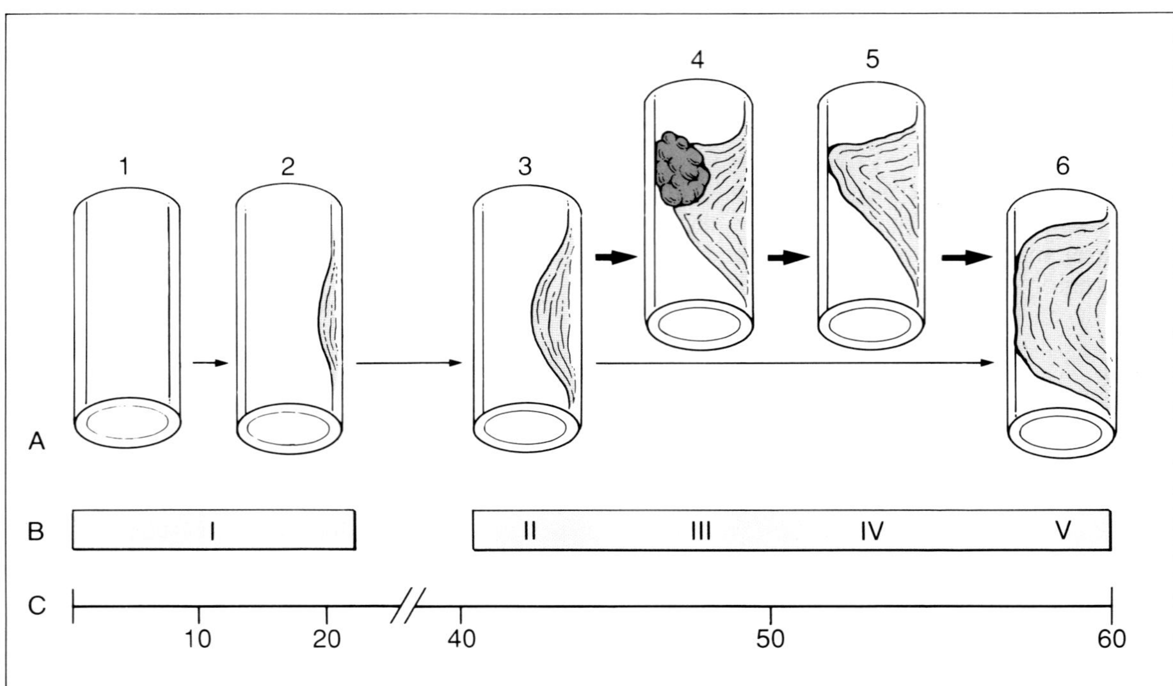

1 normal coronary artery
2 early atheromatous plaque
3 moderately large atherosclerotic plaque
4 ulcerated plaque with fresh thrombus
5 atheromatous plaque with organized thrombus
6 occlusion

Fig. 30.3 Progression of atheromatous plaque correlated with clinical manifestations. (A) Morphology of atheromatous plaque. (B) Clinical manifestations. Asymptomatic atheromatous plaque can usually be identified in routine autopsies in the second decade (I). The plaque may enlarge without causing symptoms (II). Ulceration of the plaque with thrombus formation (*broad arrows*) can lead to acute or subacute symptoms of ischemic heart disease, eg, unstable angina (III). Alternatively, the plaque may slowly enlarge (*thin arrow*) without undergoing ulceration (III). Either sequence may progress to severe narrowing or occlusion of the affected artery, with clinical manifestations ranging from stable angina to acute myocardial infarction or sudden death (IV and V). (C) Age at which the various clinical manifestations usually appear. (Adapted with the permission of the American College of Cardiology from Fuster V, Chesebro JH: Role of platelets and thrombosis in coronary atherosclerotic disease and sudden death. *J Am Coll Cardiol* 1985; 5:6:175B)

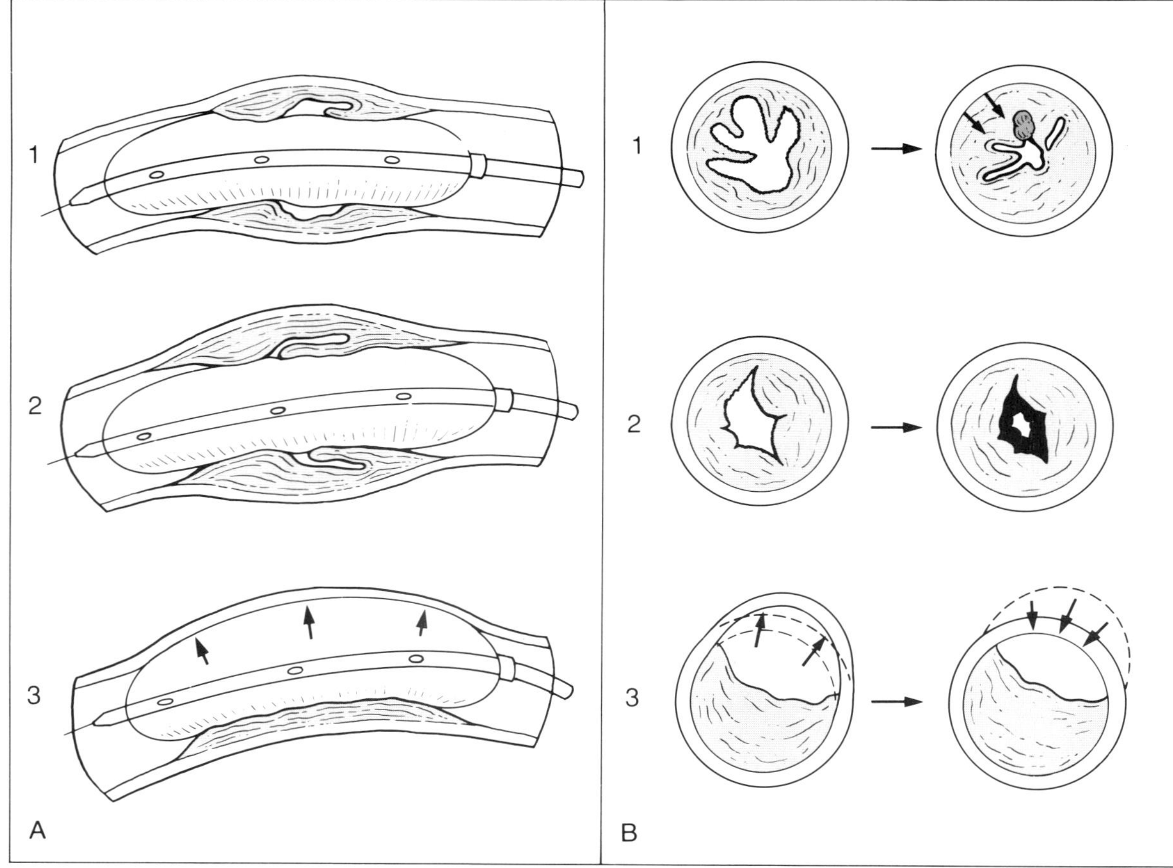

Fig. 30.4 Mechanism of coronary artery balloon angioplasty. Schematic representation of events as viewed in (A) longitudinal and (B) transverse planes. (1) Tight concentric stenosis. Expansion of the angioplasty balloon produces tears and fractures within the arteriosclerotic plaque. Some of these passages allow blood to flow through the stenotic segment. (2) Tight concentric stenosis. Extension of the tears and fractures into the media further enlarges the lumen. However, injury to the media may set the stage for thrombus formation (*black*) and subsequent restenosis. (3) Eccentric stenosis. Overstretching the uninvolved arterial wall results in further enlargement of the lumen. This transient overcorrection quickly disappears as the overstretched arterial wall regains its tone.

relative studies have shown excellent correlation between the clinical manifestations of ischemic heart disease and the morphologic features of the plaque (Fig. 30.3; see also Chapter 20).

PRINCIPLES OF PTCA

Clinical and experimental observations indicate that luminal enlargement produced by PTCA in humans results from microtrauma to the atheromatous plaque. Three major events appear to be involved in successful coronary angioplasty (Fig. 30.4):

1. The inflated balloon produces tears, fractures, or cracks in the plaque, resulting in enlargement of the lumen.
2. The inflated balloon disrupts the plaque at the point of least resistance; dissection through the intima into the media enlarges the lumen. With further inflation, the media and adventitia may stretch to conform to the outer dimensions of the inflated balloon.
3. In patients with eccentric atherosclerotic lesions, the dilated balloon may stretch the normal arterial wall in the vicinity of the plaque, resulting in a transient enlargement of the lumen. The initial increment in luminal diameter typically disappears over a period of hours, days, or weeks as the overstretched arterial wall regains its normal tone.

To sum up, successful coronary angioplasty PTCA is the result of a moderately severe injury to the arterial wall, and treatment failures—both acute occlusion and late restenosis—reflect the biological response to this trauma (see below).

TECHNIQUE OF PTCA

The principle of PTCA can be briefly summarized as follows: a specially designed balloon catheter is introduced percutaneously (usually via the femoral artery) and is advanced under fluoroscopic guidance until its tip is beyond the stenosis and the balloon straddles the stenotic segment. The balloon is then inflated for a short period of time (Fig. 30.5). These steps can be repeated one or more times until the stenosis is relieved.

The equipment used for PTCA is shown in Figs. 30.6 and 30.7. The angioplasty procedure is illustrated schematically in Fig. 30.8. The initial step is to introduce the guide catheter into

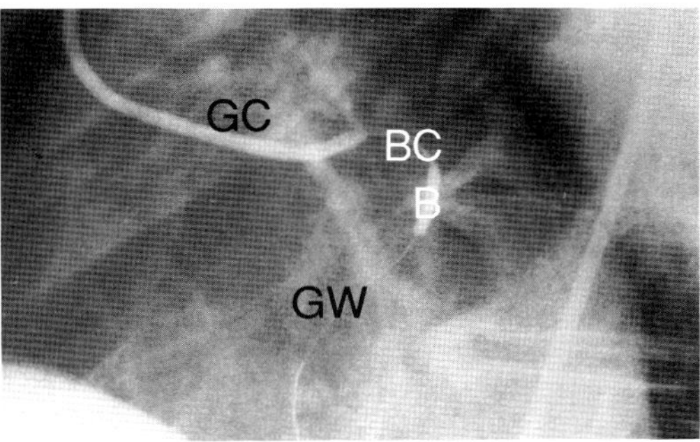

Fig. 30.5 Technique of PTCA. The coaxial system used for this procedure consists of a guide catheter (GC), guidewire (GW), and balloon catheter (BC). The guide catheter, which is large enough to accommodate the balloon catheter and guidewire, is advanced until its end hole faces the ostium of the main coronary artery to be catheterized. The balloon catheter is then passed over the guidewire and advanced until the balloon (B) straddles the stenotic segment. The balloon is then inflated for a period long enough to correct the stenosis (usually 30 to 90 seconds).

FIG. 30.6 EQUIPMENT USED FOR PTCA

Item	Comment
Imaging equipment	Standard single or biplane cine angiographic equipment. Biplane fluoroscopy desirable but not essential. Film, videotape, or digital recording.
Guide catheters	Similar to those used for coronary arteriography, but with wider diameter to accommodate balloon catheter. Usually have metallic marker at tip for fluoroscopic localization. 8 french (8F) is most popular size for femoral approach.
Balloon catheters	Balloon is at tip of catheter. End hole allows insertion over guidewire. Small shaft diameter (4F or less) allows test injections with guidewire in place. Composition of balloon: polyvinyl chloride, polyethylene. Standard length: 20 mm. Inflated diameter: 1.5 to 4 mm.
Guidewires	Teflon-coated steel. Wide variety of designs. Tip can be custom-angulated. Diameter: 0.014", 0.016", or 0.018". Length: 175cm, with distal 25 cm having increased flexibility.
Miscellaneous	Connectors, adapters, stopcocks, pressure monitors

Fig. 30.6 Equipment used for PTCA.

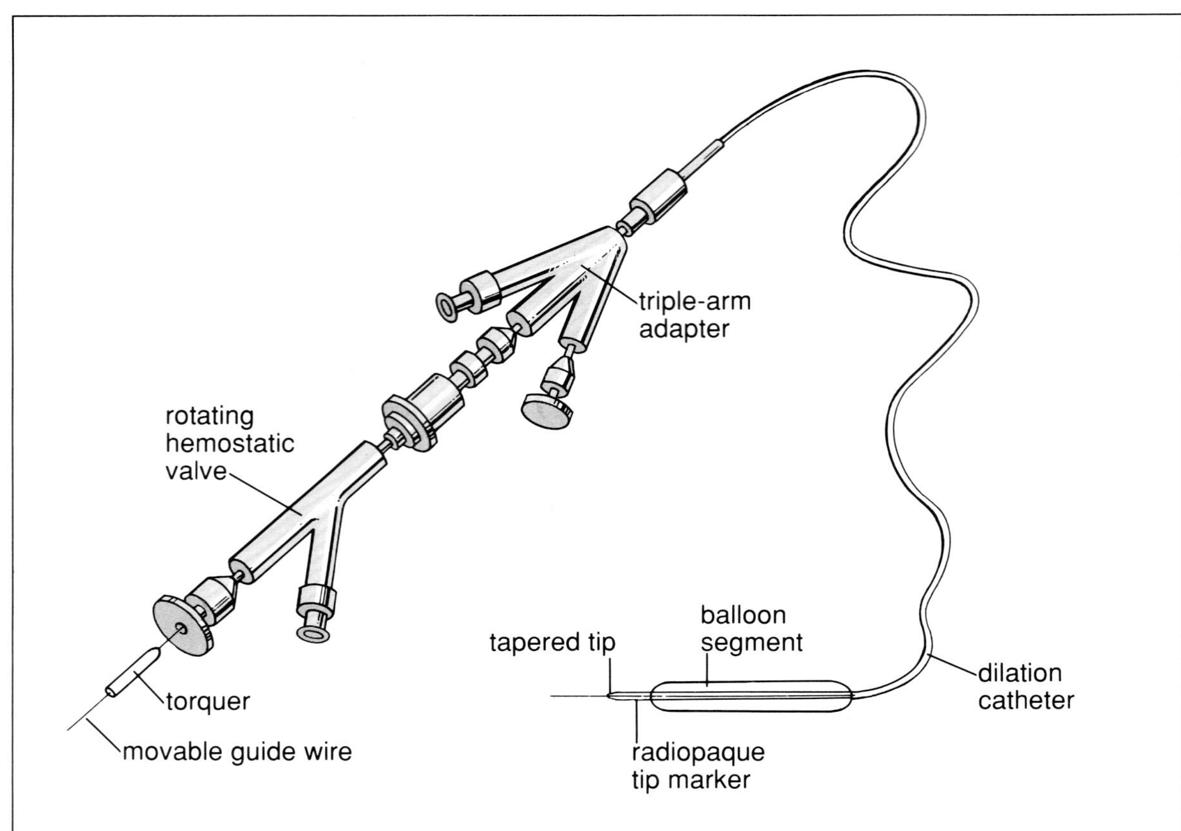

Fig. 30.7 Catheter-connector system for PTCA. The system used in our laboratory (ACS Simpson–Robert model, Advanced Cardiovascular Systems, 1500 Salado Drive, Mountainview, CA) is illustrated.

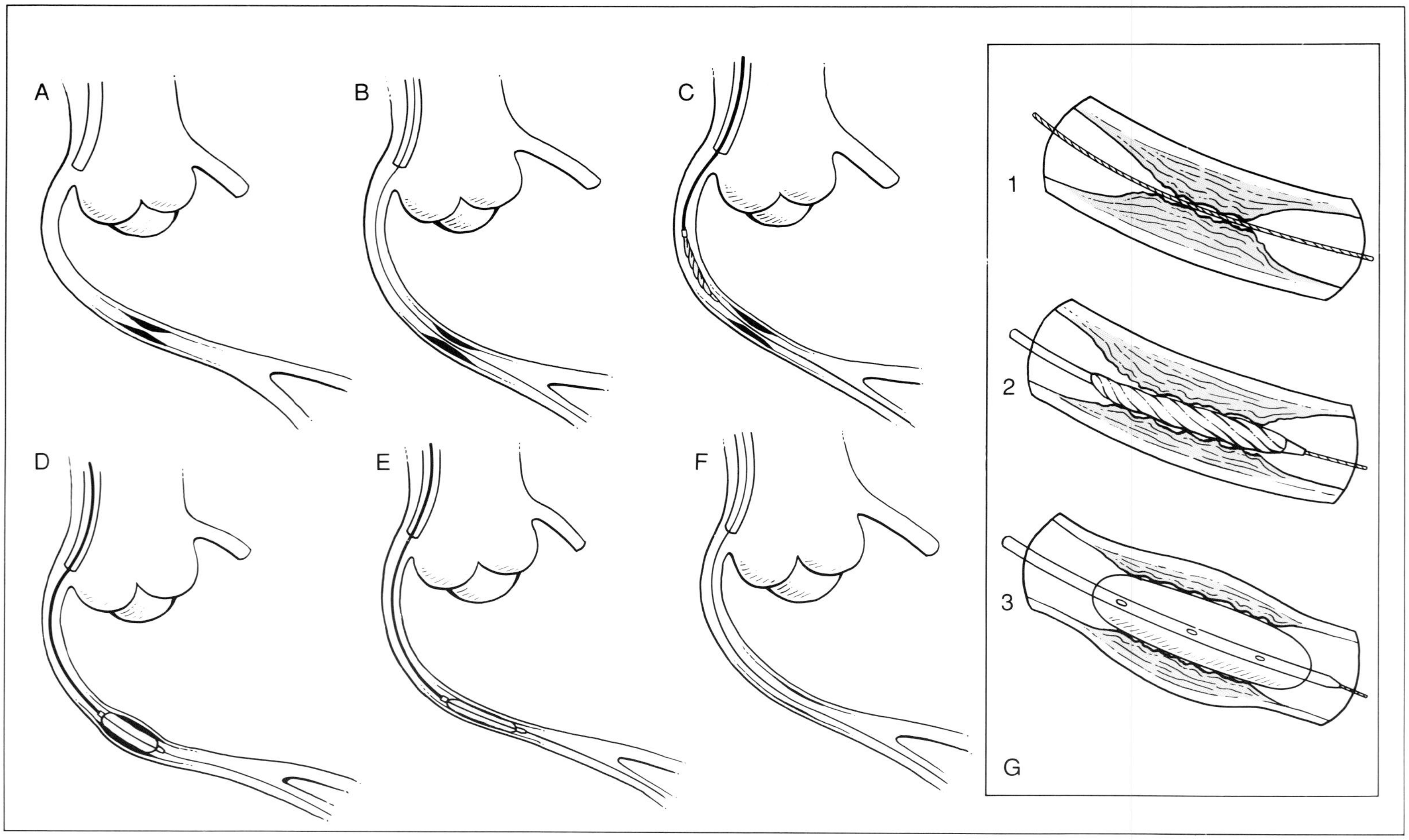

Fig. 30.8 Technique of PTCA. The maneuvers used to dilate a stenosis of the distal right coronary artery are shown schematically. (A) The guide catheter is positioned at the ostium of the right coronary artery. (B) The guidewire is passed through the guide catheter and through the stenosis. (C) The balloon catheter is passed over the guidewire. (D) The balloon catheter is positioned within the stenotic segment. (E) The balloon is inflated. (F) After the stenosis is relieved, the balloon catheter and guidewire are withdrawn. (G) Details of angioplasty: (*1*) Guidewire traversing stenosis. (*2*) Tip of balloon catheter positioned just beyond stenosis. (*3*) Angioplasty balloon inflated.

the ostium of the right or left coronary artery. The deflated balloon catheter is then introduced through the guide catheter and advanced until its tip is in the distal segment of the guide catheter. The guidewire is then advanced through the balloon catheter into the artery to be dilated. The course of the radiopaque guidewire is monitored fluoroscopically. When the tip of the guidewire is well beyond the stenosis (previously localized by coronary arteriography), the balloon catheter is passed over the guidewire and positioned so that the balloon (marked by radiopaque dots) lies within the stenotic segment (Fig. 30.9). The balloon is then inflated for a period of 30 to 90 seconds. The angioplasty procedure is monitored with frequent test injections. One or more additional dilatations may be necessary before the stenosis is significantly relieved or abolished.

Two or more balloons may be needed to treat a severe, noncompliant stenosis in a large coronary artery. The first balloon is used to cross and partially dilate the stenotic segment, after which a second, larger balloon is introduced to dilate it further. (Positioning of the second balloon catheter may be facilitated by the use of a long exchange wire.) Special techniques may be necessary if the stenosis occurs at a bifurcation. In such cases a second balloon catheter is used to minimize the risk of inadvertently occluding the branch artery while the main trunk is being dilated (Figs. 30.10 and 30.11). (Special tech-

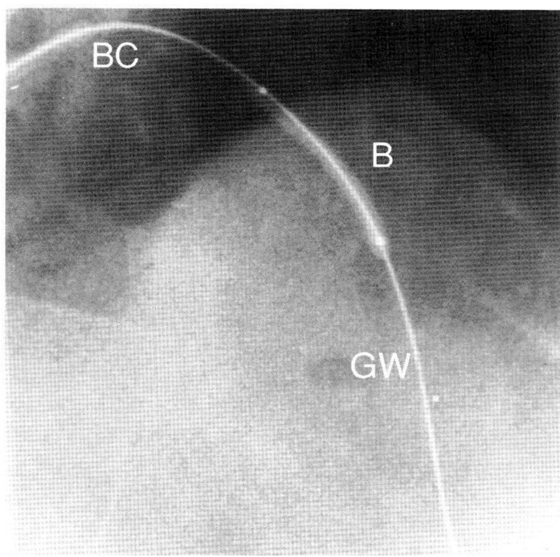

Fig. 30.9 PTCA. Cine frame (right anterior oblique projection) shows the inflated balloon (B) in the left anterior descending coronary artery. The metallic dots indicate the position of the balloon and serve as a guide during fluoroscopy. (BC = balloon catheter; GW = guidewire)

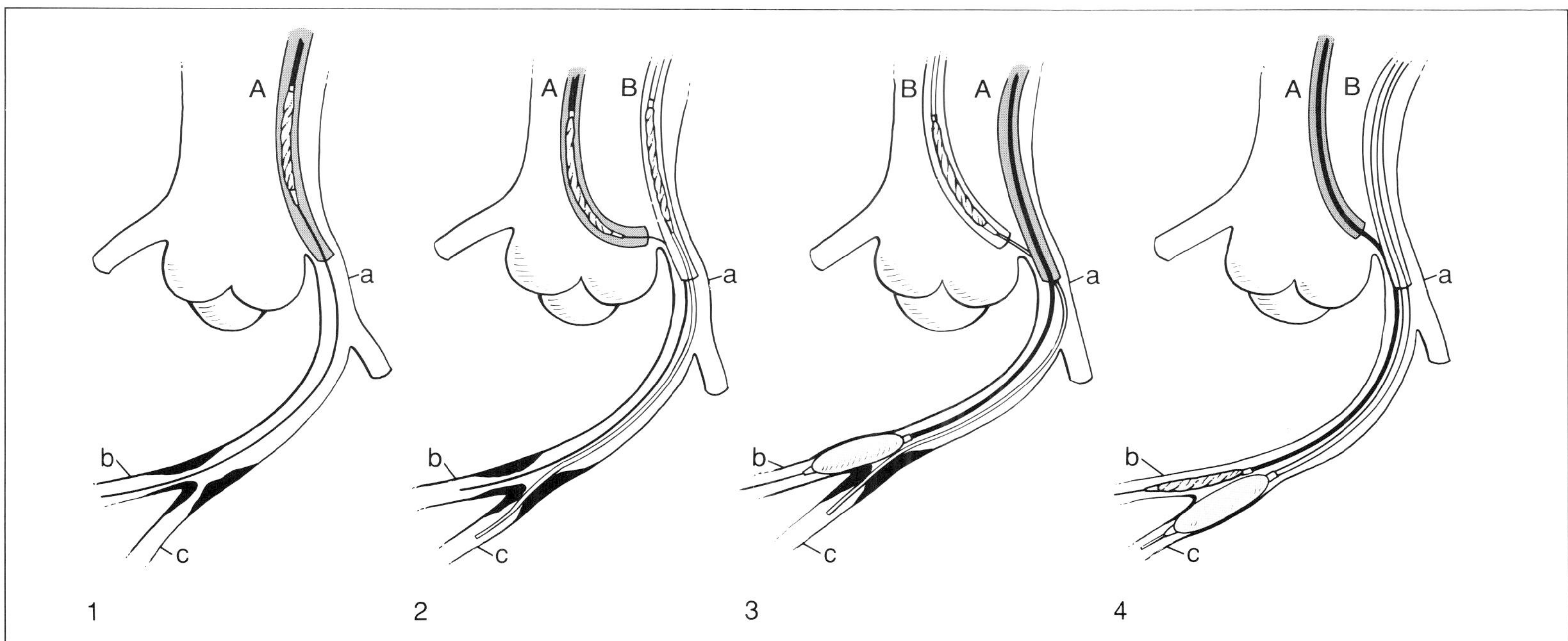

Fig. 30.10 Double balloon catheter technique for stenosis at bifurcation of two large arteries. PTCA of a stenosis at the junction of the left anterior descending (LAD) artery and its first diagonal branch is shown schematically (*1*) *System A* is inserted and its guidewire is passed beyond the stenosis of the LAD. (*2*) A second system (*system B*) is inserted. Its guidewire has been passed beyond the stenosis of the first diagonal artery. (3) The balloon of *system A* is inflated to dilate the stenotic segment of the LAD. (*4*) The balloon of *system B* is inflated to dilate the stenotic segment of the first diagonal artery.

a left main coronary artery
b left anterior descending artery
c first diagonal branch

niques for restoring luminal patency in totally obstructed coronary arteries are discussed in a subsequent section.)

The balloons used for PTCA are currently made of polyvinyl chloride or polyethylene. In general, the balloon should have an inflated diameter slightly greater than the "normal" diameter of the artery to be dilated (ie, the diameter of an adjacent unaffected segment or a branch of comparable size). Relatively large balloons (up to 4 mm in diameter) may be needed to dilate a stenotic bypass graft, whereas relatively small balloons (down to 2 mm in diameter) are used to dilate stenoses of the native coronary arteries.

Alternative access routes (eg, brachial artery) can be employed when the femoral arteries cannot be utilized. A variety of guide catheters with special shapes, sizes, and configurations have been developed to facilitate transbrachial PTCA.

The success of PTCA depends on many factors, including the morphology of the arteries, the equipment available, and the skill of the operator. A complete selection of guide catheters, balloon catheters, guidewires, and related items should be available in any cardiac laboratory in which these procedures are performed.

INDICATIONS FOR PTCA

At the present time, the range of indications for coronary angioplasty is much broader than when the procedure was introduced in 1978. At first, PTCA was offered as an alternative to CABG in symptomatic patients with a discrete, proximal, subtotal stenosis involving only a single artery. Today, PTCA is generally regarded as the procedure of choice in any patient with an approachable lesion causing symptomatic or subclinical myocardial ischemia, irrespective of the site, the number of vessels involved, the degree of stenosis, or the morphology of the lesion. Whereas symptomatic myocardial ischemia severe enough to warrant bypass surgery was once considered a prerequisite for angioplasty, PTCA is now being used to supplement medical therapy, or as an alternative to medical therapy, in patients who would not ordinarily be considered candidates for bypass surgery.

PTCA may be considered as an alternative to other forms of therapy in any patient with clinical or laboratory evidence of myocardial ischemia and angiographic evidence of significant coronary artery stenosis. From the anatomic standpoint, PTCA is usually performed in patients with single or multiple discrete lesions in a single vessel or multiple discrete lesions in two or more vessels (Fig. 30.12). The lesion (or lesions) may be located proximally or distally. None of the various morphological types of stenosis (see below; see also Chapter 20) is regarded as a definite contraindication to PTCA. However, certain situations are associated with an excessively high risk for complications or failure. For example, if the territory likely to be revascularized after successful PTCA is smaller than the territory that would be revascularized after CABG, the latter would ordinarily be considered the procedure of choice. Conditions in which the procedure is unlikely to be successful (eg, diffuse coronary artery disease, chronic total occlusion, excessively tortuous vessels, or poor left ventricular function) are relative contraindications to PTCA.

PATIENT ASSESSMENT

Patients with stable angina with reduction of luminal diameter by 60 to 90 percent in at least one artery are regarded as candidates for PTCA. In making this assessment, caliper or electronic measurements do not appear to be any more reliable than visual inspection. The stenosis should be evident on projections that best display the affected vessel; it should be clearly seen in at least two views. An accurate estimate of luminal narrowing (which is ordinarily made by visually comparing the stenotic segment with an adjacent normal segment or with a normal vessel of comparable size) may not be possible in some instances, eg, in patients with diffuse disease of the left main coronary artery. A useful rule of thumb is that the diameter of the latter is usually greater than that of the left anterior descend-

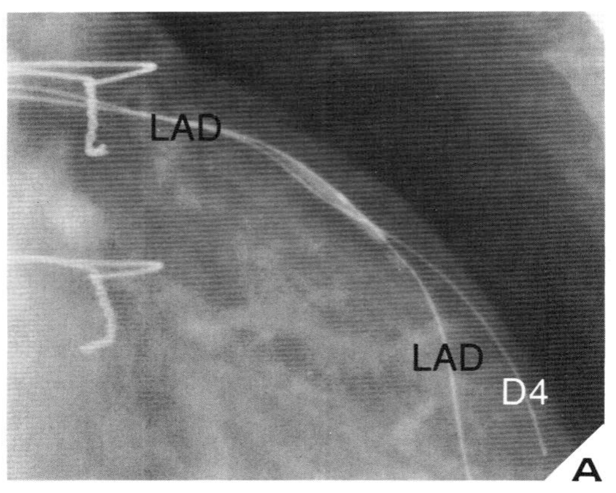

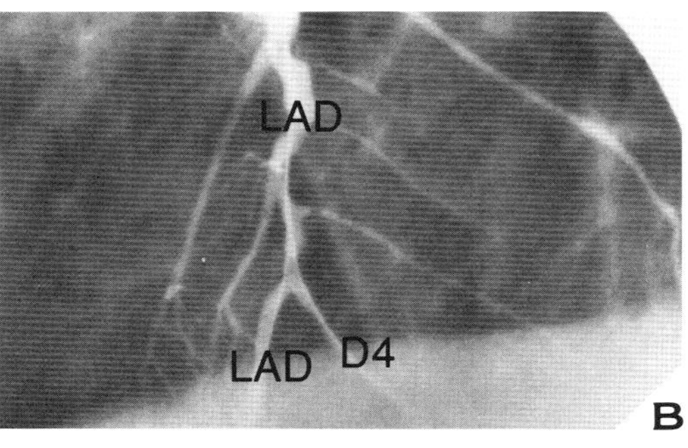

Fig. 30.11 PTCA using double balloon technique. (A) Before angioplasty (RAO projection). Both systems are in place. The guidewire of system 1 is in the left anterior descending artery (LAD). The guidewire of system 2 is in the fourth diagonal artery (D4). (B) Coronary arteriogram obtained during angioplasty procedure (RAO-Cr projection).

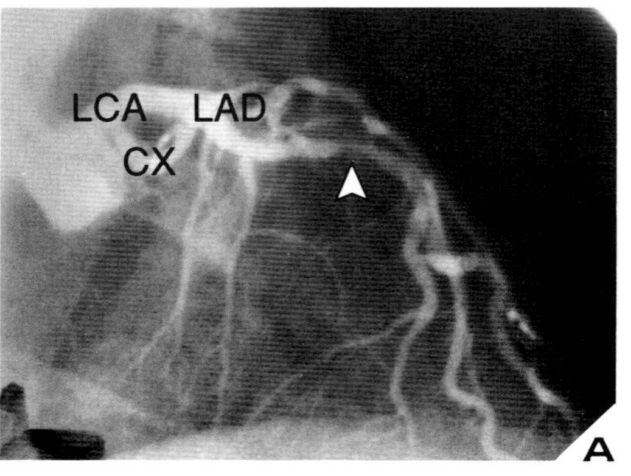

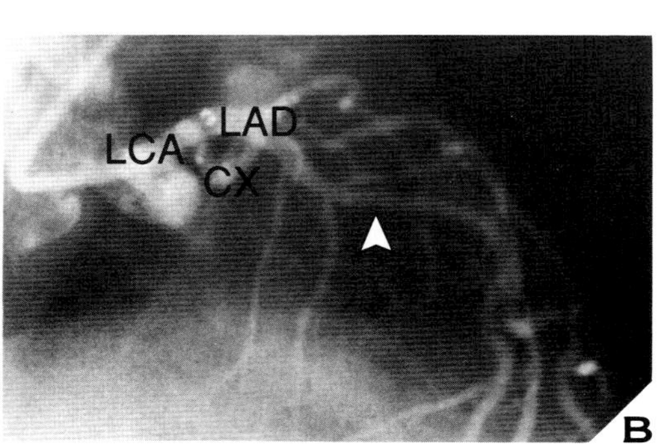

Fig. 30.12 PTCA for localized stenosis of left anterior descending artery. Left coronary arteriogram (LAO-Cr projection) (A) before and (B) after angioplasty. Note the short eccentric stenosis (*arrow*) of the left anterior descending artery (LAD), which is well separated from the large branches arising from this artery. The location and morphology of this lesion make it ideally suited for PTCA. (LCA = left coronary artery; CX = circumflex artery)

ing or circumflex arteries. Calcifications of the arterial wall (when present) provide additional reference points for estimating the degree of stenosis.

The relationship of the stenotic segment to the remainder of the coronary arterial tree should be carefully assessed, since technical modifications may be necessary if branches arise from the stenotic segment or if there are important side branches in the vicinity of the stenosis (Fig. 30.13). Stenoses located at an important bifurcation (eg, the distal right coronary artery) or at the take-off of the marginal branches of the circumflex artery require a special approach. PTCA is more likely to be unsuccessful in a vessel with a significant normal angulation than in one that is straight or only minimally curved.

The morphology of the stenotic segment is an important predictor of success or failure of PTCA. There are two main varieties: *circumscribed (uncomplicated) stenoses* and so-called *complicated stenoses*. Circumscribed stenoses, which are typically very short (less than 10 mm), are characterized by concentric, smooth borders and a triangular shape (Fig. 30.14A). Angioplasty has a very high success rate in such lesions. Complicated stenoses are usually eccentric, with irregular margins (Figs. 30.13A and 30.14B). Extraluminal accumulations of contrast material (which can simulate ulcerations) are caused by rupture of the atherosclerotic plaque. Filling defects, which represent thrombus, are characteristic features of complicated stenoses (Fig. 30.15); the latter are much less amenable to PTCA than circumscribed stenoses. The stenosis is usually of the complicated type in patients with unstable angina and in those with a recent or evolving infarct.

Increasingly, PTCA is being employed in patients with acute myocardial infarction. Coronary arteriography usually demonstrates complete or almost complete thrombotic occlusion of the infarct-related artery in such cases. However, anatomic studies indicate that, on average, 80 percent of the diameter reduction is caused by severe preexisting atherosclerotic stenosis; therefore, such lesions are theoretically suitable for PTCA. (The role of "rescue" PTCA in acute myocardial infarction and the technique of performing angioplasty in completely occluded vessels are discussed in a subsequent section.)

Stenoses occurring in aorto–coronary venous bypass grafts are usually uncomplicated circumscribed stenoses with smooth borders. The morphology of stenoses in long-standing venous

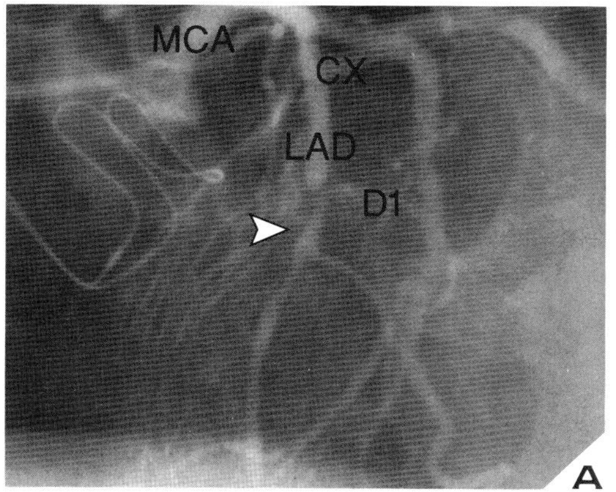

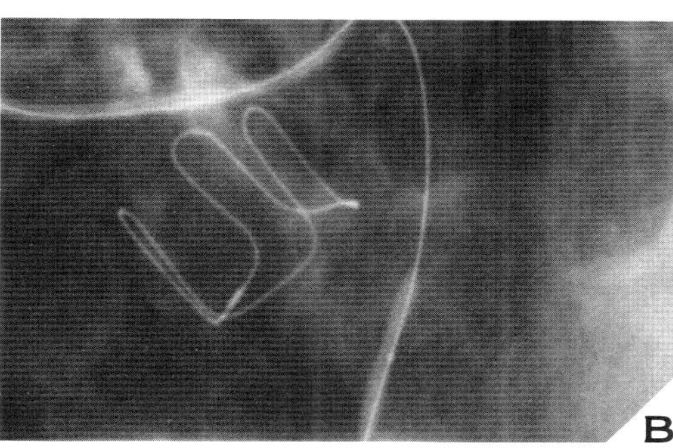

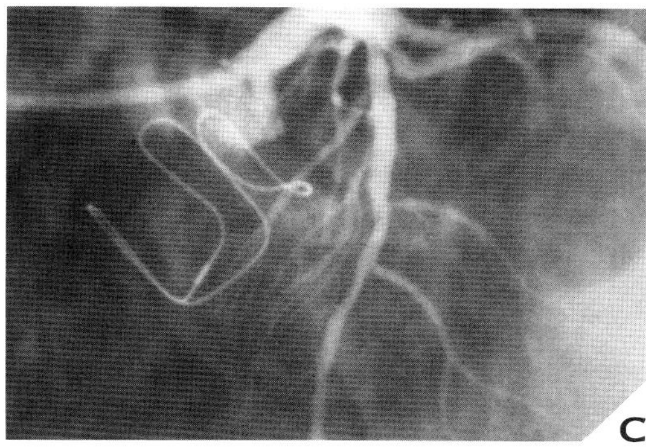

Fig. 30.13 PTCA of complicated stenosis. (A) Before angioplasty. LAO projection of left coronary arteriogram shows an irregular tubular stenosis (*arrow*) of the middle segment of the left anterior descending (LAD) artery. A large first diagonal artery (D1) arises from the narrowed segment. (B) Balloon in position. (C) Immediately after angioplasty. Patency of the stenotic segment of the LAD has been restored. There is a localized dissection along the right side of the dilated segment. Significant narrowing of the origin of the first diagonal artery persists. (MCA = left main coronary artery; CX = circumflex artery)

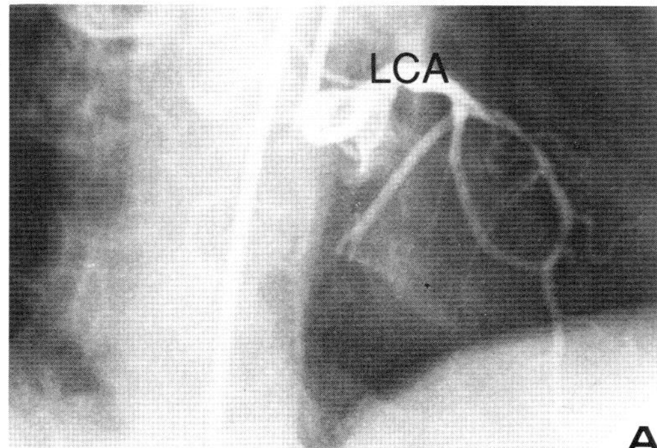

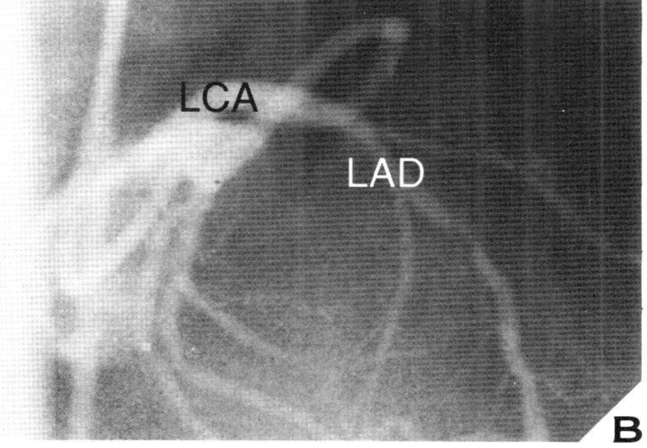

Fig. 30.14 Uncomplicated versus complicated stenosis. Coronary arteriograms (RAO projecton) of two patients with stenosis of the left anterior descending artery (LAD). (A) Circumscribed stenosis. The smooth triangular appearance of the short stenotic segment is typical of a chronic uncomplicated stenosis. (B) Complicated stenosis. The area of narrowing is eccentric with irregular borders. (LCA = left coronary artery)

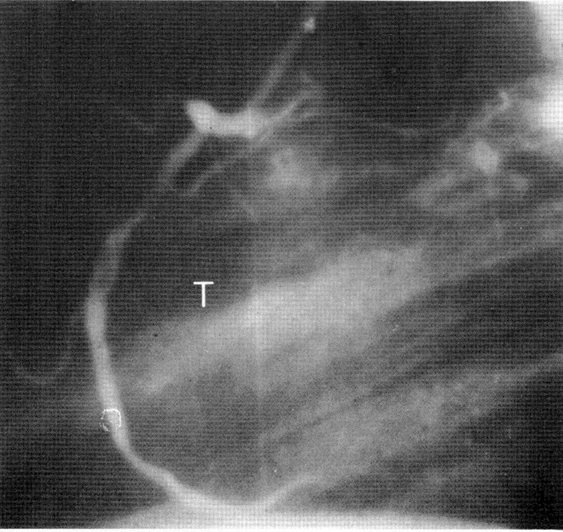

Fig. 30.15 Complicated stenosis of right coronary artery. Lateral projection of right coronary arteriogram demonstrates a 90 percent stenosis of the middle segment of the main coronary artery. Just beyond the stenosis is a filling defect [thrombus (T)] which reduces the diameter of the lumen by about 70 percent.

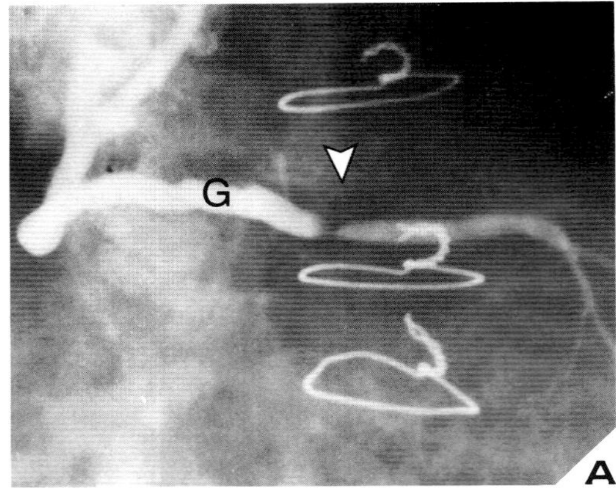

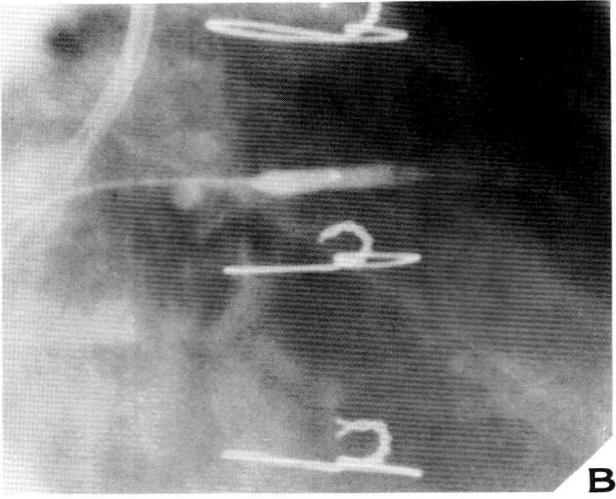

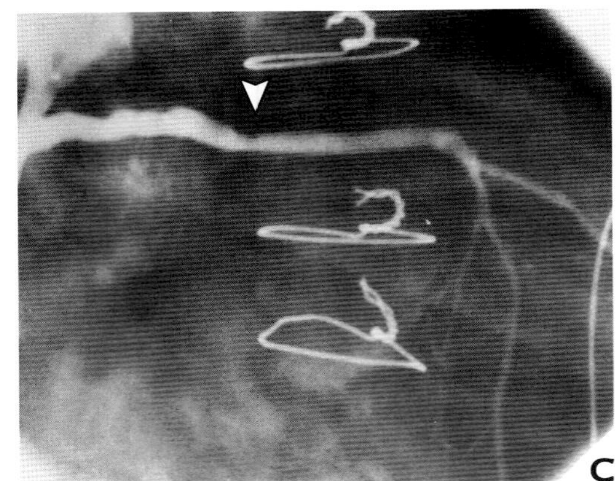

Fig. 30.16 Successful PTCA of stenotic CABG. (A) Selective left coronary arteriogram (RAO projection) shows a very tight (90 percent) circumscribed stenosis with triangular margins (*arrow*) in the middle portion of the venous graft (G), which supplies the territory of the left anterior descending artery. (B) The inflated balloon is in place. (C) Post-angioplasty arteriogram shows complete relief of the stenosis. Note irregularity (*arrow*) of superior margin of the dilated segment, indicating that the intima has been ruptured.

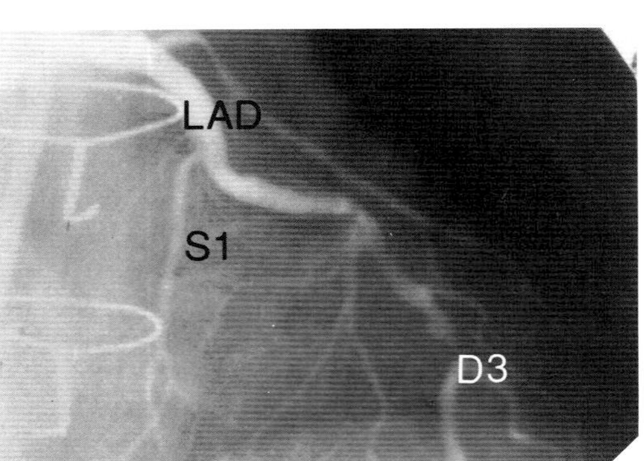

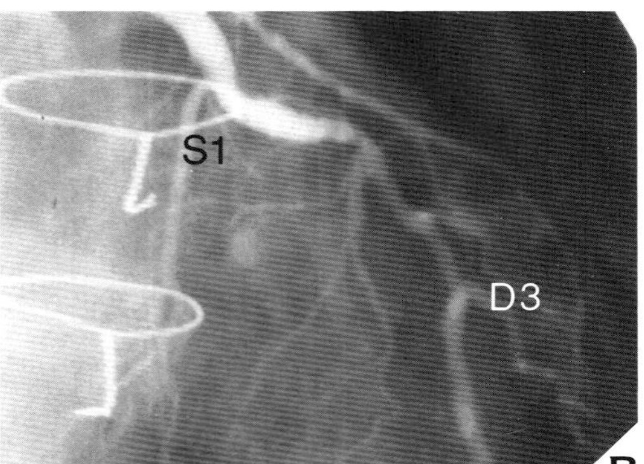

Fig. 30.17 Successful angioplasty of high-grade stenosis. (A) Pre-angioplasty arteriogram shows a 95 percent stenosis of the left anterior descending artery (LAD) just proximal to the origin of the third diagonal artery (D3). The triangular configuration suggests a stable stenosis. (B) Immediately after PTCA, continuity of the LAD has been restored. There is a residual 30 percent stenosis. The smooth borders of the dilated segment suggest that the mechanism of angioplasty was compression of the plaque plus dilatation of the normal arterial wall. (S1 = first septal artery)

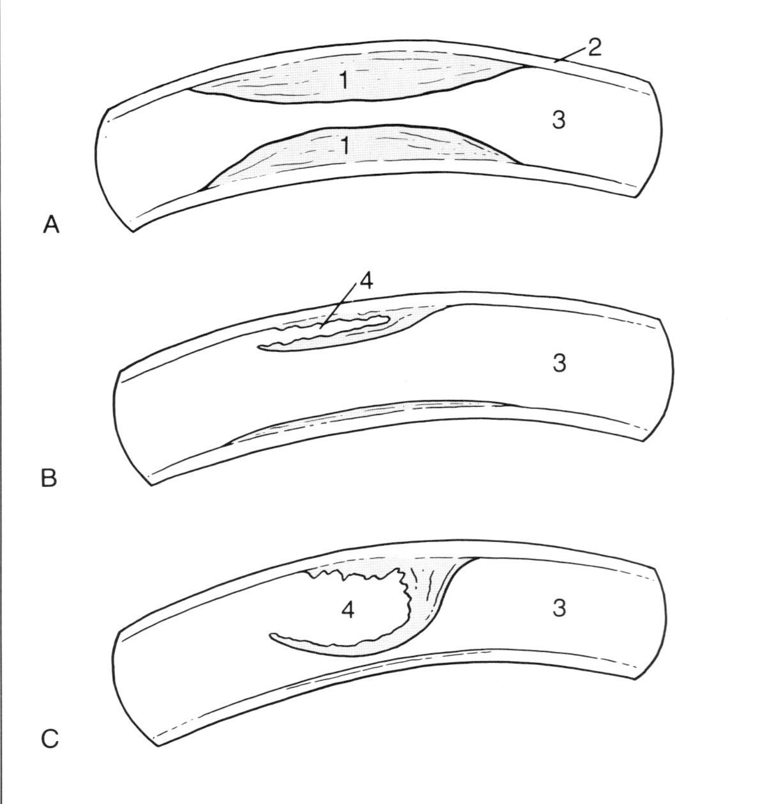

1 atheromatous plaque	3 arterial lumen
2 muscular wall of artery	4 dissection

Fig. 30.18 Localized dissection caused by PTCA. (A) Before angioplasty. (B,C) After angioplasty. (B) The inflated balloon disrupts the atheromatous plaque and the adjacent arterial wall, creating a localized pocket in the arterial wall (false channel). Contrast material that accumulates in the false channel remains in it after it has disappeared from the arterial lumen. (C) If the pocket is wide enough it may comprise the true lumen.

grafts, which commonly occur at the junction of the venous graft with the native coronary artery, is similar to that seen in the native coronary arteries. Such lesions are usually successfully treated by PTCA (Fig. 30.16). (The angiographic evaluation of aorto–coronary bypass grafts is discussed later in this chapter.)

IMMEDIATE POSTPROCEDURAL ASSESSMENT

Immediately after PTCA a variety of morphologic patterns can be identified angiographically. Common patterns include:

1. Mild to moderate coronary artery narrowing with apparent intimal disruption (Fig. 30.17). Stretching of the normal arterial wall with compression of the atheromatous plaque is believed to be responsible for relief of the stenosis in these patients.
2. Extravasation of contrast material for a short distance into the media or adventitia, suggesting a localized dissection (Fig. 30.18). Occasionally there is irregularity of the border of the stenotic segment, with contrast material extending for a short distance into the arterial wall. This finding indicates rupture of the plaque with formation of short tracts extending into the intima and media.
3. A longitudinal intraluminal lucency measuring 3 to 15 mm in length produced by a medial tear with intramural dissection (Fig. 30.19). The intraluminal lucency represents material that has been detached from the normal arterial wall and/or part of the atheromatous plaque. The detached elements are separated from the outer portion of the arterial wall by opacified blood in the false channel, resulting in a variable degree of stenosis of the natural lumen. The depth of the dissection varies from case to case. Rupture of the artery, resulting in epicardial hemorrhage, may occur in extreme cases.
4. A transverse intraluminal lucency suggesting a transverse dissection (Fig. 30.20). The lucency represents a flap formed by the atherosclerotic plaque or arterial wall caused by the angioplasty. In some instances the trans-

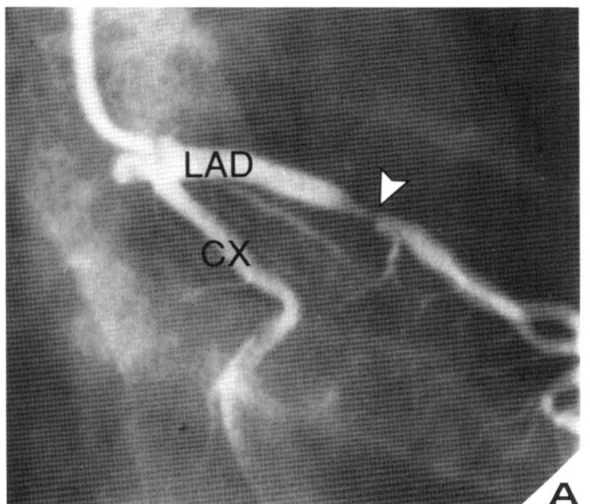

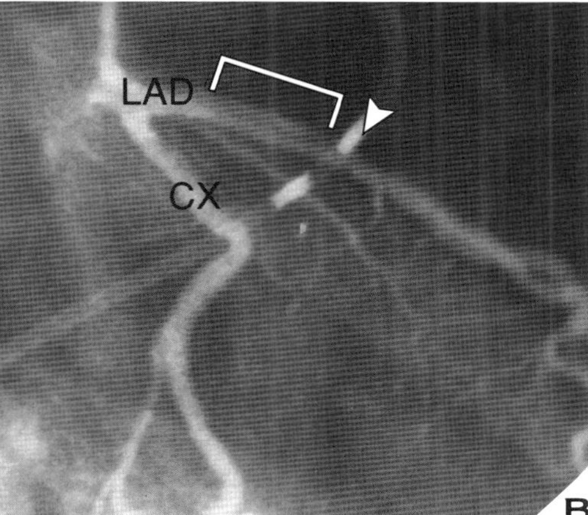

Fig. 30.19 Longitudinal dissection caused by PTCA. (A) Left coronary arteriogram (RAO projection) before PTCA demonstrates 80 percent stenosis (*arrow*) of the left anterior descending (LAD) artery. (B) Immediately after angioplasty there is considerable relief of the obstruction, with a residual 30 percent stenosis. However, dissection has occurred proximal to the dilated segment. The filling defect (*brace*) extending proximally from the area of the previous stenosis (*arrow*) represents the displaced plaque and a portion of the media. Opacified blood fills the false channel in the arterial wall. The false channel encroaches on the true lumen, producing a 50 percent stenosis. (C) Schematic representation of longitudinal dissection. *Left*: longitudinal section. *Right*: transverse section.

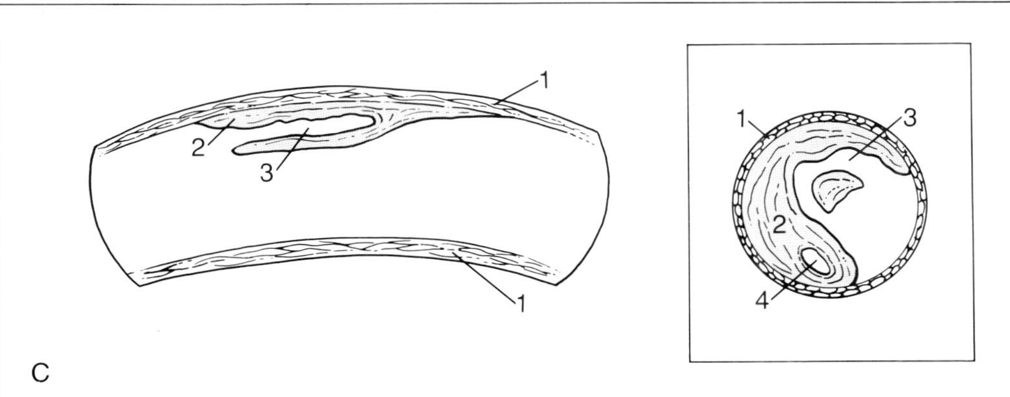

1 muscular arterial wall
2 atheromatous plaque
3 dissection
4 new channel formed by cracking of the atheromatous plaque

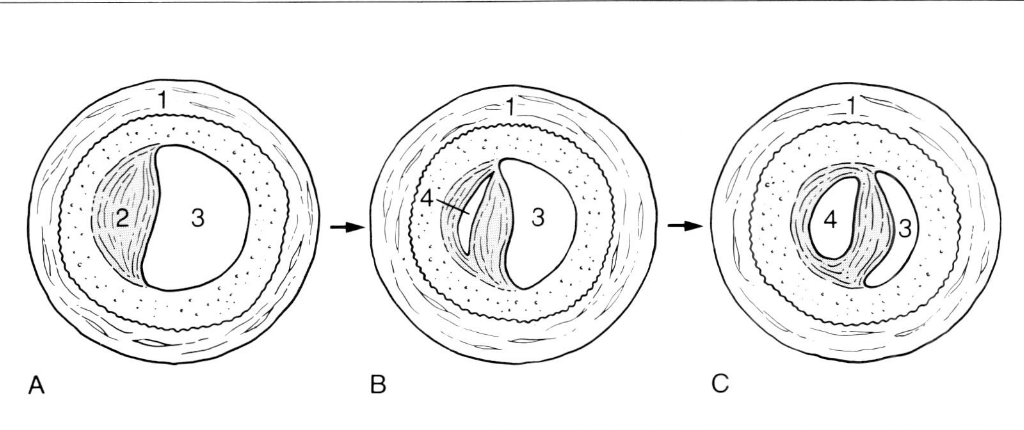

Fig. 30.20 Transverse dissection caused by PTCA. The atheromatous plaque and the adjacent arterial wall may be disrupted transversely, creating a flap that is displaced into the true lumen. (A) Before angioplasty. (B,C) After angioplasty. (A) Early dissection. (C) Late dissection.

1 arterial wall
2 atheromatous plaque
3 arterial lumen
4 false channel formed by rupture of atheromatous plaque and adjacent arterial wall.

verse intimal flap almost completely obstructs the natural lumen. If this occurs, the vessel may be more stenotic than before.

5. Luminal obstruction, which can result from thrombotic occlusion or an extreme form of transverse dissection. (The former is the most likely cause of complete post-procedural obstruction in patients undergoing PTCA for acute myocardial infarction.)

PTCA IN COMPLETE CORONARY ARTERY OCCLUSION

Patients with a completely occluded coronary artery who are not in acute distress (acute myocardial infarction) can benefit from PTCA. In general, balloon angioplasty is suitable only for occlusions less than 4 weeks old; however, laser angioplasty has recently been used to reopen chronically occluded coronary arteries.

The technique for opening a totally occluded artery is similar to that employed in conventional PTCA (Figs. 30.21 and 30.22). A guidewire is advanced to the site of the occlusion and an attempt is made to negotiate the passage. Once the guidewire has passed beyond the obstruction, an arteriogram is obtained to determine whether a significant degree of patency has been achieved; if the lumen is large enough to accept a balloon catheter, the latter is passed over the guidewire and the artery is dilated in the usual way. Special ultra-low profile balloons and over-the-wire laser systems have been developed to facilitate angioplasty of totally occluded coronary arteries.

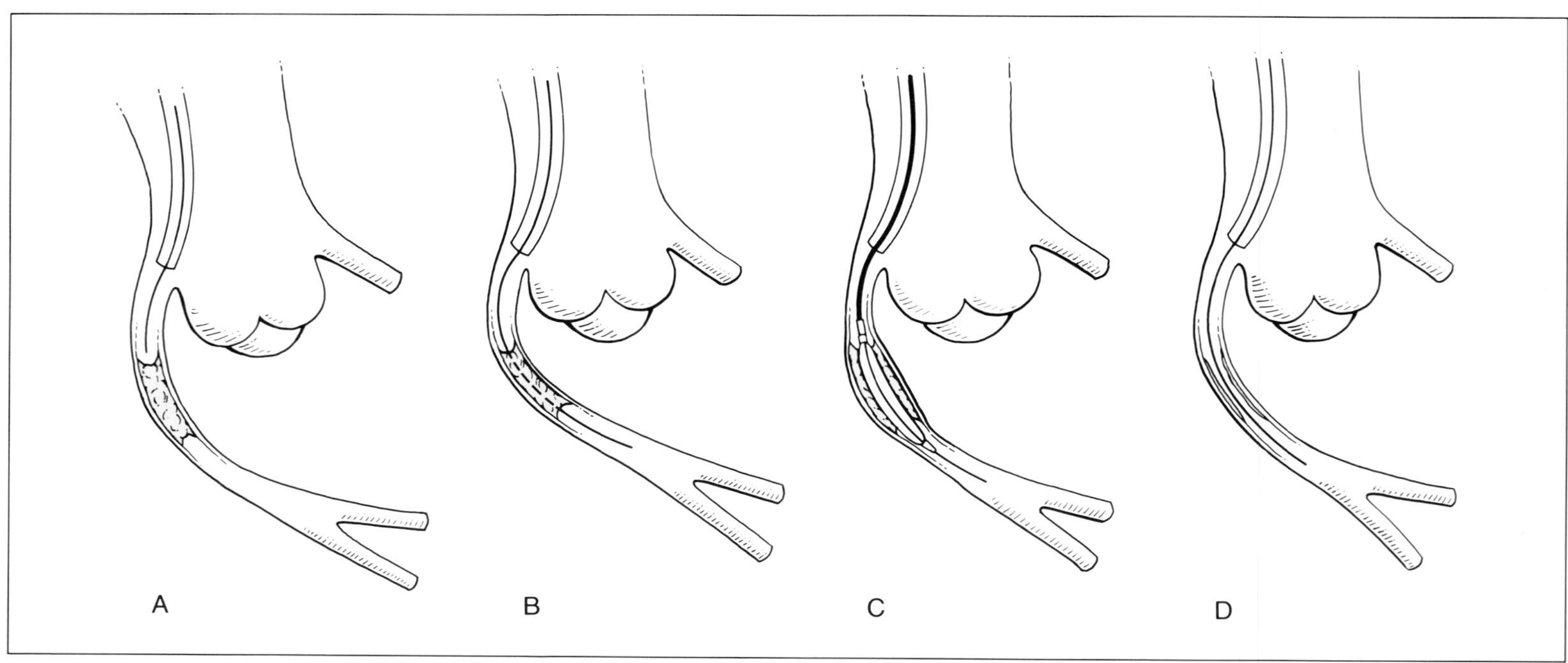

Fig. 30.21 Technique of PTCA for completely occluded artery. Technique for opening a completely occluded middle segment of the right coronary artery. (A) The guidewire is positioned just proximal to the occlusion. (B) The guidewire is advanced through the occluded segment. (C) Balloon angioplasty is performed in the usual way. (D) After angioplasty an adequate lumen is restored.

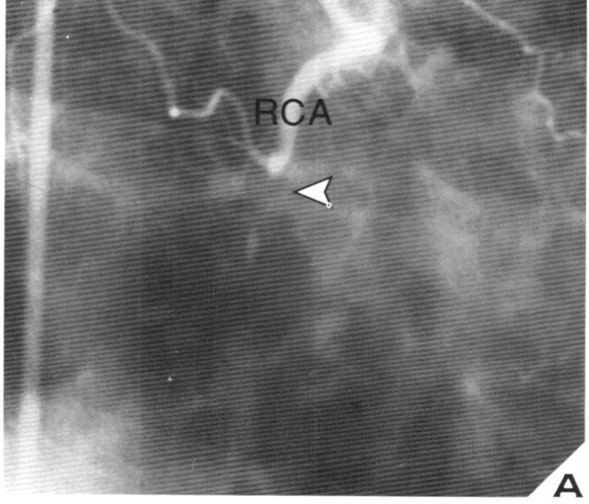

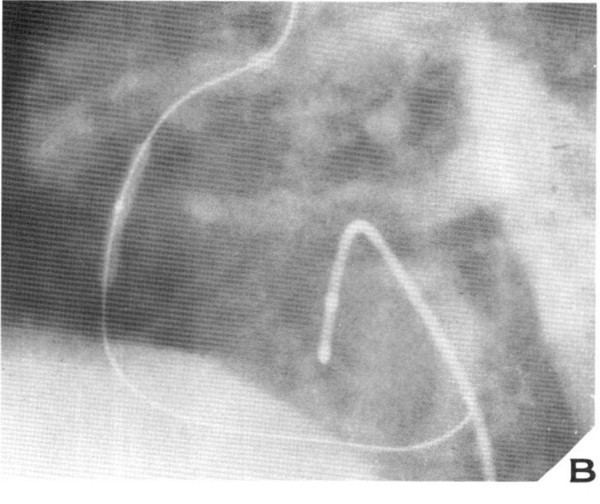

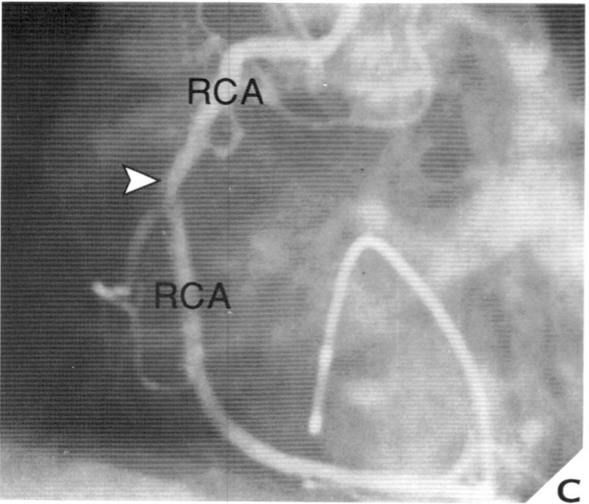

Fig. 30.22 Successful angioplasty of occluded right coronary artery. (A) Right coronary arteriogram (RAO projection) demonstrates complete occlusion (*arrow*) of middle segment of right coronary artery (RCA). Note triangular configuration of obstruction. PTCA was performed using the technique illustrated in the previous figure. (B) The inflated balloon is in place. (C) Coronary arteriogram obtained immediately after PTCA demonstrates a residual 20 percent stenosis with a small dissection (*arrow*).

ACUTE COMPLICATIONS OF CORONARY ANGIOPLASTY

Etiology and Risk Factors

Significant acute complications occur in approximately 5 percent of patients undergoing PTCA, a complication rate significantly higher than that associated with diagnostic coronary arteriography. The most serious acute complications are complete coronary closure and (rarely) coronary artery perforation or rupture (Fig. 30.23) resulting in pericardial tamponade. Factors associated with an increased risk of acute intra- or postprocedural coronary closure include female gender, a stenotic segment longer than 2 cm, stenosis at a bend of 45° or greater, stenosis at a branching point, stenosis associated with a thrombus or filling defect, unstable angina, and an evolving infarction. Residual stenosis or the presence of an intimal tear or dissection on the postprocedural arteriogram is associated with a greatly increased risk of acute closure. (The presence of acute stenosis is usually determined visually. In the past, it was customary to obtain pressure gradients across the dilated segment, in which case a residual gradient of 20 mm Hg or more was considered unsatisfactory.)

Postprocedural bleeding (prolonged bleeding or hematoma formation at the puncture site or retroperitoneal hemorrhage) is not uncommon and may in part be related to the systemic heparinization that is required for PTCA. Other intra- and postprocedural complications include transient arrhythmias, systemic hypertension, pulmonary edema, and renal failure.

Treatment

The development of new technology has made it possible to avoid emergency bypass surgery in many patients who develop acute postprocedural coronary artery occlusion secondary to thrombosis or dissection. During the early years of PTCA, approximately 75 percent of patients who developed acute closure during or immediately after PTCA required urgent bypass surgery. However, the advent of intracoronary stents (Fig. 30.24) and other innovative techniques (eg, laser angioplasty) has greatly decreased the need for emergency bypass surgery. When the occlusion is detected during the angioplasty procedure, prolonged balloon inflation (3 to 5 minutes) may help maintain arterial patency. By using a catheter with a flow-through balloon, it is possible to keep the balloon inflated for up to 30 minutes without producing severe ischemia.

RESULTS OF PTCA

Native Coronary Arteries

The success of PTCA is judged by two criteria. First, there must be a significant decrease in the stenosis (increase in diameter of at least 20 percent when compared with the initial coronary arteriogram). Second, the final diameter must be at least 50 percent of normal. Assessment of the final diameter must be as accurate as possible. There are many methods of assessing the severity of residual stenosis (eg, hand-held calipers, computer-assisted techniques, videodensitometry); however, none has proved more accurate than careful visual assessment (Fig.

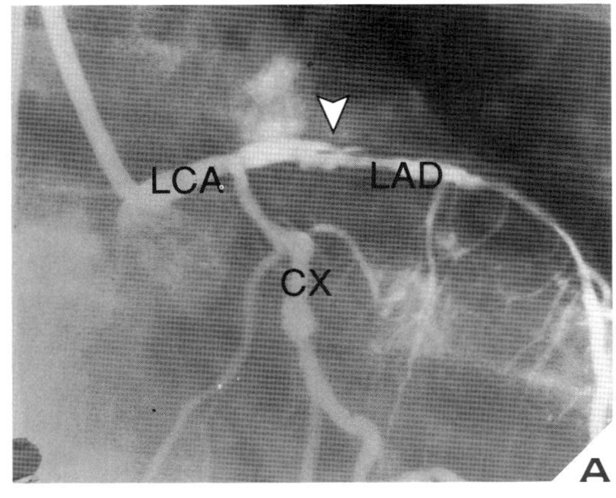

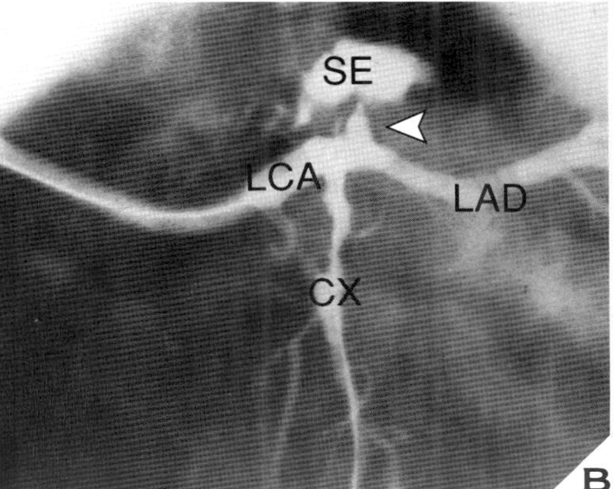

Fig. 30.23 Coronary artery perforation caused by PTCA. (A) RAO and (B) LAO projections of left coronary arteriogram reveal extravasation (*arrows*) of contrast material from the superior aspect of the left anterior descending artery (LAD). The extravasated contrast material is collecting in the subepicardial space (SE). (LCA = left main coronary artery; CX = circumflex artery).

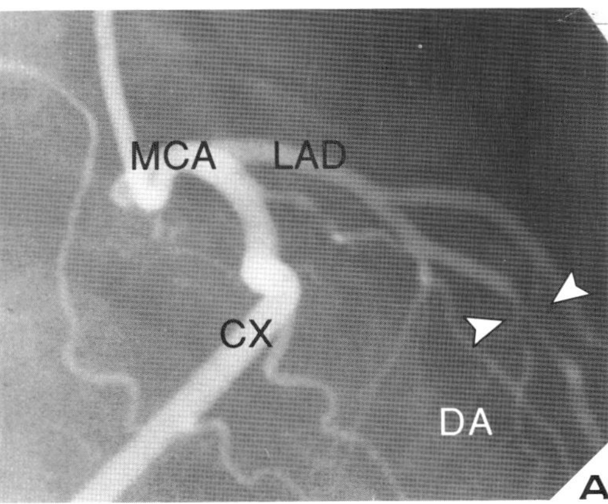

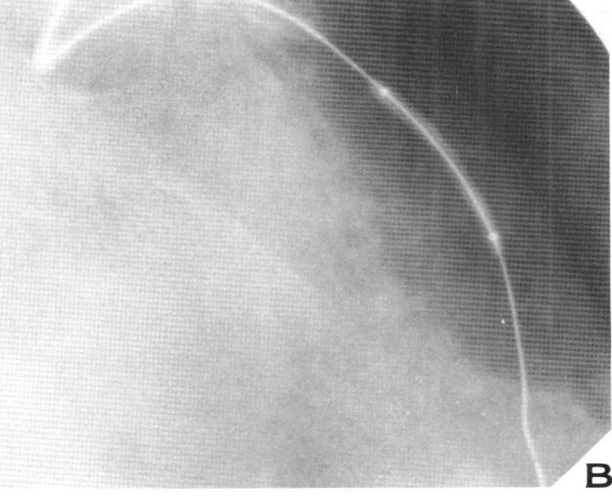

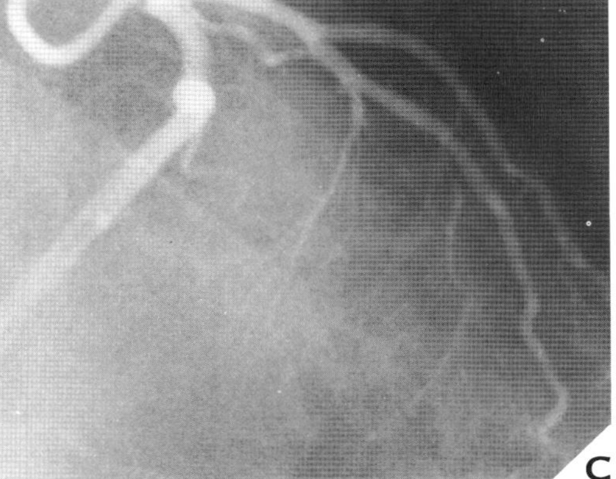

Fig. 30.24 Treatment of acute post-PTCA coronary artery closure with a stent. (A) Coronary arteriogram obtained before insertion of the stent (LAO projection). The middle segment of the left anterior descending artery (LAD) and one small diagonal branch (DA) are markedly narrowed (*arrows*). (B) Before dilatation. The stent (note characteristic irregularity of its border) is in place. The angioplasty balloon is inside the stent. (C) End result. The position of the stent is indicated by a brace. The LAD is widely patent. The stenosis of the diagonal branch is unchanged. (MCA = left main coronary artery; CX = circumflex artery)

30.25). It is important to distinguish true luminal widening from false channels and blind pouches resulting from dissection. Although false channels and blind pouches may *appear* to increase the caliber of the dilated segment, they do not result in a significant increase in flow. In general, luminal irregularities suggestive of dissection, but not associated with an ischemic episode or evidence of decreased flow, have a good prognosis (ie, they are not associated with an increased incidence of late restenosis).

The initial success rate of elective PTCA is about 90 percent. However, late restenosis is relatively frequent. Published series indicate that restenosis (defined as a loss of 50 percent or more of the initial gain in diameter or a residual stenosis of 50 percent or more) occurs in 20 to 40 percent of cases within 6 months after PTCA. Restenosis is most likely to occur after treatment of lesions involving (in order of frequency) the right coronary artery, left anterior descending artery, and circumflex artery. Restenosis is more common in patients with multiple stenotic segments than in those with an isolated stenosis, and is more likely to occur in long lesions (greater than 15 mm) than in short, circumscribed stenoses. Restenosis is unlikely when the residual stenosis is 10 percent or less; however, it is relatively common when the residual stenosis is 40 percent or more. Other factors associated with an increased risk of restenosis include angioplasty of the origin of a major branch, tortuosity and/or angulation of the treated artery, and the presence of residual thrombus at the time of angioplasty.

The chain of events culminating in restenosis is initiated at the time of PTCA; indeed, restenosis can be considered a mechanism of healing and remodeling of the iatrogenic arterial injury. The mechanical distortion produced by the inflated balloon causes cracking, splitting, and/or tearing of the deep layers of the arterial wall, which in turn exposes collagen fibers and leads to deposition of platelet aggregates and fibrin thrombi (Fig. 30.26). The propensity for thrombus formation is increased in small-diameter arteries with high shearing forces and high flow rates. Thrombus formation leads to acute occlusion in up to 5 percent of cases, and is especially likely to occur in arteries that have not been adequately dilated according to the criteria described above. Organization of mural thrombus with smooth muscle proliferation, possibly under the influence of platelet-derived growth factors, plays a major role in later restenosis (Fig. 30.27).

The functional result after PTCA is affected by multiple factors, including gender (females have a worse prognosis), the presence of collateral channels to or from the occluded artery, the degree of tortuosity of the occluded artery, the amount of myocardium at risk, the status of the other coronary arteries

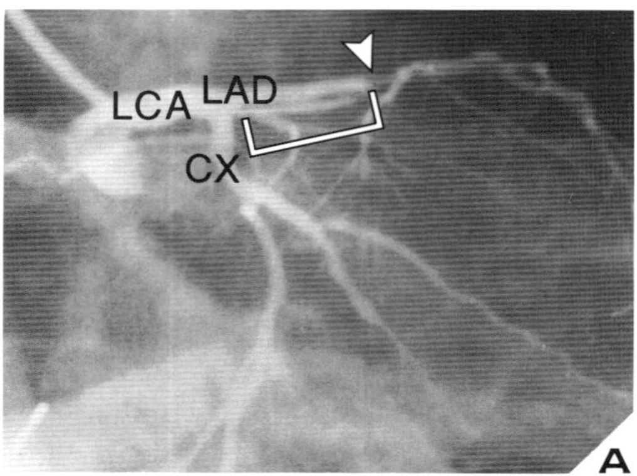

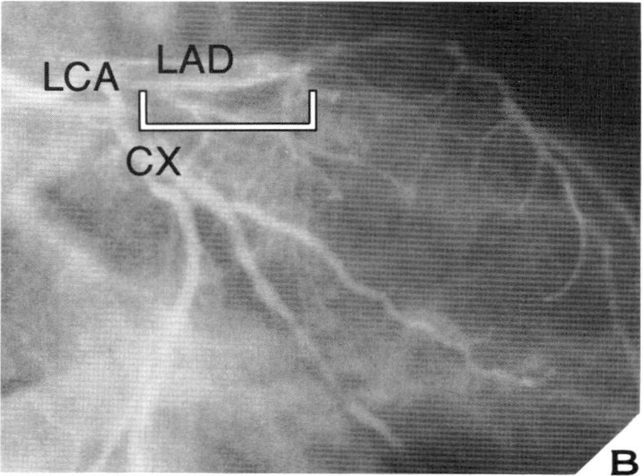

Fig. 30.25 Dissection and residual stenosis after PTCA. (A) Early phase of left coronary arteriogram (RAO projection) demonstrates a 40 percent residual stenosis (*arrow*) of the left anterior descending artery (LAD). The long, narrow collection of contrast material (*brace*) proximal to the stenosis represents a dissection. The false lumen is opacified and is separated from the true lumen by a negative shadow which represents a flap. (B) Late phase. The false channel (*brace*) is still opacified. The negative image is wider than before, and represents the composite image of the flat and unopacified blood flowing in the true lumen. (LCA = left main coronary artery; CX = circumflex artery)

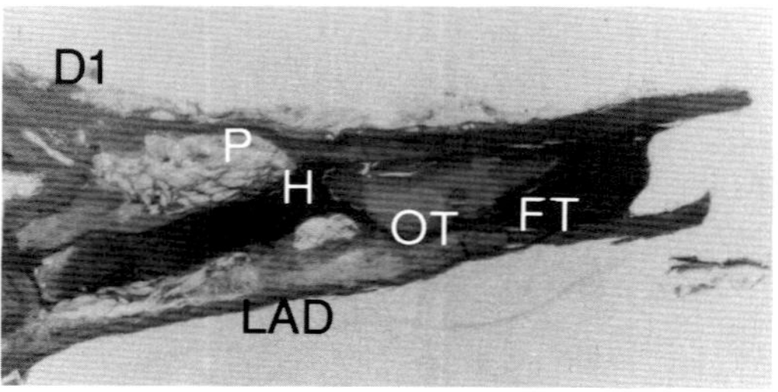

Fig. 30.26 Death after unsuccessful PTCA of the left anterior descending artery. Autopsy specimen of left anterior descending artery (LAD). In this longitudinal section the left main coronary artery is to reader's right. The LAD is completely obstructed by fresh intramural hemorrhage (H), fresh intraluminal thrombus (FT), and partially organized intraluminal thrombus (OT). The first diagonal branch (D1) is completely occluded by chronic atheromatous plaque (P).

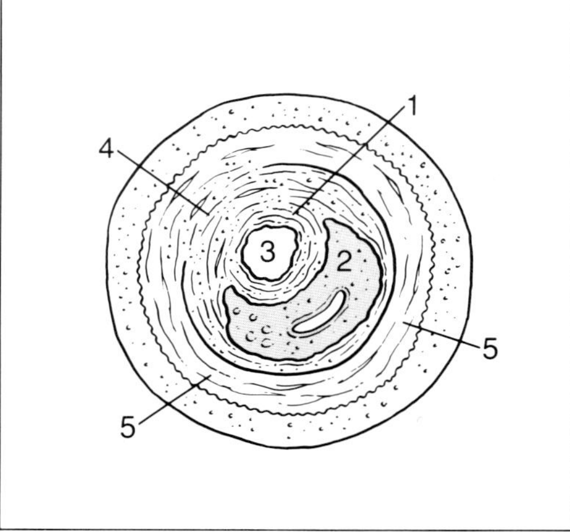

1 intimal proliferation
2 atheromatous plaque
3 arterial lumen
4 damaged media and intima
5 undamaged media

Fig. 30.27 Late restenosis after coronary angioplasty. Diagrammatic representation of a typical post-angioplasty restenosis occurring several months after balloon dilatation of an eccentric atheromatous plaque. The markedly narrowed lumen is mainly due to hypertrophy of fibromuscular tissue on the side opposite the compressed atheromatous plaque. Fibrous tissue on the surface of the compressed atheromatous plaque aggravates the stenosis. It is important to remember that restenosis, represents a healing process. Not only does the angioplasty balloon compress and fragment the atheromatous plaque, but it overstretches the arterial wall and disrupts the normal intima and media. Within the first 24 hours after angioplasty, the dominant pathologic features are tears in the plaque, endothelial exfoliation, platelet aggregation on the surface of the plaque, and intraluminal thrombus formation. By the second week, smooth muscle cells can be seen migrating from the media towards the intima, where they subsequently proliferate. At the same time, intraluminal thrombus undergoes organization by connective tissue, further narrowing the lumen. After 3 months, smooth muscle proliferation and collagen deposition are the predominant pathologic features; however, residual thrombus can still be seen. Active vasoconstriction of the stretched plaque-free portion of the arterial wall ("recoil reinstitution of tone") is also believed to play a contributory role in postangioplasty restenosis.

(patients with multiple-vessel disease have a worse prognosis), and coexisting pathology (eg, left ventricular hypertrophy, systemic hypertension, diabetes).

Coronary Artery Bypass Grafts

Stenosis of saphenous vein grafts (see below) is more common than restenosis of stenotic native coronary arteries initially treated with PTCA. (In one series, significant narrowing was present in 61.2 percent of vein grafts studied 16 months after bypass surgery.) PTCA has been successfully used to treat stenotic saphenous vein grafts. The initial success rate (approximately 90 percent) and complication rate (7.1 percent) are comparable to those of PTCA of native coronary arteries. Serious postprocedural complications are more common when PTA is performed in patients with "elderly" vein grafts. In one series, the postprocedural myocardial infarction rate was 12.5 percent for vein grafts that had been in place for 36 months or less and 28.2 percent for vein grafts that had been in place for more than 36 months (Platko et al, 1989).

SURGICAL REVASCULARIZATION

The aorta-to-coronary artery bypass graft, introduced in 1967, is widely used to treat patients with myocardial ischemia caused by obstructive coronary artery disease. The goal of bypass surgery is to provide additional blood supply to the vascular territory distal to the occluded or stenotic segment. The most widely employed bypass procedure utilizes a free peripheral vein graft harvested at the time of the bypass procedure. Other surgical revascularization techniques entail direct anastomosis of a systemic artery (left or right internal mammary or gastroepiplotic artery) to the recipient coronary artery. Coronary bypass surgery requires cardiopulmonary bypass and aortic cross-clamping. The use of external cardiac cooling and cold cardioplegia provide better surgical exposure and minimize the risk of intraoperative myocardial damage.

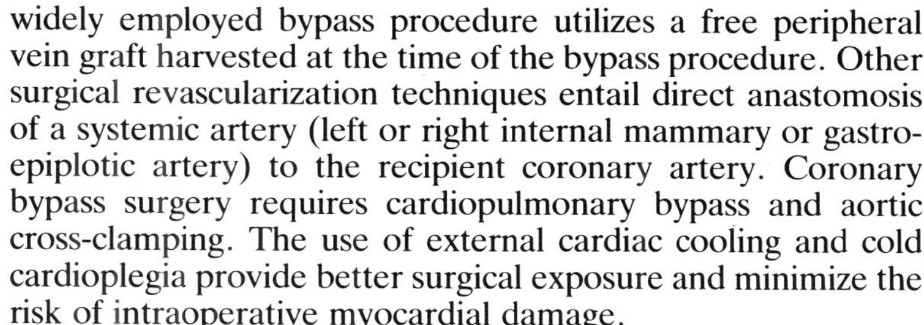

PRINCIPLES

In the standard aorto-coronary bypass operation utilizing a venous graft, a suitable length of the patient's right or left saphenous vein is harvested and inserted between the ascending aorta and the recipient coronary artery (Fig. 30.28). To avoid possible obstruction by the venous valves, the distal end of the graft is connected to the aorta and the proximal end to the recipient coronary artery. The distal connection is usually made in side-to-side fashion. However, some surgeons prefer to construct a "sequential" anastomosis consisting of one or two side-to-side anastomoses and a distal end-to-side anastomosis (Fig. 30.29). When the internal mammary artery is employed, it is necessary to dissect the artery from its normal course along the inner aspect of the anterior chest wall and connect it to the recipient coronary artery (Fig. 30.30). Both internal mammary arteries can be harvested at the same session or at two separate sessions, often many years apart.

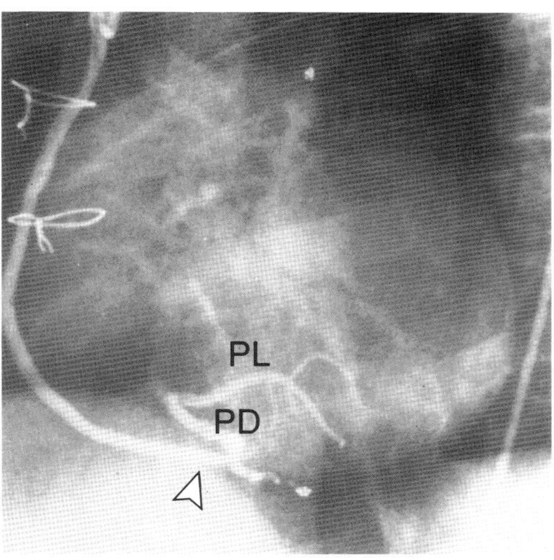

Fig. 30.28 CABG with distal end-to-side anastomosis. Selective injection of saphenous vein graft (*arrow*) connecting ascending aorta with midportion of posterior descending artery (LAO projection). The graft is uniform in caliber, indicating the absence of significant intimal hyperplasia. Note the dense opacification of the posterior descending (PD) artery and the posterolateral (PL) artery and its branches, indicating excellent perfusion of the myocardial segments supplied by these vessels.

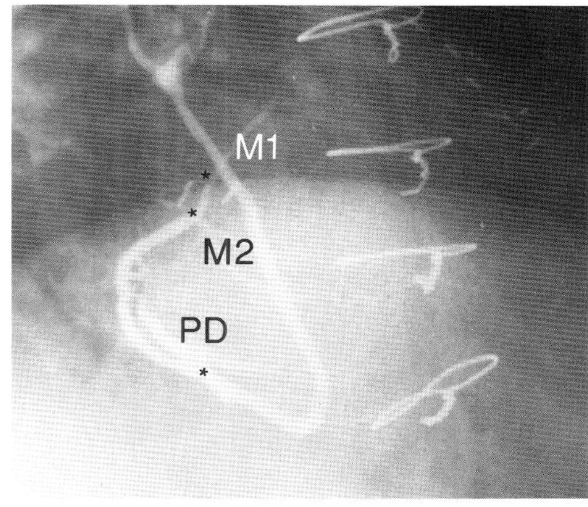

Fig. 30.29 CABG with sequential anastomoses. Selective injection of saphenous vein graft (RAO projection). The graft appears as a large channel which is connected in side-to-side fashion to the middle portion of the posterior descending artery (PD); in side-to-side fashion to the second marginal artery (M2); and in end-to-side fashion to the first marginal artery (M1). Each of the anastomoses is indicated by a *

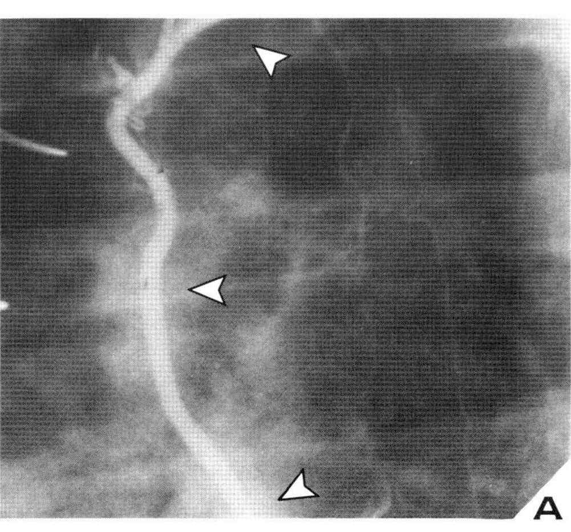

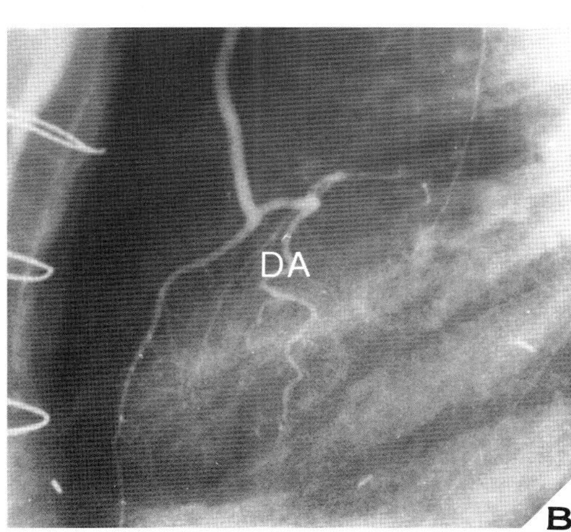

Fig. 30.30 Aorto–coronary bypass using left internal mammary artery. (A) LAO and (B) lateral projections of selective injection of selective left internal mammary arteriogram show a patent end-to-side anastomosis between the internal mammary artery (*arrows*) and the left anterior descending artery. The internal mammary artery, which normally runs along the anterior chest wall, is displaced posteriorly. The native LAD is well opacified in both antegrade and retrograde fashion. (DA = diagonal artery)

Postoperatively the vein graft acts as a conduit, conducting oxygenated blood to the myocardial territory that is supplied by the stenotic or obstructed native coronary artery. In about 25 percent of cases, the amount of the ischemic myocardium that exhibits enhanced perfusion postoperatively exceeds that normally supplied by the native artery. Therefore, after surgical revascularization, myocardial contractility may be improved in cardiac segments adjacent to those supplied by the obstructed native coronary artery or bypass graft.

NATURAL HISTORY OF BYPASS GRAFTS

The patency rate of bypass grafts during the first few postoperative weeks is 80 to 95 percent. Early stenosis or occlusion is usually related to technical factors (eg, luminal construction, recipient artery too small, hematoma at the anastomotic site, dissection) (Fig. 30.31).

Saphenous vein grafts are subjected to systemic arterial pressure, which typically results in intimal hyperplasia (Fig. 30.32). According to some reports, intimal hyperplasia can be detected as soon as 1 month after surgery. It may progress, resulting in stenosis and eventually occlusion (Fig. 30.33). Follow-up arteriographic studies have shown that 30 percent of vein grafts exhibit significant stenosis 1 year after surgery. Late stenosis and occlusion affects about 0.4 to 3 percent of grafts per year. The patency rates at 5 and 10 years are 55 and 45 percent, respectively.

The most important factors responsible for late stenosis and occlusion of saphenous vein grafts are accelerated atherosclerosis in the graft and the size of the recipient artery. (When the recipient artery is 1 mm in diameter, only 50 percent of vein grafts are still patent at 1 year.) After an initially successful revascularization procedure, the recipient coronary artery continues to be affected by the underlying atherosclerotic process. Therefore, a recipient artery that was widely patent at the end of the first postoperative year may subsequently undergo progressive stenosis with decreased flow. In some instances the atherosclerotic process in the recipient artery progresses very rapidly.

Pooled series indicate that 90 percent of mammary artery grafts are patent after 7 years. The long-term patency rate for gastroepiploic artery grafts (introduced in 1987) is not yet known.

IMAGING AFTER BYPASS SURGERY

Postoperatively, myocardial ischemia is manifested clinically by chest pain and ECG changes. Although thallium perfusion scans may provide useful information, coronary arteriography

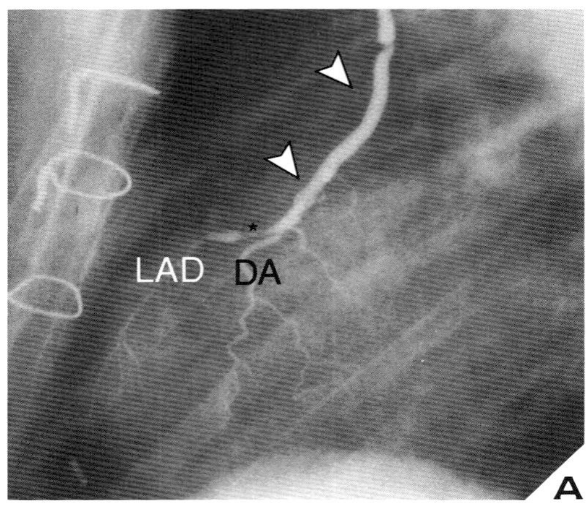

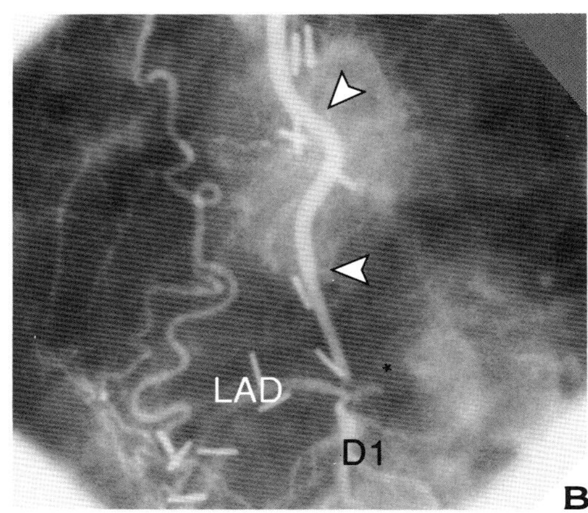

Fig. 30.31 Early failure of bypass graft. Angiographic findings in two different patients. (A) Selective injection of saphenous vein graft (*arrows*) connected sequentially to the left anterior descending artery and a diagonal artery (DA) shows poor distal perfusion owing to the small size of the recipient artery. There is a high-grade stenosis (*) in the portion of the graft between the first and second anastomoses. (B) Selective internal mammary arteriogram in a patient with sequential anastomoses to the left anterior descending (LAD) and the first diagonal (D1) arteries shows marked stenosis (*) at the connection between the internal mammary artery (*arrows*) and the diagonal artery, with poor opacification of the graft beyond this point. The stenosis at the graft–artery junction is probably due to fibrosis caused by the sutures.

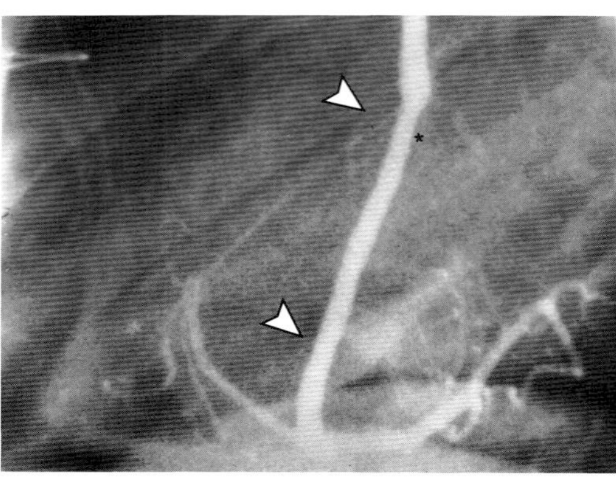

Fig. 30.32 Atherosclerosis of bypass graft. Selective injection of saphenous vein graft (*arrows*) reveals deformity (*) of the posterior border of the midportion of the graft. This appearance is compatible with early atherosclerotic degeneration of the arterialized vein graft.

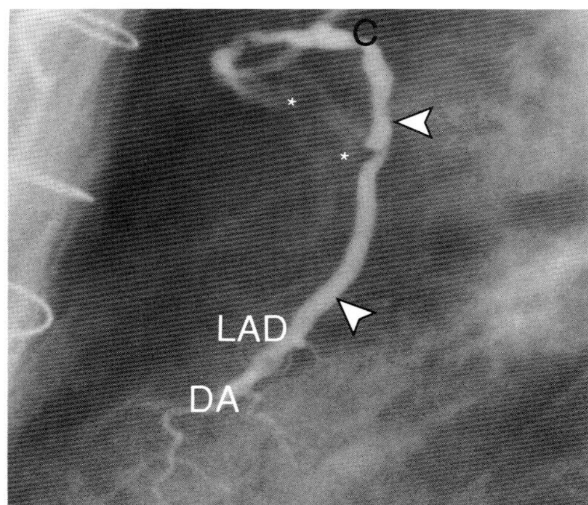

Fig. 30.33 Stenosis of vein graft secondary to atherosclerosis. Selective injection (lateral projection) of saphenous vein graft (*arrows*) connected to the left anterior descending artery (LAD) demonstrates two sharply defined eccentric defects (*) in the proximal and middle segments of the graft, causing significant (60 to 70 percent) stenosis. This appearance is compatible with advanced atherosclerosis of the vein graft. The distal connection of the graft is widely patent. (C = catheter in aorta; DA = diagonal artery)

remains the definitive study in patients with signs and symptoms of myocardial ischemia after surgical revascularization procedures.

Plain Films

Postoperative chest films reveal the typical appearance of a medial sternotomy. Some surgeons implant metallic markers to indicate the site of the aortic attachment of the saphenous vein graft. In patients with internal mammary artery grafts, metallic clips often indicate the course of the transposed artery (Fig. 30.34).

Not infrequently, a pseudoaneurysm of the ascending aorta may form as a result of extravasation at the cannulation site used for cardiopulmonary bypass. Plain films show dilatation and deformity of the ascending aorta, with filling in of the retrosternal clear space (Fig. 30.35). Contrast-enhanced CT confirms the diagnosis.

Nuclear Medicine

Thallium perfusion scanning is not as sensitive for detecting myocardial ischemia in patients who have undergone revascularization surgery as it is in those who have not been

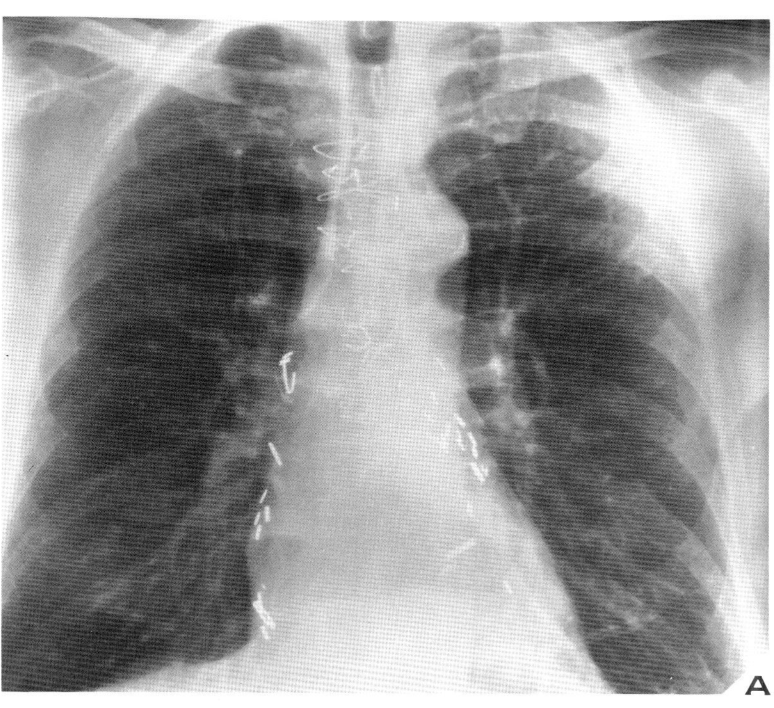

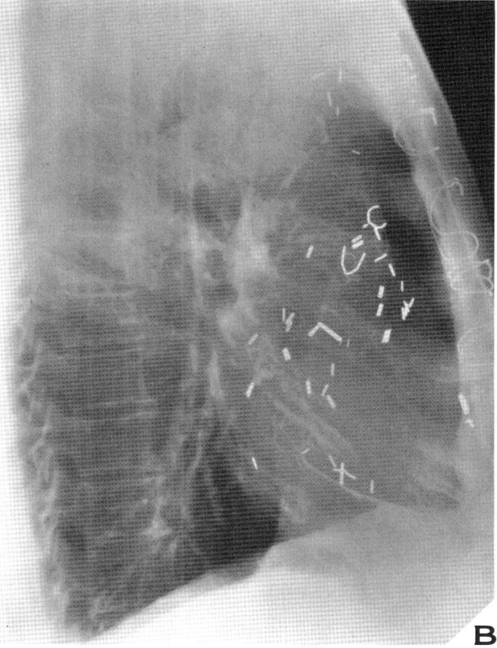

Fig. 30.34 Bilateral internal mammary artery bypass grafts. (A) Posteroanterior and (B) lateral chest films show many metallic clips along the right and left borders of the cardiovascular silhouette. The clips indicate the course of the right and left internal mammary arteries, which have been detached from the anterior chest wall and connected to the right coronary and left anterior descending arteries. Note the wires in the median sternotomy.

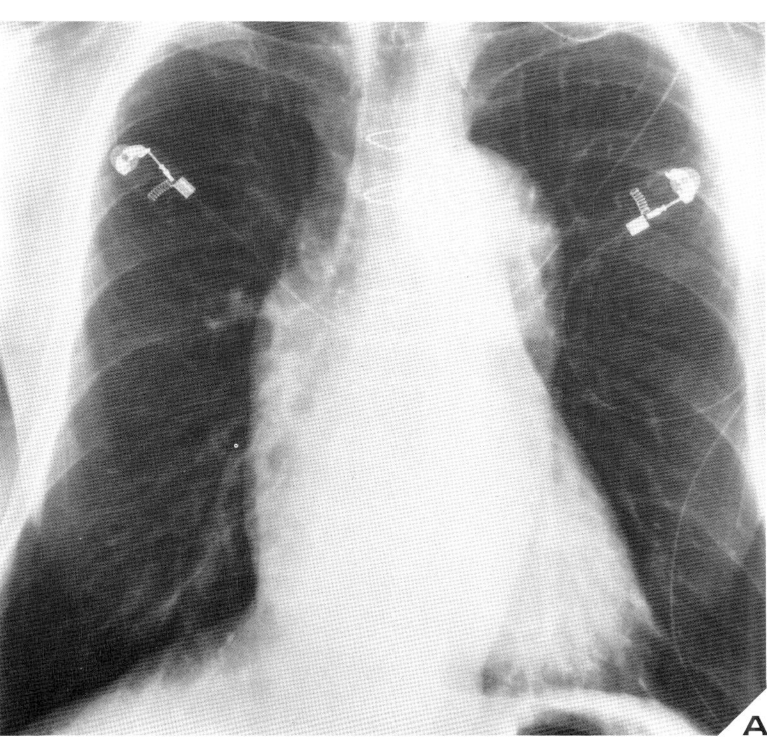

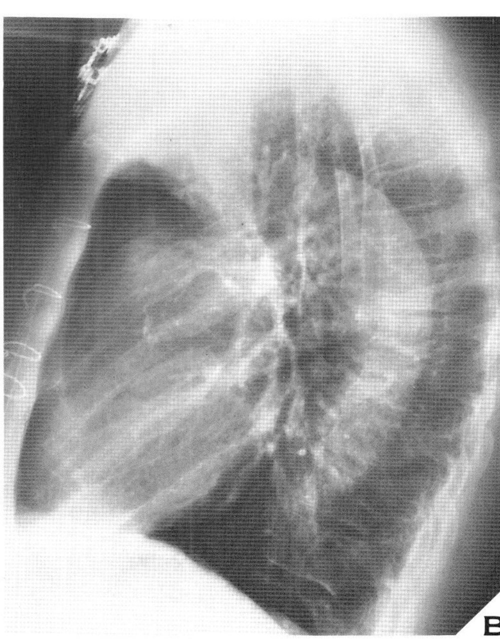

Fig. 30.35 Pseudoaneurysm of aorta after CABG. (A) Postero–anterior and (B) lateral chest films show deformity and enlargement of the ascending aorta, which projects to the right and anteriorly, encroaching on the retrosternal space. The aortic arch and descending thoracic aorta appear normal. The patient's previous films showed that the ascending aorta had been progressively enlarging ever since an aorta–coronary saphenous vein bypass graft 1 year earlier. At operation there was a false aneurysm of the aorta at the site where a cannula had been inserted for cardiopulmonary bypass.

operated on. (In general, thallium perfusion scans are more reliable after angioplasty or thrombolytic therapy.) The scintigraphic criteria for ischemia after revascularization surgery are similar to those previously described for acute or chronic ischemic heart disease (see Chapter 20).

Angiography

Postoperative angiographic evaluation after surgical revascularization procedures entails a thorough assessment of the native coronary circulation as well as the bypass graft or native systemic (internal mammary or gastroepiploic) arteries used to revascularize the myocardium (Fig. 30.36). Although the technique is similar to that previously described for conventional coronary arteriography (see Chapter 21), special catheters may be needed to selectively opacify the vein graft or native systemic artery. It is essential to verify the patency of the vein graft or native systemic artery, as well as that of the recipient coronary artery. Occasionally it is necessary to employ multiple projections to adequately delineate the connections, the size of the graft and the recipient artery, and the rate of opacification of the recipient artery.

The aortic connection is usually made to the anterior (rarely the lateral or posterior) aspect of the ascending aorta (Fig. 30.37); therefore, it may be slightly to the left or right of the midline. Some surgeons routinely implant metallic markers at the site of the aortic connection to facilitate postoperative angiography. It may also be helpful to refer to the operative note when planning the angiographic procedure. In some instances it is useful to obtain a preliminary left ventriculogram or thoracic aortogram in the LAO or lateral projection. Although

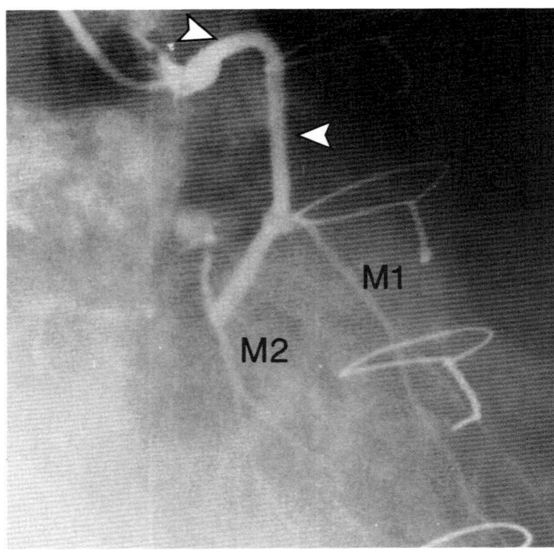

Fig. 30.36 Stenosis of recipient arteries after CABG. Selective injection of saphenous vein graft (*arrows*) demonstrates patent sequential anastomoses to the first (M1) and second (M2) marginal arteries, both of which are very poorly opacified. Comparison with the preoperative arteriogram indicated that there had been marked progression of the atherosclerotic process in the recipient arteries.

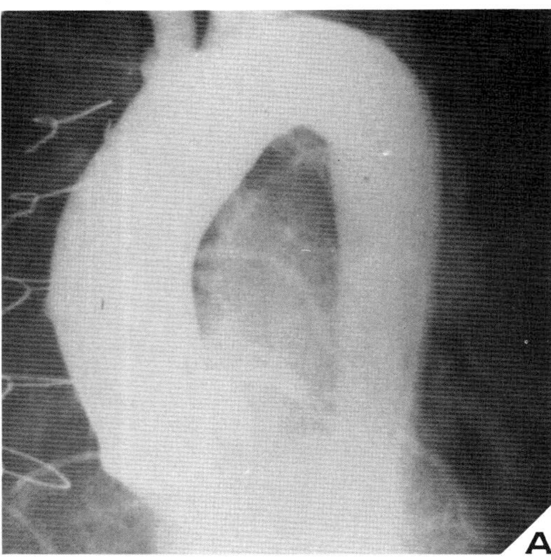

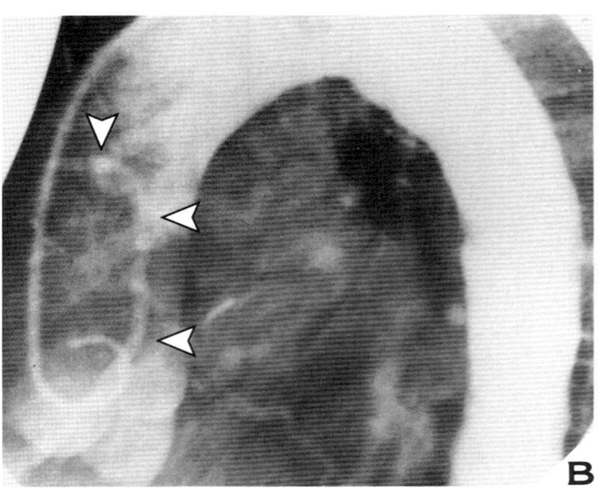

Fig. 30.37 Angiographic demonstration of proximal connection of CABG. (A) Frontal and (B) lateral projections of thoracic aortogram show the saphenous vein graft (*arrows*) arising from the anterior wall of the aorta and coursing into the area of the left anterior descending artery.

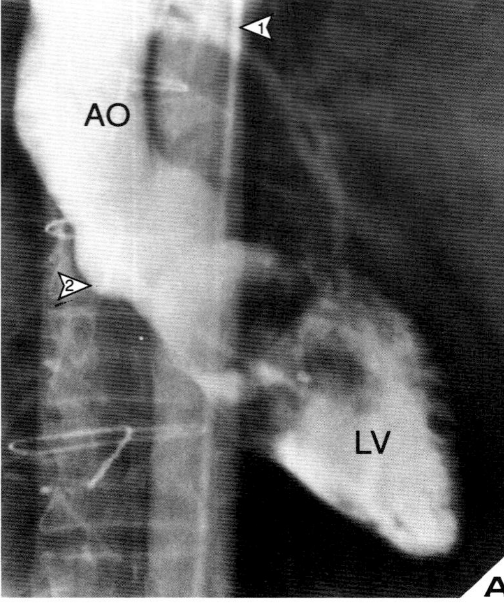

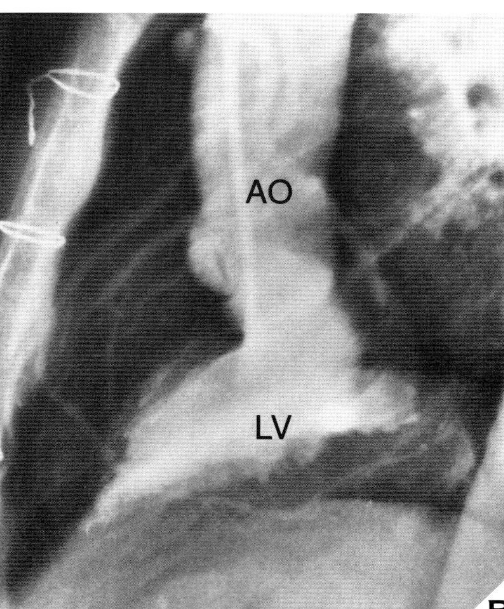

Fig. 30.38 Demonstration of CABG by left ventriculography. (A) Frontal and (B) lateral projections of left ventriculogram demonstrate three patent saphenous vein grafts connecting the aorta to the right coronary artery (*arrow 1*), left anterior descending artery, and marginal branches (*arrow 2*). Obtaining a preliminary left ventriculogram or aortogram to locate the site of the aortic connection facilitates selective angiography. (LV = left ventricle; AO = aorta)

neither ventriculography nor aortography adequately depicts the origin and course of the graft, the preliminary study may facilitate its selective catheterization (Figs. 30.37 and 30.38).

Because vein grafts connected to the right coronary artery and its branches are oriented directly downward, they may require the use of a straight catheter (Fig. 30.39). In general, the standard right coronary "Judkins" catheter can be used for vein grafts connected to the left coronary system (Fig. 30.40). However, some aorta–left coronary bypass grafts have an initial upward loop that requires the use of a special catheter with an upward hook at its tip ("left bypass graft configuration").

The left internal mammary artery (IMA) is usually used for myocardial revascularization procedures. (The right IMA can also be utilized, although this option is less extensively employed.) The left IMA is usually connected to the left anterior descending artery or to a diagonal artery (Figs. 30.41 and 30.42). IMA grafts can usually be studied with a standard right coronary "Judkins" catheter, which is introduced via the right or left femoral artery. With the patient supine, the catheter is passed into the ipsilateral subclavian artery under fluoroscopic guidance and the orifice of the IMA is "hooked" with the "nose" of the catheter. (A specially shaped "IMA" catheter, which has a more sharply angled nose than the standard right "Judkins" catheter, may facilitate this maneuver.) If the IMA cannot be cannulated, a flush subclavian arteriogram (obtained after inflating a blood pressure cuff to occlude the ipsilateral branchial artery) may provide the needed information. Finally, a selective internal mammary arteriogram obtained after retrograde catheterization of the IMA via the ipsilateral brachial artery may succeed when other techniques have failed. IMA

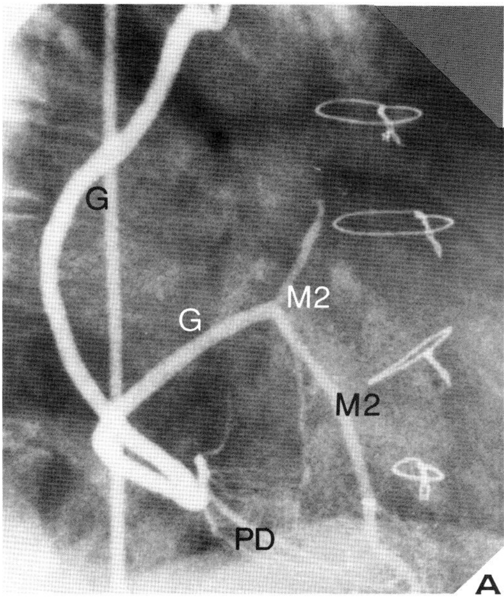

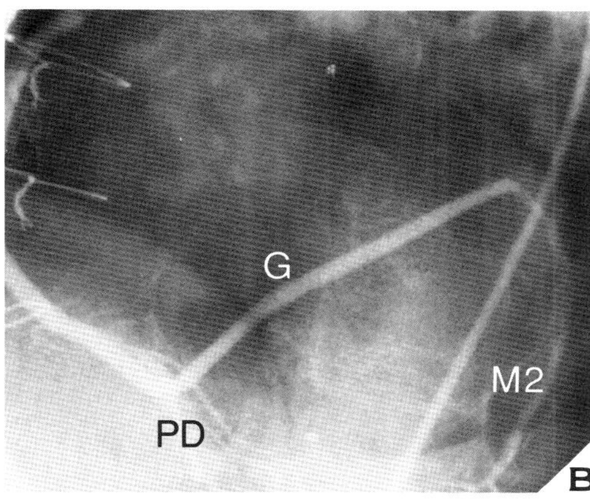

Fig. 30.39 Selective angiogram of CABG to branches of right coronary artery. Selective angiograms of the saphenous vein graft (G) in (A) LAO and (B) RAO projections demonstrate sequential connections of the graft to the middle segment of the posterior descending (PD) and second marginal (M2) arteries. (A third more distal anastomosis is not demonstrated.)

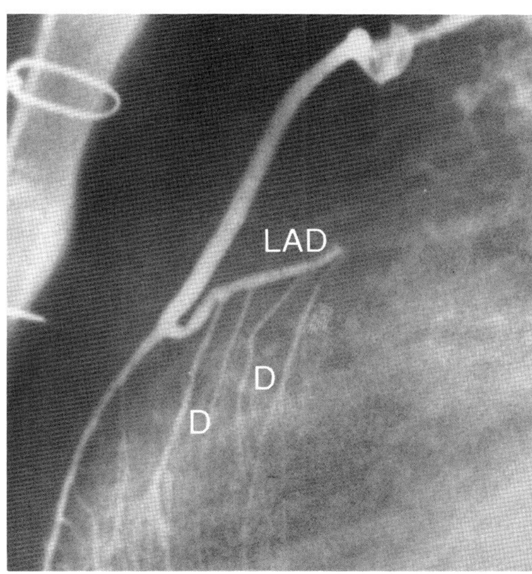

Fig. 30.40 Selective angiogram of CABG to left anterior descending artery. Lateral projection demonstrates a widely patent end-to-side anastomosis between the saphenous vein graft and the middle segment of the left anterior descending artery (LAD). (D = diagonal branches)

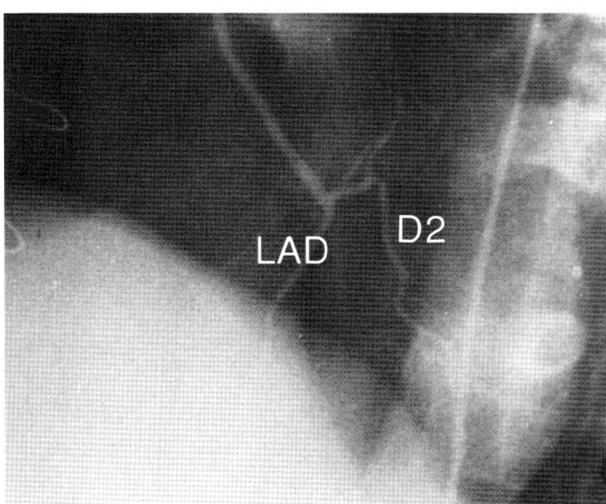

Fig. 30.41 Selective arteriogram of internal mammary artery graft. LAO-Cr projection demonstrates an end-to-side anastomosis between the transposed internal mammary artery and the middle segment of the left anterior descending artery. The recipient artery is well visualized by both antegrade and retrograde flow. (D2 = second diagonal artery)

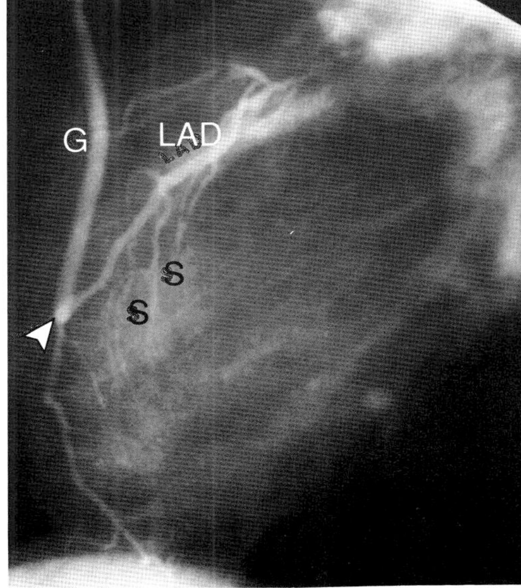

Fig. 30.42 Selective arteriogram of internal mammary artery graft. Lateral projection. The internal mammary artery (G) has been extensively mobilized and no longer follows its usual course along the posterior aspect of the anterior chest wall. The anastomosis (*arrow*) between the graft and the middle segment of the left anterior descending artery (LAD) is widely patent. (S = septal arteries)

studies with conventional contrast material are often accompanied by considerable pain, which can be decreased or entirely alleviated by using a low-osmolality contrast agent.

Careful morphologic analysis will enable one to identify the portions of the myocardium that are well perfused and those that are poorly perfused or unperfused. The bypass graft can be occluded anywhere along its course (Fig. 30.43). The site of occlusion is usually close to the aortic connection; occasionally it is at or near the connection with the recipient artery. In patients with sequential anastomoses, the angiographer must take pains to demonstrate the connection with each branch. If the proximal portion of the graft is occluded and the connection or connections to the recipient artery are patent, retrograde filling of the distal portion of the graft may occur under certain hemodynamic conditions.

The status of the native coronary arteries is accurately depicted by coronary arteriography. In some patients the proximal segments of all the native coronary arteries are occluded; in such cases myocardial perfusion is entirely dependent on the graft.

In the past, angiographic evaluation of the postoperative patient usually included left ventriculography to assess left ventricular morphology and contractility. Left ventriculography is no longer performed routinely, as nuclear imaging and echocardiography usually provide the necessary information. Postoperative left ventriculography is particularly helpful when a preoperative study is available for comparison.

TREATMENT OF ACUTE MYOCARDIAL INFARCTION

Acute myocardial infarction is usually caused by thrombotic occlusion of the infarct-related artery. The resulting ischemia leads to progressive myocardial necrosis, which typically extends from the subendocardial region to the epicardium. Cell death can occur within 20 to 30 minutes after the acute event. The rate at which necrosis proceeds depends on the elapsed time after the interruption of blood flow, the myocardial oxygen demand, and the degree of myocardial hypoperfusion. A decrease in myocardial function (which results in decreased oxygen demand) may slow the rate of necrosis. However, the ultimate extent of myocardial necrosis is determined by the loss of blood supply, and will not be altered unless adequate myocardial perfusion is restored.

The initial goal of therapy is to reduce the rate of myocardial necrosis by decreasing oxygen demand while increasing tissue oxygenation. The latter is accomplished by stimulating the collateral circulation or increasing flow through the infarct-related artery ("reperfusion"). Recent data clearly indicate the benefits of immediate myocardial reperfusion therapy. Although myocardial damage caused by reperfusion techniques ("reperfusion injury") can decrease the amount of potentially salvageable myocardium, most investigators agree that the potential benefits of an aggressive therapeutic approach warrant the risks.

THROMBOLYTIC THERAPY OF ACUTE MYOCARDIAL INFARCTION

Thrombolytic Drugs

Thrombus formation within the coronary arterial tree stimulates the release of serum and endothelial thrombolytic factors; thrombolytic drugs augment this natural thrombolytic activity. Five thrombolytic drugs either are approved for clinical use or are undergoing clinical trials to determine their efficacy in myocardial reperfusion. Three thrombolytic agents [streptokinase, urokinase, and anisoylated plasminogen streptokinase activator complex (ASPAC)] have a nonspecific effect

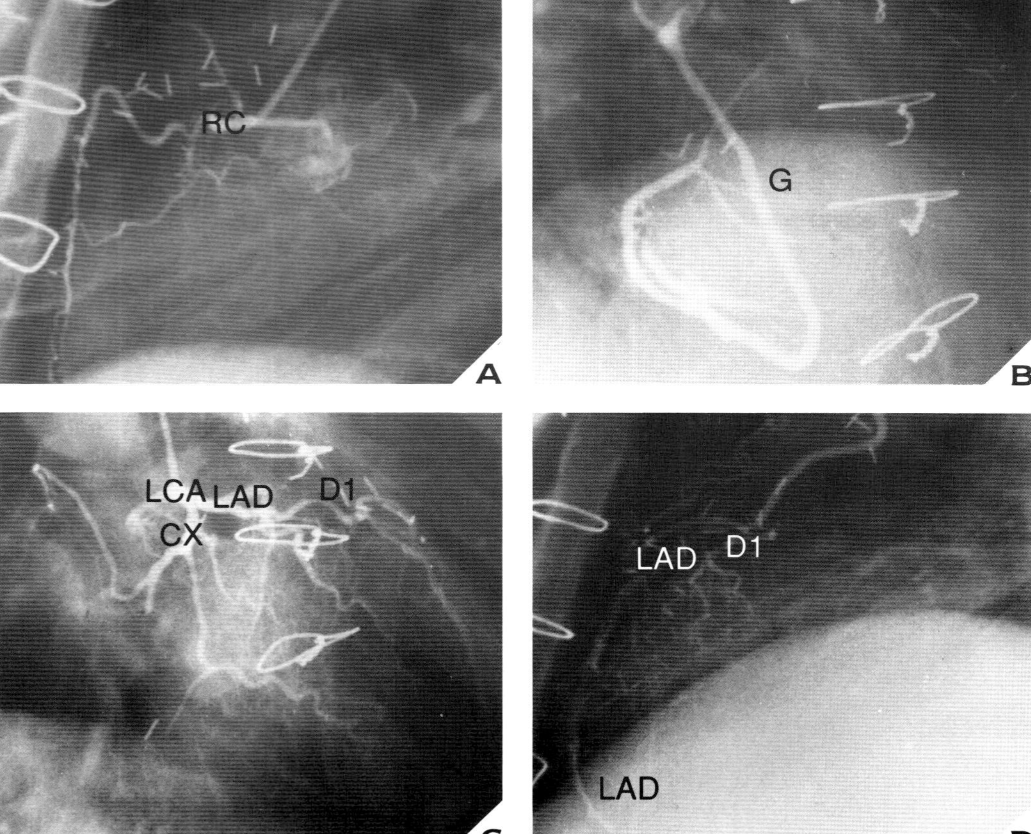

Fig. 30.43 Atherosclerotic narrowing of internal mammary artery bypass graft. (A–D) Postoperative angiographic studies in an asymptomatic patient. (A) Selective right coronary (RC) arteriogram (lateral projection) demonstrates complete occlusion of the native right coronary artery. (B) Selective injection of aorta-right coronary bypass graft (G) (RAO projection) shows a widely patent anastomosis, with excellent revascularization of the middle and distal portions of the right coronary artery. (C) Selective left coronary arteriogram (RAO projection) shows severe stenosis of the left anterior descending (LAD) and first diagonal (D1) arteries. (D) Selective left internal mammary arteriogram (lateral projection) shows that the stenoses have been bypassed by the arterial graft, which is connected to the LAD and first diagonal arteries. However, perfusion of the distal LAD is markedly decreased owing to severe stenosis of the internal mammary artery graft. A thallium scan demonstrated underperfusion of the anterolateral wall of the left ventricle.

on fibrinolysis, ie, they do not directly convert plasminogen to plasmin. Two thrombolytic agents, recombinant tissue-type plasminogen activator (rt-PA) and pro-urokinase, have a relatively specific effect on fibrinolysis.

Streptokinase activates the fibrinolytic process indirectly by forming a strong complex with plasminogen, which in turn converts the inactive proenzyme and enzyme into effective plasminogen activators. High doses of streptokinase (about 350,000 units) are usually needed to overcome baseline immunological inhibition before fibrinolytic activity can proceed. When compared with relatively "clot-specific" agents such as rt-PA, streptokinase is only moderately effective in establishing early patency of the infarct-related artery.

Urokinase, like streptokinase, is a naturally occurring enzyme which has a nonspecific effect on fibrinolysis. Large doses (2 to 3 million units) are needed for a therapeutic effect.

ASPAC is a thrombolytic agent with an affinity for fibrin (ie, it is clot selective). Its thrombolytic efficiency at an intravenous dose of 30 mg is similar to that of streptokinase administered directly into the occluded coronary (ie, the initial patency rate is approximately 75 percent).

rt-PA is a naturally occurring serum protease found in vascular endothelium. A synthetic single-chain preparation with a half-life of 1 to 3 minutes is now undergoing clinical trials. rt-PA is inactive by itself. However, in the presence of fibrin it forms a complex with plasminogen, accelerating its conversion to plasmin, which lyses fibrin on the surface of the thrombus. The specific fibrinolytic action of rt-PA and its preferential site of action on the surface of the thrombus probably account for its relatively great thrombolytic efficiency (70 to 75 percent) when compared with an intravenous dose of a nonselective agent such as streptokinase. Unlike streptokinase and urokinase, rt-PA is associated with a significant bleeding risk when used in patients with underlying vascular damage (eg, ulcerated plaque).

Pro-urokinase (single-chain urokinase plasminogen activator) is a precursor of urokinase. Unlike urokinase, it has a selective fibrinolytic activity comparable to that of rt-PA. However, its relatively great propensity for allergic and idiosyncratic reactions has limited its clinical use.

At present, the thrombolytic agents most extensively used in the treatment of acute myocardial infarction are streptokinase and rt-PA. Recent cooperative studies indicate that both agents yield similar results. However, because of its lower cost streptokinase is more widely used.

Route of Administration

When thrombolytic therapy was first introduced, the thrombolytic agent (streptokinase) was infused through an indwelling coronary arterial catheter, which was positioned with its tip as close as possible to the occluding thrombus. More recently, the intravenous route has gained an increasing number of adherents. Although cooperative studies have shown that intraarterial administration of the thrombolytic agent is more effective in achieving clot dissolution, these studies have not shown that the degree of improvement in left ventricular function was similar with both techniques.

Clinical Efficacy

The benefit—if any—of thrombolytic therapy is determined by such end points as re-opening of the infarct-related artery (reperfusion), improvement in left ventricular function, and increased survival rate.

Reperfusion of the infarct-related artery has been reported to occur in 75 percent of patients with acute myocardial infarction after early (within 4 hours after the onset of symptoms) intraarterial infusion of streptokinase. A similar reperfusion rate has been reported after early intravenous treatment with the newer thrombolytic agents. In general, thrombolysis can be detected angiographically in 60 to 65 percent of patients undergoing thrombolytic therapy. Coronary arteriograms obtained during and within 1 hour after intraarterial administration of the thrombolytic agent clearly show the efficacy of this therapeutic approach (Fig. 30.44). A number of studies have shown that thrombolytic therapy is most effective in patients whose pre-

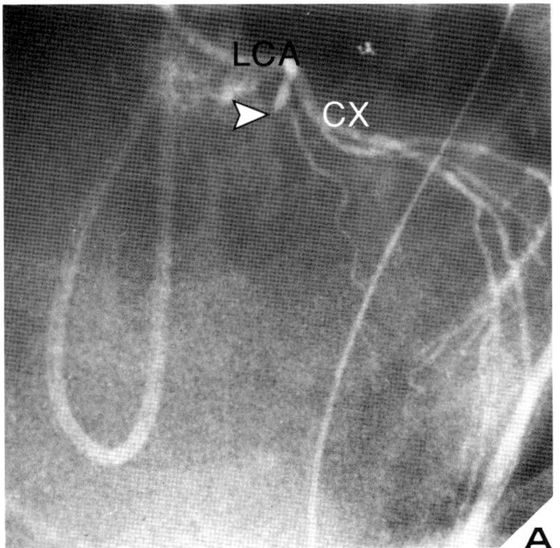

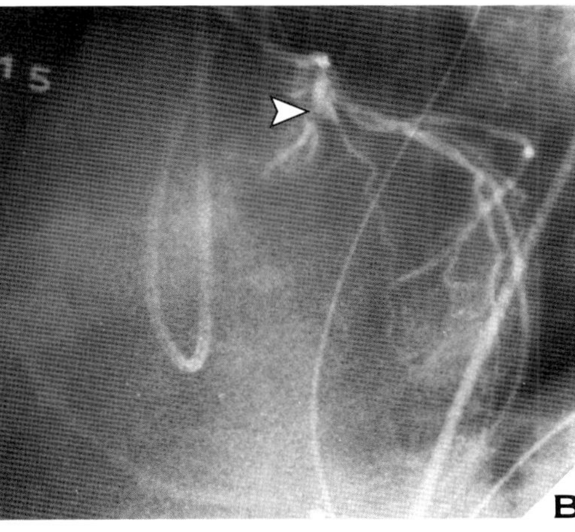

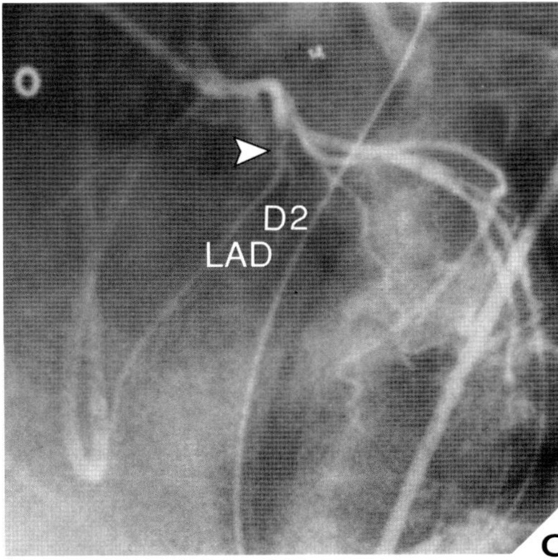

Fig. 30.44 Treatment of acute myocardial infarction by intraarterial administration of streptokinase. Left coronary arteriogram (left anterior oblique projection) obtained 2 hours after onset of symptoms. (A) Before streptokinase administration. The proximal segment of the left anterior descending artery (LAD) is occluded beyond the origin of the first diagonal branch. The triangular configuration at the site of occlusion (*arrow*) is characteristic of thrombotic obstruction. (B) Fifteen minutes after administration of 200,000 units of streptokinase. The LAD is patent; however, its distal segment is poorly perfused. (C) One hour after streptokinase administration the LAD and its second diagonal branch (D2) are visualized, although poorly opacified. (LCA = left main coronary artery; CX = circumflex artery)

treatment arteriograms show an abrupt cut-off or horizontal margin at the site of occlusion, a configuration that usually indicates acute thrombosis (see Fig. 21.30) or mural irregularity proximal to the occluded segment (see Fig. 21.28), which usually indicates ulceration of the atheromatous plaque with hemorrhage and subsequent thrombosis. PTCA is unlikely to be successful in patients in whom the proximal margin of the occluded segment has a smooth triangular configuration, an appearance typical of a chronic stenosis which has progressed to complete occlusion (see Fig. 21.29). About one third of patients undergoing thrombolytic therapy exhibit significant residual stenosis or occlusion of the infarct-related artery. Some of these patients may be candidates for PTCA or surgical revascularization; the remainder are treated medically.

A number of published reports have documented that left ventricular function is improved in patients with acute myocardial infarction who are treated with thrombolytic agents immediately after the onset of symptoms heralding the acute event. In general, the most dramatic improvement in global left ventricular function is seen when treatment is begun within 1 hour after the onset of symptoms. Some improvement is seen in patients treated within the first 3 hours, and minimal improvement can be demonstrated in patients treated within 3 to 6 hours. Patients with anterior wall infarcts exhibit a greater degree of functional improvement than those with inferior wall infarcts. Ventricular dilatation appears to be less pronounced when there is patency of the infarct-related artery secondary to spontaneous thrombolysis or successful thrombolytic therapy.

Published studies indicate that the early reocclusion rate after thrombolytic therapy is about 15 percent (range 5 to 30 percent). The early reocclusion rate is highest in patients with significant residual stenosis (greater than 50 percent) (Fig. 30.45) or persistent thrombus (Fig. 30.46) at the site of occlusion. The frequency of late stenosis and reocclusion is unknown.

There is growing evidence that early thrombolytic therapy decreases the early and late mortality of acute myocardial infarction. When combined with anticoagulant therapy, the mortality rate 3 years after acute myocardial infarction is 20 percent less than in patients treated with anticoagulant therapy alone. Early thrombolytic therapy appears to decrease the frequency of ventricular arrhythmias.

To sum up, intravenous thrombolytic therapy is now regarded as the treatment of choice in patients with acute myocardial infarction under 75 years of age who present soon after the onset of symptoms and for whom there is no contraindication to thrombolytic therapy. Although intra-arterial and intravenous thrombolytic therapy are both effective, the intravenous approach avoids catheterization and is therefore applicable to a larger number of patients. Thrombolytic therapy is most beneficial when started within 6 hours after the onset of symptoms, and ideally should be started within 3 hours. However, there is still a measurable therapeutic benefit when therapy is started after 6 hours.

URGENT ("RESCUE") PTCA

Although the success rate of early thrombolytic therapy is about 75 percent, alternative methods of myocardial revascularization may be of benefit in the failures (eg, patients with persistent occlusion or severe stenosis of the infarct-related artery resulting in progression of the infarction). In this group, the strategy

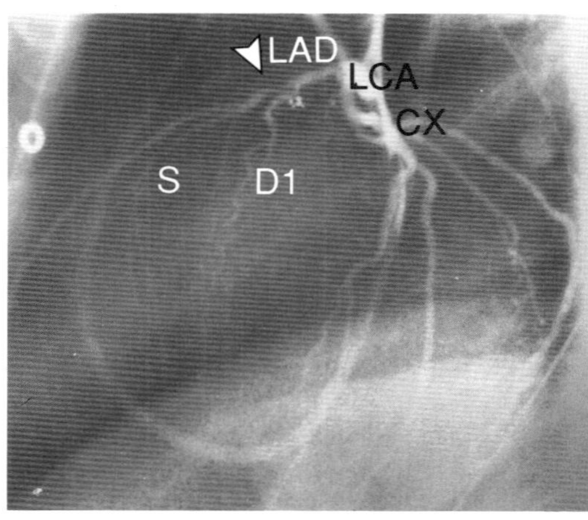

Fig. 30.45 Treatment of acute myocardial infarction by intra-arterial administration of streptokinase. Same patient as in previous figure. Lateral projection of left coronary arteriogram obtained immediately after intra-arterial administration of 200,000 U streptokinase shows adequate opacification of the left anterior descending artery (LAD) and a septal branch (S). There is significant stenosis (*arrow*) of the LAD just beyond the origin of the first diagonal branch (D1). (CX = circumflex artery; LCA = left coronary artery)

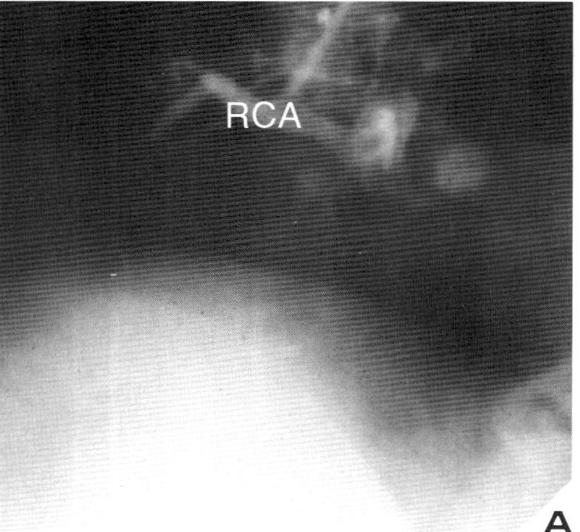

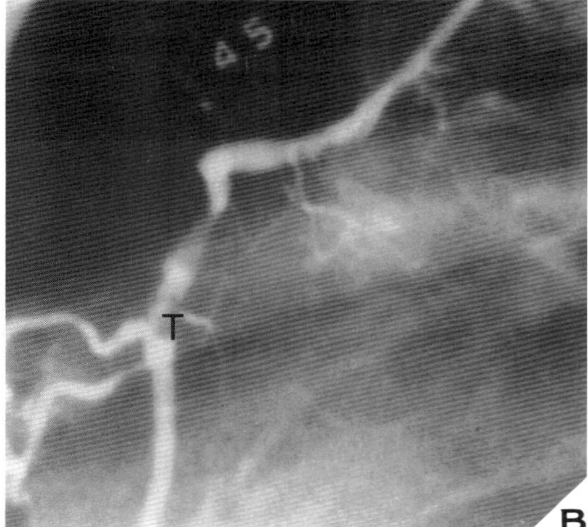

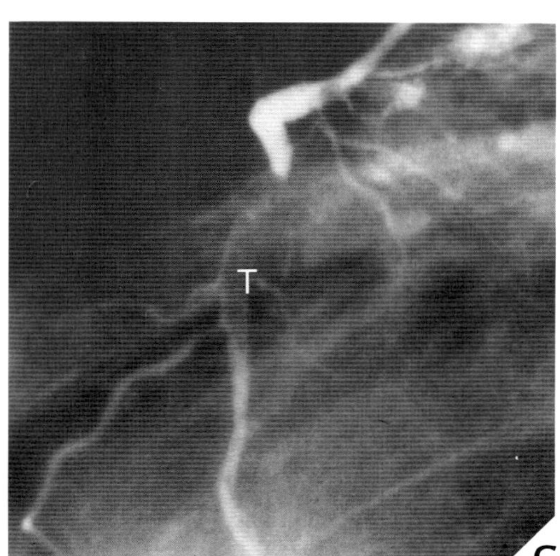

Fig. 30.46 Intra-arterial thrombolytic therapy of acute myocardial infarction. Right coronary arteriogram (lateral projection) obtained 4 hours after onset of symptoms of acute posterobasal myocardial infarction. (A) Before administration of streptokinase. The proximal segment of the right coronary artery (RCA) is occluded. The domed appearance at the site of obstruction is characteristic of thrombosis. (B) During streptokinase infusion (total dose 240,000 units). The right coronary artery is now patent; however, there is a persistent intraluminal filling defect (T). (C) At the end of the infusion, the large thrombus (T) is seen to better advantage. There is significant residual stenosis.

of urgent ("rescue") PTCA is frequently employed. In the Mayo clinic series (Lavie et al, 1990), urgent PTCA restored patency of the infarct-related artery in 71 percent of patients with complete occlusion and in 90 percent of those with severe residual stenosis. Although many patients treated with urgent PTCA had a decreased ejection fraction, the 4-year survival rate was very gratifying. When rescue PTCA is ineffective, emergency coronary artery bypass surgery may be the only alternative.

CIRCULATORY ASSIST DEVICES

Although intra-aortic counterpulsation can slightly increase cardiac output in patients with shock, the main application of this form of circulatory assist is to increase coronary artery flow in patients with severe myocardial ischemia. Intra-aortic counterpulsation is mainly used to support patients with severe pain, acute infarction, or borderline hemodynamic status until definitive revascularization therapy can be carried out.

In this technique, a specially designed balloon catheter is positioned in the descending thoracic aorta and attached to a pump (Figs. 30.47 and 30.48). With this device, diastolic flow can be increased by up to 40 mL per stroke; because coronary artery filling occurs during diastole, coronary flow is increased. Systolic "unloading" of up to 40 mL per stroke increases the effectiveness of left ventricular contraction. Cardiac catheterization and angiographic studies can be performed while the counterpulsion device is actively pumping (the nonpulsatile "flutter mode" should be used when angiographic catheters are being manipulated past the balloon). Contraindications to intra-aortic balloon counterpulsion include aortic insufficiency, aortic aneurysm, and severe aorto–iliac disease.

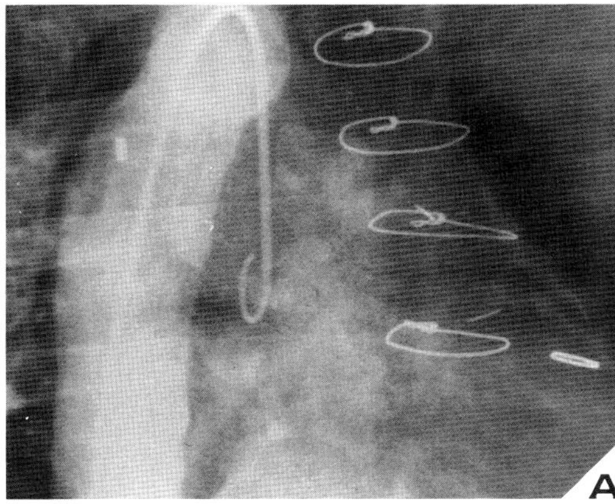

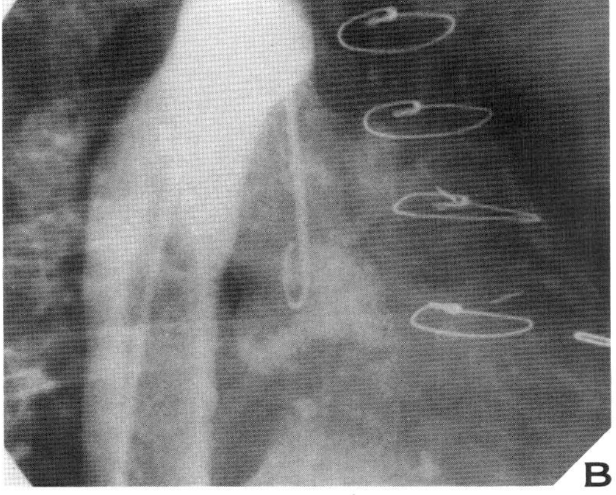

1 aorta
2 intra-aortic balloon catheter
3 inflated balloon

Fig. 30.47 Intra-aortic balloon counterpulsion. (A,B) Right anterior oblique projection of thoracic aortogram in systole (A) and diastole (B). During diastole the balloon is inflated to increase mean aortic pressure, thereby increasing coronary perfusion. During systole the balloon is deflated, lowering pressure in the descending aorta and thus enhancing left ventricular performance. (C) Diagrammatic representation of intra-aortic balloon counterpulsion system.

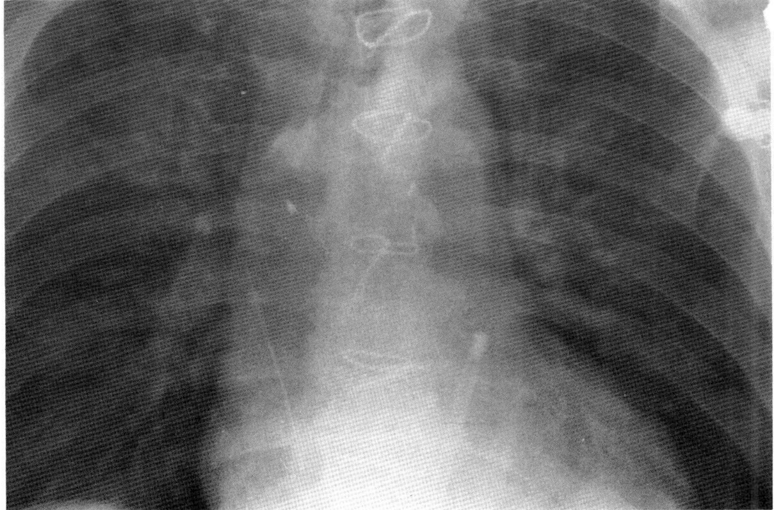

Fig. 30.48 Intra-aortic balloon counterpulsion. Frontal chest film shows the tip of the balloon catheter in the descending thoracic aorta. This patient, who had sustained two myocardial infarctions, was in congestive heart failure (note bilateral pulmonary edema) and was being evaluated for a second surgical revascularization procedure.

CHAPTER 31

Balloon Valvuloplasty, Embolization Therapy, and Valve Replacement

BALLOON VALVULOPLASTY

After its introduction as a treatment for pulmonic valvular stenosis (Kan, 1982) and aortic stenosis (Labadabi, 1983), transcatheter balloon valvuloplasty has gained increasing acceptance as an alternative to valve replacement for certain types of valvular stenosis. Balloon valvuloplasty is now regarded as the treatment of choice for pulmonic valvular stenosis; however, it is not as widely used in the treatment of aortic and mitral stenosis. At present, valve replacement remains the treatment of choice for patients with aortic stenosis severe enough to cause clinically significant left ventricular dysfunction. Balloon valvuloplasty is employed when valve replacement is not feasible, when it poses an unacceptably high risk, or when the patient's life expectancy is too short to warrant surgery (eg, patients with metastatic cancer). Balloon valvuloplasty has assumed a limited role in the treatment of mitral stenosis. The best results are obtained in the relatively small number of patients with disease limited to the commissures or leaflets. Balloon valvuloplasty is relatively ineffective in patients with involvement of the subvalvular apparatus or heavy calcification of the leaflets.

AORTIC VALVULOPLASTY

INDICATIONS

Balloon valvuloplasty is most often performed in patients with severe aortic stenosis for whom valve replacement is associated with an unacceptably high risk. The typical candidate for balloon valvuloplasty is an elderly patient with calcific aortic stenosis who presents with severe congestive heart failure. In this setting, balloon valvuloplasty is often employed as a temporizing measure; valve replacement is performed once the patient's

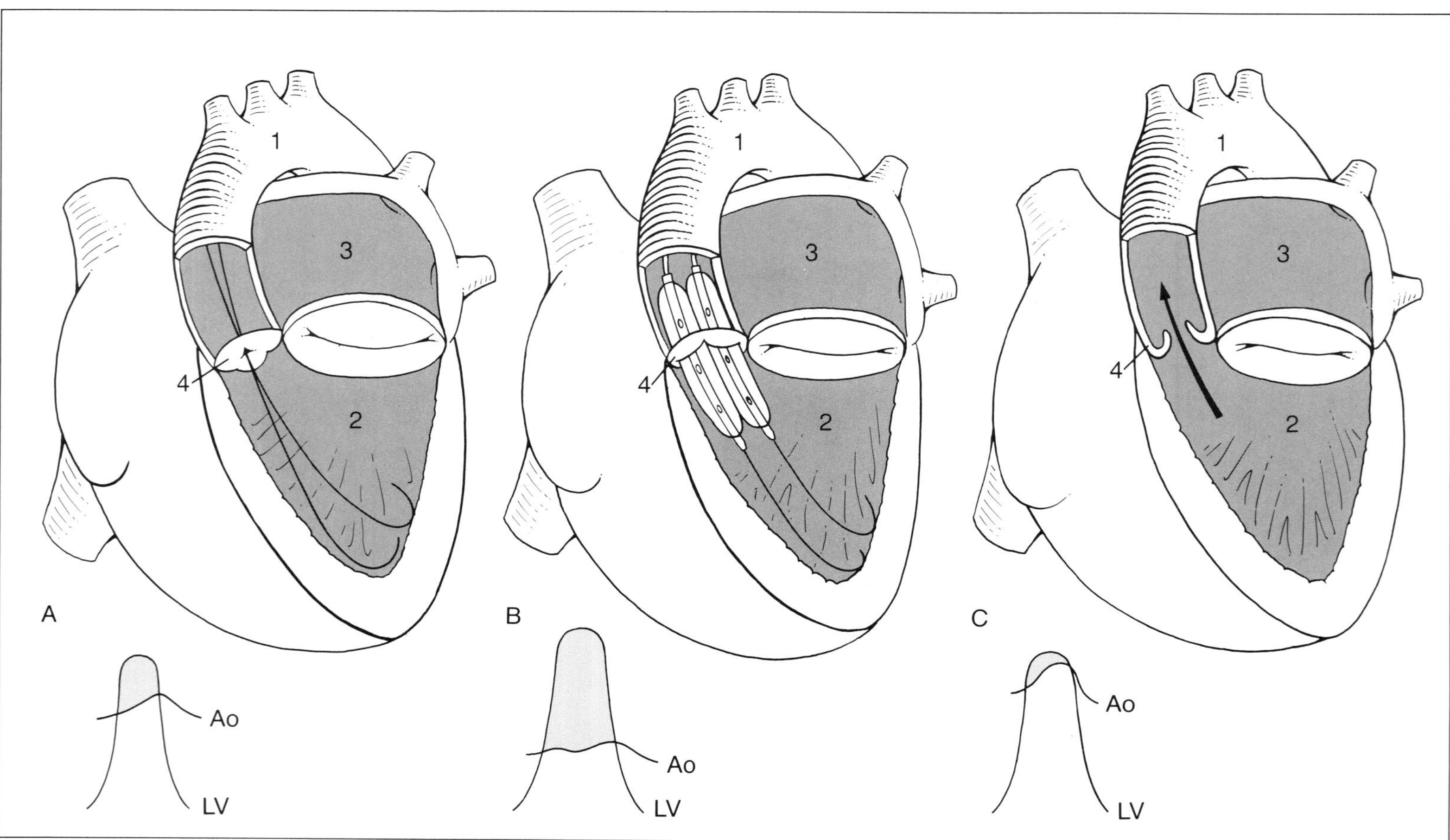

Fig. 31.1 Percutaneous aortic balloon valvuloplasty (two-balloon technique). (A) Two catheters have been introduced from the ascending aorta into the left ventricle through the stenotic aortic valve. (B) Two balloons are positioned in the area of the aortic valve and inflated. (C) Final result of balloon valvuloplasty resulting in a modest decrease in the gradient across the aortic valve.

1 aorta
2 left ventricle
3 left atrium
4 aortic valve

condition has improved. Balloon valvuloplasty is also an alternative to valve replacement in children and teenagers with congenital stenosis of the aortic valve. In such cases it may be necessary to repeat the procedure from time to time.

TECHNIQUE

The technique of balloon valvuloplasty is essentially the same as that of balloon angioplasty, introduced as a treatment for peripheral artery disease by Dotter (1964) and for coronary artery stenosis by Grüntzig (1976) (see Chapter 21). In the standard technique, the balloon catheter is introduced into a femoral artery and passed retrogradely across the aortic valve (Fig. 31.1). Alternatively, the balloon catheter can be introduced into a peripheral vein and passed into the left ventricle via a transseptal puncture; it is then advanced antegradely across the aortic valve. Once the balloon is in place, it is inflated for 5 to 30 seconds (Figs. 31.1 and 31.2). If necessary, it is reinflated after an interval of not less than 3 minutes. The size of the balloon is determined from angiographic or echocardiographic measurements of the aortic valve orifice. Two balloons can be used simultaneously to dilate larger valves (Fig. 31.1).

Balloon valvuloplasty of aortic stenosis is considered successful when the residual peak systolic left ventricular gradient is less than 50 mm Hg and/or the aortic valve area is greater than 1 cm^2 per square meter of body surface. The gradient may increase in the days and weeks after the valvuloplasty procedure. In Labadabi's series (1983), the mean residual gradient increased from 25 mm Hg to 32 mm Hg after an interval of 3 to 6 months.

MECHANISM OF VALVULOPLASTY

In patients with congenital aortic valvular stenosis or a stenotic bicuspid aortic valve, inflating the balloon ruptures the fused commissures, relieving the stenosis; by overinflating the balloon it is possible to dilate the annulus as well. In patients with calcification of the leaflets, the inflated balloon fractures the calcific deposits; after successful balloon valvuloplasty the leaflets have a hinge-like motion, resulting in improved mobility and a decrease in the functional stenosis of the valve orifice (Fig. 31.3). Fracturing the calcific nodules may fail to improve valve mobility or to relieve the stenosis in patients with fused commissures caused by inflammatory (rheumatic) valvulitis. It is also

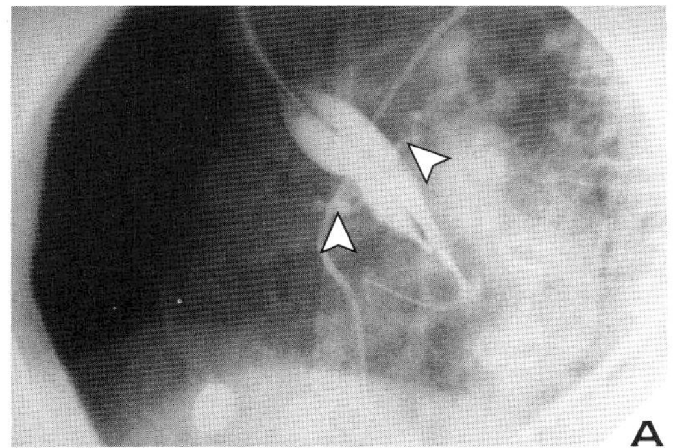

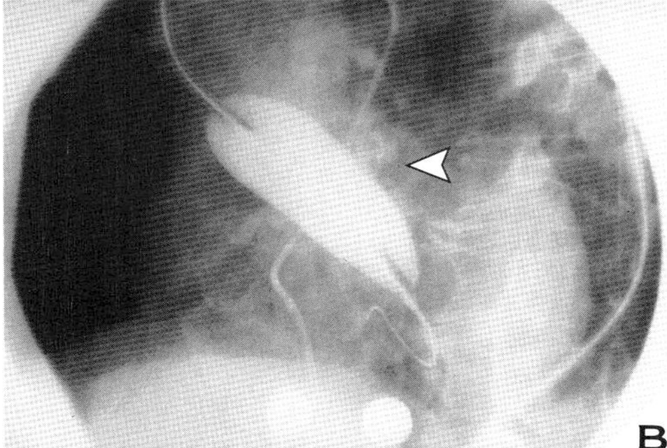

Fig. 31.2 Aortic balloon valvuloplasty. Cine frames (LAO projection) during valvuloplasty procedure in a patient with calcific aortic stenosis. (A) Shortly after inflation the balloon has a "waist" caused by the stenotic aortic valve. (B) Two seconds later the "waist" is gone, indicating that the stenosis has been relieved. Pressure measurements revealed a marked decrease in the gradient across the aortic valve when compared with the prevalvuloplasty gradient. (Calcification of the aortic leaflets is indicated by *arrows* in A and B.)

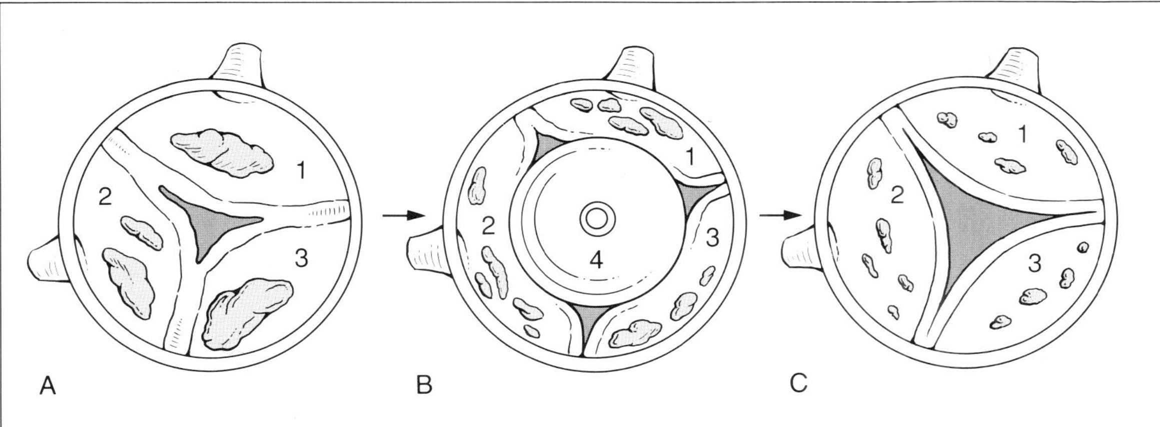

Fig. 31.3 Mechanism of balloon valvuloplasty of a calcified trifoliate valve. (A) Before balloon valvuloplasty the commissures are fused and there are calcific deposits in the leaflets, which have limited mobility. (B) After inflation of the balloon. The commissural adhesions have been disrupted and the calcified deposits are fragmented. (C) the balloon catheter has been removed. The commissures are wider and the leaflets have greater mobility.

1 leaflet of right coronary cusp
2 leaflet of left coronary cusp
3 leaflet of noncoronary cusp
4 balloon

likely to be unsuccessful in patients with congenitally bicuspid valves (Fig. 31.4), which are often heavily calcified; the results of aortic valvuloplasty in such patients are much worse than in those with trifoliate valves that are not heavily calcified.

COMPLICATIONS

Serious complications and death occur in a small percentage of cases. During valvuloplasty of a trifoliate valve, blood can still flow through the commissures with the inflated balloon in place, whereas the balloon completely occludes the valve orifice of a bicuspid valve; therefore, the risk of death and myocardial infarction is theoretically increased in patients with bicuspid valves. In one series there were two deaths in 60 aortic balloon valvuloplasties, both in patients with bicuspid aortic valves (Isner, 1987). Other acute complications of balloon aortic valvuloplasty include acute aortic insufficiency and embolization of valve debris. Injury to the mitral valve has been reported in children undergoing antegrade aortic valvuloplasty. Complications at the femoral arterial puncture site include groin hematoma, arteriovenous fistula, and pseudoaneurysm formation. Aortic insufficiency of variable severity is the rule after balloon valvuloplasty, with an average increase of one grade in the severity of the aortic insufficiency in most published series. Stated another way, any preexisting aortic insufficiency may be exacerbated by a successful balloon valvuloplasty.

RESULTS

Postprocedural angiograms rarely demonstrate any significant change in valvular morphology, even after successful balloon valvuloplasty; however, catheterization data obtained 15 minutes after the final dilatation reveal significant improvement in left ventricular function (decreased systolic stress, increased

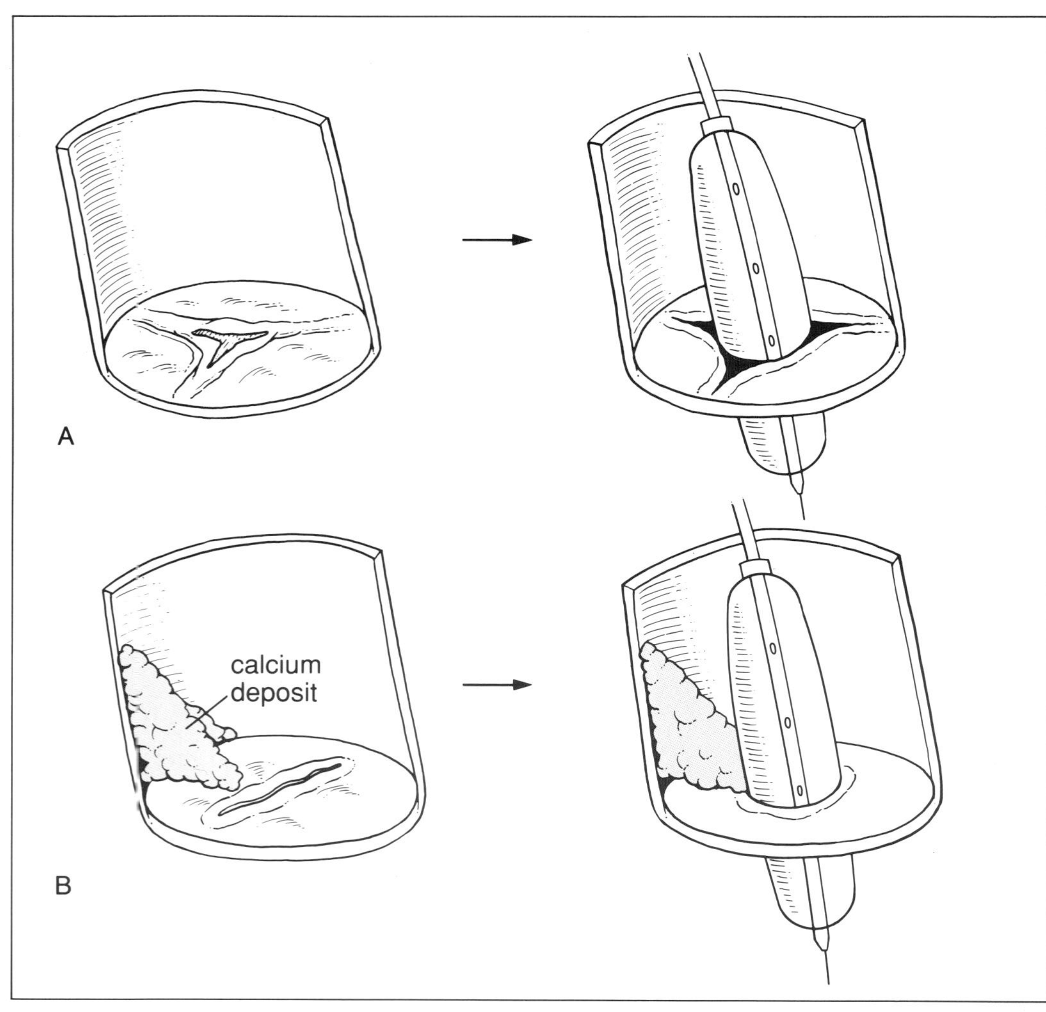

Fig. 31.4 Mechanism of balloon valvuloplasty of a bicuspid aortic valve. (A) Tricuspid (trifoliate) aortic valve. In a stenotic trifoliate valve, the inflated balloon causes cracks in the calcium deposits in the leaflets, resulting in improved mobility of the leaflets. (B) Bicuspid (bifoliate) aortic valve. Balloon valvuloplasty is often unsuccessful in patients with a congenitally bicuspid valve owing to the wider attachment of the leaflets and the tendency for the calcific deposits to extend into the adjacent aortic wall. Note that the inflated balloon completely occludes the valve orifice, increasing the risk of sudden death during valvuloplasty in patients with stenotic bicuspid valves.

ejection fraction, decreased end diastolic volume, decreased end systolic volume, decreased end diastolic pressure) and a decrease in the severity of the aortic stenosis (decreased systolic gradient, increased valve area).

Echocardiography is very useful for assessing the results of balloon valvuloplasty. Both the motion of the leaflets and the size of the annulus are clearly demonstrated on conventional echocardiography. With the addition of Doppler or color Doppler imaging, it is possible to quantitate the degree of aortic insufficiency (or recurrent stenosis, if present).

In general, successful aortic balloon valvuloplasty is accompanied by subjective improvement. Most patients report a decrease in the severity or complete disappearance of their symptoms. In children with congenital aortic stenosis, follow-up studies indicate a significant decrease in the gradient across the aortic valve, which is usually maintained for 2 to 3 years, after which repeat balloon valvuloplasty may be necessary. The long-term results are less rewarding in patients with acquired aortic stenosis; restenosis after about 6 months is the rule in such cases. In one large series, only 30 percent of adult patients still had a significantly decreased gradient across the aortic valve 10 months after the valvuloplasty procedure (Isner, 1988).

To sum up, balloon aortic valvuloplasty for acquired aortic valvular stenosis is reasonably safe; although it may provide significant symptomatic improvement for a period of months, there is no convincing evidence that it prolongs life. For this reason balloon aortic valvuloplasty cannot be regarded as an alternative to valve replacement, and should be considered only in patients for whom surgery is contraindicated. However, if one clearly understands the risks and benefits, balloon aortic valvuloplasty can be offered as a palliative procedure in carefully selected cases (eg, a fragile elderly patient with severe aortic stenosis). Indeed, it can be lifesaving in a moribund patient with severe congestive heart failure.

PULMONIC VALVULOPLASTY

Percutaneous balloon valvuloplasty has become a standard technique in the treatment of isolated pulmonic valvular stenosis, which accounts for 9 percent of all cases of congenital heart disease in children and adults. Clinical and experimental studies have shown that temporary total occlusion of the pulmonic valve is well tolerated by the hypertrophied right ventricle.

Balloon valvuloplasty is usually successful in patients with fusion of the commissures (Fig. 31.5; see also Fig. 16.47). However, it is relatively ineffective in patients with dysplastic pulmonic valves, in whom the stenosis is caused by thickened, immobile leaflets.

TECHNIQUE

The procedure is usually performed via a femoral venous approach. Both femoral veins are catheterized. One catheter is positioned in the right ventricle to allow hemodynamic monitoring, and the other is advanced into the left pulmonary artery. A guidewire is then advanced into the left lower lobe pulmonary artery, avoiding excessive slack in the right atrium or right ventricle. The balloon catheter is introduced over the guidewire and the balloon is positioned in the pulmonic valve orifice.

The correct balloon size is determined by measuring the annulus of the pulmonic valve on the lateral view of the pulmonary angiogram and correcting for magnification. The best results are obtained when the diameter of the balloon is 20 to 40 percent larger than that of the annulus. Because this is difficult to accomplish with a single balloon when the annulus is large, two balloons are usually employed in teenagers and adults. When two balloons are employed, it is desirable to use shorter balloons to avoid excessive dilatation of the right ventricular outflow tract.

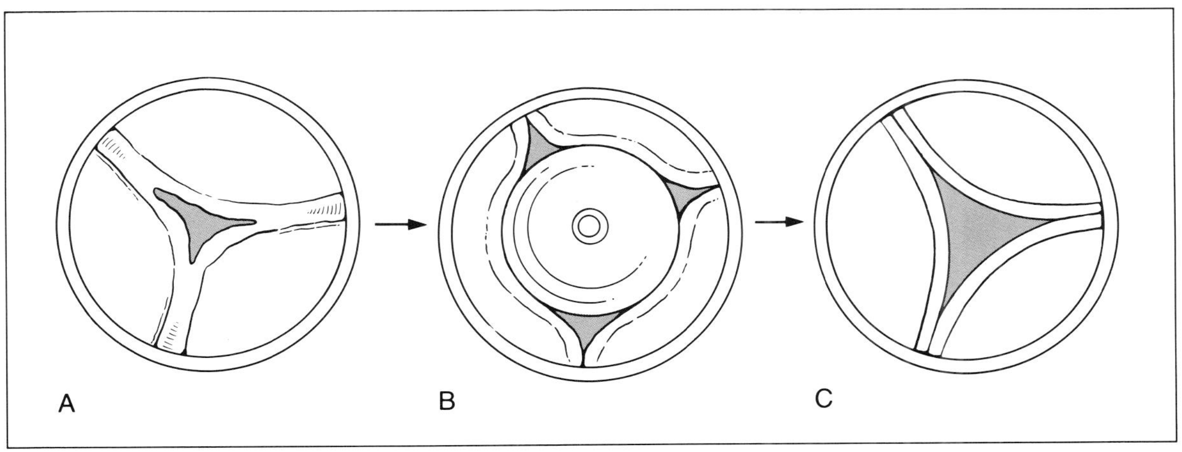

Fig. 31.5 Mechanism of balloon valvuloplasty of congenital pulmonic stenosis. (A) Stenotic pulmonic valve (viewed from above), showing fusion of the commissures. (B) Inflating the balloon disrupts the fibrotic adhesions, widening the commissures. (C) After removal of the balloon the leaflets are freely mobile.

RESULTS

The immediate results of pulmonic valvuloplasty are excellent. There is usually an immediate reduction in the transvalvular pressure gradient; restenosis within 2 years is rare. Enlargement of the pulmonic valve can be appreciated angiographically (Fig. 31.6; see also Fig. 16.48). After the procedure, echocardiography demonstrates widely patent commissures and free mobility of the leaflets. Complications are rare, although perforation of the right ventricular outflow tract and arrhythmias have been reported. Significant pulmonic insufficiency is a potential complication when balloon valvuloplasty is performed in patients with dysplastic pulmonary valve leaflets.

MITRAL VALVULOPLASTY

For many years surgical commissurotomy has been a standard treatment for rheumatic mitral stenosis. Balloon mitral valvuloplasty, introduced in 1982, has supplanted surgical commisurotomy at some major medical centers. As with the surgical technique, the mechanism of balloon mitral valvuloplasty is the mechanical disruption of the fibrous tissue bridging the commissures between the anterior and posterior mitral leaflets (Fig. 31.7). The success of the procedure depends on the mobility and thickness of the leaflets and the presence (or absence) of calcification. Another major prognostic factor is the presence (or absence) of subvalvular disease, manifested by shortness and/or fusion of the chordae tendinae and pericommissural fibrosis. Significant subvalvular disease is present in 30 to 70 percent of candidates for surgical commissurotomy or balloon valvuloplasty.

PATIENT SELECTION

At present, balloon valvuloplasty is employed mainly in symptomatic patients with mitral stenosis secondary to rheumatic heart disease; many authors prefer it to surgery (commissurotomy or valve replacement) in such cases. Careful assessment of the angiographic and echocardiographic findings is important in selecting suitable candidates for balloon mitral valvuloplasty. (Transesophageal echocardiography is particularly helpful for this purpose.)

A semiquantitative echocardiographic assessment, which takes into account the size of the mitral annulus, the mobility and thickness of the leaflets, the extent of the subvalvular disease, and the degree of calcification of the commissures, has been shown to correlate with the success rate and has been helpful in patient selection. The best results of valvuloplasty are achieved in patients with mobile, pliable mitral leaflets and minimal commissural calcification. A mobile mitral leaflet exhibits a domed appearance during diastole, with increased mobility of the midportion of the leaflet throughout the cardiac cycle. Balloon valvuloplasty is unlikely to succeed if the thickness of one or both mitral leaflets is significantly (more than 1 mm) greater than that of a normal aortic leaflet. The success rate is decreased in patients with calcification at the level of the commissures. The best results can be anticipated in patients with pliable, uncalcified valves; however, some degree of functional and symptomatic improvement can be expected even in patients with stiff, calcified valves.

Balloon mitral valvuloplasty is contraindicated in patients with left atrial thrombus. Mitral insufficiency of more than mild degree is a relative contraindication to the procedure.

TECHNIQUE

The valvuloplasty procedure can be performed in a number of ways, most of which entail transseptal catheterization of the left atrium. After the balloon catheter has been passed across the atrial septum, the balloon is positioned within the mitral annulus and inflated for about 15 seconds (Fig. 31.7). The balloon is

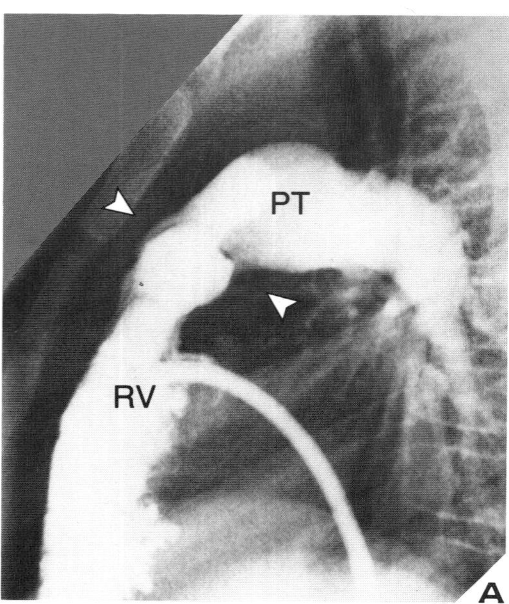

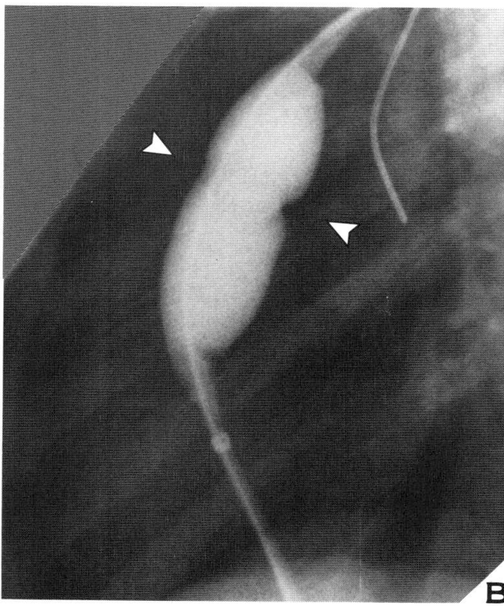

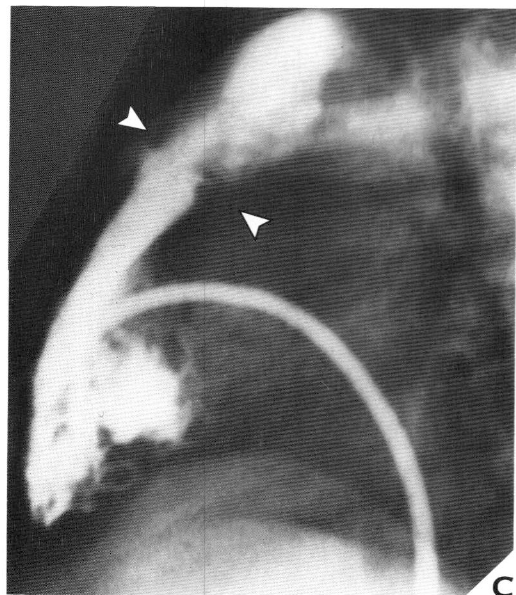

Fig. 31.6 Balloon valvuloplasty of congenital pulmonic stenosis. Cine right ventriculogram (lateral projection). (A) Before valvuloplasty (systole). The opening of the valve leaflets is restricted owing to fusion of the commissures (note domed appearance); however, the annulus is of normal size. Note poststenotic dilatation of the pulmonary trunk (PT). (B) Frame obtained before completion of the valvuloplasty shows the balloon straddling the pulmonic valve. The "waist" (*arrows*) in the balloon indicates that stenosis has not been completely relieved. (C) After completion of the valvuloplasty the orifice of the pulmonic valve (*arrows*) is significantly larger. (RV = right ventricle)

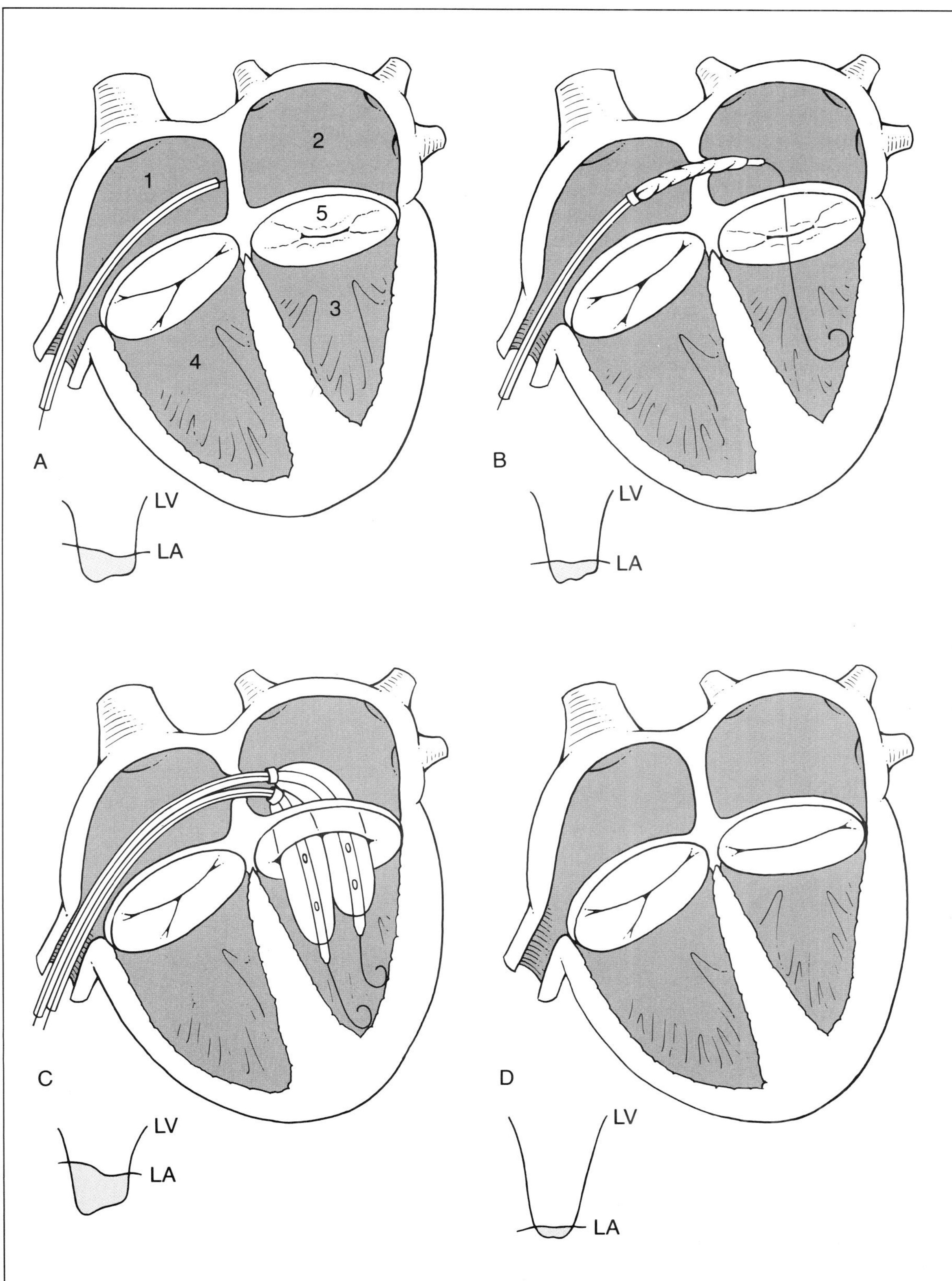

Fig. 31.7 Percutaneous balloon valvuloplasty of rheumatic mitral stenosis (transseptal technique). (A) Before performation of the atrial septum. The catheter (introduced via a femoral vein puncture) is positioned in the right atrium. Note thickening of the mitral leaflets and fusion of the commissures. (B) After perforation of the atrial septum. The guidewire has been passed across the mitral valve into the left ventricle. The balloon catheter is being advanced over the guidewire. (C) The inflated balloon straddles the mitral valve. A second balloon has been introduced. (D) After a period of inflation sufficient to disrupt the fused commissures, both balloons have been removed. The commissures are now open and the leaflets are more pliable.

1	right atrium	3	left ventricle
2	left atrium	4	right ventricle
		5	mitral valve

then inflated one to four times under fluoroscopic guidance to a maximum pressure of 4 to 5 atmospheres (ie, four to five times atmospheric pressure), or until the stenotic "waist" disappears (Fig. 31.8).

The size of the balloon used for mitral valvuloplasty depends on the size of the anatomic mitral annulus (determined echocardiographically). Using a balloon with a diameter much greater than that of the mitral annulus increases the risk of post-procedural mitral insufficiency and can even rupture the annulus. The best results are achieved when the diameter of the balloon is 80 to 90 percent of that of the mitral annulus. The largest valvuloplasty balloon that can be introduced percutaneously is 20 mm in diameter; since the adult mitral annulus usually exceeds 20 mm, it is usually necessary to employ a two-balloon technique.

Balloon mitral valvuloplasty is judged to be successful when follow-up echocardiography demonstrates a 25 percent or greater increase in mitral valve area, or when the final valve area is greater than 1.5 cm^2 per square meter of body surface.

COMPLICATIONS

Potential complications of balloon mitral valvuloplasty include the creation of a large atrial septal defect, usually caused by excessive dilatation of the iatrogenic septal defect in an effort to accommodate a relatively large valvuloplasty balloon (Fig. 31.9 see appendix); left ventricular perforation with cardiac tamponade, which can result when a high distending pressure is used to dilate a very tight mitral valve; short-term hemodynamic deterioration caused by balloon occlusion of the mitral valve orifice; systemic embolization of left atrial thrombus or mitral valve debris; and restenosis. The rate of early and late restenosis after balloon valvuloplasty is much lower than that associated with aortic valvuloplasty.

RESULTS

Successful balloon valvuloplasty improves the patient's hemodynamic status by increasing the area of the mitral valve orifice, thus increasing cardiac output at a lower pulmonary capillary pressure. The morbidity and mortality of balloon valvuloplasty are less than those of commissurotomy or valve replacement. Not only is convalescence shorter but the balloon technique avoids the hazards associated with anticoagulation, which is required after mitral valve replacement. The early and long-term results of balloon mitral valvuloplasty are promising. Restenosis is rare in the first 3 months after the procedure, and 93 percent of patients gain some degree of symptomatic relief.

ANGIOPLASTY OF STENOTIC PULMONARY ARTERIES

Stenoses of the pulmonary arteries occur in tetralogy of Fallot, congenital rubella syndrome, and Williams syndrome, and as a complication of surgical procedures (eg, palliative shunts).

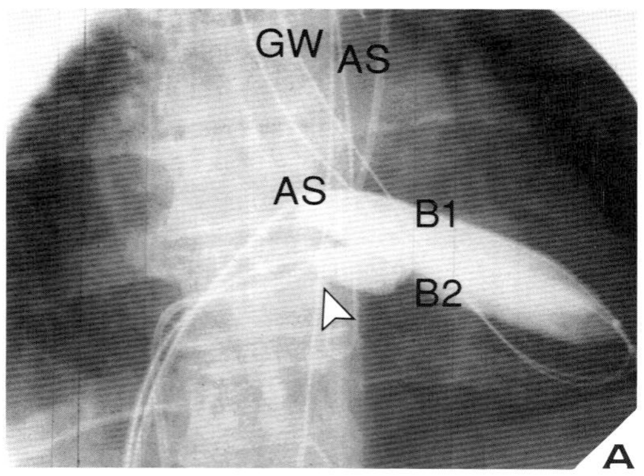

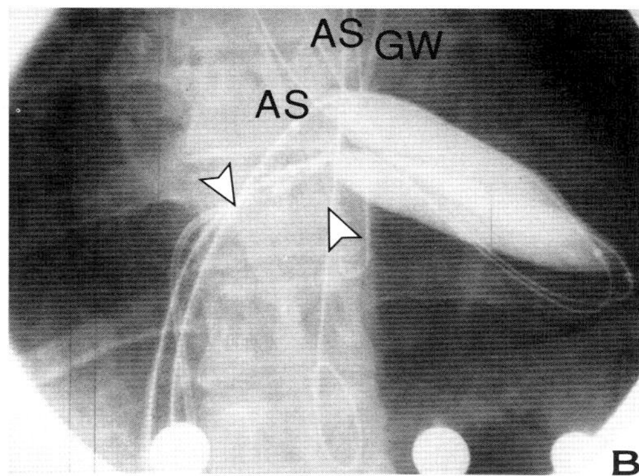

Fig. 31.8 Percutaneous mitral valvuloplasty (transseptal double balloon technique). (A) Early phase (frontal projection). The inflated balloons (B1 and B2) straddle the mitral valve (note "waist" in midportion of B2 produced by the stenotic valve). The distal parts of the balloons are in the left ventricle. The proximal parts of the balloons are in the area of the atrial septostomy (AS), which may result in a significant residual iatrogenic atrial septal defect. The tips of the guidewires (GW) are in the ascending aorta, an arrangement that serves to stabilize the balloons during the procedure. (B) At the end of the procedure both balloons have a uniform diameter, indicating that the stenosis has been relieved.

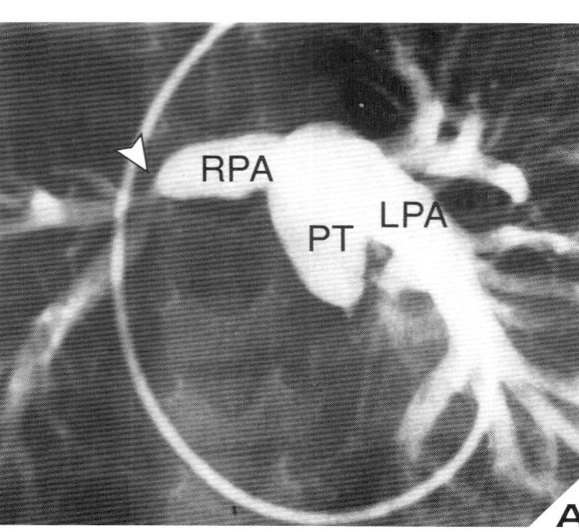

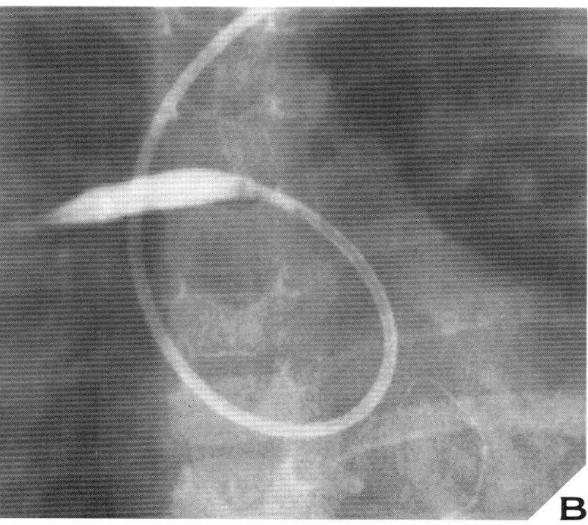

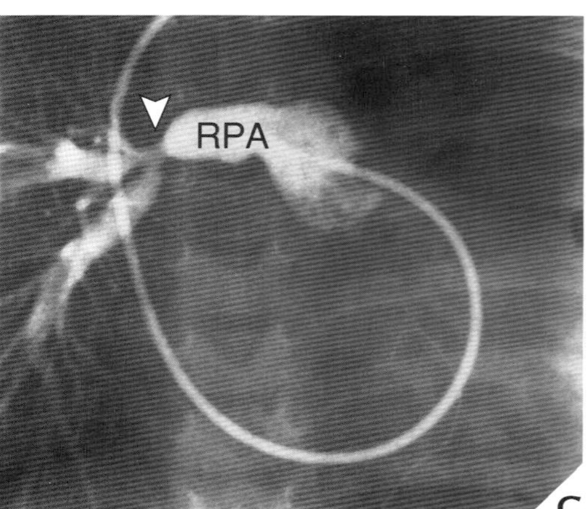

Fig. 31.10 Balloon dilatation of right pulmonary artery. (A) Selective pulmonary arteriogram (frontal projection) in a patient with tetralogy of Fallot shows stenosis (*arrow*) at the origin of the arteries supplying the right lower and middle lobes and absence of the artery to the right upper lobe. (B) During the angioplasty procedure. The distal end of the inflated balloon is just beyond the stenotic segment. (C) Selective right pulmonary arteriogram obtained immediately after the angioplasty demonstrates significant enlargement of the stenotic segment (*arrow*). (PT = pulmonary trunk; RPA = right pulmonary artery; LPA = left pulmonary artery)

Balloon angioplasty has been used since 1980 to treat pulmonary artery stenoses, which are difficult to enlarge surgically. The technique is similar to that employed for pulmonic valvuloplasty (see above) (Figs. 31.10 and 31.11). Pooled data from different centers indicate that the overall success rate is approximately 50 percent.

The best results are obtained when angioplasty is performed at an early age, preferably under 2 years. Ideally, the angioplasty balloon should have a diameter two to four times that of the stenotic segment. For patients who require multiple dilatations, the angioplasty procedure should be staged, allowing an interval of a few weeks between dilatations to permit healing. When used to treat patients with postoperative stenosis, the angioplasty procedure should be deferred until at least 4 weeks after surgery.

EMBOLIZATION PROCEDURES

Various embolization procedures have been devised to occlude abnormal connections in the cardiovascular system.

INTRACARDIAC SHUNTS

ATRIAL SEPTAL DEFECT

Permanent closure of atrial septal defects (ASDs) by means of a percutaneously introduced double umbrella ("clamshell") device has been achieved in a growing number of teenagers and adults. The percutaneous technique is suitable for centrally located (fossa ovalis type) ASDs that are not associated with other malformations (eg, partial anomalous pulmonary venous drainage). Because the umbrella must be somewhat larger than the ASD, the maximum diameter of the septal defect must be accurately measured with a calibrated balloon.

PATENT DUCTUS ARTERIOSUS

Patent ductus arteriosus (PDA) can also be closed with percutaneous catheter techniques. In the most widely utilized technique, catheters are passed into the pulmonary trunk and aorta and connected to form a loop across the ductus arteriosus. A plug of polyvinyl plastic is introduced through the femoral arterial limb of the loop and pushed into the ductus with a thick catheter (Fig. 31.12). In a recent modification, a femoral venous catheter is used to form the loop.

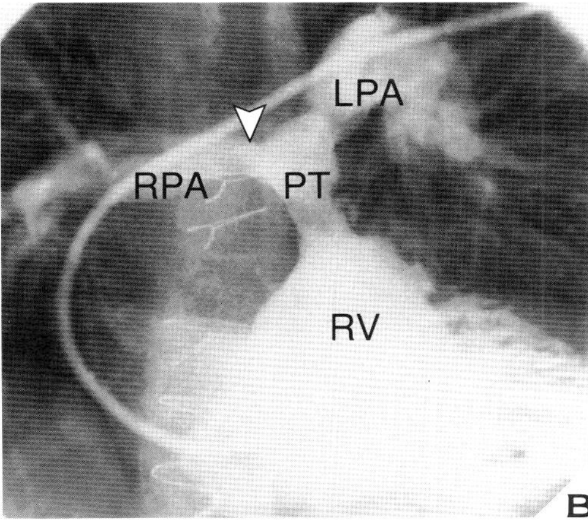

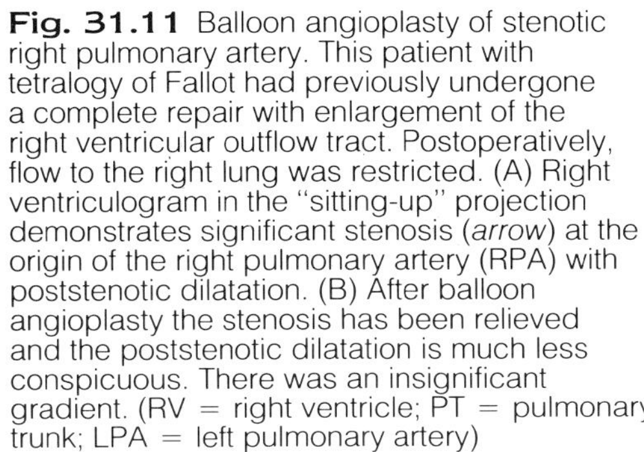

Fig. 31.11 Balloon angioplasty of stenotic right pulmonary artery. This patient with tetralogy of Fallot had previously undergone a complete repair with enlargement of the right ventricular outflow tract. Postoperatively, flow to the right lung was restricted. (A) Right ventriculogram in the "sitting-up" projection demonstrates significant stenosis (*arrow*) at the origin of the right pulmonary artery (RPA) with poststenotic dilatation. (B) After balloon angioplasty the stenosis has been relieved and the poststenotic dilatation is much less conspicuous. There was an insignificant gradient. (RV = right ventricle; PT = pulmonary trunk; LPA = left pulmonary artery)

Fig. 31.12 Percutaneous catheter closure of patent ductus arteriosus. This technique entails the use of two catheters. One catheter is passed from the right ventricle into the left pulmonary artery and positioned at the pulmonary opening of the ductus arteriosus. The second is passed retrogradely from the femoral artery into the descending thoracic aorta and postitioned at the aortic opening of the ductus. A loop is then formed between the two balloons. Polyvinyl plastic is then introduced into the loop; when the plastic material solidifies it forms a plug, completely occluding the ductus arteriosus.

Ao aorta
LPA left pulmonary artery
1 pulmonary artery catheter
2 aortic catheter
3 patent ductus arteriosus

An important limitation of the catheter technique is that the ductus may be too large or too small for the plug to remain fixed in place. Moreover, it is suitable only for adults or older children whose femoral arteries are large enough to allow passage of the plug. Because the mortality and morbidity of ductus ligation are extremely low, even in infants, the "plug" technique has not gained wide acceptance.

CLOSURE OF AORTOPULMONARY COLLATERALS BEFORE SURGERY

Certain congenital defects (eg, tetralogy of Fallot, pulmonary atresia with ventricular septal defect) are commonly associated with a systemic collateral blood supply to the lungs. Although these collaterals are essential for survival, they may pose formidable technical problems when the underlying defect is corrected surgically. The thin-walled, tortuous arteries not only are difficult to approach and ligate through a median sternotomy, but the large pulmonary venous return may flood the operative field even during cardiopulmonary bypass.

A percutaneous catheter technique has been devised to obliterate aortopulmonary collaterals. In this technique, a special balloon catheter is introduced through a femoral artery and passed into the thoracic aorta. Each collateral is then catheterized in turn. The balloon is then inflated to temporarily stop the blood flow and a metallic spring coil is introduced through the catheter (Fig. 31.13). As fibrin accumulates on the coil, the

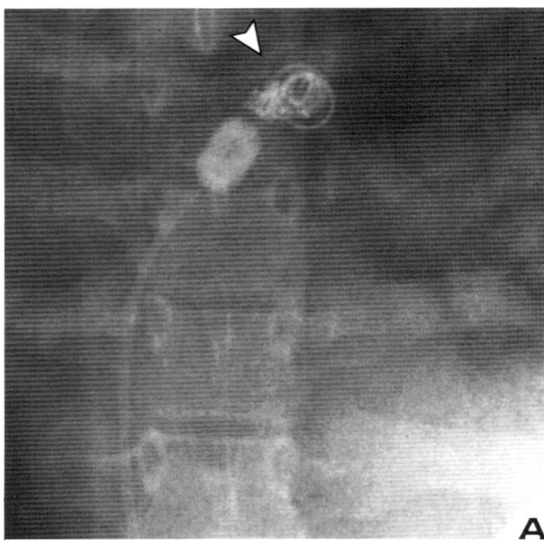

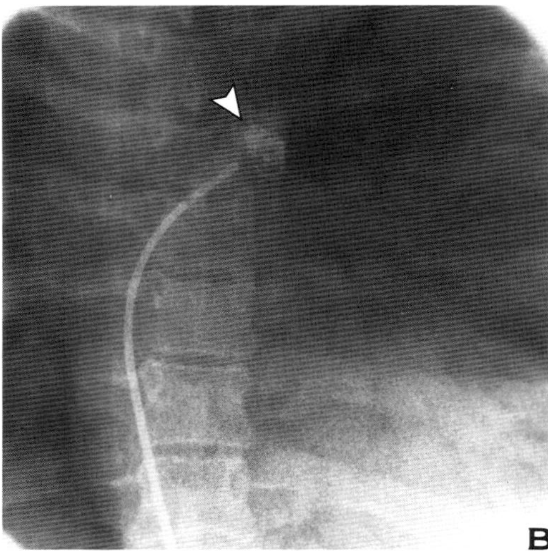

Fig. 31.13 Embolization of aortopulmonary collaterals with spring coil technique. Several large aortopulmonary collateral arteries arising from the descending thoracic aorta were demonstrated angiographically in this patient with tetralogy of Fallot and a right aortic arch. (A) A balloon catheter has been introduced via the arterial catheter into the aortopulmonary collateral. The balloon was then inflated to decrease blood flow through the collateral. Several spring coils (*arrow*) were then introduced through the catheter and delivered to a position distal to the balloon. (B) After formation of a thrombus on the surface of the coils, the balloon was deflated and the catheter removed, leaving the coils in place. In time, thrombus formation will lead to complete occlusion of the collateral.

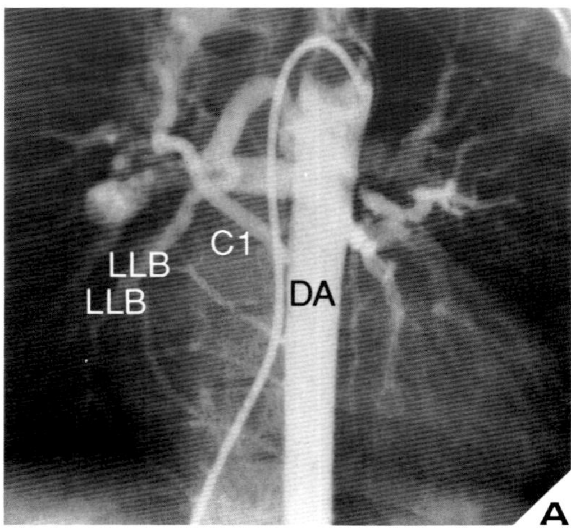

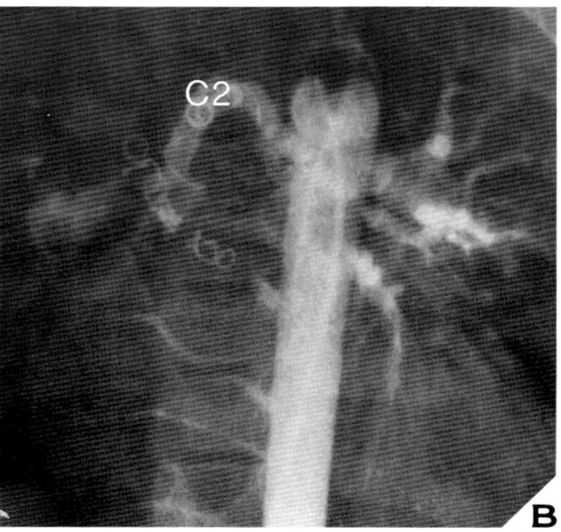

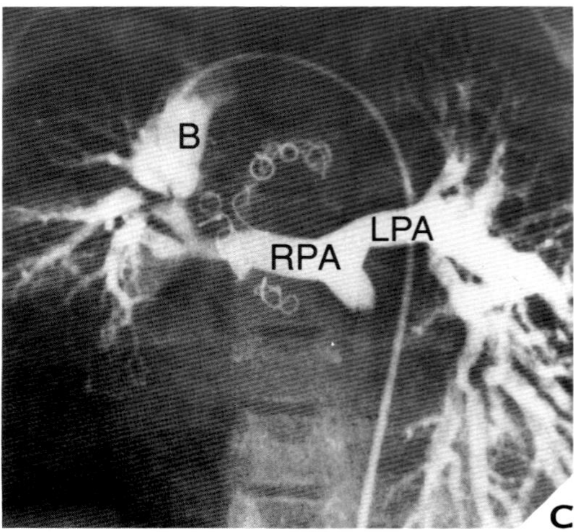

Fig. 31.14 Emoblization of aortopulmonary collateral with spring coil technique. (A) Thoracic aortogram (frontal projection) in a patient with tetralogy of Fallot and pulmonary atresia who had previously undergone a palliative shunt demonstrates large aortopulmonary collateral arteries (C1 and C2) arising from the upper descending thoracic aorta (DA) and connecting with lower lobe branches (LLB) of the right pulmonary artery. (B) Thoracic aortogram obtained after the embolization procedure demonstrates that the inferior collaterals have been occluded and the flow in the large superior collateral (C2) has been significantly decreased. (C) Selective injection through the Blalock (right subclavian to right pulmonary artery) anastomosis (B) demonstrates abnormal arborization of the middle and lower lobe branches of the right pulmonary artery owing to persistent flow through large aortopulmonary collaterals supplying this portion of the lung. (LPA = left pulmonary artery)

collateral artery is progressively occluded by thrombus (Figs. 31.14 and 31.15). Alternative methods employing detachable balloons or plastic (bucrylate) have also been used to obliterate aortopulmonary collaterals.

OCCLUSION OF ARTERIOVENOUS FISTULAS

Arteriovenous fistulas can be occluded by a variety of embolization techniques. The most common method employs detachable balloons; because the feeding arteries are usually numerous, it may be necessary to use several balloons to completely occlude the blood supply to the lesion (Fig. 31.16). The balloon occlusion technique can be used to decrease the blood flow before surgery. If the balloon occlusion technique is used in lieu of surgery (ie, as a permanent solution), several sessions may be needed to obliterate additional feeding arteries that may appear after the first, second, or third session.

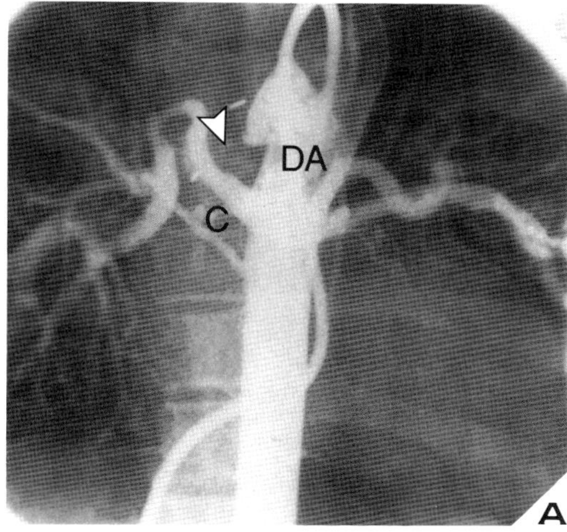

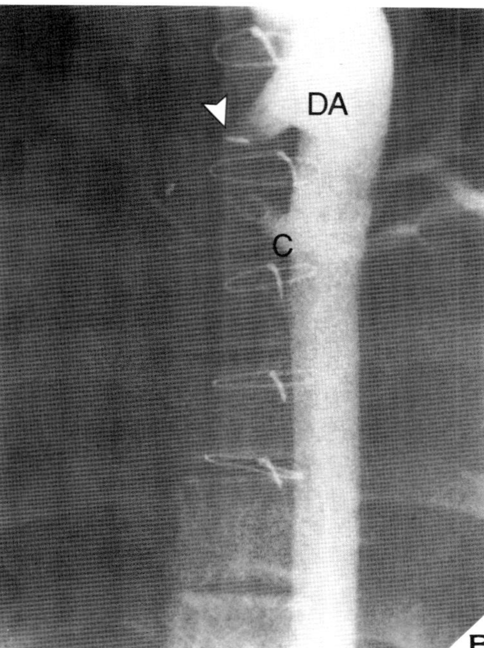

Fig. 31.15 Embolization of aortopulmonary collateral with spring coil technique. This patient with pulmonary atresia and a ventricular septal defect had previously undergone a right Blalock anastomosis and occlusion of a large aortopulmonary collateral (*arrow*). (A) Thoracic aortogram (frontal projection) demonstrates a large aortopulmonary collateral (C) arising from the right border of the descending thoracic aorta (DA). Note short stenotic segment in the intramediastinal portion of the collateral and connecting with branches supplying the right lower lobe. The patient subsequently underwent complete correction of the cardiac malformation. (B) Repeat thoracic aortogram obtained immediately after embolization procedure demonstrates no flow through the large collateral (C) seen in A, indicating that it is completely occluded (*arrow* indicates spring coil).

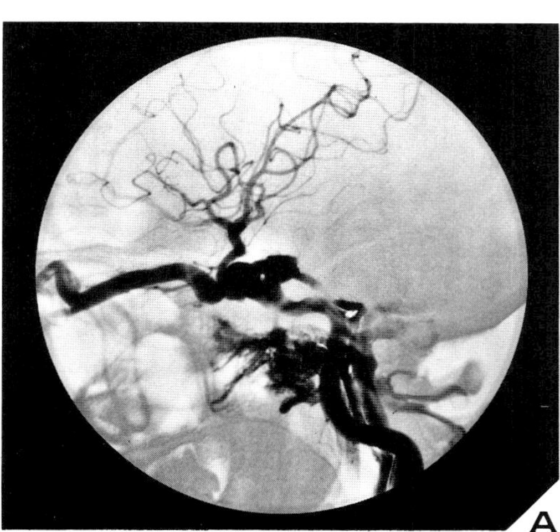

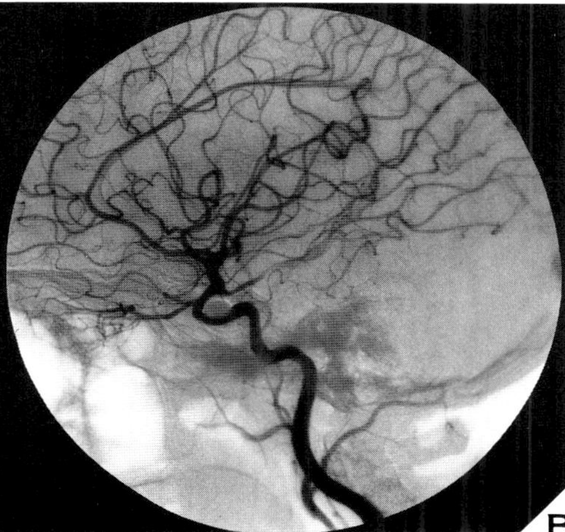

Fig. 31.16 Embolization of posttraumatic carotid–cavernous sinus fistula. (A) Early arterial phase of left internal carotid arteriogram demonstrates early opacification of intracranial venous channels indicating the presence of an arteriovenous fistula. The abnormal connection is between the internal carotid artery and the cavernous sinus. Note opacification of the cavernous sinus, ophthalmic vein, and superior petrosal sinus. (B) Repeat internal carotid arteriogram after occlusion of the fistula by a percutaneously introduced balloon shows patency of the left internal carotid artery and its intracranial branches; no early venous filling is seen. (Courtesy of Jiri Vitik, MD, Birmingham, AL)

PROSTHETIC VALVES

Surgical replacement of malfunctioning cardiac valves is now a routine procedure. Two varieties of valve are in current use: biologic (homograft or xenograft) and mechanical.

BIOLOGIC VALVES

Both human and porcine aortic valves have been extensively used as prostheses. Some biologic valves are mounted on a cloth-covered metallic ring. Examples of biologic valves include the Carpenter–Edwards valve, which is mounted on a wire device (Figs. 31.17 and 31.18), and the Hancock valve, which is mounted on a ring (Fig. 31.19). In general, biologic valves can be expected to function adequately for about 8 to 10 years, after which they usually show signs of deterioration, resulting in insufficiency or (rarely) stenosis. Rupture of an aged prosthetic valve can lead to massive regurgitation.

MECHANICAL VALVES

Mechanical valves are of two types: high profile and low profile. At present the great majority of the mechanical valves used in cardiac surgery are of the latter type.

LOW PROFILE VALVES

The most commonly employed designs are the Bjork–Shiley and the St. Jude.

Bjork–Shiley Valve

The Bjork–Shiley valve is an eccentric monocuspid disk which is attached to a metallic base ring by a hook (Fig. 31.20). The base ring is sutured to the annulus of the native valve, so that its displacement (base ring tilt) during the cardiac cycle matches that of the vessel or cardiac chamber to which it is attached (Fig. 31.21). The mean base ring tilt of a Bjork–Shiley valve positioned in the aortic orifice is 3.4° (SD, 1.5°; range 0–12°) (Fig.

Fig. 31.17 Carpenter–Edwards bioprosthetic valve. The valve (viewed from above) is supported by a serpentine wire stent which is covered by cloth. The longer part of the cloth-covered support represents the outlet and the shorter part the inlet.

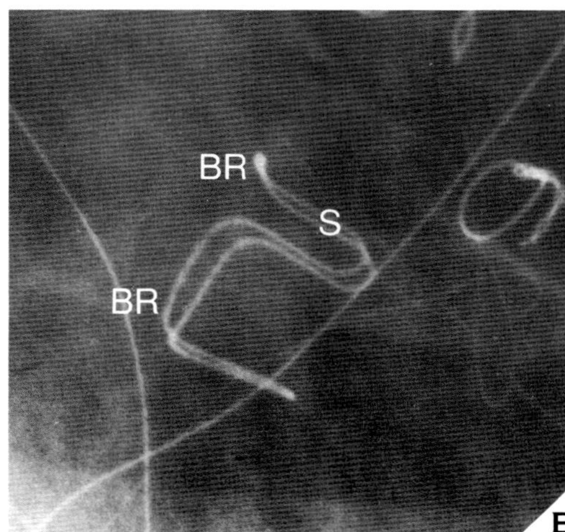

Fig. 31.18 Carpenter–Edwards bioprosthetic valve in mitral position. Cine frames in RAO projection. (A) Systole. The base ring forms a uniform line. (B) Diastole. The space between the borders of the base ring (BR) is within normal limits (see Fig. 31.21). The *arrow* indicates the direction of blood flow from left atrium to left ventricle. (S = support of the prosthesis)

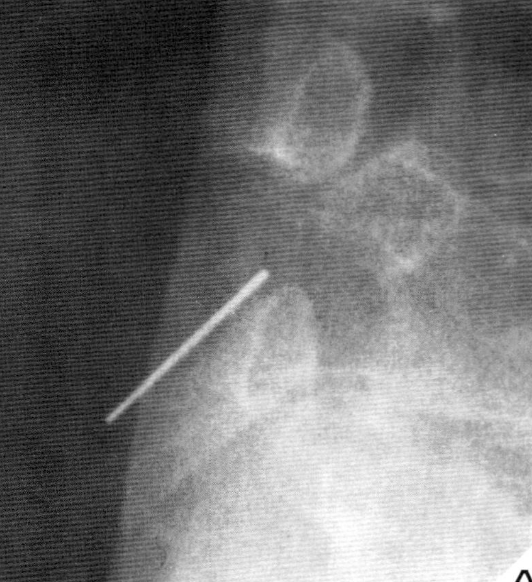

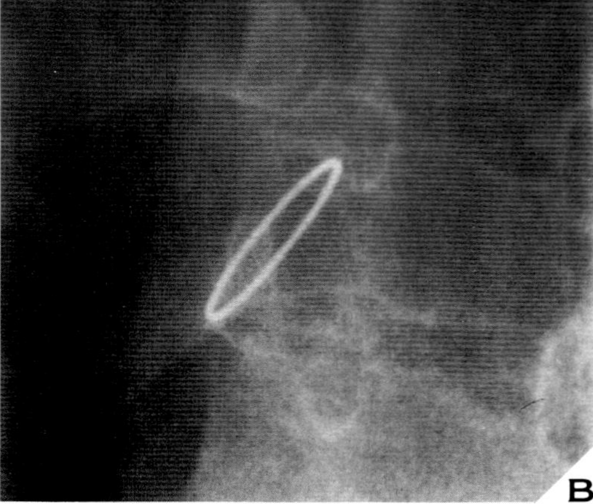

Fig. 31.19 Hancock bioprosthetic valve in aortic position. (A) Seen in profile. (B) Maximum opening of the borders. The degree of tilting of the base ring is within normal limits (see Fig. 31.21).

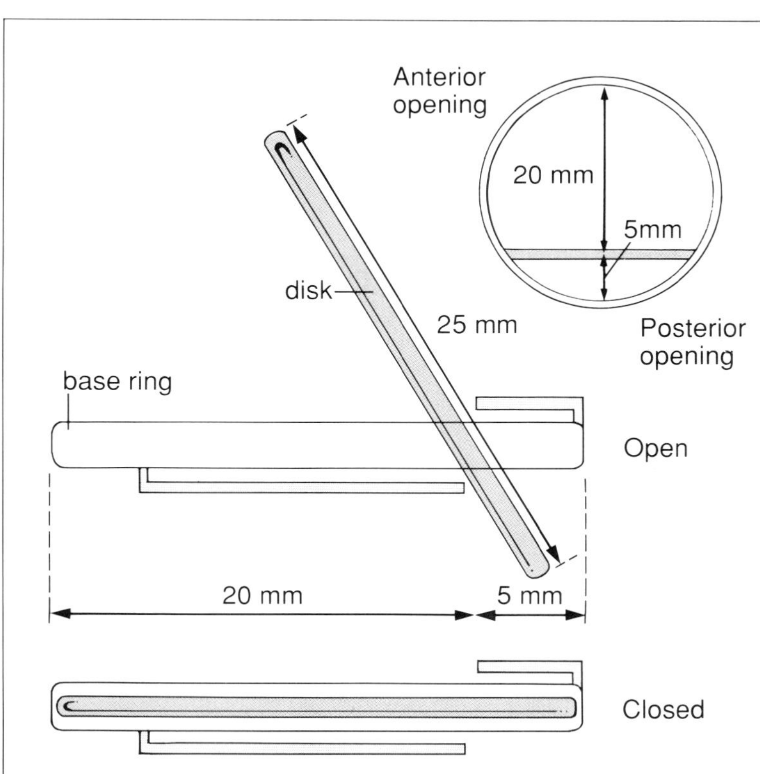

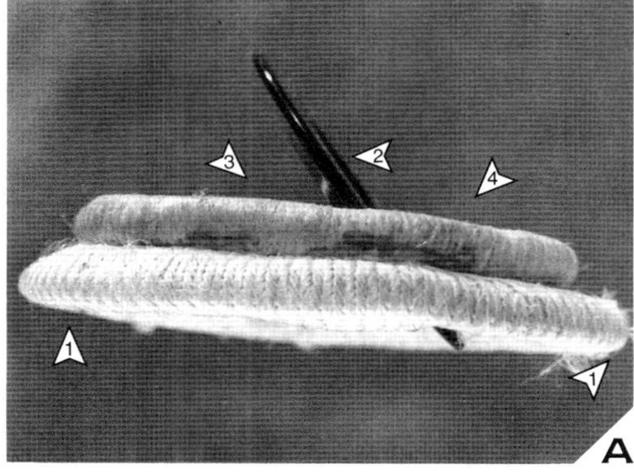

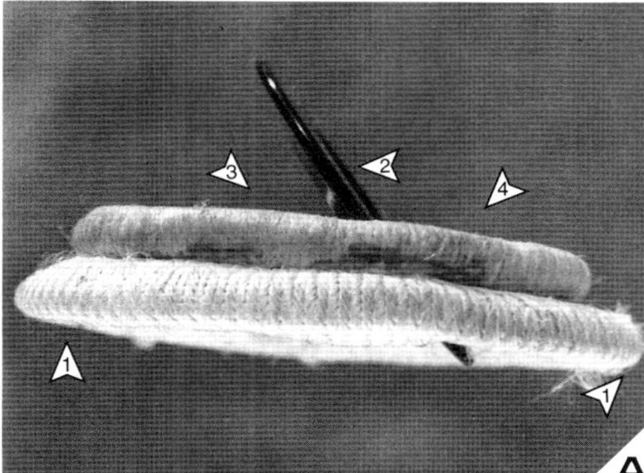

1 base ring
2 disk
3 large opening
4 small opening

Fig. 31.20 Bjork–Shiley mechanical prosthetic valve. (A) The prosthesis (viewed from the side) consists of a base ring and disk. The latter is anchored to the base ring by a specially devised hook. In the closed position the disk is parallel to the base ring and occludes the entire valve orifice. In the open position (shown here) the disk forms a 60° angle with respect to the base ring. (B) Owing to the asymmetrical placement of the hook that anchors the disk, the valve has two openings (one large and one small) when it is in the open position. The large anterior opening measures 20 mm in diameter; the small posterior opening measures 5 mm in diameter. The Bjork–Shiley valve can be used in place of any cardiac valve.

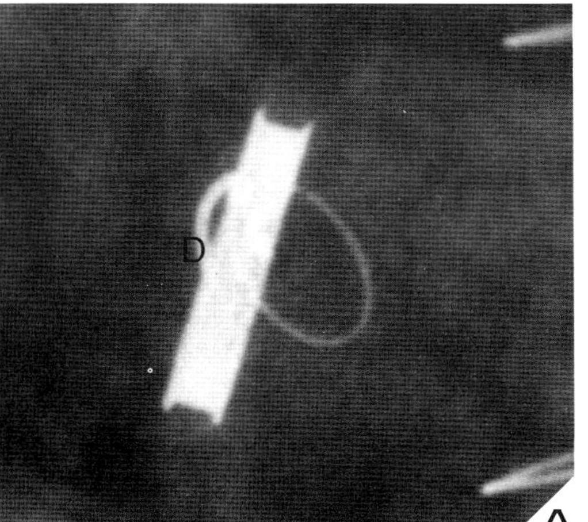

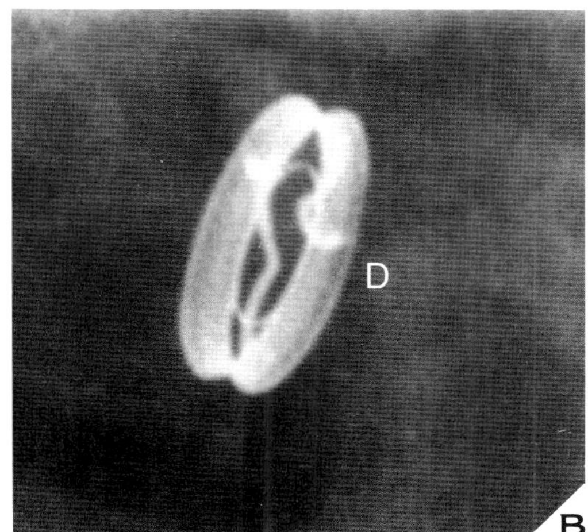

Fig. 31.21 Measuring the base ring tilt of a prosthetic valve. The base ring tilt of any prosthetic valve can be determined as follows (a Bjork–Shiley valve in the mitral position is illustrated here). *Step 1.* Cinefluoroscopy is performed in multiple projections. A frame showing the base ring in profile (ie, superimposition of the near and far sides of the base ring) at one extreme of valve motion is selected for further analysis. *Step 2.* The projected base ring diameter is measured (A). *Step 3.* The frame showing the maximum separation between the opposite sides of the base ring is selected and the distance between the near and far sides (d) is measured (B). *Step 4.* The base ring tilt is equal to the arc tangent of the quotient d/D. The displacement of the base ring (in degrees) can be read from the accompanying chart (C). (d/D is shown along the horizontal axis and base ring tilt along the vertical axis.)

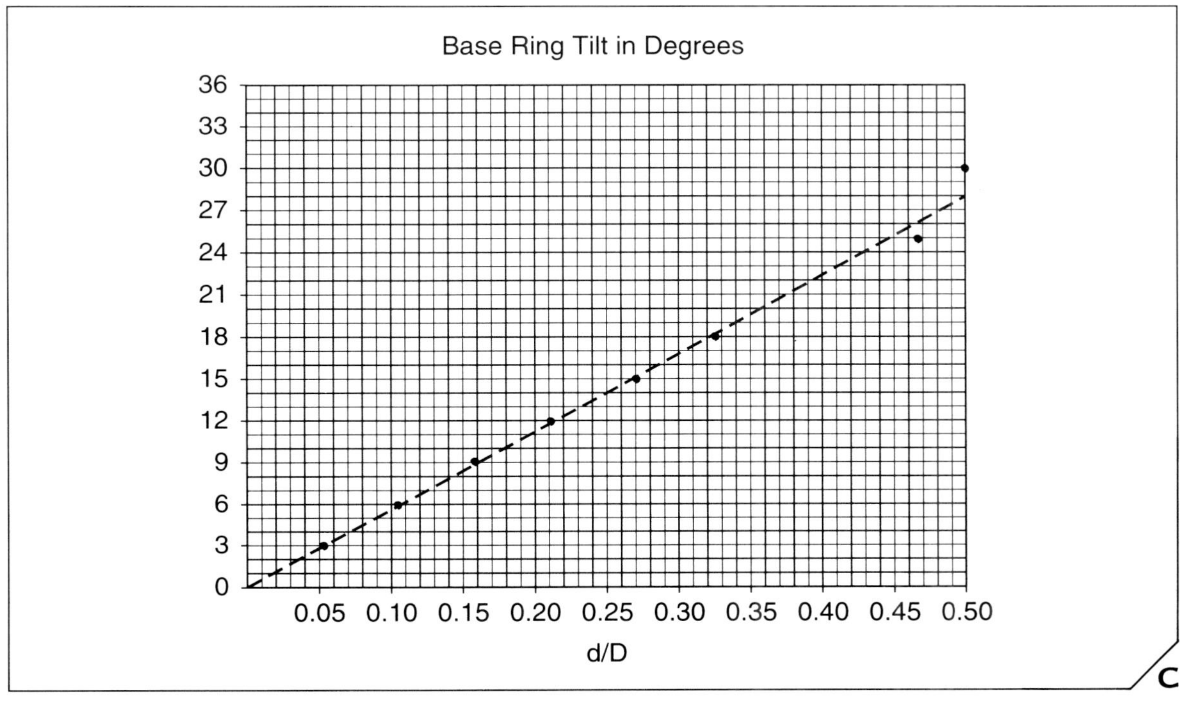

31.22). The mean base ring tilt of a Bjork–Shiley valve in the mitral position is 5.3° (SD 2.6°, range 1–15°) (Fig. 31.23).

Complications Insufficiency of the Bjork–Shiley and other prosthetic valves is usually caused by disruption of the sutures that attach the base ring to the native annulus. In such cases the base ring tilt is greater than normal. The degree of base ring tilt is highly variable and depends on the number and precise location of the disrupted sutures. Comparison with baseline postoperative radiographs is very helpful in such cases.

Malfunction of the disc results in varying degrees of functional obstruction. In a normally functioning valve, the maximum separation between the disk and the base ring is about 60°. (If cardiac output is decreased, the separation can be as little as 50°.) Restricted opening of the valve with functional stenosis is usually due to thrombosis (Fig. 31.24). If the obstruction is severe, restricted excursion of the disc can often be detected fluoroscopically (Fig. 31.25). Immediate valve replacement may be lifesaving in such cases.

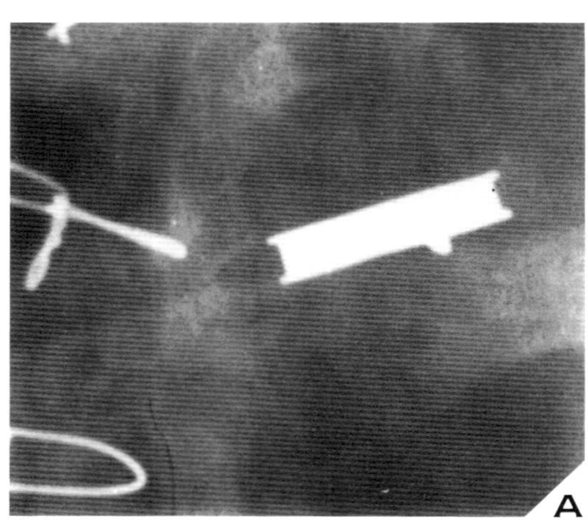

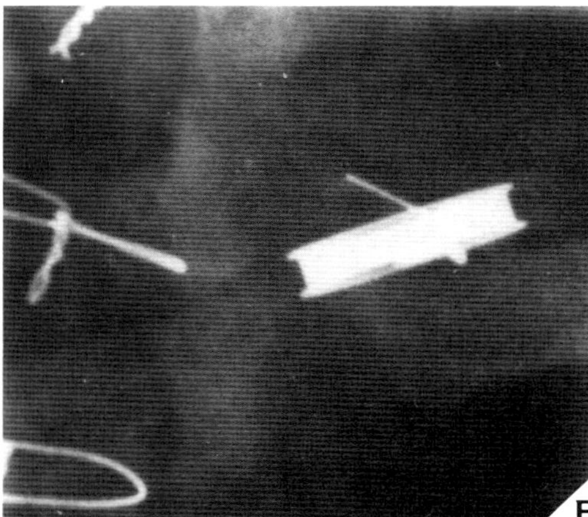

Fig. 31.22 Normally functioning Bjork–Shiley valve in aortic position. (A, B) Cine frames in LAO projection. (A) In the closed position the disk is parallel to the base ring and is obscured. (B) In the open position the disk forms a normal 60° angle with the base ring. The larger of the two openings in the valve lies beneath the acute angle formed by the disk and the base ring.

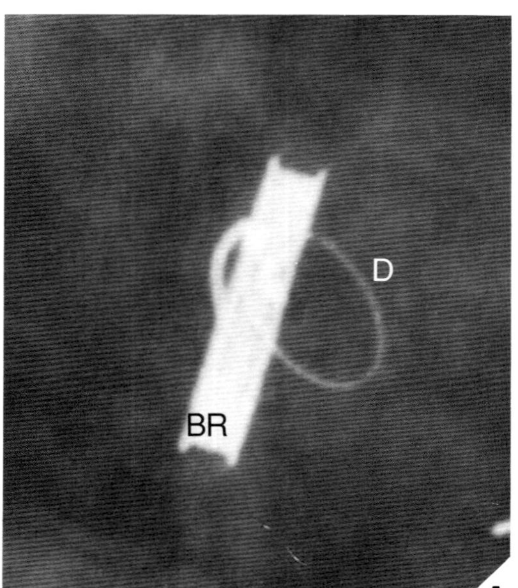

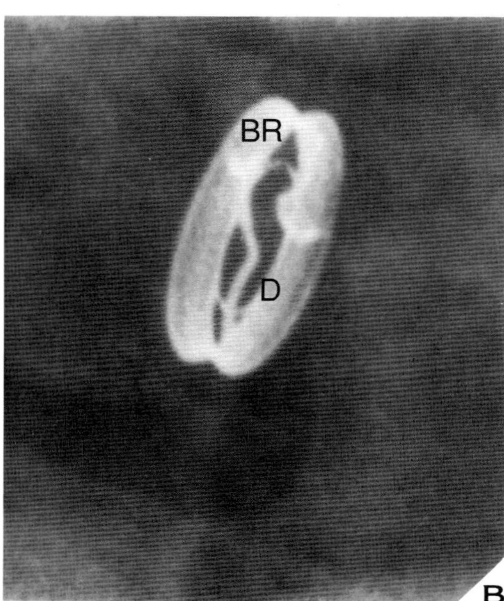

Fig. 31.23 Assessing base ring tilt. Cine frames in RAO-Cr projection in patient with Bjork–Shiley valve in the mitral position. (A) The borders of the base ring (BR) overlie each other and are seen in profile. (B) There is exaggerated displacement (*brace*) of the borders of the base ring. The displacement measured 16°. (D = disk)

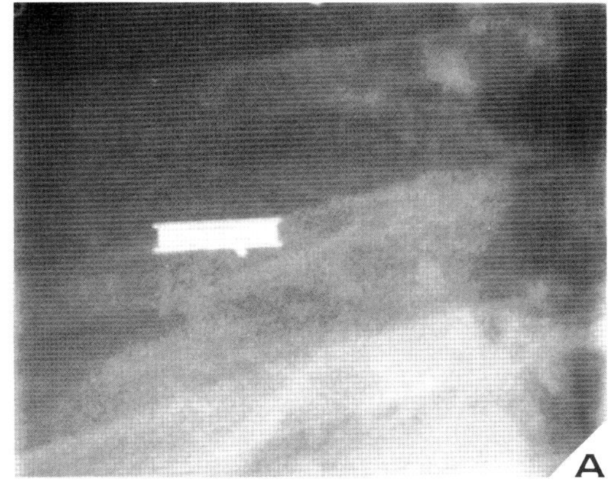

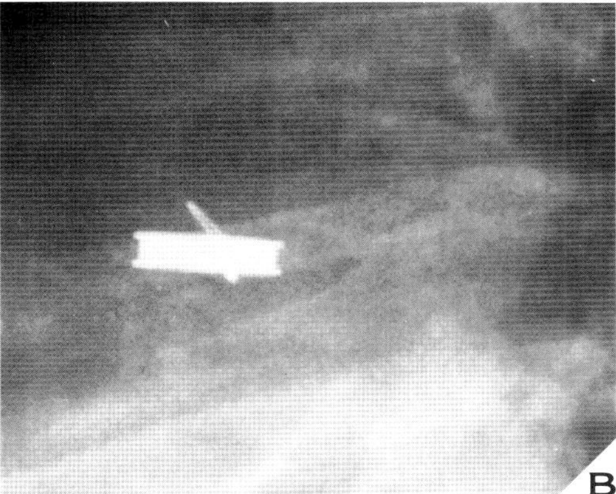

Fig. 31.24 Stenosis of Bjork–Shiley valve. (A, B) Frames of cinefluoroscopic examination of Bjork–Shiley valve in the aortic position (obtained in the lateral projection with cranio-caudal angulation to show the base ring in profile). With the valve in the open position (B) the angle between the disk and the base ring measures less than 60°. The clinical findings were consistent with stenosis of the prosthetic valve.

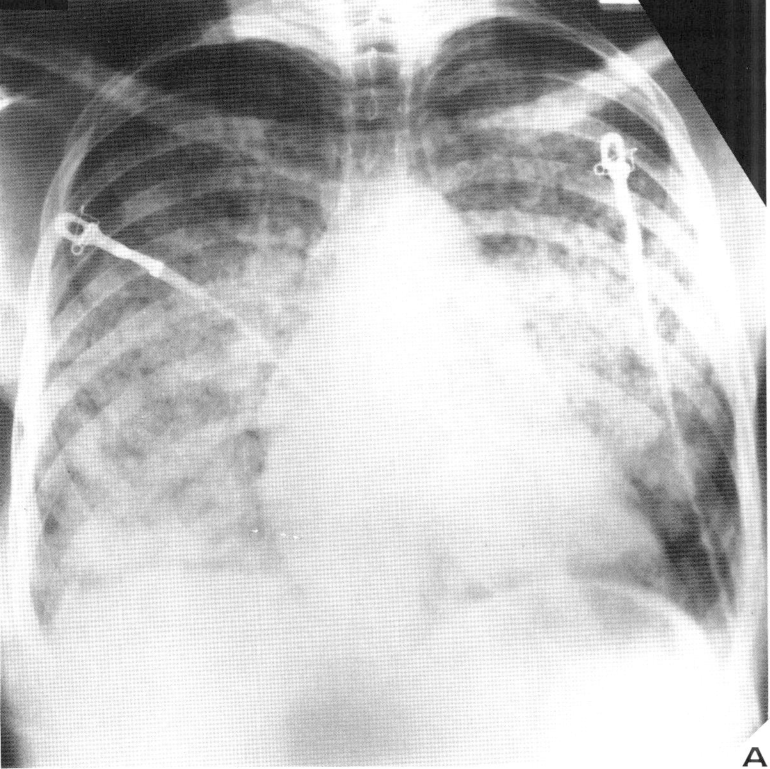

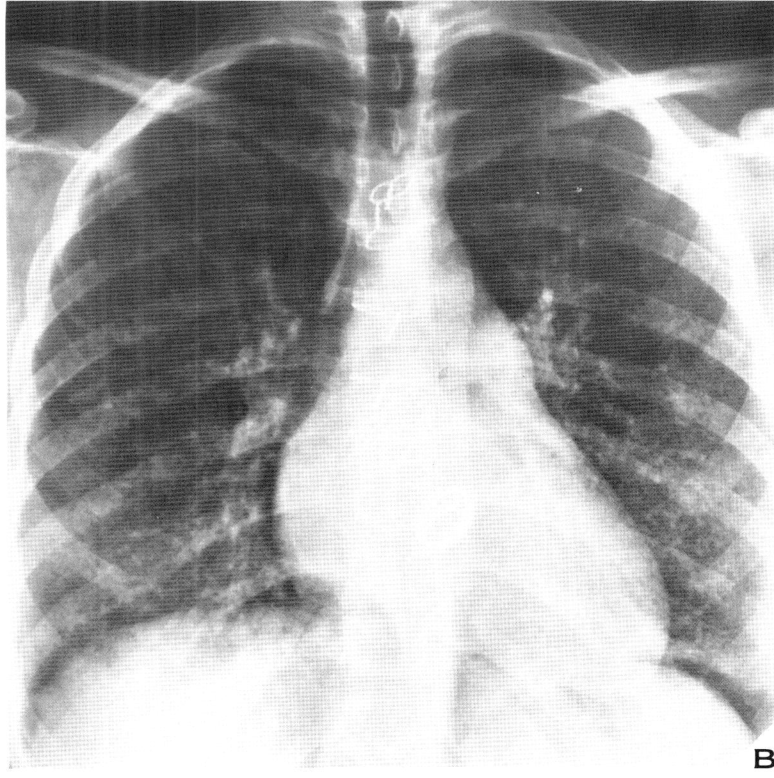

Fig. 31.25 Stenosis of Bjork–Shiley valve secondary to thrombosis. This patient presented at the emergency room with severe shortness of breath. Several years before he had undergone mitral valve replacement for mitral insufficiency. For the past few months he had not complied with his anticoagulation regimen. (A) Frontal chest film demonstrates alveolar pulmonary edema with a typical butterfly distribution. The left atrium is moderately enlarged. Fluoroscopic examination revealed markedly restricted opening of the valve, with only 14° of separation between the disk and the base ring. At operation, there was a large thrombus which prevented proper opening of the valve. The thrombosed prosthesis was replaced with another Bjork–Shiley valve. (B) Repeat chest film (obtained 7 days after the second valve replacement) shows almost complete resolution of the pulmonary edema.

St. Jude Valve

The St. Jude valve is a symmetrical bileaflet device consisting of a ring that supports two semilunar leaflets. The latter are attached to a hook such that the leaflets are perpendicular to the supporting ring when the valve is open and parallel to it when the valve is closed (Fig. 31.26). Because the valve material is not very radiopaque, neither the ring nor the leaflets can be identified fluoroscopically when viewed en face. However, the ring can be identified as a line when the valve is seen in profile. When the valve is in open position, the leaflets typically appear as two parallel lines (depending on the orientation of the X-ray beam, they may have a V-shaped configuration) (Fig. 31.27). Normal and abnormal tilting of the base ring can also be evaluated fluoroscopically by means of the technique described for the Bjork–Shiley valve.

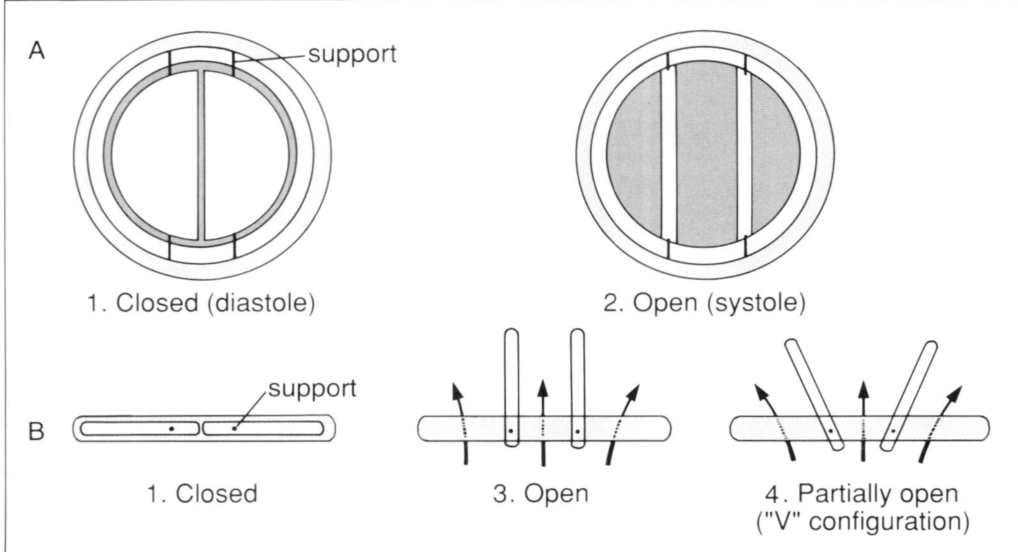

Fig. 31.26 St. Jude valve, viewed from above (A) and from the side (B). The prosthetic valve cosists of two leaflets which are attached to the base ring. In the closed position the leaflets are parallel to the base ring; in the open position the leaflets are perpendicular to the base ring. With the prosthetic valve in the closed position the leaflets are superimposed (B). Depending on the degree of opening and the obliquity of the X-ray beam, the leaflets may have a "V" configuration.

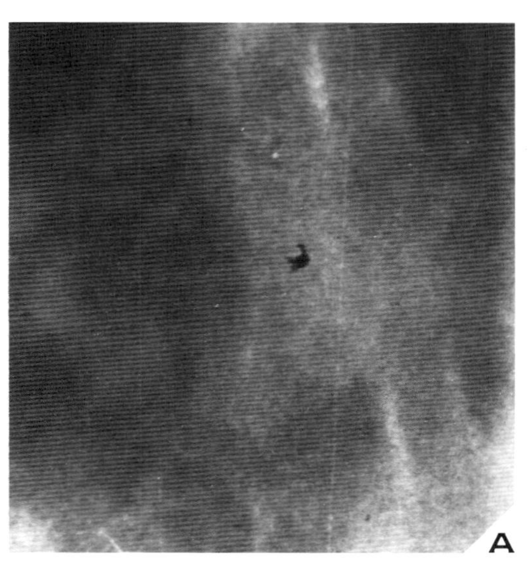

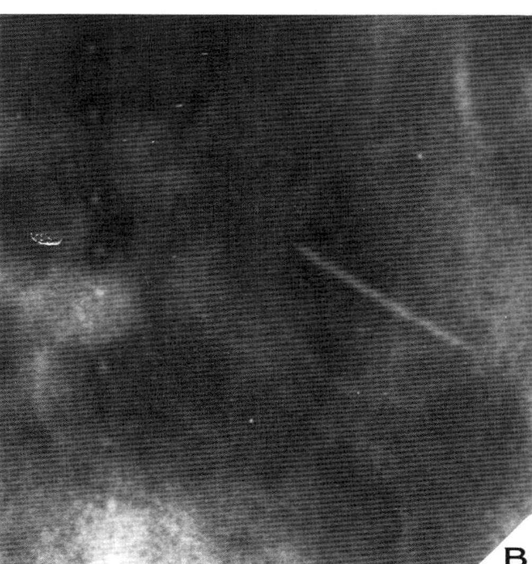

Fig. 31.27 Stenosis of St. Jude valve. Diagrammatic representation of prosthetic valve in mitral position. (A) Systole (closed position). The septal leaflet is stationary. The mural leaflet moves normally. (B) Diastole.

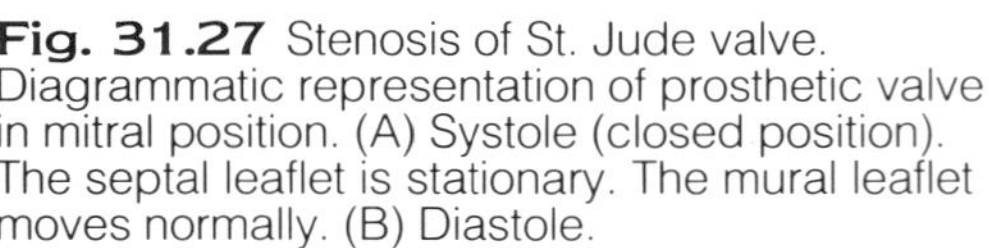

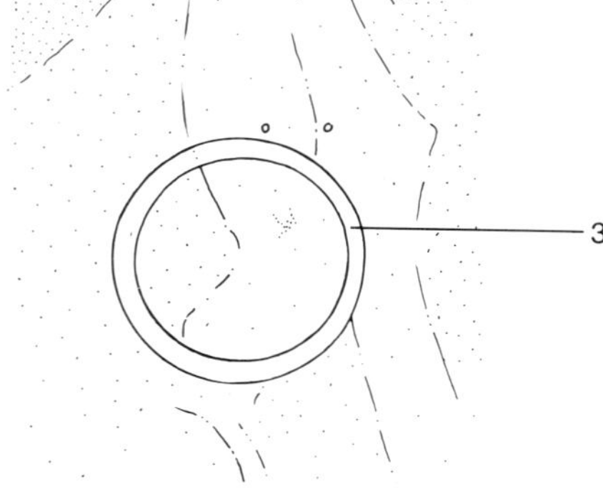

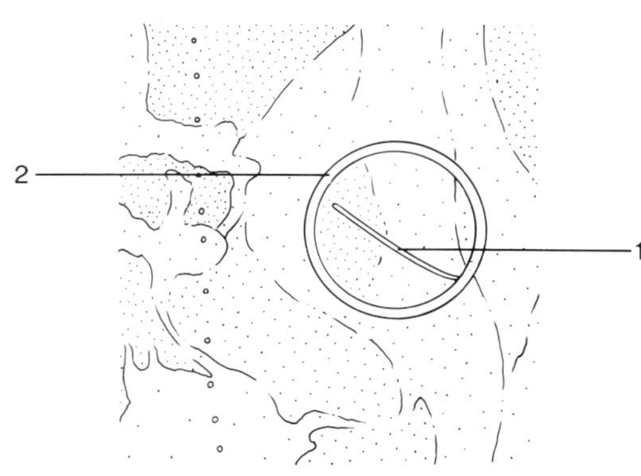

EXTERNAL CONDUITS

The surgical repair of some congenital malformations requires the insertion of a prosthetic tube between the ventricular cavity and the pulmonary trunk or the aorta. External prostheses used for this purpose typically consist of a corrugated plastic tube containing a biologic valve which is supported by a metallic ring (valved external conduit) (Fig. 31.28). Pulmonic atresia with ventricular septal defect is the most common indication for this type of repair; postoperatively, the prosthetic tube conducts the entire right ventricular output to the pulmonary arteries (see Chapter 16). Other important applications include the insertion of a conduit between the left ventricle and the pulmonary trunk in patients with corrected transposition of the great arteries with pulmonic stenosis (Fig. 31.29) and the insertion of a conduit between the left ventricle and the descending thoracic aorta in patients with severe aortic stenosis or left ventricular outflow obstruction (Fig. 31.30).

The inner surface of the prosthesis is progressively covered by fibrin and is eventually endothelialized; by the end of the first postoperative year the neointima usually covers the entire inner surface of the conduit. Excessive proliferation or peeling away of the neointima can result in obstruction.

The usual life of an external conduit is about 10 years, after which malfunctioning of the valve (often associated with calcification) or stenosis of the tube may necessitate replacement.

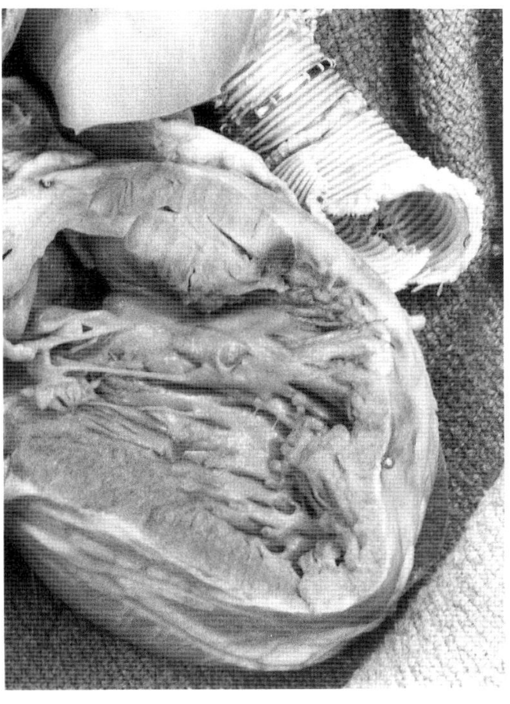

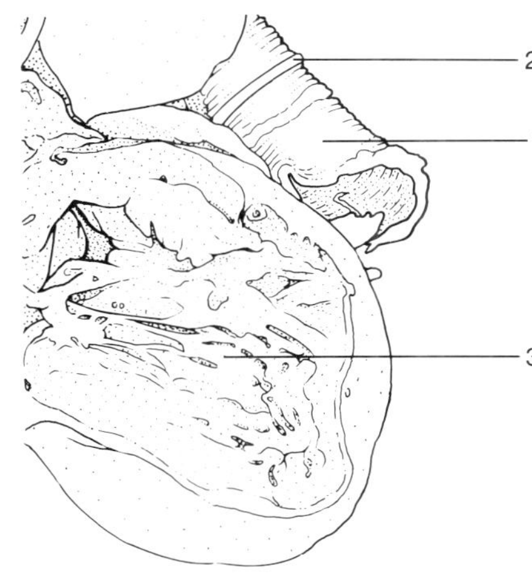

Fig. 31.28 Valved external conduit. Autopsy specimen from patient with tetralogy of Fallot and pulmonary atresia. The conduit, which is made from corrugated dacron, connects the right ventricle and the pulmonary trunk. The metallic ring is the external support of the Hancock valve (prosthetic porcine valve).

1 external conduit
2 ring for prosthetic valve
3 right ventricle

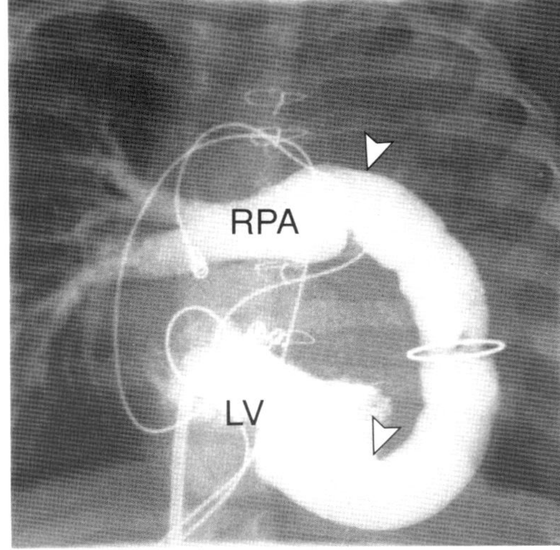

Fig. 31.29 Valved external conduit. Frontal projection of left ventriculogram demonstrates an external conduit which has been inserted between the morphologic left ventricle (LV) and the pulmonary trunk in a patient with corrected transposition of the great arteries associated with atrial situs solitus, inverted ventricles, discordant atrioventricular connection, discordant ventriculoarterial connection, and severe stenosis of the left ventricular outflow tract. The proximal and distal margins of the conduit are indicated by *arrows*. The metallic ring indicates the position of the prosthetic valve in the midportion of the conduit. (RPA = right pulmonary artery)

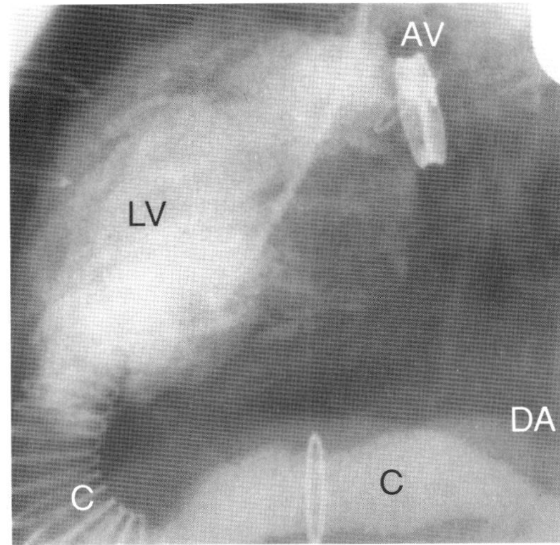

Fig. 31.30 External conduit. Lateral projection of left ventriculogram demonstrates a valved external conduit (C) which has been inserted between the apex of the left ventricle (LV) and the descending thoracic aorta (DA) in a patient with severe left ventricular tract stenosis. The metallic ring indicates the position of the prosthetic Hancock valve. In addition, the patient has had a Bjork–Shiley valve inserted in the mitral position. (AV = aortic valve)

IMAGING AND INVASIVE DIAGNOSIS

The external conduit is radiolucent and cannot be identified on plain films. However, the metallic ring supporting the valve serves to indicate its location (Fig. 31.31). A nonvalved conduit often appears radiographically as a retrosternal "mass." Degenerative changes such as calcification of the valve (Fig. 31.31) or of the conduit itself (Fig. 31.32) are readily apparent on plain films. Pseudoaneurysm formation, which is commonly associated with extensive calcification, can also be detected radiographically (Fig. 31.33).

CT is the best method for identifying the position, patency, and relations of the prosthesis to adjacent bony and soft tissue structures. Precise knowledge of the relationship of the external conduit and the sternum is of paramount importance if a second medial sternotomy is contemplated, since nicking the conduit when opening the sternum can lead to an exsanguinating hemorrhage (Fig. 31.34).

If necessary, angiography can be performed to assess the patency of the conduit (Fig. 31.35). Because of its ability to evaluate blood flow noninvasively, MRI is likely to play an increasing role in the evaluation of external conduits and their complications.

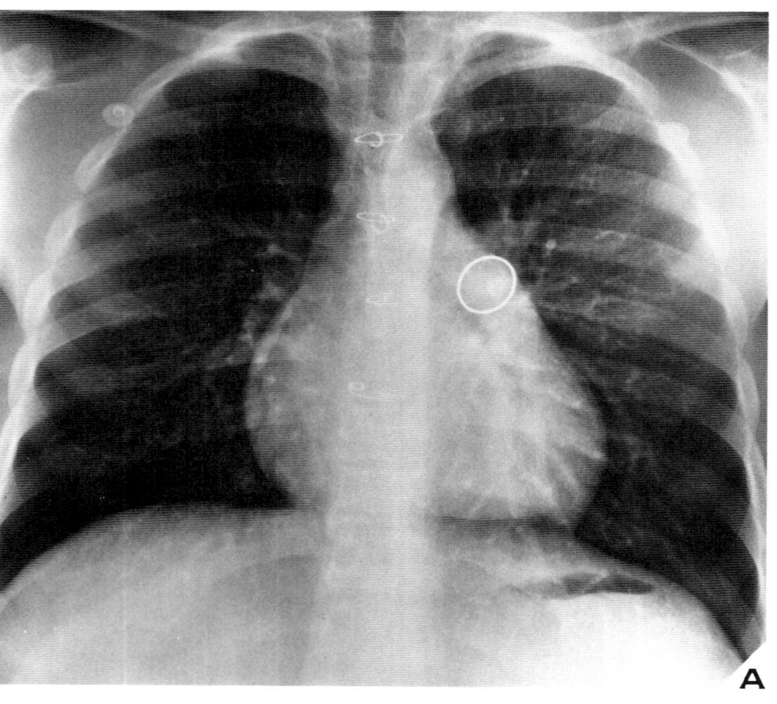

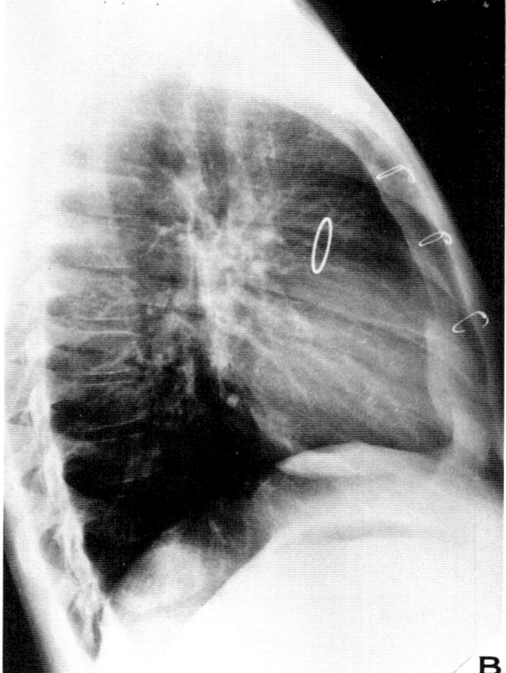

Fig. 31.31 Calcification of prosthetic valve in external conduit. Several years earlier this patient with tansposition of the great arteries underwent a procedure in which blood was rerouted from the left ventricle to the aorta and a valved external conduit was inserted between the right ventricle and the pulmonary trunk. (A) Frontal and (B) lateral chest films show the metallic ring supporting the Hancock prosthesis. Calcification within the prosthetic valve can be seen in A. Heart size and pulmonary vascularity are both normal. The patient was asymptomatic.

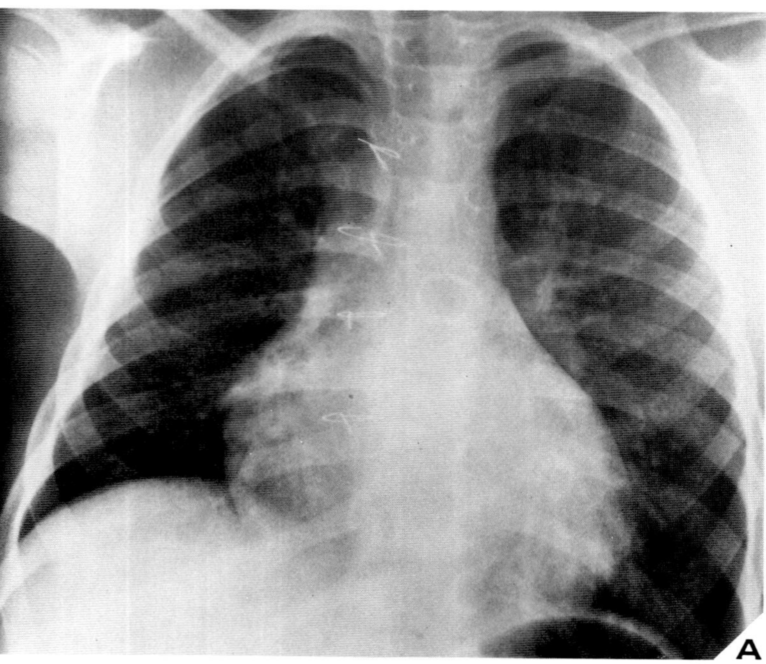

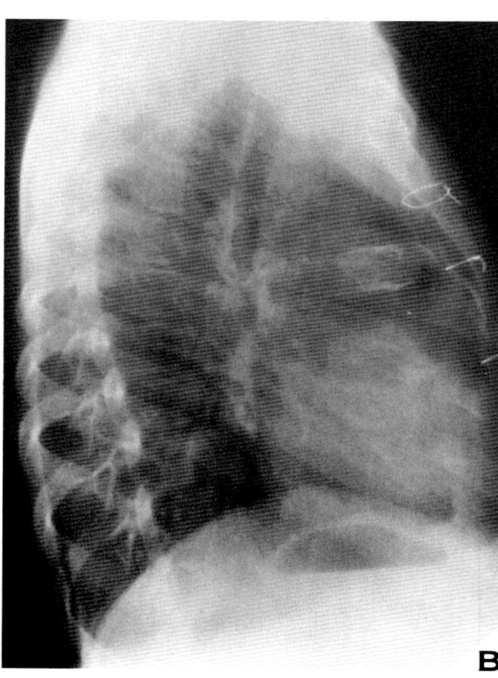

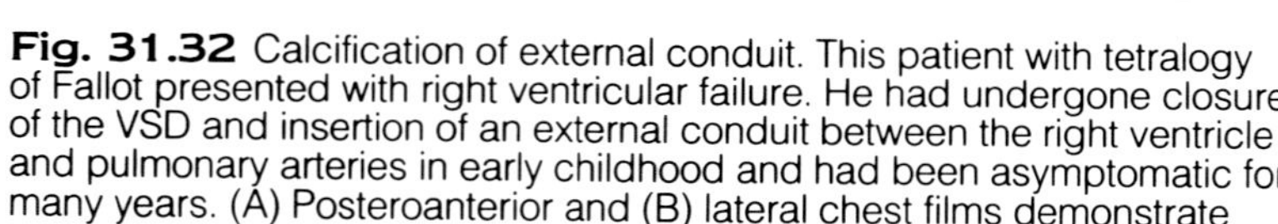

Fig. 31.32 Calcification of external conduit. This patient with tetralogy of Fallot presented with right ventricular failure. He had undergone closure of the VSD and insertion of an external conduit between the right ventricle and pulmonary arteries in early childhood and had been asymptomatic for many years. (A) Posteroanterior and (B) lateral chest films demonstrate extensive calcification of the external conduit, particularly in the segment close to the pulmonary connection. Note the right atrial and right ventricular enlargement indicating right ventricular failure secondary to obstruction of the conduit.

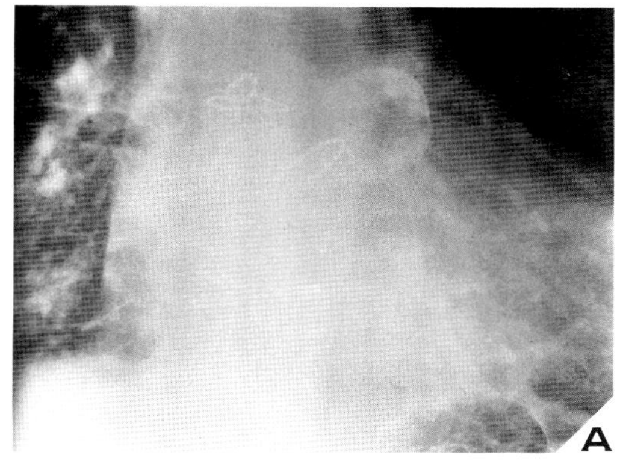

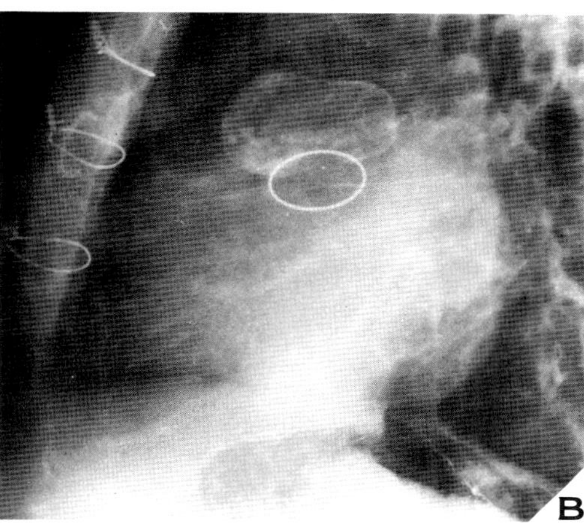

Fig. 31.33 Pseudoaneurysm after insertion of valved external conduit. (A) Posteroanterior and (B) lateral chest films demonstrate an oval calcification overlying the metallic ring that supports the Hancock valve. Thoracotomy revealed a patent, extensively calcified pseudoaneurysm which communicated with the pulmonary trunk through a very short channel.

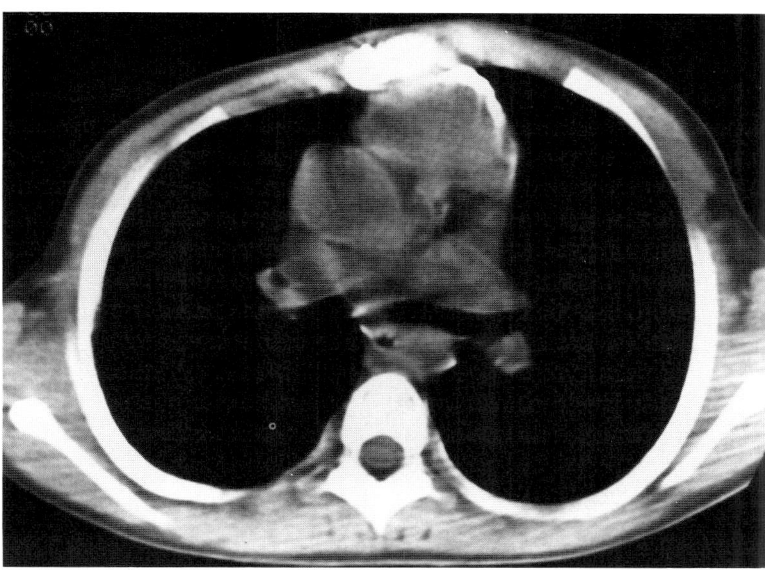

Fig. 31.34 External conduit eroding the sternum. Ungated CT scan at the level of the left atrium in a patient with tetralogy of Fallot. The external conduit conducting the right ventricle with the pulmonary arteries has eroded the posterior aspect of the sternum.

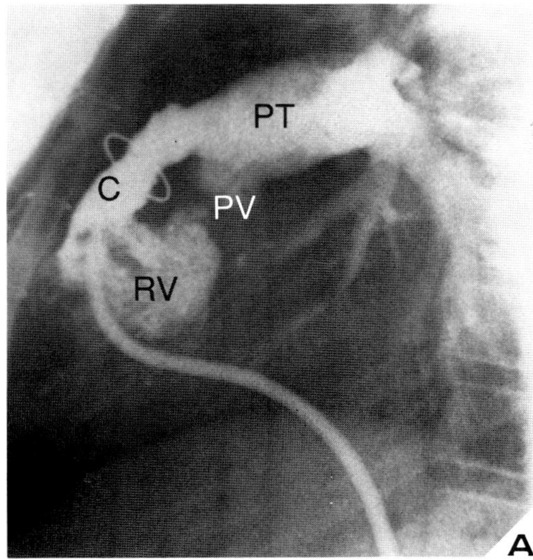

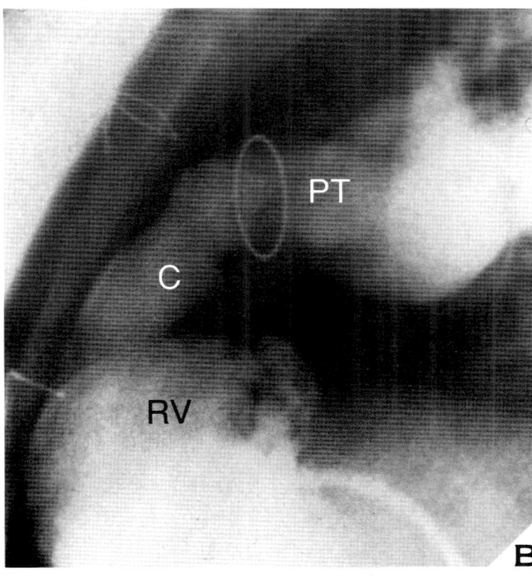

Fig. 31.35 Stenosis of external conduit. Angiographic findings in two patients with severe subpulmonic stenosis. (A) Lateral projection of right ventriculogram shows stenosis of the external conduit (C) connecting the right ventricle (RV) with the pulmonary trunk (PT) (compare diameter of its lumen with that of the pulmonary trunk). (B) In this patient the conduit is widely patent. The inferior aspect of the conduit is in contact with the anterior chest wall. (PV = native pulmonic valve)

CHAPTER 32

Cardiac Transplantation

INTRODUCTION

In this innovative surgical technique the patient's diseased or defective heart is replaced with a new heart (heterograft) from a donor. The first successful human heart transplant was performed by Christiaan Barnard in Cape Town, South Africa, in 1967. The first successful heart transplant in the United States was performed by the Stanford University team in 1968.

In the early years most patients who survived the surgical procedure died within days or weeks from acute rejection of the transplant. Today, 76 percent of heart transplant recipients survive for 2 years or longer. This dramatic increase in long-term survival reflects advances in immunosuppressive therapy—the introduction of cyclosporine (1980) in particular—rather than refinements in surgical technique.

The success of heart transplantation depends on close matching between the donor and recipient, meticulous surgical technique, and sophisticated postoperative management.

SELECTION OF THE RECIPIENT

The typical candidate for cardiac transplantation is a man or woman under 50 years of age with end-stage heart disease (New York Heart Association Class IV) whose life expectancy is 6 months or less. In one large series, the mean life expectancy without transplantation was 45 days (Baumgartner et al, 1979). Eighty to 90 percent of candidates for heart transplantation have ischemic heart disease or idiopathic cardiomyopathy. Less frequent indications include cardiac amyloidosis, hypertrophic cardiomyopathy, severe myocarditis, cardiac tumors, and complex congenital malformations. The latter category includes conditions for which total correction is very risky (eg, hypoplastic left ventricle, overriding of the atrioventricular valves, tricuspid atresia with left ventricular failure, univentricular atrioventricular connection with severe insufficiency of the atrioventricular valve and left ventricular failure) or has been unsuccessful. Heart–lung transplants have been performed in a small number of cases, mainly in patients with fixed pulmonary hypertension (primary or secondary).

Absolute contraindications to cardiac transplantation include diabetes mellitus, active peptic ulcer disease, a history of pulmonary infarction within the previous 2 months, severe pulmonary hypertension (pulmonary arterial resistance greater than 6 to 8 Wood units per square meter of body surface), severe bronchitis or pulmonary emphysema, alcoholism, severe psychiatric disease, liver disease, collagen or vascular disease, or any other systemic disorder that would contraindicate the use of immunosuppressive therapy or prevent compliance with the postoperative regimen.

THE DONOR

The potential donor is usually a victim of blunt or penetrating head trauma who has been declared legally dead (as defined by generally recognized criteria for brain death). Most heart donors are from 12 to 40 years of age. (Ideally, a male donor should be less than 35 years of age, a female less than 40 years of age.) Because the risk of significant coronary artery disease increases with age, it is necessary for donors older than 35 years of age to undergo complete coronary arteriography. The optimal size of the donor heart is determined by the size of the recipient; however, a close match is not essential, since in most instances the recipient's pericardial cavity has already enlarged to accommodate a hypertrophied, dilated heart. For this reason, technical problems in inserting the transplant are unlikely even when the donor's body weight is 30 to 40 percent greater than the recipient's.

The potential donor must satisfy a number of other conditions. He or she should not have preexisting heart disease. The donor should be clinically stable and should not require doses of inotropic drugs to maintain adequate cardiac output. The heart to be transplanted should not have been traumatized or otherwise damaged (eg, as a result of a severe closed chest injury, prolonged cardiac arrest, or intracardiac injections). Finally, there should be no evidence of septicemia at the time of organ procurement.

The risk of rejection is related to the antigenic compatibility of donor and recipient. Both the donor and the potential recipient must have the same ABO blood type. A close human leukocyte antigen (HLA) match has been reported to be associated with a lower incidence of accelerated atherosclerosis. However, a poor HLA match is not an absolute contraindication. Many centers require a lymphocytotoxic cross-match between donor lymphocytes and recipient serum to screen for antibodies that might cause acute hyperacute rejection.

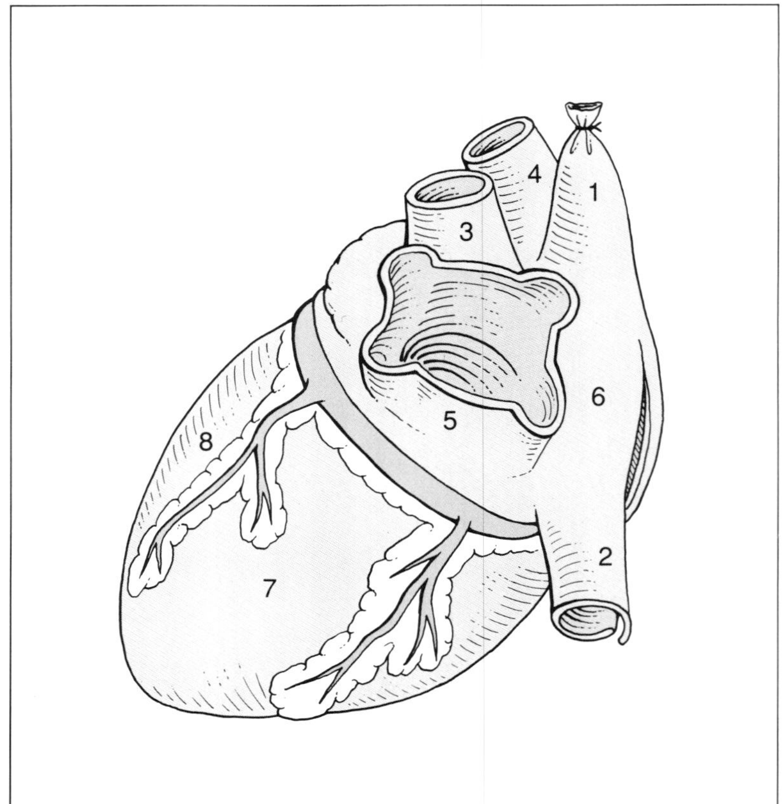

1	superior vena cava	5	left atrium
2	inferior vena cava	6	right atrium
3	aorta	7	right ventricle
4	pulmonary trunk	8	left ventricle

Fig. 32.1 The donor heart. The superior and inferior vena caval connections with the right atrium are left intact. The left atrium is intact except for a small segment at the entrance of the pulmonary veins. The aorta is sectioned at the level of the ascending segment, just below the origin of the right innominate artery. The pulmonary trunk is sectioned at the level of the bifurcation.

PROCUREMENT, PRESERVATION, AND TRANSPORTATION OF THE DONOR HEART

The procurement, transportation, and insertion of the donor heart must be meticulously organized. This is necessary to minimize the ischemic period, which is measured from the moment when the donor's aorta is clamped to the moment when the recipient's aorta is unclamped and the transplanted heart is directly perfused via the coronary arterial system. The best results are achieved when the ischemic period is 4 hours or less.

The first step in harvesting the donor heart is to divide the superior and inferior venae cavae. The pulmonary veins are transected at the edge of the pericardium and the pulmonary arteries are sectioned distal to the bifurcation. Finally, the aorta is cross-clamped and divided just below the origin of the innominate artery (Fig. 32.1).

Unless the donor and recipient are at the same hospital, it is necessary to bring the donor heart to the recipient. As soon as the donor heart is removed it is placed in a sterile bag containing Ringer's lactate solution which has been chilled to 4°C. The bag containing the donor heart is suspended in stockinette within a large plastic container, which is doubly wrapped with sterile plastic bags and placed within an ice cooler. The procurement team then leaves for the recipient's hospital by the most expeditious route.

Close communication between the surgical teams in both hospitals will minimize the interval between the time when the recipient heart is removed and the time when the donor heart arrives in the operating room. The recipient surgeon is notified when the donor cardiectomy is begun, when the procurement team leaves the donor hospital, and when the procurement team is 10 minutes away from the recipient hospital. Thus informed, the recipient surgeon can determine when to make the incision and when to institute cardiopulmonary bypass.

THE TRANSPLANTATION PROCEDURE

When the donor heart arrives, the ventricular segment of the recipient heart (including the atrioventricular and ventriculoarterial valves and the proximal portions of the great arteries) is removed. The superior and inferior pulmonary veins of the donor heart are sutured to the recipient's left atrium and the venae cavae of the donor heart are sutured to the recipient's right atrium. The aortic and pulmonary arterial anastomoses are then performed (Fig. 32.2). The aortic clamps are then released.

In most instances the transplanted heart begins to beat

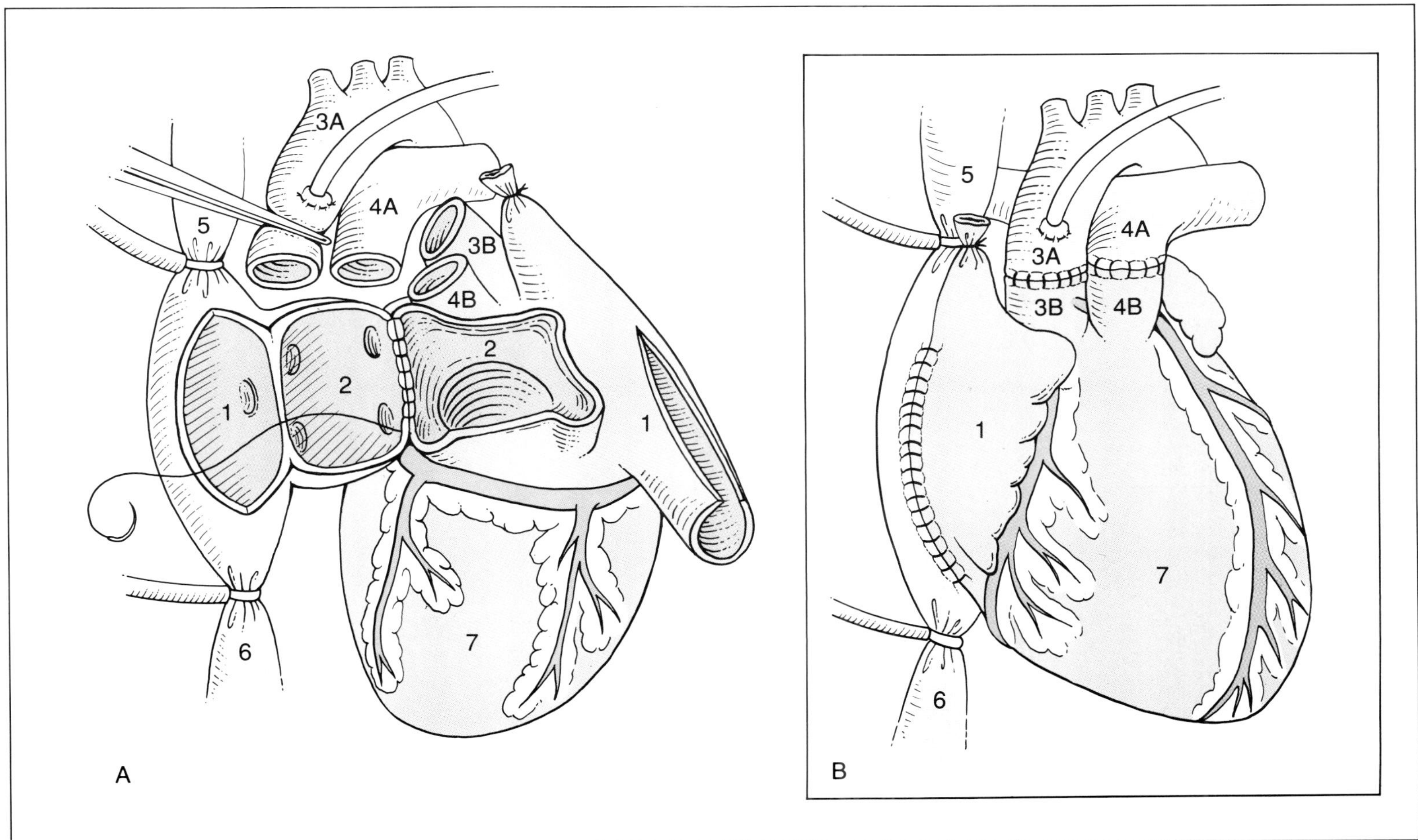

Fig. 32.2 Insertion of the donor heart (orthotopic transplant). (A) The recipient right and left atria are seen en face. A portion of the donor left atrium has been connected to the recipient left atrium. Later, the donor right atrium will be connected to the recipient right atrium. Finally, the aortas and pulmonary trunks will be connected. (B) The completed operation (note the suture lines connecting the donor and recipient aorta and the donor and recipient pulmonary trunk). The bypass cannula has not yet been removed from the recipient aorta.

1	right atrium	**4B**	donor pulmonary trunk
2	left atrium	**5**	superior vena cava
3A	recipient aorta	**6**	inferior vena cava
3B	donor aorta	**7**	ventricular myocardium
4A	recipient pulmonary trunk		

spontaneously when the aortic clamps are released. If it fails to start, it is stimulated mechanically and electrically. If these maneuvers are unsuccessful, the patient remains on cardiopulmonary bypass and a mechanical heart is inserted. The chest is then closed and the patient is taken from the operating room. The mechanical heart remains in place until a new donor heart is available.

In the technique known as heterotopic heart transplantation, which is employed in patients with severe pulmonary hypertension, the native heart is left in situ and the donor heart is surgically connected to the native heart in parallel fashion. In most instances the donor heart is placed in the right hemithorax, with its apex directed anteriorly and to the right. The right atrium and left atrium of the donor heart are connected directly to the corresponding chambers of the native heart. The pulmonary trunks of the native heart and the donor heart are connected via an external conduit. Finally, an end-to-side anastomosis is made between the ascending aorta of the native heart and that of the donor heart (Figs. 32.3 and 32.4).

PRE- AND POSTOPERATIVE CARE

Multidrug immunosuppressive therapy (cyclosporine, prednisone, and dipyramidole or azathioprine) is begun before the insertion of the heterograft and continued for life. [The usual maintenance regimen consists of cyclosporine (10 mg/kg/day), prednisone (0.2 to 0.3 mg/kg/day), and azathioprine (2 to 2.5 mg/kg/day).] Anticoagulants are administered from the second to the fourteenth postoperative day. Chest films are obtained at frequent intervals (daily for the first 7 to 10 days, then every other day) to detect pulmonary infection.

EARLY COMPLICATIONS

PULMONARY INFECTION

Any lung infiltrate is evaluated with appropriate diagnostic tests (eg, sputum culture, bronchoalveolar lavage, bronchoscopic biopsy, percutaneous needle biopsy). Viruses are responsible for about two thirds of postoperative lung infections; bacterial, fungal, and protozoan infections account for the rest. Bacterial infections (usually caused by gram-positive cocci) typically occur early in the postoperative period. Infections caused by viruses (eg, cytomegalovirus, *Herpes simplex*, *Varicella zoster*) and opportunistic fungi (eg, aspergillus, candida) predominate later on. Once a pulmonary infection has been identified, aggressive antimicrobial therapy is begun.

HYPERACUTE AND ACUTE REJECTION

Rejection of the heterograft is one of the most serious complications of cardiac transplantation; it is the major cause of postoperative morbidity and mortality. Rejection may be either hyperacute or acute.

Hyperacute rejection, which occurs in the first few hours after transplantation, is usually caused by ABO incompatibility or by lymphotoxic antibodies in the heterograft. Histologically, there is endothelial injury and intravascular thrombosis, with ischemic damage of variable degree. Hemodynamic studies reveal rapidly deteriorating systolic function. The clinical picture is that of intractable congestive heart failure, usually leading to death.

Acute rejection, a cellular phenomenon, is far more common than hyperacute rejection. The clinical manifestations of acute rejection typically appear 10 to 14 days after surgery. Although

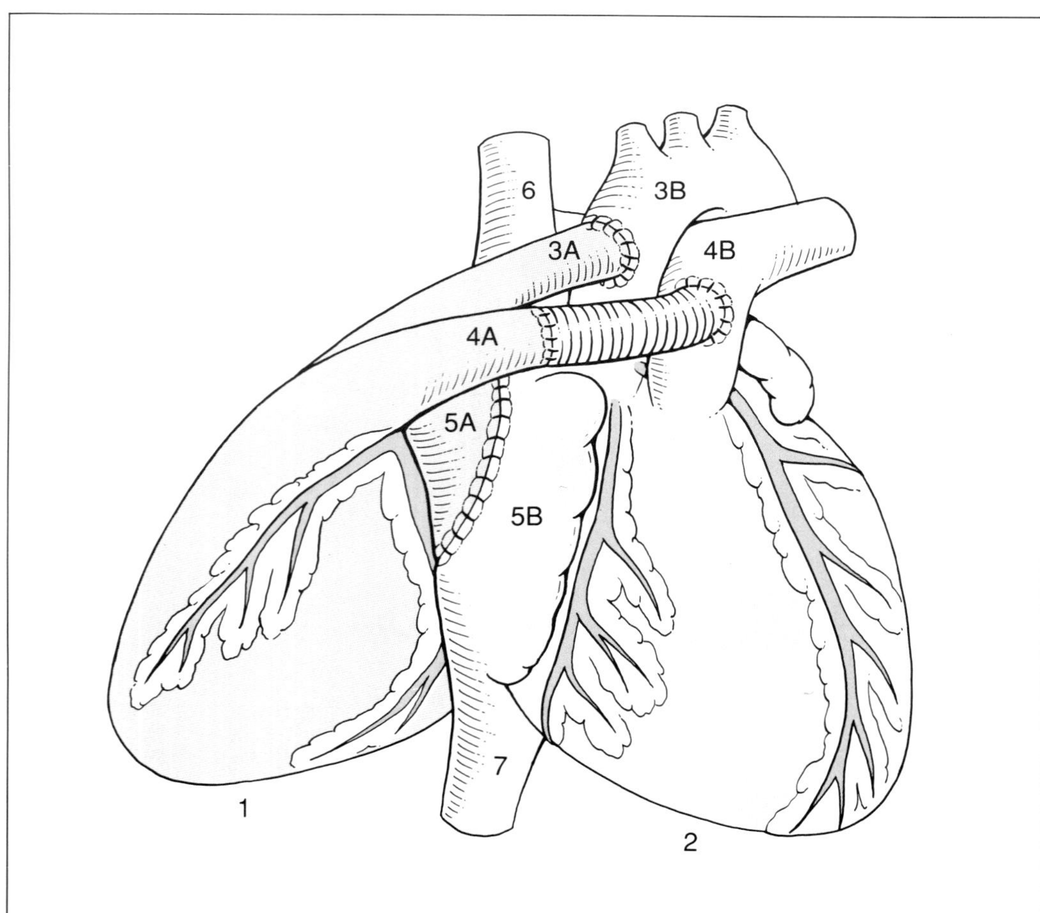

Fig. 32.3 Heterotopic cardiac transplantation. The completed procedure as viewed from the anterior aspect. The right atrium of the native heart is connected to the right atrium of the donor heart; the donor left atrium and native left atrium are connected in similar fashion. The pulmonary trunk of the donor heart is connected to the native pulmonary trunk by means of a conduit. A second conduit connects the ascending aorta of the donor heart with the native ascending aorta.

1	donor heart	5A	donor right atrium
2	native heart	5B	native right atrium
3A	donor ascending aorta	6	native superior vena cava
3B	native ascending aorta	7	native inferior vena cava
4A	donor pulmonary trunk		
4B	native pulmonary trunk		

acute rejection can occur at any time after surgery, the risk is greatest during the first 2 postoperative months. Signs and symptoms include fever, anxiety, lethargy, low back pain, atrial or ventricular arrhythmias, gallop rhythm, pericardial rub, and jugular venous distension. The ECG findings are nonspecific. The most reliable laboratory test is cytoimmunologic monitoring of the peripheral lymphocyte populations and their precursors, which has a sensitivity of 80 percent and a specificity of 80 percent in the diagnosis of early rejection. The diagnosis of acute rejection is confirmed by transcatheter endocardial biopsy. The severity of the rejection process is graded as mild, moderate, or severe according to histologic criteria (Fig. 32.5).

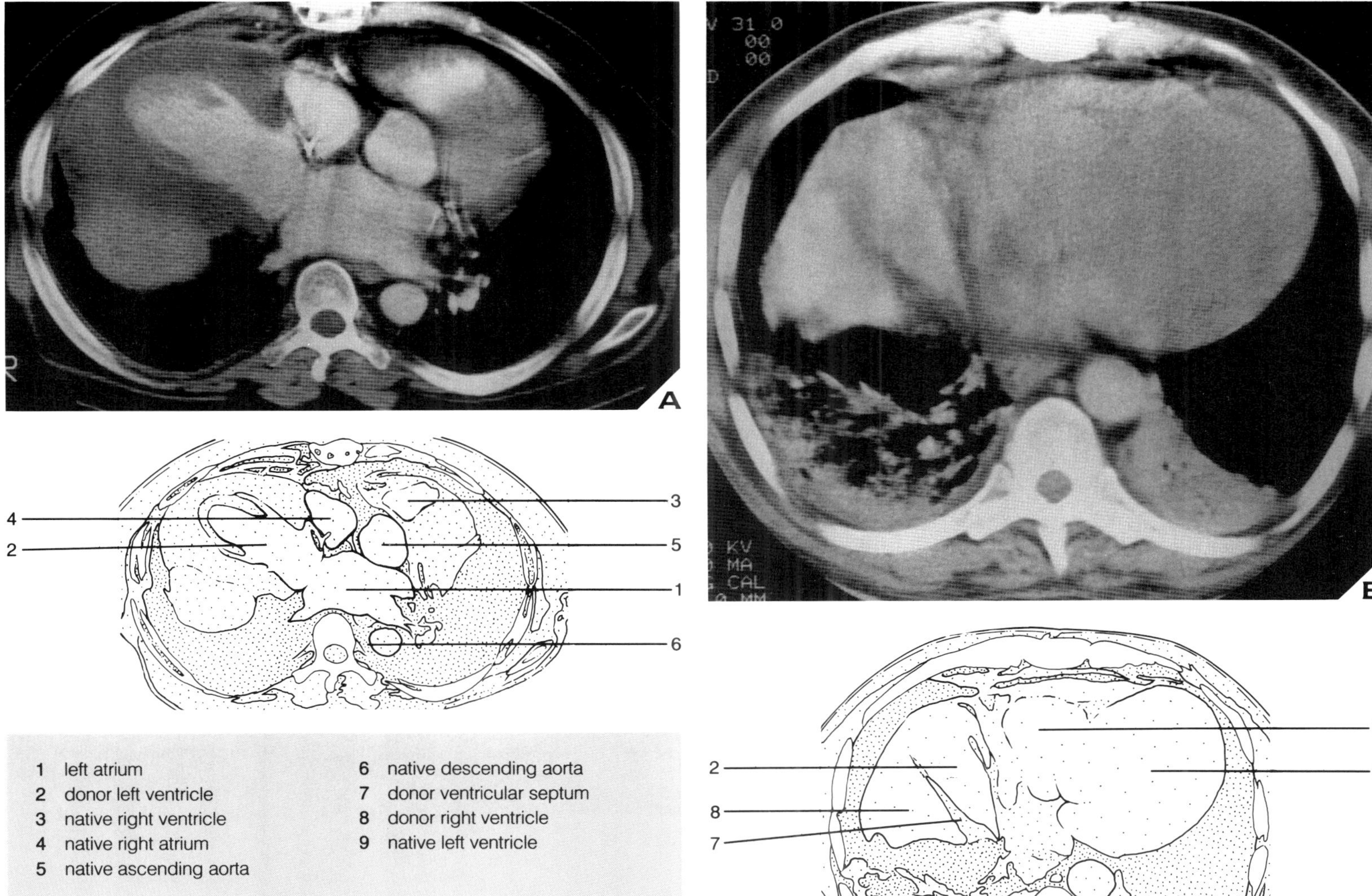

1	left atrium	6	native descending aorta
2	donor left ventricle	7	donor ventricular septum
3	native right ventricle	8	donor right ventricle
4	native right atrium	9	native left ventricle
5	native ascending aorta		

Fig. 32.4 Heterotopic cardiac transplant. (A, B) Contrast-enhanced CT scans. (A) Section at the level of the right atrium demonstrates the common left atrium constructed from the donor and native left atria, the donor left ventricle, and a portion of the native right atrium. Only a small portion of the native right ventricle is included in this section. (B) Section at the level of the ventricles shows the opacified donor right and left ventricles. There is segmental atelectasis in both lower lobes.

FIG. 32.5 HISTOLOGIC CLASSIFICATION OF SEVERITY OF REJECTION ACCORDING TO FINDINGS ON ENDOCARDIAL BIOPSY

Severity	Criteria
Mild	Few perivascular small lymphocytes.
Moderate	More intense; cellular infiltrate extending into interstitium.
Severe	Heavy cellular infiltrate; focal or diffuse myonecrosis, vasculitis with hemorrhage.

Fig. 32.5 Histologic classification of severity of rejection according to findings on endocardial biopsy.

The clinical manifestations tend to appear relatively late, often long after evidence of rejection is evident histologically. Because acute rejection is most effectively managed when treatment is begun in its incipient phase, transcatheter endocardial biopsies are routinely obtained at frequent intervals, beginning on the fifth postoperative day. Subsequently, endocardial biopsies are obtained every 7 days for the first 3 postoperative weeks, every other week for the next 6 weeks, and every 3 or 4 months thereafter.

OTHER COMPLICATIONS

Less common complications of the early postoperative period include hemorrhage at the operative site, accelerated systemic hypertension, and urinary tract infection.

LATE COMPLICATIONS

Ninety percent of rejection episodes occur during the first year after heart transplantation. However, it is clear from immunologic studies of long-term survivors that long-term immunosuppression is necessary to prevent fatal acute rejection episodes, which may occur years after transplantation surgery. Other problems encountered in long-term recipients include accelerated obstructive coronary artery disease in the donor heart secondary to proliferative arteriopathy ("graft arteriosclerosis") and the development of neoplastic disease.

CORONARY ARTERY DISEASE

Coronary artery obstruction of varying severity occurs in 40 percent of transplant recipients who survive 5 years or longer. Obstructive coronary artery disease in transplant recipients is of two distinct pathologic types: atherosclerotic and proliferative. The former, which may progress to complete occlusion of the affected vessels, is similar to the atherosclerotic process observed in native hearts. However, the latter lesion, which often leads to rapidly progressive coronary artery stenosis, is uniquely associated with the transplanted heart.

Microscopically, proliferative arteriopathy is characterized by subintimal cell proliferation. The disease process tends to be diffusely distributed throughout the affected vessels. There is a distinct predilection for small epicardial arteries, which may be markedly narrowed or obliterated. Not infrequently the arteriopathy extends proximally to involve major branches of the coronary arterial tree. Rarely, intramyocardial branches are affected.

The pathogenesis of transplant-related proliferative arteriopathy ("graft arteriosclerosis") is believed to be an immunologically mediated injury of the intima, which results in complement and platelet activation and the release of mitogenic factors. (There is no convincing evidence that it is caused by rejection.) The resulting neointimal thickening may cause severe narrowing of the affected vessels, leading to ischemic heart disease. Proliferative arteriopathy is the usual cause of accelerated coronary artery disease in transplant recipients. It commonly leads to severe ischemic heart disease and/or myocardial infarction. Acute myocardial infarction secondary to occlusion of intramyocardial branches can occur in patients with normal epicardial arteries.

Proliferative arteriopathy tends to occur more frequently in patients in whom coronary artery disease was the cause of heart

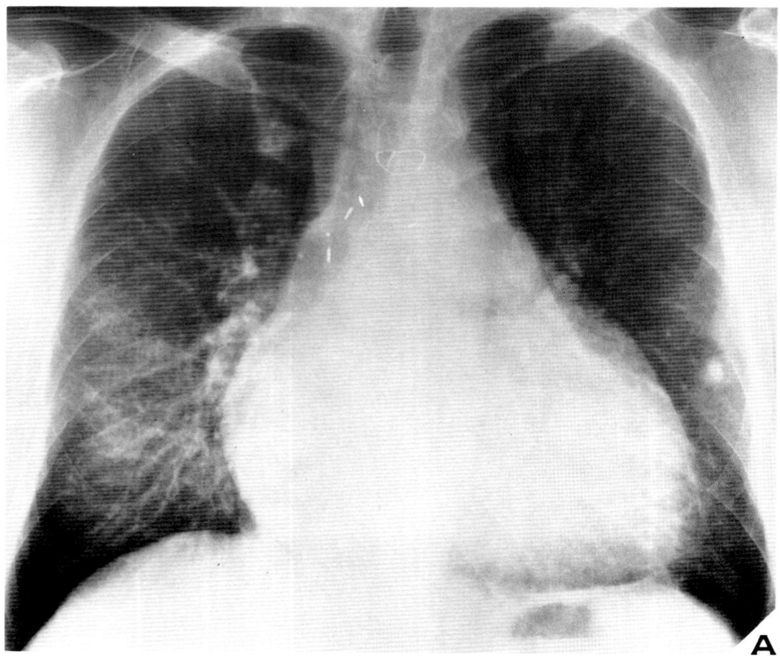

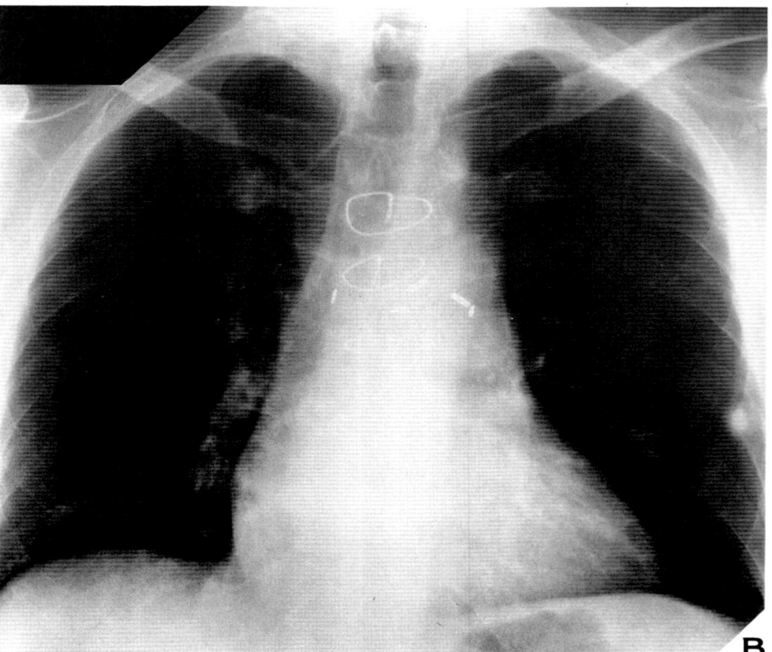

Fig. 32.6 Successful orthotopic cardiac transplant. (A) Preoperative chest film shows cardiomegaly with left ventricular and left atrial enlargement and pulmonary venous hypertension (note cephalization pattern). (B) Two months after cardiac transplantation the donor heart is of normal size. There is slight right atrial enlargement. The left ventricle, aortic arch, pulmonary trunk, and superior vena caval contour are normal. The pulmonary vasculature is normal.

failure than in those in whom it was due to cardiomyopathy. It is also more frequent when the donor was over 35 years of age. There is no significant correlation with the age, family history, lipid profile, or blood glucose level of the recipient.

Patients with ischemic heart disease secondary to proliferative arteriopathy typically present with congestive heart failure resulting from impaired myocardial contractility or with signs and symptoms of acute myocardial infarction. Because the donor heart is denervated, chest pain is uncommon.

Follow-up care of transplant recipients must include routine annual coronary arteriography, which is necessary to detect accelerated coronary arteriosclerosis in its earliest stages. Retransplantation is the only treatment option for patients with extensive, severe involvement of intramyocardial arteries; however, coronary bypass surgery may suffice in patients with occlusion of large epicardial coronary arteries.

NEOPLASTIC DISEASE

Various types of neoplastic disease occur with greatly increased frequency in heart transplant recipients. B-cell lymphoma is the most common, occurring at a frequency 34-fold greater than in the general population. Other reported neoplasms include skin cancer (squamous cell and basal cell carcinoma), myelogenous leukemia, and adenocarcinoma of the colon with liver metastases. The incidence of malignant disease in transplant recipients is 3 percent after 1 year and 25 percent after 5 years. Risk factors for post-transplant lymphoma include idiopathic cardiomyopathy, age at transplantation less than 40 years, and retransplantation.

Malignancy is the cause of death in 1 to 2 percent of heart transplant recipients. Early diagnosis is essential for prolonging survival.

CORONARY–RIGHT VENTRICULAR FISTULA

Coronary–right ventricular fistulas, which represent iatrogenic connections produced at the time of endocardial biopsy, are not uncommon in transplant recipients and are readily demonstrated by selective coronary arteriography (see Fig. 21.62). Such fistulas are too small to cause significant right ventricular overload and are well tolerated; therefore, surgical correction is unnecessary.

IMAGING AND INVASIVE DIAGNOSIS

PLAIN FILMS

Postoperative chest films typically demonstrate prominence of the right atrial contour, which represents the large composite right atrium created by joining the right atria of the donor and recipient hearts (Fig. 32.6). In the early postoperative period, the cardiothoracic ratio may be significantly increased owing to the presence of pericardial fluid. Relatively large accumulations of pericardial fluid are quite common owing to the disparity in size between the donor heart and the recipient's pericardial sac (Fig. 32.7). Occasionally a large postoperative pericardial effusion may result from obliteration of the pericardial window or obstruction of the drains. Cardiac tamponade can occur in such cases.

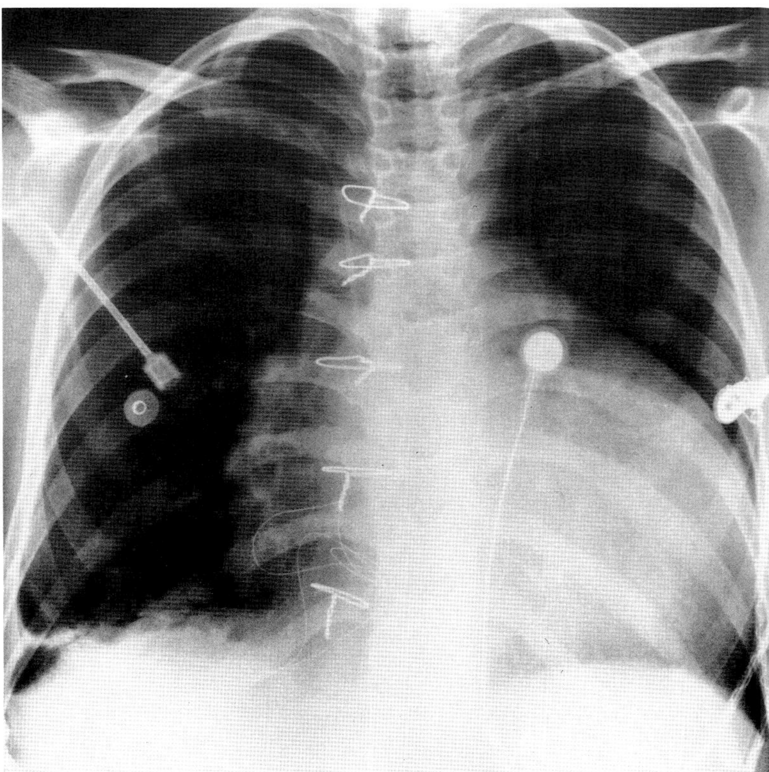

Fig. 32.7 Large postoperative pericardial effusion. Ten days after cardiac transplantation the cardiac silhouette is enlarged. The contours do not correspond to the normal configuration of the heart. There is a significant accumulation of fluid in the pericardial space owing to the discrepancy between the normal-sized donor heart and the enlarged recipient pericardium.

Myocardial edema secondary to acute rejection can cause significant cardiac enlargement; however, cardiomegaly is a late manifestation. The appearance of a new lung infiltrate in the second postoperative week or later usually signals an opportunistic infection and warrants an aggressive diagnostic approach (Fig. 32.8). The appearance of mediastinal widening or lymphadenopathy after the first postoperative year is suggestive of a lymphoproliferative disorder (Fig. 32.9).

Long-term corticosteroid administration frequently leads to the deposition of large amounts of mediastinal, epicardial, and intrapericardial fat, an appearance that can simulate enlargement of the cardiovascular silhouette or a mediastinal disease process. CT or MRI can be performed to exclude cardiac or mediastinal pathology in such cases (see below).

ECHOCARDIOGRAPHY

The postoperative morphologic alterations are clearly shown by echocardiography. After an uncomplicated cardiac transplantation, both atria are larger than normal. The posterior atrial wall and adjacent pericardium are usually thick, producing a radiographic appearance that can be mistaken for tumor or hemorrhage. Localized or generalized pericardial thickening, as well as loculated pericardial effusions and pericardial tamponade, are clearly depicted by echocardiography, particularly when a transesophageal approach is employed.

Functional changes associated with early rejection can be detected by echocardiography before clinical manifestations appear. Left ventricular dilatation and mitral insufficiency are suggestive of rejection (Fig. 32.10, Appendix). Left ventricular isovolumic relaxation time, a parameter that reflects increased diastolic stiffness and correlates with elevation of the end diastolic pressure, is prolonged in hearts undergoing rejection. Left ventricular mass and left ventricular wall thickness are also increased in such cases. The ability of cyclosporine to prevent and suppress rejection episodes is clearly demonstrated by echocardiography.

COMPUTED TOMOGRAPHY

CT clearly depicts the morphology of the donor heart and its connections with recipient structures (see Fig. 32.4). Pericardial, mediastinal, and pulmonary pathology (eg, accumulations of fluid and other material in the pericardial space, lymphomatous infiltration, lymphadenopathy), as well as accumulations of fat simulating disease, are clearly demonstrated by CT (Figs. 32.11 and 32.12).

MAGNETIC RESONANCE IMAGING

The internal structure of the donor heart and its connections with the recipient heart are clearly shown in spin–echo images; function can be evaluated by cine MRI (Fig. 32.13). A major

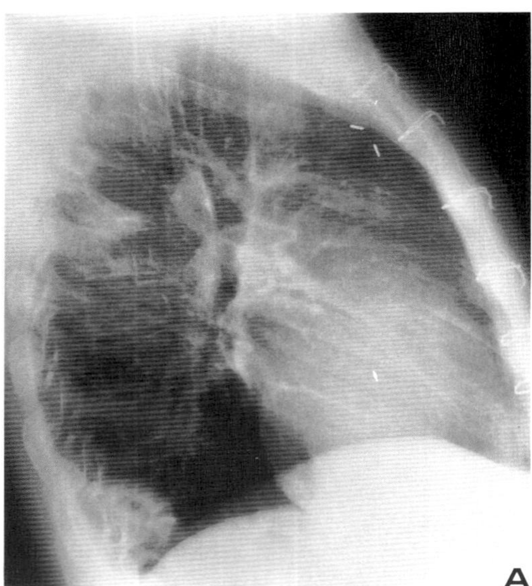

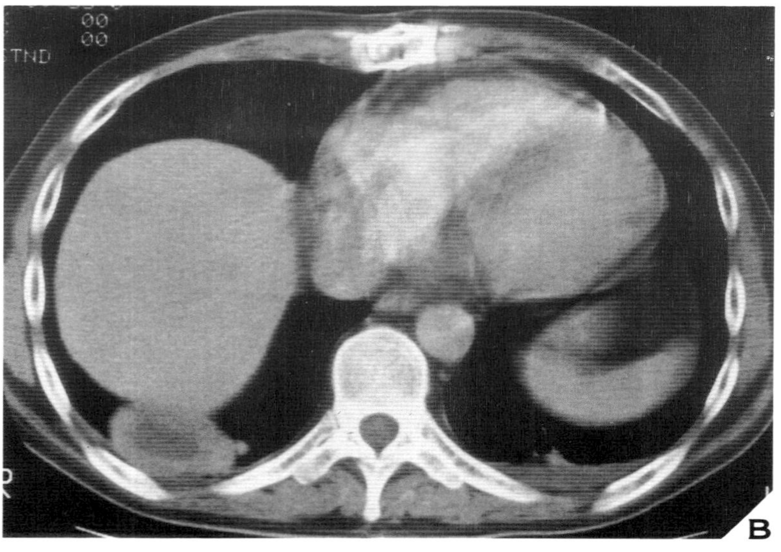

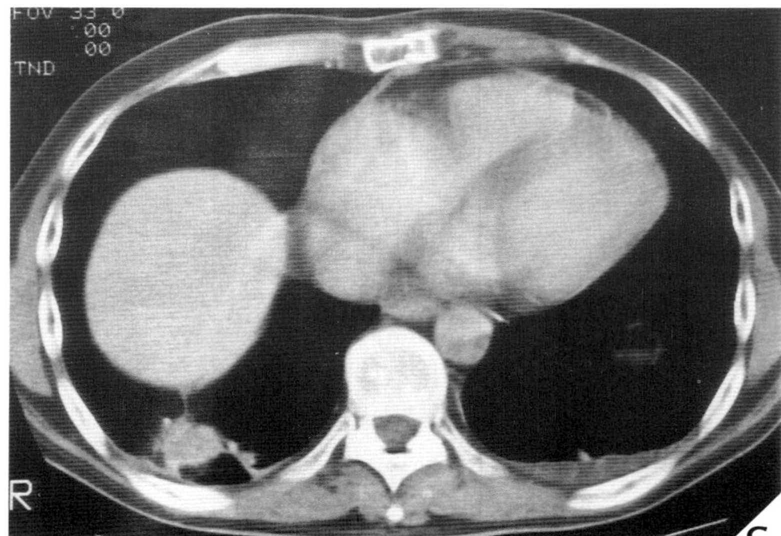

Fig. 32.8 Opportunistic lung infection (aspergillosis) after cardiac transplantation. (A) Lateral chest film obtained 6 months after cardiac transplantation shows a rounded density in the right posterior costophrenic sulcus. (B ,C) CT scans demonstrate a discrete mass adjacent to the pleural surface, with localized pleural thickening. Note decreased attenuation (B, C) and cavitation (C) within the mass. Open lung biopsy revealed an aspergilloma.

advantage of MRI over CT is its ability to detect both acute and chronic ischemia. Spin–echo images demonstrate increased signal intensity in transplant recipients with ischemic myocardium secondary to proliferative arteriopathy or coronary atherosclerosis; the findings are similar to those seen in an ischemic native heart (see Chapter 4).

At present, MRI does not play a role in the diagnosis of rejection. During the early stage of rejection the myocardial signal is not significantly altered. MRI has been reported to show increased myocardial thickness in hearts undergoing rejection; however, this finding is not sufficiently sensitive or specific to warrant the routine use of MRI to detect early rejection. Whether MR spectroscopy can identify metabolic changes that denote early rejection remains to be seen.

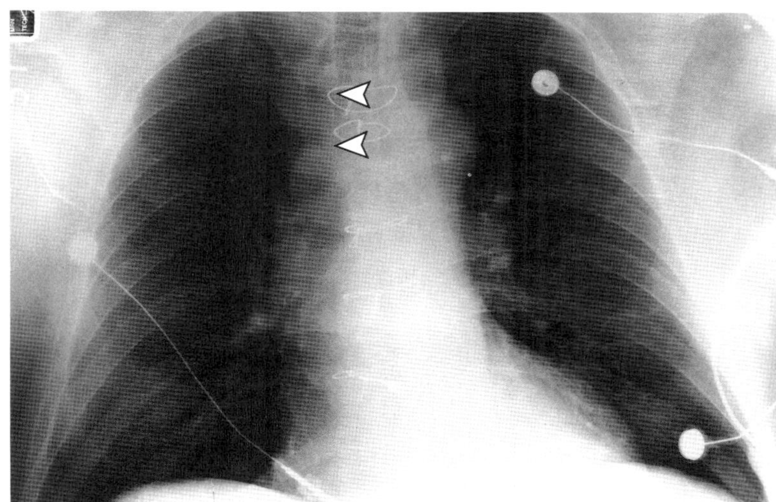

Fig. 32.9 Lymphoproliferative disease (B-cell lymphoma) after cardiac transplantation. Frontal chest film obtained 5 years after transplant demonstrates widening of the upper mediastinum. Note nodularity (*arrows*) of the mediastinal contour, which was not evident on previous chest films. A biopsy revealed B-cell lymphoma.

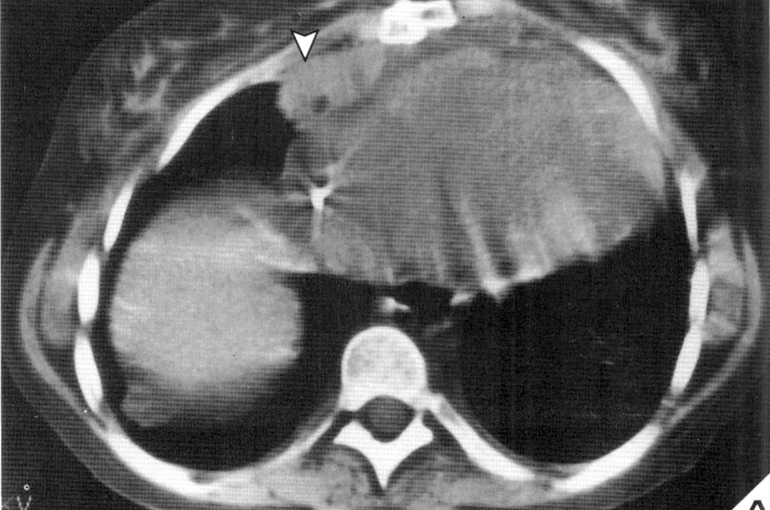

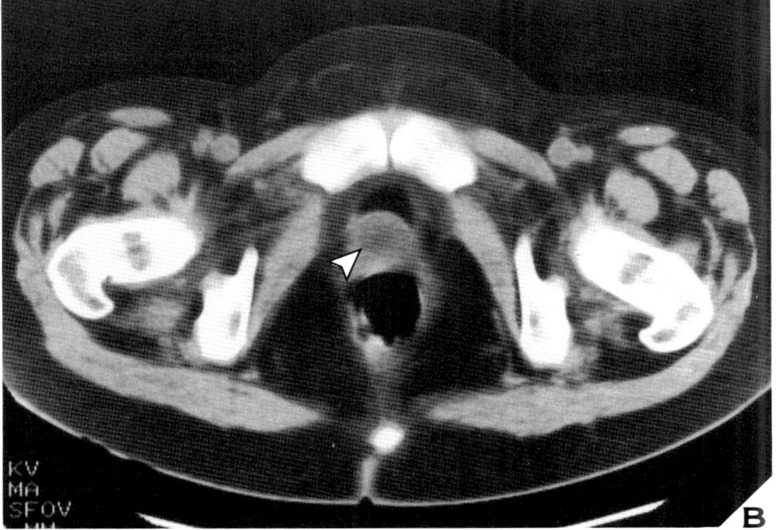

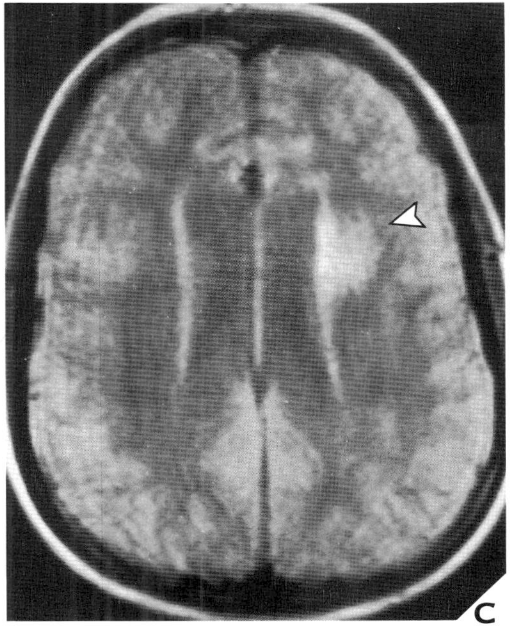

Fig. 32.11 Lymphoproliferative disorder (B-cell lymphoma) after cardiac transplantation. (A) Contrast-enhanced CT scan at the level of the heart demonstrates an intrapericardial mass (*arrow*) adjacent to the anterolateral wall of the right ventricle. There is a small pericardial effusion. (B) CT scan at the level of the pelvic outlet demonstrates a soft tissue mass (*arrow*) between the rectum and the bladder. (Air has been introduced into the bladder.) There were other masses in the bowel wall and retroperitoneum. (C) MRI of brain (TR 2500 millisec, TE 30 millisec) demonstrates an area of increased signal without mass effect (*arrow*) adjacent to the left lateral ventricle.

NUCLEAR MEDICINE

Nuclear ventriculography can be used to evaluate the morphology and function of the donor heart. Right and left ventricular size and function are accurately assessed with this technique (Fig. 32.14, Appendix). Evidence of both systolic and diastolic dysfunction (eg, decreased ejection fraction, increased duration of maximum filling) have been observed in otherwise normal left ventricles.

Myocardial uptake and clearance of ^{201}Tl (thallium) are normal in patients with normally functioning transplants; abnormal patterns characteristic of myocardial ischemia or infarction are seen in patients with obstructive coronary artery disease (see Chapters 4A and 20).

Various scintigraphic techniques have been used in an effort to detect acute rejection, with varying degrees of success. In general, thallium uptake and clearance are normal in patients

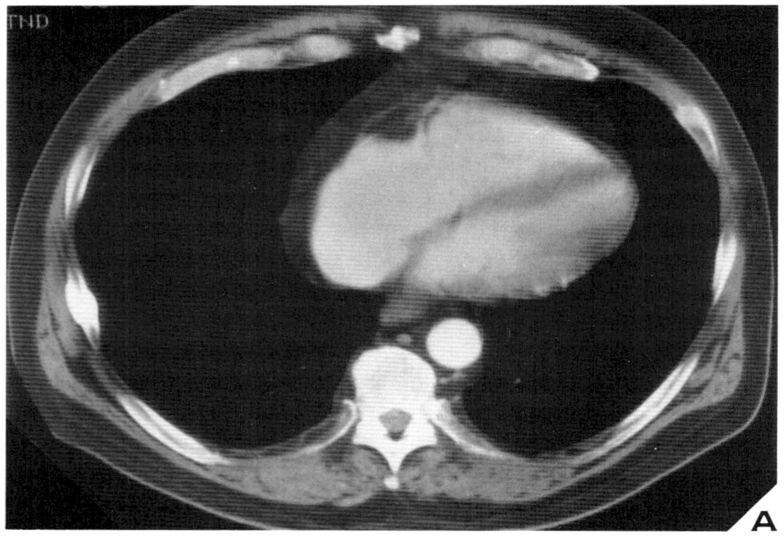

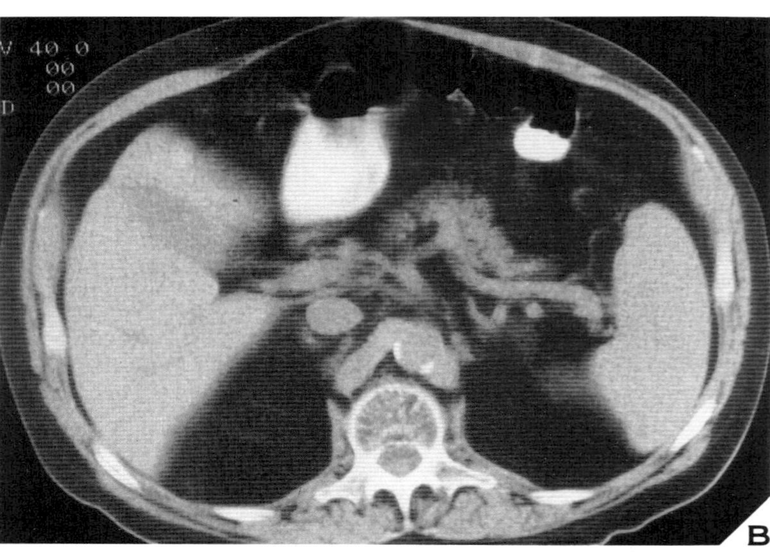

Fig. 32.12 Fat accumulation after cardiac transplantation. (A) Contrast-enhanced CT at the level of the heart demonstrates a large amount of epicardial fat anterior and lateral to the heart which displaces the fibrous pericardium posteriorly. (B) Unenhanced CT scan at the level of the celiac axis. The vessels supplying the spleen and pancreas are exquisitely outlined by the large amount of extraperitoneal fat. Note the large fat collections medial to the liver and spleen.

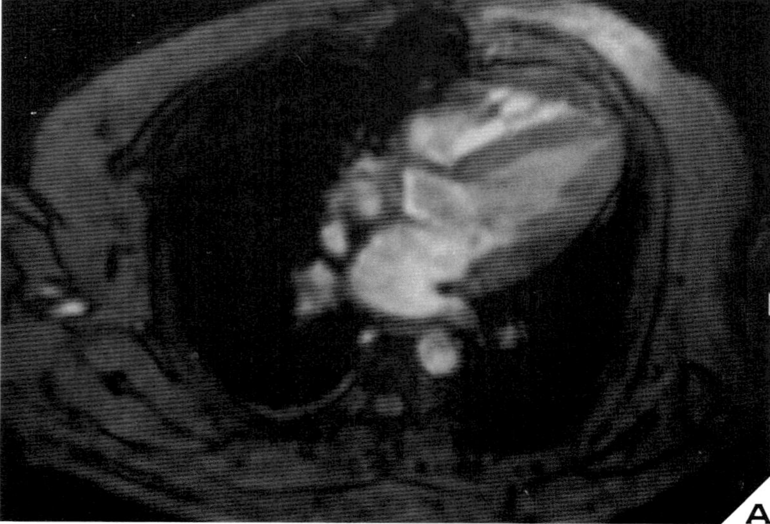

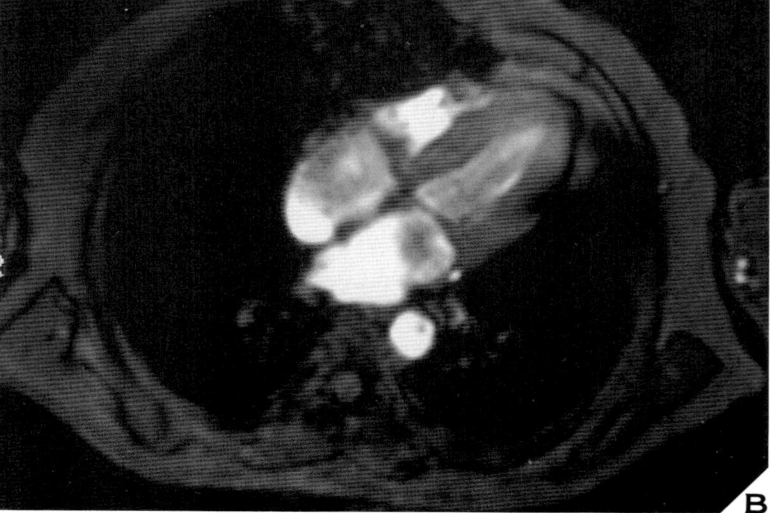

Fig. 32.13 Successful cardiac transplant (MRI findings). Cine MRI (TR 500 millisec, TE 13 millisec, flip angle 45°) in LAO projection in (A) systole and (B) diastole demonstrates normal left ventricular function and normally functioning atrioventricular valves. The deformity of the left atrial contour represents the suture line between the donor left atrium and recipient left atrium.

undergoing acute rejection. Nuclear ventriculography demonstrates impaired diastolic function of the left ventricle in hearts undergoing rejection; however, this and other functional parameters are better assessed by echocardiography. The most reliable scintigraphic test for rejection employs the ^{111}In-labeled F(ab) fragment of murine monoclonal anti-myosin (see also Chapters 4A and 20); myocardium undergoing rejection is very avid for this antibody. Published data indicate that the F(ab) technique is highly sensitive for acute rejection, with no false negatives reported thus far.

CORONARY ARTERIOGRAPHY AND LEFT VENTRICULOGRAPHY

Coronary artery obstruction, a relatively frequent complication of cardiac transplantation, is best evaluated by means of selective coronary arteriography. As noted earlier, stenosis due to atherosclerosis and proliferative arteriopathy ("graft arteriosclerosis") are both encountered in the transplanted heart.

Obstructing lesions angiographically indistinguishable from those caused by atheromatous plaque in the usual type of coronary atherosclerosis are not uncommon. In the transplanted heart, coronary atherosclerosis characteristically involves the proximal segments of the major coronary arteries. As in native hearts, stenotic lesions caused by coronary atherosclerosis are typically eccentric, with marginal irregularities, and may progress to complete occlusion.

In patients with proliferative arteriopathy, a lesion uniquely associated with transplanted hearts, coronary arteriography demonstrates concentric narrowing with minimal marginal irregularity. There is usually a gradual transition between the affected segment and the adjacent normal segment. The stenosis typically involves a long segment or an entire vessel (Fig. 32.15). Small epicardial branches are frequently occluded. When major epicardial arteries are affected, there is a predilection for their distal segments. The angiographic diagnosis of proliferative arteriopathy is straightforward when major coronary arteries are affected; however, unless one takes pains to review the patient's previous coronary angiograms, it is easy to overlook occlusion of small epicardial arteries, which may not be well-opacified even in normal individuals (Fig. 32.16).

Left ventriculography is seldom employed to evaluate heart transplants, since key parameters of myocardial function (eg, left ventricular relaxation and contractility) can be assessed by noninvasive modalities such as echocardiography or MRI (see Fig. 32.10, Appendix, and Fig. 32.13).

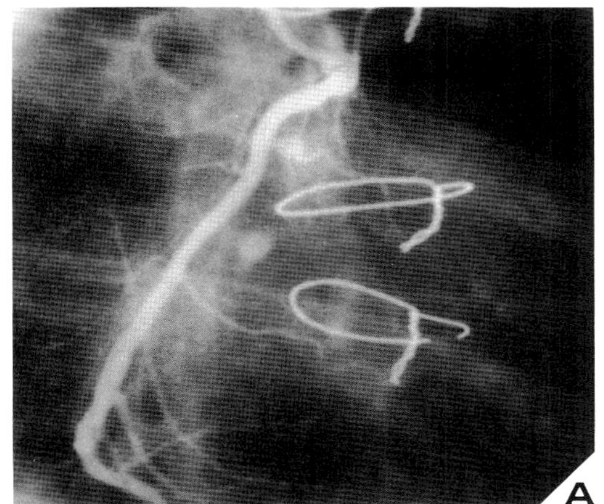

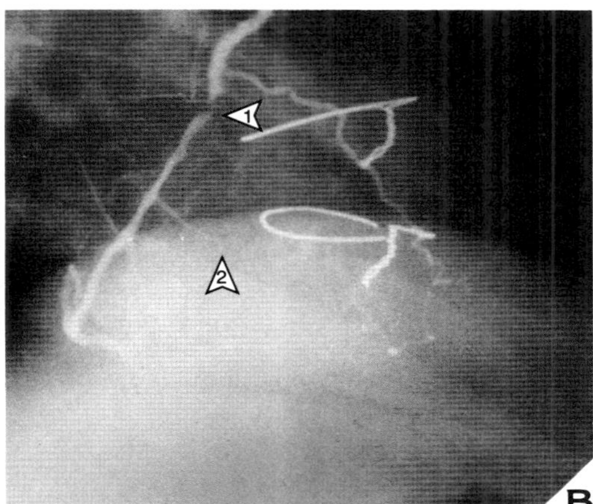

Fig. 32.15 Accelerated arteriosclerosis of coronary arteries secondary to proliferative arteriopathy ("graft arteriosclerosis"). (A ,B) Selective right coronary arteriograms (RAO projection). (A) One year after cardiac transplantation the right coronary artery is normal. (B) Four years after cardiac transplantation. There is narrowing of the middle and distal segments of the right coronary artery, with a single area of severe (95 percent) stenosis (*arrow* 1). The middle portion of the second marginal artery is also occluded (*arrow* 2).

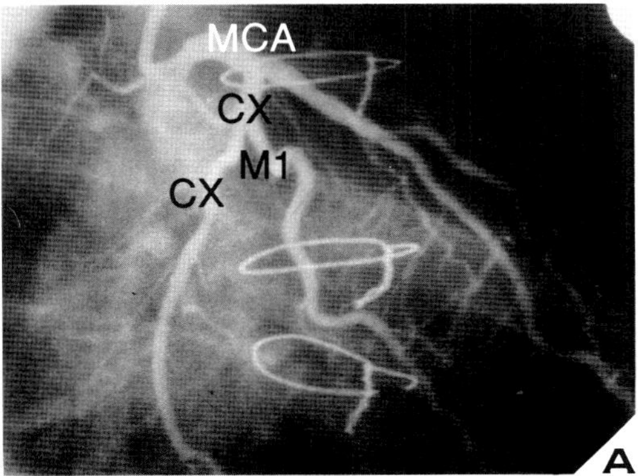

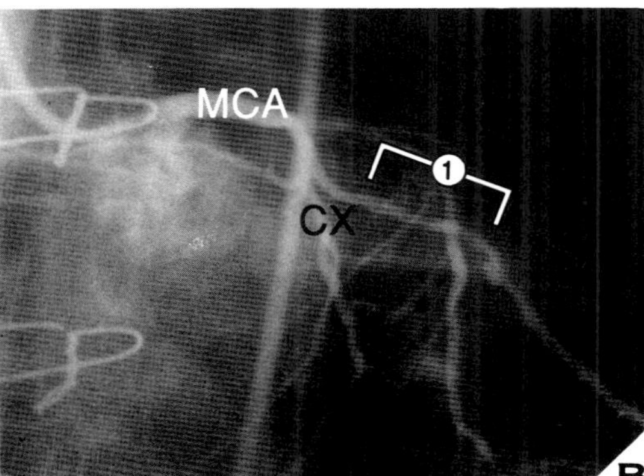

Fig. 32.16 Accelerated arteriosclerosis of coronary arteries secondary to proliferative arteriopathy ("graft arteriosclerosis"). Same patient as in Figs. 32.14 and 32.15. (A) Two years after heart transplantation. Selective left coronary arteriogram (RAO projection). One year after cardiac transplantation the left anterior descending artery, the circumflex (CX) artery, and the first marginal (M1) artery are normal. (B) Four years after cardiac transplantation. Selective left coronary arteriogram (RAO-Cr projection) demonstrates diffuse narrowing of the middle segment of the LAD, with one area of severe (90 percent) stenosis. The proximal portion of the first marginal artery is diffusely narrowed (up to 50 percent stenosis) with irregular borders (*brace* 1). Re-transplantation was performed shortly afterward. (MCA = left main coronary artery)

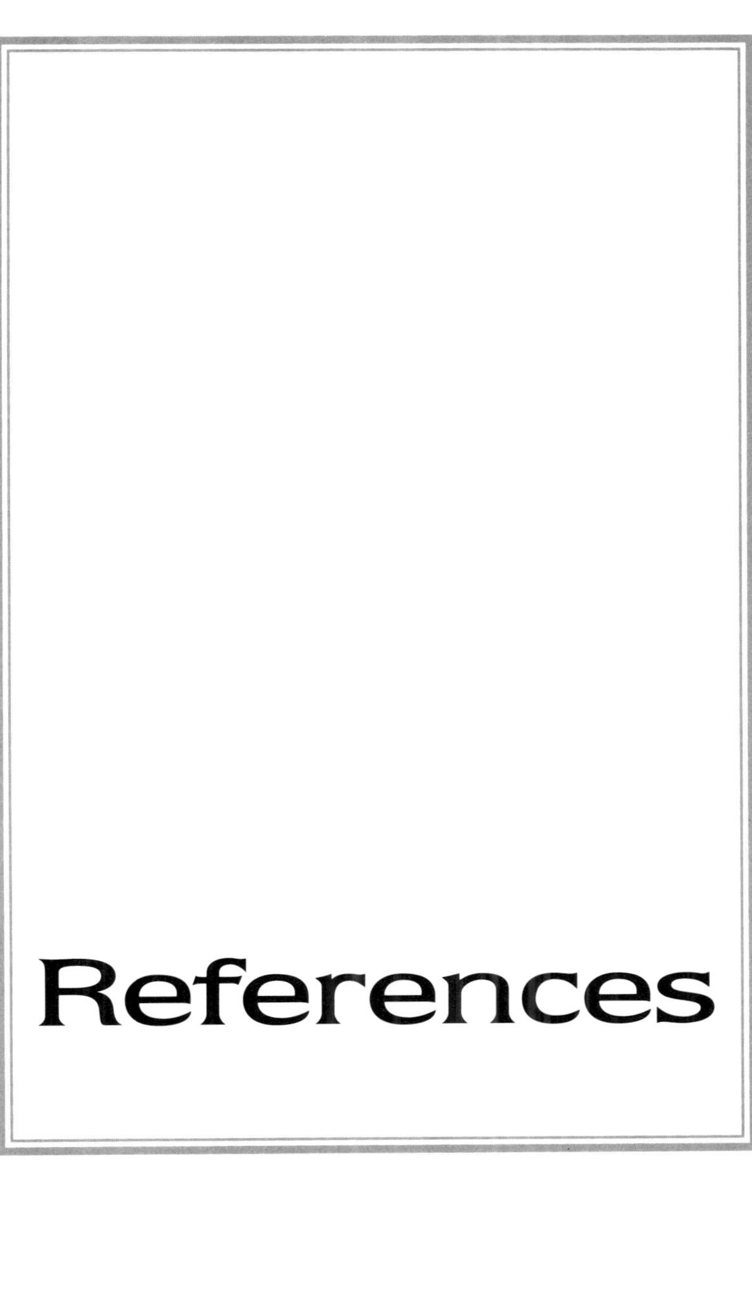

References

GENERAL REFERENCES

Amplatz K, Moller JH, Castaneda WR: *Radiology of Congenital Heart Disease.* New York: Thieme Medical Publishers, Inc, 1986.

Braunwald E: *Heart Disease. A Textbook of Cardiovascular Medicine.* 3rd ed. Philadelphia: WB Saunders Co., 1988.

Gillette PC: Cardiac dysrhythmias in infants and children. In Allen Engle MA, ed. *Pediatric Cardiovascular Disease.* Philadelphia: FA Davis, 1981:79.

Doyle EF, Engle MA, Gersony WM, Rashkind WJ, Talner NS, Eds: *Pediatric Cardiology.* New York: Springer-Verlag, 1985.

Jefferson K, Rees S: *Clinical Cardiac Radiology.* 2nd ed. London: Butterworths, 1980.

Kassner EG, ed: *Iatrogenic Disorders of the Fetus, Infant, and Child.* New York: Springer-Verlag, 1985.

Kirklin JW, Barratt–Boyes B: *Cardiac Surgery.* New York: John Wiley & Son, 1986.

Moss AF, Adams FM, Emmanoulides GS, eds: *Heart Disease in Infants, Children and Adolescents.* Baltimore: Williams & Wilkins, 1977.

Rowe RD, Freedom RM, Mehrizi A, eds: *The Neonate with Congenital Heart Disease.* 2nd ed. Philadelphia: WB Saunders, 1981.

Soto B, Pacifico AD: *Angiocardiography in Congenital Heart Malformations.* New York: Futura Publishing, 1990.

Spindola–Franco H, Fish BG: *Radiology of the Heart: Cardiac Imaging in Infants, Children and Adults.* New York: Springer-Verlag, 1985.

CHAPTER REFERENCES

CHAPTER 1: NONINVASIVE RADIOLOGIC TECHNIQUES AND ELECTROCARDIOGRAPHY

CHEST RADIOGRAPHY, FLUOROSCOPY, COMPUTED TOMOGRAPHY

Eldredge WJ, Flicker S: Evaluation of congenital heart disease using cine-CT. *Am J Cardiac Imag* 1987; 1:38.

Jefferson K: *Clinical Cardiac Radiology.* London: Butterworths, 1970.

Joseph PM, Berdon WE; Baker DH, et al: Upper airway obstruction in infants and small children. *Radiology* 1976; 121:143.

Lipton MJ: Quantitation of cardiac function. *Radiol Clin No Am* 1985; 23:613.

Sethna DH, Bateman TM, Whiting JS, Forrester JS: Comprehensive and quantitative cardiac assessment using cine-CT: Description of a new clinical diagnostic modality. *Am J Cardiac Imag* 1987; 1:18.

ELECTROCARDIOGRAPHY

Anderson RH, Ho SY, Becker AE: The clinical anatomy of cardiac conduction system. In Rowlands DJ, ed. *Recent Advances in Cardiology.* New York: Churchill Livingstone, 1984: 1.

Bigger JT: Mechanisms and diagnosis of arrhythmias. In Brunwald E, ed. *Heart Disease.* Philadelphia: WB Saunders, 1980: 630.

Chou TC: *Electrocardiolography in Clinical Practice.* 2nd ed. Baltimore: Williams & Wilkins, 1983.

Fisch CH: Electrocardiography and vectorcardiography. In Brunwald E, ed. *Heart Diseases.* 3rd ed. Philadelphia: WB Saunders, 1988:180.

Gillette PC: Cardiac dysrhythmia in infants and children. In Allen Engle MA, ed. *Pediatric Cardiovascular Disease.* Philadelphia: FA Davis, 1981: 79.

Marriott H: *Practical Electrocardiography.* 8th ed. Baltimore: Williams & Wilkins, 1988.

Myerburg R, Castellanos A: Cardiac arrest and sudden cardiac death. In Brunwald E, ed. *Heart Disease.* 3rd ed. Philadelphia: WB Saunders, 1988:742.

Zipes DP, Jalife J: *Cardiac Electrophysiology from Cell to Bedside.* Philadelphia: WB Saunders, 1990.

CHAPTER 2: ECHOCARDIOGRAPHY

Anderson RH, Macartney FJ, Shinebourne EA, et al: *Pediatric Cardiology.* New York: Churchill Livingstone, 1987: 65.

Feigenbaum H: *Echocardiography.* 4th ed. Philadelphia: Lea & Febiger, 1986.

Hatle L, Angelsen B: *Doppler Ultrasound in Cardiology.* Philadelphia: Lea & Febiger, 1985.

Helmcke F, Nanda NC, Hsiung MC, et al: Color Doppler assessment of mitral regurgitation with orthogonal planes. *Circulation* 1987; 75:175.

Nanda NC: *Atlas of Color Doppler Echocardiography.* Philadelphia: Lea & Febiger, 1989.

Nanda NC: Congenital heart disease. In Nanda NC, ed.: *Atlas of Color Doppler Echocardiography.* Philadelphia: Lea & Febiger, 1989.

Nanda NC: *Textbook of Color Doppler Echocardiography.* Philadelphia: Lea & Febiger, 1989.

Nishimura RA, Miller FA, Callahan MJ, et al: Doppler echocardiography: Theory, instrumentation, technique, and application. *Mayo Clin Proc* 1985; 60:321.

Omoto R: *Color Atlas of Real Time Two-dimensional Doppler Echocardiography.* Tokyo: Shindan-To-Chiryo, 1984.

Perry GJ, Helmcke F, Nanda NC, et al: Evaluation of aortic insufficiency by Doppler color flow mapping. *J Am Coll Cardiol* 1987; 9:952.

Ritter SB: Transesophageal echocardiography in children. New peephole to the heart. Editorial Comments. *J Am Coll Cardiol* 1990; 16:447.

Sciller NB, Shah PM, Crawford M, et al: Recommendations for quantitation of the left ventricle by two-dimensional echocardiography. *J Am Soc Echo* 1989; 2:358.

Tajik AJ, Seward JB, Hagler DJ, et al: Two-dimensional real-time ultrasonic imaging of the heart and great vessels: Technique, image orientation, structure identification, and validation. *Mayo Clin Proc* 1978; 53:271.

CHAPTER 3: INVASIVE DIAGNOSTIC PROCEDURES

Balter S, Sones M, Brancato R: Radiation exposure to the operator performing cardiac angiography with U-arm system. *Circulation* 1979; 58:925.

Baxley WA, Soto B: Hemodynamic evaluation of patients with mechanical prosthesis in both mitral and aortic position. *Am J Cardiol* 1980; 45:542.

Braunwald E, Ross J, Sonnenblick EH: *Mechanism of Contraction of the Normal and Failing Heart.* 2nd ed. Boston: Little, Brown, and Co, 1976.

Gertz EW, Wisneski JA, Gould RG, et al: Improved radiation protection for physicians performing cardiac catheterization. *Am J Cardiol* 1982; 50:1283.

Gomes AS, Baker JD, Paredero VM, et al: Acute renal dysfunction after major arteriography. *AJR* 1985; 145:1249.

Lassen EC, Berry CC, Talner LB, et al: Pretreatment with corticoids to alleviate reactions to intravenous contrast material: A randomized multi-institutional study. *N Engl J Med* 1987; 317:845.

Lister G, Talner NS: Oxygen transport in congenital heart disease. In Engle MA, ed. *Pediatric Cardiovascular Disease.* Philadelphia: FA Davis, 1981:129.

Parfrey PS, Griffiths SA, Barrett BJ: Contrast material induced renal failure in patients with diabetes mellitus, renal insufficiency, or both. *N Engl J Med* 1989; 320:143.

Reagan K, Bettman MA, Finkelstein BA, et al: Double-blind study of a new nonionic contrast agent for cardiac angiography. *Radiology* 1988; 167:409.

Rudolph A: *Congenital Disease of the Heart.* Chicago: Year Book Medical Publishers, 1974.

Rueter FG: Physician and patient exposure during cardiac catheterization. *Circulation* 1978; 58:134.

Schwab SJ, Hlatky MA, Pieper KS: Contrast nephrotoxicity: A randomized controlled trial of a nonionic and an ionic radiographic contrast agent. *N Engl J Med* 1989; 320:149.

Stacul F, Carraro M, Magnaldi S, et al: Contrast agent nephrotoxicity: Comparison of ionic and nonionic contrast agents. *AJR* 1987; 149:1287.

Weber KT, Janicki JS, Shroff SG, et al: The mechanics of ventricular function. *Hosp Prac* May 1983; 113.

CHAPTER 4: MAGNETIC RESONANCE IMAGING

Aisen AM, Chenevert TL: MR spectroscopy: Clinical perspective. *Radiology* 1989; 173:593.

Bittner V, Cranney GB, Lotan CS, et al: Overview of cardiovascular nuclear magnetic resonance imaging. *Cardiol Clin* 1989; 7:631.

Council on Scientific Affairs of the American Medical Association: Report of the Magnetic Resonance Imaging Panel. Fundamentals of magnetic resonance imaging. *JAMA* 1987; 258:3417.

Council on Scientific Affairs of the American Medical Association: Report of the Magnetic Resonance Imaging Panel. Present state of the art and future potential. *JAMA* 1988; 259:253.

Cranney GB, Lotan CS, Pohost GM: Evaluation of aortic regurgitation by magnetic resonance imaging. *Curr Prob Cardiol* 1990; 15:87.

Gangarosa RE, Minnis JE, Nobbe J, et al: Operational safety issues in MRI. *Magn Reson Imaging* 1987; 5:287.

Klipstein RH, Firmin DN, Underwood SR, et al: Blood flow patterns in the human aorta studied by magnetic resonance. *Br Heart J* 1987; 58:316.

Lim TH, Saloner D, Anderson CM: Current applications of magnetic resonance vascular imaging. *Cardiol Clin* 1989; 7:661.

Lotan CS, Cranney GB, Bouchard A, et al: The value of cine nuclear magnetic resonance imaging for assessing regional ventricular function. *J Am Coll Cardiol* 1989; 14:1721.

Nazarian GK, Julsrud PR, Elman RL, et al: Correlation between magnetic resonance imaging of the heart and cardiac anatomy. *Mayo Clin Proc* 1987; 62:573.

Pettigrew RI: Dynamic cardiac MR imaging. Technique and applications. *Radiol Clin No Am* 1989; 27:1183.

Schaefer S, Massie B, Weiner MW: Magnetic resonance spectroscopy of the heart. *Cardiol Clin* 1989; 7:697.

Stehling MJ, Howseman AM, Ordidge RJ, et al: Whole-body echo-planar MR imaging at 0.5 T. *Radiology* 1989; 170:257.

CHAPTER 4A: NUCLEAR CARDIOLOGY

Berman DS, ed: A symposium: Technetium-99m myocardial perfusion imaging agents and their relation to thallium-201. *Am J Cardiol* 1990; 66:1E.

Callahan RF, Froelich JW, McKusick KA, et al: A modified method for in vivo labelling of red blood cells with Tc99-m: Concise communication. *J Nucl Med* 1982; 23:315.

Dilsizian V, Rocco TP, Freedman NMT, et al: Enhanced detection of ischemic but viable myocardium by the reinjection of thallium after stress-redistribution imaging. *N Engl J Med* 1990; 323:141.

Gould KI, Westcott RJ, Albro PC, et al: Noninvasive assessment of coronary stenoses by myocardial imaging during pharmacologic coronary vasodilation: II. Clinical methodology and feasibility. *Am J Cardiol* 1978; 41:279.

Hendel RC, McSherry B, Karimeddini M, et al: Diagnostic value of a new myocardial perfusion, agent, Teboroxime (SQ 30,217), utilizing a rapid planar imaging protocol: Preliminary results. *J Am Coll Cardiol* 1990; 16:855.

Johnson LL, Seldin DW, Becker LC, et al: Antimyosin imaging in acute transmural myocardial infarctions: Results of a multicenter clinical trial. *J Am Coll Cardiol* 1989; 13:27.

Kiat H, Berman DS, Maddahi J, Yang LDL, et al: Late reversibility of tomographic myocardial thallium-201 defects: An accurate marker of myocardial viability. *J Am Coll Cardiol* 1988; 12:1456.

Leppo JA, O'Brien J, Rothendler JA, et al: Dipyridamolel-thallium-201 scintigraphy in the prediction of future cardiac events after acute myocardial infarction. *N Engl J Med* 1984; 310:1014.

Passamani E, Davis KB, Gillespie MJ, et al: A randomized trial of coronary artery bypass surgery: Survival in patients with low ejection fraction. *N Engl J Med* 1985; 312:1665.

Pohost GM, Zir LM, Moore RH, et al: Differentiation of transiently ischemic from infarcted myocardium by serial imaging after a single dose of thallium-201. *Circulation* 1977; 55:294.

Schelbert HR, Phelps ME, Hoffman E, et al: Regional myocardial blood flow, metabolism, and function assessed noninvasively with positron emission tomography. *Am J Cardiol* 1980; 80:1269.

Verani MS, Mahmarian JJ, Hixson JB, et al: Diagnosis of coronary artery disease by controlled coronary vasodilation with adenosine and thallium-201 scintigraphy in patients unable to exercise. *Circulation* 1990; 82:80.

CHAPTER 18: ACQUIRED VALVULAR DISEASE

AORTIC VALVE

Agatston AS: Doppler diagnosis of valvular aortic stenosis. *Echocardiography* 1986; 3:3.

Bommer WJ, Navis BS, Miller L: Quantitation of aortic regurgitation with two-dimensional Doppler echocardiography. *Am J Cardiol* 1981; 47:412.

Cranney GB, Lotan CS, Pohost GM: Evaluation of aortic regurgitation by magnetic resonance imaging. *Curr Prob Cardiol* 1990; 15:89.

Fenoglio JJ, Marcalista HA, DeCastro CM: Congenital bicuspid aortic valve after age 20. *Am J Cardiol* 1977; 39:164.

Hatle L, Anderson BA, Tromdal A: Noninvasive assessment of aortic stenosis by Doppler ultrasound. *Br Heart J* 1980; 43:284.

Hunt D, Baxley WA, Kennedy JW, et al: Quantitative evaluation of cine aortography in the assessment of aortic regurgitation. *Am J Cardiol* 1973; 31:696.

Kitabatake A, Ito H, Inove M, et al: A new approach of noninvasive evaluation of aortic regurgitant fraction by two-dimensional Doppler echocardiography. *Circulation* 1985; 72:523.

Klatte EC, June H, Burney B: Radiographic manifestation of aortic stenosis and aortic valvular insufficiency. *Semin Roentgenol* 1979; 14:122.

Mennel RG, Joyner CR, Thompson PD: The preoperative and operative assessment of aortic regurgitation. Cine aortography versus electromagnetic flow meter. *Am J Cardiol* 1972; 29:360.

Passik CS, Ackermann DM, Bluth JR, et al: Temporal causes in the changes in the cause of aortic stenosis: Surgical pathological study of 646 cases. *Mayo Clin Proc* 1987; 62:119.

Perry GJ, Helmcke F, Nanda NC, et al: Evaluation of aortic insufficiency by Doppler color flow mapping. *Am J Cardiol* 1987; 9:952.

Perry J, Nanda NC: Recent advances in color Doppler evaluation of valvular regurgitation. *Echocardiography* 1987; 4:503.

Pflugfelder PW, Landzberg JS, Cassidy MM: Comparison of cine MR imaging with Doppler echocardiography for the evaluation of aortic regurgitation. *AJR* 1989; 152:729.

Skjaerpe T, Hegrenaes L, Hable L: Noninvasive estimation of valve area in patients with aortic stenosis by Doppler ultrasound and two-dimensional echocardiography. *Circulation* 1985; 72:810.

Subramanian R, Olson LJ, Edwards WD: Surgical pathology of combined aortic stenosis and insufficiency: A study of 213 cases. *Mayo Clin Proc* 1985; 60:247.

Szamosi A, Wassberg B: Radiologic detection of aortic stenosis. *Acta Radiol* 1983; 24:201.

MITRAL VALVE

Green CE, Kelly MJ, Higgins CH: Etiologic significance of enlargement of the left atrial appendage in adults. *Radiology* 1982; 142:21.

Helmcke F, Nanda NC; Hsiung MC, et al: Color Doppler assessment of mitral regurgitation with octogonal planes. *Circulation* 1987; 75:175.

Khandheria BK, Tajik AG, Relder GS, et al: Doppler color flow imaging: A new technique for visualization and characterization of the blood flow jet in mitral stenosis. *Mayo Clin Proc* 1986; 61:623.

Olson LJ, Subramanian R, Ackerman DM: Surgical pathology of the mitral valve: Study of 712 cases spanning 21 years. *Mayo Clin Proc* 1987; 62:22.

CHAPTER 19: DISORDERS OF THE MYOCARDIUM

Becker AE, Carusso G: Myocardial disarray. A critical review. *Br Heart J* 1982; 47:527.

Bitter AV, Cranney GB, Lotan CS, et al: Overview of cardiovascular nuclear magnetic resonance imaging. *Cardiol Clin* 1989; 7:631.

Cohen J, Effat H, Goodwin JF, et al: Hypertrophic obstructive cardiomyopathy. *Br Heart J* 1964; 26:16.

Edward WD: Cardiomyopathy. *Hum Pathol* 1987; 18:625.

Fuster V, Gersh BJ, Gioliana ER, et al: The natural history of idiopathic dilated cardiomyopathy. *Am J Cardiol* 1987; 47:525.

Johnson RA, Palacios I: Dilated cardiomyopathies of the adult. *N Engl J Med* 1982; 307:1051.

Johnson RA, Palacios I: Dilated cardiomyopathies in the adults (second of two parts). *N Engl J Med* 1982; 307:1119.

Maron BJ, Gottiener JS, Ebstein SE: Patterns and significance of distribution of left ventricular hypertrophy in hypertrophic cardiomyopathy. *Am J Cardiol* 1981; 48:418.

Wigle ED: Hypertrophic cardiomyopathy. A 1987 viewpoint. Editorial. *Circulation* 1987; 75:311.

CHAPTER 20: ISCHEMIC HEART DISEASE: CLINICAL FEATURES AND NONINVASIVE DIAGNOSIS

ISCHEMIC HEART DISEASE: GENERAL, IMAGING

Ambrose JA, Winters SL, Stern A, et al: Angiographic morphology and the pathogenesis of unstable angina pectoris. *J Am Coll Cardiol* 1985; 5:609.

Armstrong WBF, O'Donald J, Dillon JC, et al: Complimentary value of 2-dimensional exercise echocardiography to routine treadmill exercise test. *Ann Int Med* 1986; 105:829.

Bartel AG, Chen JT, Peter RH: The significance of coronary calcification detected by fluoroscopy. A report of 360 patients. *Circulation* 1974; 49:1247.

Bergmann SR, Herrero P, Markham J, et al: Noninvasive quantitation of myocardial blood flow in human subjects with oxygen-15. Labelled water and positron emission tomography. *J Am Coll Cardiol* 1989; 14:639.

Buja LM, Witherston JT: The role of coronary artery lesions in ischemic heart disease: Insights from recent clinical, pathological, coronary arteriography, and experimental studies. *Hum Pathol* 1987; 18:451.

Foster V, Chesebro JH: Coronary artery sclerotic disease: Pathogenesis and thrombotic therapy. *Learning Center Highlights* Spring 1986; 10.

Goldschleger N, Selzer A, Cohn K: Treadmill stress test as indicator of presence and severity of coronary artery disease. *Ann Intern Med* 1976; 85:277.

Hamby RI: Angina pectoris: A clinical–electrocardiographic correlative study in 510 patients. *Cardiovasc Clin* 1977; 8:79.

Kelley MJ, Huang AK, Langou RA: Correlation of fluoroscopically detected coronary artery calcification with exercise stress testing in asymptomatic men. *Radiology* 1978; 129:1.

Kennel WB, Feineleib M: Natural history of angina pectoris in the Framingham Study: Prognosis and survival. *Am J Cardiol* 1972; 29:154.

Martin CN, McConahay DR: Maximal treadmill exercise electrocardiography: Correlation with coronary arteriography and cardiac hemodynamics. *Circulation* 1972; 46:956.

Sakuma H, Takeda K, Hirano T: Plain chest radiography with computed radiography: Improved sensitivity for the detection of coronary artery calcification. *AJR* 1988; 151:27.

Shub C: Stable angina pectoris: I Clinical patterns. *Mayo Clin Proc* 1990; 65:233.

Shub C: Stable angina pectoris: II Cardiac evaluation and diagnostic testing. *Mayo Clin Proc* 1990; 65:243.

Souza AS, Breem PR, Elliott LP: Chest film detection of coronary artery calcification. The value of the CAC triangle. *Radiology* 1978; 129:7.

ACUTE MYOCARDIAL INFARCTION

Bates RJ, Beutles S, Resneskow L, et al: Cardiac rupture: Challenge in diagnosis and management. *Am J Cardiol* 1977; 40:429–37.

Becker LC, Ambrosio G: Myocardial consequences of reperfusion. *Prog Cardiovasc Dis* 1987; 30:23.

Cerquira MD, Jacobson AF: Assessment of myocardial viability with SPECT and PET imaging. *AJR* 1989; 153:477.

DeWood MA, Spores J, Notske R, et al: Prevalence of total occlusion during the early hours of transmural myocardial infarction. *N Engl J Med* 1980; 303:897.

Helmcke F, Mahan E, Nanda C, et al: Two-dimensional echocardiography and Doppler color flow mapping in the diagnosis and prognosis of ventricular septal rupture. *Circulation* 1980; 81:1775.

Kaul S, Lilly DR, Gascho JA, et al: Prognostic utility of the exercise thallium-201 test in ambulatory patients with chest pain: Comparison with cardiac catheterization. *Circulation* 1988; 77:745.

Keating ED, Cross SA, Schlamowitz RA, et al: Mural thrombi in myocardial infarction. Prospective evaluation by two-dimensional echocardiography. *Am J Med* 1983; 74:989.

Khan AH, Haywood LJ: Myocardial infarction in nine patients with radiologically patent coronary arteries. *N Engl J Med* 1974; 291:427.

Khaw BA, Mattia JA, Melincoff G, et al: Monoclonal antibody to cardiac myosin: Imaging of experimental myocardial infarction. *Hibridoma* 1984; 3:11.

Killip T, Kimball JT: Treatment of myocardial infarction in a coronary care unit. A two-year experience with 250 patients. *Am J Cardiol* 20; 1967:457.

Lavie CJ, Gersh BJ: Acute myocardial infarction. Initial manifestation, management, and prognosis. *Mayo Clin Proc* 1980; 65:531.

Marder VJ, Sherry S: Thrombolytic therapy: Current status. *N Engl J Med* 1988; 318:1585.

Miller DD, Elmaleh DR, McKusick KA, et al: Radiopharmaceuticals for cardiac imaging. *Radiol Clin No Am* 1985; 23:765.

Oliva PB, Breckinridge JC: Arteriographic evidence of coronary arterial spasm in acute myocardial infarction. *Circulation* 1977; 56:366.

Quereshi SA, Rissen T, Gray KE: Survival after subacute cardiac rupture. *Br Heart J* 1982; 47:180.

Rativ O, Phelps ME, Huang SC, et al: Positron tomography with deoxyglucose for estimating local myocardial glucose metabolism. *J Nucl Med* 1982; 23:577.

Volpi A, Maggioni A, Franzosi MG, et al: In-hospital prognosis of patients with acute myocardial infarction complicated by primary ventricular fibrillation. *N Engl J Med* 1987; 317:257.

VENTRICULAR ANEURYSM AND MURAL THROMBUS

Burton NA, Stinson EB, Oyer PE, et al: Left ventricular aneurysm. Preoperative risk factors and long term postoperative result. *J Thorac Cardiovasc Surg* 1979; 77:65.

Grondin P, Kretz J, Bical O: Natural history of saccular aneurysm of the left ventricle. *J Thorac Cardiovasc Surg* 1979; 77:57.

Kiefer SK, Flaker GC, Martin RH, et al: Clinical improvement after ventricular aneurysm repair. Prediction by angiography and hemodynamic variables. *J Am Coll Cardiol* 1983; 2:30.

Lackner K. Thurn P: Computed tomography of the heart: ECG-gated and continuous scans. *Radiology* 1981; 140:413.

Olearchyk AS, Lemole GM, Spagna PM: Left ventricular aneurysm. *J Thorac Cardiovasc Surg* 1984; 88:544.

Spindola–Franco H, Kronacher N: Pseudo-aneurysm of the left ventricle. *Radiology* 1978; 127:29.

Tomada H, Hoshiai M, Furuya H, et al: Evaluation of left ventricular thrombus with computed tomography. *Am J Cardiol* 1981; 48:573.

CHAPTER 21: ISCHEMIC HEART DISEASE: INVASIVE DIAGNOSIS

CORONARY ARTERIOGRAPHY: ANATOMY AND TECHNIQUE

James TN: *The Anatomy of the Coronary Arteries*. New York: Harper and Row, 1961.

Judkins MP: Percutaneous transfemoral selected coronary arteriography. *Radiol Clin No Am* 1968; 6:467.

Sones FM, Shirey EK: Cine coronary arteriography. *Mod Conc Cardiovasc Dis* 1962; 31:735.

Soto B, Russell RO Jr, Moraski RE: *Radiographic Anatomy of the Coronary Arteries*. Mt. Kisco, NY, Futura Publishing, 1976.

CORONARY ARTERY STENOSIS AND ISCHEMIC HEART DISEASE

Bourassa MG, Lesperance J, Campeau L, et al: Fate of left ventricular contraction following aortocoronary venous graft. Early and late postoperative modifications. *Circulation* 1972; 46:724.

Fuster V, Steele PM, Chesebro JH: Role of platelets and thrombosis in coronary atherosclerotic disease and sudden death. *J Am Coll Cardiol* 1985; (suppl 175B) 5:6.

Henzlova MJ, Nath H, Bucy RP, et al: Coronary artery to right ventricle fistula in heart transplant recipients: A complication of endomyocardial biopsy. *J Am Coll Cardiol* 1989; 14:258.

Khuri SF, Warner KG, Marston W, et al: Intraoperative assessment of the physiological significance of coronary stenosis in humans. *J Thorac Cardiovasc Surg* 1986; 92:79.

Miller SW, Boucher CA: Assessing the adequacy of myocardial perfusion in man: Anatomical and functional technique. *Radiol Clin No Am* 1985; 23:589.

Rogers WJ, Smith LR, Oberman A, et al: Invasive measurements relating to long-term survival post-myocardial infarction. *Circulation* 1979; 60:32.

Rogers WJ, McDaniel HG, Mantle JO, et al: Hemodynamic Measurements. In Warner GS, ed. *Myocardial Infarction: Measurements and Intervention.* Boston: Martinus Nijhoff, 1982: 159.

CHAPTER 22: DISORDERS OF THE PERICARDIUM

Burstow DJ, Oh JK, Bailey KR, et al: Cardiac tamponade: Characteristic Doppler observations. *Mayo Clin Proc* 1989; 64:312.

Choe YE, Im JG, Park JH, et al: The anatomy of the pericardial space: A study in cadavers and patients. *AJR* 1987; 149:693.

Feigin DS, Fenoglio JJ, McAllister HA, et al: Pericardial cysts. A radiological–pathological correlation and review. *Radiology* 1977; 125:15.

Gale ME, Kiwak MG, Gale DR: Pericardial fluid distribution: CT analysis. *Radiology* 1987; 162:161.

Haynes JK, Tajik AJ, Osbourne MJ: Two-dimensional echocardiographic diagnosis of pericardial cysts. *Mayo Clin Proc* 1983; 58:60.

Moncada R, Baker M, Salinas M: Diagnostic role of computed tomography in pericardial heart disease: Congenital defects, thickening, neoplasms, and effusion. *Am Heart J* 1982; 103:263.

Nishimura RA, Connolly DC, Parkin TW, et al: Constrictive pericarditis: Assessment of current diagnostic procedures. *Mayo Clin Proc* 1985; 60:397.

Olson MC, Posnik HB, McDonald V, et al: Computed tomography and magnetic resonance imaging of the pericardium. *RadioGraphics* 1989; 9:633.

Sechtem U, Tscholakoff D, Higgins CB: MRI of the normal pericardium. *AJR* 1986; 147:239.

Soto B, Shine MS, Arciniegas JC, et al: The septal arteries in the differential diagnosis of constricted pericarditis. *Am Heart J* 1984; 108:332.

Torrance DJ: Demonstration of subepicardial fat as an aid in the diagnosis of pericardial effusion or thickening. *AJR* 1955; 74:850.

CHAPTER 23: INFECTIVE ENDOCARDITIS

Himelman RB, Chung WS, Chernoff DN, et al: Cardiac manifestations of human immunodeficiency virus infection: A two-dimensional echocardiographic study. *J Am Coll Cardiol* 1989; 13:1030.

Jaffe W, Morgan D, Pearlman AS, et al: Infective endocarditis. 1983–1988. Echocardiographic findings and factors influencing morbidity and mortality. *J Am Coll Cardiol* 1990; 15:1227.

Jussenhoven EJ, Van Herwertern LA, Roelandt J, et al: Detailed analysis of aortic valve endocarditis: Comparison of precordial, esophageal, and epicardial two-dimensional echocardiography with surgical findings. *J Clin Ultrasound* 1986; 14:209.

Keys TF: Antimicrobial prophylaxis for patients with congenital or valvular heart disease. *Mayo Clin Proc* 1982; 57:171.

Lutas EM, Roberts RB, Dereux RB, et al: Relation between the presence of echocardiographic vegetation and the complication rate in infective endocarditis. *Am Heart J* 1986; 112:107.

Martin RP: The diagnostic and prognostic role of cardiovascular ultrasound in endocarditis. Bigger is not better. (Editorial). *J Am Coll Cardiol* 1990; 15:123A.

Miller SW, Dinsmore MD: Aortic root abscess resulting from endocarditis: Spectrum of angiographic findings. *Radiology* 1984; 153:357.

Mugge A, Daniel WG, Frank G, et al: Echocardiography in infective endocarditis. Reassessment of prognostic implication of vegetation size determined by the transthoracic and transesophageal approach. *J Am Coll Cardiol* 1989; 14:631.

Nishimura RA, Connolly DC, Parkin TW, et al: Constrictive pericarditis: Assessment of current diagnostic procedures. *Mayo Clin Proc* 1985; 60:397.

Stewart JA, Silimperi D, Harris B, et al: Echocardiographic documentation of vegetative lesions in infective endocarditis: Clinical implications. *Circulation* 1980; 61:374.

Thompson RL: Staphylococcal infective endocarditis. *Mayo Clin Proc* 1982; 57:106.

Van Scoy RE: Culture-negative endocarditis. *Mayo Clin Proc* 1982; 57:149.

Wilson WR, Giuliani ER, Danielson GK, et al: General considerations in the diagnosis and treatment of infective endocarditis. *Mayo Clin Proc* 1982; 57:81.

Wilson WR, Giuliani ER, Danielson GK: Management of complications of infective endocarditis. *Mayo Clin Proc* 1982; 57:162.

CHAPTER 24: CARDIAC MANIFESTATIONS OF LUNG DISEASE

PRIMARY AND SECONDARY PULMONARY HYPERTENSION

Gefter WB, Hatabu H, Dinsmore BJ, et al: Pulmonary vascular cine NMR imaging: A noninvasive approach to dynamic imaging of the pulmonary circulation. *Radiology* 1990; 176:761.

Haworth SG: Understanding pulmonary arterial disease in young children. *Int J Cardiol* 1987; 15:101.

Heath D, Smith P, Gosney J, et al: The pathology of the early and late stage of pulmonary hypertension. *Br Heart J* 1987; 58:204.

Meyrick B, Reid L: Pulmonary hypertension. Anatomic and physiological correlates. *Clin Chest Med* 1983; 4:199.

Nicod P, Peterson K, Levine M, et al: Pulmonary arteriography in severe chronic pulmonary hypertension. *Ann Int Med* 1987; 107:565.

Rich S, Tantzker DR, Ayres SM, et al: Primary pulmonary hypertension. The national prospective study. *Ann Int Med* 1987; 107:216.

White RD, Winkler ML, Higginson CB: MR imaging of pulmonary arterial hypertension and pulmonary emboli. *AJR* 1987; 149:15.

PULMONARY EMBOLISM

Alderson PO, Martin EC: Pulmonary embolism. Diagnosis with multiple imaging modalities. *Radiology* 1987; 164:297.

Benotti JR, Dalen JE: The natural history of pulmonary embolism. *Clin Chest Med* 1984; 5:403.

Bettmann MA, Salzman EW: Current concepts in the diagnosis of pulmonary embolism. *Mod Concepts Cardiovasc Dis* 1984; 53:1.

Buckner CB, Walker CW, Purnell GL: Pulmonary embolism: Chest radiographic abnormalities. *J Thorac Imag* 1989; 4:23.

Cooperative study: Urokinase pulmonary embolism trial. Phase II. Results. *JAMA* 1974; 229:1606.

Dalen JE, Harper JS: Natural history of pulmonary embolism. *Prog Cardiovasc Dis* 1975; 17:259.

Goldhader SZ, Hennekens CH, Evans DA, et al: Factors associated with corrected and modern diagnosis of major pulmonary embolism. *Am J Med* 1982; 73:822.

Haeger K: Problems of acute deep venous thrombosis. The interpretation of signs and symptoms. *Angiology* 1969; 20:219.

Hull RD, Hirsh J, Carter CJ, et al: Diagnostic value of ventilation-perfusion lung scanning in patients with suspected pulmonary embolism. *Chest* 1985; 88:819.

Kerr IH, Simon G, Sutton GC: The value of the plain radiography in acute massive pulmonary embolism. *Br J Radiol* 1971; 44:751.

Mills SR, Jackson DC, Alder RA, et al: The incidence, etiologies, and avoidance of complications of pulmonary angiography in a large series. *Radiology* 1980; 136:295.

Posteraro RH, Sostman HD, Spritzer CE, et al: Cine-gradient-refocused MR imaging of central pulmonary emboli. *AJR* 1989; 152:465.

Rosenow EC, Osmundson PJ, Brown ML: Pulmonary embolism. *Mayo Clin Proc* 1981; 56:161.

Spies WG, Burstein SP, Dillehay GL, et al: Ventilation-perfusion scintigraphy in suspected pulmonary embolism: Correlation with pulmonary angiography and refinement of criteria for interpretation. *Radiology* 1986; 159:383.

CHAPTER 25: CARDIOVASCULAR MANIFESTATIONS OF SYSTEMIC DISORDERS

RHEUMATIC AND CONNECTIVE TISSUE DISEASES

Baggenstoss AH, Titus JL: Rheumatic and collagen disorders of the heart. In Gould SE, ed. *Pathology of Heart and Blood Vessels*. 3rd ed. Springfield, IL: Charles C. Thomas, 1968: 649.

Bluestone R, Pearson CM: Anklyosing spondylitis and Reiter's syndrome. Their interrelationship and association with HLAB27. *Adv Int Med* 1977; 22:1.

Bulkley BH, Roberts WC: Anklyosing spondylitis and aortic regurgitation: Description of the characteristic cardiovascular lesion from study of 8 necropsy patients. *Circulation* 1973; 48:1014.

Csnoka GW, Litchfield JW, Oates JK: Cardiac lesions in Reiter's disease. *Br Med J* 1961; 1:263.

Elkayam U, Weiss S, Laniado S: Pericardial effusion and mitral valve involvement in systemic lupus erythematosus: Echocardiographic study and rheumatic disease. *Ann Rheum Dis* 1977; 36:349.

Kirk J, Cosh J: The pericarditis of rheumatoid arthritis. *Q J Med* 1969; 38:397.

Lebowitz WB: The heart in rheumatoid arthritis (rheumatoid disease). A clinical and pathological study of 62 cases. *Ann Int Med* 1963; 58:102.

Paulus HE, Pearson CM, Pitts W: Aortic insufficiency in five patients with Reiter's syndrome: A detailed clinical and pathological study. *Am J Med* 1972; 53:464.

Roberts WC, Hollingsworth JF, Bulkley BH, et al: Combined mitral and aortic regurgitation in anklyosing spondylitis: Angiographic and anatomical features. *Am J Med* 1974; 56:237.

Tucker CR, Fowles RE, Calin A: Aortitis and anklyosing spondylitis: Early detection of aortic root abnormalities with two-dimensional echocardiography. *Am J Cardiol* 1982; 49:680.

SYSTEMIC HYPERTENSION

Cohn JN, Limas CJ, Gauguiha NH: Hypertension and the heart. *Arch Int Med* 1974; 1:969.

Kaplan NM: Systemic hypertension: mechanisms and diagnosis. In Braunwald E, ed. *Heart Disease*. 3rd ed. Philadelphia: WB Saunders, 1980:853.

CARDIAC MANIFESTATIONS OF RENAL DISEASE

Gottlieb MN, Braunwald E: Renal disorders in heart disease. In Braunwald E, ed. *Cardiac Disease*. Philadelphia: WB Saunders, 1980: 1854.

Lazarus JM, Lowrie EG, Hampers CL, et al: Cardiovascular disease in uremic patients on hemodialysis. *Kidney Int* 1975; 7:S167.

Linder A, Charra B, Sherrard DJ, et al: Accelerated arteriosclerosis in prolonged maintenance hemodialysis. *N Engl J Med* 1974; 290:697.

CARDIAC EFFECTS OF RADIATION THERAPY

Applefeld MM, Wiernik PH: Cardiac disease after radiation therapy for Hodgkin's disease. Analysis of 48 patients. *Am J Cardiol* 1983; 51:1679.

Botti RE, Driscoll TE, Pearson OH, et al: Radiation myocardial fibrosis simulating constricted pericarditis. *Cancer* 1968; 22:1254.

Carmel RJ, Kaplan HS: Mantle radiation in Hodgkin's disease. *Cancer* 1976; 37:2813.

ENDOCRINE AND NUTRITIONAL DISORDERS

Kannel WB, Hjortland M, Castelli WP: The role of diabetes in congestive heart failure. The Framingham Study. *Am J Cardiol* 1974;34.

Kerber RE, Sherman B: Echocardiographic evaluation of pericardial effusion in myxedema. Incidence and biochemical and clinical correlation. *Circulation* 1975; 52:823.

Seneviratne BIB: Diabetic cardiomyopathy. The preclinical phase. *Br Med J* 1977; 1:144.

Williams GA, Braunwald E: Endocrine and nutritional disorders and heart disease. In Braunwald E, ed. *Heart Disease. A Text of Cardiovascular Medicine*. Philadelphia: WB Saunders, 1980: 1826.

DISORDERS OF CONNECTIVE TISSUE, MUSCLE, AND THE CENTRAL NERVOUS SYSTEM

Bowers D: Pathogenesis of primary abnormalities of the mitral valve in the Marfan's syndrome. *Br Heart J* 1969; 31:679.

Bulkley BH, Stollerman GN: Connective tissue disease of the cardiovascular system. In Braunwald E, ed. *Heart Disease*. Philadelphia: WB Saunders, 1980: 1724.

Caben WR, Rexa MG, Kovik RB, et al: Mitral valve prolapse in conduction defects in Ehlers-Danlos syndrome. *Arch Int Med* 1977; 137:1227.

Cannon PG: The heart and lungs in myotonic muscular dystrophy. *Am J Med* 1962; 32:765.

Cote M, Davignon A, Elias G, et al: Hemodynamic findings in Friedreich's ataxia. *J Can Sci Neurol* 1976; 3:333.

Criscitello MG, Ronan JA, Besterman EM, et al: Cardiovascular abnormalities in osteogenesis imperfecta. *Circulation* 1965; 31:255.

Gauthier EJ: Cardiac disease in Friedreich's ataxia. *Ann Int Med* 1964; 60:892.

Josephson ME, Caracta AR, Gallagher JJ, et al: Site of conduction disturbances in a family with myotonic dystrophy. *Am J Cardiol* 1973; 32:114.

Krovetz LJ, Lorincz AE, Schiebler GL: Cardiovascular manifestations of the Hurler syndrome. Hemodynamic and angiocardiographic observation in fifteen patients. *Circulation* 1965; 31:132.

Madison WM, Bradley E, Castillo A: Ehlers-Danlos syndrome with cardiac involvement. *Am J Cardiol* 1963; 11:689.

McDonald GR, Schaff HV, et al: Surgical management of patients with the Marfan's syndrome and dilatation of the ascending aorta. *J Thorac Cardiovasc Surg* 1981; 81:110.

Murdock JL, Walker BA, Halpern Bl, et al: Life expectancy and causes of death in the Marfan's syndrome. *N Engl J Med* 1972; 286:804.

Renteria BG, Ferrans VJ, Roberts WC: The heart in the Hurler syndrome. Gross, histological and ultrastructural observation in five necropsy cases. *Am J Cardiol* 1976; 38:487.

Roberts WC, Honig HS: The spectrum of cardiovascular disease in the Marfan syndrome: A clinical-morphologic study of 18 necropsy patients and comparison to 151 previously reported necropsy patients. *Am Heart J* 1982; 104:115.

Soulen RL, Fishman Ek, Pyeritz RE, et al: Marfan syndrome: Evaluation with MR imaging versus CT. *Radiology* 165; 697:165.

ACQUIRED IMMUME DEFICIENCY SYNDROME (AIDS)

Acierno LJ: Cardiac complications of the acquired immunodeficiency syndrome (AIDS). A review. *J Am Coll Cardiol* 1989; 13:1144.

Cammarosano C, Lewis W: Cardiac lesion in acquired immunodeficiency syndrome (AIDS). *J Am Coll Cardiol* 1985; 5:703.

Cohen IS, Anderson DW, Virmani R, et al: Congestive cardiomyopathy in associated with acquired immunodeficiency virus infection, a 2-dimensional echocardiographic study. *J Am Coll Cardiol* 1989; 13:1030.

Corboy JR, Fink L, Miller WT: Congestive cardiomyopathy in association with AIDS. *Radiology* 1987; 165:139.

Himelman RB, Chung WS, Chernoff DN, et al: Cardiac manifestations of human immunodeficiency virus infection: A two-dimensional echocardiographic study. *J Am Coll Cardiol* 1989; 13:1030.

CHAPTER 26: NEOPLASTIC DISEASE

Amparo EG, Higgins CB, Farmer D: Gated MRI of cardiac and paracardiac masses: Initial experience. *AJR* 1984; 143:1151.

Attum AA, Johnson GS, Masri Z, et al: Malignant clinical behavior of cardiac myxomas and "myxoid imitators." *Ann Thorac Surg* 1987; 44:217.

Bini RM, Westaby S, Bargeron LM, et al: Investigation and management of primary cardiac tumors in infants and children. *J Am Coll Cardiol* 1983; 2:351.

Bogren HG, DeMaria AN, Mason DT: Imaging procedures in the detection of cardiac tumors with emphasis on echocardiography: A review. *Cardiovasc Intervent Radiol* 1980; 3:107.

Carney JA, Hruska LS, Beauchamp GD, et al: Dominant inheritance of the complex of myxomas, spotty pigmentation and endocrine overactivity. *Mayo Clin Proc* 1986; 61:165.
Freedberg RS, Kronzon I, Rumancik WM: The contribution of magnetic resonance imaging to the evaluation of intracardiac tumors diagnosed by echocardiography. *Circulation* 1988; 77:96.
Fueredi GA, Knechtges TE, Czarnecki DJ: Coronary angiography in atrial myxoma: Findings in nine cases. *AJR* 1989; 152:737.
Lund JT, Ehman RL, McAllister HA, Fenoglio JJ: *Tumors of the Cardiovascular System*. Washington, DC: Armed Forces Institute of Pathology, 1978.
McCarthy PM, Piehler JM, Schaff HV: The significance of multiple, recurrent and complex cardiac myxomas. *J Thorac Cardiovasc Surg* 1986; 91:389.
Reese IJ, Cooley DA, Frazier OH, et al: Cardiac tumor. Clinical spectrum and prognosis of lesions other than classical benign myxoma in 20 patients. *J Thorac Cardiovasc Surg* 1984; 88:439.
Steiner RM, Bulle MI, Cumpel F, et al: The diagnosis of intracardiac metastasis of colon carcinoma by radioisotopes and roentgenogram study. *Am J Cardiol* 1970; 26:300.
Tsuchiya F, Kohno A, Saitoh R, et al: CT findings in atrial myxoma. *Radiology* 1984; 151:139.
Van der Hauwaert LG: Cardiac tumors in infants and childhood. *Br Heart J* 1971; 33:125.
Winkler M, Higgins CB: Suspected intracardiac masses: Evaluation with MR imaging. *Radiology* 1987; 165:117.

CHAPTER 27: DISEASES OF THE THORACIC AORTA

DISSECTION

Edwards WD, Edwards JE: Dissecting aortic aneurysm associated with congenital bicuspid valve. *Circulation* 1978; 57:1022.
Erbel R, Engberding R, Daniel W, et al: Echocardiography in diagnosis of aortic dissection. *Lancet* March 4, 1989; 457.
Goldman AP, Kotler MN, Scanlon MH, et al: The complementary role of magnetic resonance imaging: Doppler echocardiography and computed tomography in the diagnosis of dissecting thoracic aneurysms. *Am Heart J* 1986; 111:970.
Shuford WH, Sybers RG, Weens HS: Problems in the aortographic diagnosis of dissecting aneurysm of the aorta. *N Engl J Med* 1969; 280:225.
Slater EE, De Sanctis RW: The clinical recognition of dissecting aortic aneurysm. *Am J Cardiol* 1976; 60:625.
Soto B, Harmon MA, Ceballos R, et al: Angiographic diagnosis of dissecting aneurysm of the aorta. *AJR* 1972; 116:146.
Thorsen MK, San Dretto MA, Lawson TL, et al: Dissecting aortic aneurysms: Accuracy of computed tomographic diagnosis. *Radiology* 1983; 148:773.
Yamaguchi T, Guthaner DF, Wexler L: Natural history of the false channel of Type A aortic dissection after surgical repair: CT study. *Radiology* 1989; 170:743.

ANEURYSM

DeBakey ME, Cooley DA, Crawford ES, et al: Aneurysms of the thoracic aorta. *J Thorac Cardiovasc Surg* 1958; 36:393.
Eisen S, Elliott LP: The roentgenology of cystic medial necrosis of the ascending aorta. *Radiol Clin No Am* 1968; 6:437.
Finkelmeir BA, Mentzer RM, Kaiser DL, et al: Chronic traumatic thoracic aneurysm. *J Thorac Cardiovasc Surg* 1982; 84:257.
Higgins CB, Reinke RT: Nonsyphilitic etiology of linear calcification of the ascending aorta. *Radiology* 1964; 113:609.
Szamosi A: Radiological detection of aneurysms involving the aortic root. *Radiology* 1981; 138:551.

TAKAYASU'S DISEASE

Lupi–Herrera E, Sanchez G, Marcushamer J, et al: Takayasu's arteritis: Clinical study of 107 cases. *Am Heart J* 1977; 93:94.
Park JH, Han MC, Kim SH, et al: Takayasu's arteritis: Angiographic findings and results of angioplasty. *AJR* 1989; 153:1069.
Subramanyan R, Joy J, Balakrishnan KG: Natural history of aorto-arteritis [Takayasu's disease]. *Circulation* 1989; 80:429.

CHAPTER 28: TRAUMA TO THE HEART AND GREAT VESSELS

INJURIES TO THE GREAT VESSELS

Fishbond G, Robbins D, Osborn DJ, et al: Trauma to the thoracic aorta and great vessels. *Radiol Clin No Am* 1973; 11:543.
Gundry SR, Burney RE, Mackenzie JR: Traumatic pseudo-aneurysms of the aorta. An anatomical and radiological correlation. *Arch Surg* 1984; 119:1055.
Gundry SR, Williams S, Burney R, et al: Indication for aortography. Radiography after blunt chest trauma: A reassessment of the radiographic findings associated with traumatic rupture of the aorta. *Invest Radiol* 1983; 18:230.
Hurst JW, Symbas PN, Becker AE: Traumatic disease of the cardiovascular system. In Hurst JW, ed. *Atlas of the Heart*. New York: Gower Medical Publishing, 1988: 10.2.
Kirsh MM, Behrendt DM, Orringer MB, et al: The treatment of acute traumatic rupture of the aorta. *Ann Surg* 1976; 184:308.
Marnocha KE, Maglinte DDT: Plain-film criteria for excluding aortic rupture in blunt chest trauma. *AJR* 1985; 144:19.
Marnocha KE, Maglinte DDT, Woods J, et al: Mediastinal-width bar chest-width ratio in blunt chest trauma: A reappraisal. *AJR* 1984; 142:275.
Milne ENC, Pistolesi M, Niniati M, et al: The vascular pedicle of the heart and vena azygous. The normal subject. *Radiology* 1984; 152:1.
Soulen RL, Freeman E: Radiologic evaluation of traumatic heart disease. *Radiol Clin North Am* 1971; 9:285.
Tisnado J, Tsai FY, Als A, et al: A new radiographic sign of acute traumatic rupture of the thoracic aorta: Displacement of the nasogastric tube to the right. *Radiology* 1977; 125:603.

CARDIAC INJURY

Demuth WE: High velocity bullet wound of the thorax. *Am J Surg* 1968; 115:616.
Dodd GD, Budzik RF: Identification of retained firearm projectiles on plain radiographs. *AJR* 1990; 154:471.
Gay W: Blunt trauma to the heart and great vessels. *Surgery* 1982; 91:507.
Jones EW, Helmsworth J: Penetrating wounds of the heart. Thirty years experience. *Arch Surg* 1968; 96:671.
Netter FH: Penetrating heart wounds. In *The CIBA Collection of Medical Illustrations. Vol. 5. Heart*. Edison, NJ: CIBA Pharmaceutical Company, 1978: 253.
Quadros CL, Hutchinson JE, Mogtader AH: Laceration of the mitral papillary muscle and the aortic root as a result of blunt trauma to the chest. *J Thorac Cardiovasc Surg* 1984; 88:134.
Soulen RL, Freeman E: Radiologic evaluation of traumatic heart disease. *Radiol Clin No Am* 1971; 9:285.

CHAPTER 29: ACQUIRED HEART DISEASE IN CHILDREN

RHEUMATIC FEVER

Bland EF Rheumatic fever: The way it was. *Circulation* 1987; 76:1190.
Jones' Criteria: Revised for guidance in the diagnosis of rheumatic disease. *Circulation* 1965; 32:664.
Jones TD: The diagnosis of rheumatic fever. *JAMA* 1944; 126:481.
Keith JD: Rheumatic fever and rheumatic heart disease. In Keith JD, Rowe RD, Vlad P, eds. *Heart Disease in Infancy and Childhood*. New York: McMillan Publishing, 1978: 203.
Markowitz H: The decline of rheumatic fever, role of medical intervention. *J Pediatr* 1985; 106:545.
Massell BV, Fyler DC, Roy SB: The clinical picture of rheumatic fever. Diagnosis and immediate prognosis, course and therapeutic implications. *Am J Cardiol* 1958; 1:436.

McIntosh R, Wood CL: Rheumatic infections occurring in the first three years of life. *Am J Dis Child* 1935; 49:835.

Rosenthal A, Czoniczer C, Massell BF: Rheumatic fever under 3 years of age. A report of 10 cases. *Pediatrics* 1968; 41:612.

ACUTE GLOMERULONEPHRITIS

Kirkpatrick JA, Fleisher DS: The roentgen appearance of the chest in acute glomerulonephritis in children. *J Pediatr* 1964; 64:492.

Macpherson RI, Banerjee AK: Acute glomerulonephritis: A chest film diagnosis? *J Can Assoc Radiol* 1974; 25:58.

SYSTEMIC HYPERTENSION IN CHILDREN AND ADOLESCENTS

Friedman WF: Acquired heart disease in infancy. In Braunwald E, ed. *Heart Disease*. 3rd ed. Philadelphia: WB Saunders, 1988: 819.

Kaplan NM: Systemic hypertension. In Braunwald E, ed. *Heart Disease*. 3rd ed. Philadelphia: WB Saunders, 1988: 819.

Rocchini AP: Childhood hypertension: Etiology, diagnosis and treatment. *Pediatr Clin No Am* 1984; 31:1259.

CARDIAC INFECTIONS: ENDOCARDITIS, PERICARDITIS, MYOCARDITIS

Ablemann WH: Viral myocarditis and its sequelae. *Annu Rev Med* 1973; 24:145.

Boyle JD, Pearce ML, Guze LB: Purulent pericarditis: Review of literature and report of eleven cases. *Medicine* 1967; 107:404.

Bradley EC: Acute benign pericarditis. *Am Heart J* 1964; 67:121.

Carrio I, Berna L, Ballester M, et al: Indium III antimycin scintigraphy to assess myocardial damage in patients with suspected myocarditis and cardiac rejection. *J Nucl Med* 1988; 29:1893.

Gerzen P, Granath A, Holmgren B, et al: Acute myocarditis. A followup study. *Br Heart J* 1972; 34:575.

Gore I, Saphir O: Myocarditis: A classification of 1402 cases. *Am Heart J* 1947; 34:827.

Hermans PE: The clinical manifestation of infective endocarditis. *Mayo Clin Proc* 1982; 57:15.

Johnson ChM, Rhodes KH: Pediatric endocarditis. *Mayo Clin Proc* 1982; 57:86.

Keith JD: Pericarditis. In Keith JD, Rowe RD, Vlad P, eds. *Heart Disease in Infancy and Childhood*. 3rd ed. New York: McMillan Publishing, 1978: 245.

McGuinness GA, Schieken RM, Maguire GF: Endocarditis in the newborn. *Am J Dis Child* 1980; 134:577.

KAWASAKI DISEASE (MUCOCUTANEOUS LYMPH NODE SYNDROME)

Bissett GS III, Strife JL, McCloskey J: MR imaging of coronary artery aneurysms in a child with Kawasaki disease. *AJR* 1989; 152:805.

Frey EE, Matherne GP, Mahoney LT, et al: Coronary artery aneurysms due to Kawasaki disease: Diagnosed with ultrafast CT. *Radiology* 1988; 167:725.

Fujiwara A, Hamashima Y: Pathology of the heart in Kawasaki disease. *Pediatrics* 1978; 61:100.

Kato H: Cardiovascular problems in Kawasaki's disease. In Doyle EF, Engle MA, Gersony WM, eds. *Pediatric Cardiology*. New York: Springer-Verlag, 1985: 1074.

Kawasaki T, Kosaki F, Okawa S, et al: A new infantile acute febrile mucocutaneous lymph node syndrome (MLN) prevailing in Japan. *Pediatrics* 1974; 54:271.

Kuribayashi S, Ootaki M, Tsuji M, et al: Coronary angiographic abnormalities in mucocutaneous lymph node syndrome: Acute findings and long-term follow-up. *Radiology* 1989; 172:629.

Williamson MR, Williamson SL, Siebert JJ: Indium-111 leukocyte scanning localization for detecting early myocarditis in Kawasaki disease. *AJR* 1986; 146:255.

MUSCLE AND CONNECTIVE TISSUE DISORDERS

Bacon PA, Gibson DG: Cardiac involvement in rheumatoid arthritis: An echocardiographic study. *Ann Rheum Dis* 1974; 33:20.

Bruno L, Tredici S, Mangiavavacchi M, et al: Cardiac, skeletal and ocular abnormalities in patients with Marfan's syndrome and in their relatives. *Br Heart J* 1984; 51:220.

Bulkley BH, Roberts WG: Ankylosing spondylitis and aortic regurgitation: Description of the characteristic cardiovascular lesion from study of eight necropsy patients. *Circulation* 1973; 48:1014.

Doherty NE, Siegel RJ: Cardiovascular manifestation of systemic lupus erythematosus. *Am Heart J* 1985; 110:1257.

Hartop J, Tsipouras P, Hanley JA, et al: Cardiovascular involvement of osteogenesis imperfecta. *Circulation* 1986; 73:54.

Johnson GL, Vine DL, Gottrill CM, et al: Echocardiographic mitral valve deformity in mucopolysaccharidosis. *Pediatrics* 1981; 67:401.

Liberthson RR, Homey C, Fallon JT, et al: Systemic lupus erythermatosus and heart disease. *Primary Cardiol* 1983; 9:77.

Murdock JL, Walker BA, Halpern BI, et al: Life expectancy and causes of death in Marfan syndrome. *N Engl J Med* 1972; 286:804.

Rawsthorne L, Ptacin MJ, Choi H, et al: Lupus valvulitis necessitating double valve replacement. *Arthritis Rheum* 1981; 24:561.

Renteria VG, Ferrans VJ, Roberts WC: The heart in the Hurler syndrome: Gross, histologic and ultrastructural observations in five necropsy cases. *Am J Cardiol* 1976; 38:487.

Roberts WC, Hollingsworth JF, Bulkley BH, et al: Combined mitral and aortic regurgitation in ankylosis spondylitis. Angiographic and anatomical features. *Am J Med* 1974; 56:237.

Stollerman GH: Rheumatic and heritable connective tissue disease of the cardiovascular system. In Braunwald E, ed. *Heart Disease*. 3rd ed. Philadelphia: WB Saunders, 1978: 1706.

Thomas D, Hill W, Geddes R, et al: Early detection of aortic dilatation in ankylosing spondylitis using echocardiography. *Aust NZ J Med* 1982; 12:10.

POMPE'S DISEASE (GLYCOGENOSIS TYPE II)

Boxer RA, Fishman M, LaCorte MA, et al. Cardiac imaging in Pompe disease. *J Comput Asst Tomogr* 1986; 10:857.

Dickinson DF, Houlsby WT, Wilkinson JL: Unusual angiographic appearances of the left ventricle in 2 cases of Pompe's disease (glycogenosis type II). *Br Heart J* 1979; 41:238.

Rees A, Elbl F, Minhs K, et al: Echocardiographic evidence of outflow tract obstruction in Pompe's disease (glycogen storage disease of the heart). *Am J Cardiol* 1976; 37:1103.

INFANTS OF DIABETIC OR PREDIABETIC MOTHERS

Friedman WF. Acquired heart disease in infancy. In Braunwald E, ed. *Heart Disease*. 3rd ed. Philadelphia. WB Saunders, 1988: 1012.

ENDOCARDIAL FIBROELASTOSIS

Condon V: The heart and great vessels. In Silverman FN, ed. *Caffey's Pediatric X-Ray Diagnosis*. 8th ed. Chicago: Year Book Medical Publishers, 1985: 999.

Engle MA, Ehlers KH: Endocardial anomalies of the left heart. *Dis Chest* 1955; 5:380.

Factor SM: Endocardial fibroelastosis: Myocardial and vascular alterations associated with viral-like nuclear particles. *Am Heart J* 1978; 96·791.

Friedman WF: Acquired heart disease in infancy. In Braunwald E, ed. *Heart Disease*. 3rd ed. Philadelphia: WB Saunders, 1988: 1012.

ENDOMYOCARDIAL FIBROSIS (EMF)

Davies JNP, Bold JD: The pathology of endocardial fibrosis in Uganda. *Br Heart J* 1955; 17:337.

Wynne J, Braunwald E: The cardiomyopathies and myocarditides. In Braunwald E, ed. *Heart Disease*. 3rd ed. Philadelphia: WB Saunders, 1988:1435.

CHAPTER 30: TREATMENT OF ISCHEMIC HEART DISEASE BY SURGERY AND CATHETER TECHNIQUES

PERCUTANEOUS TRANSLUMINAL CORONARY ANGIOPLASTY (PTCA)

Anderson HV, King III SB: Coronary artery laser therapy. *AJR* 1988; 150:995.

Brown BG, Olson EL, Dodge HT: Percutaneous transluminal coronary angioplasty and subsequent restenosis: Quantitative and qualitative methodology for their assessment. *Am J Cardiol* 1987; 60:34B.

Connor AR, Vlietstra RE, Schaff HV: Earlier and late results of coronary artery bypass after failed angioplasty. Actuarial analysis of late cardiac events and comparison with initially successful angioplasty. *J Thorac Cardiovasc Surg* 1988; 96:191.

Davies MJ, Woolf N, Robertson WB: Pathology of acute myocardial infarction with particular reference to occlusive coronary thrombi. *Br Heart J* 1976; 38:659.

Fuster V, Steele PM, Chesebro JH: Role of platelets and thrombosis in coronary artery sclerotic disease and sudden death. *J Am Coll Cardiol* 1985; 5:175B.

Gruentzig AR, Senning A, Siegenthaler WE: Non-operative dilatation of coronary artery stenosis: Percutaneous transluminal coronary angioplasty. *N Engl J Med* 1979: 301:61.

Holmes DR, Vlietstra RE: Percutaneous transluminal coronary angioplasty: Current status and future trends. *Mayo Clin Proc* 1986; 61:865.

King SB III: Prediction of acute closure in percutaneous transluminal coronary angioplasty. *Circulation* 1990; 81 (suppl IV):IV.

Roberts WC, Buja LM: The frequency and significance of coronary arterial thrombi and other observations in fatal acute myocardial infarction. The study of 107 necropsy patients. *Am J Med* 1972; 52:425.

Roubin GS, King SB III, Douglas JS: Restenosis and percutaneous transluminal coronary angioplasty: The Emory University Hospital experience. *Am J Cardiol* 1987; 60:39B.

Roubin GS, King SB III, Douglas JS, et al: Intracoronary stenting during percutaneous transluminal coronary angioplasty. *Circulation* 1990; 81 (suppl IV): IV.

SURGICAL REVASCULARIZATION

Campeau L, Lesperance J, Bourassa MG: Natural history of saphenous vein aortocoronary bypass grafts. *Mod Concepts Cardiovasc Dis* 1984; 53:59.

FitzGibbon GM, Leach AJ, Keon WG, et al: Coronary bypass graft fate. Angiographic study of 1179 vein grafts early, one year, and five years after operation. *J Thorac Cardiovasc Surg* 1986; 91:773.

Goldman S, Copeland J, Moritz T: Internal mammary artery and saphenous vein graft patency. Effects of aspirin. *Circulation* 1990; 82 (suppl IV):237.

Goldman S, Copeland J, Moritz T, et al: Saphenous vein graft patency one year after coronary bypass surgery and effects of antiplatelet therapy. *Circulation* 1989; 80:1190.

Kaiser GC: CABG: Lessons from the randomized trials. *Ann Thorac Surg* 1986; 42:3.

McNamara JJ, Bjerke HS, Chung GKT, et al: Blood flow in sequential vein grafts. *Circulation* 1979; 60 (suppl I):33.

Morris JJ, Smith LR, Glower DD, et al: Clinical evaluation of single versus multiple mammary artery bypass. *Circulation* 1990; 82 (suppl IV):214.

Reeder G, Bresnahan JF, Holmes DR: Angioplasty for aortocoronary bypass graft stenosis. *Mayo Clin Proc* 1986; 61:14.

Tector AJ, Schmall TM, Janson B, et al: The internal mammary artery graft: Its longevity after coronary bypass. *JAMA* 1981; 246;2181.

TREATMENT OF ACUTE MYOCARDIAL INFARCTION

DeFeyter PJ, van Eenige MJ, van der Wall MJ, et al: Effects of spontaneous and streptokinase-induced recanalization on left ventricular function after myocardial infarction. *Circulation* 1983; 67:1039.

DeWood MA, Motske RN, Hensley GR, et al: Intra-aortic balloon contra pulsations with and without reperfusion for myocardial infarction shock. *Circulation* 1980; 61:1105.

Ellis SG: Interventions in acute myocardial infarctions. *Circulation* 1990; 81 (suppl IV):43.

Goldberg S, Greenspan AJ, Urban PL, et al: Reperfusion arrhythmia: A marker of restoration of antegrade flow during intracoronary thrombolysis for acute myocardial infarction. *Am Heart J* 1983; 105:26.

Kennedy JW, Ritchie JL, Davis KB, et al: Western Washington randomized trial of intracoronary streptokinase in acute myocardial infarction. *N Engl J Med* 1983; 309:1477.

Lavie CJ, Gersh BJ, Chesebro JH: Reperfusion in acute myocardial infarction. *Mayo Clin Proc* 1990; 65:549.

Leiboff RH, Katz RJ, Wasserman AG, et al: A randomized angiographically controlled trial of intracoronary streptokinase in acute myocardial infarction. *Am J Cardiol* 1984; 53:404.

Marx M, Levin DC: Coronary thrombolytic therapy: State of the art. *AJR* 1986; 147:1.

Reduto LA, Smalling RW, Freund GC, et al: Intracoronary infusion of streptokinase in patients with acute myocardial infarction: Effects of reperfusion on left ventricular performance. *Am J Cardiol* 1981; 48:403.

Rogers WBJ, Mantle JA, Hood WBP, et al: Prospective randomized trial of intravenous and intracoronary streptokinase in acute myocardial infarction. *Circulation* 1983; 68:1051.

Serruys PW, Suryapranata H, Simoons ML, et al: Intracoronary thrombosis in patients with acute myocardial infarction: The Netherlands randomized trial and current status. *Circulation* 1987; 76 (suppl II):63.

CHAPTER 31: BALLOON ANGIOPLASTY, EMBOLIZATION THERAPY, AND VALVE REPLACEMENT

BALLOON VALVULOPLASTY: HISTORIC, AORTIC VALVE

Dotter CT, Judkins MP: Transluminal treatment of atherosclerotic obstruction: Description of a new technique and a preliminary report of its application. *Circulation* 1964; 30:654.

Gruentzig AR, Senning A, Siegenthaler WE: Non-operative dilatation of coronary-artery stenosis: Percutaneous transluminal coronary angioplasty. *N Engl J Med* 1979; 301:61.

Isner JM, Salem DN, Desnoyers MR, et al: Treatment of calcific aortic stenosis by balloon valvuloplasty. *Am J Cardiol* 1987; 59:313.

Isner JM, Salem DN, Desnoyers MR, et al: Dual balloon technique for valvuloplasty of aortic stenosis in adults. *Am J Cardiol* 1988; 61:583.

Kennedy KD, Hauck AJ, Edwards WD, et al: Mechanisms of reduction of aortic valvular stenosis by percutaneous transluminal balloon valvuloplasty. Report of five cases and review of the literature. *Mayo Clin Proc* 1988; 63:769.

Lababidi Z, Wu J, Waltz JT: Percutaneous balloon aortic valvuloplasty: Results in 23 patients. *Am J Cardiol* 1984; 53:194.

Rocchini AP, Beekman RH, Shachar GB, et al: Balloon aortic valvuloplasty: Results of the valvuloplasty and angioplasty of Congenital Anomalies Registry. *Am J Cardiol* 1990; 65:784.

BALLOON VALVULOPLASTY: PULMONIC VALVE

Cooke JP, Seward JD, Holmes DR: Percutaneous balloon valvulotomy for pulmonic stenosis in an adult. *Mayo Clin Proc* 1987; 62:306.

Kan JS, White RI, Mitchell SE, et al: Percutaneous balloon valvuloplasty: A new method for treating congenital pulmonary-valve stenosis. *N Engl J Med* 1982; 307:540.

BALLOON VALVULOPLASTY: MITRAL VALVE

Block BC, Palacios IF, Jacobs M, et al: The mechanism of successful mitral valvulotomy in humans. *Am J Cardiol* 1987; 59:178.

Chen CH, Wang X, Wang Y, et al: Value of two-dimensional echocardiography in selecting patients and balloon sizes for percutaneous balloon mitral valvuloplasty. *J Am Coll Cardiol* 1989; 14:1651.

Inoue K, Owaki T, Nakamura T, et al: Clinical applications of transvenous mitral commissurotomy by a new balloon catheter. *J Thorac Cardiovasc Surg* 1984; 87:394.

Lock JE, Khalilullah M, Shrivastava S: Percutaneous catheter commissurotomy in rheumatic mitral stenosis. *N Engl J Med* 1985; 313:1515.

Wilkins GT, Weyman A, Abascal V: Percutaneous balloon dilatation of the mitral valve: An analysis of echocardiographic variables related to outcome and the mechanism of dilatation. *Br Heart J* 1988; 60:299.

ANGIOPLASTY OF STENOTIC PULMONARY ARTERIES

Lock JE, Castaneda–Zuniga WR, Fuhrman BP, et al: Balloon dilatation angioplasty of hypoplastic and stenotic pulmonary arteries. *Circulation* 1983; 67:962.

EMBOLIZATION PROCEDURES

Barth KH, White RI, Kaufman SL, et al: Embolotherapy of pulmonary arterial venous malformations with detachable balloons. *Radiology* 1982; 142:599.

Fellows KE: Therapeutic catheter procedures in congenital heart disease: Current status and future prospects. *Cardiovasc Intervent Radiol* 1984; 7:170.

Lasjaunias P, Rodesch G, Druvost P, et al: Treatment of vein of Galen aneurysm malformation. *J Neurosurg* 1989; 7:746.

Stannard MW, Fellows KE: Therapeutic catheter procedures. *Prog Pediatr Radiol* 1980; 7:237.

White RI, Lynch–Nyham A, Terry P, et al: Pulmonary arterial venous malformations. Technique and long term outcome of embolotherapy. *Radiology* 1988; 169:663.

White RI, Mitchell SE, Barth KH, et al: Angioarchitecture of pulmonary arterial venous malformations: An important consideration before embolotherapy. *AJR* 1983; 140:681.

PROSTHETIC VALVES AND EXTERNAL CONDUITS

Agrawal KC, Edwards WD, Feldt RH, et al: Pathogenesis of non-obstructive fibrous peels in right-sided porcine valved extracardiac conduit. *J Thorac Cardiovasc Surg* 1982; 83:584.

Green CE, Glass–Royal M, Bream PR, et al: Cine fluoroscopy evaluation of peri prosthetic valve regurgitation. *AJR* 1988; 151:455.

Kan JS, Marvin WJ, Bass JL, et al: Balloon angioplasty-branch pulmonary artery stenosis: Results from the valvuloplasty and angioplasty of Congenital Anomalies Registry. *Am J Cardiol* 1990; 65:798.

Kitamura S, Sato K, Naito Y: Closure of patent ductus arteriosus by transfemoral catheter method. *Chest* 1976; 70:631.

Kotler MN, Mintz GS, Panidis I, et al: Non-invasive evaluation of normal and abnormal prosthetic valve function. *J Am Coll Cardiol* 1983; 2:151.

Mills NL, King TD: Non-operative closure of left to right shunts. *J Thorac Vasc Surg* 1976; 72:371.

Park SC, Neches WH, Zuberbuhler JR: Clinical use of blade atrial septostomy. *Circulation* 1977; (suppl III); 55:172.

Ross DN, Summerville J: Correction of pulmonary atresia with a homograft aortic valve. *Lancet* 1966; 2:1446.

Silver MD, Butany J: Mechanical heart valves. Methods of examination, complications, and modes of failure. *Hum Pathol* 1987; 18:577.

Steiner RM, Mintz GS, Morse D, et al: The radiology of cardiac valve prostheses. *RadioGraphics* 1988; 8:277.

Zuberbuhler JR, Dankner E, Zoltun R, et al: Tissue adhesive closure of aortic-pulmonary communications. *Am Heart J* 1974; 88:41.

CHAPTER 32: CARDIAC TRANSPLANTATION

Adey C, Nath P, Soto B: Heterotopic heart transplantation: A radiographic review. *RadioGraphics* 1987; 7:151.

Allen M, Naasz CA, Popp RL, et al: Noninvasive assessment of donor and native heart function after heterotopic heart transplantation. *J Thorac Cardiovasc Surg* 1988; 95:75.

Anderson JL, Fowles RE, Biever CP, et al: Idiopathic cardiomyopathy, age, and suppressor-cell dysfunction as risk determinants of lymphoma after cardiac transplantation. *Lancet* 1978; 2:1174.

Austin JH, Schulman LL, Mastrobattista A: Pulmonary infection after cardiac transplantation: Clinical and radiological correlation. *Radiology* 1989; 172:259.

Baumgartner WA, Augustine S, Borkon AM, et al: Present expectations in cardiac transplantation. *Ann Thorac Surg* 1987; 43:585.

Billingham ME: Diagnosis of cardiac rejection by endomyocardial biopsy. *J Heart Transplant* 1982; 1:25.

Carrio I, Berna L, Ballester M, et al: Indium III antimyosin scintigraphy to assess myocardial damage in patients with complete myocarditis and myocardial rejection. *J Nucl Med* 1988; 29:1893.

Couetil JP, McGoldrick JP, Wallwork J, et al: Malignant tumors after heart transplantation. *J Heart Transplant* 1990; 9:622.

Eichenspurner H, Haberl R, Angermann C, et al: New methods for noninvasive monitoring of rejection after heart transplantation. *Texas Heart Inst J* 1988; 15:7.

Frist W, Yasuda D, Segall G, et al: Noninvasive detection of human cardiac transplant rejection with Indium-III antimyosin [FAB] imaging. *Circulation* 1987; 76 (suppl V):81.

Gao S, Alderman EL, Schroeter JS: Progressive coronary luminal narrowing after cardiac transplantation. *Circulation* 1990; 82 (suppl IV):269.

Hanto DW, Frizzerd G, Kzimier A: Epstein-Barr virus immunodeficiency, and B-cell lymphoproliferation. *Transplantation* 1985; 39:461.

Henry DA, Corcoran HL, Lewis TD, et al: Orthotopic cardiac transplantation: Evaluation with CT. *Radiology* 1989; 170:343.

Kinlen L, Sheil AGR, Peto J, et al: Collaborative United Kingdom-Australian study of cancer in patients treated with immuno-suppressive therapy drugs. *Br Med J* 1979; 2:1461.

Konertz W, Sheikhzadeh A, Weyand M, et al: Heterotopic heart transplantation. *Texas Heart Inst J* 1988; 15:159.

Krikorian JG, Anderson JL, Biever CP, et al: Malignant neoplasms following cardiac transplantation. *JAMA* 1978; 240:639.

Levett JM, Karp RM: Heart transplantation. *Surg Clin No Am* 1985; 65:613.

Olivari MT, Kubo SH, Braunlin EA, et al: Five years experience with triple-drug immunosuppressive therapy in cardiac transplantation. *Circulation* 1990; 82 (suppl IV):276.

Pennock JL, Oyer PE, Reitz BA, et al: Cardiac transplantation in perspective for the future. Survival complications: Rehabilitation and costs. *J Thorac Cardiovasc Surg* 1982; 83:168.

Petrossian GA, Nichols AB, Marboe CC: Relation between survival and development of coronary artery disease and anti-HLA antibodies after cardiac transplantation. *Circulation* 1989; 80 (suppl III):122.

Uretsky BF, Murali S, Reddy S, et al: Development of coronary artery disease in cardiac transplant patients receiving immuno-suppressive therapy with cyclosporine and prednisone. *Circulation* 1987; 76:827.

Valantine HA, Fowler MB, Hunt, SA, et al: Changes in Doppler echocardiographic indexes of left ventricular function as a potential marker of acute cardiac rejection. *Circulation* 1987; 76 (suppl V):86.

Weyand M: Heterotopic heart transplantation. Current indications for the procedure, with results in ten patients. *Texas Heart Inst J* 1988; 15:159.

Wisenberg G, Pflugfelder PW, Kostuk WJ, et al: Diagnostic applicability of magnetic resonance imaging in assessing human cardiac allograft rejection. *Am J Cardiol* 1987; 60:130.

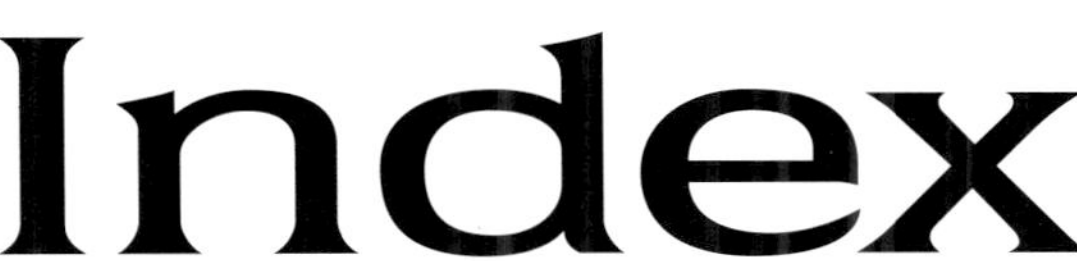

Index

Note: numbers in **boldface** refer to Figure numbers

COLOR APPENDIX

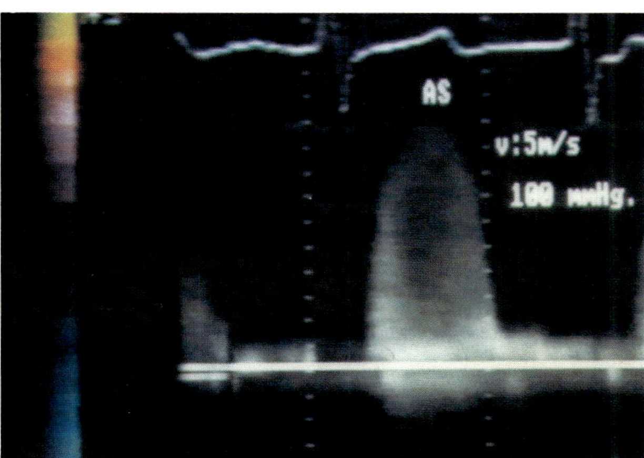

Fig. 2.12 Spectral wave form by continuous Doppler in aortic stenosis from suprasternal approach. The vertical axis measures the velocity of the blood through the aortic orifice during systole (5 meters per second). The calculated gradient through the aortic valve is 100 mm Hg. (AS = aortic stenosis; V = velocity of blood through the aortic valve; mm Hg = pressure.measured in millimeters of Hg)

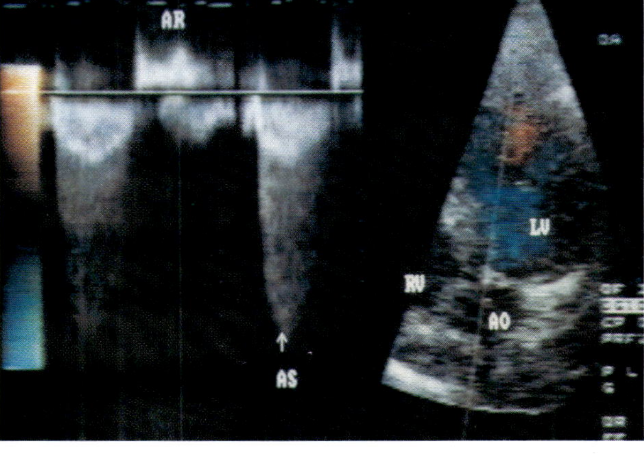

Fig. 2.13 Spectral wave form of Doppler, demonstrating high velocity through the aortic valve. (left) From an apical window, aortic insufficiency is demonstrated on top of the baseline and the stenosis is towards the lower part in the opposite direction. (right) Continuous-wave Doppler beam directed through the area of the aortic valve. The blue color signals indicate laminar velocity during systole, located before the site of obstruction. (AR = aortic regurgitation; AS = aortic stenosis; CD = continuous Doppler)

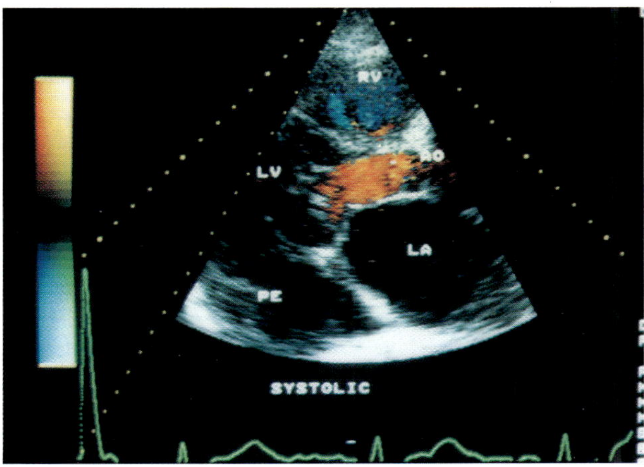

Fig. 2.14 Long-axis view of the heart from the parasternal window. Systolic frame. Red signal in LV represents the laminar blood flow towards the aorta. The red and blue signals to the right of the septum represent the turbulent jet produced by blood passing through the ventricular septal defect.

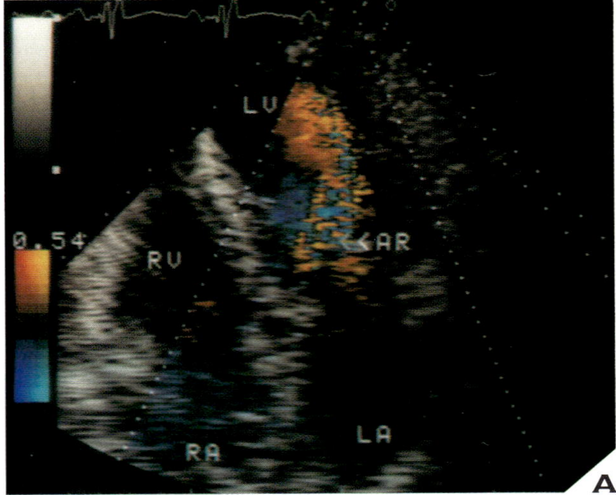

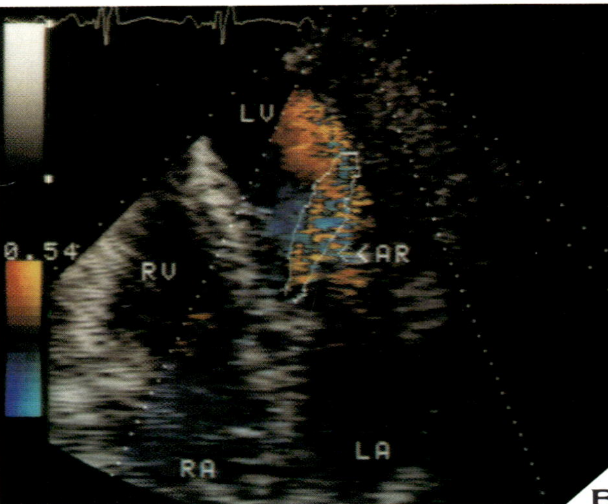

Fig. 2.17 Color Doppler depicting aortic insufficiency; 2-D echocardiogram in four-chamber projection from apical window in diastolic frames. (A) Mosaic color signal is seen in the left ventricular outflow tract, indicating aortic insufficiency. (B) Planimetry of the area of the aortic insufficiency indicates Grade III insufficiency. (AR = aortic insufficiency)

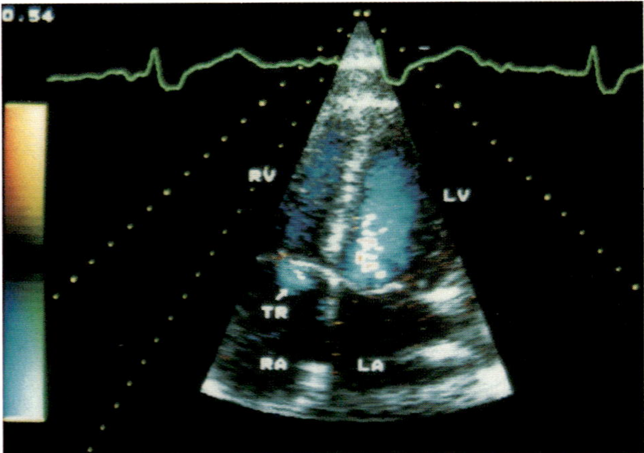

Fig. 2.18 Tricuspid insufficiency. Four-chamber view and apical approach were used. Color Doppler demonstrates blue signals in right atrium during systole, indicating mild tricuspid insufficiency (TR). Note that the mitral valve is competent.

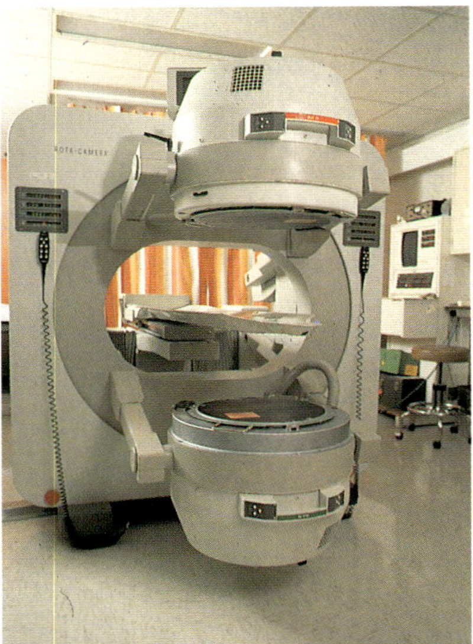

Fig. 4A.3
A SPECT camera.

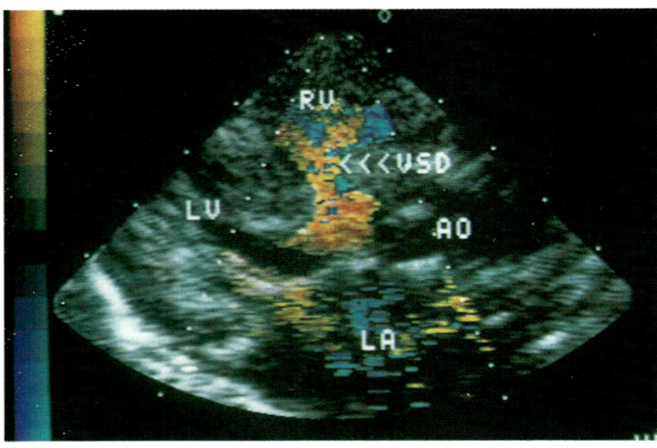

Fig. 9.6 Muscular outlet VSD. Color Doppler image (apical long axis projection) of 2-dimensional echocardiogram demonstrates ventricular septal defect (VSD) with turbulent flow in right ventricle secondary to the left to right shunt.

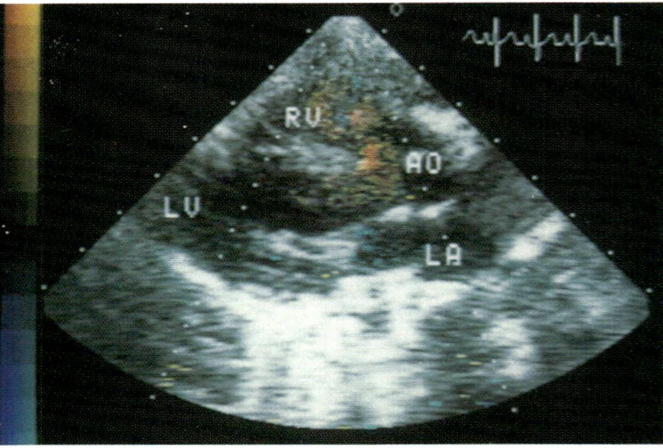

Fig. 11.9 Tetralogy of Fallot (echocardiographic features). Long-axis projection through a paracardial window shows the aorta overriding the ventricular septal defect. Both ventricles connect with the aortic valve.

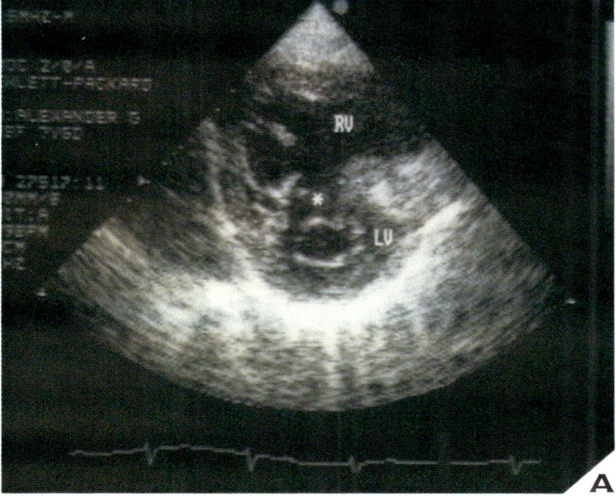

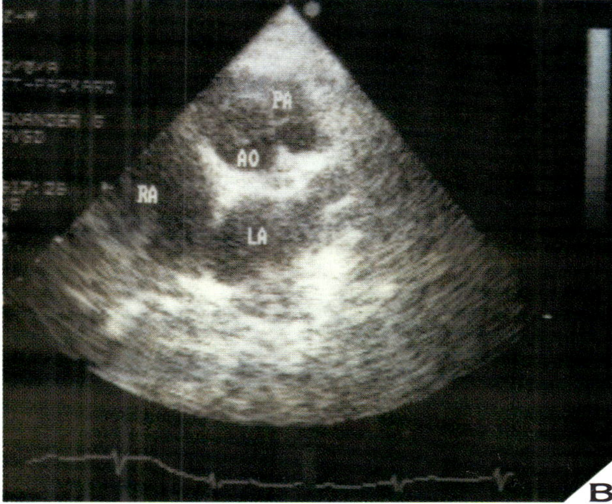

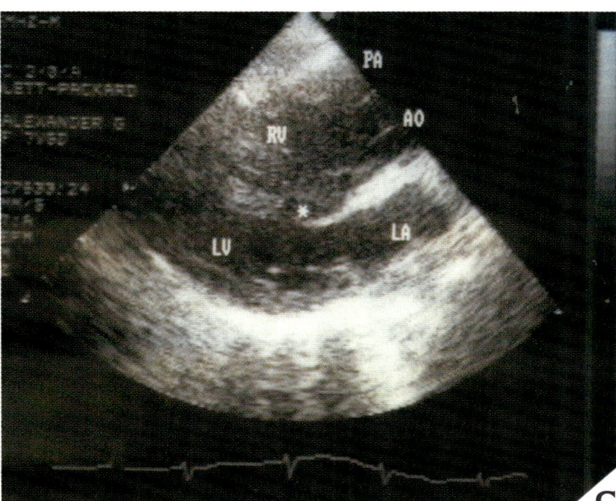

Fig. 11.28 Double-outlet right ventricle (echocardiographic findings). Short-axis views via a parasternal window at the level of the ventricles (A) and atria (B). The atria are normally related and are located posterior to the aorta and pulmonary trunk. The ventricles are connected via a muscular VSD (*). (C) Long-axis view. The morphologic right ventricle is anterior and supports the aorta and pulmonary trunk (PA).

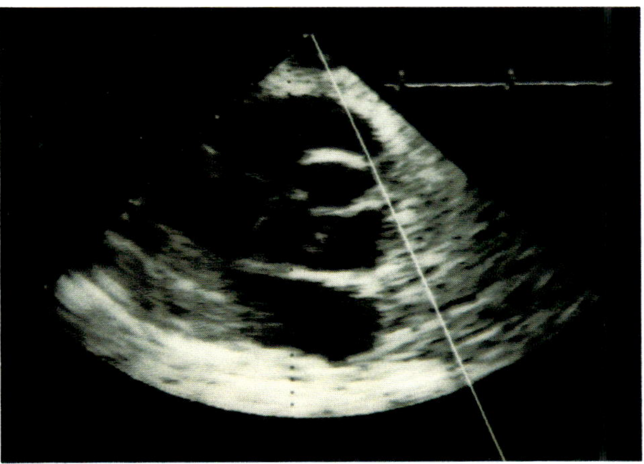

Fig. 11.37 Pulmonary atresia with VSD (echocardiographic features). Short-axis projection shows absence of right ventricular outlet. The right ventricle is connected to the aorta via a large VSD.

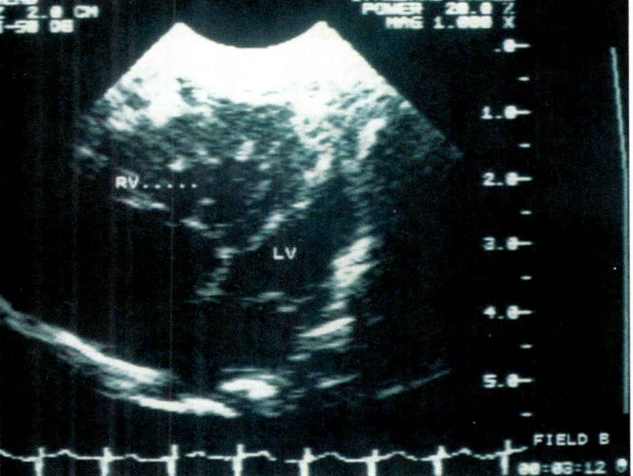

Fig. 11.43 Pulmonary atresia with intact ventricular septum (echocardiographic findings). Four-chamber parasternal view. The left atrium and left ventricle are in continuity and are of normal size. The aortic valve is related to the left ventricle. The right ventricle is very small.

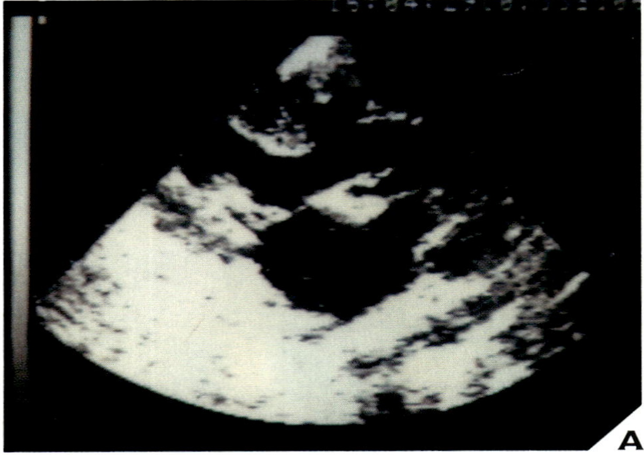

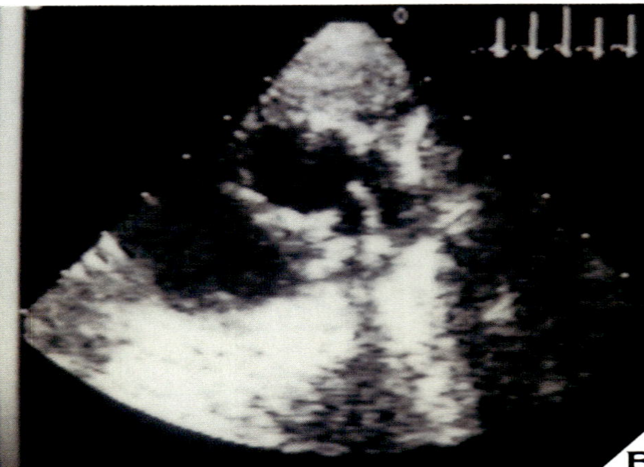

Fig. 11.49 Truncus arteriosus (echocardiographic features). Long-axis (A) and short-axis (B) projections. The left ventricle is connected to the truncal valve. The truncus arteriosus, located immediately above the truncal valve, divides into left and right pulmonary arteries and continues as the aorta.

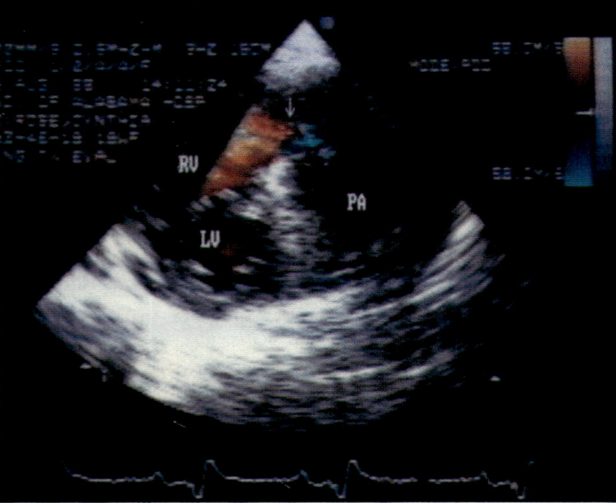

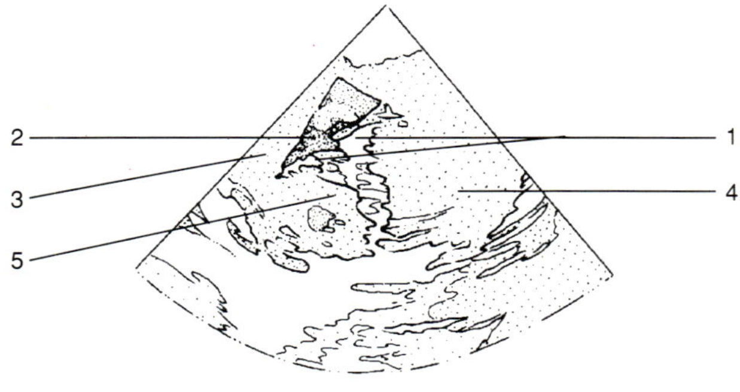

1 deformed pulmonic valve	4 pulmonary trunk
2 turbulent flow	5 left ventricle
3 right ventricle	

Fig. 13.9 Isolated absence of the pulmonic valve leaflets. Color-flow Doppler echocardiography (short axis section) shows severe turbulence in the right ventricle during diastole, indicating severe pulmonic insufficiency. The dysplastic pulmonic valve leaflets are represented by a short echogenic ridge. The pulmonary trunk is markedly dilated.

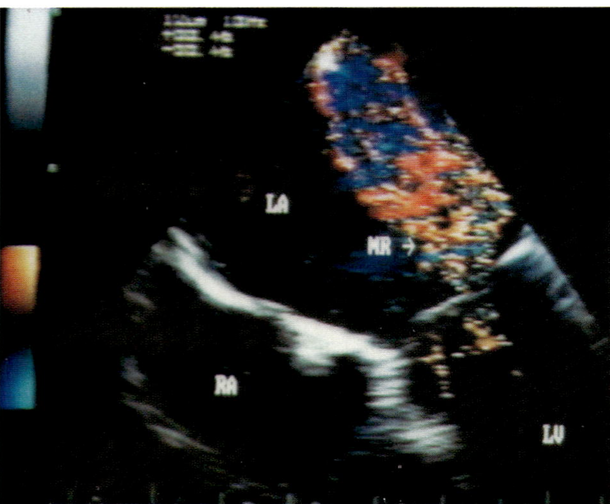

Fig. 13.13 Congenital mitral insufficiency. Color-flow Doppler echocardiogram (four-chamber view via parasternal window; in systole) shows left ventricular and left atrial enlargement. Note marked turbulence (MR) in the left atrium, indicating severe mitral insufficiency.

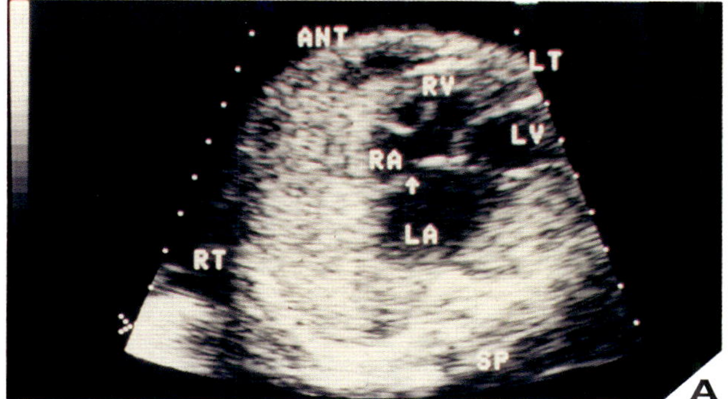

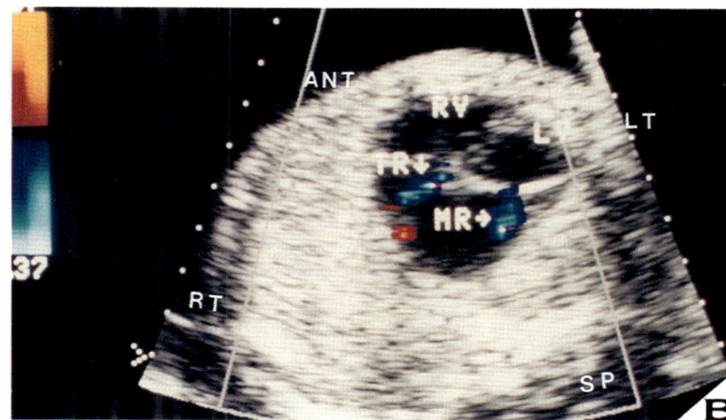

Fig. 15A.14 Severe aortic stenosis. (A) Four-chamber view demonstrates enlargement of the left ventricle and left atrium. The atrial septum (*arrow*) is bulging from left to right. (B) Color Doppler flow mapping in the same fetus demonstrates blue regurgitant jets in the atrium, indicating the presence of both mitral (MR) and tricuspid (TR) insufficiency. (RT = right; LT = left; ANT = anterior; SP = spine)

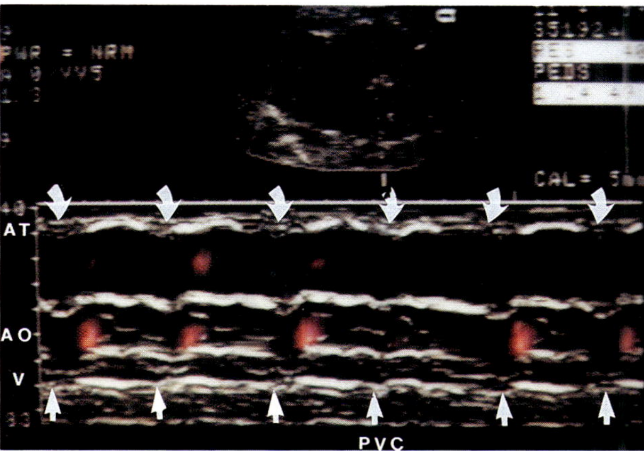

Fig. 15A.22 Premature ventricular contraction. Color M-mode echocardiogram. The M-mode cursor passes first through the posterior (left) atrium (AT), then through the aortic root (AO), and finally through the wall of the right ventricle (V). The ventricular motion (*straight arrows*) precedes the atrial motion (*curved arrows*) during the premature beat. There is a compensatory pause after the premature beat. The red color in the central portion of the figure represents flow in the aortic root during systole. The premature beat is followed by opening of the aortic valve; however, because the ventricle has not had sufficient time to completely fill for this ejection, there is very little color.

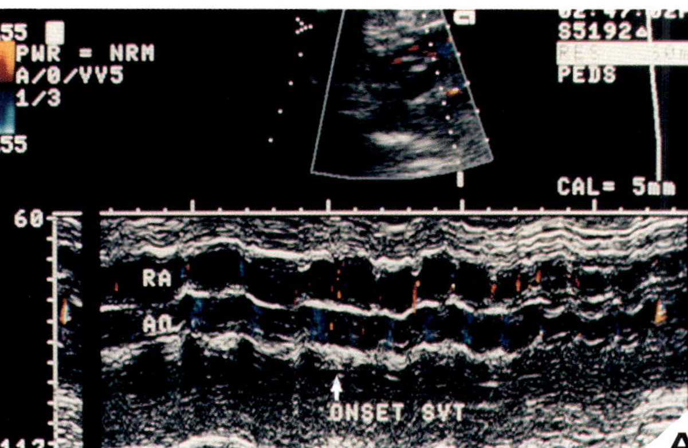

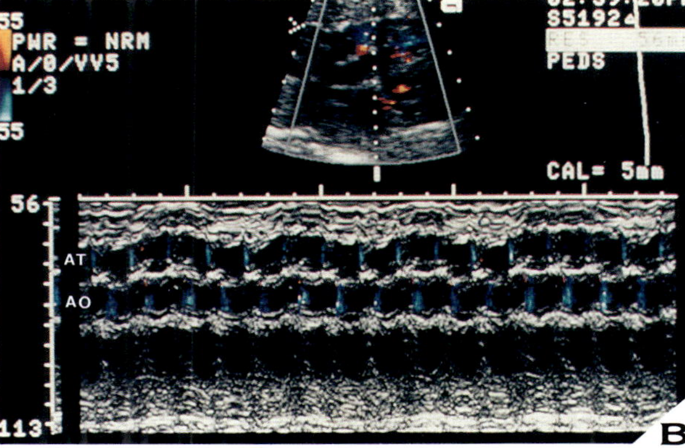

Fig. 15A.24 Supraventricular tachycardia (SVT). (A) Color M-mode echocardiogram at the onset of SVT (*arrow*). Without color, fetal movement would make interpretation very difficult. (B) Stable SVT. Both atrial and ventricular flow are away from the transducer and are shown in blue.

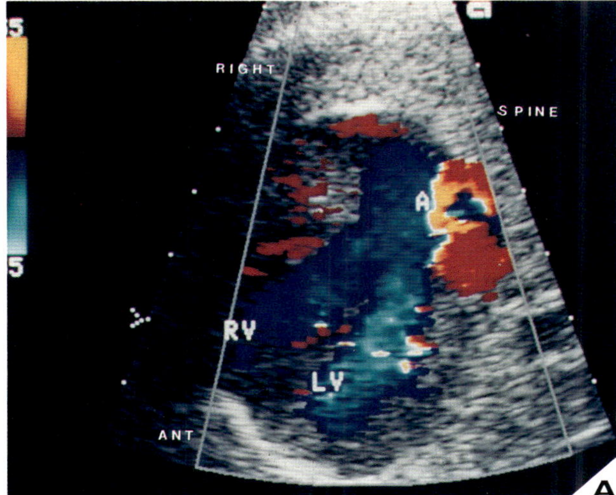

Fig. 15A.31 Color flow Doppler imaging: effect of transducer position on color encoding. (A) With the fetus oriented so that the apex of the heart is pointed away from the transducer, diastolic flow is encoded as blue. (B) With the fetus oriented so that the apex is pointed away from the transducer, diastolic flow is encoded in red.

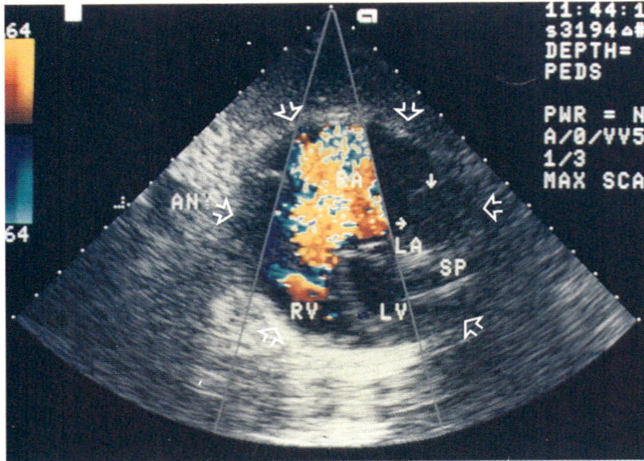

Fig. 15A.32 Tricuspid insufficiency with secondary congestive heart failure. Transverse section of the fetal chest (outlined by *open arrows*) shows very little amniotic fluid around the fetus. The heart occupies almost the entire thorax in this scanning plane, leaving very little room for the lungs. The right ventricle and right atrium are massively enlarged. The color flow map demonstrates the turbulence of the regurgitant flow across the tricuspid valve into the right atrium. The arrows indicate the location of the interatrial septum. (SP = fetal spine)

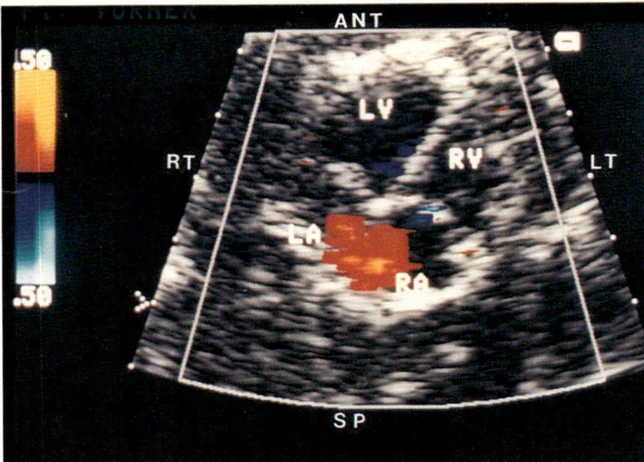

Fig. 15A.33 Normal right to right shunting through the foramen ovale. In this normal fetus, oriented with the apex pointing towards the transducer, the flow from the right atrium to the left atrium is encoded as red. In addition, there is a trivial blue jet tricuspid insufficiency.

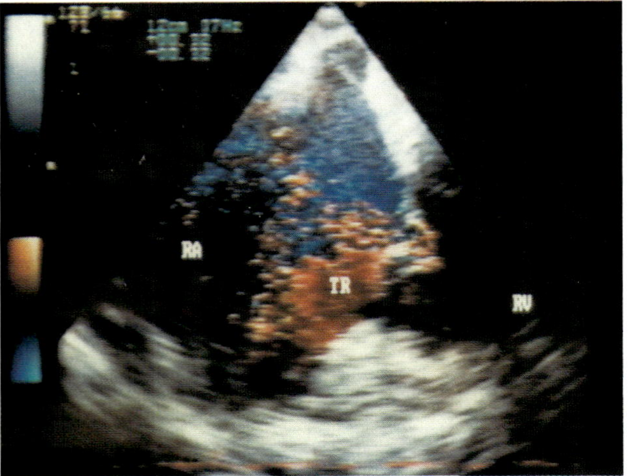

Fig. 16.29 Severe tricuspid insufficiency following repair of tetralogy of Fallot. Color Doppler image of echocardiogram in the long axial projection (in systole) demonstrates severe turbulence in the right atrium caused by the regurgitant jet. Color, indicating turbulence, is present in almost half the right atrial cavity.

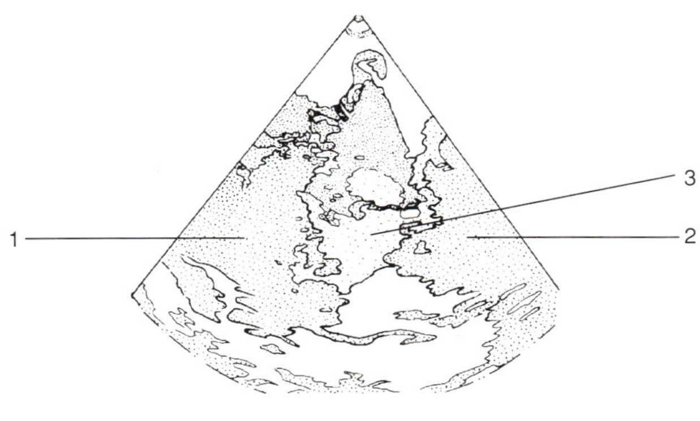

1 right atrium
2 right ventricle
3 regurgitant jet through incompetent tricuspid valve

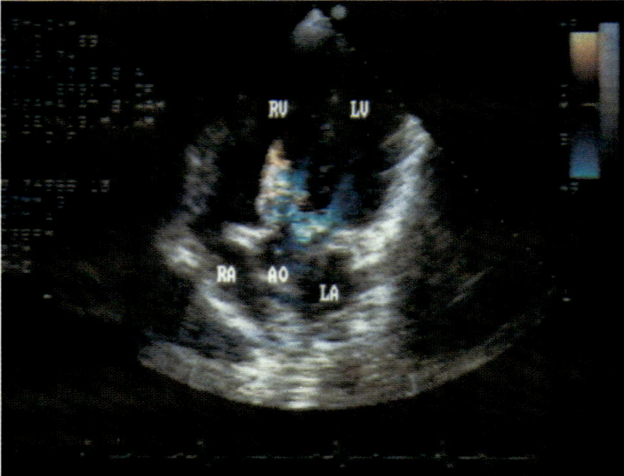

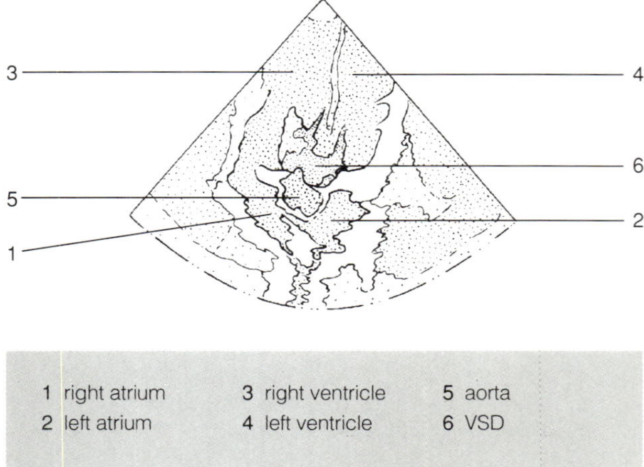

1 right atrium
2 left atrium
3 right ventricle
4 left ventricle
5 aorta
6 VSD

Fig. 16.30 Residual VSD after complete repair of tetralogy of Fallot. Color Doppler image of echocardiogram (four-chamber view) demonstrates significant turbulence in the right ventricle produced by blood passing across the VSD from the left ventricle. The VSD is closely related to the aortic valve.

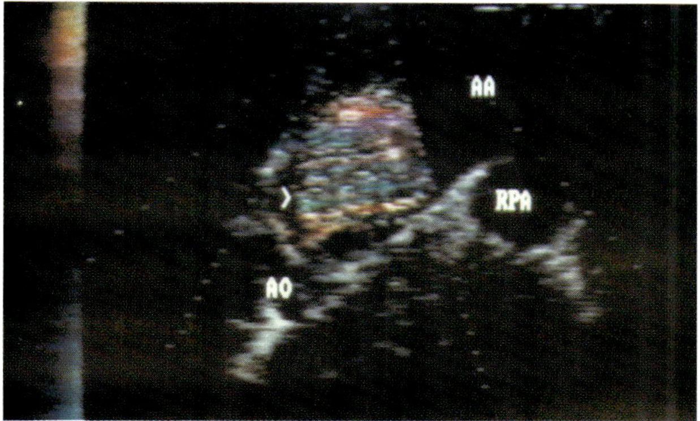

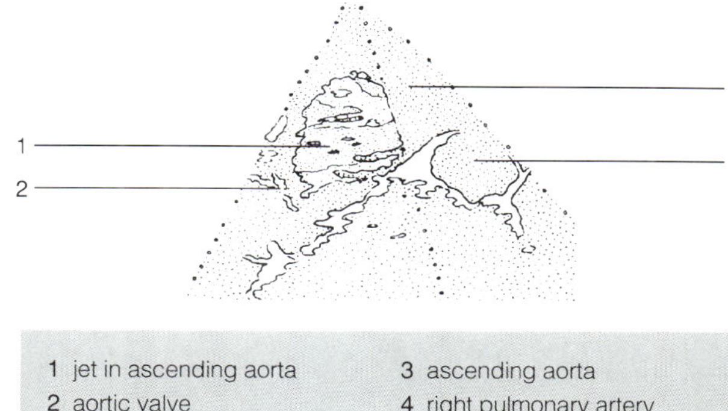

1 jet in ascending aorta	3 ascending aorta
2 aortic valve	4 right pulmonary artery

Fig. 18.8 Severe aortic stenosis. Two-dimensional color Doppler electrocardiogram (right parasternal view of ascending aorta). The mosaic pattern of blood within the jet reflects turbulent flow beyond the stenotic valve. The base of the jet is very narrow, indicating severe aortic stenosis.

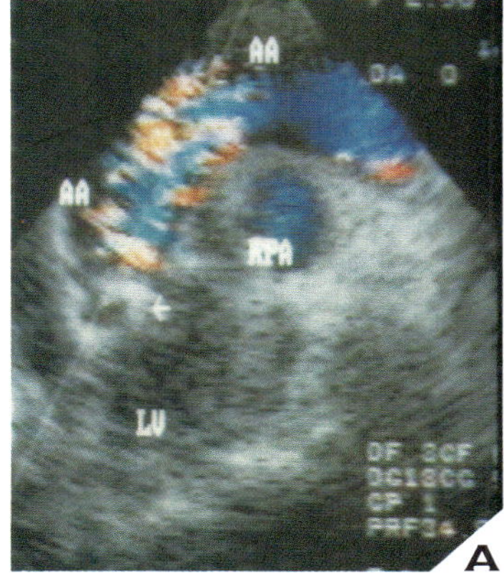

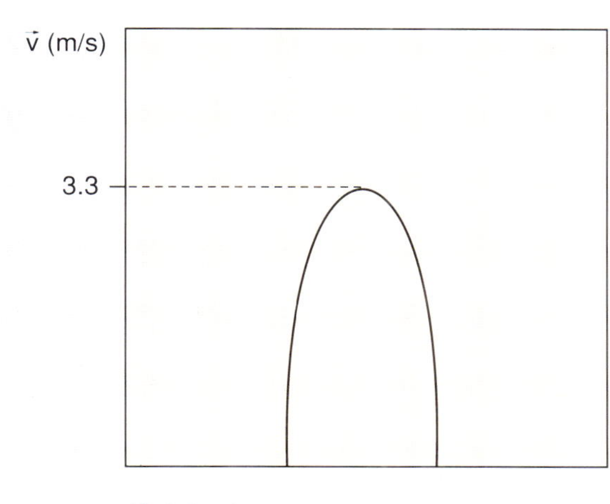

v̄: 3.3 m/s
Δ: 44 mm Hg

B

Fig. 18.9 Aortic stenosis. Two-dimensional color Doppler (A) and diagrammatic representation of the corresponding continuous wave Doppler recording (B) of poststenotic jet. The velocity of the jet was 3.3 meters/second and the calculated instantaneous peak gradient was 44 mm Hg.

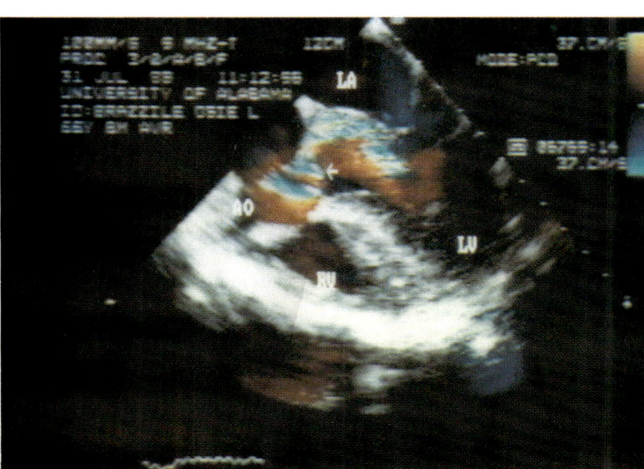

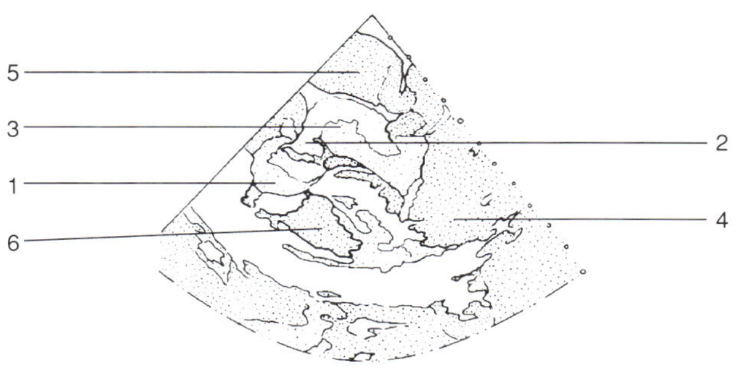

Fig. 18.21 Aortic insufficiency secondary to aortic valve prolapse. Transesophageal color Doppler echocardiogram. Frontal long axial scan demonstrates an eccentric mosaic-pattern jet in the left ventricular outflow tract originating at the aortic valve, indicating aortic regurgitation. A prolapsed aortic valve leaflet is also seen.

1 aorta	4 left ventricle
2 prolapsed aortic valve leaflet	5 left atrium
3 regurgitant jet in left ventricular outflow tract	6 right ventricle

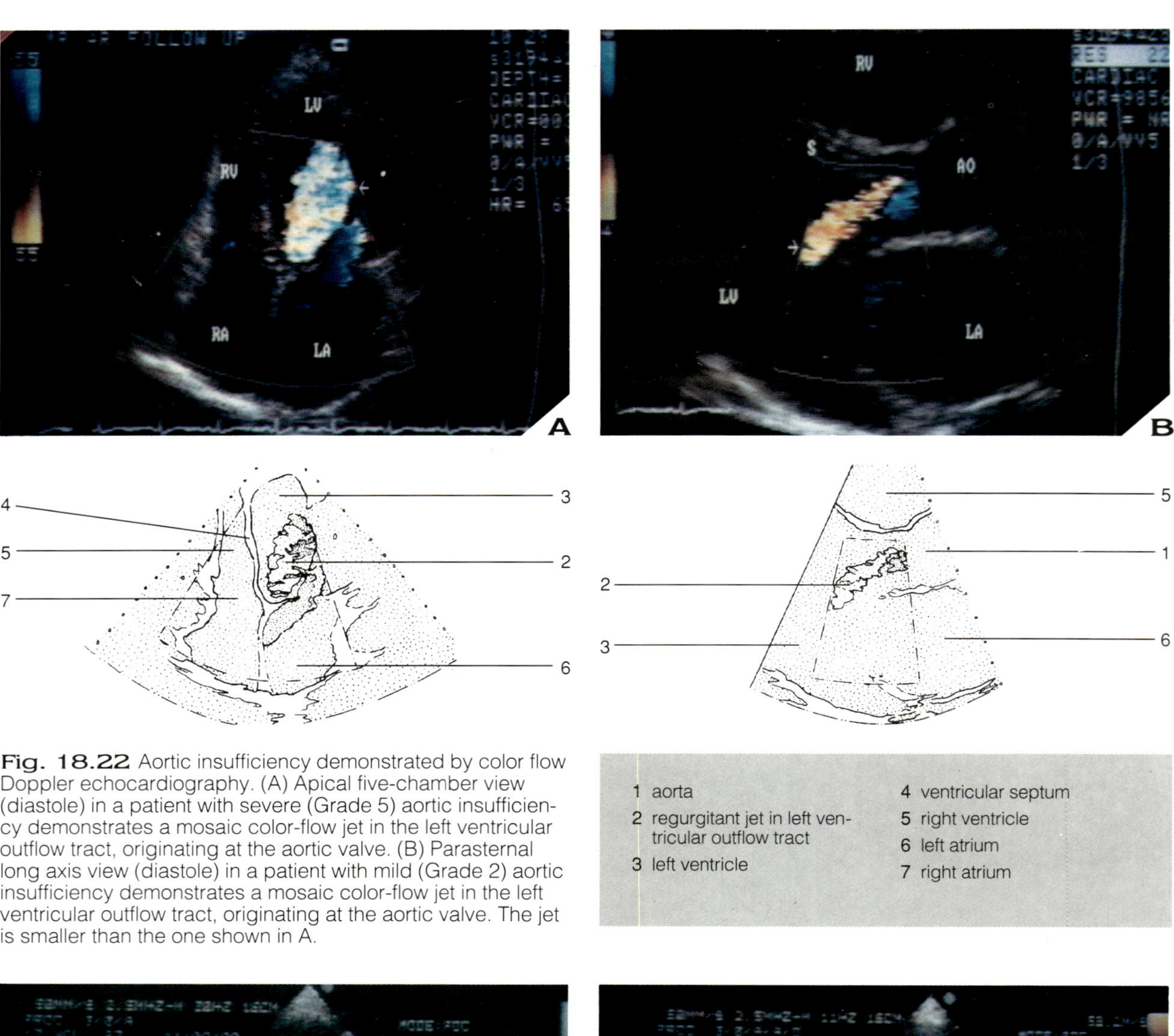

Fig. 18.22 Aortic insufficiency demonstrated by color flow Doppler echocardiography. (A) Apical five-chamber view (diastole) in a patient with severe (Grade 5) aortic insufficiency demonstrates a mosaic color-flow jet in the left ventricular outflow tract, originating at the aortic valve. (B) Parasternal long axis view (diastole) in a patient with mild (Grade 2) aortic insufficiency demonstrates a mosaic color-flow jet in the left ventricular outflow tract, originating at the aortic valve. The jet is smaller than the one shown in A.

1 aorta
2 regurgitant jet in left ventricular outflow tract
3 left ventricle
4 ventricular septum
5 right ventricle
6 left atrium
7 right atrium

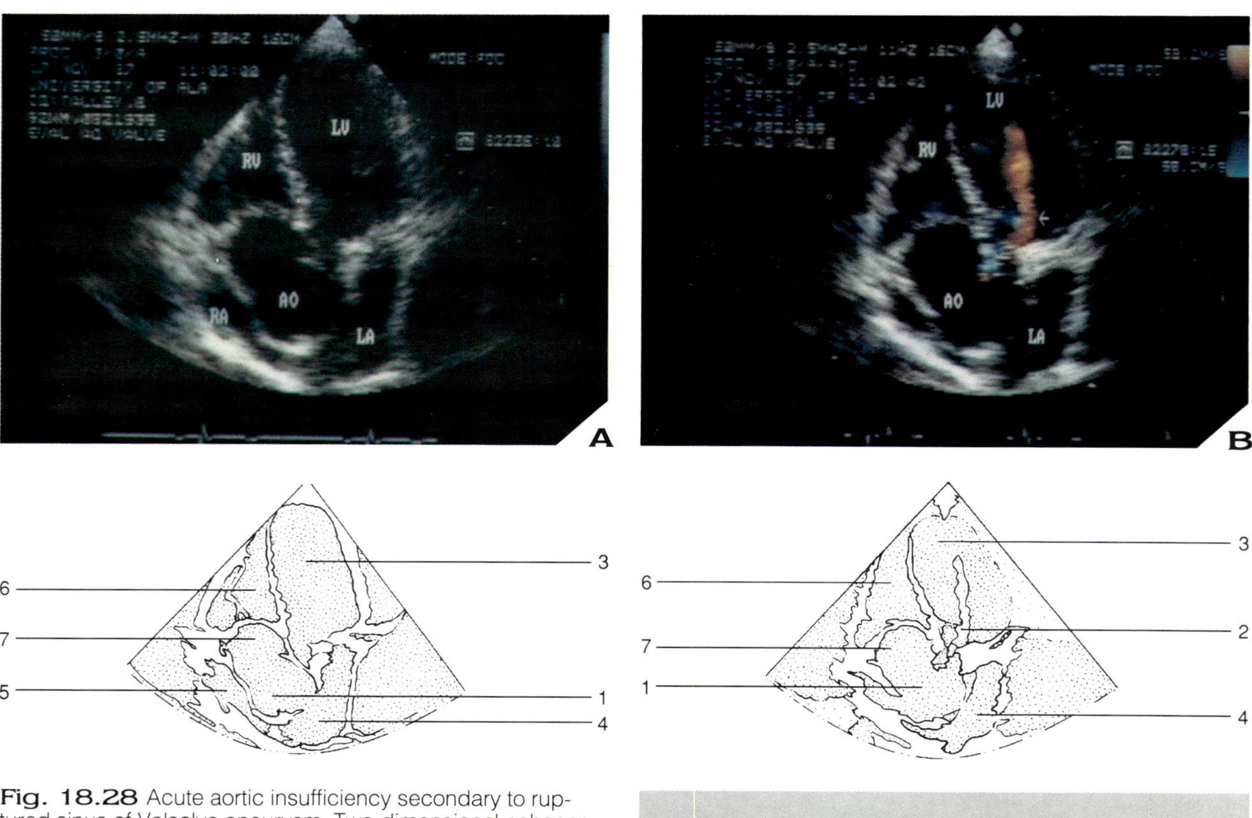

Fig. 18.28 Acute aortic insufficiency secondary to ruptured sinus of Valsalva aneurysm. Two-dimensional echocardiogram (apical five-chamber view) without (A) and with (B) color Doppler imaging. Note the regurgitant jet into the left ventricular outflow tract in B. The aortic root is markedly dilated. The aneurysmally enlarged right coronary sinus protrudes into the right ventricle.

1 dilated aortic root
2 regurgitant jet in left ventricular outflow tract
3 left ventricle
4 left atrium
5 right atrium
6 right ventricle
7 aneurysm of right coronary sinus of Valsalva

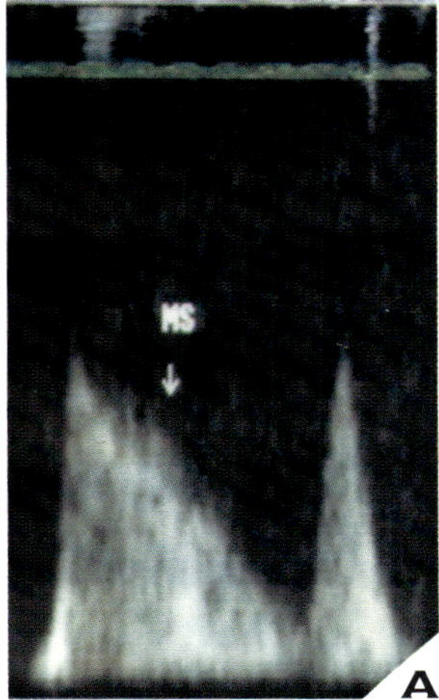

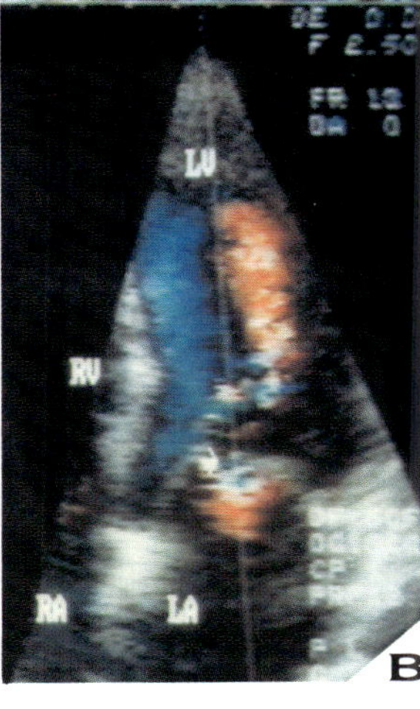

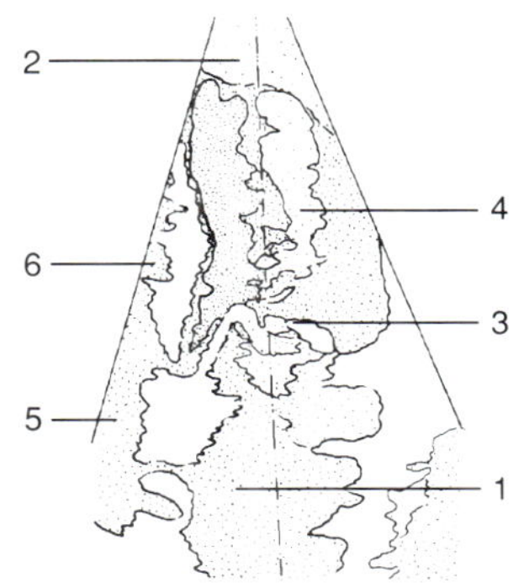

1 left atrium
2 left ventricle
3 domed, stenotic mitral valve
4 turbulent flow
5 right atrium
6 right ventricle

Fig. 18.40 Mitral stenosis. (A) Color Doppler guided continuous wave echocardiography shows findings typical of mitral stenosis. Left atrial emptying is prolonged (100 milliseconds; normal, 20 to 60 milliseconds) and the slope of the run-off curve is abnormally flat. The time needed to decrease the left atrium–left ventricle gradient by 50 percent from its baseline value at the beginning of diastole ($T_{1/2}$) is abnormally long. (B) Two-dimensional color Doppler echocardiogram during diastole (four-chamber view) shows restricted opening of the leaflets with doming of the mitral valve and turbulent flow in the left ventricle.

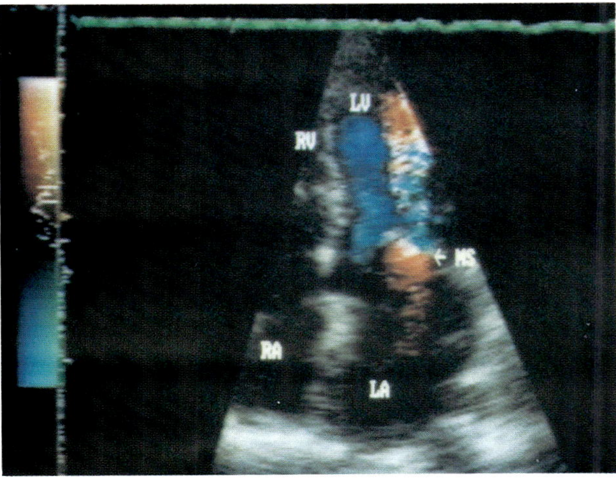

Fig. 18.41 Mitral stenosis. Transthoracic two-dimensional echocardiogram with color Doppler imaging, during diastole (apical four-chamber view). Note the mosaic pattern of the jet originating at the level of the mitral valve. The turbulent jet is directed towards the apex of the left ventricle.

1 left atrium
2 left ventricle
3 stenotic mitral valve
4 jet (turbulent flow)
5 right atrium
6 right ventricle

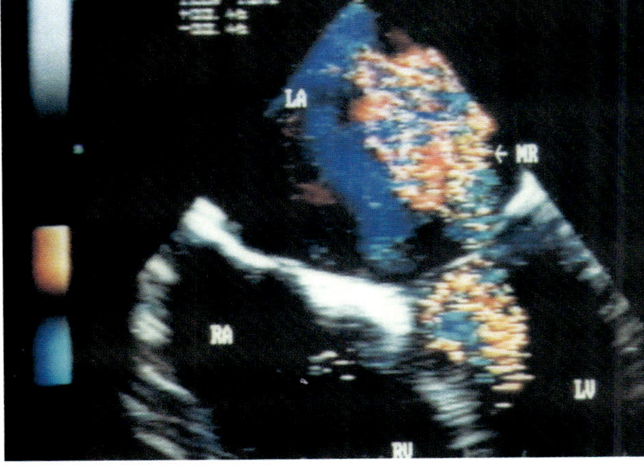

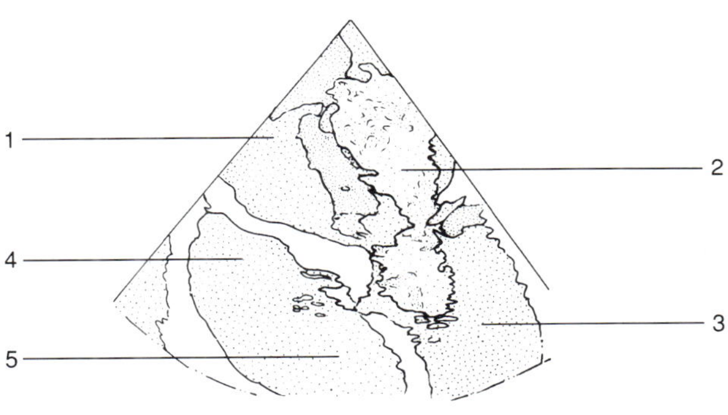

Fig. 18.52 Severe mitral insufficiency demonstrated by color Doppler. Transesophageal echocardiogram (long-axial four-chamber view, in systole) demonstrates a mosaic pattern color-flow jet extending from the mitral valve into the left atrium. The large area occupied by the turbulent jet indicates severe mitral insufficiency.

1 left atrium
2 regurgitant jet
3 left ventricle
4 right atrium
5 right ventricle

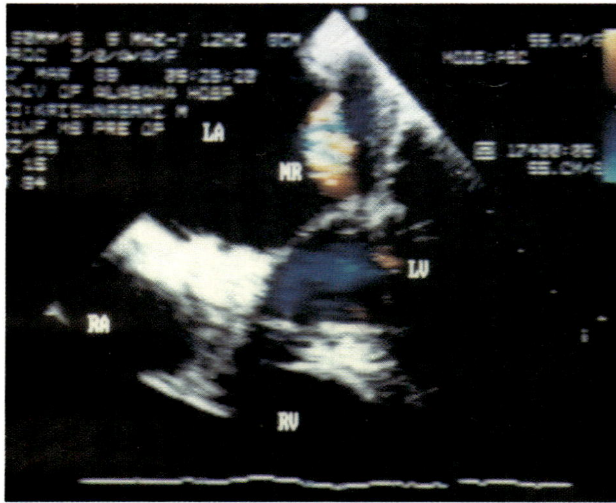

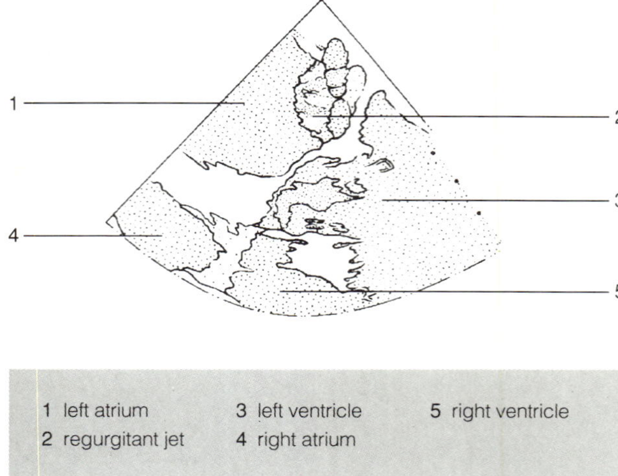

1 left atrium
2 regurgitant jet
3 left ventricle
4 right atrium
5 right ventricle

Fig. 18.53 Mild mitral insufficiency demonstrated by color Doppler technique. Transesophageal echocardiogram with color Doppler imaging. Frontal long-axial four-chamber view (in systole) demonstrates a mosaic jet within the left atrium. Its apex is at the mitral valve orifice. The regurgitant jet occupies a relatively small area, indicating mild mitral insufficiency.

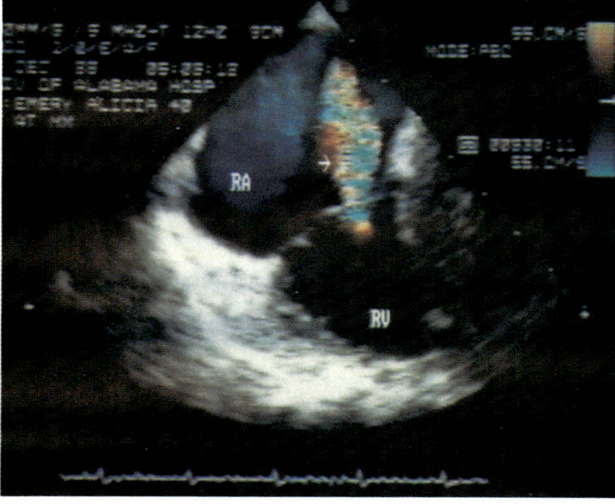

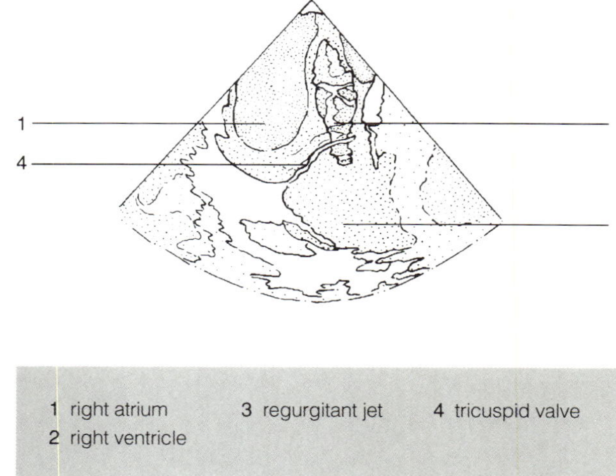

1 right atrium
2 right ventricle
3 regurgitant jet
4 tricuspid valve

Fig. 18.63 Tricuspid insufficiency. Parasternal two-chamber color Doppler image through the right atrium and right ventricle demonstrates turbulence originating at the tricuspid valve and extending into the middle of the right atrium.

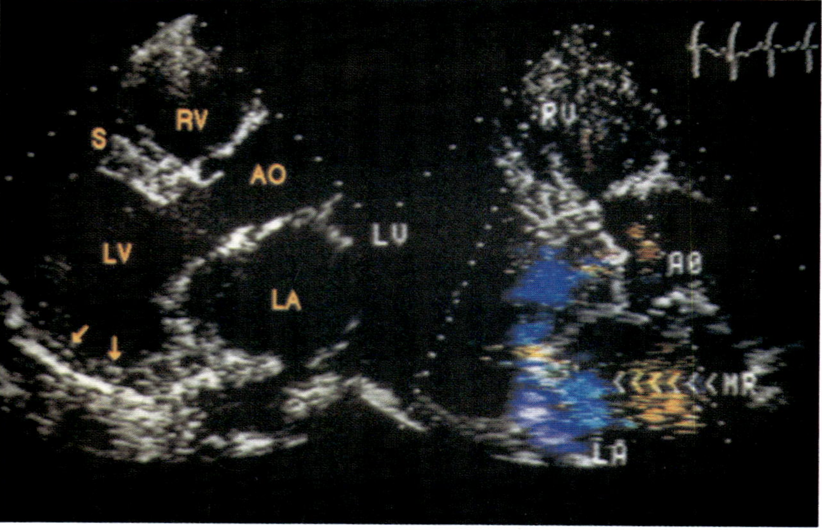

Fig. 20.10 Old myocardial infarction (echocardiographic findings). (left) Long axial view via left parasternal window (in systole) demonstrates a deformity (*arrows*) of the posteroinferior aspect of the left ventricle (LV), immediately beneath the mitral valve; the deformed segment expands during systole. (right) Color Doppler image in systole (same projection). The blue signal in the left atrium (LA) indicates regurgitant blood flow due to mitral insufficiency (MR) (AO = aorta; RV = right ventricle; S = ventricular septum)

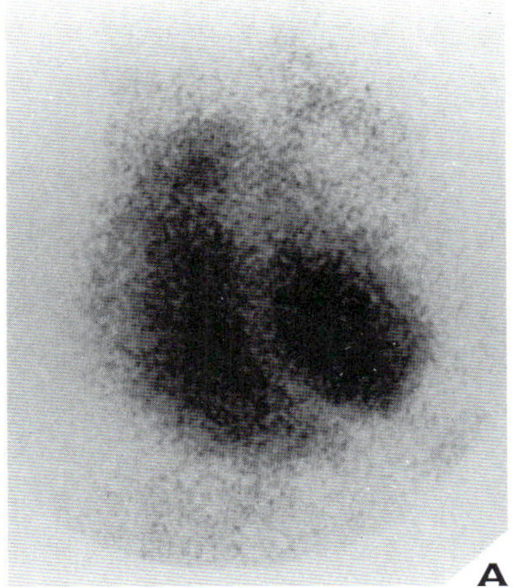

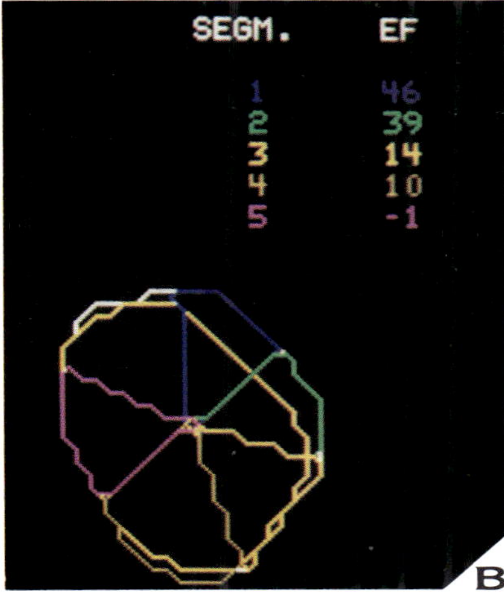

Fig. 20.11 Gated radionuclide angiography. Resting study following intravenous administration of 25 mCi ^{99m}Tc-labeled red blood cells (right anterior oblique projection). (A) Analog display of ventricular activity. (B) Computer-generated tracing of left ventricular contours (by segments) in systole and diastole. Note the globally diminished contractility of the entire left ventricular wall, which is particularly dramatic in the septal, apical, and inferolateral segments.

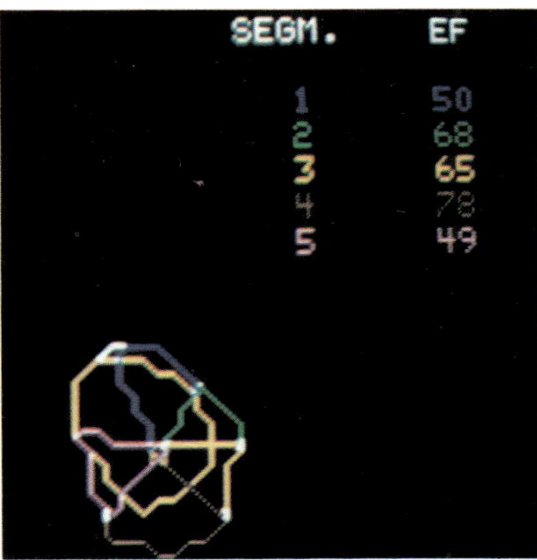

Fig. 20.12 Gated radionuclide angiography. Resting study in right anterior oblique projection following intravenous administration of 25 mCi of ^{99m}Tc-labeled red blood cells. Note superimposition of computer-generated contours of septum and anterolateral wall (segment 5), indicating segmental akinesis. The ECG was compatible with previous myocardial infarction secondary to occlusion of the left anterior descending coronary artery.

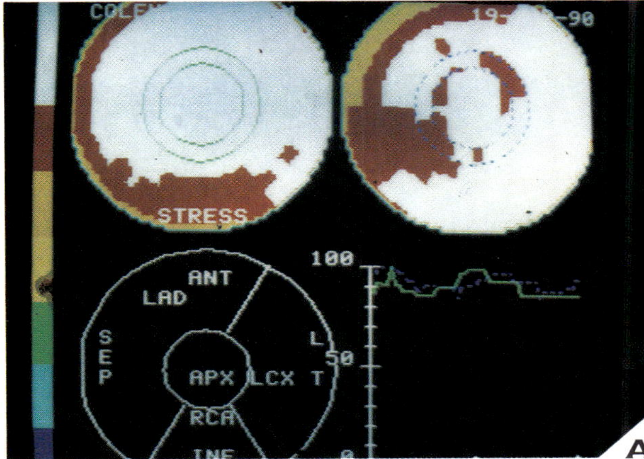

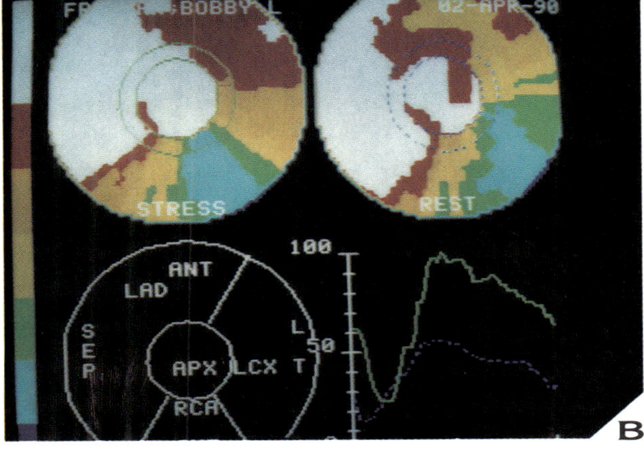

Fig. 20.16 Normal and abnormal thallium exercise stress test. (A and B) SPECT with color-coded "bulls-eye" display. (A) Normal study. Both the stress (left) and resting (right) studies demonstrate uniform distribution of the radiopharmaceutical (^{201}Tl), manifested by a uniform distribution of counts. (B) Myocardial infarction. Note markedly decreased uptake in posterolateral and inferior segments of the left ventricle. There is no change with exercise. This pattern is compatible with an old infarct with scarring (fibrous replacement) of the affected myocardium. (White and red indicate normal myocardial perfusion; blue and red indicate decreased myocardial perfusion.) In the accompanying graphic display (A and B, bottom right), the green line indicates the expected number of counts in the posteroinferior segment of the left ventricle and the blue line indicates the actual number of counts.

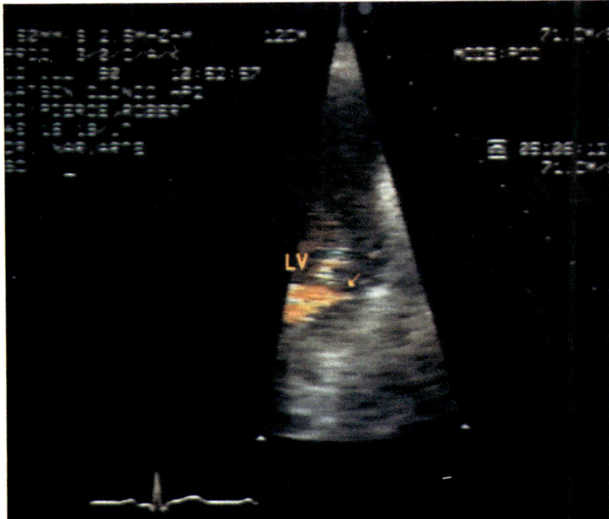

Fig. 20.29 Left ventricular aneurysm (echocardiographic findings). Same patient as shown in Fig. 20.28. Long axial view via apical window shows deformity of the inferolateral segment of the left ventricle (LV). Flowing blood can be seen to enter the mouth of the aneurysm (*arrow*) during systole on this color Doppler image.

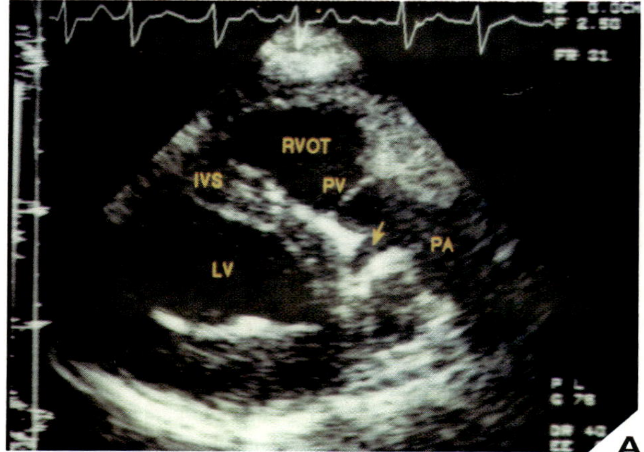

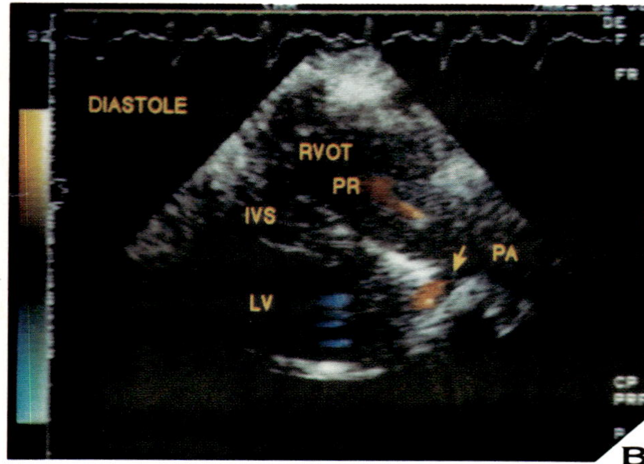

Fig. 20.39 Anomalous origin of the left coronary artery from the pulmonary trunk (echocardiographic findings). (A and B) Short-axis views obtained via a parasternal window. One wall of the pulmonary trunk (PA) is interrupted (*arrow*) at the origin of the anomalous left coronary artery. Diastolic flow (red) from the left coronary artery into the pulmonary trunk can be seen on the color Doppler image (B). (LV = left ventricle; IVS = ventricular septum; RVOT = right ventricular outflow tract)

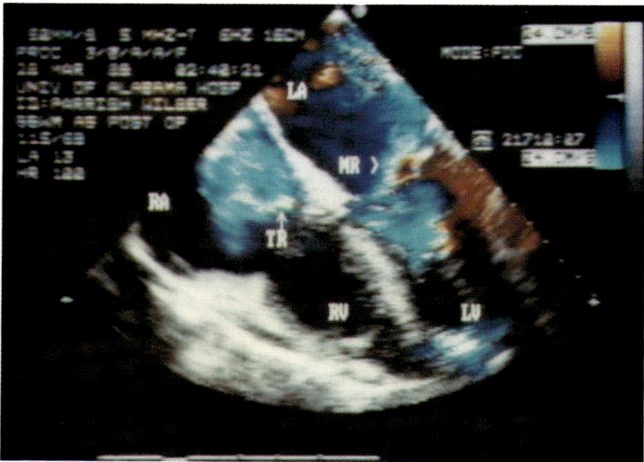

Fig. 23.10 Bacterial endocarditis involving mitral and tricuspid valves. Four-chamber view of color Doppler image at the level of atrioventricular valves (in systole). The blue color in the right atrium (RA) indicates turbulent flow produced by the regurgitant jet (TR) through the incompetent tricuspid valve during systole. The smaller area of blue color (MR) in the left atrium indicates the regurgitant jet through the incompetent mitral valve. (RV = right ventricle; LV = left ventricle)

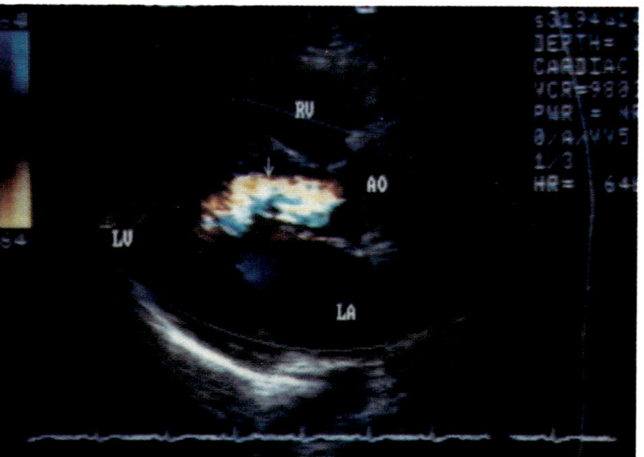

Fig. 23.11 Bacterial endocarditis with aortic insufficiency. Color Doppler echocardiogram. Long axial view (via parasternal window) in diastole demonstrates moderate enlargement of the left atrium (LA). The mosaic color (*arrow*) in the left ventricular outflow tract indicates regurgitant flow through the incompetent aortic valve during diastole. (AO = aorta; LV = left ventricle; RV = right ventricle)

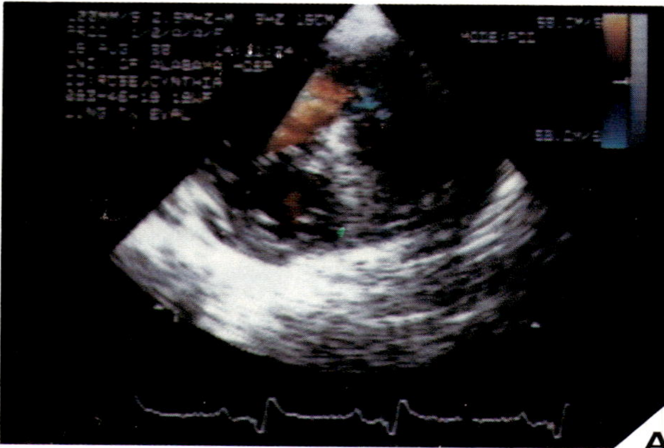

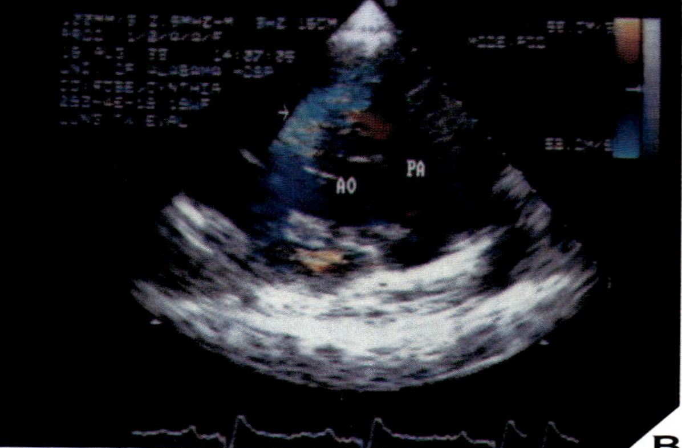

Fig. 24.7 Echocardiographic findings in chronic cor pulmonale. (A and B) Color Doppler images in short axis projection (diastole) show marked dilatation of the pulmonary trunk. Note turbulent flow in the right ventricular outflow tract indicating pulmonic valvular insufficiency.

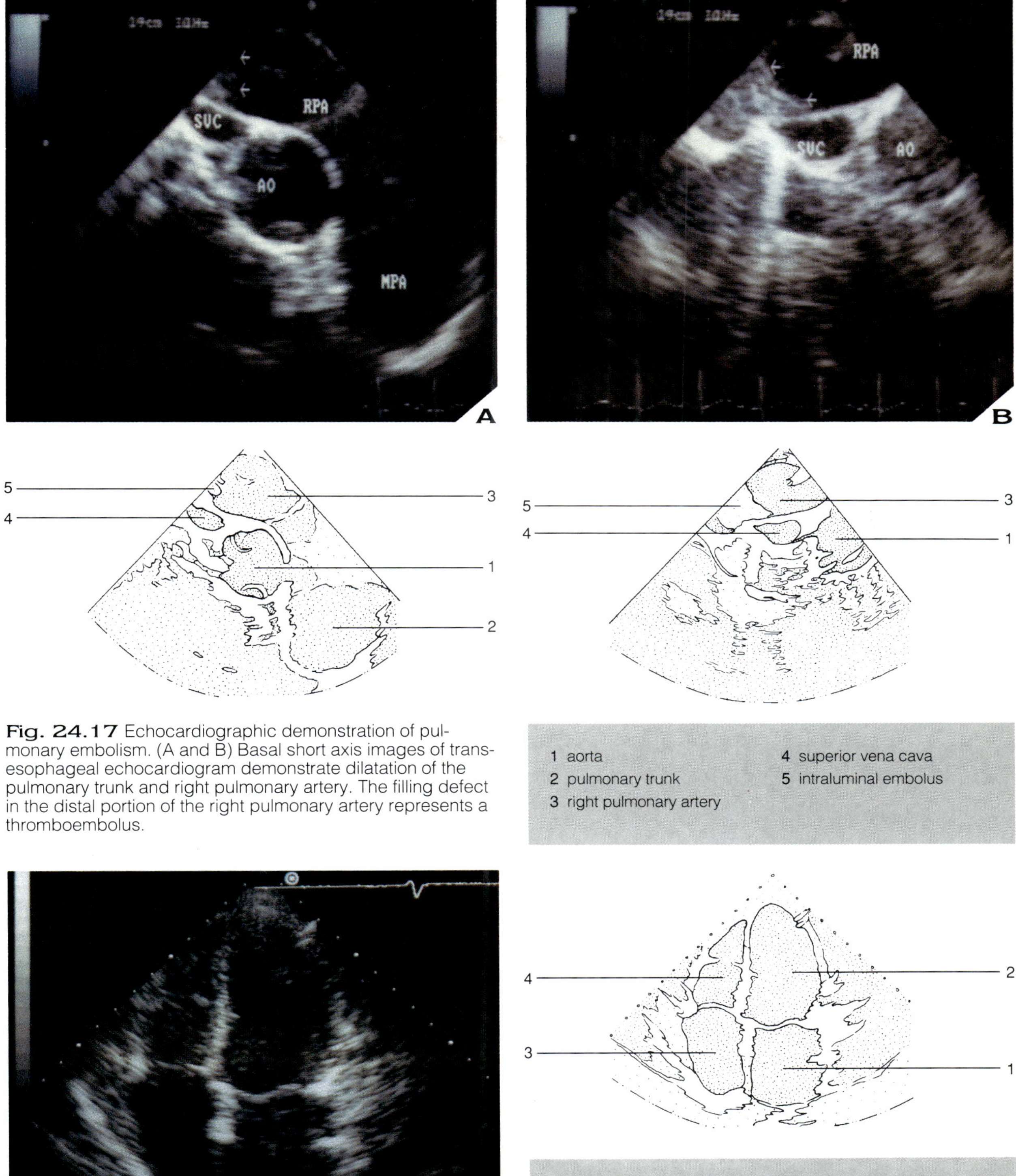

Fig. 24.17 Echocardiographic demonstration of pulmonary embolism. (A and B) Basal short axis images of transesophageal echocardiogram demonstrate dilatation of the pulmonary trunk and right pulmonary artery. The filling defect in the distal portion of the right pulmonary artery represents a thromboembolus.

1 aorta
2 pulmonary trunk
3 right pulmonary artery
4 superior vena cava
5 intraluminal embolus

1 left atrium
2 left ventricle
3 right atrium
4 right ventricle

Fig. 24.28 Echocardiographic findings in primary pulmonary hypertension. Apical four-chamber view demonstrates enlargement of the right atrium. The tricuspid and mitral valves are within normal limits. The filling defect in the right atrium represents a mural thrombus, a common finding in patients with primary pulmonary hypertension.

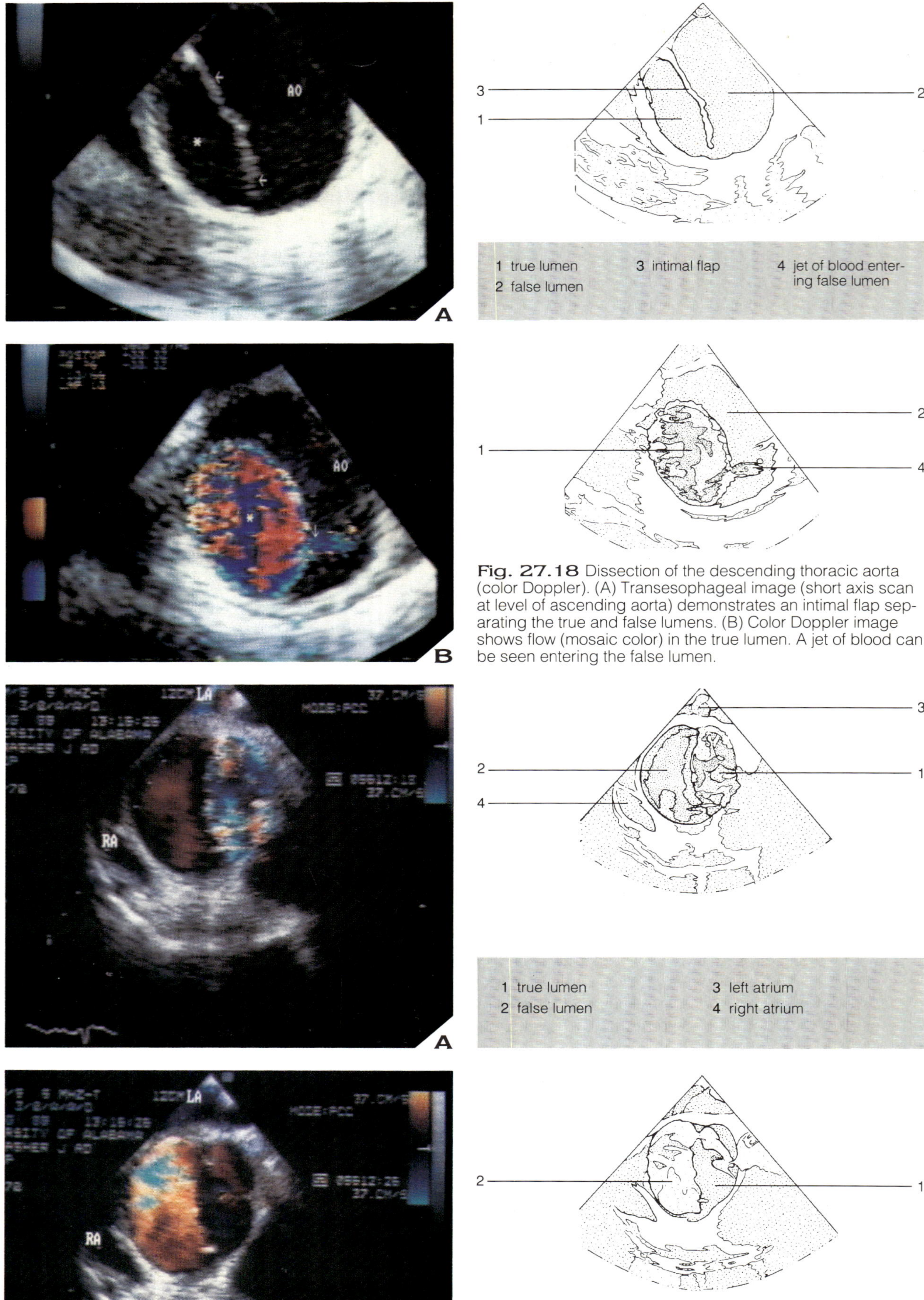

Fig. 27.18 Dissection of the descending thoracic aorta (color Doppler). (A) Transesophageal image (short axis scan at level of ascending aorta) demonstrates an intimal flap separating the true and false lumens. (B) Color Doppler image shows flow (mosaic color) in the true lumen. A jet of blood can be seen entering the false lumen.

Fig. 27.19 Dissection of ascending aorta (color Doppler). (A and B) Transesophageal scans of ascending aorta at two different phases of cardiac cycle show the true and false lumens separated by an intimal flap. Color Doppler mapping demonstrates different flow patterns in each channel: the true lumen is uniformly filled by mosaic color, whereas the false lumen appears red.

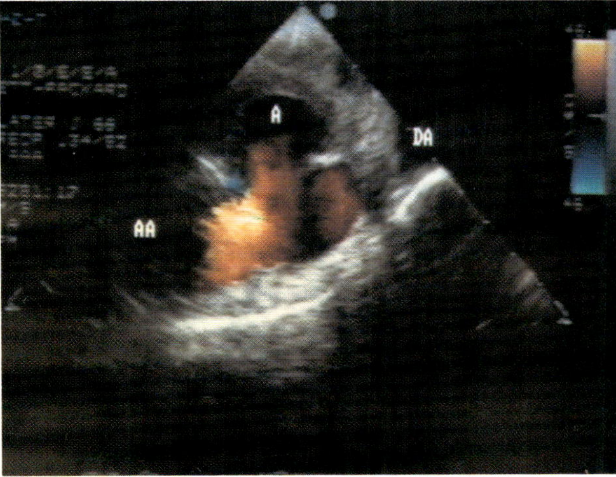

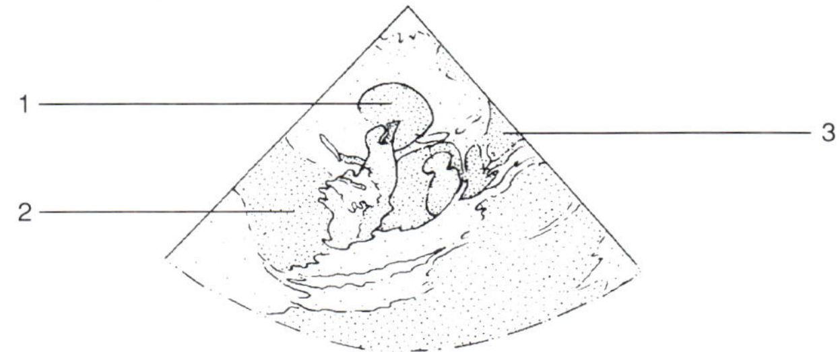

1 aneurysm of aortic arch
2 ascending aorta
3 descending aorta

Fig. 27.40 Aortic arch aneurysm (echocardiographic findings). Transesophageal scan of aortic arch demonstrates a large aneurysm arising from the inferior wall of the aortic arch. Color Doppler imaging indicates blood flow entering the aneurysm. Portions of the normal ascending and descending aorta are also visualized.

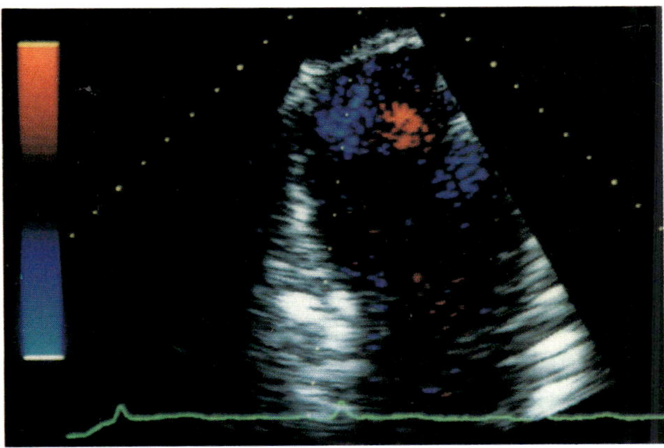

Fig. 27.42 Aneurysm of the descending thoracic aorta (echocardiographic findings). Two-dimensional echocardiogram obtained via a supraclavicular window demonstrates an aneurysm of the descending thoracic aorta. The aneurysm measures 6 cm in diameter.

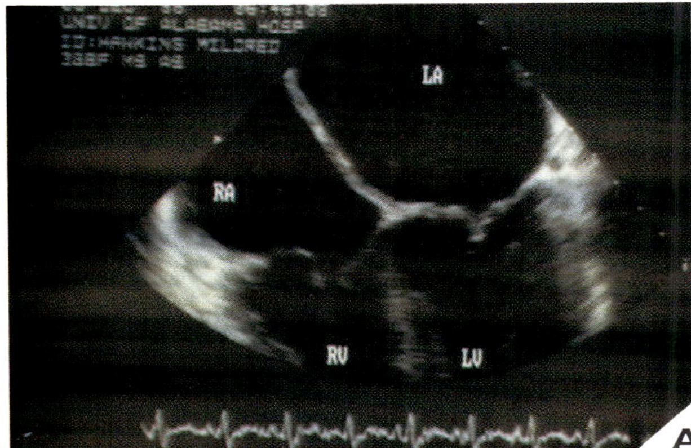

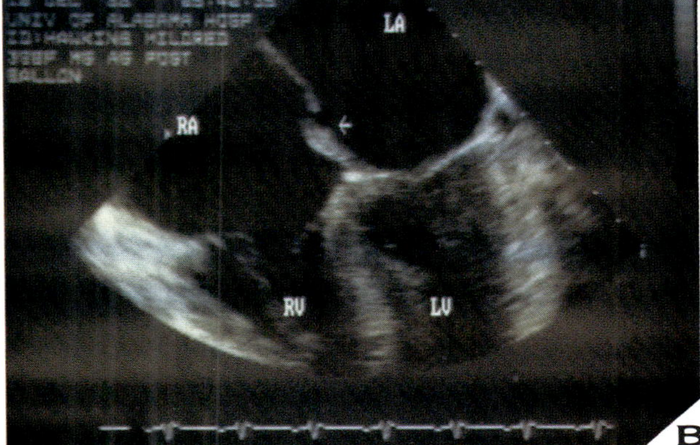

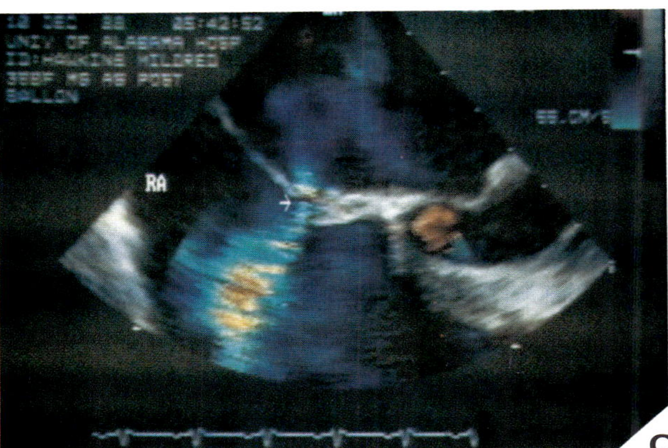

Fig. 31.9 Iatrogenic atrial septal defect after mitral balloon valvuloplasty. (A–C) Four-chamber transesophageal echocardiograms. (A) Before valvuloplasty the atrial septum is intact. Note the marked thickening of the mitral leaflets. (B,C) After valvuloplasty there is a small iatrogenic atrial septal defect (*arrow*). Systolic flow through the ASD is seen on the color Doppler image (C). (LA = left atrium; RA = right atrium; LV = left ventricle; RV = right ventricle)

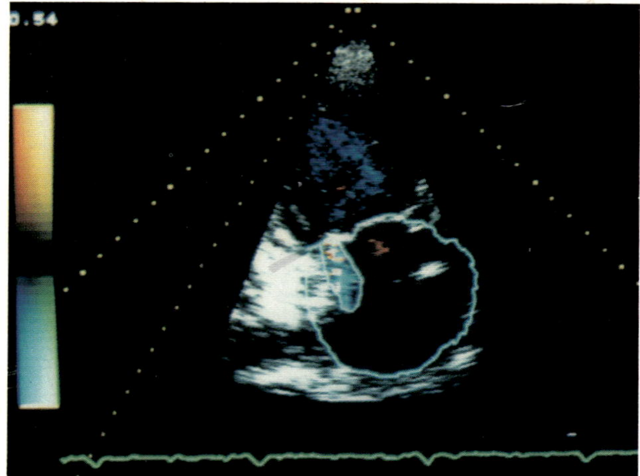

Fig. 32.10 Acute rejection. Color Doppler echocardiogram (apical four-chamber view) demonstrates dilatation of the left atrium and left ventricle. Note moderate mitral insufficiency, which was not evident on previous postoperative studies. Left ventricular systolic function was normal. Endocardial biopsy revealed acute rejection.

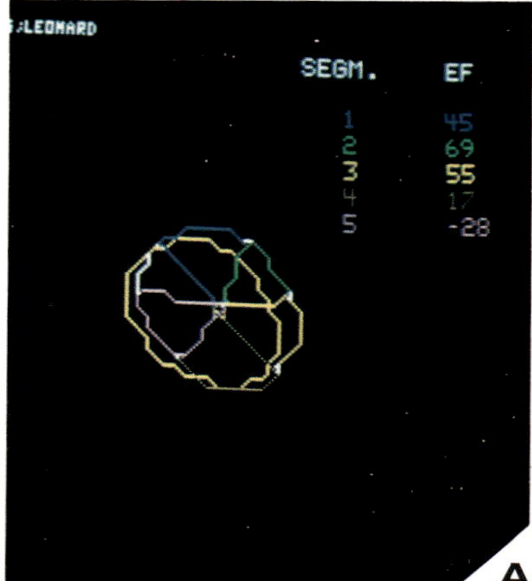

Fig. 32.14 Ischemic cardiomyopathy secondary to accelerated arteriosclerosis (demonstrated by nuclear ventriculography). (A and B) Computer-generated diagrams of left ventriculogram in LAO projection (^{99}Tc-labeled RBCs, 24 mCi). (A) Study obtained 3 years after cardiac transplantation demonstrates dilatation of the left ventricle with poor contraction of all segments and akinesis of the ventricular septum. The measured ejection fraction was 40 percent. Coronary arteriography revealed diffuse stenosis of the left anterior descending artery and stenosis of the middle and distal segments of the right coronary artery (see Figs. 32.15 and 32.16). Re-transplantation was performed several months later. (B) Study obtained several months after the second cardiac transplant demonstrates hypokinesis of the septum; however, the other left ventricular segments contract normally. The measured ejection fraction was 60 percent.